PRINCIPLES AND PRACTICE OF
PSYCHIATRIC NURSING

THIRD EDITION

PRINCIPLES
AND
PRACTICE
OF
PSYCHIATRIC
NURSING

GAIL WISCARZ STUART, Ph.D., R.N., C.S.

Associate Professor, College of Nursing, Graduate Program:
Assistant Professor, College of Medicine,
Department of Psychiatry and Behavioral Sciences:
Medical University of South Carolina,
Charleston, South Carolina

SANDRA J. SUNDEEN, R.N., M.S.

Chief Psychiatric Nurse, Mental Hygiene Administration
Maryland Department of Health and Mental Hygiene, Baltimore, Maryland;
Adjunct Assistant Professor, University of Maryland School of Nursing.
Baltimore, Maryland; Adjunct Assistant Professor,
Salisbury State College,
Salisbury, Maryland

with illustrations

THE C. V. MOSBY COMPANY
ST. LOUIS · WASHINGTON, D.C. · TORONTO   1987

MOSBY

A TRADITION OF PUBLISHING EXCELLENCE

Editor: Linda Duncan
Assistant Editor: June Heath
Project Editor: Patricia Gayle May
Designer: Nancy Steinmeyer
Editing and Production: Editing, Design & Production, Inc.

Artwork for the part and chapter openers is by M.C. Escher.
Reprinted with permission of John W. Vermeulen on behalf of the
Escher heirs. Photographs courtesy National Gallery of Art,
Washington, D.C.

THIRD EDITION

Previous editions copyrighted 1979, 1983

International Standard Book Code: 0-8016-4792-4

Printed in the United States of America

The C.V. Mosby Company
11830 Westline Industrial Drive, St. Louis, Missouri 63146

GW/VH/VH   9 8 7 6 5 4 3 2 1   03/C/312

CONTRIBUTORS

BEVERLY A. BALDWIN, R.N., M.S.

Assistant Professor, Project Director,
Gerontology Training Program,
University of Maryland School of Nursing,
Baltimore, Maryland

E. SUSAN BATZER, R.N., M.S., C.S.

Psychotherapist and Consultant,
Fallston, Maryland;
Program Coordinator,
Psychiatric Emergency Service,
Baltimore County, Maryland

RUTH WILDER BELL, R.N., D.N.Sc.

Chairperson, Department of Nursing,
Towson State University,
Towson, Maryland

SANDRA G. BENTER, R.N., M.S., C.S.

Doctoral Candidate,
Catholic University School of Nursing,
Washington, D.C.;
Visiting Assistant Professor,
Towson State University School of Nursing,
Towson, Maryland;
Psychotherapist and Consultant,
Pikesville, Maryland

THERESA S. FOLEY, Ph.D., R.N., C.S.

Assistant Professor,
University of Michigan School of Nursing
Ann Arbor, Michigan

KATHRYN G. GARDNER, R.N., M.S.

Psychiatric Nurse Consultant,
Rochester General Hospital;
Director of Group Psychotherapy
Research Team,
Department of Psychiatry,
University of Rochester,
Rochester, New York

BARBARA A. GRIMES

Doctoral Candidate,
University of Michigan School of Nursing,
Ann Arbor, Michigan

PATRICIA E. HELM, M.S.N., C.S.

West Haven Veterans Administration Medical Center
West Haven, Connecticut

JEANETTE LANCASTER, R.N., Ph.D., F.A.A.N.

Dean and Professor,
Wright State University–Miami Valley School of Nursing,
Dayton, Ohio

WADE LANCASTER, Ph.D.

Assistant Professor of Marketing,
College of Business and Administration,
Wright State University,
Dayton, Ohio

MICHELE T. LARAIA, R.N., M.S.N.

Assistant Professor and Research Coordinator,
Department of Psychiatry and Behavioral Sciences,
Medical University of South Carolina,
Charleston, South Carolina

PAULA CHELES La SALLE, R.N., M.S., C.S., C.C.M.H.C.

Psychiatric Nurse Clinical Specialist,
Howard County General Hospital,
Columbia, Maryland

RITA J. LAUTZ, R.N., Ph.D., C.S.

Psychotherapist,
Bel Air, Maryland;
Consultant,
Psychiatric Emergency Service,
Baltimore County, Maryland

FRANCES G. LEHMANN, M.S.N., R.N., C.S.

Frances G. Lehmann Health Consultants,
Indianapolis, Indiana

HELEN R. PEDDICORD, R.N., M.S.

Director of Residential Services,
Regional Institute for Children and Adolescents,
Rockville, Maryland

SUSAN G. POORMAN, R.N., M.S.N., C.S., C.S.E.

Assistant Professor, School of Nursing,
University of Pittsburgh;
Psychotherapist and Consultant,
Pittsburgh, Pennsylvania

AUDREY REDSTON-ISELIN, R.N., M.A., C.S.

Clinical Specialist, Children's Service,
Soudview Throgs Neck Community Mental Health Center,
Albert Einstein College of Medicine,
Yeshiva University,
Bronx, New York;
Psychotherapist and Consultant,
White Plains and New York, New York

RITA L. RUBIN, R.N., M.S., C.S.

Clinical Nurse Specialist,
Child and Adolescent Psychiatric Nursing,
Sheppard-Pratt Hospital,
Towson, Maryland;
Psychotherapist and Consultant,
Reisterstown, Maryland

KAY SIENKILEWSKI, R.N., M.S.

Director of Nursing,
Sprinfield Hospital Center,
Sykesville, Maryland

PREFACE

In writing the first edition of this text, we felt much like pathfinders traversing unexplored frontiers. Our first edition reflected both a departure and an evolution. It was a departure from all other texts of psychiatric nursing that organized nursing care, either overtly or covertly, around the medical model and its classifications of psychiatric disorders. Our text was an evolution in that it attempted to identify and refine, for psychiatric nurses, the distinct body of knowledge that is nursing.

The second edition of our text continued to be a departure and an evolution, but also a consolidation. Although departing from a traditional approach, we continued to use nursing's conceptual model, the nursing process, as the basis for defining and describing the practice of psychiatric nursing.

This third edition takes one more step down the path of psychiatric nursing science by laying plans for exploring the frontiers ahead. The strengths of this new edition include extensive revisions that reflect progress in both nursing and the broader field of psychiatry. Specifically, nursing research has been integrated and applied in each chapter. Advances in biological psychiatry have been explored relevant to identified patient problems and treatment. A separate chapter on psychopharmacology has been added to this edition to develop greater understanding of this important treatment modality, as well as to underscore the role of the psychiatric nurse in managing psychopharmacological interventions with patients. Continuing from previous editions, this third edition strengthens and consistently applies a nursing model for practice and demonstrates the way in which it can be used in a variety of mental health settings. NANDA diagnoses and the latest proposed Draft of the DSM-III-R in Development are integrated and utilized throughout the text. And, most important, the critical role of psychiatric-mental health nurses in health education is identified and described with suggested implementation in the various chapters related to clinical nursing problems.

A separate chapter of the text is devoted to our conceptual model of health-illness phenomena, in which theory and practice are integrated and elements of the model are clearly identified, explained, and interrelated. Within this model, nursing and medical diagnoses are presented as being distinct, but complementary, rather than contingent or redundant. Knowledge of both, however, is viewed as being necessary for practice. Thus throughout the text the medical model is presented as

a complement, and occasional supplement, to the nursing process model that strives to preserve its unique identity. If this sounds less than absolute, it is because this is a less than absolute endeavor. It is a responsive, emerging, and exciting charting of unexplored territories that we engage in with all of our peers and colleagues who are practicing, teaching, and learning the art and science of psychiatric nursing. Our book is a part of all of you together and a challenge to each of you individually to contribute to the future direction of the principles and practice of psychiatric nursing.

Part One, Principles of Psychiatric Nursing, has a sharpened focus on the professional dimensions of psychiatric nursing practice. It presents a refined analysis of our conceptual model of health-illness phenomena that provides a framework for the nursing therapeutic process. Unit I defines concepts and theories of care. Chapter 1 critically analyzes the roles and functions of psychiatric nurses from the many perspectives of historical evolution, contemporary practice, levels of performance, and issues of professional autonomy. Chapter 2 continues to explore models of psychiatric care, while introducing the medical model and a brief perspective of the nursing model used in this text. Chapter 3 describes a nursing model of health-illness phenomena that is inclusive and holistic, yet discrete and relevant to nursing practice. This model views health and illness as a continuum of adaptation and provides an organizing framework for the application of the nursing process. Chapter 4 presents a comprehensive analysis of the elements of the nurse-patient relationship, including the effective use of self, the therapeutic communication process, the phases of the nurse-patient relationship, responsive and action dimensions, therapeutic impasses, and supervision. Chapter 5 describes the phases and needed documentation of the nursing process with application demonstrated in a clinical case analysis. The Standards of Psychiatric and Mental Health Nursing Practice are integrated throughout this discussion. Chapter 6 describes elements of the comprehensive psychiatric evaluation including the mental status examination, psychiatric examination, and new technological approaches to biological evaluation. Chapter 7 presents legal and ethical aspects of psychiatric nursing care, and Chapter 8 stimulates the reader to analyze future challenges facing psychiatric nursing practitioners.

The first three chapters of Unit II describe primary, secondary and tertiary prevention levels of nursing intervention. Chapters 12 through 21 have all been revised, reorganized, and strengthened from a nursing perspective. Each explores a category of maladaptive coping responses, including the nursing problems of anxiety, alterations in self-concept, disturbances of mood, self-destructive behavior, disruptions in relatedness, problems with the expression of anger, impaired cognition, and substance abuse. Other new chapters discuss psychophysiological illness and variations in sexual response. At the beginning of each of these chapters, a continuum of adaptive and maladaptive coping responses is presented relative to the chapter's nursing problem. Each phase of the nursing process is then applied and synthesized with the conceptual model. A consistent approach is used in formulating nursing diagnoses and comparing them with relevant medical diagnoses. Nursing research is used to provide a rationale for nursing interventions. Principles and nursing actions for the interventions are clearly discussed and concisely summarized in each of these chapters. Evaluation is addressed in light of effectiveness, efficiency, and areas in need of further study. The strength of this integrated approach is that it can be applied in any nursing care setting to patients who are responding to any type of stressor, whether physical, psychological, or sociocultural. Thus it is as useful to nurses working on medical units of general hospitals, long-term care facilities, and community health agencies, as it is to nurses working in psychiatric facilities. The last two chapters in Part One, Chapters 22 and 23, address updated analyses of somatic therapies and psychopharmacology.

Part Two, Practice of Psychiatric Nursing, has similarly been divided into two units. The first unit describes psychiatric nursing practice in specific settings including inpatient, community mental health, and the general hospital. Unit II addresses specialized treatment approaches including behavior modification, group and family approaches, child and adolescent psychiatric nursing, intervening in family abuse, violence and sexual assault, care of the chronic mentally ill, and gerontological psychiatric nursing. All of Part Two reflects the most current thinking on the treatment settings, modalities, and roles of psychiatric nursing.

We have also tried to clarify content and reinforce learning throughout the text. To this end, each chapter contains behaviorally stated learning objectives, expanded illustrations and tables, summaries of important points, directions for future nursing research, suggested cross-references, updated references, and more extensive annotated suggested readings. This edition of our book is also accompanied by an instructor's manual, which is complete with learning objectives, lecture outlines, chapter glossaries, thought-provoking discussion questions, and multiple-choice test questions that include both theoretical aspects and clinical applications of the text's content.

Visually, this third edition continues to incorporate the artwork of M.C. Escher. Over the past four years his drawings have continued to stimulate and intrigue us, as we believe that they truly reflect the complexity of human behavior and one's own perceptual responses. We have come to identify with the precision, balance, and creative perspective of his work, and hope to realize these same qualities in this latest edition of our text.

We end this preface to our third edition with a note of expectancy and a stirring "call to action," complete with images of flying banners, quickened steps, and an assertive stance. Books such as ours make a certain impact on the field by their very presence, but Sir William Osler once observed, "What I read, I forget. What I hear, I remember. What I see, I know." It is therefore imperative that nurses communicate the nature and quality of the art and science of psychiatric nursing through their words, actions, and performance. To such a vision, we dedicate this third edition of our book.

Gail Wiscarz Stuart
Sandra J. Sundeen

CONTENTS

PART TWO
PRACTICE OF PSYCHIATRIC NURSING

I Settings

PART ONE

PRINCIPLES
OF PSYCHIATRIC NURSING

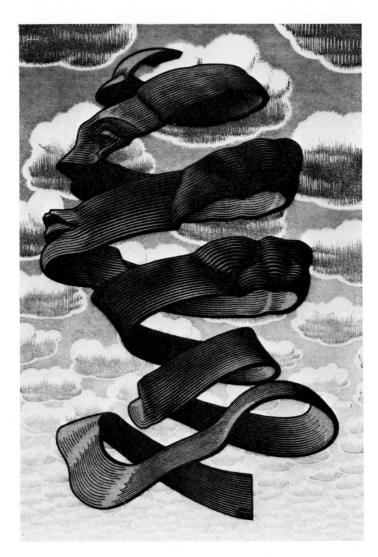

UNIT I
CONCEPTS AND THEORIES

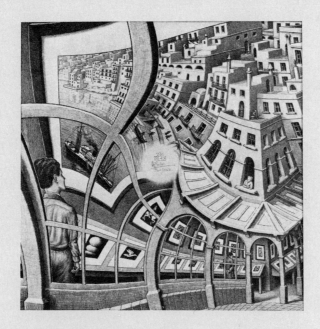

The philosophies of one age have become the absurdities of the next, and the foolishness of yesterday has become the wisdom of tomorrow.

Sir William Osler

CHAPTER 1

ROLES AND FUNCTIONS OF PSYCHIATRIC NURSES

LEARNING OBJECTIVES

After studying this chapter, the student should be able to:

- describe the early history of psychiatric nursing.

- discuss the evolution of a psychiatric nursing role, including the specific contributions of Peplau.

- relate the influence of the social environment on psychiatric nursing.

- describe the nature, scope, and setting of psychiatric nursing practice.

- identify direct and indirect psychiatric nursing care functions using the concepts of primary, secondary, and tertiary prevention.

- analyze factors that contribute to effective interdisciplinary team functioning.

- discuss the leadership capabilities needed by psychiatric nurses.

- analyze the way in which the psychiatric nurse's level of performance is affected by each of the following factors: laws, qualifications, practice setting, and personal competence and initiative.

- assess the purpose and importance of the American Nurses' Association Standards of Psychiatric–Mental Health Nursing Practice.

- evaluate the position of psychiatric nursing on the six characteristics of the scale of professionalization.

- critique problematic areas for psychiatric nursing and formulate recommendations for future growth.

- identify directions for future nursing research.

- select appropriate readings for further study.

Evolutionary perspectives

The function of nursing or caring for the sick has existed since the beginning of civilization. Family members, servants, friends, neighbors, and religious groups have all cared for the ill or infirm throughout the course of history. Before 1860 the emphasis in psychiatric institutions was on custodial care, and this was provided by attendants who were prepared to maintain control of the patients. Frequently these attendants were little more than jailers or cellkeepers with very little training, and psychiatric care was poor. Nursing, as a profession, began to emerge in the late nineteenth century.

■ Early history

In 1873 Linda Richards graduated from the New England Hospital for Women and Children in Boston. She developed better nursing care in psychiatric hospitals and organized nursing services and educational programs in state mental hospitals in Illinois. Basic to her theory of care was Richard's premise: "It stands to reason that the mentally sick should be at least as well cared for as the physically sick."[14] For these activities she is called the first American psychiatric nurse.

The first school to prepare nurses to care for the mentally ill opened at McLean Hospital in Waverly,

Massachusetts, in 1882. It was a two-year program, but few psychological skills were addressed. The care was mainly custodial because nurses filled the function of caring for the physical needs of patients. Until the end of the nineteenth century little changed in the role of psychiatric nurses. They had limited special training in psychiatry, and they primarily adapted the principles of medical-surgical nursing to the psychiatric setting. They attended to the physical needs of patients, such as medications, nutrition, hygiene, and ward activities. At that time, psychological care consisted of being kind and tolerant to the patients.

One important contribution of Linda Richards was her ability to assess both the physical and emotional needs of her patients. In this early period of nursing history the emotional and physical needs of patients were separated. Nursing education reflected this division, and nurses were taught either in the general hospital or in the psychiatric hospital. Johns Hopkins was the first school of nursing to include a fully developed course for psychiatric nursing in the curriculum. This occurred in 1913, and thereafter other schools began to do likewise. It was not until the late 1930s that nursing education viewed the importance of psychiatric knowledge in general nursing care related to all illnesses.

An important factor influencing the history of psychiatric nursing was the development of various somatic therapies, including insulin shock therapy (1935), psychosurgery (1936), and electroconvulsive therapy (1937). These all required the medical-surgical skills of nurses. Although these therapies did not foster the patient's insight, they did control his behavior and make him more amenable to psychotherapy. Somatic therapies also increased the demand for improved psychological treatment for those patients who did not respond.

As nurses became more involved with these therapies, they began their struggle to define their role as psychiatric nurses. An editorial that appeared in the *American Journal of Nursing*[16] in 1940 described the conflict between nurses and physicians as nurses attempted to implement what they saw as appropriate nursing care for the psychiatric patient. This conflict was to continue for many years in the perpetuation of sex-role stereotyping and continues to demand attention in present nursing practice.[39] Another article published in 1933[40] described how psychiatrists were looking for experienced psychiatric nurses to work in psychiatric hospitals. A superintendent of nursing from a state hospital identified the three most pressing needs at that time as (1) more nurses, (2) better prepared nurses, and (3) cooperation and understanding of the nursing organizations.

The period after World War II was one of major growth and change in psychiatric nursing. Because of a large number of service-related psychiatric problems and the increase in treatment programs offered by the Veterans Administration, there was an increased need for psychiatric nurses with advanced preparation. The content of psychiatric nursing had now become an integral part of the generic nursing curriculum, and its principles were applied to other areas of nursing practice, including general medicine, pediatric, and public health nursing. Graduate nursing programs, however, were few in number.

In 1946 Congress passed the National Mental Health Act which authorized the creation of the National Institute of Mental Health (NIMH) and a program for (1) training professional psychiatric personnel, (2) conducting psychiatric research, and (3) aiding the development of mental health programs at the state level. The purpose of the National Institute of Mental Health, located in Bethesda, Maryland, is to research the origins of mental illness and possible methods of treatment. It is also the administrative body that distributes training funds and research grants. Psychiatric nursing was one of the professions specified in the act that paved the way for federal funding of nursing education. Collegiate programs developed at both the baccalaureate and graduate levels. At about the same time the nursing profession endorsed the development of graduate programs that focused on clinical practice in nursing. By 1947 eight graduate programs in psychiatric nursing had been initiated.

Basic nursing programs also continued to grow and change. Many nursing leaders questioned the practice of having specialized hospitals offer training programs to prepare nurses to care for a particular type of patient, such as psychiatric hospitals training psychiatric nurses. The trend was to combine the basic knowledge and various skills needed by nurses into one general education program.

In 1948 Brown's report on "Nursing for the Future" recommended the elimination of basic schools of nursing in mental hospitals. The report stated, "We recommend that hospitals for the mentally ill still conducting schools of nursing consider means whereby they can relinquish their schools and, as a substitute, make their clinical facilities more widely available for affiliating students (from general training schools)."[7:136] It also recommended the use of the psychiatric hospital in advanced courses of instruction for graduate nurse specialists. This report was given additional support in 1950 when the National League for Nursing (NLN) required that a school had to provide an experience in psychiatric nursing to be accredited.

■ Role emergence

It was in this developmental period that the role of psychiatric nurses began to emerge. In 1947 Weiss[61] published an article in the *American Journal of Nursing* that reemphasized the shortage of psychiatric nurses and attempted to describe how psychiatric nurses differ from general duty nurses. She described "attitude therapy" as the nurse's directed use of attitudes that contributes to the patient's recovery. In implementing this therapy, the nurse observes the patient for minute and fleeting changes, demonstrates acceptance, respect, and understanding of the patient as a fellow human being, and promotes the patient's interest and participation in reality. She stressed the need to treat each patient as an individual with unique problems. It was also her belief that only physicians should attempt to interpret the patient's behavior and the physician would prescribe the appropriate attitude needed by the nurse based on the patient's problem. More independent functions were described by Santos and Stainbrook[52] in 1949. They believed that nurses should perform "psychotherapeutic tasks" and understand concepts related to therapy, such as transference. They were vague, however, about the exact nature of the nurse's functions.

An article by Bennett and Eaton[6] appeared in the *American Journal of Psychiatry* in 1951 and identified three problems affecting psychiatric nurses: the scarcity of qualified psychiatric nurses, the partial use of their abilities, and the fact that "very little real psychiatric nursing is carried out in otherwise good psychiatric hospitals and units." They described the following functions and responsibilities of the chief psychiatric nurse:

1. To have policy-making authority independent of the psychiatric staff members, hospital administrators, and general nursing staff
2. To decide psychiatric nursing policies
3. To develop all rules and regulations of the department
4. To train an auxiliary staff of assistants to conform to his or her standards

The role of the nurse in insulin treatment, electroconvulsive therapy, and lobotomy was discussed. Two additional areas were also included—community activities and psychotherapy. They believed it was the responsibility of the psychiatric nurse to join mental health societies, consult with welfare agencies, work in outpatient clinics, practice preventive psychiatry, engage in research, and help educate the public. They took a stand supporting the nurse's participation in individual and group psychotherapy. Bennett and Eaton state, "Despite the fact that most psychiatrists seem to ignore the role of the psychiatric nurse in psychotherapy, all nurses in psychiatric wards do psychotherapy of one kind or another by their contacts with patients."[6:170] They urged that psychotherapy should be used purposefully and believed that nurses, like psychologists and social workers, should be used in "team psychotherapy." Many of the issues raised in the article would be debated years later.

■ **NURSING THERAPY.** The most controversial issue, however, was that of nurses conducting psychotherapy. Mellow[35] wrote in the *American Journal of Nursing* of the work she did with schizophrenic patients at Boston State Hospital in 1951. She defined these activities as "nursing therapy" and delineated three phases in the treatment process. The task in phase 1 was to establish contact with the patient and enter his life as a partner in the establishment of a therapeutic symbiotic relationship. In phase 2 the nurse allows the patient to relive his symbiotic attachment to a maternal figure and helps him resolve it. The final task of phase 3 is to help the patient manage his separation anxieties as he assumes more responsibility for his own life. In 1952 Tudor[59] published a study, "Sociopsychiatric Nursing Approach to Intervention in a Problem of Mutual Withdrawal on a Mental Hospital Ward," in which she described the nurse-patient relationships she es-

tablished, which were characterized by unconditional care, few demands, and the anticipation of her patients' needs.

As nurses engaged in these kinds of activities, many questions arose. Are these activities therapeutic or are they therapy? What is a therapeutic relationship or a one-to-one nurse-patient relationship? How does it differ from psychotherapy? These questions were addressed by Dr. Hildegard Peplau, a dynamic nursing leader whose ideas and beliefs would shape the future of psychiatric nursing.

In 1952 Peplau[41] published a book, *Interpersonal Relations in Nursing,* in which she described the skills, activities, and role of psychiatric nurses. It was the first systematic, theoretical framework developed for psychiatric nursing. She defined nursing as a "significant, therapeutic process" and believed the nurse-patient relationship was characterized by four overlapping and interlocking phases—orientation, identification, exploitation, and resolution. As she studied the nursing process in nurse-patient situations, she saw various roles emerge. These included the nurse as a resource person, a teacher, a leader in local, national, and international situations, a surrogate parent, and a counselor. She stated, "Counseling in nursing has to do with helping the patient remember and to understand fully what is happening to him in the present situation, so that the experience can be integrated with rather than dissociated from other experiences in life."[41:64]

The use of the nursing process in defining a role for psychiatric nurses was further evident when, in 1953, the National League for Nursing published "A Study of Desirable Functions and Qualifications for Psychiatric Nurses."[42] This report identified the following desirable functions:

1. Collecting significant data relating to the identification of problems (e.g., observing behavior, recording observations)
2. Making inferences and/or judgments based on these data and leading to action (e.g., interpreting the behavior of the patient, seeking to understand patients' needs)
3. Acting or intervening on the basis of inferences (e.g., clarifying with a patient the meaning of a procedure, discussing and acting to solve problems in a work situation)
4. Evaluating the entire process in terms of whether problems identified have been solved (e.g., mutually evaluating experiences and learning)

As nurses continued to describe their qualifications, skills, activities, and responsibilities, the role of the psychiatric nurse began to gain substance and definition.

Evolutionary Timeline in Psychiatric Nursing

Social environment		Psychiatric nursing
	1873	Linda Richards graduated from the New England Hospital for Women and Children
	1882	First school to prepare nurses to care for the mentally ill opened at McLean Hospital in Massachusetts
American Journal of Nursing first published	1900	
Clifford Beer's book, *A Mind That Found Itself,* published	1908	
Florence Nightingale died	1910	
	1913	Johns Hopkins was first school of nursing to include a course on psychiatric nursing in its curriculum
	1920	First psychiatric nursing textbook, *Nursing Mental Disease* by Harriet Bailey, published
Electroconvulsive therapy developed	1937	
National Mental Health Act passed by Congress, creating National Institute of Mental Health (NIMH) and providing training funds for psychiatric nursing education	1946	
	1950	National League for Nursing (NLN) required that schools of nursing must provide an experience in psychiatric nursing to be accredited
	1952	Hildegard Peplau published *Interpersonal Relations in Nursing*
Maxwell Jones published *The Therapeutic Community*	1953	
Development of major tranquilizers	1954	
	1962	Hildegard Peplau published "Interpersonal Techniques: The Crux of Psychiatric Nursing"
Community Mental Health Centers Act passed	1963	*Perspectives in Psychiatric Care* published; *Journal of Psychiatric Nursing and Mental Health Services* published
	1973	*Standards of Psychiatric–Mental Health Nursing Practice* published; Certification of psychiatric mental health nurse generalists established by the American Nurses' Association
Report of the President's Commission on Mental Health	1978	
	1979	*Issues in Mental Health Nursing* published; Certification of psychiatric mental health nurse specialists established by the American Nurses' Association
Mental Health Systems Act passed	1980	*Nursing: A Social Policy Statement* published by the American Nurses' Association
Mental Health Systems Act repealed	1981	
	1982	*Revised Standards of Psychiatric and Mental Health Nursing Practice* published
National Center for Nursing Research created in National Institute of Health (NIH)	1985	*Standards of Child and Adolescent Psychiatric and Mental Health Nursing Practice* published
	1987	*American Journal of Psychiatric Nursing* published

Two significant developments in psychiatry in the 1950s would affect nursing's role for years to come. The first was Jones'[26] publication of *The Therapeutic Community* in 1953, which encouraged using the patient's social environment to provide a therapeutic experience. The patient was to be an active participant in his or her own care and become involved in the daily problems of the community. All patients were to help solve problems, plan activities, and develop the necessary rules and regulations. Their independence was increased as they gained control over many of their own personal activities. The environment fostered trust, self-direction, and individual dignity, and patients became aware of how their behavior affected others. Therapeutic communities became the preferred environment for psychiatric patients.

The implications of this development were explored in a 1954 article by Gregg.[22] She stated that the work of the psychiatric nurse was to "help create an environment in which the patient will have an opportunity to develop new behavior patterns that will enable him to make a more mature adjustment to life." This involved the creation of "nurse-patient relationships that promote emotional growth and are consistent with the therapeutic plan of the doctor-patient relationship." Gregg contrasted this environment to those which are custodial or protective and those which emphasize conformity and acceptable routines. To establish a therapeutic environment, she believed the patient had to be allowed to express conflict, the staff had to try to understand him, and that there had to be an opportunity for learning and growth through the development of interpersonal relationships.

The idea of the therapeutic community received support in the second significant development in psychiatry—the use of psychotropic drugs in the early 1950s. This allowed more patients to become treatable and required fewer environmental constraints such as locked doors and straightjackets. It also required more personnel to provide therapy and allowed for the expansion of roles of various psychiatric practitioners, including nurses.

■ **EMERGING FUNCTIONS.** An article by Maloney[30] published in 1962 raised the question of whether the psychiatric nurse does have independent functions. She reviewed the spectrum of nursing philosophies and descriptions of roles and functions. One clear area of independent functioning was identified in the management and supervision of the patient's environment. This function, however, was able to be either therapeutic or mechanical and clerical depending on the nurse's goals in implementation.

Hays[23] conducted a review of the literature in 1958 and reported that the following functions of psychiatric nurses were described: dealing with patients' problems of attitude, mood, feeling-tone, and interpretation of reality; exploration of disturbing and conflicting thoughts and feelings; using positive feelings of the patient toward the therapist to bring about psychophysiological homeostasis; counseling patients in emergencies, including panic and fear; and strengthening the well part of patients. She reported that the nurse-patient relationship was referred to by a variety of terms, including the "therapeutic use of self," "therapeutic nurse-patient relationship," "psychiatric nursing therapy," "supportive psychotherapy," "rehabilitation therapies," and "nondirective counseling." The distinction between these terms and the exact nature of the nurse's role remained hazy.

Once again Peplau[43] would clarify psychiatric nursing's position and direct its future growth. In an article entitled "Interpersonal Techniques: The Crux of Psychiatric Nursing" published in 1962, she identified the heart of psychiatric nursing to be in the role of counselor or psychotherapist. The other functions of mother surrogate, technician, manager, socializing agent, and health teacher were seen as subroles. Within this article she differentiated between general practitioners who were staff nurses working on psychiatric units and psychiatric nurses who were specialists and expert clinical practitioners with graduate degrees in psychiatric nursing.

Thus, from an undefined role involving primarily physical care, psychiatric nursing was evolving a role of clinical competence based on interpersonal techniques and use of the nursing process. The expanding ideas and clinical experiences of psychiatric nurses would receive an even larger forum with the publication of two new nursing journals in 1963—*Perspectives in Psychiatric Care* and the *Journal of Psychiatric Nursing and Mental Health Services*. Both of these journals continue to explore elements of psychiatric nursing practice, although the name of the latter journal was changed in 1981 to the *Journal of Psychosocial Nursing and Mental Health Services*. In 1979, a third journal, *Issues in Mental Health Nursing*, and in 1986 yet a fourth journal, *American Journal of Psychiatric Nursing*, were published, providing nurses with additional vehicles in which to exlore the emerging psychiatric nursing role.

■ **Social-environmental influences**

An evolutionary perspective on psychiatric nursing practice would be incomplete without a discussion of its relationship to the larger social environment. A major factor in this regard is the 35 years of federal support for psychiatric nursing education which has advanced the practice of psychiatric-mental health nursing in this country. Programs started with federal funds have increased the numbers of new master's degree psychiatric nursing programs, thus providing greater numbers in practice; baccalaureate nursing programs have placed greater emphasis on the integration of mental health concepts into their curricula; and many continuing education programs which focus on psychiatric-mental health content have been developed.

The more current focus of psychiatric nursing is on primary prevention and implementing care and consultation in the community. This was stimulated by the Community Mental Health Centers Act of 1963, which made federal money available to states to plan, construct, and staff community mental health centers. This legislation was prompted by the growing awareness of the value of treating people in the community and preventing hospitalization whenever possible. It also encouraged the formation of multidisciplinary treatment teams as the skills and expertise of many professions were joined to alleviate illness and promote mental health. This team approach continues to be negotiated at present. The issues of territoriality, professionalism, authority structure, consumer rights, terminology, functioning, labeling, and the use of paraprofessionals are still being debated throughout the country.

The 1978 report of the President's Commission on Mental Health[49] tried to address some of the complex problems and inadequacies of the existing mental health services system. The report emphasized the continued need for community-based services that would provide the following:

1. A range of diagnostic, treatment, rehabilitative, and supportive services that would include long-term and short-term care
2. Easy access and continuity of care
3. Coordination with the network of other human services, such as education, health, income, and social services to provide comprehensive care
4. Adaptation to meet changing circumstances and the needs of special population groups
5. Adequate financing with public and private funds

The report focused on the need to broaden the base of knowledge about the nature and treatment of mental disabilities and called attention to the maldistribution, homogeneity, and tension among mental health professionals that ultimately work to the disadvantage of the patient. Increased mental health funding was proposed in an effort to solve some of these problems.

The Mental Health Systems Act of 1980 was passed to give substance to these recommendations, with particular focus on services for children, youth, the elderly, minority populations, and the chronic mentally ill. It was signed by President Carter who regarded it as landmark legislation because, while it reaffirmed the goal of providing comprehensive mental health services for the United States, it also established a federal role in mental health in the 1980s.

■ **PRESENT CONSTRAINTS.** This necessary and commendable role seemed less certain, however, with the change to the Reagan administration in 1981. The Mental Health Systems Act was repealed almost immediately after President Reagan took office. In October of that year, the new Federal Fiscal Budget for 1982 went into effect, in which the funds for psychological and social health services, as well as for the education of health care professionals, had been severely cut. The remaining money was to be dispensed primarily through block grants to the states. Instead of the previous 25 categorical grants for health and human services, there are now four block grants awarded to each state:

1. Alcohol, drug abuse, and mental health
2. Maternal and child care
3. Primary care
4. Prevention and health services

The major concerns related to block grants are that

1. There will not be sufficient funds available for the needed services, and states will not make up the deficits to support these essential programs
2. Some health concerns are best handled through a national approach
3. Lack of guidelines and responsibility may lead to inefficient use of funds, inadequate programs, and neglect of groups most in need

Thus the bywords of "fewer services, economic constraints, and less federal regulation" have come to replace those of "comprehensive care, right to health, and government subsidy." Consequently the concern is that the most needy, who are least likely to receive equitable health care from state to state, will not have the advocacy that the federal government has historically provided as a basic right.

Since 1946 the social environment has greatly changed. At the present time, psychiatric nursing faces drastic cutbacks in federal funding for nursing education, retrenchment in various health care services, and compensation ceilings, amid cries of nursing shortages and unserved patient needs. As a result of the federal cutbacks in funding nursing education and the phasing down in general of clinical training in the psychiatric-mental health nursing field, Chamberlain predicted the following consequences and problems:

1. Closure of some graduate programs
2. Schools of nursing will need to accommodate more part-time enrollments
3. Greater recruitment efforts must be made to attract nurses into psychiatric mental health nursing
4. More attention must be paid to the undergraduate curriculum so that students will have a knowledge and clinical experience base in working with the mentally ill
5. Education, research, and service must develop workable and long-standing linkages
6. The peer review system instituted by NIMH for its grant applications should be maintained for the quality control it brings to nursing curricula.[8]

The picture does not look bright for the mental health field. Psychiatric nurses must take a pro-active stance by becoming involved in the political and legislative process in their own localities. As power shifts to the states, nurses need to establish political advocacy groups to influence the legislative bodies that now have responsibility for allocating mental health funds. The challenges to nursing are many; the future is less than clear.

Contemporary practice

Psychiatric nursing is an interpersonal process that strives to promote and maintain behavior that contributes to integrated functioning. The patient or client system may be an individual, family, group, organization, or community. The American Nurses' Association Division on Psychiatric and Mental Health Nursing defined psychiatric and mental health nursing as follows*:

A specialized area of nursing practice employing theories of human behavior as its science and purposeful use of self as its art. It is directed toward both preventive and corrective impacts upon mental disorders and their sequelae and is concerned with the promotion of optimal mental health for society, the community, and those individuals who live within it.[2:5]

The National Institute of Mental Health officially recognizes psychiatric and mental health nursing as one of the four core mental health disciplines, along with psychiatry, psychology, and social work. The present practice of psychiatric nursing is based on a number of

*Quotations in this chapter are from the American Nurses' Association, Division on Psychiatric and Mental Health Nursing Practice: Statement on psychiatric and mental health nursing practice, Kansas City, Mo., 1976. Reprinted by permission.

underlying premises or beliefs. See the accompanying box that describes some of the major philosophical beliefs of psychiatric nursing practice.

■ Roles and activities

The psychiatric nurse uses knowledge from the psychosocial and biophysical sciences and theories of personality and human behavior to derive a theoretical framework on which to base his or her practice. The choice of a conceptual model and theoretical framework is an individual one for each nurse. Various theories of psychiatric care are briefly described in Chapter 2 and a nursing model of health-illness phenomena is presented in Chapter 3.

Some nurses might base their practice on a psychoanalytical framework, others might adopt a family systems orientation, whereas still others may use a behavioral theoretical model. The nurse's choice of a model will depend on personal philosophy, educational background, setting, and experience in working with patients. Powers[48] believes that one criterion for the selection of a theory base should be its fit as an organized frame of reference for developed nursing models. The selected theoretical framework, she believes, should encompass the following commonalities of nursing models:

1. A holistic view of people, with usually three major interdependent subsystems or components
2. People as systems in dynamic interaction with the environment
3. People developing over time
4. People adapting continuously to both internal and external forces or variables

The theoretical model selected by the nurse can then be utilized as a framework for nursing practice.

■ **PRACTICE SETTINGS.** Psychiatric nurses may practice in settings that vary widely in purpose, type, location, and administration. They may be employed by an agency or self-employed in a private practice. Nurses who are employed by an agency are remunerated for their services on either a salaried or fee-for-service basis. The majority of nurses work in such organized settings, and the administrative policies of these organizations can either foster or limit the full utilization of the nurse's potential. Nurses who are self-employed receive remuneration for their services through third-party payment and direct patient fees. Some of these self-employed specialists maintain staff privileges with institutional facilities.

The settings in which nurses work can focus on either acute or long-term care. Some examples of settings include psychiatric hospitals, community mental

Philosophical Beliefs of Psychiatric Nursing Practice

■ The individual has intrinsic worth and dignity. Each person is worthy of respect by his nature and presence alone.

■ The goal of the individual is one of growth, health, autonomy, and self-actualization.

■ Every individual has the potential to change and the desire to pursue personal goals.

■ The person functions as a holistic being who acts on, interacts with, and reacts to the environment as a whole person. Each part affects the total response, which is greater than the sum of each separate component.

■ All people have common, basic, and necessary human needs. Maslow[31] categorized these needs as physical, safety, love and belonging, esteem, and self-actualization. Physical needs include physiological requirements such as food, water, and air. Safety needs pertain to the necessity of a secure physical environment that is free from threat. Love and belonging needs include the desire for intimacy and relatedness. Esteem needs refer to the desire for self-respect and recognition from others that one is a worthwhile and valuable person. Self-actualization needs include the desire for self-fulfillment as one concentrates on realizing one's own potential.

■ All behavior of the individual is meaningful. It arises from personal needs and goals and can only be understood from the person's internal frame of reference and within the context in which it occurs.

■ Behavior consists of perceptions, thoughts, feelings, and actions. These occur in a sequential manner; from one's perceptions thoughts arise, emotions are felt, and actions are conceived. Disruptions may occur in any of these areas and be evident in distorted perceptions, impaired thought processes, alterations in the expression of emotions, and maladaptive or inappropriate actions.

■ Individuals vary in their coping capacities. These are dependent on genetic endowment, environmental influences, nature and degree of stress, and available resources. All individuals have the potential for both health and illness.

■ Illness can be a growth-producing experience for the individual. The goal of nursing care is to maximize the person's positive interactions with his environment, promote his level of wellness, and enhance his degree of self-actualization.

■ All people have a right to an equal opportunity for adequate health care regardless of sex, race, religion, ethics, or cultural background. Nursing care is based on the needs of individuals, families, and communities and mutually defined goals and expectations.

■ Mental health is a critical and necessary component of comprehensive health care services.

■ The individual has the right to participate in decision making regarding his physical and mental health. The person has the right to self-determination. This right allows the individual the choice of changing present behavior or continuing it without modification. It is the decision of the individual to pursue health or illness.

■ An interpersonal relationship has the potential for producing change and growth within the individual. It is the vehicle for the application of the nursing process and the attainment of the goal of nursing care.

health centers, general hospitals, community health agencies, outpatient clinics, homes, schools, prisons, health maintenance organizations, private organizations, crisis care units, day and night care centers, offices, camps, and industrial centers.

■ FUNCTIONS. Within these settings, psychiatric nurses may assume various roles. They may be staff nurses, administrators, consultants, in-service educators, clinical practitioners, researchers, or program evaluators. Thus the settings of practice range from institutional to community based to independent practice, and the corresponding roles can include both direct and indirect nursing functions. The American Nurses' Association has identified nine major activities involved in the practice of psychiatric nursing.[2] (See box on Psychiatric Nursing Activities.)

The distinction of direct and indirect nursing care functions can more specifically describe the various functions or activities engaged in by psychiatric nurses. **"Direct nursing care functions** presume that the nurse's actions and reflections are focused on a particular client or family and that the nurse has personal responsibility and is accountable to the client or family for the outcome of such actions."[2:15] **Indirect nursing care functions** are those in which some other person actually carries out the patient's care. The nursing responsibilities inherent in these roles require the qualifications of a psychiatric and mental health nursing specialist. All of the direct and indirect nursing functions are actions for which the nurse is directly responsible. They are done whether or not the patient is under medical care and in any setting agreed on by the nurse and the patient.

In projecting future roles of psychiatric nurses, Slavinsky envisions the creation of a new primary care role for psychiatric nurses developed in liaison with community health nurses, using a system of mutual referral and consultation.[53] This primary care role would involve three functions: (1) assessment, (2) direct patient care, and (3) case management. Such a role would combine both the direct and indirect care functions previously described as nurses attempt to meet the needs of patients in a more humane and effective way.

■ **PRIMARY PREVENTION.** The concepts of primary prevention, secondary prevention, and tertiary prevention provide a framework for discussing these activities.[57] Primary prevention is a community concept that involves lowering the incidence of illness in a community by altering the causative factors before they have an opportunity to do harm. It is a concept that precedes disease and is applied to a generally healthy population. It includes health promotion, illness prevention, and protection against disease. Within this area lie many of nursing's independent functions that have as their goal decreasing the vulnerability of individuals to illness and

---

**Psychiatric Nursing Activities
Identified by the
American Nurses' Association***

1. Providing a therapeutic milieu
2. Working with the here-and-now problems of clients
3. Using the surrogate parent role
4. Caring for the somatic aspects of the client's health problems
5. Teaching factors related to emotional health
6. Acting as a social agent
7. Providing leadership to other personnel
8. Conducting psychotherapy
9. Engaging in social and community action related to mental health

*American Nurses' Association, Division on Psychiatric and Mental Health Nursing Practice: Statement on Psychiatric and mental health nursing practice, Kansas City, Mo., 1976, The Association.

---

strengthening their capacity to withstand stressors. Direct nursing care functions in this area include:

1. Health teaching regarding principles of mental health
2. Affecting changes in improved living conditions, freedom from poverty, and better education
3. Consumer education in such areas as normal growth and development and sex education
4. Initiating appropriate referrals before mental disorder occurs based on assessment of potential stressors and life changes
5. Assisting patients in a general hospital setting to avoid future psychiatric problems
6. Working with families to support family members and group functioning
7. Becoming active in community and political activities related to mental health

■ **SECONDARY PREVENTION.** Secondary prevention involves the reduction of actual illness by early detection and treatment of the problem. Following are direct nursing care functions in this area:

1. Intake screening and evaluation services
2. Home visits for preadmission or treatment services
3. Emergency treatment and psychiatric services in the general hospital
4. Providing a therapeutic milieu
5. Supervising patients receiving medication
6. Suicide prevention services
7. Counseling on a time-limited basis
8. Crisis intervention
9. Psychotherapy with individuals, families, and groups of various ages ranging from children to older adults
10. Intervening with communities and organizations based on an identified problem

■ **TERTIARY PREVENTION.** Tertiary prevention involves reducing the residual impairment or disability resulting from the illness. Direct nursing care functions in this area include the following:

1. Promoting vocational training and rehabilitation
2. Organizing aftercare programs for patients discharged from psychiatric facilities to facilitate their transition from the hospital to the community
3. Providing partial hospitalization options for patients

In addition to these direct nursing care functions,

psychiatric nurses engage in indirect activities that affect all three levels of prevention. These activities include educating nursing personnel in in-service, continuing, generic, or advanced educational programs; administrating in mental health settings to facilitate the provision of optimal nursing care; supervising nursing personnel to improve the quality of nursing services; consulting with colleagues, other professionals, consumer groups, community care givers, and local and national agencies; and researching clinical nursing problems.

■ Interdisciplinary mental health teams

An essential part of contemporary practice is cooperation and collaboration with other health care providers. Nurses may be members of three different types of teams: *unidisciplinary,* having all team members of the same discipline; *multidisciplinary,* having members of different disciplines who each provide specific services to the patient; and *interdisciplinary,* having members of different disciplines involved in a formal arrangement to provide patient services while maximizing educational interchange. Most organized mental health settings employ an interdisciplinary team approach, which requires highly coordinated and frequently interdependent planning based on the separate and distinct roles of each of the team members (Fig. 1-1).

■ Physicians, whether or not they are the team leaders, carry the medical responsibility for diagnosis, medical orders, medication, admission, and discharge, and the accountability for medical treatment.

■ Activity therapists are accountable and responsible for activity programming, although aspects of it may be shared with nurses.

■ Social workers are accountable and responsible for family casework and social placement.

■ Psychologists are accountable and responsible for psychological assessment and testing.

■ Nurses are accountable and responsible for the patient's milieu and for implementing the nurs-

ing process with all of its ramifications, ranging from assessment and planning care, providing a safe environment, dealing with the daily activity of patients, and evaluating the outcome of care.

■ **BARRIERS TO TEAM FUNCTIONING.** Interdisciplinary collaboration and functioning may or may not proceed smoothly. Given and Simmons describe seven barriers to interdisciplinary team formation: educational preparation, role ambiguity and incongruent expectations, authority, power, status, autonomy, and personal characteristics of members.[21] Benfer has identified three specific problems related to team functioning:

1. Problems identifying roles and functions
2. Difficulties in resolving overlapping roles
3. Communication problems within the team[5]

If the roles and functions of the various team members are not clarified and agreed on, then confusion, crossing of boundaries, resentment, and underutilization of health professionals are likely to occur. Some overlapping of roles and functions among psychiatric professionals is to be expected, since all mental health disciplines have access to the same body of knowledge on which professional education and improvement of practice are based. Thus, all the mental health team's members may be competent in providing psychotherapy, although some may prefer group therapy, others individual therapy, and still others family therapy. Only those team members who possess the necessary education, experience, and credentials can be considered qualified to handle ethically responsible psychotherapy. For nurses, psychotherapy should be undertaken only by a psychiatric clinical nurse specialist educated at the master's level.

The issue of various team members moving toward an individual psychotherapy approach has many implications. Ruch identifies a number of problems that can result when this approach is used in conjunction with assigning patients an individual therapist.[51] It can lead

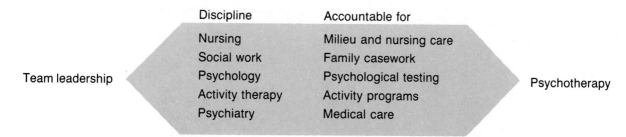

Fig. 1-1. Roles assumed by mental health team members. (Modified from Benfer, B.: Perspect. Psychiatr. Care 18(4):167, 1980.)

to unhealthy competition by team members to establish equally significant relationships with the patient. It might also lead to a disruption of the psychotherapeutic process, or can cause the patient to be very confused. Finally, he suggests that when a patient has several close relationships with team members it will be less likely that the patient will develop an efficacious therapeutic alliance. Ruch concludes that formal psychotherapy is best left to one member of the team who can then coordinate other interpersonal interventions.

In addition to a discrete role description, certain personal characteristics essential to teamwork are seen in the professional members who are able to tolerate frustration and are flexible in their adjustment to new situations. Appropriate members and adequate time are also important to the interdisciplinary team functioning. Table 1-1 summarizes these elements.

■ **JOINT COMMISSION ON INTERPROFESSIONAL AFFAIRS.** Partially in response to vested interests among mental health professionals and lack of cooperation, the Joint Commission on Interprofessional Affairs (JCIA) was founded in 1974. The members are representatives of the American Nurses' Association, the American Psychiatric Association, the American Psychological Association, and the National Association of Social Workers. Each organization has three representatives, and the commission meets three times a year to discuss legislation, reimbursement, education, and patient care issues related to mental health. JCIAs goal is to promote interprofessional trust, communication, and cooperation among mental health practitioners.

JCIA recommends that a variety of ways be pursued to facilitate communication and resolution of problems at national, state, and local levels, including such undertakings as joint meetings, regular exchange of information, exchange of formal liaison representatives, and organization of local and statewide interprofessional groups.

A major effort of the commission has been the development of the following guidelines for interprofessional ethics:

1. Seek to achieve interprofessional unity and cooperation.
2. Recognize and respect the autonomy and specialized competency of each profession.
3. Know the facts before speaking or issuing public positions about interprofessional issues and utilize the facts in a responsible and appropriate fashion.
4. Attempt to resolve issues through direct discussion, debate, and negotiation.
5. Pursue joint actions toward mutually acceptable goals.

Utilization of these guidelines should enhance the effectiveness of each of the professions in the delivery of mental health services. JCIA is presently working on case examples regarding autonomy, consultation, collaboration and supervision in relation to legal responsibilities, assessment and diagnosis, treatment planning, and service delivery to determine how the professions can better work together.

TABLE 1-1

ANALYSIS OF INTERDISCIPLINARY TEAMS

Personal qualities vital to interdisciplinary team function	Activities necessary for interdisciplinary team function
Accept differences/perspectives of others	Establish new professional interaction patterns
Function interdependently	Accept changes in authority and status
Negotiate role with other team members	Develop modes of conflict resolution and decision making
Form new values, attitudes, and perceptions	
Tolerate constant review and challenge of ideas	
Take risks	
Possess personal identity and integrity	
Accept team philosophy of care	

From Given, B., and Simmons, S.: Nurs. Forum **16**(2):165, 1977.

■ Leadership skills

Knowledge and strategies that enable psychiatric nurses, individually and collectively, to exercise leadership and management in the settings in which they work must be developed. It will not only impact on the care patients receive, but it will also serve to strengthen and expand the contribution of psychiatric nursing to the larger health care system.

Various theories have been developed regarding the complex social and psychologic phenomena involved in leadership. Most of the studies in this area, however, have focused on men in business organizations. Yet there is much to be gained from greater insight into the factors that promote or inhibit effective leadership among nurses.

One might approach this area from two different perspectives: examine the individual who is occupying a position of leadership or explore leadership as a transactional process. The former approach would include the styles and functions of leadership, whereas the latter would include the conditions, processes, and contexts of leadership as a social role or transaction (Table 1-2).[36]

Dumas has noted the following:

Those processes occurring in the groups in which or with which nurses work are of special significance. Pressures to conform to the image of the kind, nurturing, self-sacrificing angel of mercy (the analogue of the good mother) pose a perplexing dilemma for nurse leaders. Those who conform often find themselves deluged by bids from subordinates and colleagues in other disciplines for special attention or assistance to help them deal with the stresses of organizational life. These demands often exceed the responsibilities of their formal positions and drain time and energy that should be used for work tasks. Those who resist run the risk of the opposite stereotype—the cold, rigid, inconsiderate authoritarian leader (the rejecting, depriving, bad mother). There are big prices to pay in either instance.[15:712-713]

■ **CHANGE AGENTS.** There is no question but that psychiatric nurses must utilize their leadership skills and work as change agents to a greater degree than is presently being done. This need derives from the imperative of providing adequate, humane, and socially acceptable care to mental health consumers. To this end, nurses can initiate change; assist in change by supporting, participating, or implementing it; engage in joint ventures for planned change; and evaluate completed change. To do this, however, the following key characteristics are needed by the psychiatric nurse[32]:

1. The ability to take risks. This means to develop the ability to calculate potential risks surrounding the implementation of the change and then to decide whether or not these risks are indeed worth taking.
2. A commitment to the efficacy of the change. The change agent must develop a commitment to investigating the worth, value, effectiveness, and necessity of the change before initiating it.
3. Three areas of competence: knowledge of nursing that combines research findings and basic science information, clinical competence, and interpersonal relationship and communication skills.

This last characteristic requires the use not only of facilitative communication skills, but also confrontation when appropriate, a skill that nurses have tended to avoid using. Confrontation can only be justified as a precursor to negotiations, which are a foundation for change. It is a process that has two phases. The first requires an assault on the system to be changed. The second requires reconciliation to mend strained relationships or to create new ones. Smoyak believes:

Confrontations are in order when the goals are resolving an issue, improving health care systems, defining changing work roles, revamping licensing and practicing acts, gaining and keeping suitable salary schedules, attaining and maintaining control over professional practice, or any other professional issue, locally defined and carried out, on which there is consensus among nurses who are affected by the issue. They are in order when the group has gathered facts, may have tried other means, and has decided on collective action.[55:1635]

One result of such nursing initiative is that nursing licensure statutes have undergone considerable change and scrutiny in the last decade. Although not all states have revised their nurse practice acts, those which have show nurses assuming responsibility for more complex patient care that involves major independent decision making. Another positive sign is the 1980 publication of the American Nurses' Association entitled, *Nursing: A Social Policy Statement,*[3] which defines and establishes the scope of nursing practice and nursing's social responsibility.

Yet such statements and definitions cannot actually determine the scope of practice, relationships between nurses and other health professionals, needs of the consumer, or interaction between nursing and the government in formulating and implementing health-related policy. Only nurses working together through political processes can make these determinations. Although the impact of nurses on the quality and quantity of health care may be phenomenal, it is largely untapped. Nurses have the potential to be significant forces in the process of shaping the health care future of our society, if they

TABLE 1-2

THE NATURE OF EFFECTIVE LEADERSHIP

Conditions of effective leadership	Social processes underlying effective leadership	Styles of leadership	Functions of effective leadership
Recipient of communication must be able to understand it	Respect expressed *by* leader breeds respect *for* leader	Authoritarian style characterized by firmness, self-assurance, and domination of others	Leaders facilitate adaptive capacity of social systems
Person must have resources and ability to comply with directive	Leader must demonstrate competence in performing own roles	Democratic style characterized by responsiveness, participation, and mutual interaction	Leaders are alert to unanticipated consequences of previous collective action
Person must believe action is consistent with personal beliefs and values	Leader should be in continuing touch with what is going on in work group	Bureaucratic style characterized by strict, adhered to rules	Leaders are both present oriented and future oriented
Person must perceive directive as consistent with purposes and values of organization	Although leader has access to power that coerces, he seldom makes use of it	Laissez-faire style characterized by lack of direction and control	Leaders represent group to its environment
		Paternalistic style characterized by benevolent control	Leaders evaluate resources for system and cope with problems of their allocation
			Leaders express aspirations that evoke resonance among members of group
			Leaders mobilize, guide, coordinate, and control efforts of group members
			Leaders symbolize, extend, and deepen collective unity among members of system
			Leaders enunciate values and ideals of group and give people pride in their group identity
			Leaders arbitrate and mediate inevitable conflicts that emerge in social interaction, so that most members of group believe justice has been done most of time
			Leaders serve as scapegoats for larger group

Modified from Merton, R.: Am. J. Nurs. **69:**2614, 1969.

can learn to use their power and resources in the political arena—one of the truly most important targets for nursing actions.

Level of performance

The description of various nursing activities and functions is also indicative of the wide variation in levels of performance. Not all psychiatric nurses are able to perform each of these functions. Individual nurses have primary responsibility and accountability for their own practice and one aspect of accountability is that nurses define and adhere to the legitimate scope of their practice. Four major factors play a role in determining the level at which the nurse functions and the types of activities he or she engages in.

■ Laws

The first and primary factor affecting the level of nursing practice is the law. Each state has its own nurse practice act, which regulates entry into the profession and defines the legal limits of nursing practice that must be adhered to by all nurses. At present, there are three general patterns of nurse practice acts: regulatory acts, expanded definition acts, and delegatory acts. Some acts recognize advanced practice of nurses, while others do not. Nurses should become familiar with the nurse practice act of their own state and define and limit their practice accordingly.

■ Qualifications

The second factor is the qualifications of the nurse, including education, work experiences, and certification status. The American Nurses' Association has identified two types of practitioners: nurses who are generalists and are called psychiatric and mental health nurses, and nurses who are specialists and are called psychiatric and mental health nurse specialists.[2]

■ **EDUCATION AND EXPERIENCE.** The recommended educational preparation for the generalist role is a baccalaureate degree in nursing. One also needs to demonstrate the profession's standards of knowledge, experience, and quality of care through formal review processes. The majority of nurses working in psychiatry are generalists. They provide most of the care for most of the people served by nursing.

In contrast, specialization involves adding to the generic base of nursing practice an organized and systematized body of knowledge and competencies within a discrete area of nursing, applied through specialized practice. The specialist in psychiatric and mental health nursing is characterized by graduate education, supervised clinical experience, and depth of knowledge, com-

petence, and skill in practice. This increased depth of knowledge is reflected in the specialist's more refined ability to apply this knowledge to the solution of mental health problems. The minimum level of preparation for the specialist is a master's degree in psychiatric nursing, which is characterized by academically supervised clinical practice and study in the theoretical bases for therapeutic intervention.

Currently there are over 60 master's degree programs in psychiatric nursing and over 6,000 psychiatric and mental health nurses have master's degrees. In addition, there are 30 doctoral programs in nursing (Table 1-3). They focus on either research and theory development in nursing or advanced development of the nurse-therapist role with research focused on specific clinical problems. The first type of program usually leads to a Doctor of Philosophy (Ph.D.) degree, whereas the second results in a Doctor of Nursing Science (D.N.Sc.) degree. Doctorally prepared nurses contribute to the advancement of knowledge in the field of psychiatric and mental health nursing through research and scholarship.

Another qualification is the nurse's relevant work experience. Although work experience does not replace education, it does provide an added and necessary dimension to one's level of competence and ability to function therapeutically. Gardner[20] believes that one's role should be determined by the education, experiential level, and personal assets of the nurse. She suggests defining the role of the psychiatric nurse in an ambulatory setting based on three levels of practice. Table 1-4 summarizes the requirements and responsibilities of each level of practice. The nurses identified in Level 3 of this table are clinical nurse specialists. They are nurses with a master's degree in psychiatric nursing who possess advanced knowledge and expertise in psychiatric care and principles of supervision and consultation. Additional elements of this advanced nursing role are explored by Critchley and Maurin.[10]

■ **CERTIFICATION.** The final qualification is the certification process, which is a formal review of the clinical practice of the nurse that has evolved within the American Nurses' Association.

The objectives of this process as described by Tousley are to

1. Assure the public of quality care
2. Provide credentials to expedite employment and third-party reimbursement for services rendered
3. Expand opportunities for vertical and horizontal mobility and career advancement
4. Attain greater prestige and peer recognition for achieving clinical expertise
5. Improve clinical practice[58]

TABLE 1-3

DOCTORAL PROGRAMS IN NURSING, 1984–1985

Institution	Degree	Institution	Degree
AL U. of Alabama in Birmingham Birmingham, AL 35294	D.N.S.	**NY** Adelphi University Garden City, NY 11530	Ph.D.
AZ U. of Arizona Tucson, AZ 85721	Ph.D.	**NY** New York University New York, NY 10003	Ph.D.
CA U. of California, San Francisco San Francisco, CA 94143	D.N.S.	**NY** Teachers College, Columbia University New York, NY 10027	Ed.D.
CA U. of San Diego San Diego, CA 92110	D.N.S.	**NY** U. of Rochester Rochester, NY 14642	Ph.D.
CO U. of Colorado Denver, CO 80262	Ph.D.	**OH** Case Western Reserve University Cleveland, OH 44106	Ph.D.
DC Catholic University of America Washington, DC 20064	D.N.Sc.	**OR** Oregon Health Sciences University Portland, OR 97201	Ph.D.
FL U. of Florida Gainesville, FL 32610	Ph.D.	**PA** Pennsylvania State U. University Park, PA 16802	Ph.D.
FL U. of Miami Coral Gables, FL 33124	Ph.D.	**PA** U. of Pennsylvania Philadelphia, PA 19104	D.N.Sc.
GA Medical College of Georgia Augusta, GA 20912	Ph.D.	**PA** U. of Pittsburgh Pittsburgh, PA 15261	Ph.D.
IL Rush University Chicago, IL 60612	D.N.Sc.	**PA** Widener University Chester, PA 19013	D.N.
IL U. of Illinois at the Medical Center Chicago, IL 60612	Ph.D.	**RI** U. of Rhode Island Kingston, RI 02881	Ph.D.
IN Indiana University Indianapolis, IN 46223	D.N.S.	**SC** U. of S. Carolina Columbia, SC 29008	Ph.D.
KS U. of Kansas Kansas City, KS 66103	Ph.D.	**TX** Texas Woman's University Denton, TX 76204	Ph.D.
MD U. of Maryland Baltimore, MD 21201	Ph.D.	**TX** U. of Texas at Austin Austin, TX 78712	Ph.D.
MA Boston University Boston, MA 02215	D.N.S.	**UT** U. of Utah Salt Lake City, UT 84112	Ph.D.
MI U. of Michigan Ann Arbor, MI 48104	Ph.D.	**VA** George Mason U. Fairfax, VA 22030	D.N.S.
MI Wayne State University Detroit, MI 48202	Ph.D.	**VA** U. of Virginia Charlottesville, VA 22903	Ph.D.
MN U. of Minnesota Minneapolis, MN 55455	Ph.D.	**WA** U. of Washington Seattle, WA 98195	Ph.D.
		WI U. of Wisconsin-Madison Madison, WI 53792	Ph.D.
		WI U. of Wisconsin-Milwaukee Milwaukee, WI 53201	Ph.D.

TABLE 1-4

LEVELS OF PRACTICE FOR PSYCHIATRIC NURSES IN AMBULATORY SETTINGS

	Level 1	Level 2	Level 3
Educational requirements	No formal education is necessary other than current state licensure	Baccalaureate degree in nursing	Master's degree in psychiatric nursing
Experience requirements	Minimum of 1 year experience in acute psychiatric nursing care	Minimum of 2 years of experience in acute psychiatric care settings	Advanced knowledge and expertise in psychiatric care and principles of supervision and consultation
Nature of practice	Supportive treatment	Supportive treatment	Insight treatment
Therapeutic functions	Communicating with other professionals and agencies relative to patient care	Primary responsibility for supportive therapy	Primary responsibility for insight-oriented psychotherapy
	Assisting in assessment and data collection	Assessment of patient functioning	Responsibility for patients cared for by nurses in levels 1 and 2 of practice
	Assisting patient to use environmental resources	Initiation and attendance at all conferences regarding patients	Assessment of patient pathology
	Assisting in community primary prevention programs	Assignment to interdisciplinary teams responsible for delivery of primary mental health care in ambulatory units	Supervision of other health team members
			Participation in primary community prevention programs
			Responsibility for obtaining supervision consultation
			Responsible for assumption of nursing leadership

Modified from Gardner, K.: J. Psychiatr. Nurs. **15**:26, 1977.

Within psychiatric nursing there are two levels of certification: the **generalist** who may be a staff nurse, and the **specialist** in either adult or child and adolescent psychiatric nursing. As of May 1982, there were 679 certified nurse generalists, 717 certified nurse specialists in adult psychiatric mental health nursing, and 66 certified nurse specialists in child and adolescent psychiatric mental health nursing.

To become a certified generalist the psychiatric nurse must demonstrate expertise in practice, knowledge of theories concerning personality development and behavior patterns in treating mental illness, and the relationship of such treatments to nursing care. Special requirements include

1. Two years' experience within the preceding four years prior to application
2. Current work in direct nursing care for a minimum of four hours per week

Certification as a specialist requires that the nurse evidence a "high degree of proficiency in interpersonal skills, in the use of the nursing process, and in psychiatric, psychological, and milieu therapies."[2:11-12] Following are six requirements for certification in psychiatric and mental health nursing:

1. Current involvement in direct clinical nursing practice at least 4 hours per week
2. A master's or higher degree in nursing, with a

specialization in psychiatric and mental health nursing *or* one may apply for individual consideration if one possesses a baccalaureate degree in nursing and a master's degree in a related field, such as psychology, sociology, social work, human relations, or counseling and guidance, *or* a master's or higher degree in nursing, plus a baccalaureate in any field and a diploma in nursing.

3. Practice in psychiatric and mental health nursing after receiving a master's degree with direct patient/client contact for either 8 hours a week for 2 years *or* 4 hours a week for 4 years
4. Access to clinical supervision or consultation
5. Experience in at least two different treatment modalities
6. At least 100 hours of supervision/consultation by a certified member of the core mental health disciplines (clinical specialist in psychiatric and mental health nursing, psychiatrist, psychologist, or psychiatric social worker) after receiving a master's degree

On successful completion of the certification examination and written documentation, the nurse is identified as Certified (C.) if a generalist, or a Certified Specialist (C.S.) in psychiatric mental health nursing. Although any specialist nurse may be certified, it is expected that the nurse who is self-employed in the practice of psychotherapy will obtain certification to assure the public of his or her ability to perform as a competent nurse psychotherapist.

■ Setting

The third factor influencing the psychiatric nurse's level of performance is the setting in which he or she practices. According to Peplau, the role nurses assume in any psychiatric mental health setting depends upon the

1. Competence brought to work as a consequence of basic or post-basic nursing education
2. Definition of mental illness that prevails in a given setting
3. Extent of consensus about whether each profession should or should not have any discrete and unique roles or whether there can be overlap
4. Cost of certain kinds of care, the difference in status and salary levels, and the number of persons needed and available to provide certain kinds of care[44]

A basic consideration is the philosophy of the health care system and the way in which the setting defines mental illness. From this definition will emerge the work of the patient and the role of the nurse as illustrated in Table 1-5. If the setting is that of an organization, additional constraints may be imposed on the nurse due to administrative policies, staff norms, or nursing service expectations.

A study done by Sloboda[54] determined that inpatient nurses ranked their functions as primarily those of a "nurse clinician" followed by "change agent" and finally "therapist." Nurses in outpatient settings ranked all three functions fairly equally. Lieb, Underwood, and Glick[29] suggest that inpatient staff nurses are limited in providing primary therapy because of the ready supply of other professionals and a concern for appropriate preparation. The nurse's relationship with other health professionals thus emerges as an important influence on level of functioning.

Traditional settings for psychiatric nurses include psychiatric facilities, community mental health centers, the general hospital, and private practice. With the movement toward early discharge and increased community care, however, alternative treatment settings are emerging, such as home health care agencies, business and industry, and health maintenance organizations.

Wojdowski and Hartnett describe the inception, growth, and structure of a formal acute psychiatric service within a large health maintenance organization (HMO) in which psychiatric nurse clinicians were valued for their special expertise.[62] They noted that the new service reduced the overload on the more traditional outpatient facility and increased patient satisfaction. In addition, the HMO experienced a low psychiatric hospitalization rate once the service was in operation which contributed to the overall cost-effectiveness of the organization.

The present economic environment of the health care system in this country suggests that new opportunities will emerge for psychiatric nurses in nontraditional settings. Nurses should assess mental health needs and practically and creatively identify settings and strategies that will be most effective in promoting health and preventing illness.

■ Personal initiative

The fourth and final factor affecting the nurse's level of functioning is the personal competence and initiative of the individual nurse. These personal qualities will determine how the nurse interprets his or her role and the success of its implementation. The importance of this final factor should not be ignored, since without a realization of clinical competence and the assumption

TABLE 1-5

DIFFERENT DEFINITIONS OF MENTAL ILLNESS AND THEREFORE OF THE WORK OF THE PATIENT AND THE ROLE OF THE NURSE

Definition	Work of the patient	Role of the nurse
Socially unacceptable behavior of the patient has previously been "rewarded"; he has unfortunately been "conditioned" to behave in these ways	Submit to treatment using behavior modification (reconditioning) techniques	Surveillance of patient following treatment plan; pass out rewards; general nursing routine care
Unacceptable behavior is the result of genetic inheritance	Submit to whatever ameliorative treatment of symptoms is ordered	Surveillance and custody; reporting; general nursing routine care
Unacceptable behavior is due to a biochemical imbalance	Submit to tests and prescribed treatment drugs to rectify the imbalance	Surveillance; reporting; pass medications, such as tranquilizers, stimulants, lithium, hormones, etc.; observe effects; general nursing routine care
Unacceptable behavior is due to some unknown but adverse brain activity	Submit to prescribed treatment (electrostimulation, electroshock, lobotomy, etc.)	Surveillance; reporting; pretreatment and posttreatment "preparation"; general nursing (and surgical nursing) care
Unacceptable behavior reflects problems in living with people and lack in intellectual and interpersonal competencies to understand and solve those problems	Participate in psychotherapy sessions and in ad hoc talking sessions with the available professionals, to investigate, understand, and resolve those problems and in the process gain new intellectual and interpersonal competencies on an experiential/educative basis	Use all "activities of daily living" as a basis for observation, discussion, and intervention in ways that enhance the patient's intellectual and interpersonal competencies to change his own behavior; also general nursing care. Using "situational counseling" to aid patients involved in disputes, violence, and other grossly unacceptable behavior to investigate the problem inherent in the acting-out situation. Referral for other professional services, such as clergy, and coordination and follow-up on discharge
The unacceptable behavior is due to "lack of insight" into intrapsychic causes	Seek psychoanalysis for those who can afford it	

From Peplau, H.: Int. Nurs. Rev. **25**(2):45, 1978.

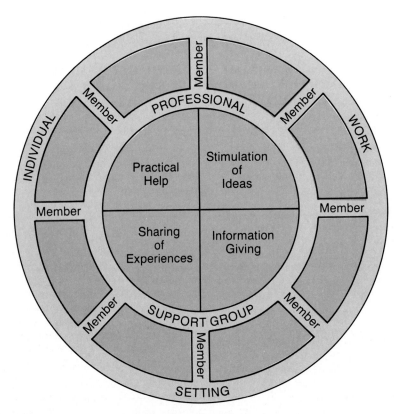

Fig. 1-2. Professional support group model. (From Johnson, R., et al.: The professional support group: a model for psychiatric clinical nurse specialists, J. Psychosoc. Nurs. 20(2):9, 1982.)

of professional initiative, the nurse will be significantly limited in performance.

■ **BURNOUT AND SUPPORT.** In recent years, the nursing literature has described a phenomenon known as job burnout, defined as a "syndrome of physical and emotional exhaustion, involving the development of negative self-concept, negative job attitudes, and loss of concern and feeling for clients."[46] It may lead to physical illness, irritability, cynicism, fatigue, and withdrawal from one's nursing work. At an extreme, it might also produce harmful patient contact through physical or verbal abuse or nontherapeutic communication.

Burnout results from prolonged stress that causes a depletion of a nurse's personal resources. Some of the common sources of stress for psychiatric nurses are conflict with one's supervisors or co-workers, job dissatisfaction, inappropriate nurse-patient ratios, high patient acuity, authority not equal to one's responsibility, lack of participation in decisions affecting one's work, inadequate staff support, lack of promotion potential, low salary, lack of autonomy, and numerous organizational constraints.

One study of stress among nurses in four specialty areas reported that psychiatric nurses found that they experienced intense interpersonal involvement and frequent conflicts with patients, families, physicians, and colleagues.[11] They also experienced less social affirmation and recognition than intensive care nurses and less assistance than operating room nurses. The authors conclude that these findings are noteworthy, especially in view of the fact that psychiatric nurses are expected to provide psychosocial assistance and support to their patients, and to some degree, their peers.

Another recent study measured specific aspects of occupational stress as perceived by psychiatric nurses.[13] The authors of the study found that stressors inherent in the nursing role produced low levels of stress, but that stressors inherent in the organizational system produced high levels of stress. In fact, 50% of the high stresses and all the top ten identified stresses were organizational in nature. The single most stressful experience involved not being notified of changes before they occurred.

Given the seriousness of the problem, it is important to plan and implement stress management strategies for psychiatric nurses. Evans and Lewis claim the best cure for burnout is prevention.[17] They suggest that measures should be instituted to provide a supportive environment for psychiatric nurses. Attention should be paid to the number and mix of staff, delegation of unessential paperwork, open communication, recognition of nurses' contributions, opportunity to influence one's work context, involvement in unit decision making, encouragement of professional activities, and the provision of new work roles or responsibilities. They believe that "support, understanding, receptivity and flexibility are all keys to providing an environment in which professional practice and personal growth can flourish.[17:173]

A final strategy for enhancing the personal growth and competence of the psychiatric nurse is the use of support groups to both prevent and alleviate staff burnout. They have been described in the nursing literature for both staff nurses[19] and clinical nurse specialists.[25] Fig. 1-2 presents a model of a professional support group developed by Johnson and co-workers.[25] The four major purposes of this group are to: (1) provide practical help to one another, (2) stimulate ideas, (3) share professional experiences, and (4) share relevant information. Possible group activities are described in Table 1-6.

In conclusion, these four factors together account for variations in levels of nursing practice. Specifically, these variations will be evident in regard to the following:

- Assessment and data collection
- Analysis of data
- Application of theory
- Breadth and depth of knowledge base, especially clinical, psychosocial, and pathophysiological theories relating to nursing diagnosis and treatment
- The range of nursing techniques
- Need for, kind, and extent of supervision by other nurses in practice
- Evaluation of effects of practice
- Identification of relationships among phenomena, nursing actions, effects (outcomes for the patients)[3:19-20]

TABLE 1-6

PROFESSIONAL SUPPORT GROUP ACTIVITIES

Purposes	Related activities
Practical help	Case presentations Evaluating record-keeping methods Interventions for staff performance problems Standardized nursing care plan development Position title changes
Stimulation of ideas	Educational meeting reports Individual role components discussion
Sharing of experiences	Discussion of difficult work experiences Description of successful interventions
Sharing information	Exchange of continuing education brochures Distribution of articles Update on new laws Sharing of institutional policies Suggestions of resources for additional information for problem solving

From Johnson, R., et al.: J. Psychosoc. Nurs. Ment. Health Serv. **20**(2):9, 1982.

All nurses who are practicing with patients, however, are expected to address the phenomena that form the core of nursing practice. These are identified and described in the *Standards of Psychiatric and Mental Health Nursing Practice.*

STANDARDS OF PSYCHIATRIC AND MENTAL HEALTH NURSING PRACTICE

INTRODUCTION

The purpose of *Standards of Psychiatric and Mental Health Nursing Practice* is to fulfill the profession's obligation to provide a means of improving the quality of care. The standards reflect the current state of knowledge in the field and are therefore provisional, dynamic, and subject to testing and subsequent change. Since standards represent agreed-upon levels of practice, they have been developed to characterize, to measure, and to provide guidance in achieving excellence in care.*

The standards presented here are a revision of the standards enunciated by the Division on Psychiatric and Mental Health Nursing Practice in 1973. They apply to any setting in which psychiatric and mental health nursing is practiced, and to both generalists and specialists in psychiatric and mental health nursing. Standards V-F (psychotherapy) and X (community health systems) apply specifically to the specialist. The standards are written within the framework of the nursing process, which includes data collection, diagnosis, planning, treatment, and evaluation.*

The treatment or intervention phase of the nursing process is elaborated upon in order to highlight the specific interventions or nursing care activities commonly carried out by psychiatric and mental health nurses: therapeutic interventions, health teaching, activities of daily living, somatic therapies, therapeutic environment, and psychotherapy. In addition to the standards concerned with the nursing process are standards that address professional performance, such as use of theory, peer review, continuing education, interdisciplinary team collaboration,

community health systems, and research. Accountability of the provider to the client, client rights, and client advocacy are implicit throughout the standards.

A rationale is provided for each standard, and criteria are developed to measure each standard. The criteria are divided into *structure, process,* and *outcome.* They are intended to provide a means by which attainment of the standard may be specifically measured. The criteria for each standard are not exhaustive.

Standards of Psychiatric and Mental Health Nursing Practice should be used in conjunction with the following ANA publications: (1) *Standards of Nursing Practice,* (2) *Statement on Psychiatric and Mental Health Nursing Practice,* (3) *Nursing: A Social Policy Statement,* and (4) *Code for Nurses with Interpretive Statements.*

PROFESSIONAL PRACTICE STANDARDS

STANDARD I. THEORY
The nurse applies appropriate theory that is scientifically sound as a basis for decisions regarding nursing practice.
Rationale

Psychiatric and mental health nursing is characterized by the application of relevant theories to explain phenomena of concern to nurses, and to provide a basis for intervention and subsequent evaluation of that intervention. A primary source of knowledge for practice rests on the scholarly conceptualizations of psychiatric and mental health nursing practice and on research findings generated from intradisciplinary and cross-disciplinary studies of human behavior. The nurse's use of selected theories provides comprehensive, balanced perceptions of clients' characteristics, diagnoses, or presenting conditions.

From American Nurses' Association, Division on Psychiatric and Mental Health Nursing Practice: Standards of psychiatric and mental health nursing practice, Kansas City, Mo., 1982, The Association. Reprinted by permission.
*From American Nurses' Association: A plan for implementation of the standards of nursing practice, Kansas City, Mo., 1974, The Association, p. 4.

STANDARDS OF PSYCHIATRIC AND MENTAL HEALTH NURSING PRACTICE—cont'd.

STANDARD II. DATA COLLECTION

The nurse continuously collects data that are comprehensive, accurate, and systematic.

Rationale

Effective interviewing, behavioral observation, and physical and mental health assessment enable the nurse to reach sound conclusions and plan appropriate interventions with the client.

STANDARD III. DIAGNOSIS

The nurse utilizes nursing diagnoses and/or standard classification of mental disorders to express conclusions supported by recorded assessment data and current scientific premises.

Rationale

Nursing's logical basis for providing care rests on the recognition and identification of those actual or potential health problems that are within the scope of nursing practice.

STANDARD IV. PLANNING

The nurse develops a nursing care plan with specific goals and interventions delineating nursing actions unique to each client's needs.

Rationale

The nursing care plan is used to guide therapeutic intervention and effectively achieve the desired outcomes.

STANDARD V. INTERVENTION

The nurse intervenes as guided by the nursing care plan to implement nursing actions that promote, maintain, or restore physical and mental health, prevent illness, and effect rehabilitation.

Rationale

Mental health is one aspect of general health and well-being. Nursing actions reflect an appreciation for the hierarchy of human needs and include interventions for all aspects of physical and mental health and illness.

STANDARD V-A. INTERVENTION: PSYCHOTHERAPEUTIC INTERVENTIONS

The nurse uses psychotherapeutic interventions to assist clients in regaining or improving their previous coping abilities and to prevent further disability.

Rationale

Individuals with and without mental health problems often respond to health problems in a dysfunctional manner. During counseling, interviewing, crisis or emergency intervention, or daily interaction, nurses diagnose dysfunctional behaviors, engage clients in noting such behaviors, and assist the client in modifying or eliminating those behaviors.

STANDARD V-B. INTERVENTION: HEALTH TEACHING

The nurse assists clients, families, and groups to achieve satisfying and productive patterns of living through health teaching.

Rationale

Health teaching is an essential part of the nurse's role with those who have mental health problems. Every interaction can be utilized as a teaching-learning situation. Formal and informal teaching methods can be used in working with individuals, families, groups, and the community. Emphasis is on understanding principles of mental health as well as on developing ways of coping with mental health problems. Client adherence to treatment regimens increases when health teaching is an integral part of the client's care.

STANDARD V-C. INTERVENTION: ACTIVITIES OF DAILY LIVING

The nurse uses the activities of daily living in a goal-directed way to foster adequate self-care and physical and mental well-being of clients.

Rationale

A major portion of one's daily life is spent in some form of activity related to health and

STANDARDS OF PSYCHIATRIC AND MENTAL HEALTH NURSING PRACTICE—cont'd.

well-being. An individual's developmental and intellectual levels, emotional state, and physical limitations may be reflected in these activities. Nurses are the primary professional health care providers who interact with clients on a day-to-day basis around the tasks of daily living. Therefore, the nurse has a unique opportunity to assess and intervene in these processes in order to encourage constructive changes in the client's behavior so that each child, adolescent, and adult can realize his potential for growth and health or maintain that level previously achieved.

STANDARD V-D. INTERVENTION: SOMATIC THERAPIES

The nurse uses knowledge of somatic therapies and applies related clinical skills in working with clients.

Rationale

Various treatment modalities may be needed by clients during the course of illness. Pertinent clinical observations and judgments are made concerning the effect of drugs and other somatic treatments used in the therapeutic program.

STANDARD V-E. INTERVENTION: THERAPEUTIC ENVIRONMENT

The nurse provides, structures, and maintains a therapeutic environment in collaboration with the client and other health care providers.

Rationale

The nurse works with clients in a variety of environmental settings such as inpatient, residential, day care, and home. The environment contributes in positive and negative ways to the state of health or illness of the client. When it serves the interest of the client as an inherent part of the overall nursing care plan, the setting is structured and/or altered.

STANDARD V-F. INTERVENTION: PSYCHOTHERAPY

The nurse utilizes advanced clinical expertise in individual, group, and family psychotherapy, child psychotherapy, and other treatment modalities to function as a psychotherapist, and recognizes professional accountability for nursing practice.

Rationale

Acceptance for the role of psychotherapist entails primary responsibility for the treatment of clients and entrance into a contractual agreement. This contract includes a commitment to see a client through the problem presented or to assist the client in finding other appropriate assistance. It also includes an explicit definition of the relationship, the respective role of each person in the relationship, and what can be realistically expected of each person.

STANDARD VI. EVALUATION

The nurse evaluates client responses to nursing actions in order to revise the data base, nursing diagnoses, and nursing care plan.

Rationale

Nursing care is a dynamic process that implies alterations in data, diagnoses, or plans previously made.

PROFESSIONAL PERFORMANCE STANDARDS

STANDARD VII. PEER REVIEW

The nurse participates in peer review and other means of evaluation to assure quality of nursing care provided for clients.

Rationale

Evaluation of the quality of nursing care through examination of the clinical practice of nurses is one way to fulfill the profession's obligation to ensure that consumers are provided excellence in care. Peer review and other quality assurance procedures are utilized in this endeavor.

Roles and functions of psychiatric nurses **27**

STANDARDS OF PSYCHIATRIC AND MENTAL HEALTH NURSING PRACTICE—cont'd.

STANDARD VIII. CONTINUING EDUCATION

The nurse assumes responsibility for continuing education and professional development and contributes to the professional growth of others.

Rationale

The scientific, cultural, social, and political changes characterizing our contemporary society require the nurse to be committed to the ongoing pursuit of knowledge that will enhance professional growth.

STANDARD IX. INTERDISCIPLINARY COLLABORATION

The nurse collaborates with other health care providers in assessing, planning, implementing, and evaluating programs and other mental health activities.

Rationale

Psychiatric nursing practice requires planning and sharing with others to deliver maximum mental health services to the client and the community. Through the collaborative process, different abilities of health care providers are utilized to communicate, plan, solve problems, and evaluate services delivered.

STANDARD X. UTILIZATION OF COMMUNITY HEALTH SYSTEMS

The nurse participates with other members of the community in assessing, planning, implementing, and evaluating mental health services and community systems that include the promotion of the broad continuum of primary, secondary, and tertiary prevention of mental illness.

Rationale

The high incidence of mental illness in our contemporary society requires increased effort to devise more effective treatment and prevention programs. Nurses must participate in programs that strengthen the existing health potential of all members of society. Such concepts as primary prevention and continuity of care are essential in planning to meet the mental health needs of the community. The nurse uses organizational, advisory, advocacy, and consultative skills to facilitate the development and implementation of mental health services.

STANDARD XI. RESEARCH

The nurse contributes to nursing and the mental health field through innovations in theory and practice and participation in research.

Rationale

Each professional has responsibility for the continuing development and refinement of knowledge in the mental health field through research and experimentation with new and creative approaches to practice.

The question of professional autonomy

Psychiatric nurses as a group displayed certain personal qualities in a study reported by Mlott.[37] He found that they possessed adequate defenses, a good self-concept, adequate but flexible impulse control, the ability to trust others, and tolerance. They viewed events as products of their own actions and sought information relevant to problems they encountered. He also reported that they were better adjusted and more active, striving, independent, effective, self-confident, persevering, and determined than other nurse subspecialties. His study paints a rather rosy picture of psychiatric nurses as competent, effective, and confident mental health professionals. However, are they truly professionalized?

The professional status of nursing has been a long-debated issue both within nursing and among observers and scholars outside of nursing. Often, in the nursing literature, one sees defensive assertions or soothing assurances that yes, indeed, nursing really is a profession. However, outside the field, nursing is described as a semiprofession, subprofession, or marginal profession. One can only conclude that there is no consensus, and the question is far from resolved. It is helpful, however, to analyze psychiatric nursing's present position on the professionalization continuum because, in so doing, conflicts and roadblocks to future growth can be identified.

Viewed as a continuum, professionalization "is the evidence of a continuous attempt of a group in any community or society to gain more and more control over certain resources related to an occupational area."[60] The attainment of professional status necessarily involves a struggle. Society alone has the power to grant it, and consensus for it must exist in the body politic. The six characteristics of the scale of professionalization identified by Moore[38] are comprehensive in scope and developmental in nature. They suggest the following sequencing or process of professionalization:

1. **Occupation.** The requirement that the work be a full-time undertaking by a group of individuals.
2. **Calling.** A personal commitment or intention to pursue a stable career in the occupation. It incorporates socialization into the culture of the profession with its values, norms, and symbols.
3. **Organization.** The formation of an association by members because of their recognition of common occupational interests. The organization concerns itself with the occupation's status as a profession, the tasks of its members, the ways

to raise the quality of applicants, and political action.
4. **Education.** Preparation by intense study of a systematic "body of theory." This body of theory is a system of abstract propositions that describe in general terms the classes of phenomena which make up the profession's focus of interest and is then practically applied. Theory construction through systematic research is a distinctive professional activity as characterized in the role of researcher-theoretician. In this way, the profession creates, organizes, and transmits its knowledge. The minimal educational requirement is the baccalaureate degree, although many professions have considerably longer educational requirements. A spirit of rationality prevails among the members, as evidenced in its ongoing commitment to learning and the processes of reasoning and the assumption of a critical attitude toward its theory and knowledge base.
5. **Service orientation.** Characterized by rules of competence, conscientious performance, and loyalty or service. Rules of competence require the accreditation of educational programs, establishment of a licensing system, and maintenance and improvement of standards through continuing education. Rules of conscientious performance refer to self-discipline and self-regulation. Rules of service require that the professionals serve the clients' interests first, placing it over personal gain or commercial profit.
6. **Autonomy.** Legitimate control over one's own work. Autonomy is the ultimate value for professionals characterized by professional authority. The outcome of autonomy and authority is power, prestige, and status accorded by society, which in turn expects exemplary behavior from the profession.

Psychiatric nursing has amply met the first two characteristics. The remaining four, however, appear to be problematic.[56]

■ Organization

The American Nurses' Association was founded in 1896. It is the major professional organization, but approximately only 25% of all licensed nurses belong to it. American Nurses' Association members, furthermore, represent various educational backgrounds and, consequently, various interpretations of the tasks and roles of nursing. They disagree on the uniqueness of their contribution as health care team members, their educational programs and their legal rights and responsibilities.[1] The American Nurses' Association has a specialty subgroup, the Council on Psychiatric and Mental Health Nursing. In 1973 it published the *Standards of Psychiatric and Mental Health Nursing Practice* and revised them in 1982. The *Statement on Psychiatric and Mental Health Nursing Practice*,[2] which defines psychiatric nursing, identifies types of practitioners, and describes the scope of practice, was published in 1976. Both of these publications have served to clarify and refine the role, tasks, and functioning of psychiatric nurses.

Since 1948, the American Nurses' Association has had an economic security program, with one of its goals being to upgrade the economic position of registered nurses. To do this, it engages in collective bargaining activities. The majority of nurses appear to accept the validity and necessity of collective action to attain economic goals. What remains in conflict are the mechanism and scope of issues appropriately covered by collective bargaining agreements, specifically, the inclusion of patient care issues in negotiations and the leadership dilemma of a professional organization functioning as a collective bargaining agent.

Underlying the position of the American Nurses' Association toward collective bargaining is the conviction that nurses must speak for nursing. This is a more fundamental issue than the single aspect of salary or scheduling. It is the basis for the difference between a professional organization and a union, and it has particular significance for nursing because of its long history of domination by other groups. No one group represents a majority of nurses; neither is the economic security program the primary purpose of the American Nurses' Association. However, unless nursing accepts its responsibility to control its own practice and to have nurses speak for nursing, the economic security issue may end up being the end, not just the means.

Cleland[9] has described a professional collective bargaining model. She believes that the labor contract can become the legal instrument through which the profession can implement standards of care. To do so, the labor contract should include negotiated clauses relating to wages, hours, and conditions of work. To gain control of nursing practice, she believes the contract should contain provisions on (1) shared governance, (2) individual accountability, and (3) collective professional responsibility. Clearly, the model she advocates is a professional one that would necessitate the active participation and support of nurses. Before it can be widely undertaken, however, nurses need to collectively decide if they wish to be professionals.

■ **NETWORKING AND NURSING.** In addition to supporting its formal organizations, nursing would also benefit from another strategy—networking. Networks are groups of individuals drawn together by common frustrations and concerns for the purpose of supporting and helping one another. Networks range from informal friendships, to small groups providing professional contacts and advancement, to large, open groups providing emotional support.

Nursing's prevailing inbreeding, infighting, and impotence have been noted in the literature. The history of nursing documents the profession's preoccupation with internal disagreements, inconsistencies, and deficiencies. Furthermore, nurses often feel disenfranchised and alienated from nursing peers in other positions, and this frequently results in conflict among nurse administrators, educators, practitioners, and researchers. To counter this phenomenon, nurses should identify with their peers, feel trusted by their colleagues, and pledge loyalty to other members of their own profession.

One structural mechanism to assist in this process is the formation of networks that can help nurses to unite and value their profession. Meisenhelder believes that nursing networking is needed on three levels.[34] Networking at the grass roots or staff nurse level is crucial to the unity and survival of the profession, as nurses work toward caring for one another and having an influence on their work environment. She believes that a supportive staff network can extend beyond affirmation of the members and become an influential force in managing daily nursing care.

The next level of networking is at the leadership level where nursing leaders can similarly unite for a common goal of increased power in the health care system. Nurses at this level are in an excellent position to make a significant contribution to the self-esteem of their fellow professionals through support and affirmation of both their abilities and their potential. The final level includes informational networks that are a requisite for effective political action. Herein lies a dormant element of nursing power that is often described but seldom activated.

■ **Education**

A major challenge to psychiatric nursing in the area of education is the need for a well-defined body of nursing knowledge. The question "Is psychiatric nursing unique?" has preoccupied the profession for some time now.

McMurrey explores the subject of unique nursing knowledge by attempting to answer three questions: (1) What is unique knowledge? (2) Does nursing have a unique knowledge base? and (3) Is a unique knowledge base essential to nursing?[33] She argues that knowledge becomes unique because of the unique perspective of the discipline in which that knowledge is incorporated. She further cautions that if nursing does not define its focus, it cannot become an autonomous profession, and therefore one of two things will occur. Either the functions that have been associated with nursing will be taken over by others, or, in their search for definition, nurses will assume roles within other disciplines, such as psychology or medicine. There is some evidence that both of these trends are already taking place in the field of psychiatric nursing.

Nursing's contribution is an outcome of a unique manner of problem conceptualization, the utilization of theoretical models to explain behavior, and a nursing process approach to individuals, families, and communities. Lego[28] asserts that knowledge determines uniqueness, and nursing is distinguished by a holistic approach, crisis orientation, and knowledge of general health matters. The existence of this psychiatric nursing textbook, which incorporates existing nursing research, is organized around a nursing model of health-illness phenomena, and views the nursing process as the basis for practice, is evidence of the distinct body of knowledge that is nursing. It is the combination of this knowledge base, clinical skills, holistic viewpoint, and behavioral focus that makes the psychiatric nurse's contribution a valuable and unique one.

■ **NURSING RESEARCH.** The development of conceptual models by nursing leaders further attests to the validity of viewing nursing as a unique profession. These theoretical models contribute to the knowledge base of nursing education, the framework for nursing practice, and the direction for nursing research. Over 50% of federally supported nursing research projects deal with investigations into nursing practice, and the development of doctoral programs in nursing suggests that "the science of nursing is coming of age."[4] The momentum in nursing research is steadily increasing, as is evident in the establishment of a National Center for Nursing Research in the National Institute of Health; the development of programs for the preparation of nurse scientists (Table 1-3); increasing support of federal and interstate agencies; increased acceptance of long-term, research-oriented goals toward enlarging nursing's body of knowledge; development of centers for nursing research; a rise in the number of consortia and collaborative efforts; change in the nature and number of avenues for reporting research (Table 1-7); and changes in the direction of research from a limited number of studies on curricula, administration, and personal attributes of nurses to more extensive clinical studies that apply the new nursing science to practice.

Along with these advances, however, have emerged a number of problems identified by Feldman[18]: the need for financial support often outweighs available money; as the quantity of doctoral programs have increased, the quality may have suffered; there are still too few research journals in existence and too few research papers accepted; a rush to produce research has led to inferior quality in some cases; many nurses do not appreciate research, are unable to interpret research findings, and do not use them in practice; and some nurses do not participate in research because they view it as costly, time consuming, and demanding in preparation, or because they have poor self-images and are reluctant to ask for help and expose themselves to possible criticism. Rather than simply identifying problems, Feldman[18] offers possible solutions to enhance nursing's growth in this area. All of the following are applicable to psychiatric nursing:

1. **Funding.** If the nursing profession truly supports nursing science, it must contribute to nursing's evolution. Hospital nursing services, professional nursing organizations, and educational facilities should encourage research by contributing a percentage of their income to this endeavor. Also, positions should exist for nurse researchers to be hired in clinical and educational settings.

2. **Collaboration.** Collaboration takes many forms and may occur in developing research questions, designing and implementing studies, providing forums for developing theory and reporting investigative work, and establishing networks for sharing all kinds of information. Symposia must continue to increase, involving nurses at all levels, in all types of practice. A nationwide research network could be established using computers; the technology is available to set up an international network by satellite.

3. **Education.** The process of educating nurses to perform research must be stepped up to meet the demands of a developing science. This involves additional recruitment but not at the expense of quality. Doctoral programs in nursing must have a core of productive nurse scientists who can serve as role models and mentors to students in the in-depth study of specific problems. This would enhance theory development by encouraging greater concentration on concerns of highest priority. It would also involve students in the research process in such a way that their enthusiasm and creativity would be nurtured. However, doctoral preparation for re-

search is just the beginning; postdoctoral work will enable the scientist to pursue particular areas of need and interest and to more fully develop the researcher role.

4. **Marketing.** Enhancing the usefulness of nursing research requires changing the present climate to one of increased receptivity, valuing, learning, and involvement in the process and outcomes of research studies. To accomplish this, Feldman proposes an intensive effort in "marketing" research. She describes the strategies useful in marketing products as segmenting the market, identifying common characteristics within each of the target segments, identifying the needs of those markets, and developing a marketing plan to appeal to the target markets. She then describes how this approach can be adapted to the problem of increasing receptivity to research among nursing professionals.

5. **Reporting.** Increased reporting of research in journals designed for that purpose is advocated. However, new ideas are needed about ways to communicate findings in a fashion acceptable to clinical practitioners. Additionally, prestige must be given to the replication of selected studies, and replication studies must be reported as readily as originals.

The importance of this final suggestion, reporting, should not be minimized. To attain full professional status, the body of nursing knowledge must be accepted as legitimate by other professionals, as well as by society. Many people outside of nursing and some within nursing, still have no concept of this body of knowledge nor of the unique expertise of nursing. To overcome this, psychiatric nurses need to write and publish more and in a greater variety of journals and texts, including multidisciplinary journals and consumer publications. A recent study by Kalisch and Kalisch examined the quality of news about psychiatric nurses in the nation's newspapers.[27] They found that there is inadequate dissemination of psychiatric nursing information to the public via the news media, as well as deficiencies in the quality of reported information.

Nurses should also increase their visibility by attending and presenting papers at the meetings of their colleagues, including psychiatrists, psychologists, and social workers. A more assertive and self-confident public stance is both necessary and appropriate for the psychiatric nurse, since knowledge of the role of psychiatric

nurses has been found to be correlated with an accepting attitude and greater utilization among other mental health professionals.[12] The gradual implementation of each of these proposed solutions by psychiatric nurses will promote the creation, organization, and transmission of the distinct body of science that is nursing.

■ Service orientation

There is consensus that nursing is characterized by explicit rules of competence and strong rules of loyalty or service. The rules of performance, however, pertain to self-regulation and accountability for practice that must be demonstrated individually and collectively. The mechanisms within psychiatric nursing to accomplish this include state licensure, certification, primary nursing as a mode of staffing, nursing audit, implementation of standards of practice, and peer review. Sometimes these mechanisms appear more structural than functional.

The dichotomy between nursing theory and nursing practice is somewhat addressed in the literature, and is implied in the sometimes adversarial roles of nursing educators and administrators. Often what is learned in theory is not implemented in practice. For example, direct and indirect psychiatric nursing care functions, although impressive, are often carried out sporadically and inconsistently. One study examined what functions psychiatric nurses employed in an inpatient setting considered to be important and how well nurses were able to perform them.[47] The results indicated the following 5 as the "most important" functions of the 46 listed:

1. To assess patients' emotional needs
2. To respond to patients' crises
3. To intervene to reduce panic of disturbed patients
4. To make sure patients' rights are safeguarded
5. To assess the effect of somatic therapies on patients

Although these functions implied the use of the nursing process, the items to "develop a nursing care plan" and "implement a nursing care plan" were ranked as numbers 18 and 15, respectively. Items related to leadership functions ranked low—providing leadership was ninth, initiating improvements was eleventh, participating in policy making was twenty-fourth, and political involvement was twenty-ninth. Psychotherapy activities were numbered 34, 36, and 38, and research activities were 32, 41, and 46. The ability ratings corresponded closely with the importance ratings. The same questionnaire was given to a group of psychiatrists and psychologists. Significantly, they gave a lower rank-

TABLE 1-7

**OVERVIEW OF CONTEMPORARY NURSING JOURNALS PUBLISHED
IN THE UNITED STATES (1900-1987)***

Journal title	Year of first issue					
	1900-1915	1916-1931	1932-1947	1948-1963	1964-1979	1980-1987
Am. J. Nurs.	•					
Nurs. Outlook	•					
R.N.			•			
Briefs			•			
A.A.N.A.J.			•			
Nurses' Lamp				•		
Perspect. Psychiatr. Care				•		
J. Psychosoc. Nurs. Ment. Health Serv.				•		
J. Nurs. Educ.				•		
Nurs. Forum				•		
Regan Rep. Nurs. Law				•		
A.O.R.N.J.				•		
J. Pract. Nurs.				•		
J. Nurse Midwife				•		
Imprint				•		
Occup. Health Nurs.				•		
Nurs. Res.				•		
Cardiovasc. Nurs.					•	
Nurs. Clin. North Am.					•	
Am. Nurse					•	
Image					•	
J. Nurs. Care					•	
J. Neurosurg. Nurs.					•	
J. Contin. Educ. Nurs.					•	
Superv. Nurse					•	
J. Nurs. Admn.					•	
Nursing '87					•	
Heart Lung					•	
J.O.G.N. Nurs.					•	
Matern. Child Nurs. J.					•	
Crit. Care Med.					•	
Crit. Care Update					•	
J. Am. Assoc. Nephrol. Nurses Tech.					•	
A.P.N.J.					•	
J.E.N.					•	
J. Gerontol. Nurs.					•	
Nurse Pract.					•	
Pediatr. Nurs.					•	
Iss. Com. Ped. Nurs.					•	
M.C.N.					•	
Nurse Educ.					•	
Nurses Drug Alert					•	
Nurs. Adm. Q.					•	
Ad. Nurs. Sci.					•	
Cancer Nurs.					•	

TABLE 1-7—cont'd

OVERVIEW OF CONTEMPORARY NURSING JOURNALS PUBLISHED IN THE UNITED STATES (1900-1987)*

Journal title	Year of first issue					
	1900-1915	1916-1931	1932-1947	1948-1963	1964-1979	1980-1987
Today's O.R. Nurse					●	
Crit. Care Q.					●	
Iss. Mental Health Nurs.					●	
Nurs. Lead					●	
Res. Nurs. Health					●	
Topics Clin. Nurs.					●	
West J. Nurs. Res.					●	
J. Enterostomal Ther.					●	
Oncology Nurs. Forum					●	
Nephrology Nurse					●	
School Nurse					●	
Life Support Nurse					●	
Emerg. Nurse Legal Bull.					●	
Nurs. Law Ethics						●
Geriatric Nurse						●
Nurs. Health Care						●
Nurs. Insights						●
The Dean's List						●
Modern Nurse Magazine						●
Professional Nurse						●
Adv. Nurs. Sci.						●
Nurs. Econ.						●
J. Prof. Nurs.						●
Am. J. Psychiatr. Nurs.						●

*From Binger, J.: Image **13**(3):67
*State nurses' association journals are not included here.

ing, compared with that of the nurses, to nurses' ability to assess emotional needs and develop and implement a nursing care plan, despite the importance they placed on those items. This study raises many questions about the role of the nurse and the contrast between theory and practice.

Traditionally, one response to this perceived dichotomy was an attempt to place blame on either the "ivory-towered" educators, the "nonsupportive" nurse administrators, or the "impersonal" hospital organization. However, this type of response is characterized by a passivity and a noticeable lack of accountability. What is needed at present is for psychiatric nurses to assume an active posture of accountability to oneself, one's patients, one's colleagues, one's profession, the public, and nurse administrators.

Accountability means to be answerable to someone for something. It focuses responsibility on the individual nurse for his or her actions, or perhaps, lack of actions:

Organized nursing services and the professional association carry the leadership responsibility for development, implementation, and evaluation of nursing care systems which assure relevant, high quality nursing to consumers. Individual nurses have primary responsiblity and accountability for their own practice, and thus activities to monitor and improve the quality of nursing care form an intrinsic part of the individual's practice.

In the field of psychiatric and mental health nursing, nurses have a particular obligation to define, supervise, and evaluate nursing care. Nursing standards provide authoritative measures for determining the quality of nursing care a client receives, whether services are provided solely by a professional nurse or by a professional nurse and nursing assistants.[22]

The preconditions of accountability, therefore, include ability, responsibility, andd authority. Finally, accountability includes formal review processes and requirements, but also an attitude of integrity and vigilance—"a quality of the heart and mind of those professionals who are competent and determined that every psychiatric patient will have the best problem-resolving assistance possible."[45]

■ Autonomy

Autonomy implies self-determination, independence, shared power, and authority, and professionals are not likely to achieve it without having met the previous characteristics of professionalization. It is the socially sanctioned condition that allows for the definition and control over a work domain, achieved through a negotiated process. For psychiatric nursing, attaining autonomy means being able to define the domain of nursing and being able to exercise control over psychiatric nursing practice.[56] This idea of shaping destiny, rather than letting outside forces be in control, is the crux of power viewed as a positive force and strength or the capacity to attain goals. Power can be viewed as both a means to an end and a product, the instrument used to attain full professional status and the outcome of achieving professionalization. It involves a conscious decision to identify goals, plan strategy, assume responsibility, exercise authority, and be held accountable.

Autonomy, at an individual level of analysis, has two major and interrelated components. The first is **control over nursing tasks,** which means:

1. Having the opportunity for independent thought and action
2. Having appropriate utilization of one's time, skills, and ability by being able to eliminate, refuse, and delegate nonnursing tasks
3. Having the authority and responsibility for implementing goals related to quality nursing care
4. Being able to initiate changes and innovations in one's practice

The second component of autonomy is that of **participation in decision making.** It requires the nurse's participation in the following:

1. Determining and implementing standards of quality nursing care
2. Decisions affecting one's nursing job context, including salary, staffing, and professional growth

3. Institutional policies, procedures, and goals

This characteristic of autonomy is particularly problematic for nursing. Most nurses are employed in hospitals in which authority rests primarily with administrators, physicians, and trustees.[50] Furthermore, nurses are frequently expected to do tasks they are overqualified to do, such as housekeeping, dietary, and clerical duties. This results in the underutilization of their many important skills. Nurses are thus caught in the crosswind. They staff the units around the clock, make important clinical decisions, and shoulder major responsibility for coordinating and managing the patient care units; but they lack the legitimate decision-making authority as to the allocation of hospital resources. Because nurses are not compensated on a fee-for-service basis, they are not viewed as a source of revenue by hospital administrators and therefore lack a most critical base for power. It is not surprising that if nurses do not have a role in hospital decision making, then they will have only a limited ability to exercise control of their practice.

Recommendations from two national studies of nursing, the National Commission on Nursing sponsored by the American Hospital Association and the Institute of Medicine's Study of Nursing, reflect this problem and call for increased decision-making authority for nurses and collaborative relationships with physicians in providing care. In addition, the new Joint Commission on Accreditation of Hospitals (JCAH) Nursing Service Standards extend the current provision for nursing staff communication with a hospital's governing body to include appropriate communication "with those levels of management involved in policy decisions affecting patient care services in the hospital."[24]

Nurses should not expect, however, that autonomy and power will be given to them. It is obtained in a negotiated process with other health professionals, consumers, and society at large. It requires increased access to concrete resources, demonstration of expertise, and acknowledgment by other professionals, which is evidenced in interdependent collaboration. Nurses are not yet fully accepted as professionals by other disciplines and often do not function at their full potential. Yet psychiatric nursing is practiced largely in collaboration, coordination, and cooperation with a variety of other professionals working with and on behalf of the patient. Nurses will progress in this area as they are able to communicate with other professionals and as their clinical skills demand recognition and respect. As nurses view themselves in a positive way, they will increase their ability to assert themselves and function effectively.

Benfer[5] has some specific suggestions in this regard. She believes that psychiatric nurses must first assess patients based on their own conceptualization of the patient's emotional difficulties, rather than first checking with the psychiatrist or other team members for their conceptualization. When the nurse has completed her assessment, she must then be able to articulate that information both orally and in writing. This requires an assertiveness in putting forth ideas, observations, and beliefs about treatment, because unless psychiatric nurses define their own role, others will define it for them. Benfer does not believe nurses have done very well in explaining their framework for practice and communicating to other mental health team members what the nursing process is and how it is utilized.

Nurses also have a team teaching function to share their knowledge, experience, and perceptions with other team members so that the result is more skilled practitioners. Although nurses have often taught interns and residents, this teaching has seldom been given adequate recognition and importance. Furthermore, some nurses may feel threatened at the thought of teaching other professionals. However, teaching and learning are continuous experiences in life, and nurses have a contribution to make in this area.

Finally, for interdisciplinary teams to function well, the members must view themselves as equals. Benfer believes that this is one of the most elusive and difficult issues affecting nurses who must be helped to strengthen their self-concepts by identifying their expertise and the ways in which they can contribute to the common purpose of the team.

Thus, the movement toward professionalization contains complex issues for all psychiatric nurses. Many of these issues are interwoven and all of them are familiar, since they have been repeatedly addressed by nurses over many decades. The prize is professional autonomy, but its attainment, at present, remains a question.

■ SUGGESTED CROSS-REFERENCES ■

This chapter serves as a foundation for formulating principles of psychiatric nursing, and implementing psychiatric nursing practice. As such, it is related to all other chapters of this text.

DIRECTIONS FOR FUTURE RESEARCH

The following are some of the nursing research problems raised in Chapter 1 that merit further study by psychiatric nurses:

1. The way in which block grants have affected the programs and services for mental health and mental illness in this country
2. Factors associated with the recruitment of nursing students into the field of psychiatric nursing
3. The impact psychiatric nurses have on the legislative branch of government at the local, state, and national levels
4. The amount of nursing care in the areas of primary, secondary, and tertiary prevention performed by psychiatric nurses relative to their qualifications, roles, and settings
5. Structural and process characteristics of effective mental health teams
6. Factors that promote and inhibit effective leadership among psychiatric nurses
7. The degree to which psychiatric nurses act as change agents, promoting innovations in their practice settings
8. The perceptions by other mental health professionals and the public of the doctoral degree in nursing
9. The level of public understanding of certification, the types of psychiatric nurse practitioners, and their functions
10. The nontraditional settings and the parameters of practice of psychiatric nurses
11. The extent of and factors contributing to psychiatric nursing "burnout" and ways to effectively deal with this phenomenon
12. The manner in which the *Standards of Psychiatric and Mental Health Nursing Practice* are implemented in various psychiatric settings
13. The formal and informal networks that support psychiatric nurses
14. The level of integration and application of nursing research in the major textbooks of psychiatric nursing
15. The extent to which psychiatric nurses have contributed publications or presentations in multidisciplinary journals or forums
16. The effectiveness of mechanisms to assure accountability in psychiatric nursing practice
17. The degree to which psychiatric nurses exercise control over their nursing tasks and participate in the decision-making structure of the organizations in which they work

■ SUMMARY ■

1. Nursing began to emerge as a profession in the nineteenth century. Linda Richards was the first American psychiatric nurse, and the first school for psychiatric nurses opened in 1882. The National Mental Health Act of 1946 provided funds for nursing education. A critical development within the profession occurred with the publication of Peplau's book in 1952 in which she presented a theoretical framework for psychiatric nursing. By 1962 psychiatric nursing had evolved a role of clinical competence based on interpersonal techniques and use of the nursing process. Counseling was a primary nursing function.

The Community Mental Health Centers Act of 1963 influenced the movement of the practice of psychiatric nursing into the community and the formation of multidisciplinary treatment teams. Other influences included the 1978 President's Commission on Mental Health, the Mental Health Systems Act of 1980, and the present environment of fiscal restraint, retrenchment, and budgetary cuts.

2. Psychiatric nursing is an interpersonal process that strives to promote and maintain behavior which contributes to integrated functioning. The patient or client system may be an individual, family, group, organization, or community. It may be practiced in a variety of settings. Various direct and indirect nursing functions were described based on the model of primary, secondary, and tertiary prevention.

3. An essential part of contemporary practice is cooperation and collaboration with other health care providers. The role functions of various team members and barriers to effective team functioning were discussed.

4. The development of knowledge and strategies enabling nurses to exercise leadership and management in the settings in which they work is essential. Characteristics of psychiatric nurses as change agents and the nature of effective leadership were described.

5. Four major factors that help to determine the levels of function and types of activities a nurse engages in are the law; qualifications, including education, work experiences, and certification status; practice setting; and personal competence and initiative. Job burnout and support systems were analyzed.

6. The *Standards of Psychiatric and Mental Health Nursing Practice* as identified by the American Nurses' Association were presented.

7. The question of whether psychiatric nurses are truly professionalized was addressed. The following problematic areas were explored:

a. Organization, including lack of support for the American Nurses' Association, disagreement over tasks and roles, questions related to collective bargaining issues, and the need for the formation of networks that can help nurses unite and value their profession

b. Education, specifically the need for a well-defined body of nursing knowledge, problems and advances in nursing research, and the need for greater visibility of psychiatric nurses through publishing and presentations

c. Service orientation, focusing on the issues of self-regulation, accountability, and the theory-practice dichotomy

d. Autonomy, with its elements of self-determination, power, authority, and status as evidenced in control over nursing tasks and participation in decision making in nursing care, job context, and institutional policies and goals

■ REFERENCES ■

1. American Nurses' Association: Educational preparation for nurse practitioners and assistants to nurses: a position paper, New York, 1965, The Association.
2. American Nurses' Association, Division on Psychiatric and Mental Health Nursing Practice: Statement on psychiatric and mental health nursing practice, Kansas City, Mo., 1976, The Association.
3. American Nurses' Association: Nursing: a social policy statement, Kansas City, Mo., 1980, The Association.
4. Andreoli, K., and Thompson, C.: The nature of science in nursing, Image **9**(2):37, 1977.
5. Benfer, B.: Defining the role and function of the psychiatric nurse as a member of the team, Perspect. Psychiatr. Care **18**(4):166, 1980.
6. Bennett, A., and Eaton, J.: The role of the psychiatric nurse in the newer therapies, Am. J. Psychiatry **108**:167, Sept. 1951.
7. Brown, E.: Nursing for the future, New York, 1948, Russell Sage Foundation.
8. Chamberlain, J.: The role of the federal government in development of psychiatric nursing, J. Psychosoc. Nurs. Ment. Health Serv. **21**(4):11, 1983.
9. Cleland, V.: The supervisor in collective bargaining, J. Nurs. Adm. **4**(4):33, 1974.
10. Critchley, D., and Maurin, J.: The clinical specialist in psychiatric mental health nursing: theory, research and practice, New York, 1985, John Wiley and Sons.
11. Cronin-Stubbs, D., and Brophy, E.: Burnout: can social support save the nurse? J. Psychosoc. Nurs. Ment. Health Serv. **23**(7):9, 1985.
12. Davidson, K., et al.: A descriptive study of the attitudes of psychiatrists toward the new role of the nurse therapist, J. Psychiatr. Nurs. **16**(11):24, 1978.
13. Dawkins, J., Depp, F., and Selzer, N.: Stress and the psychiatric nurse, J. Psychosoc. Nurs. Ment. Health Serv. **23**(11):9, 1985.
14. Doona, M.: At least as well cared for . . . Linda Richards and the mentally ill, Image **16**(2):51, 1984.
15. Dumas, R.: Expanding the theorectical framework for effective nursing, Nurs. Clin. North Am. **13**(4):707, 1978.
16. Editorial, Am. J. Nurs. **40**:23, 1940.
17. Evans, C., and Lewis, S.: Nursing administration of psychiatric-mental health care, Rockville, Md., 1985, Aspen Systems Corp.
18. Feldman, H.: Nursing research in the 1980's: Issues and implications, Adv. Nurs. Sci. **3**(1):85, 1980.

19. Forsyth, D., and Cannady, N.: Preventing and alleviating staff burnout through a group. J. Psychosoc. Nurs. Ment. Health Serv. **19**(9):35, 1981.

20. Gardner, K.: Levels of psychiatric nursing practice in an ambulatory setting, J. Psychiatr. Nurs. **15**:26, Sept. 1977.

21. Given, B., and Simmons, S.: The interdisciplinary health-care team: fact or fiction? Nurs. Forum **16**(2):165, 1977.

22. Gregg, D.: The psychiatric nurse's role, Am. J. Nurs. **54**:848, 1954.

23. Hays, D.: Suggested clinical practice of psychiatric nurses recorded in the literature between 1946 and 1958. In Psychiatric nursing 1946 to 1974: A report on the state of the art, New York, 1975, American Journal of Nursing Co.

24. JCAH Perspectives, 1985. 5,4,4.

25. Johnson, R., et al.: The professional support group: a model for psychiatric clinical nurse specialists, J. Psychosoc. Nurs. Ment. Health Serv. **20**(2):9, 1982.

26. Jones, M.: The therapeutic community: a new treatment method in psychiatry, New York, 1953, Basic Books, Inc.

27. Kalisch, P., and Kalisch, B.: Psychiatric nurses and the press: a troubled relationship, Perspect. Psychiatr. Care **22**(1):5, 1984.

28. Lego, S.: Nurse psychotherapists: how are we different? Perspect. Psychiatr. Care **11**(4):144, 1973.

29. Leib, A., Underwood, P., and Glick, I.: The staff nurse as primary therapist: a pilot study, J. Psychiatr. Nurs. **14**:11, Oct. 1976.

30. Maloney, E.: Does the psychiatric nurse have independent functions? Am. J. Nurs. **62**:61, June 1962.

31. Maslow, A.: Motivation and personality, New York, 1954, Harper & Row, Publishers, Inc.

32. Mauksch, I.G., and Miller, M.H.: Implementing change in nursing, St. Louis, 1981, The C.V. Mosby Co.

33. McMurrey, P.: Toward a unique knowledge base in nursing, Image **14**(1):12, 1982.

34. Meisenhelder, J.: Networking and nursing, Image **14**(3):77, 1982.

35. Mellow, J.: Nursing therapy, Am. J. Nurs. **68**:2365, 1968.

36. Merton, R.: The social nature of leadership, Am. J. Nurs. **69**:2614, Dec. 1969.

37. Mlott, S.: Personality correlates of a psychiatric nurse, J. Psychiatr. Nurs. **14**(2):19, 1976.

38. Moore, W.: The professions: roles and rules, New York, 1974, Russell Sage Foundation.

39. Moscato, B.: The traditional nurse-physician relationship. In Kneisl, C.R., and Wilson, H.S., editors: Current perspectives in psychiatric nursing, vol. 1, St. Louis, 1976, The C.V. Mosby Co.

40. Noyes, A.: Nursing needs in the state mental hospitals, Am. J. Nurs. **33**:787, 1933.

41. Peplau, H.: Interpersonal relations in nursing, New York, 1952, G.P. Putnam's Sons.

42. Peplau, H.: Historical development of psychiatric nursing. A preliminary statement on some facts and trends, 1956. (Mimeographed.)

43. Peplau, H.: Interpersonal techniques: the crux of psychiatric nursing, Am. J. Nurs. **62**:53, June 1962.

44. Peplau, H.: Psychiatric nursing: role of nurses and psychiatric nurses, Int. Nurs. Rev. **25**(2):41, 1978.

45. Peplau, H.: The psychiatric nurse—accountable? To whom? For what? Perspect. Psychiatr. Care **18**(3):128, 1980.

46. Pines, A., and Maslach, C.: Characteristics of staff burnout in mental health settings, Hosp. Community Psychiatry **29**:233, 1978.

47. Plutchik, R., Conte, H., Wells, W., and Karasu, T.: Role of the psychiatric nurse, J. Psychiatr. Nurs. **14**(9):38, 1976.

48. Powers, M.: Universal utility of psychoanalytic theory for nursing practice models, J. Psychiatr. Nurs. **18**(4):28, 1980.

49. Report to the president from the President's Commission on Mental Health, vol. 1, Washington, D.C., 1978, U.S. Government Printing Office.

50. Roemer, M., and Friedman, J.: Doctors in hospitals: medical staff organization and hospital performance, Baltimore, 1971, The Johns Hopkins University Press.

51. Ruch, M.: The multidisciplinary approach: when too much is too many, J. Psychosoc. Nurs. **22**(9):18, 1984.

52. Santos, E., and Stainbrook, E.: Nursing and modern psychiatry, Am. J. Nurs. **49**:107, 1949.

53. Slavinsky, A.: Psychiatric nursing in the year 2000: from a nonsystem of care to a caring system, Image **16**(1):17, 1984.

54. Sloboda, S.: What are mental health nurses doing? J. Psychiatr. Nurs. **14**:24, 1976.

55. Smoyak, S.: The confrontation process, Am. J. Nurs. **74**(9):1632, 1974.

56. Stuart, G.: How professionalized is nursing? Image **13**(1):18, 1981.

57. Sundeen, S.J., et al.: Nurse-client interaction: implementing the nursing process, ed. 3, St. Louis, 1985, The C.V. Mosby Co.

58. Tousley, M.: Certification as a credential: what are the issues? Perspect. Psychiatr. Care **20**(1):23, 1982.

59. Tudor, G.: Sociopsychiatric nursing approach to intervention in a problem of mutual withdrawal on a mental hospital ward, Psychiatry **15**(2):193, 1952.

60. Unschuld, P.: Medico-cultural conflicts in Asian settings: an exploratory theory, Soc. Sci. Med. **9**:304, 1975.

61. Weiss, M.O.: The skills of psychiatric nursing, Am. J. Nurs. **47**:174, 1947.

62. Wojdowski, P., and Hartnett, K.: The HMO question: can a large health maintenance organization deliver acute psychiatric nursing services? J. Psychosoc. Nurs. Ment. Health Serv. **23**(9):23, 1985.

■ ANNOTATED SUGGESTED READINGS ■

*Aiken, L. (editor): Nursing in the 1980s: crises, opportunities and challenges, Philadelphia, 1982, J.B. Lippincott.

This is an interdisciplinary analysis by leading experts in nursing and health care of the issues, dilemmas, and challenges facing nursing in the 1980s and the likely consequences of nursing actions. It is a highly recommended source book for all nurses.

*American Nurses' Association: Professionalism and the empowerment of nursing, Kansas City, Mo., 1982, The Association.

This compilation of papers presented in the 1982 ANA convention addresses power and professionalism in a world of many health needs and few health dollars.

*American Nurses' Association, Division on Psychiatric and Mental Health Nursing Practice: Statement on psychiatric and mental health nursing practice, Kansas City, Mo., 1976, The Association.

This is the official statement of the American Nurses' Association, which includes a definition and description of setting, types of practitioners, and list of functions. This pamphlet is a resource for all psychiatric nurses.

*American Nurses' Association, Division on Psychiatric and Mental Health Nursing Practice: Standards of psychiatric and mental health nursing practice, Kansas City, Mo., 1982, The Association.

In this publication the ANA presents the standards of psychiatric nursing, each of which is accompanied by a rationale and structure, process, and outcome criteria. The criteria provide a means by which attainment of the standards may be specifically measured.

*Berger, M.S., et al.: Management for nurses, ed. 2, St. Louis, 1980, The C.V. Mosby Co.

The concepts of leadership and management are the focus of this excellent text. It is a compilation of thought-provoking articles on structural, personnel, and economic factors and their influence on organization functioning. Worthwhile reading for all nurses.

*Christman, L., and Counte, M.: Hospital organization and health care delivery, Boulder, Co., 1981, Westview Press.

An overview of hospitals, as organizations, is described in this text which is ideal for students. Topics include models of organizations, conflict, leadership, communication, change, performance, and future perspectives. Recommended reading because all nurses need to know more about the organizations in which they work.

*Critchley, D., and Maurin, J.: The clinical specialist in psychiatric mental health nursing: theory, research and practice, New York, 1985, John Wiley and Sons.

This book is intended for clinical nurse specialists and presents more advanced discussions of theory and practice in the field.

Ducanis, A., and Golin, A.: The interdisciplinary health care team, Germantown, Md., 1980, Aspen Systems Corp.

Research findings and theoretical concepts are incorporated in this book on interdisciplinary health care team functioning.

It should prove helpful reading to both practicing and student nurses.

*Evans, C., and Lewis, S.: Nursing administration of psychiatric-mental health care, Rockville, Md., 1985, Aspen Systems Corp.

This book provides guidelines and assistance to nurses responsible for the administration of psychiatric-mental health nursing care. It is the only book to do so in psychiatric nursing and has much to offer all employed nurses, not only those in administration.

*Fagin, C.: Psychiatric nursing at the crossroads; quo vadis? Perspect. Psychiatr. Care **19**(3-4):99, 1981.

The author discusses two phases in the development of psychiatric nursing. The first phase is prior to 1952 when psychiatric nursing acquired recognition as a specialty in nursing and a second phase, which establishes future directions for psychiatric nursing.

*Fagin, C.: Nursing as an alternative to high-cost care, Am. J. Nurs. **82**:56, Jan. 1982.

This address summarizes available research that supports nursing effectiveness and economic viability. Competition and substitution are the key concepts in Fagin's position. A notable need that emerges from this paper is to document the effectiveness and costs of psychiatric nursing care. One might consider this paper as a mandate for action by all nurses.

*Greenleaf, N., editor: The politics of self-esteem, Nurs. Digest, **6**:1, Fall, 1978.

This is a compilation of 13 articles and an annotated bibliography that focus on the politics and self-esteem of women, particularly nurses. They explore the issues of biology, work, and the psychology of sex roles and suggest some strategies for change. This is important reading for all nurses.

Hamilton P.A.: Health care consumerism, St. Louis, 1982, The C.V. Mosby Co.

The author, a nurse, demonstrates the depth and breadth of what consumers are saying and feeling about health care in America. Both providers and consumers of health care can benefit from reading this book, which covers the issues of the consumer's role, cost, quality, rights, and ethics in the health care domain. It is not specific to psychiatric care, but provides valuable basic background.

Hardy, M., and Conway, M.: Role theory: perspectives for health professionals, New York, 1978, Appleton-Century-Crofts.

This collection of articles integrates principles of role theory and research and presents a framework from which one can determine role identity and related stressors. Its scholarly approach and thorough bibliography make it a useful reference for advanced study on roles.

*Kolin, P.C., and Kolin, J.L.: Professional writing for nurses in education, practice, and research, St. Louis, 1980, The C.V. Mosby Co.

The ability to communicate well in writing is a prime requisite for nurses. This book addresses the wide range of written communication used by nurses from patient records to writing for publication. A good resource text.

*Lancaster, J., and Lancaster, W.: Concepts for advanced

---

*Asterisk indicates nursing reference.

nursing practice: the nurse as change agent, St. Louis, 1982, The C.V. Mosby Co.

This book identifies, describes, and provides practical ways for dealing with key issues currently facing nursing. It is a collection of articles divided into three major sections, all of which serve to conceptualize the role of the nurse as an agent of change.

*Lego, S.: The one-to-one nurse patient relationship. In Psychiatric nursing 1946 to 1974: a report on the state of the art, New York, 1975, The American Journal of Nursing Co.

The author discusses the history and trends, assesses published research, and summarizes patterns in the literature that have reflected and promoted one-to-one psychiatric nursing. The bibliography is quite extensive, and this is an excellent resource article.

*Lysaught, J.: Action in affirmation toward an unambiguous profession of nursing, New York, 1980, McGraw-Hill.

This is a follow-up study of the 1970 recommendations of the National Commission for the Study of Nursing and Nursing Education. It is a status report on the pursuit of the goal of nursing as an "unambiguous" profession.

*Mauksch, I.G., and Miller, M.H.: Implementing change in nursing, St. Louis, 1981, The C.V. Mosby Co.

This is a valuable resource to all nurses who view their role as change agents. The text covers the nature of change, the nurse's role in change, strategies for implementing it, and ways to make successful change permanent. Valuable learning here for all nurses.

*McConnell, E.: Burnout in the nursing profession, St. Louis, Mo., 1982, The C.V. Mosby Co.

This source presents the complete picture of burnout in professional nursing. A very good source for this critical problem.

*Milio, N.: Promoting health through public policy. Philadelphia, 1981, F.A. Davis Co.

This useful text describes how public policy evolves and its consequences for the health of Americans. The documentation throughout is excellent, and its depth and substance make this a valuable book for all nurses to read.

*Moscato, B.: The traditional nurse-physician relationship. In Kneisl, C.R., and Wilson, H.S., editors: Current perspectives in psychiatric nursing, vol. 1, St. Louis, 1976, The C.V. Mosby Co.

The author examines sex-role stereotyping as one element inherent in the traditional nurse-physician relationship. She uses a transactional analysis framework to identify limitations in this relationship and suggests supervision, support, and self-exploration to expand nursing roles beyond tradition.

*Pearlmutter, D.: Recent trends and issues in psychiatric-mental health nursing, Hosp. Community Psychiatry **36**(1):56, 1985.

An excellent overview of the field is presented in this article which highlights history, practice, education, and research issues. Highly recommended reading!

*Peplau, H.: Interpersonal relations in nursing, New York, 1952, G.P. Putnam's Sons.

This book presents the first theoretical framework for the practice of psychiatric nursing. It describes phases and roles in psychiatric nursing, psychological tasks, influences in nursing situations, and methods for studying nursing as an interpersonal process. It had a major impact on psychiatric nursing and is a "classic" in nursing literature.

*Peplau, H.: Some reflections on earlier days in psychiatric nursing, J. Psychosoc. Nurs. **20**:(8): 1982.

This historical review covers some of the facts of psychiatric nursing up to 1950. An interesting look at nursing's past.

President's Commission on Mental Health: Report to the president, vol. 1, Washington, D.C., 1978, U.S. Government Printing Office.

This is a government report of a 1-year study commissioned by President Carter to review the mental health needs of the nation. It was completed in April 1978, and volume 1 contains recommendations to the president on how the nation might best meet those needs.

*Puetz, B.: Networking for nurses, Rockville, Md., 1983, Aspen Systems Corp.

Any nurse interested in career advancement or encouraging others toward that goal will find this book helpful. The author describes strategies for networking, personal growth, and mentoring.

*Smoyak, S., and Rouslin, S. (editors): A collection of classics in psychiatric nursing literature, Thorofare, N.J., 1982, Slack Inc.

This is a truly classic collection of 37 articles written by the luminaries in psychiatric nursing. It provides a clear sense of the field's early history.

*Styles, M.: On nursing: toward a new endowment, St. Louis, 1982, The C.V. Mosby Co.

This text proposes and utilizes a process for securing nursing's professional identity. It is creatively written as a conversation with the reader and the ideas cause one to think, evaluate, and mature in one's conceptions.

*Wieczoiek, R.: Power, politics and policy in nursing, New York, 1985, Springer Publishing Co.

Numerous perspectives on nursing and power are presented in this timely book. It is an important contribution to our professional literature with implications for all nurses.

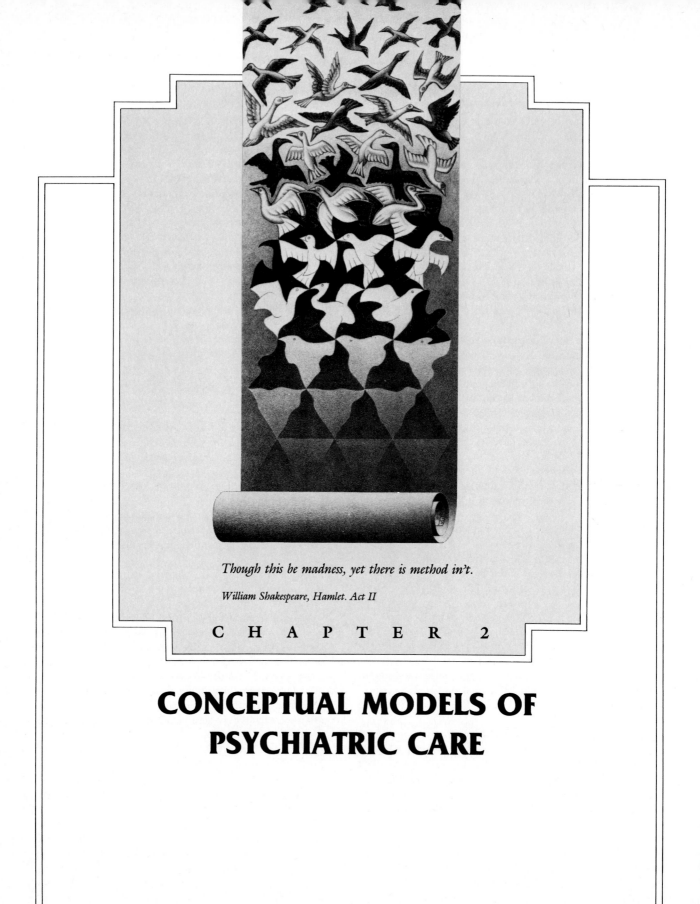

Though this be madness, yet there is method in't.

William Shakespeare, Hamlet. Act II

C H A P T E R   2

CONCEPTUAL MODELS OF PSYCHIATRIC CARE

LEARNING OBJECTIVES

After studying this chapter, the student should be able to:

- discuss the concepts of mental health and mental illness.

- describe the purpose of using a conceptual model as a framework for professional practice.

- compare and contrast eight models of mental health care: psychoanalytical, interpersonal, social, existential, communication, behavioral, medical, and nursing.

- identify major theorists associated with each model.

- describe the roles of the therapist and the patient within the context of each model.

- analyze the therapeutic process as it is experienced within each of the models.

- critique the advantages and disadvantages of the various models.

- compare and contrast the nursing diagnosis and the medical diagnosis.

- identify directions for future nursing research.

- select appropriate readings for further study.

Most people believe that they can recognize normal and abnormal behavior in themselves and their associates. In fact, this is true to an extent. Although a person may be unwilling or unable to admit to a serious disturbance of feelings or behavior, most are aware of feeling "nervous" or "irritable" or "depressed" from time to time. This awareness results from a comparison of present behavior to an internalized norm or behavioral self-expectation. Mild or transient disruptions in behavior or feelings are usually experienced as anxiety and resolved by the utilization of coping mechanisms. Each person learns a repertoire of these adaptive mechanisms as he moves through the developmental process. Some are consciously recognized and selected, as when an angry person goes for a walk to "cool down" before confronting the object of the anger. Others are unconscious and take place without the person's awareness. An example of this is the displacement of anger to a spouse when the person is really angry at a supervisor at work. A more complete discussion of conscious and unconscious means of coping with anxiety will be found in Chapter 12.

Personal coping mechanisms are not always adequate to control anxiety. When the person is unable to cope alone, he faces the difficult decision to seek help from another person. The helping person may be a friend or relative, a nonprofessional counselor, or a mental health professional. The choice may depend on the severity of the problem. A young girl wondering how to act on her first date may discuss her concerns with her mother, her older sister, her best friend, or her favorite teacher as she tries to learn new ways to cope with an unfamiliar situation. On the other hand, a woman who is so frightened of crowds that she refuses to leave her house needs to seek help from a professional therapist. Frequently, significant others are instrumental in assisting the troubled person to identify what type of help to consider. Seriously disturbed people may not recognize their need for help. Others may be frightened of the need to see a psychiatrist or other health professional or may think that they will be labeled as "crazy." These people need encouragement and support to reach out for help.

Normalcy may be defined on the basis of the individual's own feelings of anxiety or discomfort. It may also be defined based on the cultural mores, norms, and value system in the society of which the individual is a member. Observable behavior that deviates from the norm may be labeled as deviant or sick, and social pressure may be applied to convince the individual to seek help. In this case, "help" implies the modification of behavior in the direction of compliance with social norms. Clinical example 2-1 gives a brief description of normal behavior that at first appeared deviant.

Behavior may also be defined as normal or deviant for political reasons. Thomas Szasz[22] is a theorist who believes that certain types of behavior are labeled "crazy" for the convenience of society and the political system, even though the behavior may be acceptable to the person involved. According to this frame of reference, the

---

CLINICAL EXAMPLE 2-1

Early in the fall semester a black male exchange student from Africa was brought to the psychiatric emergency room. He had been walking around the campus carrying a spear and had been apprehended by the university security patrol. His speech was heavily accented and they could not understand his explanation of his behavior. Later evaluation revealed that in his culture one never went walking at night without a spear to defend against attack by wild beasts or hostile neighboring tribes. He was sent back to his dormitory after being convinced that his spear was not appropriate to the culture of the American college campus.

---

institutionalization of a woman who had been walking nude through her neighborhood could be interpreted as the political system's response to the discomfort of the neighbors. In the Soviet political system, citizens who criticize the government may be labeled mentally ill and hospitalized. In the view of the leadership, such behavior is definitely deviant.

These examples demonstrate that the definition of normal behavior is in no way simple or obvious. Does normality mean conformity? Does it mean an ability to control anxiety? Does it mean acceptability to significant others? Depending on one's frame of reference, it could mean any, all, or none of these. Perhaps the most generally accepted definition of normal behavior at the present time is that the individual is able to function adequately in activities of daily living and to feel reasonably satisfied with his life-style. This is far from precise, but human behavior covers such a range that an exact description of normal behavior is probably impossible. Behavior must be viewed on a continuum with a wide variation of what is accepted as normal. If this is not the case, individual behavior could be unreasonably restricted with resulting limitations on creativity and personal growth. Mental health nurses can often be most helpful by trying to understand the patient's view of his behavior and assisting him to change behaviors that he has defined as unsatisfactory.

Most mental health professionals practice within the framework of a conceptual model. A model is a means of organizing a complex body of knowledge, such as concepts related to human behavior. Utilization of a model assists the practitioner to function rationally and allows for evaluation of the individual's effectiveness as a therapist. Organization of data also facilitates much needed research into human behavior.

At the present time scientific knowledge of behavior is limited. Therefore it is difficult to view any particular conceptual model as right or wrong. Unfortunately, adherents of one model or another do, at times, become embroiled in conflicts about which framework is most accurate. In reality, the only measure of the value of any approach to mental health care is the satisfaction of the person who receives the care. It has not been proved whether the patient's response to care results from the theoretical model utilized or from the relationship with the therapist, irrespective of the model.

In the remainder of this chapter, an overview will be presented of several conceptual models that are commonly utilized by contemporary mental health professionals. The models to be discussed include psychoanalytical, interpersonal, social, existential, communication, behavioral, medical, and nursing models. Information to be discussed relative to each model is the definition of behavioral deviations, the therapy process, the role of the patient, the role of the therapist, and identification of representative theorists. Since it is impossible to provide a thorough exploration of even one of these complex theories in a single chapter, the reader is referred to the annotated suggested readings, which include several basic references for each theoretical framework.

Psychoanalytical model

Psychoanalytical theory was first conceptualized by Sigmund Freud in the late nineteenth and early twentieth centuries. It not only encompassed the nature of deviant behavior but also proposed an entirely new perspective on human development. Many of Freud's ideas were controversial, particularly in the Victorian society into which they were introduced. Sexuality was a central concept in his developmental theory. The emotional response to the assertion that children are sexual beings for a time overshadowed the broader implications of Freudian theory. The effort to observe human behavior objectively was a great contribution of the early psychoanalysts, as was the identification of a mental structure. Such concepts as id, ego, and superego and the ego defense mechanisms are still widely accepted and utilized by many therapists. Most people readily accept the existence of an unconscious level of mental functioning. Due to limitations of space, the psychoanalytical theory of psychosexual development will not be presented here. The focus will be on the analytical method of intervening in deviant behavior, realizing that this must be based on an understanding of the norm. Readers interested in exploring psychoanalytical theories of psychosocial development are referred to the works of Freud and Erik Erikson, a contemporary psychoanalytical theorist and to the discussion in Chapter 30.

■ Psychoanalytical view of behavioral deviations

Psychoanalysts trace disrupted behavior in the adult back to earlier developmental stages. At each stage of development, there is a task to be accomplished. For instance, the child at the anal stage must learn to accept limits on his behavior and become more independent. If there is undue emphasis on any stage or unusual difficulty in dealing with the associated conflicts, there is a fixation of psychological energy (libido) at that point in an attempt to deal with anxiety. This leaves less libido available to the ego for other tasks, since energy is utilized to maintain repression of early conflicts. At times of stress, when the anxiety level rises, the individual may regress behaviorally to the level of the fixation, utilizing the defenses which were effective at that time. Unfortunately, these are childhood defenses that may not be appropriate to the adult situation. However, since the childhood conflict was not resolved, the adult is not free to implement mature problem-solving techniques.

For example, a young woman was never able to resolve her competitive feelings toward her mother for her father's attention. She repressed this conflict from the phallic stage of development. In addition, she projected her feelings of jealousy and anger to her mother and was never able to relate to her openly. As she reached maturity, she was never able to develop close relationships with other women. She suspected that they were always competing with her for the attention of males. At the same time, her relationships with men were dependent and childlike with constant demands that they prove their devotion to her. Basically, she was lonely and unhappy.

According to psychoanalysts, neurotic symptoms arise when so much energy must be invested to control anxiety that there is serious interference with functional ability. Incidentally, everyone is neurotic to some extent according to this conceptual model. Everyone carries the burden of childhood conflicts and is influenced in adulthood by childhood experiences. For this reason, psychoanalysts in training must undergo a personal analysis so that their neurotic behavior will not hinder their objectivity as therapists.

Symptoms are representative in a symbolic way of the original conflict. For instance, compulsive hand washing may represent the individual's attempt to cleanse himself of impulses that were labeled as unclean by the mothering person during the anal stage of development. This characteristic of a neurotic symptom occurs through the utilization by the ego of the mechanisms of condensation and displacement. Thus the meaning of the behavior is hidden from the conscious awareness of the individual, who is usually upset about these uncontrollable thoughts, actions, and feelings.

Freud developed most of his theories around neurotic symptoms. His theory is less well formulated in the area of psychosis, and it was found that people with psychotic behavior were not responsive to classical psychoanalytical therapy. This position has in more recent times been modified by psychoanalytical theorists such as Harold Searles and Frieda Fromm-Reichmann who have had success in working with psychotic patients. In essence, the psychotic symptom is seen as occurring when the ego must invest most or all of the libido at hand in an effort to defend against primitive id impulses. This leaves little, if any, energy to deal with external reality. This leads to the use of symbolization and the lack of reality testing ability seen in psychosis.

■ Psychoanalytical process

Psychoanalysis as developed by Freud utilizes the methods of free association and dream analysis to effect reconstruction of the personality. Free association refers to the verbalization of thoughts as they occur without any conscious screening or censorship. Of course, there is always unconscious censorship of thoughts and impulses that are threatening to the ego. The psychoanalyst searches for patterns in the material that is verbalized and in the areas that are unconsciously avoided. The latter areas are identified by comparison to the therapist's knowledge of basic themes of human conflict. Conflictual areas that are not discussed or recognized by the patient are identified as resistances. Additional insight into the nature of the resistances can be derived from the analysis of the patient's dreams, which symbolically communicate areas of intrapsychic conflict.

The therapist attempts to assist the patient to recognize intrapsychic conflicts through the use of interpretation. Interpretation involves explaining to the patient the meaning of dream symbolism and the significance of the issues that are discussed or avoided. The process is complicated by the inevitable occurrence of transference. This refers to the patient's development of strong positive or negative feelings toward the analyst. These feelings are unrelated to the present behavior or characteristics of the analyst. They represent the patient's past response to a significant other, usually a parent. The therapist's reciprocal response to the patient is called countertransference. The transference provides the motivation for a patient to work in therapy. Strong positive transference causes the patient to want to please the therapist and to accept interpretations of his behavior. Strong negative transference may impede the progress of therapy as the patient actively resists the therapist's interventions. Countertransference can also interfere with therapy if the analyst is unaware of it or unable to deal with it.

Since the therapist can temporarily replace the significant other of the patient's early life experience, previously unresolved conflicts can be brought into the therapeutic situation and worked through to a healthier resolution. This releases previously cathected (invested) libido for mature adult functioning. The person is able to conduct his life according to an accurate assessment of external reality and is also able to relate to others uninhibited by neurotic conflicts. Psychoanalytical therapy is a long-term proposition. The patient is seen frequently, usually five times a week and usually over a period of several years. It is therefore time consuming and expensive.

■ Roles of the patient and the psychoanalyst

The respective roles of the patient and the psychoanalyst were explicitly defined by Freud. The patient was to be an active participant, freely revealing all thoughts exactly as they occurred and describing all dreams. The analytical patient frequently is in a recumbent position during therapy to induce relaxation, which facilitates free association. This also places the patient in a vulnerable position vis-a-vis the therapist, helping to recreate the childhood situation.

The psychoanalyst is a shadow person. Whereas the patient is expected to reveal all his thoughts and feelings, the analyst reveals nothing personal. This is to allow the transference to develop uncontaminated by the reality of the therapist as a person. The analyst usually conducts the therapeutic session outside of the direct line of vision of the patient, so that nonverbal responses do not influence the patient's verbalizations. Verbal responses are noncommittal for the most part and brief so as not to interfere with the associative flow. For instance, the analyst might respond with "Uh huh," "Go on," or "Tell me more." The therapist departs from this communication style when an interpretation of behavior is made. Interpretations are presented for the patient to accept or reject, but rejections are attributed to the operation of resistance. Likewise, any frustration that the patient expresses toward the analyst is interpreted as part of the transference. All the patient's behavior can be defined within the context of the psychoanalytical therapy model. By termination of therapy, the patient should be able to view the analyst realistically as another adult,

having worked through his conflicts and dependency needs.

■ Other psychoanalytical theorists

Much of Freud's basic theory is still utilized by psychotherapists. The theorists who followed him have modified and built on the original psychoanalytical theories. Even some of Freud's contemporaries who later severed relationships with him reveal the basic influence of psychoanalytical theory in their own work. Most prominent among those who left Freud to form their own schools are C.G. Jung, who developed the idea of the "collective unconscious," and Alfred Adler, who evolved the concept of the "inferiority complex."

Several contemporary theorists who are viewed to be psychoanalytical in orientation are listed below with a brief statement identifying their major contribution or area of study:

- Erik Erikson—expanded Freud's theory of psychosocial development to encompass the entire life cycle; identified an epigenetic progression of developmental tasks; described behavioral disturbances resulting from failure to accomplish developmental tasks
- Anna Freud—expanded psychoanalytical theory in the area of child psychology; further developed the concept of the mechanisms of defense
- Melanie Klein—extended use of psychoanalytical techniques to work with young children through development of play therapy
- Karen Horney—focused on psychoanalytical theory relative to neurotic behavior; related behavior to cultural and interpersonal factors; rejected Freud's view of feminine sexuality
- Frieda Fromm-Reichmann—utilized psychoanalytical techniques with psychotic individuals; expanded the psychoanalytical theory of psychotic behavior
- Karl Menninger—applied the concept of dynamic equilibrium to mental functioning; expanded the concept of coping; developed levels of dysfunction

The unique contributions of these theorists can best be understood by reading their works. This, too, will foster an appreciation for the continuing relevance of many aspects of psychoanalytical theory.

Interpersonal model

The origin of the interpersonal model of psychotherapy can be traced clearly to psychoanalytical thought. Karen Horney, Erich Fromm, and Wilhelm

Reich have been identified as the first theorists who attempted to incorporate sociocultural influences on human behavior into the psychoanalytical model.[6] However, the theorist who will be presented here as most representative of the interpersonal model is Harry Stack Sullivan, a twentieth-century American therapist. In addition, attention will be given to the interpersonal nursing theory of Hildegard Peplau. Her work represents a milestone in the conceptualization of the psychotherapeutic role of the nurse in the context of the interpersonal relationship.

■ Interpersonal view of behavioral deviations

Interpersonal theorists believe that behavior evolves within the context of interpersonal relationships. Whereas Freudian theory emphasizes the intrapsychic experience of the individual, interpersonal theory shifts the focus to the social or interpersonal experience. Sullivan, like Freud, traced a progression of psychological development. In fact, the psychoanalytical influence can be seen in some of Sullivan's terminology. For instance, the "self-system" bears marked resemblance to the "ego."

Sullivan also places emphasis on early life experiences as extremely influential to the individual's later mental health. He believes that anxiety is first experienced empathically when the infant perceives the anxiety of the mothering person. Later, anxiety is associated with disapproval from significant others. The self-system develops in the context of approval and disapproval. Disapproval causes anxiety because it includes a threat of rejection by the significant other. Security operations are developed to deal with anxiety-provoking areas of disapproval. The most anxiety-laden experiences are dissociated, meaning that they are excluded from the awareness of the self. Note the similarity to the psychoanalytical concept of repression.

If a child is given only disapproving messages about the self, a negative self-system develops. Interestingly, Sullivan states that "... one can find in others only that which is in the self."[10:310] Therefore a person who sees himself as untrustworthy will view others with suspicion. The person is then not only burdened with a lack of self-approval, but is also handicapped in establishing supportive relationships with others, which could, theoretically, help modify his self-concept.

Sullivanian theory states that the individual bases his behavior on two complex drives: the drive for satisfaction and the drive for security. Satisfaction refers to the basic human drives, including hunger, sleep, lust, and loneliness.[10] Security relates to culturally defined needs, such as conformity to the social norms and value

system of one's particular ethnic group. Sullivan states that when the nature of a person's self-system interferes with his ability to attend to his needs for either satisfaction or security, he is mentally ill.[10]

When Peplau defined nursing as an interpersonal process, she also discussed the importance of basic human needs. She believes that needs must be met if a healthy state is to be achieved and maintained. Health is defined as "forward movement of personality and other ongoing human processes in the direction of creative, constructive, productive, personal and community living."[16:2] Lack of growth, for whatever reason, implies impaired health. The two interacting components of health are physiological demands and interpersonal conditions.[16] These may be viewed as parallel to the drives of satisfaction and security identified by Sullivan. Clinical example 2-2 may clarify this perspective on behavioral deviation.

> ### CLINICAL EXAMPLE 2-2
>
> Ms. Y, an attractive 26-year-old woman, appeared at a psychiatric outpatient clinic requesting therapy. She described her problem as "I can't get close to people." She said that her childhood was happy; that she had loving parents and liked her sister. Her family were devout members of a fundamentalist Protestant church, so most of her activities were church related. She had many friends during childhood and then one close girl friend in early adolescence. She thought that her fear of closeness began when she slept over at her friend's house. During the night her friend began to fondle her in a way that she interpreted as sexual. She became very frightened and felt guilty about this. She did not tell her parents because of her guilt and, in fact, had told no one before entering therapy. Although she attended college, she never dated and would participate only in superficial social contacts. She realized that this was not healthy young adult behavior and, as the behavior continued into her twenties, Ms. Y decided that she needed to seek help.

From an interpersonal frame of reference, Ms. Y was unable to fulfill her needs for friendship and sexual love. Sullivanians would perceive a lack of satisfaction because of the unfulfilled lust dynamism and a lack of security because of her fear that she had deviated from the norm of her cultural group. Her anxiety stemmed from her conviction that her parents would disown her if they heard what had happened. This belief was based on their earlier responses to childhood sexual play. The therapist decided that Ms. Y first needed to experience intimacy at a nonsexual level and this was approached in the therapeutic situation. When she began to feel comfortable sharing closeness with the therapist, she gradually tried to explore friendships and finally was able to begin dating.

■ Interpersonal therapeutic process

The interpersonal therapist, like the psychoanalyst, explores the patient's life history. The focus of this exploration is on the person's progress through the developmental stages of learning to relate productively to other people. Components of the self-system are identified, including the security operations that are used to defend the self. The therapist also notes areas the patient avoids or claims to have forgotten, since this material may have been dissociated.

The crux of the therapeutic process is the corrective interpersonal experience. The premise is that by experiencing a healthy relationship with the therapist, the patient can learn to have more satisfying interpersonal relationships in general. The therapist actively encourages the development of trust by relating authentically to the patient. This includes the expectation that the therapist share feelings and reactions with the patient. The process of therapy is essentially a process of reeducation, as the therapist helps the patient identify interpersonal problems and then encourages him to try out more successful styles of relating. For example, fear of intimacy is frequently experienced by patients. The therapist allows the patient to become close while clearly communicating that there is no threat of sexual involvement. It is believed that closeness within the therapeutic relationship builds trust, facilitates empathy, enhances self-esteem, and thus fosters growth toward healthy behavior. Peplau[16] describes this process as "psychological mothering," which includes the following steps:

1. The patient is accepted unconditionally as a participant in a relationship that fully satisfies his needs.
2. There is recognition of and response to the patient's readiness for growth as initiated by the patient.
3. Power in the relationship shifts to the patient as he is able to delay gratification and to invest energy in goal achievement.

Therapy is terminated when the patient has developed the ability to establish satisfying human relationships, thereby meeting his basic needs. Termination is viewed as a significant part of the relationship that must be experienced and shared by both the therapist and the patient. It is through this process that the patient learns that leaving a significant other involves pain but can also be an opportunity for growth.

■ Roles of the patient and the interpersonal therapist

The patient-therapist dyad is viewed as a partnership by practitioners of interpersonal therapy. Sullivan describes the therapist as a "participant observer" who should not remain detached from the therapeutic situation.[20] The therapist's role is to actively engage the patient, establish trust, and empathize. There is an active effort to provide the patient with consensual validation, thereby helping him to realize that his perceptions and concerns are in many ways similar to those of others. There is an atmosphere of uncritical acceptance to encourage the patient to speak openly. The therapist then interacts as a real person who also has beliefs, values, thoughts, and feelings. The patient's role is to share his concerns with the therapist and to participate in the relationship to the best of his ability. The relationship itself is meant to serve as a model of interpersonal relationships. As the patient matures in his ability to relate, he can then improve and broaden his other life experiences with people outside the therapeutic situation.

Interpersonal nursing roles have been identified by Peplau.[16] They include the following:

1. Stranger—the role assumed by both nurse and patient when they first meet
2. Resource person—provider of health information to a patient who has assumed the consumer role
3. Teacher—assisting the patient as learner to grow and learn from his experience with the health care system
4. Leader—assisting the patient as follower to participate in a democratically implemented nursing process
5. Surrogate—assuming roles that have been assigned by the patient, based on his significant past relationships, similar to the psychoanalytical concept of transference
6. Counselor—helping the patient integrate the facts and feelings associated with an episode of illness into his total life experience

By functioning within these various roles, which may be assumed by the nurse or assigned to others, the practitioner assists the patient to meet the goals of therapy: need satisfaction and personal growth. In addition, the therapist experiences growth as she learns about herself through her role performance. Self-awareness is essential to success as an interpersonal therapist.

Social model

The two preceding models have centered on the individual and his intrapsychic processes and interpersonal experiences as the most significant factors to be considered in psychiatric care. The social model moves beyond the individual to include consideration of the social environment as it impacts on the person and his life experience. A criticism of psychoanalytical theory, in particular, is that it was heavily influenced by Freud's Victorian, Viennese, upper middle-class, Jewish background. It has been suggested that concepts such as the oedipal complex, castration anxiety, and penis envy might not extend to other cultures and times. Likewise, his view of women very much reflects his culture and times and has been repeatedly challenged, particularly by feminists.

There are recent theorists who believe that the culture itself is instrumental in defining mental illness, prescribing the nature of therapy and determining the future of the person who has been assigned the patient role. To represent this point of view, consideration will be given to the theories of Thomas Szasz and Gerald Caplan. In addition, the community mental health plan of the 1960s will be presented as an example of a governmental effort to respond to the philosophy of the social theorists.

■ Social view of behavioral deviations

According to theorists in this group, social conditions are largely responsible for the existence of deviant behavior. Deviancy is culturally defined. Behavior that is considered to be normal in one cultural setting may be eccentric in another and psychotic in a third. This was exemplified by the experience of the African exchange student mentioned in Clinical example 2-1. With this point of view, Szasz[21] writes of the "myth of mental illness." He believes that society must find a way of managing "undesirables," so it labels them as mentally ill. People who are so labeled are usually those who are unable or refuse to conform to social norms. The response to this behavior is generally to institutionalize the person. If he then conforms to social expectations, he is considered to be recovered and is allowed to return to the community. Institutionalization, then, has the dual function of removing deviant members from the community and of exerting social control over their behavior. Szasz states, "Mental illness is coercion concealed as loss of self-control; institutional psychiatry is countercoercion concealed as therapy."[22:100]

The first part of Szasz' statement recognizes that the individual is also responsible for his behavior. The person has control over whether to conform to social expectations. The person who is called mentally ill may be a scapegoat, but the individual participates in the scapegoating process by inviting it or by allowing it to occur. Szasz objects strongly to the designation of deviant behavior as "illness." He believes that illness can occur in the body and that diseases of the body can influence behavior (e.g., brain tumors), but there is no physiological disruption that can be demonstrated to cause most deviancy.[21] He distinguishes between the biological condition that is central to illness and the social role which is the focus of deviancy.

Caplan has also approached the study of deviant behavior from a social perspective. He has extended the public health model of primary, secondary, and tertiary prevention to the mental health field. Primary prevention is the avoidance of occurrence of disease. Secondary prevention is the reduction of the duration of the illness episode, and tertiary prevention is the limitation of impairment resulting from a disease process.[7] Caplan has focused particularly on primary prevention, since much attention has been given in the past to the secondary and tertiary levels. Lack of understanding of causation of deviant behavior has hindered the development of primary prevention techniques.

Caplan believes that social situations can predispose the person to mental illness. These situations include such conditions as poverty, family instability, and inadequate education. Deprivation throughout the life cycle leaves the individual with limited ability to cope with stress. The person has few available environmental supports. This combination results in a predisposition to utilize pathological means of coping.

Crises are viewed as possible precipitating causes of deviant behavior. When in crisis, a person is vulnerable. If internal coping mechanisms or external supports are inadequate, the person may exhibit pathological behavior. However, a crisis may also be an opportunity for growth if there are adequate resources to help the person learn from the experience and develop improved coping mechanisms. The supports must be available through the social system.

■ Social therapeutic process

Theorists who see behavioral deviation as intertwined with the social environment believe that therapy is also influenced by this dimension. Szasz is an advocate of freedom of choice for psychiatric patients. He believes that the individual should be allowed, without coercion, to select his own therapeutic modality and therapist. This also implies a well-informed consumer who can base this decision on knowledge of available modes of therapy.[10] Szasz does not believe in involuntary institutionalization of the mentally ill and comments, "Involuntary mental hospitalization is like slavery. Refining the standards for commitment is like prettifying the slave plantations. The problem is not how to improve commitment, but how to abolish it."[22:89] He also questions whether any psychiatric hospitalization is truly voluntary. Szasz is not in favor of the recent community mental health trend that purports to place mental health care within the reach of every American. He questions the extension of the involvement of government in what he views as essentially a private concern.

Caplan, on the other hand, has been a great proponent of community psychiatry. He interpreted the 1963 announcement by President Kennedy of the government's intention to become involved in the improvement of mental health care as a challenge to psychiatry. He foresaw a new focus on the reduction of the frequency of mental health problems, which then prompted his elaboration of theories of primary prevention.[7] To a great extent this theorist concentrates on the role of the mental health professional in combating societal problems, thereby indirectly benefiting those who could be future psychiatric patients. This is accomplished through the process of consultation.

The mental health consultant indirectly helps socially deprived individuals who are at risk for developing a mental illness. Examples of such groups might be the poor or minorities. Other people who are at risk and need primary prevention services are those in crisis, for example, mothers of premature babies or the recently widowed. The consultant may intervene on a variety of levels. In consultee-centered case consultation the focus is on an individual client and that person's problems. This approach has relatively narrow impact. Consultee-centered administrative consultation provides advice on program development or on the interpersonal relationships of agency workers. Care must be taken that the focus remain on the work situation rather than an attempt to deal with workers' personal problems. The third type of consultation is program-centered administrative consultation. Attention is paid to a broader perspective of the overall program of an agency or a group of related agencies.[7]

■ **Roles of the patient and the social therapist**

In the opinion of Szasz, an individual can be helped to solve his problems only if he requests such help. The patient, then, initiates the therapeutic encounter and defines the problem to be solved. The patient also has the right to approve or disapprove of the therapeutic intervention that is recommended. Therapy is successfully completed when the patient is satisfied with the changes that he has chosen to make in his life-style. The therapist collaborates with the patient to promote change. This includes making recommendations to the patient about possible means of effecting behavioral change. It does not include any element of coercion, particularly the threat of hospitalization if the patient does not conform to the therapist's demands. The therapist's role may also include protecting the patient from social demands that he be treated against his will. Szasz feels strongly that the therapist has moral and ethical obligations which are primarily directed toward the patient.

Caplan also takes a moral approach to therapy. However, he believes that society itself has a moral obligation to provide a wide range of therapeutic services covering all three levels of prevention. The patient has a consumer role and selects the level of help that is appropriate from a wide array of available services. Ideally, the client is reached by primary preventive services and thereby avoids the need for secondary or tertiary care. The client, it is hoped, never becomes a patient. For example, a recently widowed woman may be seen by her clergyman, who has received consultative training in counseling techniques. If he is concerned about the course of her grief process, he may refer her to a crisis intervention clinic where she will receive brief psychotherapy from a mental health professional. The person receiving crisis intervention services is viewed as a client who needs support over a short period of time while coping mechanisms and environmental supports are strengthened. The widow may then be referred to a community group of widows who help each other adjust to the shock of widowhood.

Therapists may be professional or nonprofessional with professional consultation. For instance, indigenous supportive people such as clergy, police, bartenders, and beauticians can be trained to be helpful listeners and to refer people who need professional help to appropriate resources. The therapist in the social context is not tied to the office but is expected to be involved in the community. Activities may include home visits, lectures to community groups, or consultation to other agencies. The rationale for this is that the more involved the therapist is in the community, the more impact there will be on the mental health of the people. Community involvement also enhances the therapist's ability to understand patients who live in that environment.

■ **Community mental health**

A movement of the 1960s that had great significance for psychiatric care was community mental health. It marked the vigorous entry of the federal government into the field of mental health and proved to be a mixed blessing. On the positive side, public attention was brought to the inadequacies of mental health care for the majority of the population. Public funding stimulated the creation of new facilities and the training of additional mental health professionals. Impetus was given to the examination of care delivery systems and, as a result, some modifications were made. For instance, there was interest in establishing a broader range of services with greater accessibility to the community served. There was also an emphasis on making services available to groups that had previously been neglected, such as the mentally retarded, children, the poor, alcoholics, and drug abusers.

Critics of community mental health point to the enormous amount of money that was spent with no apparent significant impact on the incidence of mental illness. They view it as a bandwagon that was used by some agencies to acquire new physical facilities with little or no commitment to the community mental health philosophy. The pressure to deinstitutionalize chronically hospitalized patients sometimes resulted in the imposition of people without social skills on unprepared communities with inadequate resources. In some cases the utilization of nonprofessional mental health workers led to the suspicion that the disadvantaged were being subjected to yet another type of second-rate care.

There is no doubt that community mental health has had an impact on psychiatric care delivery. It is still too soon to evaluate the total effect in an objective manner. However, the very stimulation of scrutiny of psychiatric services must be viewed as a healthy development, even if all the results did not meet the original high expectations.

Existential model

The existential model of psychiatric care and its theorists are heavily influenced by the work of such philosophers as Sartre, Heidegger, and Kierkegaard. They are also in agreement with the theory of the I-thou relationship as described by the religious philosopher Martin Buber. The focus is generally on the importance of the individual's experience in the here and now with much less attention being given to the person's past history than is the case with other theoretical models. Among the earliest existentialistic psychiatric thinkers were Karl Jaspers and Ludwig Binswanger. Many contemporary theorists espouse this point of view, including Frederick S. Perls, founder of gestalt therapy; William Glasser, founder of reality therapy; Albert Ellis, rational-emotive therapy; Carl Rogers, particularly in his later work with encounter groups;

and R.D. Laing, who combines his existentialist philosophy with an iconoclastic view similar to that of Szasz.

■ Existentialist view of behavioral deviations

Existentialist theorists tend to believe that behavioral deviations result when the individual is out of touch with himself or his environment. This alienation is the result of inhibitions or restrictions that the person has placed on himself. As a result, he is not free to choose from among all possible alternative behaviors. A deviant behavior is frequently a way of avoiding more socially acceptable, and therefore more responsible, behavior.

The person who is alienated from himself experiences feelings of helplessness, sadness, and loneliness. Lack of self-awareness and self-approbation prevents participation in authentic and rewarding relationships with others. Theoretically, the person has innumerable choices in terms of behavior. However, Heidegger[10] noted that people tend to avoid being real and instead yield to tradition and the demands of others. This belief has been accepted by the existentialist practitioners of mental health care.

Black[5] has described the psychiatric patient as a person who has either lost or never found the values that can give meaning to his existence. Hence the world seems absurd to him, and its demands appear invalid. Rather than accept the painful realities of life, he gives up. His lack of commitment may lead to a hazy identity and a sense of unreality, which extends to his perception of other people.

■ Existential therapeutic process

There are several therapies that are basically existential. These include logotherapy and gestalt, rational-emotive, reality, and encounter group therapy. Basic to all of them is the assumption that the patient needs to be able to choose freely from what life has to offer. Although the approaches are somewhat different, the goal is generally to return the patient to an authentic awareness of his being. Laing[15] describes the process of going mad and then returning to sanity. Going mad is compared to death, movement backward, an altered sense of time, self-absorption, and a return to the womb. Recovery is compared to return to life, forward movement, restoration of temporal meaning, the growth of a new ego, and "an existential rebirth." It is the work of therapy for the patient, with the help of the therapist, to find his way from the alienation of madness to the relatedness of a full life.

The existential therapeutic process focuses on the

encounter. The encounter is not merely the meeting of two or more persons but is their appreciation of the total existence of each other. As Binswanger has stated, "encounter is a being-with-others in *genuine presence*, that is to say, in the present which is altogether continuous with the *past* and bears within it the possibilities of a *future*."[10:377] This temporal orientation that takes note of the patient's life as a process of becoming is also basic to most existential theories. Through the encounter, the patient is helped to accept and understand his past, live fully in the present, and look forward to the future.

The actual process of therapy differs somewhat depending on the specific theory being practiced. Following are several of the better known existentially based theories with a brief statement concerning the therapeutic process of each. For further information, the reader is encouraged to explore the writings of these theorists.

- Rational-emotive therapy (Albert Ellis)—an active-directive, cognitively oriented therapy. Confrontation is used to force the patient to assume responsibility for his behavior. The patient is encouraged to accept himself as he is, not because of what he does. He is taught to take risks and try out new behavior. Action is emphasized for both the patient and the therapist.[11]
- Logotherapy (Viktor E. Frankl)—a future-oriented therapy; "the patient is actually confronted with and oriented toward the meaning of his life."[12:153] This search for meaning (*logos*) is viewed as a primary life force. This includes meaning in the spiritual sense. Without a sense of meaning, life becomes an "existential vacuum." The aim of therapy is to help the patient become aware of his responsibleness. In essence, the patient is guided to take control of his own life and to determine its meaning for himself.
- Reality therapy (William Glasser)—central themes are the need for identity reached by loving, feeling worthwhile, and behaving responsibly. The patient is helped to recognize his life goals and the way he keeps himself from accomplishing his goals. He is made aware of the alternatives available to him. Another focus of therapy is the development of the capacity for caring, through the warm acceptance of the therapist. Temporal orientation is to the present. The patient is directed to talk about any topic but to focus on behavior rather than feelings.[13]
- Gestalt therapy (Frederick S. Perls)—emphasizes the here and now. The patient is encouraged to identify feelings by enhancing self-awareness. There is focus on body sensations as they reflect feelings. The increased awareness makes the patient more sensitive to other aspects of his existence. Self-awareness is expected to lead to self-acceptance. The patient is assisted to deal with unfinished business by becoming aware of the totality of his responses. More attention is focused on the "how" and "what" of behavior, rather than the "why."[13]
- Encounter group therapy (William C. Schutz, Carl Rogers)—focuses on the establishment of intimate interactions in a group setting. Therapy is oriented to the here and now. The patient is expected to assume responsibility for his own behavior. Feeling is stressed; intellectualization discouraged. Group exercises in relating are frequently utilized. Group members are encouraged to honestly and openly share their thoughts and feelings, thus becoming more self-aware.[13]

■ Roles of the patient and the existential therapist

The existential theorists emphasize that the therapist and the patient are equal in their common humanity. The therapist is to act as a guide to the patient who has gone astray in his search for authenticity. The therapist is frequently very direct in pointing out areas where the patient should consider changing. However, there is also a focus on caring and warmth. The therapist as well as the patient is to be open and honest. The therapeutic experience is a model for the patient, during which he can test new behaviors prior to risking them in his daily life.

The patient is expected to assume and accept responsibility for his behavior. Dependence on the therapist is generally not encouraged. In this sense, the patient is treated as an adult. Frequently there is a de-emphasis of illness. The patient is viewed as a person who is alienated from himself and others, but for whom there is hope if he can trust and follow the directions of the therapist. The patient is always active in therapy, working to meet the challenge presented by the therapist.

Communication model

A sophisticated system of communication is one of the characteristics that distinguishes human beings from lower orders of animal life. In the eyes of communication theorists, all behavior communicates something. The understanding of the meaning of behavior is based on the clarity of communication between the actor (sender) and observer (receiver). Disruptions in behavior may, then, be viewed as disturbances in the communication process. This point of view is appealing in an information-oriented culture such as the contemporary United States. The prevalence of the use of media for the dissemination of information demonstrates the increasing utilization of communication techniques. At the same time, breakdown in successful transmission of information causes anxiety and frustration.

Theorists who have particularly emphasized the importance of communication are Eric Berne, the founder of transactional analysis, and Paul Watzlawick and his associates who have studied the pragmatics of human communication.

■ Communications view of behavioral deviations

All behavior is communication, whether verbal or nonverbal. Therefore deviant behavior may be viewed as an attempt to communicate. The message may be masked or distorted; the route may be indirect, but the end result of behavior is still the transmission of a message to others who are able to perceive it.

According to Berne,[4] people communicate from the frame of reference of one of three ego states: parent, adult, or child. These terms do not refer to actual status in life, but refer to the concept that the person acts like a parent, for instance. A communication unit is referred to as a transaction. *Complementary transactions* occur when the message that is directed from one ego state to another is responded to as implicitly expected so the ego state which is addressed actually responds:

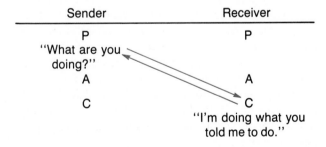

For instance, the sender's parent addresses the receiver's child and then the receiver's child responds to the sender's parent. Problems occur when transactions are crossed. As an example, the sender's adult may address the receiver's adult, but receive a response from the receiver's parent to the sender's child, for instance, "Bring me a glass of milk, please" followed by "Get it yourself, I'm busy." This type of transaction results in a communication block. The four most common crossed communications are the following:

1. Adult to adult—child to parent (the transference reaction)

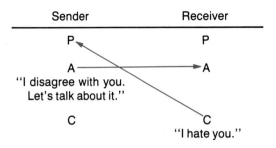

2. Adult to adult—parent to child (countertransference)

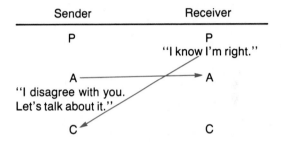

3. Child to parent—adult to adult (exasperating)

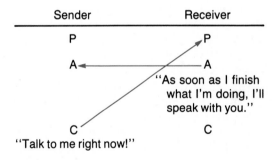

4. Parent to child—adult to adult (impudent)

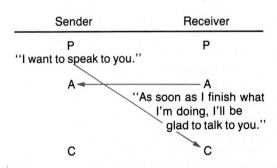

In some transactions an ulterior motive is operating. For example, the adult may appear to be addressing the other's adult but may expect a response from the parent or child. In other ulterior transactions there may be superficial social and deeper psychological levels of meaning operating at the same time. According to Berne, the basis of transactional analysis is "rigorous analysis of single transactions into their component specific ego states."[4:20]

Berne further believes that people respond to three drives or hungers: (1) stimulus hunger—the need for sensation, (2) recognition hunger—the need for special interpersonally experienced sensations, and (3) structure hunger—the need to organize. The last drive leads the person to structure his time. He describes six basic types of social behavior that help to provide the needed structure: (1) withdrawal; (2) rituals, which are responses to custom and characterized by strokes or units of recognition; (3) activities, or work; (4) pastimes; (5) games; and (6) intimacy.[4] Two of these in particular, games and intimacy, require further elaboration. He describes games as "sets of ulterior transactions, repetitive in nature, with a well-defined psychological payoff." "Payoff" refers to the feelings that are aroused by the game. Each participant receives a payoff, although the feelings may differ. The other elements of the game are the "con," or bait, which involves the other player; the switch, in which the initiator changes the rules or the character of the game; and the cross-up, in which the other player feels confused and becomes aware of the switch. All these factors are necessary for a game to be played. Intimacy refers to an open relationship in which game playing is avoided. Structure is also accomplished by way of a script, which Berne identifies as a "'life plan' which derives from childhood ideas." Deviant behavior, then, indicates that the person is relating through game playing rather than intimacy and may be living out a script that is irrelevant to his adult life.

Watzlawick[23] and other communications pragmatists believe that deviant behavior is based on disrupted communication patterns. They have identified several such patterns. The first is an effort not to communicate, which is self-defeating because it is impossible. A second is a lack of congruity in levels of communication. In this case the focus is on the content of the message, but the real issue involves the relationship between the communicators. When a person makes a statement about himself, the other may confirm, reject, or disconfirm it. Disconfirmation denies the reality of the other.

Imperviousness is a situation in which each person assumes he understands and is understood when this is not actually the case. Discrepancies in punctuation occur when one party has less information than the other but does not know it, leading to different perceptions of reality. The person who exhibits the self-fulfilling prophecy generally behaves as he expects others to respond to him, thus reinforcing his (usually negative) self-concept.

Human relationships are either symmetrical or complementary. Symmetry implies equality; whereas complementarity implies difference. One disruption in this area is called symmetrical escalation, which occurs when the participants strive to be "more equal." A disruption of complementarity is folie à deux, in which each partner confirms the pathologic condition of the other. For instance, a rigid, controlling mother and a passive, compliant child may depend on each other for role confirmation.[23] Watzlawick also presents the concept of the pragmatic paradox, which is demonstrated by the double bind. (See Chapter 17.)

■ Communications therapeutic process

Because communications theorists locate the disruption in behavior within the communication process, interventions are made in patterns of communication. This may take place with individuals, groups, or families. The communication pattern is first assessed and the disruption diagnosed. The patient is then helped to recognize his own disrupted communication. In this sense, there is a definite education component to communication therapy.

Transactional analysts assist patients to recognize ego states in themselves and others and to identify crossed transactions. Analysis of games is an important part of therapy. The patient is helped to see what games he plays repeatedly. He is then assisted to find the elements of these games (i.e., What is the payoff for him? For the other person?). Games that arise during therapy are pointed out, and alternative behavior is presented. As with the existential therapies, the emphasis is on authenticity and responsibility for the self. In addition to the focus on games, the patient also works to discover his script. Once identified, the script can be modified to meet the person's adult needs and to facilitate healthy relationships.

Watzlawick and his colleagues developed the technique of the therapeutic double bind. They contend that there are two ways to induce change in therapy. One is to tell the person to change, which he probably would have done if he were able to do so. The other is to tell him not to change, which enhances his awareness of his behavior, increases tension, and may stimulate him to change. Telling the person to change by not changing creates a paradox in which any behavior is expected to result in a change. The theorists point out that this is a difficult technique to master and should only be attempted by skilled therapists who can deal with the high level of anxiety that might result.

■ Roles of the patient and the communications therapist

The communications therapist induces change in the patient by intervening in the communication process. Feedback is given about the person's success at communicating. Effective communication is reinforced, and alternatives for ineffective communication are discussed. In group or family settings, patterns are analyzed on a more complex level. The therapist also demonstrates how to relate to others clearly, without playing games or using paradoxes. Nonverbal communication is also emphasized, particularly in terms of congruence with verbal behavior.

The patient must be willing to become involved in an analysis of his style of communicating. If in transactional analysis, he frequently will have to study the communication theory. He is then asked to participate in identifying ego states, games, and scripts. The responsibility for changing rests with the patient. Significant others are often included in communication therapy to deal with their response to change in the identified patient. Change in one participant in a communication system stimulates responses in the other members. These responses are generally directed toward maintaining the status quo. Thus change is more lasting if it takes place at the system level.

Behavioral model

Behavior modification therapy is derived from learning theories. The focus is on the patient's actions, not on thoughts and feelings. It is believed by these theorists that a change in behavior will lead to a change in the cognitive and affective spheres. Behavior therapists emphasize the quantitative aspect of observable behavior. They believe that one of the strengths of this approach is the possibility of conducting research on the effectiveness of therapy. They contend that most other psychotherapies are not compatible with a scientific research process because of the high degree of subjectivity involved in defining the problem and identifying improvement. In addition, there is variation in the therapeutic behavior of psychotherapists who utilize other models. Personality style tends to individualize therapy even among therapists who share the same theoretical framework. Behavior modification therapy, on the other hand, is structured and therefore more reproducible from therapist to therapist.

Prominent theorists of behavioral therapy include H.J. Eysenck, Joseph Wolpe, and B.F. Skinner.

■ Behavior theorists' view of behavioral deviations

Since the behavioral theorists believe that all behavior is learned, deviations from the norm are viewed as habitual responses that can be modified through application of learning theory. Learning occurs when a stimulus is presented, a response occurs, and the response is reinforced. The response is strengthened by repetition of the learning sequence. The desirability of the reinforcer to the learner is also important, although even painful (aversive) reinforcers have been found to enhance a behavior more than no response at all.

From the behavioral point of view, then, deviations from behavioral norms occur when undesirable behavior has been reinforced. Clinical example 2-3 illustrates this theory.

CLINICAL EXAMPLE 2-3

Ms. J was a 45-year-old woman who was brought to the mental health center at the insistence of her family. She was actively resisting her 20-year-old son's plan to move to his own apartment by threatening to kill herself. Each time she threatened, he agreed not to move for a few more weeks, thus reinforcing her behavior. The therapeutic plan was that the son would set a date to move and do so. At the same time, Mr. J would give his wife extra attention during the difficult time of their son's leaving.

■ Behavioral therapeutic process

Behavioral therapy, as described by Wolpe,[8] includes the techniques of reciprocal inhibition. This is based on the premise that the observable behavior, or symptom, is a learned response to anxiety. The symptom is reinforced because it leads to a reduction of anxiety, even though it is not otherwise a productive behavior. Reciprocal inhibition attempts to substitute a more adaptive behavior for the symptom through the learning of an alternative means of reducing the anxiety. One such approach is desensitization or the relaxation technique. The patient establishes a hierarchy of anxiety-provoking experiences from low to high levels of anxiety. He then either actually experiences or fantasizes each experience from lowest to highest. During the fantasy he may practice relaxation exercises with the coaching of the therapist. Sometimes the patient is hypnotized. The whole process takes several therapy sessions, since the patient does not move on to the next level of the hierarchy until the anxiety associated with the lower level has been alleviated. For further discussion of this technique and an example of a hierarchy, see Chapter 12.

Another approach that has been advocated by Wolpe for the alleviation of anxiety is assertiveness training. This is useful when the patient's anxiety arises from interpersonal relationships. Assertiveness implies the ability to stand up for one's own rights while not infringing on the rights of others. It is differentiated from passive behavior, which ignores one's own rights, and aggressive behavior, which violates the other's rights. In therapy the patient identifies his usual mode of behavior. Through role play and practice he works to modify his behavior toward increased assertiveness. This, in turn, increases self-esteem and the sense of self-control, thus reducing interpersonally based anxiety.

Other behavior modification approaches include aversion therapy and the token economy system. Aversion therapy refers to the use of a painful stimulus, usually an electrical shock, to create an aversion to a stimulus. This approach has been tried as an attempt to change homosexual behavior.[8] There has been controversy over the moral-ethical aspects of utilizing a method of therapy that deliberately induces pain to change behavior. Therapists who use this approach believe the end justifies the means. Patients who accept aversion therapy generally do so of their own volition. This gives some indication of the strength of emotional pain so intense that physical pain is accepted to alleviate it.

Token economy systems are positive reinforcement programs that are frequently utilized to encourage socially acceptable behavior in chronically hospitalized patients. The person is rewarded with a token, generally a poker chip, when the desirable behavior occurs and penalized by removal of tokens when undesirable behavior takes place. When enough tokens are accumulated, they may be spent for cigarettes, snacks, grounds passes, or whatever is meaningful to the patient. This pleasurable experience reinforces the future repetition of the desired behavior. For patients with good ability for abstract thinking, points may be substituted for tokens. It is important, however, to be sure that the reward is highly desirable to the patient. This approach may also be helpful with children and acting-out adolescents.

■ Roles of the patient and the behavioral therapist

The roles of patient and therapist when a behavioral approach to treatment is used are those of learner and teacher, respectively. The therapist is an expert in behavior who can help the patient unlearn his symptoms and replace them with more satisfying behavior. The therapist utilizes the patient's anxiety as a motivational force toward learning. Behavioral objectives are devised, and careful evaluation takes place.

As a learner, the patient is an active participant in the therapy process. He must produce fantasies or practice uncomfortable behaviors. Behavior modification patients may be well versed in the rationale for the therapy, although this is in no way necessary for this approach to be used. However, the knowledgeable patient is a more cooperative patient. There are frequently homework assignments to further reinforce the teaching done in the therapeutic session. Significant others may also be enlisted to continue the therapy program at home. Therapy is considered to be complete when the symptoms are gone. There is no attempt to unearth an underlying conflict, and the patient is not encouraged to explore his past.

Medical model

The medical model refers to psychiatric care that is based on the traditional physician-patient relationship and focuses on the diagnosis of a mental illness. Subsequent treatment is based on this diagnosis. Somatic treatments, including pharmacotherapy, electroconvulsive therapy, and, occasionally, psychosurgery, are important components of the treatment process. The interpersonal aspect of this approach to treatment varies widely, from intensive insight-oriented intervention to brief, superficial medication-supervision sessions.

Much of modern psychiatric care is dominated by the medical model. Other health professionals may be utilized for specific purposes such as interagency referrals, family assessment, and health teaching, but physicians are viewed as the leaders of the team when this model is in effect. In the same way, elements of other models of care may be used in conjunction with the medical model. For instance, a patient may be diagnosed as schizophrenic and treated with phenothiazine medication but may also be on a token economy program to encourage socially acceptable behavior.

Siegler and Osmond[19] believe that the medical model performs two functions. The first is that of treating the ill. The second is to avoid the placing of blame for deviant behavior. This second function is extremely important and may account for the wide acceptance of the medical model. When illness is attributed to disease and a cause is postulated that is external to the patient and his immediate social system, the focus can be on healing rather than blaming. Viewing mental illness in this way helps to remove some of the social stigma that is otherwise attached to it.

Chamberlin, however, disputes the contention that the medical model reduces stigmatism. She believes that the labeling of behavior that results from diagnosis is destructive to the patient. Behavior takes place in the context of the social system and should be interpreted within that context. She asserts that a diagnosis of mental illness, particularly schizophrenia, creates fear and withdrawal of others from the patient.[9]

A positive contribution of the medical model has been the continuous exploration for causes of mental illness using the scientific process. Recently there have been great strides in learning about brain and nervous system functioning. This has led to a beginning understanding of the probable physiological components of many behavioral disruptions. This progress will, in turn, lead to increasingly specific and sophisticated approaches to psychiatric care.

■ Medical view of behavioral deviations

Most adherents of the medical model believe that deviant behavior is a manifestation of a disorder of the central nervous system. As Andreasen writes, "Mental illness is truly a nervous breakdown—a breakdown that occurs when the nerves of the brain have an injury so severe that their own internal healing capacities cannot repair it."[3:219] She lists several types of brain disorders that could lead to mental illness: loss of nerve cells, excesses or deficits in chemical transmission, abnormal patterns of brain circuitry, problems in the command centers, and disruptions in the movement of messages along nerves.[3]

At present, the exact nature of the physiological disruption is not well understood. It is suspected that for the psychotic disorders, such as bipolar disorder, major depression, and schizophrenia, there is an abnormality in the transmission of neural impulses. It is also believed that this difficulty occurs at the synaptic level and involves neurochemicals, such as dopamine, serotonin, and norepinephrine.

Recently a new group of neurochemicals, named endorphins and enkephalins, have attracted a great deal of interest. They have been referred to as natural opiates because they bind to opiate receptors in the brain. Their role in determining behavior is being explored.

Much research is currently taking place to better understand the nature of the brain's involvement in emotional response. Another area of research focuses on stressors and the human response to stress. Researchers are asking the question "Why do some people seem to tolerate great stress and continue to function well and others fall apart when a small problem arises?" They suspect that there may be a physiological stress

threshold which may be genetically determined. These research areas are intriguing, but for the present, not well enough defined to provide definitive guidelines for therapy.

Environmental and social factors are also considered in the medical model. They may be either predisposing or precipitating factors in an episode of illness. For example, the person who is unemployed, lonely, and lives near a bar may be predisposed by these factors to develop a drinking problem. In combination with other possible genetic and physiological predispositions this constellation of circumstances could result in alcoholism. In another instance an episode of illness in an alcoholic patient could be precipitated by the social event of separation from his wife.

■ Medical therapeutic process

The medical process of therapy is well defined and familiar to most patients. The physician's examination of the patient includes the history of the present illness, past history, social history, medical history, review of systems, physical examination, and mental status examination. Additional data may be collected from significant others, and past medical records are reviewed, if available. A preliminary diagnosis is then formulated, pending further diagnostic studies and observation of the patient's behavior. This process may take place on an ambulatory or an inpatient basis, depending on the condition of the patient.

The diagnosis is stated and classified according to the Draft of the DSM-III-R in Development (DSM-III-R)[2] of the American Psychiatric Association. The names of the various illnesses are augmented by a description of diagnostic criteria, which are tested for reliability on a group of psychiatric practitioners. Changes in the DSM reflect changes in the medical model of psychiatric care. DSM-III-R is the most up to date.[2]

According to Andreasen, one DSM-III innovation was the detailed discussion of each disorder, which was followed by a definition that included a specific set of diagnostic criteria. This edition also reorganized the classification system, adding many more classifications than were present in DSM-II. The changes were

1. The use of more objective and descriptive terminology
2. Increased focus in the diagnostic interview
3. A clearer and more objective diagnostic process

Andreasen also describes limitations in DSM-III. It failed to completely reflect a medical model by focusing on disorders, not diseases. There was no discussion of causation. Although use of the manual led to a more reliable diagnosis, it did not assist the clinician in predicting treatment, course, or outcome.[3] The Draft of the DSM-III-R in Development[2] represents an attempt to resolve these problems by including more specific diagnostic criteria, including efforts to describe the course of the illness.

A difference between DSM-III-R[2] and earlier diagnostic manuals is the use of the concept of multiaxial diagnosis. Five axes are presented as factors to be considered in formulating a psychiatric diagnosis. These five axes are presented in their entirety in Chapter 3. Axes I and II include the mental disorders. The diagnostic categories of Personality Disorders and Specific Developmental Disorders are assigned to axis II; all other diagnoses are included in axis I. This was done so that the axis II diagnoses would not be overlooked if they occurred in conjunction with the frequently more dramatic axis I conditions.[2] Axis III is used for documentation of any coexisting physical conditions. These three axes make up the diagnosis that is to be documented for any patient who receives psychiatric care. Specialized clinical settings or individuals who are conducting psychiatric research may choose to include axes IV and V as well. Axis IV documents the severity of psychosocial stressors on a scale of one to seven.[2] Axis V rates the patient's highest level of adaptive functioning in the last year.[2] The fact that axis IV and V information is not routinely included in the medical diagnosis illustrates one of the important differences between psychiatry and psychiatric nursing. These factors would always be important to include when formulating a nursing diagnosis.

After the diagnosis is formulated, treatment is instituted. The physician-patient relationship is fostered to engender trust in the physician and compliance with the treatment plan. If indicated, the therapist will also assist the patient to look at the stressful situation in his life and his usual style of coping. Other health team members may be enlisted to contribute their expertise to the patient's care. Response to treatment is evaluated on the basis of the patient's subjective assessment of how he is feeling combined with the therapist's objective observations of the occurrence of symptomatic behavior. In some cases therapy may be terminated when the patient returns to a satisfactory functional level. For instance, the person who has experienced an adjustment disorder with depressed mood may, after a short course of medication and supportive therapy, be able to return to his usual life-style. Other patients will require long-term follow-up therapy, often including pharmacotherapy. For example, the patient with bipolar disorder may need to take lithium carbonate indefinitely and also need to see a therapist for observation of behavior and periodic laboratory studies. Still other patients may receive long-term insight-oriented therapy to assist them to learn improved methods of coping with stressors.

■ Roles of the patient and the medical therapist

The roles of physician and patient have been well defined by tradition and hold true in the psychiatric setting. The physician is the healer. This role entails responsible identification of the patient's illness and instituting a treatment plan that will not be harmful to the patient. Although the patient may have input into the plan, the physician prescribes the recommended form of therapy and generally applies the power inherent in his high-status position if the patient refuses to comply with the plan. Patients are frequently not encouraged to question the physician's decision.

The patient is expected to assume the behavior of the sick role. This involves an admission that he is ill, which can be a problem in psychiatry. Patients are sometimes not aware of their disturbed behavior and may actively resist treatment, which is not congruent with the medical model. Another expectation of the patient is that he comply with the treatment program and work hard to get well. Inherent in this expectation is the anticipation that observable improvement will occur. If it does not, there are frequently suspicions expressed by caregivers and significant others that the patient is not trying hard enough. This can be frustrating to a patient who feels he is trying to get well and is disappointed at his own lack of progress. The patient may also have difficulty meeting the expectation that he let people take care of him but also that he try to help himself. These two activities are often not compatible, and it may be difficult to comply with both. The patient who is unable to respond to the therapy offered may be transferred to another physician, another mental health professional, or to a long-term custodial institution where his deviant behavior will be tolerated.

Nursing model

Since nursing is in the process of coming of age as a profession, there is still no one universally accepted theoretical model for the provision of nursing care. However, nursing theorists have proposed several models that are currently being explored and refined. These include models based on general systems theory, developmental theories, and interaction theory.[17] There are some general similarities among these nursing models. They all incorporate a holistic approach to the individual, with attention given to biological, psychological, and sociocultural needs. Nursing care delivery is viewed as a collaborative process, with both the nurse and the patient contributing ideas and energy to the therapeutic process. The focus is on the caring functions of nurses, which are distinct from, but complementary to, the curing functions of physicians.

Shaver points out that the medical model does not fit well with nursing. A human ecological model works much better. The focus is on personal behaviors, the environment, and host factors.[18] Fig. 2-1 illustrates the difference between the nursing and medical models as described by Shaver.

Nurses are experts at observing and interpreting patient's behavior. They also assist the patient to assess his own behavior, identify unfulfilling behaviors, and undertake behavioral change. Caring also implies concern about the patient's emotional response to the problem. The nurse therefore also utilizes comfort measures to ease the patient's pain, emotional as well as physical. To understand the patient as a whole person, time must be spent talking with him and establishing a therapeutic nurse-patient relationship. The nurse also acts as a patient advocate. When appropriate, the nurse represents the patient in the health care system and helps to interpret his needs to significant others and to health team members.

Some prominent nursing theorists who have been developing models for nursing care delivery include Ida Jean Orlando, Hildegard Peplau, Imogene King, Dorothea Orem, Joan Riehl, Sister Callista Roy, and Martha Rogers. The works of all of these nursing leaders are recommended to the reader to gain a broad appreciation of the issues currently being addressed in nursing. Johnston compares the congruency of nursing with other psychosocial models to clarify similarities and differences, with the hope that research related to theory-based practice will result. The concepts that are compared include the person, the environment, and health.[14] Table 2-1 shows which nursing models are most closely related to selected major psychosocial models. The remainder of this chapter reflects our philosophy of nursing. This nursing model is discussed in detail in Chapter 3.

■ Nursing view of behavioral deviations

The focus of nursing is on the individual's response to potential or actual health problems.[1] The defining characteristics of nursing as related to this focus include the *health-illness phenomena* that are encountered, the *theory base* for nursing care, the *nursing actions* that are carried out, and the *effects* that are identified as a result of nursing intervention.[1]

Behavior is viewed on a continuum from healthy, adaptive responses to maladaptive responses that are indicative of illness. The actual behavior observed is the

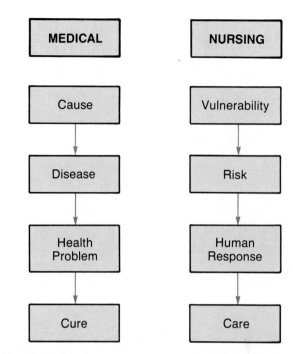

Fig. 2-1. Shaver's comparison of the biomedical and nursing models of care.

result of a number of factors. Each individual is predisposed to respond to life events in unique ways. These predispositions are biological, psychological, and sociocultural and are the sum of the person's heritage and past experiences. Behavior is the result of the combination of the predisposing factors with precipitating stressors. Stressors are life events that are perceived by the individual as challenging, threatening, or demanding. The nature of the behavioral response depends on the person's primary appraisal of the stressor and secondary appraisal of the coping resources that are available to him. The continuum of coping responses may then include actual health problems that lead to a medical diagnosis or potential health problems. Nursing intervention may take place at any point on the continuum. Nursing diagnoses may focus on behaviors associated with a medical diagnosis or other health behaviors that the patient wishes to change. A nurse may practice primary prevention by intervening in a potential health problem, secondary prevention by intervening in an actual acute health problem, or tertiary prevention by intervening to limit the disability caused by actual chronic health problems.

Human behavior is viewed from a holistic perspective. A stressor that has primary impact on physiological functioning will also affect the person's psychological and sociocultural behavior. For instance, a man who has had a myocardial infarction may also become severely

```
┌─────────────────────────────────┐
│            TABLE 2-1            │
│                                 │
│   NURSING MODELS THAT RELATE    │
│      CLOSELY TO SELECTED        │
│   MAJOR PSYCHOSOCIAL MODELS     │
```

Psychosocial model	Nursing model
Psychoanalytic/interpersonal (Freud, Sullivan, Erikson)	Interpersonal (Peplau) Self-care (Orem)
Behavioral (Watson, Skinner)	Adaptation (Roy)
Communication (Bateson, Weakland, Watzlawick)	Systems (King)
Humanistic (Maslow)	Unitary man (Rogers)

Modified from Johnston, R.L.: Individual psychotherapy: relationship of theoretical approaches to nursing conceptual models. In Fitzpatrick, J.J., Whall, A.L., Johnston, R.L., and Floyd, J.A.: Nursing models and their psychiatric mental health applications. Bowie, Md., 1982, Robert J. Brady Co.

depressed because he fears he will lose his ability to work and to satisfy his wife sexually. On the other hand, the patient who enters the psychiatric inpatient unit with a major depression may be suffering from malnutrition and dehydration because of refusal to eat or drink. The holistic nature of nursing encompasses all these facets of behavior and incorporates them into patient care planning.

■ **The nursing therapeutic process**

Psychiatric nurses base their care of patients on the nursing process, including the steps of data collection, formulation of the nursing diagnosis, planning, implementation, and evaluation. Data collection includes the eliciting of a complete health history, learning the patient's perception of his problems and their causes, and assessing strengths and weaknesses of the patient system and the social system. The nurse attempts to identify the predisposing factors and the precipitating stressors to the immediate problem. She also assesses the patient's biopsychosocial behavior in terms of norms for a person of the patient's age, sex, and sociocultural background and consults professional literature. Inferences are validated with the patient to limit the introduction of bias. Other resources for data collection include the patient's health records, significant others, and other health professionals who have provided care to the patient. Data are collected more systematically when the nurse

uses a data collection tool that incorporates information about the total health status of the individual.

The nursing diagnosis is formulated on the basis of the collected data. It is a statement of the patient's nursing problem that incorporates the behavioral disruption and the stressor or stressors which are contributing to the actual or potential disruption. The nursing diagnosis provides the focus for nursing care and thus requires the input and concurrence, when possible, of the patient. It is not adequate to take note of the patient's medical diagnosis and use that as a basis for nursing care. Each patient differs from every other, and, although there may be common needs related to the medical diagnosis, there will also be individual needs related to that person's unique life experience.

Nursing care goals are formulated on the basis of the nursing diagnosis. Generally, both long- and short-term goals are developed. Long-term goals describe the health behavior to be accomplished when the identified problem is considered to be resolved. Short-term goals are contributory to the long-term goal.

Nursing actions are planned and implemented on the basis of nursing care goals combined with knowledge and review of nursing theory. Nursing care goals must be mutually developed with understanding of the patient's own goals for his health care. Goals should be stated in behavioral terms. It is important to establish priorities for the nursing care goals that have been mutually agreed on by the nurse and patient. This avoids fragmentation in the provision of nursing care.

Nursing actions may be dependent, based on the physician's order. For example, dispensing medication is a dependent nursing function. Other nursing actions are independent. Deciding to approach a patient who appears upset and allowing him to express his feelings is an independent nursing function. There are also interdependent nursing functions. Requesting the social worker to obtain information for the patient about his medical insurance and reinforcing the social worker's explanation are interdependent functions. All these levels of nursing should be incorporated into the written nursing care plan, since all are important to the total well-being of the patient. Nursing actions should also take advantage of the patient's strengths to build on the healthy aspects of his behavior. All patients have strengths. It is a nursing challenge to discover them and capitalize on them. Well-planned nursing intervention will assist the patient to accomplish the major goals of developing insight and carrying out a plan of positive action.

Nursing actions may also include various psychotherapeutic modalities of care, depending on the nurse's level of professional experience and education. Nurses with advanced psychiatric preparation may be qualified to conduct individual, group, or family psychotherapy, psychodrama, assertiveness training, behavior modification, or other specialized therapies. Many of these therapeutic modalities may be recognized as having been mentioned earlier in this chapter. The nursing model does not preclude the use of any modality of care delivery as long as the nurse is skilled in its application and receives adequate supervision. Nursing care is always implemented with respect for the rights and dignity of the patient and with empathy for the patient as a troubled person who deserves concern and caring. To ensure the highest quality of patient care, the nursing care plan must take into account the potential contributions of the entire health care team and particularly the preferences, wants, and needs of the patient.

Nursing care is continuously evaluated and modified by the patient and the nurse as the nursing process is used. Modifications are made in each phase of the nursing care plan on the basis of the evaluation. The most important factor in the evaluation process is the patient's reaction to the nursing care. Therefore the patient must be an active participant in this process. Validation with the patient is essential to be sure that the nurse's inferences are correct. Ongoing evaluation can add flexibility to nursing care, allowing the nurse and patient to explore alternatives and make choices concerning the most helpful interventions.

Nursing care is terminated mutually by the patient and the nurse. Termination is based on the successful accomplishment of the identified goals. At other times termination results because the patient or the nurse must leave the care delivery system or because the patient chooses not to comply with the identified plan. Whatever the reason for the termination, there should be a final evaluation of the nursing care episode. This serves as a learning and growth experience for the patient and the nurse.

■ Roles of the patient and the nurse

The nurse-patient relationship is based on mutuality. The needs of the patient are the focus of the relationship. Emphasis is on the strengths of the patient as a person and his growth potential. The patient is an active participant in the nursing care and is asked for feedback about the effectiveness of that care. Modifications in the care plan result from the collaboration of the nurse and patient. Another role assumed by the patient is that of learner, as the nurse strives to make him aware of his health needs and helps him to understand the nature of his health problems.

The nurse coordinates the patient's health care experience, elicits his needs, and when necessary, interprets these needs to other mental health team members. The nurse applies knowledge of nursing theory and the biological and social sciences to the patient's health problem and utilizes this knowledge to devise a sophisticated plan of care. The nurse is also responsible for the patient understanding this plan. If he seems puzzled or is noncompliant, the nurse explores his understanding and explains the nursing care plan as needed. Most important, the nurse cares for the patient, in the fullest sense of caring. She listens to his problems nonjudgmentally and empathizes and helps him to identify and articulate his feelings. The nurse is accessible at the time a need arises and conveys a sense of availability to the patient. She engenders trust by being consistent and reliable and by maintaining confidentiality. The nurse encourages the patient to be as independent as possible but also allows dependency when this is necessary. Through the application of psychomotor and interpersonal skills, the nurse assists the patient to grow and to reach his maximal functional capabilities.

DIRECTIONS FOR FUTURE RESEARCH

The following are some of the nursing research problems raised in Chapter 2 that merit further study by psychiatric nurses:

1. The relationship between various stressors, anxiety levels, and behavioral deviations
2. Measurement of patient behavioral outcomes related to the application by nurses of psychotherapeutic techniques based on various conceptual models
3. Exploration of the ability of nurses to identify and describe the conceptual model or models that comprise the theoretical base for their practice
4. The relationship between preference for a particular conceptual model and other characteristics, such as sociocultural background, personality characteristics, and educational level
5. Conceptual models that are incorporated into curricula of graduate programs in psychiatric nursing
6. Characteristics of team relationships when members of interdisciplinary teams are homogeneous or heterogeneous in terms of preferred conceptual models of psychiatric care
7. Consumer awareness of the characteristics of various therapeutic approaches and the extent to which choice of therapist is based on understanding of the therapist's frame of reference
8. Portrayal of various therapeutic approaches in the media and how it influences the public's perception of psychiatric care

■ SUGGESTED CROSS-REFERENCES ■

The nursing model of health-illness phenomena which describes nursing and medical diagnoses is discussed in Chapter 3. The elements of the nursing process are discussed in Chapter 5 and integrated throughout the other chapters of the book. Medical diagnostic categories are integrated throughout Chapters 9 to 22. Primary intervention strategies based on the medical and behavioral models are discussed in Chapter 9. Community mental health is discussed in Chapter 25. For further discussion of crisis intervention and the consultation process, see Chapters 10 and 26. Behavior modification is discussed in Chapter 27.

SUMMARY

Model (major theorists)	View of behavioral deviation	Therapeutic process	Role of patient and therapist
Psychoanalytical (S. Freud, Erikson, Adler, Jung, Searles, A. Freud, Klein, Horney, Fromm, W. Reich, Fromm-Reichmann, Menninger)	Based on early development and inadequate resolution of developmental conflicts. Ego defenses inadequate to control anxiety. Symptoms result as effort to deal with anxiety and are related to unresolved conflicts.	Psychoanalysis uses techniques of free association and dream analysis. Interprets behavior. Uses transference to revise earlier traumatic experiences. Identifies problem areas through interpretation of patient's resistances.	Patient verbalizes all thoughts and dreams; considers therapist's interpretations. Long-term commitment to frequent therapy sessions. Therapist remains remote to encourage development of transference. Interprets patient's thoughts and dreams in terms of conflicts, transference, and resistance.
Interpersonal (Sullivan, Peplau)	Anxiety arises and is experienced interpersonally. Symptoms occur when security operations are unable to protect the self from anxiety. Basic fear is fear of rejection. Person needs security and satisfaction that result from positive interpersonal relationships.	Relationship between therapist and patient builds feeling of security. Therapist helps patient experience trusting relationship and gain interpersonal satisfaction. Patient then assisted to develop close relationships outside therapy situation.	Patient shares with therapist anxieties and feelings as he is able. Therapist develops close relationship with patient. Uses empathy to perceive patient's feelings. Uses relationship as a corrective interpersonal experience.
Social (Szasz, Caplan)	Social and environmental factors create stress, which causes anxiety, resulting in symptom formation. Unacceptable (deviant) behavior is socially defined and meets needs of social and political system.	Patient helped to deal with social system. May use crisis intervention. Environmental manipulation and enlistment of special supports also employed. Peer support encouraged.	Patient actively presents problem to therapist and works with therapist toward resolution. Utilizes community resources. Therapist explores patient's social system and helps patient use resources available. Works to create new resources when needed.
Existential (Jaspers, Binswanger, Perls, Glasser, Ellis, Rogers, Laing, Frankl)	Life is meaningful when one can fully experience and accept the self. Behavioral deviation is expression of the individual as he is thwarted in his effort to find and accept self. The self can be experienced through authentic relationships with other people.	Person aided to experience authenticity in relationships. Therapy frequently conducted in groups. Patient encouraged to explore and to accept self. Patient helped to assume control of his behavior.	Patient assumes responsibility for behavior. Participates in meaningful experiences to learn about real self. Therapist helps patient to recognize value of self. Clarifies realities of situation. Introduces patient to genuine feelings and expanded awareness.

SUMMARY

Model (major theorists)	View of behavioral deviation	Therapeutic process	Role of patient and therapist
Communication (Berne, Watzlawick)	Behavioral disruptions occur when messages are not clearly communicated. Language can be used to distort meaning. Messages may be transmitted simultaneously at several levels. Verbal and nonverbal messages may lack congruence. These conditions result in behavioral deviations.	Communication patterns analyzed. Feedback given to clarify problem areas. Family therapy frequently used to help modify lack of congruence or complementarity in communication. Transactional analysis focuses on games and learning to communicate directly without game playing.	Patient looks at communication patterns, including games. Works to clarify own communication and validate messages from others. Therapist interprets communication pattern to patient. Helps him improve communication with significant others. Teaches principles of good communication.
Behavioral (Eysenck, Wolpe, Skinner)	Behavior is learned. Deviations occur because person has formed undesirable behavioral habits. Since behavior is learned, it can also be unlearned. Deviant behavior may be perpetuated because it reduces anxiety. If so, another anxiety-reducing behavior may be substituted.	Therapy is educational process. Behavioral deviations not rewarded. More productive behaviors reinforced. Reciprocal inhibition involves substituting an acceptable behavior that reduces anxiety for deviance. Relaxation therapy and assertiveness training are behavioral approaches.	Patient practices behavioral technique used. Does homework and reinforcement exercises. Helps develop behavioral hierarchies. Therapist determines behavioral technique. Teaches patient about behavioral approach. Helps develop behavioral hierarchy. Reinforces desired behaviors.
Medical (Freud, Meyer, Kraeplin, Spitzer)	Behavioral disruptions result from a disease process, probably originating in central nervous system. Symptoms result from a combination of physiological, genetic, environmental, and social factors. Deviant behavior relates to patient's tolerance for stress.	Diagnosis of illness is based on present condition and historical information plus diagnostic studies, and treatment is related to diagnosis. Frequently includes somatic therapies in addition to various interpersonal techniques. Treatment approach adjusted depending on symptomatic response. Other mental health professionals involved when their expertise is required.	Patient practices prescribed therapy regimen. Reports effects of therapy to physician. Complies with long-term therapy if necessary. Therapist uses combination of somatic and interpersonal therapies. Diagnoses illness and prescribes therapeutic approach. May teach patient about illness.
Nursing (Orlando, Peplau, King, Orem, Rogers, Riehl, Roy)	Person is biopsychosocial entity who responds to stress in an individualized way. Behavioral disruptions affect whole person. Observable behaviors must be related to predisposing factors and precipitating stressors involved. Every person demonstrates strengths as well as weaknesses. Adaptive responses to stress (health) and maladaptive responses (illness) are on a continuum of potential behaviors.	Nursing process includes data collection, formulation of a nursing diagnosis, planning, implementation, and ongoing concurrent evaluation, resulting in modification of care plan. Plan is mutually formulated with patient. Nurse collaborates with other caregivers. Long- and short-term goals specified.	Patient collaborates in development of nursing care plan. Participates in evaluation and modification of treatment. Therapist collaborates with patient and other health team members in developing plan of care. Modifies plan based on patient feedback and own observations. May use many therapeutic modalities within nursing process framework, depending on education, experience, and available supervision.

■ REFERENCES ■

1. American Nurses' Association: Nursing: a social policy statement, Kansas City, Mo., 1980, The Association.
2. American Psychiatric Association: Draft of the DSM-III-R in Development (subject to change), as proposed by the Work Group to Revise DSM-III. American Psychiatric Association, October 1985.
3. Andreasen, N.C.: The broken brain, New York, 1984, Harper & Row, Publishers.
4. Berne, E.: What do you say after you say hello? New York, Grove Press, Inc.
5. Black, Sr. K.M.: An existential model for psychiatric nursing, Perspect. Psychiatr. Care **6**:185, July-Aug. 1968.
6. Brown, J.A.C.: Freud and the post-Freudians, Baltimore, 1961, Penguin Books, Inc.
7. Caplan, G.: Principles of preventive psychiatry, New York, 1964, Basic Books, Inc.
8. Cautela, J.: Behavior therapy. In Hersher, L., editor: Four psychotherapies, New York, 1970, Appleton-Century-Crofts.
9. Chamberlin, J.: On our own, New York, 1978, McGraw-Hill Book Company.
10. Ehrenwald, J.: The history of psychotherapy, New York, 1976, Jason Aronson, Inc.
11. Ellis, A.: Rational-emotive therapy. In Hersher, L., editor: Four psychotherapies, New York, 1970, Appleton-Century-Crofts.
12. Frankl, V.: Man's search for meaning, New York, 1959, The Beacon Press.
13. Harper, R.A.: The new psychotherapies, Englewood Cliffs, N.J., 1975, Prentice-Hall, Inc.
14. Johnston, R.L.: Individual psychotherapy: relationship of theoretical approaches to nursing conceptual models. In Fitzpatrick, J.J., Whall, A.L., Johnston, R.L., and Floyd, J.A.: Nursing models and their psychiatric mental health applications, Bowie, Md., 1982, Robert J. Brady Company.
15. Laing, R.D.: The politics of experience, New York, 1967, Ballantine Books.
16. Peplau, H.E.: Interpersonal relations in nursing, New York, 1952, G.P. Putnam's Sons.
17. Riehl, J.P., and Roy, C.: Conceptual models for nursing practice, New York, 1974, Appleton-Century-Crofts.
18. Shaver, J.F.: A biopsychosocial view of human health, Nurs. Outlook **33**:186, July-Aug., 1985.
19. Siegler, M., and Osmond, H.: Models of madness, models of medicine, New York, 1976, Harper Colophon Books.
20. Sullivan, H.S.: The psychiatric interview, New York, 1954, W.W. Norton & Co., Inc.
21. Szasz, T.S.: Ideology and insanity, Garden City, N.Y., 1970, Anchor Books, Doubleday Publishing Co.
22. Szasz, T.S.: The second sin, Garden City, N.Y., 1974, Anchor Books, Doubleday Publishing Co.
23. Watzlawick, P., Beavin, J.H., and Jackson, D.D.: Pragmatics of human communication, New York, 1967, W.W. Norton & Co., Inc.

■ ANNOTATED SUGGESTED READINGS ■

The following selections are representative works of respected psychiatric theorists. All are recommended as resources of classical approaches to psychiatry.

Adler, A.: The practice and theory of individual psychology, New York, 1929, Harcourt, Brace & Co.
Berne, E.: Transactional analysis in psychotherapy, New York, 1961, Grove Press, Inc.
Berne, E.: Games people play, New York, 1964, Grove Press, Inc.
Caplan, G.: Principles of preventive psychiatry, New York, 1964, Basic Books, Inc.
Ellis, A., and Harper, R.A.: A guide to rational living, Englewood Cliffs, N.J., 1961, Prentice-Hall, Inc.
Erikson, E.: Childhood and society, ed. 2, New York, 1963, W.W. Norton & Co., Inc.
Frankl, V.: Man's search for meaning, New York, 1959, The Beacon Press.
Freud, A.: The ego and the mechanisms of defense, New York, 1966, International Universities Press.
Freud, S.: In Strachey, J., editor: The standard edition of the complete psychological works of Sigmund Freud, London, 1953-1974, Hogarth Press.
Fromm-Reichmann, F.: Principles of intensive psychotherapy, Chicago, 1950, The University of Chicago Press.
Fromm-Reichmann, F.: In Bullard, D.M., editor: Psychoanalysis and psychotherapy, selected papers, Chicago, 1959, The University of Chicago Press.
Glasser, W.: Reality therapy: a new approach to psychiatry, New York, 1965, Harper & Row, Publishers.
Horney, K.: The collected works of Karen Horney, vols. 1 and 2, New York, 1937-1950, W.W. Norton & Co., Inc.
Jung, C.G., Mayman, M., and Pruyser, P.: The psychogenesis of mental disease, New York, 1960, Pantheon Books.
Klein, M.: The psychoanalysis of children, London, 1949, Hogarth Press.
Laing, R.D.: The politics of experience, New York, 1967, Ballantine Books.
Menninger, K.A.: The vital balance, New York, 1963, Viking Press.
*Peplau, H.E.: Interpersonal relations in nursing, New York, 1952, G.P. Putnam's Sons.
Perls, F.S.: In and out of the garbage pail, Lafayette, Calif., 1969, Real People Press.
Rogers, C.R.: Client-centered therapy, Boston, 1951, Houghton Mifflin Co.
Rogers, C.R.: Carl Rogers on encounter groups, New York, 1970, Harper & Row, Publishers, Inc.
Schutz, W.C.: Joy, New York, 1967, Grove Press, Inc.
Sullivan, H.S.: In Perry, H.S., and Gawel, M.L., editors: The interpersonal theory of psychiatry, New York, 1953, W.W. Norton & Co., Inc.
Sullivan H.S.: In Perry, H.S., and Gawel, M.L., editors: The

_____

*Asterisk indicates nursing reference.

psychiatric interview, New York, 1954, W.W. Norton & Co., Inc.

Szasz, T.: The myth of mental illness, New York, 1961, Hoeber-Harper.

Watzlawick, P., Beavin, J.H., and Jackson, D.D.: Pragmatics of human communication, New York, 1967, W.W. Norton & Co., Inc.

Wolpe, J.: The practice of behavior therapy, ed. 2, New York, 1973, Pergamon Press.

The following selections include anthologies of theoretical approaches to psychiatry. There are also several selections of interest to the nurse who is developing a conceptual approach to psychiatry.

Andreasen, N.C.: The broken brain, New York, 1984, Harper and Row, Publishers.

This is a readable book that provides current and valuable information about the anatomy and physiology of the brain, which is then applied in discussions of the biological theories of psychiatric disorders. It is recommended to students and to practicing nurses as a way of updating knowledge in this rapidly expanding area.

*Black, Sr. K.: An existential model for psychiatric nursing, Perspect. Psychiatr. Care **6**:178, July-Aug. 1968.

This article discusses the concept of the existential encounter as it applies to the therapeutic nurse-patient relationship. A basic respect for the dignity of the patient is conveyed, and the model is illustrated with a clinical example.

Brown, J.A.C.: Freud and the post-Freudians, Baltimore, 1961, Penguin Books, Inc.

This book presents a review of the works of the major post-Freudian theorists, allowing the reader to compare them with Freud and each other.

*Clark, C.C.: Combining therapeutic approaches, J. Psychiatr. Nurs. **15**:18, Oct. 1977.

This author compares and contrasts two apparently incompatible approaches to psychotherapy: psychoanalysis and behavioral therapy. She demonstrates that a combination of these approaches may be used very effectively with some patients. She also identifies several commonalities between these models.

*Clark, M.D.: Carl Rogers revisited, Can. J. Psychiatr. Nurs. **22**:14, Jan.-March 1981.

This article is a concise review of the principles of Rogers' approach to counseling. It is a good example of the application of a theoretical frame of reference to the therapy process.

*Critchley, D.L.: The adverse influence of psychiatric diagnostic labels on observation of child behavior, Am. J. Orthopsychiatry **49**:157, Jan. 1979.

The author found that informing a student nurse of a psychiatric diagnosis for a child influenced the perception of the child's behavior. Children diagnosed as not normal were not perceived to behave normally, even when the child was not, in reality, mentally ill. This demonstrates the value of nursing research in model development and also points out the dangers inherent in labeling behavior.

He also points out the problems of focusing on pathologic conditions rather than health, thereby reinforcing sick behavior.

Ehrenwald, J.: The history of psychotherapy, New York, 1976, Jason Aronson, Inc.

This is a fascinating description of the historical development of models of psychotherapy, including both mystical/religious and scientific approaches. Theories are illustrated with lengthy and informative quotes from the original theorist.

*Fitzpatrick, J.J., Whall, A.L., Johnston, R.L., and Floyd, J.A.: Nursing models and their psychiatric mental health applications, Bowie, Md., 1982, Robert J. Brady Company.

This book takes the important step of attempting to compare and correlate nursing models with mental health care models. It provides much food for thought and should stimulate lively debate. This is not a book for beginning students. A thorough knowledge of the theories is needed to comprehend the condensed presentations in this text.

Frank, J.D.: Persuasion and healing, Baltimore, 1973, The Johns Hopkins University Press.

This thought-provoking comparison of psychotherapy to other forms of persuasion, such as religious revivalism, and thought reform considers several models of psychiatric care in terms of this frame of reference. It is particularly useful for those who are engaged in psychotherapy.

Haley, J.: The art of psychoanalysis. In Haley, J.: The power tactics of Jesus Christ, New York, 1969, Avon Books.

The author takes a provocative look at psychoanalysis as a power relationship that is set up to enhance the superior position of the therapist. It is amusing reading, but very thought-provoking.

Hall, C.S., and Lindzey, G.: Theories of personality, ed. 3, New York, 1978, John Wiley & Sons, Inc.

This work is a thorough discussion of a wide range of personality theories, primarily from a psychological approach. It is particularly useful as a reference on the behavioral models of therapy.

Hall, E.: A conversation with Erik Erikson. Psychol. Today **17**:6:22, June 1983.

Erikson reflects on his developmental theory from the perspective of the final stage of the life cycle.

Harper, R.A.: The new psychotherapies, Englewood Cliffs, N.J., 1975, Prentice-Hall, Inc.

This book is a concise and clearly written overview of a variety of contemporary approaches to psychotherapy. It would be most useful as an introduction to the basic assumptions of the theories included.

Hersher, L.: Four psychotherapies, New York, 1970, Appleton-Century-Crofts.

This edited volume includes good descriptions of client-centered, rational-emotive, behavior, and psychoanalytical therapies and provides an opportunity to compare and contrast basic concepts of these theoretical approaches to psychotherapy.

*Loomis, M.E., and Wood, D.J.: Cure: the potential outcome of nursing care. Image **15**:1:4, Winter 1983.

It has been said that nurses care and physicians cure. These authors present a case for the curative function of the nurse. They present a model of health care and describe clinical decision making related to human response to actual or potential health problems.

*Mansfield, E.: A conceptual framework for psychiatric–mental health nursing, J. Psychiatr. Nurs. **18**:34, June 1980.

This article describes a conceptual model for a graduate program in psychiatric nursing. It incorporates theoretical concepts of general systems, human development, communication, and self-esteem into a nursing process model. Of particular interest are the author's suggestions about the utility of the model for generating nursing research.

*Powers, M.E.: Universal utility of psychoanalytic theory for nursing practice models, J. Psychiatr. Nurs. **18**:28, April 1980.

This author demonstrates that a nursing practice model can accommodate the adaptation of a particular theoretical concept. She applies classical psychoanalytical theory to nursing in a way that challenges the reader to agree or disagree with her assertion.

Powers, M.E.: Understanding psychological man: a state-of-the-science report. Psychol. Today **16**:5:40, May 1982.

In this article, several leading psychologists who represent most of the major schools of thought provide their views on the current state of psychology. Most of the models described in this chapter are represented with applications to trends such as psychobiology and technological advances.

*Riehl, J.P., and Roy, C.: Conceptual models for nursing practice, New York, 1974, Appleton-Century-Crofts.

This excellent discussion of the status of the development of models for nursing practice presents several nursing models in a format that allows the reader to make comparisons. It is highly recommended for nurses at all levels of experience and education.

Rosenhan, D.L.: On being sane in insane places, Science **179**:250, 1973.

This report of admission of several pseudopatients to psychiatric hospitals raises interesting questions about the implications of labeling people as mentally ill. The experiential aspect of being a psychiatric patient is also recounted. The article is worthwhile reading for any nurse.

Scheff, T.J.: Being mentally ill: a sociological theory, Chicago, 1966, Aldine Publishing Co.

The author discusses the definition of insanity from a sociological framework and presents interesting material on the experience of being a psychiatric patient and the role of society in defining the conditions of insanity.

*Shaver, J.F.: A biopsychosocial view of human health. Nurs. Outlook **33**:186, July/Aug., 1985.

The author compares the medical and nursing models of health care. She describes a biopsychosocial nursing model and provides several examples of health care interventions that are based on this model. This paper is scholarly and thought-provoking.

Siegler, M., and Osmond, H.: Models of madness, models of medicine, New York, 1976, Harper Colophon Books.

This comparison of the medical model to other models of psychiatric care presents the case for the continued use of the medical model as the most helpful framework for psychiatry.

*Slavinsky, A.T.: Psychiatric nursing in the year 2000: from nonsystem of care to a caring system. Image **16**:1:17, Winter 1984.

From the perspective of the year 2000, the author analyzes the deficiencies of the current mental health system and proposes nursing roles to improve mental health care. She makes a convincing case for the pivotal role of mental health nurses in a caring system.

*Sundeen, S.J., et al.: Nurse-client interaction, ed. 3, St. Louis, 1985, The C.V. Mosby Co.

This book provides discussion of nursing process and includes a clinical example of the utilization of this means of organizing nursing care planning.

Wolberg, L.R.: The techniques of psychotherapy, parts I and II, ed. 2, New York, 1967, Grune & Stratton, Inc.

This is an extremely thorough presentation of basic theories of psychotherapy, followed by a discussion of the practice of psychotherapy. It is an excellent resource for the experienced practitioner of psychiatric nursing. There is also a discussion of psychosocial development, including the theories of Freud, Erikson, and Sullivan.

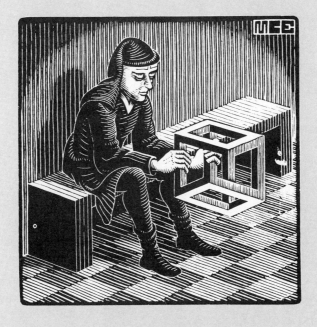

The highest wisdom has but one science, the science of the whole.

Leo Tolstoy, *War and Peace*

C H A P T E R   3

A NURSING MODEL OF HEALTH-ILLNESS PHENOMENA

LEARNING OBJECTIVES

After studying this chapter, the student should be able to:

- discuss why it is difficult to define mental health and conditions and criteria associated with it.

- relate the dimensions and prevalence of mental and addictive disorders in the United States.

- identify developmental stages and tasks of the individual and family life cycles.

- describe the concepts of cultural relativism and ethnocentrism and the implications of each for psychiatric nursing care.

- analyze a nursing model of health-illness phenomena and the components of it that result in adaptive or maladaptive coping responses.

- critique the significance of stressful life events in precipitating illness based on recent research.

- discuss the importance of one's primary appraisal of a stressor as it occurs on the cognitive, affective, physiological, behavioral, and social levels.

- describe various types of coping resources.

- discuss the importance of one's secondary appraisal of coping resources that involve cognitive, affective, physiological, behavioral, and social responses.

- distinguish between constructive and destructive coping mechanisms and between neurotic and psychotic disorders.

- compare and contrast coping responses, health problems, nursing diagnoses, and medical diagnoses.

- analyze the interrelationship between the use of the DSM-III-R medical diagnoses and the NANDA nursing diagnoses.

- identify directions for future nursing research.

- select appropriate readings for further study.

Defining mental health and illness

Since the early 1940s, the terms mental health and mental hygiene have appeared in the literature and in statements of public policy. They are now common in everyday speech and thought. However, there have been relatively few attempts to define "mental health," and little consensus exists at present.

One of the few studies to examine the dimensions of subjective mental health in American men and women reported that both men and women use the same six basic dimensions in making self-evaluations of their mental health: unhappiness, lack of gratification, strain, feelings of vulnerability, lack of self-confidence, and uncertainty.[6] Yet problems continue to exist for researchers and clinicians.

Mental health is often spoken of as a state of well-being, such as happiness, contentment, satisfaction, or achievement. These are difficult terms to apply and fluctuate according to different situations and conditions.[43] This is not to deny that happiness is a desirable consequence of mental health, but it poses problems if used as a criterion. There are similar problems with viewing

mental health statistically as the central tendency or mean of a group. What one derives in this way is "average," which may not necessarily mean "healthy."

In seeking the positive signs of mental health, Jahoda[22] suggested the following conditions:

1. The idea of any single criterion of mental health should be abandoned. Good mental health cannot be refined down to a simple concept and a simple item of behavior is not adequate.

2. The terms we use to define mental health may seem to be abstract but they should be reduced to definite operational procedures and there is a need to have scales and measures for each criterion.

3. Each of the criteria should be thought of as a continuum or as containing continua since there are unhealthy trends for an otherwise healthy person.

4. These criteria of mental health should operate at any point in time to define the state of the individual or can be thought of as indicative of trends in the individual towards health or dis-

ease. Implicit in the criteria is the concept of gradients of mental health.

5. The criteria are regarded as relatively enduring attributes of the person. They are not merely functions of a particular situation the individual may find himself in.

6. These criteria are set up as the optimum of mental health. They are not to be regarded as absolute, and the minimum standard for any individual to achieve has yet to be determined and may change with age. Each individual has his own limits and no one reaches the ideal in all the criteria. However, the assumption made is that most people can approach the optimum, and below a yet to be determined minimum, most if not all people will break down.

■ Criteria of mental health

The following six criteria were offered by Jahoda[22] as a recipe for mental health:

1. Positive attitudes toward self
2. Growth, development, and self-actualization
3. Integration
4. Autonomy
5. Reality perception
6. Environmental mastery

Positive attitudes toward self include an acceptance of self and self-awareness. There has to be some objectivity about the self and the acquisition of a realistic level of aspiration that will necessarily change with age. A healthy person must also have a sense of identity, a feeling of wholeness, a sense of belongingness, security, and meaningfulness.

Second, there is the criterion of **growth, development, and self-actualization.** Maslow and Rogers developed extensive theories on the development and realization of the human potential. Maslow describes the concept of "self-actualization," and Rogers emphasizes the "fully functioning person." Both theories focus on the entire range of human adjustment. They describe a self that is engaged in a constant quest, always seeking new growth, new development, and new challenges. Their theories focus on the total person and such considerations as whether a person is adequately in touch with his own self to free the resources that are there, whether he has free access to his feelings and emotions and can integrate them with his intellectual and cognitive functioning, whether he is immobilized by inner conflicts and stresses or can interact freely and openly with his environment, and whether he can share himself with other people and grow from such experiences.

Maslow[32] identified fifteen basic personality characteristics that distinguish "self-actualized" individuals—people moving in the direction of achieving and reaching their highest potential. Rogers[41] described seven essential personality traits of the "fully functioning person" who is similarly moving toward self-growth and fulfillment. These are presented in Table 3-1.

The third criterion involves the concept of **integration,** or the relatedness of all processes. This involves a balance between what is expressed and what is repressed, between outer and inner conflicts and drives,

TABLE 3-1

THEORIES ON DEVELOPMENT AND REALIZATION OF HUMAN POTENTIAL

Maslow's "self-actualized" individual	Rogers' "fully functioning" person
Has accurate perception of reality	Moves away from facades that are not true to self
Has a high degree of acceptance of self, others, and human nature	Moves away from others' expectations of what he "ought to be"
Exhibits spontaneity	Moves away from pleasing others who impose artificial goals on him
Is problem-centered as opposed to self-centered	
Has need for privacy	
Demonstrates high degree of autonomy and independence	Moves toward becoming autonomous, self-directing, and self-responsible
Has freshness of appreciation	
Has frequent "mystic or peak" experiences	Is open to change and exploring his potential
Shows identification with mankind	Is open to his own self and the lives of others
Shares intimate relationships with a few significant others	Trusts and values himself and dares to express himself in new ways
Has democratic character structures	
Possesses strong ethical sense	
Demonstrates unhostile sense of humor	
Possesses creativeness	
Exhibits resistance to conformity	

and a regulation of one's moods and emotions. It includes the concepts of emotional responsiveness and control and a unified philosophy of life. This consistent set of values provides a framework for a certain continuity in all responses. This criterion can at least in part be measured by the person's ability to withstand stress and cope with anxiety. The ability to withstand stress involves a strong but not rigid ego, so that a person is able to handle change and grow from it.

Autonomy is the fourth criterion of mental health. This involves self-determination, a balance between dependence and independence, and the acceptance of the consequences of one's actions. It implies that one is responsible for himself, including decisions, actions, thoughts, and feelings. Consequently, the person is able to respect the autonomy and freedom of choice in others.

The fifth criterion involves **reality perception,** the ability of the individual to test by empirical action his assumptions about the outside world. The mentally healthy person is able to change his perceptions in the light of new information. This criterion also includes the ability of empathy or social sensitivity, a respect for the feelings and attitudes of others.

The last criterion is that of **environmental mastery.** A mentally healthy person feels success in an approved role in his society or group. He can deal effectively with the world, work out his problems of living, and obtain satisfaction from life. It incorporates the idea of social competence as well. The person should have the essential quality of being able to cope with loneliness, aggression, and frustration without being overwhelmed. The mentally healthy person has the ability to respond to other individuals, to love and be loved, and to cope with others in reciprocal relationships. He should maintain the ability to make new friendships and to have satisfactory social group involvement.

Finally, a person should not be assessed against some vague or ideal notion of health. Rather, he should be seen in a group context, an age context, and an individual context. It is not a matter of how well someone fits an arbitrary age standard, but rather what is reasonable for a particular person with a specific background and life experience. Is there continuity or discontinuity with the past? Is there evidence of evolving adaptation to changing needs throughout the person's life cycle? Such a view incorporates the concept of **psychobiological resilience,** which proposes that there is a recurrent human need to weather periods of stress and change throughout life. The ability to successfully weather each period of disruption and reintegration leaves the person better able to deal with the next change. This dimension equates mental health with adaptation and mental illness with maladaptation.

■ Dimensions of mental illness

The health-illness continuum is asymmetrical. The two poles of health and illness are not equally clear. Rather, standards of mental health are less clear and less agreed on than those of mental illness. Whereas conceptions of mental health can be extended indefinitely in unbounded potential, conceptions of mental illness are bounded somewhat by greater consensus of symptoms of mental disorders that can be specified and studied.

The varied mental disorders are a major contributor to the burden of illness in the United States. They attract less public attention than do some other disorders for a number of reasons, including their relatively low mortality rates, the low social status of many of the mentally ill, and the stigma that many people attach to mental disorders. Still, both the chronicity of some of the disorders and the problems that can arise from them combine to produce great strains on affected individuals and the larger health care system.

The overall prevalence of mental and addictive disorders for all age groups in the United States is approximately 15% to 22.5%. Thus, mental disorders, alcoholism, and drug addictions profoundly disrupt the lives of 30 to 45 million people in America each year. Furthermore, mental disorders and addictive states rank third for personal health care expenditures. Conservative estimates of annual expenditures for direct health care are placed at $20 billion and of total economic costs to society at $185 billion.[1]

Research in the field has greatly improved drug and psychosocial therapies for some mental illnesses and addictions, but much work remains to be done on the prevention, diagnosis, and treatment of these disabling conditions. Yet, since 1966, the real level of federal support for research in the area has dropped markedly, even as research opportunities and available researchers have increased. For example, more than $300 is spent on research for every patient being treated with cancer, while the comparable figure for schizophrenia is $7. The recent Report of the Board on Mental Health and Behavioral Medicine, Institute of Medicine, has therefore called for a marked expansion of research support for mental illness and addictive disorders. Emerging information about brain functioning and behavioral responses to stress gives hope that the efforts of sustained research and clinical support will benefit the millions of individuals, families, and communities whose lives are touched by severe mental disorders, alcoholism, and drug addiction.

Developmental norms and stages

Knowledge of normal growth and development is essential for assessing a person's functioning, as well as for intervening with a nursing model for health-illness phenomena. Other sources[45] describe these stages in some detail, and the nurse should be familiar with normative stages, tasks, and parameters to know what issues the person has faced in the past and what challenges lie ahead. In addition to individual development, knowledge of the family cycle is also important. Many nursing interventions are directed at the family level, ranging from mobilizing their support of an individual patient to interrupting and modifying dysfunctional family patterns.

Table 3-2 summarizes the developmental stages of the individual using Erikson's theory[16] of psychosocial development and Duvall's stages[14] of the family life cycle. Streff[44] integrated Erikson's theory with that of Duvall's to define developmental tasks of the family that parallel those of the individual. Such an integrated approach allows one to view life as successive stages marked by critical developmental tasks. This aids the nurse in identifying future changes that may be potential stressors for an individual or family. By acknowledging, understanding, and anticipating them, the nurse can design and implement effective nursing care.

Cultural relativism

Mental health and illness emerge within a social context in which cultural relativism is a particularly important problem, since the content and form of mental health and mental illness will vary greatly from one culture to another. Different cultures place different kinds of stressors on people. So too, they vary in symbolic interpretation, acceptance of expression and repression, cohesion of social groups, and tolerance of deviation.

The search for a link between cultural factors and mental illness has significant roots. As early as 1897, Durkheim wondered about a connection between suicide and social conditions.[13] In the 1930s, Faris and Dunham suggested a causal relationship between schizophrenia and the living conditions in Chicago slums.[17] Leighton and co-workers documented both an overall correlation between mental illness and social disarray and correlations between specific sociocultural settings and particular types of psychiatric disorders.[30] Dohrenwend and Dohrenwend have found that while schizophrenia seems to be present in all cultures, there is considerable discrepancy in the types of schizophrenia that dominate in different cultures.[12] Likewise, Cohen demonstrated cultural factors in the etiology of depressive reactions.[11] Finally, Eisenthal has summarized these

studies and a larger sampling of the literature on this subject.[15]

The danger in ignoring cultural diversity and group norms is that one may equate deviance with illness. When social alternatives are equated with illness, an unusual life-style is regarded as sick, and aberrant behavior is taken as a sign of personal abnormality. For example, in one study that controlled for psychiatric condition and social class, it was found that nonwhite males were involuntarily hospitalized more often than white males because they were more often brought into treatment by the police. The authors concluded that the more coercive conditions under which nonwhites enter treatment determine the more severe responses to nonwhites' deviance.[42]

This can potentially be avoided if one recognizes that health-illness and conformity-deviance are two distinctly independent variables. Combining them generates four separate patterns: the healthy conformist, the healthy deviant, the unhealthy conformist, and the unhealthy deviant (Fig. 3-1). This obliges any mental health professional to attend carefully to the meaning of any apparent deviant behavior, to its significance in its social context. It may reflect an adaptation to realistic forces in a person's life or conformity to group norms.

■ Ethnocentrism

Another challenge in assessing mental health and illness arises from ethnocentrism which is marked by two assumptions:

1. "Others" should live by our own peculiar ethnic or national logic and mores.

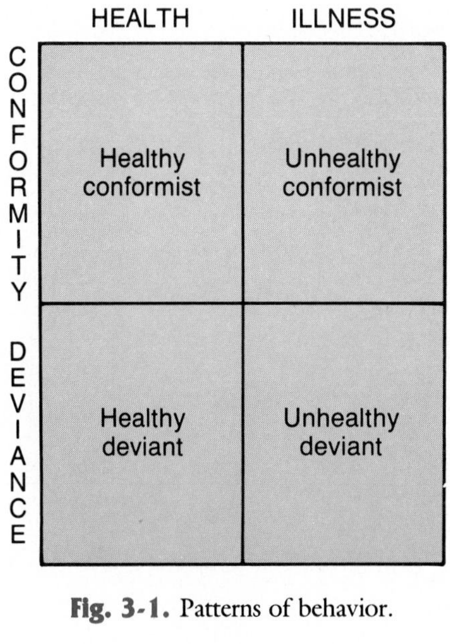

	HEALTH	ILLNESS
C O N F O R M I T Y	Healthy conformist	Unhealthy conformist
D E V I A N C E	Healthy deviant	Unhealthy deviant

Fig. 3-1. Patterns of behavior.

TABLE 3-2

DEVELOPMENTAL STAGES AND TASKS OF THE INDIVIDUAL AND FAMILY UNIT

Erikson's stage of individual psychosocial development[16]	Developmental task of the individual[45]	Duvall's stage of the family life cycle[14]	Developmental task of the family identified by Streff[44]
Trust vs. mistrust (0-2 years)	Oral needs are of primary importance Adequate mothering is necessary to meet infant's needs Acquisition of hope	Premarital-married couple	Establishing relationship Defining mutual goals Developing intimacy Developing appropriate dependence, independence, interdependence pattern Establishing mutually satisfying relationship Negotiating boundaries of couple relationship and with individuals' families of origin Discussing issue of childbearing Making decision to conceive
Autonomy vs. shame (1½-3 years)	Anal needs are of primary importance Father emerges as important figure Acquisition of will	Childbearing	Working out authority and responsibility issues Working out caretaker roles Having children Forming new unit Facilitating child's establishment of trust Acknowledging need for personal time and space while sharing with each other and child
Initiative vs. guilt (3-6 years)	Genital needs are of primary importance Family relationships contribute to early sense of responsibility and conscience Acquisition of purpose	Preschool	Continuing individual development as couple, parent, and family Experiencing changes in energy and time for individual and couple needs Promoting continued growth in each other and the relationship while encouraging child to develop autonomy and retain self-esteem Establishing own family tradition with each other and children without guilt related to breaks with traditions of families of origin
Industry vs. inferiority (6-12 years)	Active period of socialization for child as he moves from family and into society Acquisition of competence	School age	One or both spouses establishing new roles in work settings or community or changes in child-rearing practices and gaining recognition for selves and children Children in school and after-school activities, relating with peers, self-esteem being enhanced or inhibited, and interfacing with activities in family

TABLE 3-2—cont'd

DEVELOPMENTAL STAGES AND TASKS OF THE INDIVIDUAL AND FAMILY UNIT

Erikson's stage of individual psychosocial development[16]	Developmental task of the individual[45]	Duvall's stage of the family life cycle[14]	Developmental task of the family identified by Streff[44]
Identity vs. identity diffusion (13 + years)	Search for self, in which peers play important role Psychosocial moratorium is provided by society to aid adolescent Acquisition of fidelity	Teenage	Parents continue to develop roles in community and interests other than with children Children examine ways to experience freedom while expressing responsibility for actions Struggles evolve with parents as emancipation process proceeds Family's value system may be challenged Couple relationship may be strong or weak, depending on how members respond to each other's needs
Intimacy vs. isolation (adulthood)	Characterized by increasing importance of human closeness and sexual fulfillment Acquisition of love	Launching career	Parents launching young adults with rituals marking rites of passage Change in relationship with children who are becoming adults and/or in new living situations; change in couple's relationship because of children's absence and increased time with one another
Generativity vs. self-absorption (middle-age)	Characterized by productivity, creativity, parental responsibility, and concern for new generation Acquisition of care	Middle-age parents	Energy channeled into guiding next generation via family or community activities, or couple may now be dealing with issues of aging of their own parents Children of middle-age parents may be adolescent
Integrity vs. despair (old age)	Characterized by unifying philosophy of life and more profound love for mankind Acquisition of wisdom	Aging family members	Persons have achieved satisfying relationships and feel sense of accomplishment and desire to continue to live fully until death instead of existing in state of despair Aging members are coping with bereavement and may now be living alone

2. One can influence "others" to change their way of life or philosophy.[46]

If one's own views and standards are imposed on others, misdiagnosis or a therapeutic impasse might result. When this principle operates among groups of people in a society, it becomes the foundation for nationalism or racism, and can result in political friction between nations. A related problem occurs when clinicians tend to regard their theories or their psychotherapeutic techniques as universally applicable to all people in the absence of relevant research among other cultural groups. What is needed in this pluralistic world is an understanding of the nature of different peoples and the social, cultural, and political forces that shape one's perceptions, feelings, and behaviors.

Through the reflective process of analyzing one's

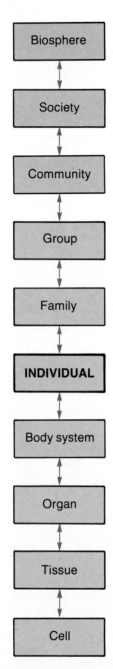

Fig. 3-2. Levels of organization that make up the social hierarchy.

own feelings and reactions to culturally diverse patients, the nurse will be able to better meet the needs of patients. Most important, the nurse must be able to view culturally diverse patients as individuals and seek a common ground of communication and understanding. In this way, the nurse will be able to accept and respect the anxieties, problems, experiences, and goals of these people and share the fundamental human bond through

which the therapeutic nurse-patient relationship is both established and maintained.

A final reason to consider racial and ethnic factors in psychiatric care has been identified through recent psychiatric research. Current findings suggest that cultural differences exist in the symptom presentations of various psychiatric disorders. Significant racial differences have also been noted among proposed biological markers for various psychiatric disorders, such as serum creatinine phosphokinase, platelet serotonin, and HLA-A2. Failure to control for race would therefore alter the interpretation of studies evaluating these markers. Finally, racial and ethnic differences in response to psychotropic medications, such as higher blood levels found among Asians, affect dosage requirements and potential side effects.[26] In light of these research findings, more care should be taken in incorporating the sociocultural needs of the patient in planning therapeutic psychiatric care.

A nursing model of health-illness phenomena

Models serve many useful purposes. They help to clarify relationships, generate hypotheses, and give perspective to an abstract idea or concept. Psychiatric nurses can practice more effectively if their actions are based on a model of health-illness phenomena that is inclusive, holistic, and yet discrete and relevant. Such a model must recognize that the presence of health or illness is an outcome of multiple characteristics of a person interacting with a number of interdependent factors in the larger social environment.

It assumes that nature is ordered as a social hierarchy or continuum from the simplest unit to the most complex (Fig. 3-2). Each level within this hierarchy represents an organized whole with distinctive properties and a level of complex integrated organization. The study of each level therefore requires unique criteria for explanation of structure and function. Additionally, each level is a component of each higher level, so that nothing exists in isolation. Thus the individual is a component of family and community. Material and information flow across levels, and each level is influenced by all the others. For this reason, one level of organization, such as the individual, cannot be characterized as a dynamic system without incorporating the other levels of the social hierarchy. The most basic level of nursing intervention is the individual level. An exploration of this level must focus on its unique aspects without forgetting its relationship to the whole because "wholeness" is part of the essence of nursing.

The model that will serve as the unifying perspective

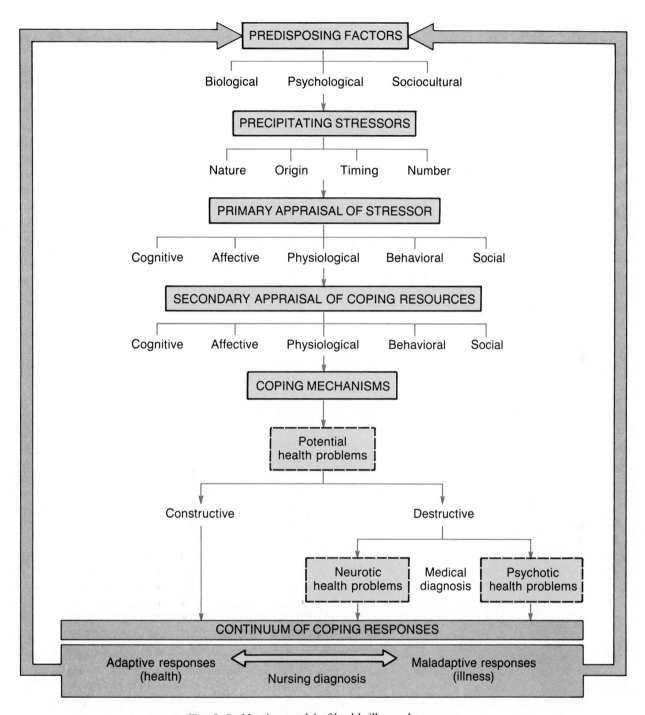

Fig. 3-3. Nursing model of health-illness phenomena.

for this text is presented at the level of the individual in Fig. 3-3. It portrays a flow of pertinent events that result in adaptive or maladaptive coping responses, the basis for the health-illness continuum. This model also serves as the focus for the application of the nursing process. Each element of it is important both in itself and in its relation to the larger hierarchy and will now be discussed.

■ **Predisposing factors**

Predisposing factors are biological, psychological, and sociocultural in nature. They may be viewed as conditioning factors that influence both the type and amount of resources one can elicit to handle stress. Genetic background, nutritional status, biological sensitivities, general health status, and exposure to biological toxins are examples of **biological** predispositions. **Psy-**

TABLE 3-3

SOCIAL READJUSTMENT RATING SCALE

Rank	Life event	Mean value
1	Death of spouse	100
2	Divorce	73
3	Marital separation	65
4	Jail term	63
5	Death of close family member	63
6	Personal injury or illness	53
7	Marriage	50
8	Fired at work	47
9	Marital reconciliation	45
10	Retirement	45
11	Change in health of family member	44
12	Pregnancy	40
13	Sex difficulties	39
14	Gain of new family member	39
15	Business readjustment	39
16	Change in financial state	38
17	Death of close friend	37
18	Change to different line of work	36
19	Change in number of arguments with spouse	35
20	Mortgage over $10,000	31
21	Foreclosure of mortgage or loan	30
22	Change in responsibilities at work	29
23	Son or daughter leaving home	29
24	Trouble with in-laws	29
25	Outstanding personal achievement	28
26	Wife begin or stop work	26
27	Begin or end school	26
28	Change in living conditions	25
29	Revision of personal habits	24
30	Trouble with boss	23
31	Change in work hours/conditions	20
32	Change in residence	20
33	Change in schools	20
34	Change in recreation	19
35	Change in church activities	19
36	Change in social activities	18
37	Mortgage or loan less than $10,000	17
38	Change in sleeping habits	16
39	Change in number of family get-togethers	15
40	Change in eating habits	15
41	Vacation	13
42	Christmas	12
43	Minor violations of the law	11

Reprinted with permission from Holmes, T., and Rahe, R.: J. Psychosom. Res. 11:213, 1967, Pergamon Press, Ltd.

chological factors include, but are not limited to, intelligence, verbal skills, morale, personality type, past experiences, self-concept, motivation, psychological defenses, and locus of control, or a sense of mastery over one's own fate.

Sociocultural characteristics that act as predisposing factors include age, education, income, occupation, social position, cultural background, religious upbringing and beliefs, political affiliation, socialization experiences, and level of social integration or relatedness. Together these factors provide a link with higher and lower levels of the hierarchy and a backdrop against which all present experiences are given meaning and value.

■ Precipitating stressors

Stressors are stimuli that the individual perceives as challenging, threatening, or demanding. They require excess energy and produce a state of tension and stress within the individual. They may be biological, psychological, or sociocultural in nature, and they may arise from one's internal or external environment. In addition to describing the **nature** and **origin** of a stressor, it is also important to assess the timing of the stressor. This **timing** has many dimensions, such as when the stressor occurred, the duration or length of time of exposure to the stressor, and the frequency with which it occurs. A final factor to be considered is the **number** of stressors experienced by the individual within a certain period of time, because events may be more difficult to deal with when they occur close together.

■ **STRESSFUL LIFE EVENTS.** One particular group of stressors that have received a good deal of attention in the health-illness literature are stressful life events. Holmes and Rahe[20] provided the major impetus to the systematic scaling of life events by measuring the correlation of major life events and physical and psychiatric illness. They developed the "Social Readjustment Rating Scale" (Table 3-3). The scale ranks important life events and assigns a specific value to each one on the basis of the amount of coping behavior needed by the individual to deal with the event. As the score of the mean value increases, the likelihood of an illness is similarly hypothesized to increase.

Rahe[40] has also developed a questionnaire called the "Schedule of Recent Experience," which assesses the occurrence of life events for the individual during specific periods of time. The schedule is used to determine the degree of change experienced by the person in a given time period by adding together the mean values of reported life events. Rahe suggests that the schedule is useful in identifying the degree and type of life change experienced.

More recent issues related to life events as stressors focus on the nature of the event and the magnitude of change it represents. There appear to be three ways of categorizing events reported in the literature. The first method is by social activity, which involves family, work, educational, interpersonal, health, financial, legal, or community crises. The second categorization includes the individual's social field. These events are defined as follows: entrances, the introduction of a new person into the individual's social field; and exits, departure of a significant other from the person's social field. A third way of classifying events is by relating them to social desirability. In terms of the currently shared values of American society, one group of events can be considered generally desirable, such as promotion, engagement, and marriage. In contrast, another and proportionately larger group of events can be viewed unfavorably, such as death, financial problems, being fired, and separation.

Unfortunately, conclusions regarding life events are far from definitive. Although they have been correlated with the onset of anxiety and disease symptoms, the methodological and theoretical aspects of research in this area have been the subject of much criticism. Intervening or mediating variables are often not taken into account in the design and execution of empirical studies. The use of unidimensional scales with questionable content validity, internal consistency, and test-retest reliability continues to be a problem. Also, the particular events in the scales may not be the most relevant to certain groups, such as students, working mothers, the elderly, or the poor.

Recent research has shown that social class and ethnic group membership affect the rating of the magnitude of the stress associated with various life events.[5] Also, the life-events approach provides no clues to the specific processes by which the events have an impact on health. In retrospective studies, sources of error in the measurement of life events include selective memory, denial of certain events, and overreporting to justify a current illness. In prospective studies, the subjective evaluation of the significance of the life event to the individual has often been neglected.

■ **LIFE STRAINS AND HASSLES.** Finally, life-events theory is built primarily on the idea of change. However, much stress arises from chronic conditions of living that are unsatisfactory, such as boredom, continuing family tension, job dissatisfaction, and loneliness. This is reflected in the work of Pearlin and Schooler,[37] who wished to explore what people considered potential life strains. In their sample of 2300 people, aged 18 to 65, the following four areas were delineated:

1. Marital strains
2. Parental strains associated with teenage and young adult children
3. Strains associated with household economics
4. Overloads and dissatisfactions associated with the work role

These findings suggest more long-term life dissatisfactions rather than major episodic events.

More recent research by Kanner and Lazarus[28] indicates that small daily hassles or stresses may be more closely linked to and may have a greater effect on one's moods and health than the major misfortunes of life. Hassles are defined by these researchers as irritating, frustrating, or distressing incidents that occur in everyday life. They may include disagreements, disappointments, and unpleasant surprises, such as losing a wallet, getting stuck in a traffic jam, or arguing with one's teenage daughter. In their research, hassles turned out to be better predictors of psychological and physical health than life events. The more frequent and intense the hassles people reported, the poorer their overall mental and physical health. Major events did have some long-term effects, and the authors suggest that these effects may be accounted for by the daily hassles they precipitate.

It has been shown that a certain amount of stress is necessary for survival, and degrees of it can challenge the individual to grow in new ways. However, too much stress that is inappropriately timed can place excessive demands on the individual and interfere with his integrated functioning. So too, it is recognized that stress does not reside within the particular life event itself or within the individual. Rather, it is in the interaction between the individual and situation. The questions that emerge, therefore, are "How much stress is too much?" and "What is a stressful life event?" These questions lead one to explore the significance of the event for the individual's need-value system. The importance of the person's perception or subjective appraisal in determining the stress values of an event has been documented and is crucially important to the implementation of therapeutic activities.

■ Primary appraisal of a stressor

Primary appraisal of a stressor refers to the processing and comprehension of the stressful situation that takes place on many levels for the individual. Specifically, it involves cognitive, affective, physiological, behavioral, and social responses. Primary appraisal is an evaluation of the significance of an event for one's well-being. It is the step in which the stressor assumes its meaning, intensity, and importance by the unique interpretation and affective significance assigned to it by the person at risk.

Cognitive appraisal is a critical part of this model of health-illness phenomena. Lazarus[27] believes cognitive factors play a central role in adaptation. They affect the impact of stressful events, the choice of coping patterns used, and the emotional, physiological, and behavioral reactions or responses. The process of cognitive appraisal mediates psychologically between the person and the environment in any stressful encounter. That is, the person evaluates whether a situation is damaging, or potentially damaging, on the basis of his understanding of the power of the situation to produce harm and the resources he has available to neutralize or tolerate the harm.

Lazarus[27] describes three types of primary cognitive appraisals to stress:

1. *Harm/loss,* referring to damage that has already occurred
2. *Threat,* referring to anticipated or future harm
3. *Challenge,* in which the focus is placed positively on potential gain, growth, or mastery, rather than on the possible risks

This last perception of challenge may play a crucial role in psychological hardiness or resistance to stress. One longitudinal study showed that people whose attitude on life could be rated high on challenge (viewing change as a challenge rather than a threat), commitment (the opposite of alienation), and control (the opposite of powerlessness), remained healthier than the others.[38] The authors conclude that stress-resistant people have a specific set of attitudes toward life, an openness to change, a feeling of involvement in whatever they are doing, and a sense of control over events. They propose that such differences in cognitive appraisal affect one's response to events. Those who view stress as a challenge are more likely to transform events to their advantage and thus reduce their level of stress. This is in contrast to more passive, avoidance, and self-defeating tactics, in which the source of stress does not go away.

Among the most important factors affecting one's cognitive appraisal are commitments and beliefs.[29] Commitments are an expression of what is important to the individual, and they underlie the choices one makes in life. Commitments can thus guide people into or away from situations that threaten, harm, or potentially may be of benefit. Beliefs also determine how a person evaluates what is happening. Beliefs about personal control and existential beliefs are particularly relevant to stress reduction, since they influence both one's emotional response and potential coping ability.

An **affective** response is the arousal of a feeling state. With regard to the primary appraisal of a stressor, the predominant affective response is a nonspecific or generalized anxiety reaction. Consistent with this is the **physiological** response associated with the "fight-or-flight" response. It involves the stimulation of the sympathetic division of the autonomic nervous system and increased activity of the pituitary-adrenal axis. The **behavioral** response of the individual at the time of primary appraisal is focused on the impact of the stressor. A range of behaviors may be evident, depending on the level of anxiety experienced by the individual and the physiologic changes he is experiencing. They are usually reactive behaviors, rather than goal-directed behaviors, at this time. Chapters 12 and 13 explore these responses in greater depth.

Finally, Mechanic[34] describes three aspects of a person's **social** response to stress and illness. The first is the search for meaning, in which individuals seek out information concerning their problem. This is a prerequisite for devising a coping strategy, because only through some formulation of what is occurring can a reasonable response be devised.

The second is social attribution, in which the person tries to identify the unique factors that contributed to the present problematic situation. Patients who view their problem as a result of their own negligence may be blocked from assuming an active, adaptive coping response. They may view their problems as a sign of their personal failure and engage in self-blame and passive and withdrawn behavior. Thus the way in which cause is conceptualized by both patients and health professionals can greatly affect successful coping.

The third social response is social comparison, in which the individual compares his own skills and capacities with those of other persons with similar problems. How a person comes to assess himself depends very much on those around him with whom comparisons are made. In many situations, feelings and self-esteem may depend as much on this comparison process as on the objective coping capacities of the individual. The outcome of this social response is an evaluation of the need for support from one's social network or social support system. Both one's predisposing factors, such as age, developmental level, and cultural background, and the particular characteristics of the precipitating stressor jointly determine one's perceived need for social support.

In summary, the way a person interprets or appraises an event is the psychological key to understanding his coping efforts in that situation and to understanding the nature and intensity of his stress response.

Unfortunately, many nurses and other health professionals ignore this fact when they presume to know how certain stressors will affect an individual and render "routine" care. Not only does this depersonalize the individual, but it also undermines the basis of nursing care. The patient's appraisal of life stressors with its cognitive, affective, physiological, behavioral, and social components must be an essential part of the nurse's assessment.

■ Secondary appraisal of coping resources

Secondary appraisal is an evaluation of one's coping resources, options, or strategies. It is a crucial feature of every stressful encounter because the outcome depends on what, if anything, can be done, as well as what is at stake. It should be noted that primary and secondary appraisals are probably not separate processes, but are often integrated into the same overall evaluation.

■ **TYPES OF COPING RESOURCES.** Mechanic[34] identifies five major coping resources that are helpful in assisting individuals in adapting to the stress of illness. These are economic assets, individual abilities and skills, defensive techniques, social supports, and motivational impetus. They incorporate all levels of the social hier-

archy represented in Fig. 3-2, and the interrelationships between the individual, family group, and society levels of the hierarchy assume critical importance at this point of the model.

Lazarus and Folkman add to these the resources of health and energy, positive beliefs, problem-solving and social skills, and social and material resources.[29] The important role played by physical well-being is well documented in the literature. Similarly, viewing oneself positively can serve as a basis of hope and can sustain one's coping efforts in the most adverse of circumstances. Problem-solving skills include the ability to search for information, analyze situations in order to identify the problem and generate alternative courses of action, weigh alternatives with respect to desired or anticipated outcomes, and select and implement an appropriate plan of action. Social skills facilitate solving problems involving other people, increase the likelihood of being able to enlist the cooperation and support of others, and in general give the individual greater control over social interactions. Finally, material resources refer to money and the goods and services that money can buy. Obviously, monetary resources greatly increase one's coping options in almost any stressful situation.

Presently, much research is being conducted re-

Dimensions of Social Networks

1. Structural characteristics
   a. Size: The number of individuals with whom the person has direct contact. Criteria used may include frequency of contact or perceptions of importance or closeness.
   b. Density: The extent to which members of a person's social network know and contact each other independent of the focal person.
2. Characteristics of component linkages
   a. Intensity: The strength of the tie as measured by feelings about the other person or exchange of reciprocal services.
   b. Durability: The degree of stability of the person's ties with another.
   c. Multidimensionality: The number of functions (advice, support, and feedback) served by a relationship.
   d. Reciprocity: The degree to which emotional and task-oriented support is both given and received by the focal person.

e. Relationship density: The degree to which the focal person's relationships serve a variety of functions.
   f. Dispersion: Geographical proximity to members of one's network.
   g. Frequency: The amount of contact through phone, letter, and face-to-face meetings.
   h. Homogeneity: The extent to which members of a network share common social attributes, such as political or religious affiliation, and socioeconomic status.
3. Normative context of the relationship
   a. Nuclear family
   b. Extended family
   c. Friend
   d. Neighbor
   e. Work acquaintance
   f. Community acquaintance

garding these coping resources.[38] Antonovsky is examining what he calls "generalized resistance resources"—characteristics of the person, group, or environment that can encourage more adaptive responses.[4] He believes knowledge and intelligence offer such a resource, since they allow people to see different ways of dealing with their stress. Two other resources he identifies are a strong ego identity and commitment to a stable and continuing social network. Thus, empirical research is lending support to the interrelationship between predisposing factors and coping resources within a strong social community.

Like primary appraisal, secondary appraisal of coping resources involves cognitive, affective, physiological, behavioral, and social responses. One's **cognitive** appraisal at this time concentrates on the availability and effectiveness of possible coping strategies. But secondary appraisal is more than a mere intellectual exercise of analyzing all the things that might be done. Rather, it is a complex evaluative process that takes into account which coping options are available, the likelihood that a given coping option will accomplish what it is supposed to, and the likelihood that one can apply a particular strategy effectively.

Affectively, the previously elicited general anxiety response becomes refined into specific dominant emotions. These may include joy, sadness, fear, anger, acceptance, distrust, anticipation, or surprise.[39] Emotions may be further classified according to type, duration, and intensity—characteristics that change over time and events. For example, when an emotion is prolonged over time it can be classified as a mood; when prolonged over a longer period of time, it can be considered to be an attitude.

Physiologic responses reflect the interaction of multiple neuroendocrine axes involving growth hormone, prolactin, adrenocorticotropic hormone (ACTH), luteinizing and follicle-stimulating hormones, thyroid-stimulating hormone, vasopressin, oxytocin, epinephrine, norepinephrine, and insulin.[33]

Behavioral responses will reflect both the emotions and physiologic changes experienced by the individual, as well as his cognitive analysis of the stressful situation. Caplan[8] described four interdigitating phases or facets of an individual's responses to a stressful event.

- Phase 1 is behavior that changes the stressful environment or enables the individual to escape from it.
- Phase 2 is behavior to acquire new capabilities for action to change the external circumstances and their aftermath.

- Phase 3 is intrapsychic behavior to defend against unpleasant emotional arousal.
- Phase 4 is intrapsychic behavior to come to terms with the event and its sequelae by internal readjustment.

Conceptualizing the individual's behavior response in terms of these phases may be helpful to the nurse.

One's **social** response is that of evaluating the actual social support available to the individual. Numerous studies have documented increased rates of psychiatric disorder and of general medical morbidity and mortality among persons who are socially isolated. So, too, research in the fields of medical sociology, epidemiology, organizational and social psychology, and experimental stress reveal that those members of the social environment who are perceived by the stressed individual as "significant others" do serve health protective and health restorative functions.

■ **SOCIAL SUPPORT SYSTEMS.** Social support for the individual begins in utero and is communicated in a variety of ways to the newborn baby, including the way he is held, fed, and comforted. As life progresses, support is increasingly derived from other members of the family, then from peers at school, work, and in the community. At times of great need, support may be provided by nurses or other health professionals. Although social support systems or social networks are commonly understood terms, they reflect a complexity of dimensions. Some of the major dimensions used to describe social networks are presented in the accompanying box.

Structural characteristics refer to properties of the overall network, characteristics of component linkages refer to properties of the individual relationships, and normative context refers to the type of relationship.[35]

Given the complexity of the concept, it is not surprising that it is defined differently by various researchers and practitioners. These definitions indicate that different types of support may be provided by social support systems. Some of the functions of social networks that have been identified are shown in Table 3-4. Although phrased differently by each theorist, five common functions of social networks may be described as:

1. Emotional support
2. Task-oriented help
3. Feedback and evaluation
4. Social relatedness and integration
5. Access to new information

The value of social networks in providing emotional support has long been recognized. Some believe it is

---

TABLE 3-4

FUNCTIONS OF SOCIAL SUPPORT SYSTEMS

Caplan[7]	House[21]	Walker et al.[47]	Weiss[48]
Emotional support	Emotional support	Emotional support	Attachment
Task-oriented assistance	Instrumental support	Material aid and services	Exchange of services
Communication of evaluation and expectation	Appraisal support	Maintenance of social identity	Guidance; social integration
Sense of belonging	Informational support	Access to new social contacts	Sense of alliance; reassurance of worth
		Diverse information	Opportunity to provide nurturance

---

the primary function and equate support with love, affection, and nurturance. Although not minimizing this contribution of social support, Caplan[7] believes that the most important contribution is in the cognitive and educational areas and in helping the person with concrete tasks. Caplan states that a supportive group of family, friends, or community members helps the individual deal with his environment:

This group or network adds to his information; helps him improve his own data collection; aids him in evaluating the situation and working out a sensible plan; and assists him in implementing his plan, assessing its consequences, and replanning in line with the feedback information. It reminds him of his continuing identity and bolsters his positive feelings about himself; assures him that his discomforts are expectable and, although burdensome, can usually be tolerated; and maintains his hope in some form of successful outcome of his efforts, which is a prerequisite to his continuing them.

In effect a supportive social network complements and supplements those specific aspects of the individual's functioning which are weakened by the effect of the stressful experience.[7:415]

Although relative importance of the functions of social support may be subject to some variation, there is strong agreement with Caplan on its effect. Two areas of its effect are particularly relevant, the relationship of social support to help seeking and to psychological adaptation. In a review article, Gourash[18] outlined the four general ways that social networks influence help seeking:

1. Buffering the experience of stress that obviates the need for help
2. Precluding the necessity for professional assistance through the provision of instrumental and affective support

3. Acting as screening and referral agents to professional services
4. Transmitting attitudes, values, and norms about help seeking

These findings have implications for primary, secondary, and tertiary prevention.

The large number of studies that address the outcome of psychological adaptation prevents discussing each one in detail. Five important review articles, however, outline the historical context and scope of research in this area. In 1974 Cassel[9] explored the topic from an epidemiological perspective and concluded that social support was an important environmental factor affecting human resistance to disease. Cobb[10] in 1976 reviewed social support around the crises of the life cycle, including pregnancy and childhood, hospitalization, recovery from illness, extensive life changes, employment termination, bereavement, aging and retirement, and the threat of death. He suggests that social support functions as a moderating variable that facilitates coping with crises in an adaptive way. Kaplan, Cassel, and Gore's[24] review in 1977 emphasized the importance of social support as protective of health but only in the presence of certain circumstances that they believe need to be better conceptualized and researched. Mueller[36] in 1980 presented a comprehensive review of the literature on social support and psychiatric disorders. Finally, Greenblatt and co-workers[19] in 1982 reviewed the patterns and characteristics of social networks that maintain health and prevent illness, explored the relationship between social networks and the course and outcome of treatment for mental illness, and described clinical network interventions that have been used to facilitate patient care and maximize performance of ex-patients in the community.

What one can conclude from all these studies is that links do exist between social support and outcome coping responses. However, a precise definition of social support, its determinants or conditions, its measurement, the nature of the support process, and the existence of a causal relationship between social support and maladaptation have yet to be established in theoretical or empirical work.

The importance of social support is well documented, but maximizing the benefit it can provide in a specific situation requires a clearer understanding of the dimensions of the social network given in the box on p. 77; the predisposing factors of the individual, including his needs and attitudes toward using his support network; the nature of the environment; the characteristics of the stressor; and the way in which all of these interact. Future research in this area will be of great value.

■ Coping mechanisms

It is at this point in the model that coping mechanisms and potential health problems emerge. As such, it is a fertile time for nursing activities directed to primary prevention. Coping mechanisms can be defined as any effort directed at stress management. They can be **task oriented** and involve direct problem-solving efforts to cope with the threat itself or **intrapsychic** or ego defense oriented with the goal of regulating one's emotional distress. A more detailed discussion of coping mechanisms used by people experiencing stress can be found in Chapter 12.

Coping mechanisms may be either constructive or destructive in nature. They can be considered **constructive** when one's anxiety is treated as a warning signal that something is wrong and the individual accepts it as a challenge to clarify and resolve the underlying problem. In this respect, anxiety can be compared to a fever—both serve as warnings that the system is under attack. Once employed successfully, constructive coping mechanisms will modify the way past experiences will be utilized to meet future threats. **Destructive** coping mechanisms, in contrast, are used to protect oneself from anxiety without resolving the conflict causing it. The mechanism is one of evasion instead of resolution.

■ MEDICAL DIAGNOSES.
Destructive coping mechanisms are often subject to medical evaluation and diagnosis. The medical diagnosis of a psychiatric health problem can be broadly differentiated as neurotic or psychotic. In the DSM-III, **neurotic disorders** are distinguished by the following characteristics[2]:

1. A symptom or group of symptoms that is distressing and is recognized as unacceptable and alien to the individual.
2. Reality testing is grossly intact.
3. Behavior does not actively violate gross social norms (although functioning may be significantly impaired).
4. The disturbance is relatively enduring or recurrent without treatment and is not limited to a transitory reaction to stressors.
5. There is no demonstrable organic cause or factor.

In situations of severest conflict, however, the person may be powerless to cope with the threat by such patterns and may be forced to deal with the conflict by distorting reality as in **psychosis.** Psychosis consists of the following characteristics[2]:

1. A severe mood disorder
2. Regressive behavior
3. Personality disintegration
4. A significant reduction in level of awareness
5. Great difficulty in functioning adequately
6. Gross impairment in reality testing

This last characteristic is critical. When there is gross impairment in reality testing, the individual incorrectly evaluates the accuracy of his or her perceptions and thoughts and makes incorrect inferences about external reality, even in the face of contrary evidence. According to the DSM-III, direct evidence of psychosis is the presence of either delusions or hallucinations without insight into their pathological nature. It is obvious, therefore, that psychotic health problems reflect the most severe level of illness and maladaptive coping responses.

Medical diagnoses are stated and classified according to the Diagnostic and Statistical Manual of Mental Disorders of the American Psychiatric Association. The names of the various illnesses are augmented with a description of diagnostic criteria, which are tested for reliability by psychiatric practitioners. The third edition of this manual, DSM-III, was published in 1980[2] and the most recent is Draft of the DSM-III-R in Development.[3]

DSM-III-R uses a multiaxial system so that attention is given to certain types of disorders, aspects of the environment, and areas of functioning that might be overlooked if one focused exclusively on the single presenting problem. The individual is thus evaluated on each of the following axes:

Axis I	Clinical Syndromes and V Codes
Axis II	Developmental Disorders and Personality Disorders

TABLE 3-5

SEVERITY OF PSYCHOSOCIAL STRESSORS (AXIS IV)

Code	Term	Adult examples	Child or adolescent examples	Code	Term	Adult examples	Child or adolescent examples
1	None	No apparent psychosocial stressor	No apparent psychosocial stressor	6	Extreme	Death of close relative, divorce	Death of parent or sibling, repeated physical or sexual abuse
2	Minimal	Minor violation of law, small bank loan	Vacation with family	7	Cata-strophic	Concentration camp experi-ence, devas-tating natu-ral disaster	Multiple family deaths
3	Mild	Argument with neighbor, change in work hours	Change in school-teacher, new school year	0	Unspec-ified	No information or not appli-cable	No information or not appli-cable
4	Moderate	New career, death of close friend, pregnancy	Chronic paren-tal fighting, change to new school, illness of close rela-tive, birth of sibling				
5	Severe	Serious illness in self or family, major financial loss, marital sepa-ration, birth of child	Death of peer, divorce of parents, ar-rest, hospi-talization, persistent and harsh parental dis-cipline				

From American Psychiatric Association: Diagnostic and statistical manual of mental disorders, ed. 3, Washington, D.C., 1980, The Association.

Axis III   Physical Disorders and Conditions
Axis IV   Severity of Psychosocial Stressors
Axis V   Global Assessment of Functioning

Axes I and II comprise the entire classification of mental disorders plus V Codes (Conditions Not Attributable to a Mental Disorder That Are a Focus of Attention or Treatment). These are listed on pages 83 to 88. The disorders listed on Axis II, Developmental Disorders and Personality Disorders, generally have an onset in childhood or adolescence and usually persist in a stable form into adulthood. Axis III allows the clinician to identify any current physical disorder or condition that is potentially relevant to the understanding or treatment of the individual. These three axes make up the diagnosis that is to be documented for any patient who receives psychiatric care.

Specialized clinical settings or individuals who are conducting psychiatric research may choose to include Axes IV and V as well. Axis IV documents the severity of psychosocial stressors on a scale of 1 to 7 as represented in Table 3-5. Avis V allows the clinician to rate an individual's psychological, social, and occupational functioning on a continuum of mental health-illness. Ratings are made on a 9-point global assessment of functioning scale (see box on page 82) for both current functioning and the highest level of functioning during the past year. Psychiatric nurses will utilize all five axes of the DSM-III-R in their work with patients and integrate the axes with the related nursing diagnoses in planning and implementing nursing care.

Global Assessment of Functioning Scale (Axis V)

Consider psychological, social, and occupational functioning on a continuum of mental health-illness.

Code

9 Good functioning in all areas, interested and involved in a wide range of activities, socially effective, generally satisfied with life, no more than everyday problems or concerns, absent or minimal symptoms (e.g., mild anxiety before an exam, an occasional "blow-up" with family member)

8 No more than slight impairment in social, occupational or school functioning (e.g., temporarily falling behind in school work); if symptoms are present, they are transient and expectable reactions to psychosocial stressors (e.g., upset by breakup with girlfriend)

7 Some difficulty in social, occupational, or school functioning, but generally functioning pretty well, has some meaningful interpersonal relationships **OR** some mild symptoms (e.g., depressed mood and mild insomnia, occasional truancy or theft within the household)

6 Moderate difficulty in social, occupational, or school functioning **OR** moderate symptoms (e.g., few friends and conflicts with peers, flat affect and circumstantial speech, occasional panic attacks)

5 Any serious impairment in social, occupational, or school functioning **OR** serious symptoms

(e.g., no friends, unable to keep a job, suicidal preoccupation, severe obsessional rituals, frequent shoplifting)

4 Major impairment in several areas, such as work or school, family relations, judgment, thinking or mood (e.g., depressed man avoids friends, neglects family, and is unable to work; child frequently beats up younger children, is defiant at home, and is failing at school) **OR** some impairment in reality testing or communication (e.g., speech is at times illogical, obscure, or irrelevant) **OR** single suicide gesture

3 Inability to function in almost all areas (e.g., stays in bed all day; no job, home, or friends) **OR** behavior is considerably influenced by delusions or hallucinations **OR** serious impairment in communication (e.g., sometimes incoherent) or judgment (e.g., acts grossly inappropriately)

2 Some danger of hurting self or others, or occasionally fails to maintain minimal personal hygiene (e.g., suicide attempts without clear expectation of death, frequently violent, manic excitement, smears feces) **OR** gross impairment in communication (e.g., largely incoherent or mute)

1 Persistent danger of severely hurting self or others (e.g., recurrent violence) **OR** persistent inability to maintain minimal personal hygiene **OR** serious suicide act with clear expectation of death

From American Psychiatric Association: Draft of the DSM-III-R in Development (subject to change), as proposed by the Work Group to Revise DSM-III. American Psychiatric Association, October 1985. Used with permission.

DSM-III-R Classification: Axes I and II Categories and Codes[3]

All official DSM-III-R codes are included in ICD-9-CM. In order to maintain compatibility with ICD-9-CM, some codes (followed by a *) are used for more than one DSM-III-R diagnosis or subtype.

A long dash following a diagnostic term indicates the need for a fifth digit subtype or other qualifying term. The term "specify" following the name of some diagnostic categories indicates qualifying terms that clinicians may wish to add in parentheses after the name of the disorder.

NOS = Not Otherwise Specified

The current severity of a diagnosis may be specified after the diagnosis as:

Mild	*Currently*
Moderate	*meets*
Severe	*diagnostic*
	criteria

In partial remission (or residual state)
In complete remission

Disorders Usually First Evident in Infancy, Childhood, or Adolescence

Developmental Disorders
Note: These are coded on Axis II.

Mental retardation
Code in fifth digit: 1 = with other behavioral symptoms (requiring attention or treatment and that are not part of another disorder), 0 = without other behavioral symptoms.

317.0x	Mild mental retardation, _____
318.0x	Moderate mental retardation, _____
318.1x	Severe mental retardation, _____
318.2x	Profound mental retardation, _____
319.0x	Unspecified mental retardation, _____

Pervasive developmental disorders
Autistic Disorder,
299.00	infantile onset, _____
299.90*	childhood onset, _____
299.90*	onset unknown or NOS, _____
299.80	Pervasive developmental disorder NOS, _____

Specific developmental disorders
Language and speech disorders

315.39	Articulation disorder
307.00*	Stuttering
307.00*	Cluttering
315.31*	Expressive language disorder
315.31*	Receptive language disorder

Academic skills disorders
315.00	Reading disorder
315.90	Expressive writing disorder
315.10	Arithmetic disorder

Motor skills disorder
315.40	Coordination disorder
315.90	Specific developmental disorder NOS

Other developmental disorders
315.90	Developmental disorder NOS

Disruptive behavior disorders
314.01	Attention deficit-hyperactivity disorder
313.81	Oppositional disorder
312.90	Conduct disorder

Eating disorders
307.10	Anorexia nervosa
307.51	Bulimic disorder
307.52	Pica
307.53	Rumination disorder of infancy
307.50	Eating disorder NOS

Tic disorders
307.23	Tourette's disorder
307.22	Chronic motor or vocal tic disorder
307.21	Transient tic disorder

Specify: single episode
recurrent episode
307.20	Tic disorder NOS

Disorders of elimination
307.60	Functional enuresis
307.70	Functional encopresis

Other disorders of infancy, childhood or adolescence
313.89	Reactive attachment disorder of infancy and early childhood
307.30	Stereotypy/habit disorder
313.23	Elective mutism
309.21	Separation anxiety disorder
313.82	Identity disorder [DELETION BEING CONSIDERED]

From American Psychiatric Association: Draft of the DSM-III-R in Development (subject to change), as proposed by the Work Group to Revise DSM-III. American Psychiatric Association, October 1985. Used with permission.

DSM-III-R Classification: Axes I and II Categories and Codes—cont'd

Organic Mental Syndromes and Disorders (Non–Substance-Induced)

Organic Mental Syndromes whose etiology or pathophysiologic process is either noted as an additional diagnosis from outside the mental disorders section of ICD-9-CM (DSM-III-R Axis III) or is unknown.

293.00	Delirium
294.10	Dementia
294.00	Amnestic syndrome
293.81	Organic delusional syndrome
293.82	Organic hallucinosis
293.83	Organic affective syndrome
	Specify: manic
	depressed
	mixed
294.80*	Organic anxiety syndrome
310.10	Organic personality syndrome
	Specify if explosive type
294.80*	Organic mental syndrome NOS

Dementias arising in the senium and presenium

	Primary degenerative dementia, senile onset
290.30	with delirium
290.20	with delusions
290.21	with depression
290.00	uncomplicated

Code in fifth digit:
1 = with delirium, 2 = with delusions,
3 = with depression, 0 = uncomplicated.

290.1x	Primary degenerative dementia, presenile onset, _____
290.4x	Multi-infarct dementia, _____

Psychoactive Substance Use Disorders
Psychoactive substance-induced organic mental disorders

	Alcohol
303.00	intoxication
291.40	idiosyncratic intoxication
291.80	withdrawal
291.00	withdrawal delirium
291.30	hallucinosis
291.10	amnestic disorder
291.20	dementia associated with alcoholism
	Barbiturate or similarly acting sedative or hypnotic
305.40	intoxication

292.00*	withdrawal
292.00*	withdrawal delirium
292.83*	amnestic disorder
292.82*	dementia
292.90*	flashback disorder
310.90*	residual disorder
	Opioid
305.50	intoxication
292.00*	withdrawal
310.90*	residual disorder
	Cocaine
305.60	intoxication
292.00*	withdrawal
292.81*	delirium
292.11*	delusional disorder
292.90*	flashback disorder
310.90*	residual disorder
	Amphetamine or similarly acting sympathomimetic
305.70	intoxication
292.00*	withdrawal
292.81*	delirium
292.11*	delusional disorder
292.90*	flashback disorder
310.90*	residual disorder
	Phencyclidine (PCP) or similarly acting arylcyclohexylamine
305.90*	intoxication
292.81*	delirium
292.11*	delusional disorder
292.90*	flashback disorder
310.90*	residual disorder
	Hallucinogen
305.30	hallucinosis
292.81*	delirium
292.11*	delusional disorder
292.90*	flashback disorder
310.90*	residual disorder
	Cannabis
305.20	intoxication
292.81*	delirium
292.11*	delusional disorder
292.90*	flashback disorder
310.90*	residual disorder
	Tobacco
292.00*	withdrawal
	Caffeine
305.90*	intoxication

DSM-III-R Classification: Axes I and II Categories and Codes—cont'd

Other drug or unspecified psychoactive substance

292.81*	delirium
292.82*	dementia
292.83*	amnestic disorder
292.11*	delusional disorder
292.12	hallucinosis
292.84*	affective disorder
294.80*	anxiety disorder
292.90*	flashback disorder
310.90*	residual disorder
305.90*	intoxication
292.00*	withdrawal
292.90*	organic mental disorder NOS

Psychoactive substance dependence disorders

303.90	Alcohol dependence
304.10	Barbiturate or similarly acting sedative or hypnotic dependence
304.00	Opioid dependence
304.20	Cocaine dependence
304.40	Amphetamine or similarly acting sympathomimetic dependence
304.50*	Phencyclidine (PCP) or similarly acting arylcyclohexylamine dependence
304.50*	Hallucinogen dependence
304.30	Cannabis dependence
305.10	Tobacco dependence
304.60	Inhalant dependence
304.90*	Polysubstance dependence
304.90*	Psychoactive substance dependence NOS

Sleep and Arousal Disorders

Note: Narcolepsy, an Axis III physical disorder, is included here for completeness.

Disorders of initiating or maintaining sleep (insomnia) or excessive daytime sleepiness

Disorders primarily of insomnia

307.42	Learned insomnia
780.52*	Childhood onset insomnia
780.52*	Restless legs sleep disorder

Disorders primarily of excessive daytime sleepiness

347.00	Narcolepsy (code on Axis III)
780.54	Idiopathic hypersomnolence disorder

Disorders of insomnia or excessive daytime sleepiness

780.52*	Myoclonic sleep disorder
780.53	Sleep-induced respiratory impairment

Specify type:
  obstructive sleep apnea
  nonobstructive sleep apnea
  nonapneic hypoventilation
  chronic obstructive pulmonary disease (COPD)

780.52*	Insomnia or excessive daytime somnolence secondary to other physical disorder
307.49	Subjective sleep disturbance without objective findings
307.40	Disorder of insomnia or excessive daytime sleepiness NOS

Disorders of the sleep-wake schedule

307.45*	Frequently changing sleep-wake schedule disorder
307.45*	Disorganized sleep-wake pattern disorder
780.55	Delayed or advanced sleep phase disorder
307.45*	Sleep-wake schedule disorder NOS

Parasomnias

307.46*	Sleepwalking disorder
307.46*	Sleep terror disorder
307.47*	Dream anxiety disorder
307.46*	Functional enuresis, nocturnal type (See also 307.60 Functional enuresis, in the childhood section)
307.47*	Parasomnia NOS

Schizophrenic Disorders

Code in fifth digit: 1 = subchronic, 2 = chronic, 3 = subchronic with acute exacerbation, 4 = chronic with acute exacerbation, 0 = unspecified.

Schizophrenia,

295.3x	paranoid, _____
	Specify if stable type
295.2x	catatonic, _____
295.1x	disorganized, _____
295.9x	undifferentiated, _____
295.6x	residual, _____

Specify: childhood onset (below 12)

DSM-III-R Classification: Axes I and II Categories and Codes—cont'd

adolescent onset (12-18)
adult (early/mid) onset
(18-44)
late onset (after 45)

Delusional (Paranoid) Disorders

297.10   Delusional (Paranoid) disorder

Specify type: persecutory
jealous
erotomanic
somatic
grandiose
other

Psychotic Disorders Not Elsewhere Classified

295.40   Schizophreniform disorder
Specify: single episode
recurrent episode
295.70   Schizoaffective disorder
Specify: bipolar
depressive
298.80   Brief reactive psychosis
297.30   Induced psychotic disorder
298.90   Psychotic disorder NOS (Atypical psychosis)

Mood (Affective) Disorders

Code manic episode in fifth digit: 4 = with psychotic features (specify mood-congruent or mood-incongruent), 2 = without psychotic features, 0 = unspecified.
Code major depressive episode in fifth digit: 4 = with psychotic features (specify mood-congruent or mood-incongruent), 3 = with melancholia, 2 = without melancholia, 0 = unspecified. Specify if chronic.

Bipolar disorders

Bipolar disorder,
296.6x   mixed, _____
296.4x   manic, _____
296.5x   depressed, _____
301.13   Cyclothymia
296.70   Bipolar disorder NOS

Depressive disorders

Major Depression,

296.2x   single episode, _____
296.3x   recurrent, _____
300.40   Dysthymia
296.82   Depressive disorder NOS

Anxiety Disorders

Panic disorder,
300.21*   with extensive phobic avoidance (Agoraphobia)
300.21*   with limited phobic avoidance
300.01   without phobic avoidance
300.22   Limited symptom attacks with phobic avoidance (Agoraphobia without panic attacks)
300.23   Social phobia
300.29   Simple phobia
300.30   Obsessive compulsive disorder
309.89   Post-traumatic stress disorder
Specify if delayed onset
300.02   Generalized anxiety disorder
300.00   Anxiety disorder NOS

Somatoform Disorders

300.81   Somatization disorder
300.11   Conversion disorder
Specify: single episode
recurrent episode
307.80   Idiopathic pain disorder
300.70*   Hypochondriasis
300.70*   Dysmorphic somatoform disorder
300.70*   Undifferentiated somatoform disorder
300.70*   Somatoform disorder NOS

Dissociative Disorders

300.14   Multiple personality disorder
300.13   Psychogenic fugue
300.12   Psychogenic amnesia
300.60   Depersonalization disorder
300.15*   Trance/possession disorder
300.15*   Dissociative disorder NOS

Gender and Sexual Disorders
Gender identity disorders

302.50   Transsexualism
Specify sexual history: asexual, homosexual, heterosexual, unspecified

DSM-III-R Classification: Axes I and II Categories and Codes—cont'd

302.89* Nontranssexual cross gender disorder
      Specify sexual history: asexual, homosexual, heterosexual, unspecified
302.60 Gender identity disorder of childhood
302.85 Gender identity disorder NOS

Paraphilias

Specify if fantasy only

302.20 Pedophilia
302.40 Exhibitionism
302.90* Paraphilic rapism [UNDER CONSIDERATION]
302.84 Sexual sadism
302.83 Sexual masochism
302.82 Voyeurism
302.81 Fetishism
302.30 Transvestic fetishism
302.10 Zoophilia
302.90* Frotteurism
302.90* Paraphilia NOS

Sexual dysfunctions

Where appropriate, specify:
  psychogenic only, biogenic only, or
  psychogenic and biogenic; specify:
  lifelong or acquired; specify:
  generalized or situational

    Sexual desire disorders
302.71 Hypoactive sexual desire disorder
302.79* Sexual aversion disorder
    Sexual arousal disorders
302.72* Female sexual arousal disorder
302.72* Male sexual arousal disorder
    Orgasm disorders
302.73 Inhibited female orgasm
302.74 Inhibited male orgasm
302.75 Premature ejaculation
    Sexual pain disorders
302.76 Functional dyspareunia
306.51 Functional vaginismus
302.70 Sexual dysfunction NOS

Other gender and sexual disorders

302.00 Ego-dystonic homosexuality
302.89* Sexual disorder NOS

Factitious Disorders

    Factitious disorder,
300.16   with psychological symptoms

301.51   with physical symptoms
300.19*   with physical and psychological symptoms
300.19* Factitious disorder NOS

Impulse Control Disorders Not Elsewhere Classified

312.31 Pathological gambling
312.32 Kleptomania
312.33 Pyromania
312.39* Trichotillomania
312.39* Impulse control disorder NOS

Adjustment Disorder

    Adjustment disorder,
309.00   with depressed mood
309.24   with anxious mood
309.28   with mixed emotional features
309.30   with disturbance of conduct
309.40   with mixed disturbance of emotions and conduct
309.23   with work (or academic) inhibition
309.83   with withdrawal
309.82   with physical complaints
309.90 Adjustment disorder NOS

Other Disorders Associated with Physical Condition

625.40 Premenstrual dysphoric disorder [UNDER CONSIDERATION]
316.00 Psychological factors affecting physical condition
    Specify physical condition on Axis III

Personality Disorders

Note: These are coded on Axis II.
301.00 Paranoid
301.20 Schizoid
301.22 Schizotypal
301.50 Histrionic
301.81 Narcissistic
301.70 Antisocial
301.83 Borderline
301.82 Avoidant
301.60 Dependent
301.40 Obsessive Compulsive
301.84 Passive Aggressive
301.89* Masochistic [UNDER CONSIDERATION]
301.89* Personality disorder NOS

DSM-III-R Classification: Axes I and II Categories and Codes—cont'd

V Codes for Conditions Not Attributable to a Mental Disorder That Are a Focus of Attention or Treatment

V65.20	Malingering
V62.89*	Borderline intellectual functioning (Note: This is coded on Axis II.)
V71.01	Adult antisocial behavior
V71.02	Childhood or adolescent antisocial behavior
V62.30	Academic problem
V62.20	Occupational problem
V62.82	Uncomplicated bereavement
V15.81	Noncompliance with medical treatment
V62.89*	Phase of life problem or other life circumstance problem

V61.10	Marital problem
V61.20	Parent-child problem
V61.80	Other specified family circumstances
V62.81	Other interpersonal problem

Additional Codes

300.90	Unspecified mental disorder (nonpsychotic)
V71.09*	No diagnosis or condition on Axis I
799.90*	Diagnosis or condition deferred on Axis I
V71.09*	No diagnosis or condition on Axis II
799.90*	Diagnosis or condition deferred on Axis II

■ Continuum of health-illness coping responses

When a particular event occurs, the person mentally processes the information. Based on specific conditioning factors, the quality of the stressor, his perception of the situation, and his analysis of his resources and needs, he will respond to the stressor. His responses theoretically can be placed on a coping continuum of health and illness.

A nursing evaluation of one's health status may be done by measuring an individual's potential and liability in three areas: (1) functional (tasks and responsibilities of daily living), (2) psychological (intellectual and emotional realms), and (3) clinical (physical components).[23] Functional status is the ability to carry out the tasks of daily living and to fulfill the challenges of one's social roles and responsibilities. Psychological status includes the person's sense of well-being, mental and emotional state, perception of the quality of life, and integration of strengths and resources toward maximizing personal potential. Clinical status incorporates the physical and biological dimensions of health including risk factors, such as cigarette smoking and pathological or disease processes. By including all three areas in one's assessment, the nurse can provide a holistic approach to the patient, and better evaluate his coping responses in light of his overall life perspective. Those responses which support integrated functioning can be viewed as adap-

tive, or healthy, responses. They lead to growth, learning, and goal achievement. Those responses which block integrated functioning can be viewed as maladaptive, or illness, responses. They can be evident as impaired thought processes, alterations in the expression of emotions, physiologic illness, inappropriate behavior, or problems in socialization.

■ NURSING DIAGNOSES

These responses to stress, whether actual or potential, are the subject of nursing diagnoses. A nursing diagnosis is the independent judgment of a nurse about a patient's behavioral response to stress. It is a statement of the patient's nursing problems, which may be overt, covert, existing, or potential, and should include both the behavioral disruption or threatened disruption and the contributing stressors.[25] Like the diagnoses, the treatments of these disruptions or maladaptive responses are a nursing function.

The accompanying box lists the nursing diagnoses identified through the 7th National Conference of the North American Nursing Diagnosis Association (NANDA). In addition to these diagnoses, the Council on Psychiatric and Mental Health Nursing of the American Nurses' Association has been developing a taxonomy on the phenomena of concern for psychiatric mental health nurses. The taxonomy they have initially proposed for the classification of human responses of concern for psychiatric/mental health nursing practice

North American Nursing Diagnosis Association (NANDA)
Approved Nursing Diagnoses

Activity intolerance
Activity intolerance, potential
Airway clearance, ineffective
Altered comfort: chronic pain
Altered growth and development
Altered sexuality patterns
Anxiety
Bowel elimination, alteration in: constipation
Bowel elimination, alteration in: diarrhea
Bowel elimination, alteration in: incontinence
Breathing pattern, ineffective
Cardiac output, alteration in: decreased
Comfort, alteration in: pain
Communication, impaired: verbal
Coping, family: potential for growth
Coping, ineffective family: compromised
Coping, ineffective family: disabling
Coping, ineffective individual
Diversional activity, deficit
Family process, alteration in
Fear
Fluid volume alteration in: excess
Fluid volume deficit, actual
Fluid volume deficit, potential
Functional incontinence
Gas exchange, impaired
Grieving, anticipatory
Grieving, dysfunctional
Health maintenance, alteration in
Home maintenance management, impaired
Hopelessness
Hyperthermia
Hypothermia
Impaired adjustment
Impaired social interaction
Impaired swallowing
Impaired tissue integrity
Ineffective thermoregulation

Injury, potential for: (poisoning, potential for; suffocation, potential for; trauma, potential for)
Knowledge deficit (specify)
Mobility, impaired physical
Noncompliance (specify)
Nutrition, alteration in: less than body requirements
Nutrition, alteration in: more than body requirements
Nutrition, alteration in: potential for more than body requirements
Oral mucous membrane, alteration in
Parenting, alteration in: actual
Parenting, alteration in: potential
Post trauma response
Potential alteration in body temperature
Potential for infection
Powerlessness
Rape trauma syndrome
Reflex incontinence
Self-care deficit: feeding, bathing/hygiene, dressing/grooming, toileting
Self-concept, disturbance in: body image, self-esteem, role performance, personal identity
Sensory-perceptual alteration: visual, auditory, kinesthetic, gustatory, tactile, olfactory
Sexual dysfunction
Skin integrity, impairment of: actual
Skin integrity, impairment of: potential
Sleep pattern disturbance
Social isolation
Spiritual distress (distress of the human spirit)
Stress incontinence
Thought processes, alteration in
Tissue perfusion, alteration in: cerebral, cardiopulmonary, renal, gastrointestinal, peripheral
Total incontinence
Urge incontinence
Urinary elimination, alteration in patterns
Urinary retention
Violence, potential for: self-directed or directed at others

From North American Nursing Diagnosis Association Classification of Nursing Diagnosis: Proceedings of the Seventh Conference, 1987, St. Louis, The C.V. Mosby Co.

TABLE 3-6

TAXONOMY FOR THE CLASSIFICATION OF HUMAN RESPONSES OF CONCERN FOR PSYCHIATRIC/MENTAL HEALTH NURSING PRACTICE

Response Class: Individual

A. Biological Response Patterns
   10. Alterations in Circulation
   11. Alterations in Elimination
   12. Alterations in Endocrine/Metabolic Functioning
   13. Alterations in Musculo/Skeletal Functioning
   14. Alterations in Nutrition/Metabolism
   15. Alterations in Neurological/Sensory Functioning
   16. Alterations in Oxygenation
   17. Alterations in Reproductive/Sexual Functioning
   18. Alterations in Physical Integrity
B. Socio/Behavioral Response Patterns
   20. Alterations in Communication
   21. Alterations in Conduct/Impulse Control
   22. Alterations in Motor Behavior
   23. Alterations in Role Performance
   24. Alterations in Self Care
   25. Alterations in Sleep/Arousal
   26. Alterations in Sexuality
C. Emotional Response Patterns
   30. Excess or Deficit of Dominant Emotions
D. Defensive Response Patterns
   40. Excess or Deficit of Defenses
E. Perceptual/Cognitive Response Patterns
   50. Alterations in Perception/Cognition
F. Value/Belief Response Patterns
   60. Alterations in Spirituality
   61. Alterations in Values

From American Nurses' Association. A Model for Identification of Psychiatric Nursing Practice Phenomena. Kansas City, Missouri: the Association, 1986.

is presented in Table 3-6. Both of these classification systems are in their developmental stages, and one can expect to see further development and growth of a taxonomy for psychiatric nursing in the future.

Coping responses to stress emerge whether or not a medical diagnosis of an existing health problem has been made. If the individual has been medically diagnosed, the treatment of the medical health problem would be primarily a medical function. It is here that the practice of medicine and nursing mesh and become complementary, while each retains its distinct focus. The practice of nursing does not require a medical diagnosis.

A nurse may implement the nursing process for maladaptive responses *whether or not* there is a diagnosis of a medical health problem. However, all health professionals have an obligation to refer a patient to another practitioner when it is in the patient's best interests.

An additional aspect of nursing care is presented by Loomis and Wood[31] in their model of clinical nursing which proposes that the potential outcome of nursing is not limited to "care" alone, but may include the possible "cure" of actual or potential health problems. They present four prototypes of health care situations to demonstrate this point.[31] The first is typical of the medical model in which a patient's actual health problem precedes his human responses. In this case, nurses collaborate with physicians in treating the physiological response to the health problem, and collaborate with the patient and his support system in treating the emotional, cognitive, behavioral, and social responses. When human responses precede health problems, nurses act to prevent potential health problems by health education, environmental change, and supporting social systems. When health problems are defined as human responses, the nursing diagnosis is the same as the medical diagnosis, and nurses assume curative functions. Finally, when a patient's health problems are interactive with his human responses, the caring and curing activities may be synonomous as nurses mediate among medical treatments, health deviations, and life-style disruptions. Thus, the overlap when intervening in health problems and human responses suggests the interdependence between nursing and medicine and the need for effective interdisciplinary collaboration.

The final outcome of the model is the emergence of health and illness behaviors. They are seen as a continuum of responses rather than discrete entities. The various elements of the model are summarized in Table 3-7. Volumes have been written in the literature with regard to each component of this model. This brief description of it was presented to reveal the organizing framework for this text. Chapters 12 to 21 explore various maladaptive responses. In the beginning of each of these chapters, a continuum of coping or health-illness will be described. This will be followed by a discussion of relevant predisposing or conditioning factors, precipitating stressors, behaviors, and coping mechanisms. Building on this theoretical knowledge, each phase of the nursing process will be applied to the specific maladaptive response. Medical diagnoses of health problems will be presented when appropriate and related to the nursing diagnoses. Through the consistent use of this framework, the art and science of psychiatric nursing practice will emerge.

TABLE 3-7

SUMMARY OF THE NURSING MODEL OF HEALTH-ILLNESS PHENOMENA

Component	Definition	Dimensions
Predisposing factors	Conditioning factors that influence both the type and amount of resources which the individual can elicit to cope with stress	Biological Psychological Sociocultural
Precipitating stressors	Stimuli that the individual perceives as challenging, threatening, or demanding and that require excess energy for coping	Nature Origin Timing Number
Primary appraisal of a stressor	An evaluation of the significance of a stressor for one's well-being in which it assumes its meaning, intensity, and importance	Cognitive Affective Physiological Behavioral Social
Secondary appraisal of coping resources	An evaluation of one's coping resources, options, and strategies	Cognitive Affective Physiological Behavioral Social
Coping mechanisms	Any effort directed at stress management	Constructive Destructive
Continuum of health-illness responses	A range of human responses reflective of one's health status	Adaptive Maladaptive

■ SUGGESTED CROSS-REFERENCES ■

This chapter serves as a foundation for formulating principles of psychiatric nursing and implementing psychiatric nursing practice. As such, it is related to all other chapters of this text.

■ SUMMARY ■

1. Lack of consensus exists on the definition of mental health. Jahoda's conditions and criteria of mental health were described, and the dimensions and prevalence of mental illnesses were discussed.

2. Developmental stages and tasks of the individual and family life cycles were identified.

3. The concept of cultural relativism was explored because the content and form of mental illness vary greatly from one culture to another. Problems posed by ethnocentrism and implications for psychiatric research were also described.

4. A nursing model of health-illness phenomena was presented at the individual level of the social hierarchy. This model serves as the focus for the application of the nursing process. It portrays six components that result in adaptive or maladaptive coping responses.

  Predisposing factors that are biological, psychological, and sociocultural in nature.

b. Precipitating stressors that vary in nature, origin, timing, and number. Research related to stressful life events was critiqued.

c. Primary appraisal of a stressor is an evaluation of the significance of an event for one's well-being that takes place on the cognitive, affective, physiological, behavioral, and social levels.

d. Secondary appraisal of coping resources is an evaluation of one's coping resources or strategies that involve cognitive, affective, physiological, behavioral, and social responses.

e. Coping mechanisms are any efforts directed at stress management and may be constructive or destructive in nature. Destructive coping mechanisms are often subject to medical diagnoses classified according to Axes I through V of the *Draft of the DSM-III-R in Development.*[3]

f. The continuum of health-illness responses is a range of human responses reflective of one's health status. These responses to stress, whether actual or potential, are the subject of nursing diagnoses. The relationships among coping responses, health problems, medical diagnoses, and nursing diagnoses were explored.

DIRECTIONS FOR FUTURE RESEARCH

The following are some of the nursing research problems raised in Chapter 3 that merit further study by psychiatric nurses:

1. Attitudes of psychiatric nurses regarding the health-illness and conformity-deviance conceptions of mental illness
2. Nurses' knowledge of developmental stages and tasks of the individual and family units
3. The role of psychiatric nurses in the delivery of mental health care to ethnic minorities
4. The prevalence of ethnocentrism among psychiatric nurses and patient care outcomes associated with it
5. The validity and reliability of tools used to collect data about coping strategies used by healthy and ill individuals
6. Methods to evaluate the effectiveness of coping strategies
7. The direct and interactive effects related to the nature, origin, timing, and number of stressors
8. Variables that intervene between stressful life events and maladaptive coping responses
9. Stressful life events, chronic strains, and daily hassles relevant to various high-risk groups
10. The role of social attribution in an individual's response to threat
11. The types of coping resources associated with adaptive responses and their mechanism of action
12. The nature of the social support system, including its determinants, measurement, the support process, and its causal effect on coping responses

■ REFERENCES ■

1. American Journal of Psychiatry: Research on mental illness and addictive disorders: progress and prospects **142**(7), July 1985.
2. American Psychological Association: Diagnostic and statistical manual of mental disorders, ed. 3, Washington, D.C., 1980, The Association.
3. American Psychological Association: Draft of the DSM-III-R in Development (subject to change), as proposed by the Work Group to Revise DSM-III. American Psychiatric Association, October 1985.
4. Antonovsky, A.: Health, stress and coping, San Francisco, 1979, Jossey-Bass.
5. Askenasy, A.R., Dohrenwend, B.P., and Dohrenwend, B.S.: Some effects of social class and ethnic group membership on judgments of the magnitude of stressful life events: a research note, J. Health Soc. Behav. **18**(4):432, 1977.
6. Bryant, F.: Dimensions of subjective mental health in American men and women, J. Health Soc. Behav. **25**(2):116, June 1984.
7. Caplan, G.: Support systems and community mental health, New York, 1974, Behavioral Publications.
8. Caplan, G.: Mastery of stress: psychosocial aspects, Am. J. Psychiatry **138**(4):41, 1981.
9. Cassel, J.: Psychosocial processes and "stress": theoretical formulation, Int. J. Health Serv. **4**:471, 1974.
10. Cobb, S.: Social support as a moderator of life stress, Psychosom. Med. **38**:300, 1976.
11. Cohen, Y.: Social structures and personality, New York, 1961, Holt, Rinehart and Winston.
12. Dohrenwend, B.P., and Dohrenwend, B.S.: Social and cultural influences on psychopathology, Annu. Rev. Psychol. 7(25):417, 1974.
13. Durkheim, E.: Suicide: a study in sociology, translated by J. Spaulding and C. Simpson, Glencoe, Ill., 1951, Free Press.
14. Duvall, E.: Marriage and family development, ed. 5, Philadelphia, 1977, J.B. Lippincott Co.
15. Eisenthal, S.: The sociological approach. In Lazare, A., editor: Outpatient psychiatry: diagnosis and treatment, Baltimore, 1979, Williams & Wilkins.
16. Erikson, E.: Childhood and society, ed. 2, New York, 1963, W.W. Norton & Co., Inc.
17. Faris, R., and Dunham, H.: Mental health in urban areas: an ecological study of schizophrenia and other psychoses, Chicago, 1939, University of Chicago Press.
18. Gourash, N.: Help-seeking: a review of the literature, Am. J. Community Psychol. **6**:499, 1978.
19. Greenblatt, M., Becerra, R., and Serafetinides, E.: Social networks and mental health: an overview, Am. J. Psychiatry **139**(8):977, Aug. 1982.
20. Holmes, T., and Rahe, R.: The social readjustment rating scale, J. Psychosom. Res. **11**:213, 1967.
21. House, J.: Work stress and social support, Reading, Mass., 1981, Addison-Wesley Publishing Co., Inc.
22. Jahoda, M.: Current concepts of positive mental health, New York, 1958, Basic Books Publishers.
23. Jordan-Marsh, M. et al.: Life-style intervention: a conceptual framework, Patient Educ. Counsel. **6**(1):29, 1985.
24. Kaplan, B., Cassel, J., and Gore, S.: Social support and health, Med. Care **15**(5):(suppl.):47, 1977.
25. Kim, M., McFarland, G., and McLane, A.: Classification of nursing diagnoses, St. Louis, 1984, The C.V. Mosby Co.
26. Lawson, W.: Racial and ethnic factors in psychiatric research, Hosp. Community Psychiatry **37**(1):50, Jan. 1986.
27. Lazarus, R.: Psychological stress and the coping process, New York, 1966, McGraw-Hill, Inc.
28. Lazarus, R.: Little hazards can be hazardous to health, Psychology Today **15**:58, July 1981.
29. Lazarus, R., and Folkman, S.: Stress, appraisal and cop-

ing, New York, 1984, Springer Publishing Co.

30. Leighton, A., et al.: Stirling county study of psychiatric disorder and sociocultural environment: my name is legion, vol. 1, New York, 1959, Basic Books Publishers.

31. Loomis, M., and Woods, D.: Cure: the potential outcome of nursing care, Image **15**(1):4, Winter 1983.

32. Maslow, A.: Motivation and personality, New York, 1958, Harper and Row Publishers.

33. Mason, J.: A re-evaluation of the concept of nonspecificity in stress theory, J. Psychol. Res. **8**:323, 1971.

34. Mechanic, D.: Illness behavior, social adaptation, and the management of illness, J. Nerv. Ment. Dis. **165**(2):79, 1977.

35. Mitchell, R., and Trickett, E.: Task force report: social networks as mediators of social support, Community Ment. Health J. **16**(1):27, 1980.

36. Mueller, D.: Social networks: a promising direction for research on the relationship of the social environment to psychiatric disorder, Soc. Sci. Med. **14A**:147, 1980.

37. Pearlin, L.I., and Schooler, C.: The structure of coping, J. Health Soc. Behav. **19**(3):2, 1978.

38. Pines, M.: Psychological hardiness: the role of challenge in health, Psychology Today **14**:34, Dec. 1980.

39. Plutchik, R., Kellerman, H., and Conte, H.: A structural theory of ego defense and emotions. In Izard, C., editor: Emotions in personality and psychopathology, New York, 1979, Plenum Press.

40. Rahe, R.: Life-change measurement as a predictor of illness, Proc. R. Soc. Med. **61**:1124, 1968.

41. Rogers, C.: On becoming a person, Boston, 1961, Houghton Mifflin Co.

42. Rosenfield, S.: Race differences in involuntary hospitalization: psychiatric versus labeling perspectives, J. Health Soc. Behav. **25**(1):14, Mar. 1984.

43. Rosow, I.: Docs: ortho and para, Am. J. Orthopsychiatry **51**(2):255, 1981.

44. Streff, M.: Examining family growth and development: a theoretical model, Adv. Nurs. Sci. **3**(4):61, 1981.

45. Sundeen, S., Stuart, G., et al.: Nurse-client interaction: implementing the nursing process, ed. 3, St. Louis, 1985, The C.V. Mosby Co.

46. Tsung-yi, L.: A global view of mental health, Am. J. Orthopsychiatry **54**(3):369, July 1984.

47. Walker, K., MacBride, A., and Vachon, M.: Social support networks and the crisis of bereavement, Soc. Sci. Med. **11**:35, 1977.

48. Weiss, R.: The provisions of social relationships. In Rubin, A., editor: Doing unto others, Englewood Cliffs, N.J., 1974, Prentice-Hall, Inc.

■ ANNOTATED SUGGESTED READINGS ■

American Journal of Psychiatry: Research on mental illness and addictive disorders: progress and prospects, **142**(7), July 1985.

This summary document reports the latest findings, statistics, and progress in mental and addictive disorders. It makes an eloquent case for the need for increased research funding in the field of psychiatric care.

*Bevilacqua, J.: Voodoo—myth or mental illness? J. Psychiatr. Nurs. **18**(2):17, 1980.

This is a fascinating clinical study of a 14-year-old Haitian girl's experience with what has been diagnosed as mental illness. The author raises many questions on etiology, interventions, and influence of voodoo and causes the reader to consider how the system that we work in perpetuates mental illness rather than relieves it.

Jordan-Marsh, M. et al.: Life-style intervention: a conceptual framework, Patient Educ. Counsel. **6**(1):29, 1985.

This excellent paper presents a conceptual framework that individuals can use to assess their life-styles and plan for health-behavior changes. It can also be used by nurses who are developing programs to teach healthy life-style choices.

*Flaskerud, J.: Community mental health nursing: its unique role in the delivery of services to ethnic minorities, Perspect. Psychiatr. Care **20**(1):37, 1982.

The author reviews shared characteristics and values of various cultural groups and describes culture-related interventions that are most appropriate to the role of community mental health nurses.

Foulks, E. et al.: Current perspectives in cultural psychiatry, New York, 1977, Spectrum Publications.

This text presents a good overview of cultural issues in psychiatry. It is recommended reading for the interested nurse.

*Hoover, R., and Parnell, P.: Stress and coping, J. Psychosoc. Nurs. Ment. Health Serv. **22**(6):16, 1984.

This article describes an interesting program of four 1-hour sessions developed to help nonpsychiatric patients gain an understanding of stress and their coping methods.

Klerman, G. et al.: A debate on *DSM-III*, Am. J. Psychiatry **141**(4):539, April 1984.

The advantages and disadvantages of the DSM-III are debated in this series of four brief articles. It is recommended reading for all psychiatric nurses who integrate and use the DSM-III in their practice.

*Knab, S.: Polish Americans, J. Psychosoc. Nurs. Ment. Health Serv. **24**(1):31, 1986.

This article focuses on how Polish Americans deal with mental health problems, including the types of services they seek and how the role of the nurse is perceived.

Lazarus, R., and Folkman, S.: Stress, appraisal and coping, New York, 1984, Springer Publishing Co.

This text compiles all of Lazarus' work on stress and coping into one understandable volume. It is definitive reading for any nurse interested in mastering the area of stress and coping in practice or research.

*Leininger, M.: Reference sources for transcultural health and nursing, Thorofare, N.J., 1984, Slack Inc.

This is a comprehensive, ready-to-use bibliography of health-related sources from transcultural nursing, anthropology, and other fields contributing to cross-cultural health care.

---

*Asterisk indicates nursing reference.

*Miller, T.: Life events scaling: clinical methodological issues, Nurs. Res. **30**(5):316, 1981.

This article examines (1) research evidence addressing the assessment of life events, (2) prominent scales for the measurement of stress in life events, and (3) various issues, problems, and implications for clinical and research application. A good review of a timely issue.

*Minrath, M.: Breaking the race barrier, J. of Psychosoc. Nurs. Ment. Health Serv. **23**(8):19, 1985.

Specific issues are addressed in this article about breaking the race barrier between white therapists and ethnic minority patients. It is one of the few psychiatric nursing articles to address this issue directly.

Ness, R., and Wintrob, R.: Folk healing: a description and synthesis, Am. J. Psychiatry **138**(11):1477, 1981.

This is an excellent review of four systems of folk healing that have evolved in different cultural groups in the United States: faith healing, rootwork, curanderism, and espiritismo.

*Orque, M., Bloch, B. and Monrrov, L.: Ethnic nursing care, St. Louis, 1983, The C.V. Mosby Co.

This book explains different cultural approaches that will improve patient care to people of various cultural backgrounds. It is worthwhile reading for all nurses.

*Panzarine, S.: Coping: conceptual and methodological issues, Adv. Nurs. Sci. 7(4):49, 1985.

Many aspects of coping are reviewed in this article with attention given to the complexity of the coping construct and the need for more rigorous clinical research in the area by nurses.

Pedersen, P., Sartorius, N., and Marsella, A.: Mental health services: the cross-cultural context, Beverly Hills, Calif., 1984, Sage Publishers.

This is advanced reading for the nurse who wishes to explore culture-general and culture-specific approaches to overcoming ethnocentrism in psychiatric-mental health care.

*Schlesinger, R.R.: Cross-cultural psychiatry: the applicability of Western Anglo psychiatry to Asian-Americans of Chinese and Japanese ethnicity, J. Psychosoc. Nurs. **19**(9):26, 1981.

This excellent study focuses on Asian-Americans of the East Asian group and investigates the applicability of Western psychiatry to this particular cultural group. Stimulating and enlightening reading.

Sue, D.: Counseling the culturally different: theory and practice, New York, 1981, John Wiley & Sons, Inc.

Attention all psychiatric nurses who are working with patients from different cultures—this book is necessary reading. It is one of the few texts devoted to this topic that approaches it from an integrated conceptual framework. Specific chapters concern Asian-Americans, blacks, Hispanics, and American Indians.

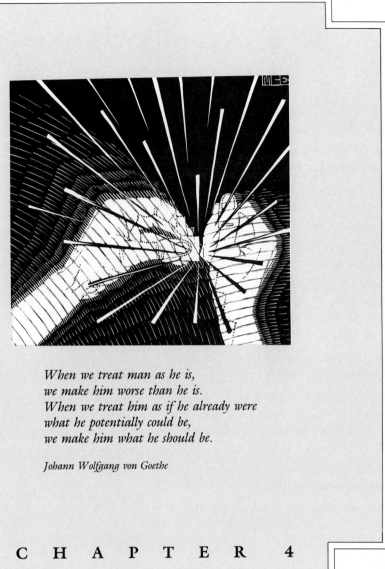

When we treat man as he is,
we make him worse than he is.
When we treat him as if he already were
what he potentially could be,
we make him what he should be.

Johann Wolfgang von Goethe

C H A P T E R   4

THE THERAPEUTIC NURSE-PATIENT RELATIONSHIP

LEARNING OBJECTIVES

After studying this chapter, the student should be able to:

- state the nature and goals of the therapeutic nurse-patient relationship.

- discuss six personal qualities needed by the nurse to be an effective helper.

- describe the tasks of the nurse and particular problems that may arise in each of the four phases of the relationship process.

- relate the relevance of communication theory to nursing.

- compare and contrast the verbal and nonverbal levels of communication in types of behavior, effectiveness, factors limiting correct interpretation, and implications for nursing care.

- identify the three elements of the communication process.

- analyze the structural and transactional analysis models of the communication process with respect to the components of each and the communication problems they reveal.

- define and give examples of 12 therapeutic communication techniques.

- describe how each of the responsive dimensions of genuineness, respect, empathic understanding, and concreteness can be demonstrated by the nurse in a therapeutic relationship.

- describe how each of the action dimensions of confrontation, immediacy, nurse self-disclosure, catharsis, and role playing can be demonstrated by the nurse in a therapeutic relationship.

- define the following therapeutic impasses and identify nursing interventions that can effectively deal with them: resistance, transference, and countertransference.

- discuss the goals of supervision and the ways in which therapy and supervision are parallel processes.

- demonstrate increasing effectiveness in using therapeutic relationship skills with psychiatric patients.

- identify directions for future nursing research.

- select appropriate readings for further study.

Nature of the relationship

The therapeutic nurse-patient relationship is a mutual learning experience and a corrective emotional experience for the patient. It is predicated on Sullivan's observation "We are all more human than otherwise." In this relationship the nurse uses personal attributes and specified clinical techniques in working with the patient to bring about insight and behavioral change. In general, the goals of a therapeutic relationship are directed toward the growth of the patient and include the following:

1. Self-realization, self-acceptance, and an increased genuine self-respect
2. A clear sense of personal identity and an improved level of personal integration
3. An ability to form intimate, interdependent, interpersonal relationships with a capacity to give and receive love
4. Improved functioning and increased ability to satisfy needs and achieve realistic personal goals

To achieve these goals, various aspects of the patient's life experiences will be explored during the course of the relationship. The nurse will allow for the patient's expression of perceptions, thoughts, and feelings and relate these to observed and reported actions. Areas of conflict and anxiety will be clarified. It is also important for the nurse to identify and maximize the ego strengths of the patient and to encourage socialization and family relatedness. Problems of communication will be corrected and maladaptive behavior patterns modified as the patient tests out new patterns of behavior and coping mechanisms.

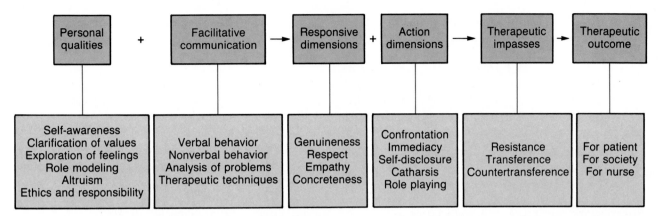

Fig. 4-1. Elements affecting the nurse's ability to be therapeutic.

■ Characteristics

The nature of the nurse-patient relationship is characterized by the mutual growth of two individuals who "dare" to become related to discover love, growth, and freedom. It is an I-thou relationship,[9] or an authentic relationship between two people who are in the process of becoming. The uniqueness of each is valued, and there is respect for differing values. There is mutual satisfaction derived and the world of each is enlarged and enriched by the other.

The communication is a dialogue or discussion, not a monologue, as deeply significant convictions are shared. The reality and worth of the patient are affirmed, which allows him to grasp and more fully define his ego identity. This requires the nurse to be open to experiences and willing to disclose aspects of his or her own being to the patient. Rogers summarizes the characteristics of helping relationships that facilitate growth in the following series of questions:

1. Can I *be* in some way which will be perceived by the other person as trustworthy, as dependable or consistent in some deep sense?
2. Can I be expressive enough as a person that what I am will be communicated unambiguously?
3. Can I let myself experience positive attitudes toward this other person—attitudes of warmth, caring, liking, interest, and respect?
4. Can I be strong enough as a person to be separate from the other?
5. Am I secure enough within myself to permit him his separateness?
6. Can I let myself enter fully into the world of his feelings and personal meaning and see these as he does?
7. Can I be acceptant of each facet of the other person which he presents to me? Can I receive

him as he is? Can I communicate this attitude? Or can I only receive him conditionally, acceptant of some aspects of his feelings and silently or openly disapproving of others?
8. Can I act with sufficient sensitivity in the relationship that my behavior will not be perceived as a threat?
9. Can I free him from the threat of external evaluation?
10. Can I meet this other individual as a person who is in the process of *becoming,* or will I be bound by his past and my past?[56:50-51]

All nurses working with patients may ask themselves these questions and must accept responsibility for the progress of the relationship. The therapeutic nurse-patient relationship is a complex one that can be analyzed in many different ways. Various elements and therapeutic dynamics of it merit further exploration. These include the nurse as helper, phases of the relationship, facilitative communication, responsive and action dimensions, therapeutic impasses, and effectiveness of the nurse. The interplay among the elements that produce a therapeutic outcome is shown in Fig. 4-1. The rest of this chapter will analyze each of these elements.

The nurse as helper

Helping others is a function of all concerned people, and it is not limited to health professionals. Neither is there a cluster of traits that describes a helping person who is universally effective. Nurses, however, as helpers, must be therapeutic in their care, since the goal of nursing is to facilitate the patient's positive adaptation as a unique individual to the stress he is experiencing.

The principal helping tool the nurse can use in her practice is herself. Thus self-analysis becomes the first building block in being able to provide quality nursing care. It has been suggested that nurses as professionals have become impersonal and detached. Is it possible that nurses are alienated from their true selves and do not allow patients the freedom to express all aspects of themselves? Jourard believes that during the socialization process into nursing, the nurse's spontaneity is destroyed and she becomes detached from her real self:

> Now, if a nurse is afraid or even ignorant of her own self, she is highly likely to be threatened by a patient's real-self expressions. . . . A nurse who is more aware of the breadth and depth of her own real self is in a much better position to empathize with her patients and to encourage (or at least not block) their self-disclosures.[35:184]

Research on counselor and teacher effectiveness suggests some essential qualities associated with being able to help others. These can be viewed as necessary characteristics for all nurses who wish to be therapeutic. It is hoped that by describing these qualities in some detail, the nurse will be able to set goals for future growth.

■ Awareness of self

There is universal agreement among theorists and practitioners that helpers need to be able to answer the question "Who am I?" The nurse who cares for the biological, psychological, and sociocultural needs of patients will be exposed to a broad range of human experiences. The nurse must learn to deal with anxiety, anger, sadness, and joy in helping patients at all intervals of the health-illness continuum.

Self-awareness has been identified as the key component of the growth-producing, psychiatric nursing experience.[39] The nurse's goal is the attainment of authentic, open, and personal communication. The nurse must be able to examine personal feelings and reactions, as well as his or her actions as a professional provider of care. A firm understanding and acceptance of self will allow the nurse to acknowledge a patient's differences and uniqueness.

A holistic nursing model of self-awareness has been identified by Campbell.[13] It consists of four, main interconnected parts—the psychological, physical, environmental, and philosophical components.

1. The *psychological* component of self-awareness includes knowledge of one's emotions, motivations, self-concept, and personality. Being psychologically self-aware means being sensitive to one's feelings and the external emotional stressors that affect those feelings.
2. The *physical* component of the self is the knowledge of personal and general physiology, one's bodily sensations, one's body image, and the physical potentials that one is capable of attaining.
3. The *environmental* aspect of the self consists of one's social environment, relationships with others, and knowledge of the relationship between humans and nature.
4. The *philosophical* component refers to the sense that one's life has meaning. A sense of meaning involving self-awareness is a personal philosophy of life and death that may or may not include a formulation of a superior being but which does take into account the world in which one lives and the ethics of the behavior that evolves from it.

Together, these components provide a model that can be used to promote the self-awareness and self-growth of both nurses and the patients for whom they care.

■ INCREASING SELF-AWARENESS.

No one ever completely knows his inner self. The Johari Window shown in Fig. 4-2 illustrates this idea.[45] Quadrant 1 is the open quadrant, which includes the behaviors, feelings, and thoughts known to the individual and those around him. Quadrant 2 is called the blind quadrant because it includes all those things which others know, but the individual does not know. Quadrant 3 is the hidden quadrant, and it includes those things which only the individual knows about himself. Quadrant 4 is the unknown quadrant, which contains aspects of the self unknown to the individual and others. Altogether, these quadrants represent the total self. The following three principles may help one understand how the self functions in this representation:

1. A change in any one quadrant will affect all other quadrants.
2. The smaller the first quadrant, the poorer the communication.
3. Interpersonal learning means that a change has taken place so that quadrant 1 is larger, and one or more of the other quadrants are smaller.[45:14]

The process of increasing self-awareness is now evident. The goal is to enlarge the area of quadrant 1, while reducing the size of the other three quadrants. The process of increasing knowledge of self is begun by **listening to oneself.** This means allowing oneself to experience genuine emotions, identify and accept personal needs, and move one's body in free, joyful, and spontaneous ways. It includes exploring one's own thoughts, feelings, memories, and impulses:

> I am most alive when I am open to all the many facets of my inner living—desires, emotions, the flow of ideas, body

sensations, relationships, reasoning, forethought, concern for others, my sense of values and all else within me. I am most alive when I can let myself experience and genuinely realize all of these facets even as I am truly feeling and expressing my wholeness.[10:276]

The next step in the process is to reduce the size of quadrant 2 by **listening to and learning from others.** Knowledge of oneself is not possible without association with other people. As a person relates to others, he broadens his perception of self. But such learning requires active listening and openness to the feedback others provide. The final step involves reducing the size of quadrant 3 by **self-disclosing,** or revealing to others important aspects of oneself. As Jourard states, "No man can come to know himself except as an outcome of disclosing himself to another person. Self-disclosure is a symptom of personality health and a means of achieving healthy personality."[35:6]

Compare *A* and *B* of Fig. 4-3. *A* represents a person with little self-awareness. His behaviors and feelings would tend to be limited in variety and scope. *B*, however, shows an individual with great openness to the world. Much of his potential is being developed and realized. He has an increased capacity for experiences of all kinds—joy, hate, work, and love. He has few defenses and can interact more spontaneously and honestly with others. This configuration represents a worthy goal for the nurse to attain for herself and others. The consequences of being attuned with the inward sense of self are greater integration of the many aspects of one's being, greater feelings of vitality, better mobilization for action, more committed choices, and more authenticity in relationships.

■ **THE NURSE AND SELF-GROWTH.** It is frequently assumed that because a nursing student has taken some courses in the behavioral sciences, she is able to use herself in a therapeutic manner in the clinical setting. Most nursing textbooks that describe the nursing process include a paragraph or two, stressing the importance of self-awareness in quality nursing care. The process and components of self-growth for the nurse are never described. A student who took the initiative to seek out this information would discover that the nursing literature is seriously lacking in references that develop in depth the concept of self-awareness and its application to the nurse. The self-concept of the patient is treated in a similarly cursory and general way. These omissions convey an implicit message to the nursing student: self-analysis is commendable, but a token assessment will suffice. To further reinforce this message, the student's curriculum is burdened with tasks and reports that allow little time for quiet contemplation leading to self-growth.

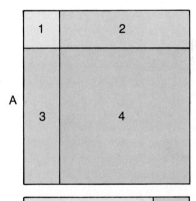

Fig. 4-2. Johari Window. Each quadrant, or windowpane, describes one aspect of the self. (From Sundeen, S.J. et al.: Nurse-client interaction: implementing the nursing process, ed. 3, St. Louis, 1985, The C.V. Mosby Co.)

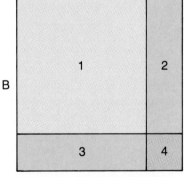

Fig. 4-3. Johari Windows showing varying degrees of self-awareness. **A,** Person with little self-understanding. **B,** Individual with great self-awareness. (From Sundeen, S.J. et al.: Nurse-client interaction: implementing the nursing process, ed. 3, St. Louis, 1985, The C.V. Mosby Co.)

It is necessary that nurses have the time to explore and define the many facets of their personalities. If nursing does involve perceiving, feeling, and thinking, nursing students should have the time and opportunity to study the basics of their experiences. Authenticity in relationships must be learned. For the nurse to do this, it is first necessary to experience openness and authenticity in relationships with instructors and supervisors. Rogers has stated that one might enhance another's personal growth by accepting this person as an individual and by viewing the world as it appears through his eyes.[56] The student and instructor can mutually participate in a relationship that accepts and respects individual differences. By acting as role models, instructors can facilitate students' self-awareness, increase their level of functioning, stimulate more self-direction, and enable them to cope more effectively with the stressors of life.

Authenticity also involves being truthful and open to exploring one's thoughts, needs, emotions, values, defenses, actions, communications, problems, and goals. In the process of becoming a nurse, the student has many new experiences providing opportunities for self-learning. Feelings about them should be focused on and discussed. The student might enter clinical settings with high ideals and unrealistic images. Perhaps she views nurses as "miracle workers" who are all knowing and all caring in their mission. During initial encounters the student may feel fearful, anxious, and inadequate, and may wonder how she will ever acquire the necessary knowledge. The student might devalue her ability and feel that she is imposing on her patients. Both her expectations and abilities should be analyzed to raise her self-esteem and reinforce her capabilities. At another time, she may identify closely with the patient and feel anger at the impersonal system and unresponsive personnel. Her anger should be identified, verbalized, and accepted. Only then can she analyze how she expresses anger and how these feelings can be resolved in a constructive manner.

It is not easy to embark on a career in nursing while still in adolescence. As a nurse, the student will be faced with many adult responsibilities. The student will be forced to face disease, bizarre behavior, complex problems, and even death when most of one's friends are focusing on youth, enjoyment, and the future. This might alienate her from some friends and trigger feelings of despair and self-doubt. Her feelings of loneliness and sadness should be shared, so that she can experience the benefit of an interpersonal relationship in working through her own needs.

The development of self-awareness by the nurse must be a self-initiated process. The nurse is an active participant in analyzing thoughts, communications, and relationships with others. Because it is difficult to be participant and observer at the same time, other ways of collecting data should be used. Tape recordings provide an opportunity for the student to review communications and study them more closely. Videotapes give feedback regarding nonverbal messages as well as tone and inflection. Maintaining a diary allows for the expression of feelings, the description of perceptions of the student's self-concept, and comments on the student's level of self-esteem.

This introspection should also be accompanied by self-disclosure. Sharing perceptions with others allows the nurse to gain new information and evolve new insights. The interaction with the analysis may be written in the form of a process recording.[69] This disciplines the nurse to look beyond the obvious and take the time to explore feelings. The instructor can review the recording with the student and identify areas that may have been overlooked or blocked.

Throughout this growing process, the student needs the support and guidance of an instructor. Together, they can analyze the student's behavior; the student can then assess personal strengths and limitations. It is often helpful to share these experiences with a peer group. Because students are all in a similar situation, they are able to empathize, criticize, and support each other as they learn, together, more about themselves.

Finally, the process of self-awareness is a painful one. It is not easy or pleasant to objectively examine one's self, particularly when what one finds conflicts with one's self-ideal. But, like many painful experiences, it presents a challenge: accept these limitations of the self or change the behaviors that support them. Choices such as this are the catalysts for growth and stimulate new responses to the question "Who am I?"

■ Clarification of values

In addition to knowing who they are, nurses should be able to describe "What is important to me?" This awareness aids the nurse in being honest with herself and avoiding the unwarranted and unethical use of patients to meet personal needs. Although the nurse-patient relationship involves mutual growth and satisfaction, the needs of the patient always take precedence. Nurses should have enough sources of satisfaction and security in their nonprofessional life to avoid the temptation of using their patient for the pursuit of personal satisfaction or security. If they do not have sufficient personal fulfillment, they should realize it, and their sources of dissatisfaction should be clarified so that they do not interfere with the success of the nurse-patient relationship.

■ **VALUE SYSTEMS.** Values are the concepts that a person holds worthy in his own personal life. They are formed as a result of one's life experiences with family, friends, culture, education, work, and relaxation. The word "value" has positive connotations, since it denotes worth or significance. Yet values also imply negatives. If we value one thing, such as honesty, then it follows that we do not value its opposite, such as dishonesty. Areas in which people are likely to hold strong values include religious beliefs, sexual preferences, family ties, other ethnic groups, and sex-role beliefs.

Value systems, however, are more than statements of what one treasures or highly regards. They provide the framework, either consciously or unconsciously, for many of one's daily decisions and actions. By being aware of one's value system, the nurse can more readily identify situations in which she is involved in a value system conflict. Clarification of values also provides some insurance against the tendency to project values onto another. Many therapeutic relationships test the nurse's values. If a patient is describing a sexual behavior that the nurse finds unacceptable, or if the patient is talking about divorce and the nurse strongly believes that marriage contracts should not be broken, or if the patient is a "born-again" Christian but the nurse has no belief in God or religion, how does the nurse respond? Can the nurse maintain personal values and still accept those of the patient? Can she empathize and help the patient problem solve, while being aware of personal values and natural tendancies to project those values?

■ **VALUE CLARIFICATION PROCESS.** Understanding one's values may be promoted by *value clarification.* It is a method developed by Raths, Harmin, and Simon[55] and adapted to nursing by Uustal,[72] whereby a person can discover his own values by assessing, exploring, and determining what one's personal values are and what priority they hold in one's personal decision making. It is a growth-producing process that promotes self-understanding and permits one to behave in ways appropriate to one's personal value priorities. Value clarification does not tell an individual what his values should be or what values he should live by. To avoid the imposition of values, value clarification focuses exclusively on the process of valuing or how people come to have the values they have.

Seven criteria have been identified by Raths to be used in determining whether a person is actually holding a value or not. These criteria should be considered in relation to a person's strongest value and tested against his own definition of a value. They are broadly grouped into the following three steps:

Choosing   1. Freely
            2. From alternatives

            3. After thoughtful consideration of the consequences of each alternative
Prizing   4. Cherishing, being happy with the choice
            5. Willing to affirm the choice publicly
Acting   6. Doing something with the choice
            7. Repeatedly, in some pattern of life[55]

The first three criteria, those of **choosing,** rely on the person's cognitive abilities; the next two criteria, **prizing,** emphasize the emotional or affective level; the last two criteria, **acting,** have a behavioral focus.

It has been found that simple exposure to the value clarification process causes change in people. Rokeach[58] contends that change takes place when the person becomes disturbed emotionally as a result of realizing the existence of certain contradictions in his value system. To eliminate the inevitable self-dissatisfaction that follows such a realization, the person will realign his values to coincide with his new self-conception.

■ **THE MATURE VALUING PROCESS.** Rogers has described the valuing process in the mature person.[56] He does not view it as an easy or simple thing. Rather, the process is complex, the choices often perplexing and difficult, and there is no guarantee that the choice made will prove to be self-actualizing. The valuing process in the mature person has the following characteristics[37]:

1. It is fluid and flexible, based on the particular moment and the degree to which the moment is experienced as enhancing, enriching, and actualizing. Values are not held rigidly but are continually changing.
2. The valuing experience is highly differentiated, that is, tied to a particular time and experience.
3. The locus of evaluation in the valuing process is firmly established within the person. It is his own experience that provides the value information. Although he is open to all the evidence that he can obtain from other sources, he views it as outside evidence that is not as significant as his own responses. The psychologically mature adult trusts and uses the wisdom of himself.
4. In the valuing process, the person is open to the immediacy of his experiences, trying to sense and clarify all its complex meanings. However, the immediate impact of the moment is colored by experiences from the past and conjecture about the future. Thus past and future are in the present moment and enter into the valuing process.

■ **Exploration of feelings**

It is often assumed that helping others requires complete objectivity and detachment from one's feelings. This is definitely not true. Complete objectivity and detachment from one's feelings describes someone who is unresponsive, false, unapproachable, impersonal, and alienated from oneself—qualities that impede or prohibit the establishment of a therapeutic relationship. What is desired is that the nurse be open to her feelings, aware of them, and in control of them so that they can be used in helping patients.

Nurses, as people, are feeling all the time, and these feelings serve an important purpose. They are barometers for feedback about ourselves and our relationships with others. They are useful, serve adaptive purposes, and are part of our learning experience. Gaylin believes:

Feelings are the instruments of rationality. . . . They are fine tunings directing the ways in which we will meet and manipulate our environment. . . . Mental illness is usually a mere disarray of the ingredients of survival. All that is necessary is rearrangement. Feelings are internal directives essential for human life.[24:3-7]

While helping others, nurses will experience many feelings—elation at seeing a patient improve, disappointment when a patient regresses, unappreciation when a patient refuses help, and anger in response to the patient who is demanding or manipulative. Feelings of power can arise when patients express strong dependence on the nurse or indicate that the nurse has influence over them. When patients express profuse gratitude to the nurse, she must wonder if the patients believe they helped themselves or whether the nurse did it for them.

If the nurse is open to her own feelings, she has access to two important pieces of information, how she is responding to the patient and how she is appearing to him. While talking to a patient, the nurse should be aware of her response to him. Despite his words, she might perceive a strong sense of despair or anger. Her feelings are valuable clues to the patient's problems and should be incorporated in her care for him. So too, the nurse should be aware of the feeling she is conveying to the patient. Is her mood one of hopelessness or contempt? If the nurse views feelings as barometers and feedback instruments, her effectiveness as a helper will

■ Ability to serve as model

Formal helping is a strong influence process and nurses do function as models to their patients, whether they want to or not. Much research has shown the power of models for acquiring socially adaptive, as well as maladaptive, behaviors. This imposes the obligation on the nurse to model adaptive and growth-producing behavior. If a nurse has a chaotic personal life, such as

one characterized by stormy intimate relationships, drug abuse, or conflictual parental ties, it will be evident in her work with patients. Not only will it decrease the effectiveness of care, but the nurse's credibility as a helper and the validity of care are likely to be questioned. The nurse may object to this with claims that she is able to separate her personal from her professional life, but in psychiatry, this is not possible because psychiatric nursing *is* the therapeutic use of self.

This is not to imply, however, that the nurse must be totally conforming to local community norms or must live an idyllic placid life. What is suggested is that the effective nurse has a fulfilling and satisfying personal life that is not dominated by conflict, distress, or denial and that his or her approach to life conveys a sense of growing and adapting.

■ Altruism

It is vital for nurses to have an idea of "Why do I want to help others?" This does not necessitate an extensive analysis of motives, but rather an awareness that one is acting for oneself, as well as for the value of the patient. Obviously, an effective helper is interested in people and tends to help out of a deep love for humanity, which is focused on a particular person or group of people. It is also true that everyone seeks a certain amount of personal satisfaction and fulfillment from their work. The goal is to maintain a balance between these two needs. Helping motives have the potential of becoming destructive tools in the hands of naive or zealous users.

Another danger lies in subscribing to an extreme view of altruism. Altruism can be defined as concern for the welfare of others. It does not mean that because one works out of a sense of altruism, one should not expect adequate compensation and recognition. It does not mean that one must practice extreme denial or self-sacrifice. The desire to help humanity is not in conflict with the desire for a satisfying life. In fact, only if the nurse's personal needs have been appropriately met can she expect to be maximally therapeutic.

Finally, a sense of altruism can also apply to more general social support and change motives. Altruism is necessary for society to survive. Activist helpers are needed who are primarily concerned with changing social conditions to meet human welfare needs. One goal of all helping professionals should be to create a people-serving and growth-facilitating society. As such, a legitimate and necessary role for the nurse is to work to change the larger structure and process of society in ways that will promote the individual's health and welfare.

■ Sense of ethics and responsibility

Personal beliefs about people and society can serve as conscious guidelines for action. When these ethical principles are shared among helpers, they are written down and codified. The Code for Nurses (see Chapter 7) reflects common values regarding nurse-patient relationships and responsibilities and serves as a frame of reference for all nurses in their judgments about patient welfare and social responsibility.

For professional psychiatric nurses, decisions are a part of one's daily functioning. Responsible ethical choice involves accountability, risk, commitment, and justice. Sigman identifies the following elements of responsible ethical behavior for the nurse[65]:

1. A moral principle exists that involves a moral obligation or duty to do or to refrain from doing something that is within the power of the person to do, or is such that the person can do otherwise.
2. Some source of responsibility is involved as well as a source of reward, praise, or punishment for responsible actions.
3. The cause of the behavior is internal to the individual, and he or she is not compelled to act by others.
4. The behavior itself is not done through igno-

rance, is respectful of the laws, maintains one's integrity and freedom of choice, and attempts to do justice.

The concept of responsible ethical choice, therefore, involves a dynamic decision-making process for the nurse that incorporates one's values, one's judgments, and one's actual choice.

Related to one's sense of ethics is the need for the nurse to assume responsibility for her own behavior. This involves knowing one's own limitations and strengths and being accountable for them. The nurse, as a member of a health care team, has the knowledge and expertise of other people readily available and should use them appropriately. Responsibility implies maturity, and as a quality of an effective nurse it is essential.

Phases of the relationship

A vital characteristic of the nurse-patient relationship is the sharing of behaviors, thoughts, and feelings to establish a context of therapeutic intimacy. Coad-Denton[17] describes this as the use of the nursing process to support the patient as he explores his areas of needs, solves problems, and acquires new coping skills. As such, it is distinct from social superficiality and imposes specific expectations on the nurse. Table 4-1 identifies seven components of relationships in general and con-

TABLE 4-1

CONTRAST BETWEEN SOCIAL SUPERFICIALITY AND THERAPEUTIC INTIMACY

Components of relationship	Social superficiality	Therapeutic intimacy
Mutual self-disclosure	Variable	Patient: self-disclosure; nurse: self-disclosure in terms of response to patient only
Focus of conversation	Unknown to participants	Known to nurse and patient
Pertinence of topic	Social, business, generalized, impersonal	Personal and relevant to nurse and patient
Relationship of experiences to topic	Sense of uninvolvement and use of indirect knowledge	Sense of involvement and use of direct knowledge
Time orientation	Past and future	Present
Use of feelings	Sharing of feelings discouraged	Sharing of feelings encouraged by nurse
Recognition of individual worth	Not acknowledged	Fully acknowledged

From Coad-Denton, A.: Therapeutic superficiality and intimacy. In Longo, D., and Williams, R., editors: Psychosocial nursing: assessment and intervention, New York, 1978, Appleton-Century-Crofts.

trasts social superficiality and therapeutic intimacy on these components.

This is not to assume, however, that these elements emerge simultaneously or at the same time. Rather, they evolve as the nurse moves through the various phases of the therapeutic relationship with the patient. Four sequential phases of the relationship process have been identified: preinteraction phase; introductory, or orientation, phase; working phase; and termination phase. Each phase builds on the preceding one and is characterized by specific tasks. These phases will be described only as they apply to the nurse working with a psychiatric patient. Other sources present detailed information on basic elements of the relationship process.[69,70]

■ Preinteraction phase

■ **CONCERNS OF NEW NURSES.** The preinteraction phase begins before the nurse's first contact with the patient. Her initial task is one of self-exploration as she analyzes her own feelings, fantasies, and fears. In her first experience working with psychiatric patients the nurse will bring with her the misconceptions and prejudices of the general public. (See accompanying box that lists some common concerns of psychiatric nursing students.) Some of these feelings and fears are common to all novices, and an overriding one is usually anxiety or nervousness, which is provoked by new experiences of any kind. A related feeling is ambivalence or uncertainty, since the nurse may see the need for working with these patients but feel unclear about his or her own ability or motivations.

This may be compounded by a threat to the nurse's role identification, which is precipitated by the informal nature of psychiatric settings. Usually psychiatric patients do not wear hospital gowns or clothing, the staff do not wear uniforms, and the staff and patients mingle in a casual, relaxed, and apparently unstructured way. A common first reaction among students is a feeling of panic when they realize that they "can't tell the patients from the staff." The student's discomfort may be made more acute if one of the patients mistakes her for a newly admitted patient. Finally, it is unsettling for many students to give up their uniform, stethoscope, and scissors, since it dramatically emphasizes that, in this nursing setting, the most important tools are one's ability to communicate, empathize, and problem solve. Without a tangible physical illness to care for with treatments and activities, new students are likely to feel acutely self-conscious and hesitant about introducing themselves to a patient and initiating a conversation.

Many nurses express feelings of inadequacy and fears of hurting or exploiting the patient. They may worry about saying the wrong thing, which might drive

---

Common Concerns of Psychiatric Nursing Students

- Acutely self-conscious
- Afraid of being rejected by the patients
- Anxious because of the newness of the experience
- Concerned about personally overidentifying with psychiatric patients
- Doubtful of the effectiveness of one's skills or coping ability
- Fearful of physical danger or violence
- Inadequate in one's therapeutic use of self
- Suspicious of psychiatric patients stereotyped as "different"
- Threatened in one's nursing role identity
- Uncertain about one's ability to make a unique contribution
- Uncomfortable about the lack of physical tasks and treatments
- Vulnerable to emotionally painful experiences
- Worried about hurting the patient psychologically

---

the patient "over the brink," or wonder if, with their limited knowledge and experience, they will be of any value. They may wonder how they can help or if they can really make a difference. Some nurses perceive the plight of psychiatric patients as hopeful, others perceive it as hopeless.

A common fear of nurses is related to the stereotype of psychiatric patients as abusive and violent. Because this is the picture portrayed by the media, many nurses are afraid of being physically hurt by a patient's outburst of aggressive behavior. Other nurses fear being psychologically hurt by a patient through rejection or silence. A final fear is related to the nurse's questioning of her own mental health. She may fear mental illness and worry that exposure to psychiatric patients might cause her to lose control of her own grasp on reality. Nurses who are working on their own crises of identity and intimacy may fear overidentifying with patients and using patients to meet their own needs.

Clinical example 4-1 contains many of the feelings and fears expressed by one nursing student in the preinteraction phase of self-analysis as reported in the notes from her diary of her psychiatric rotation.

Schoffstall has described a method that can be used preclinically in the classroom setting to assess and reduce the anxiety of students who are about to begin their clinical experience in psychiatric nursing.[62] The pur-

CLINICAL EXAMPLE 4-1

When first told that I would have a clinical psychiatric nursing experience, I received this information with a blank mind. Mental overload, denial, repression, or whatever it was made me hear the words but put off dealing with it. Then, when given a chance to sort through my thoughts and feelings, I thought more about what this experience would entail. Having never been personally involved with any people who were psychiatrically ill before, I was unable to rely on past personal experiences. I did, however, have quite a "pseudo–knowledge base" from my novels, television, and movie encounters. Do places like the hospital in "One Flew Over the Cuckoo's Nest" really exist? Was the portrayal of "Sybil" accurate? How could I possibly help someone who has so many problems, like the boy in "Ordinary People"? I'm afraid these thoughts have raised more questions in me than they have answered.

Three things scare me the most about this experience. First, I feel that the behavior of a psychiatric patient is quite unpredictable. Would they get violent or aggressive without any warning? Would this aggression be directed toward me? If so, would I be hurt? Did I provoke them and was I wrong in my actions that caused this sudden shift? The second, related to the first, is my feeling of inadequacy. I've been exposed to physically ill people and have learned how to respond to them. But, the psychologically ill are almost totally alien to me. How can I help? What if I do, or say, or infer something they could take offense to. Will I have the patience to persevere? I just don't know, and my not knowing makes me even more nervous. My third fear is how seeing and being in contact with the psychiatrically ill will affect me. Although I know it's not contagious, the more exposure and knowledge I acquire in this area, the more I may begin to doubt my own stability and sanity. I mean adolescence hasn't been easy for me, and I feel like I'm just now beginning to see things more clearly and feel better about myself. Will this experience stir up any past fears and doubts and, if so, how will I handle it? I am beginning to realize that there is a fine line between sanity and insanity and that the psychiatric patients we'll meet have been unable to gather enough resources from within to cope with their problems. Help, reassurance, and understanding are their needs. I'm hoping I can help them . . . but I'm just not sure.

poses of the exercise were to identify student concerns and anxieties, identify factors that influence the nurse-patient relationship, provide information about the experience, and discuss the subjective experiences of the patient related to hospitalization and the psychiatric diagnosis. In a group setting, students were asked to anonymously write down a specific fantasy that they had about going to a psychiatric hospital or beginning their experience in psychiatric nursing. The fantasies were then read aloud, and the group discussed the content and feelings in the responses. In a similar group discussion, they were then asked how they thought patients felt about being hospitalized. The exercise was found to be an effective way to handle the reluctance of the students to express their concerns and increase their empathy toward psychiatric patients.

■ **SELF-ASSESSMENT.** Experienced nurses benefit by analyzing additional aspects of their practice. They may ask themselves the following questions:

- Do I label patients with the stereotype of a group?
- Is my need to be liked so great that I become angry or hurt when a patient is rude, hostile, or uncooperative?
- Am I afraid of the responsibility I must assume for the relationship and do I therefore limit my independent functions?
- Do I cover feelings of inferiority with a front of superiority?
- Do I require sympathy, warmth, and protection so much that I err by being too sympathetic or too protective toward patients?
- Do I fear closeness so much that I am indifferent, rejecting, or cold?
- Do I need to feel important and keep patients dependent on me?

The type of self-analysis that characterizes the preinteraction phase is a necessary task because, to be effective, nurses should have a reasonably stable self-concept and an adequate amount of self-esteem, engage in constructive relationships with others, and face reality to help patients do likewise. If they are aware of and in control of what they convey to their patients verbally and nonverbally, nurses can function as role models to their patients. To do this, however, some nurses abandon their own personal strengths and assume a facade of "professionalism." This facade is an alienation of their authentic self and, instead of increasing their effectiveness, it immobilizes them and acts as a barrier to establishing mutuality with patients.

All nurses possess professional assets and limitations. Therapeutic use of self means using and maximizing one's assets or strengths and minimizing one's limitations. Promoting a patient's self-realization and self-acceptance is facilitated by the nurse's acceptance of self and behaving in ways congruent with her own personality. Nurses receive feedback from patients, which can help them identify their strengths and assets. Self-analysis, peer review, and supervision provide opportunities to explore feelings and fears and develop useful insights into one's professional role. The nurse who is therapeutic uses this information and relates to patients in a natural, congruent, and relaxed manner.

Additional tasks of this phase include gathering data about the patient if information is available and planning for the first interaction with the patient. The nursing assessment is begun, but most of the work related to it is accomplished with the patient in the second phase of the relationship. The nurse reviews general goals of a therapeutic relationship and considers what she has to offer to the patient.

■ Introductory, or orientation, phase

It is during the introductory phase that the nurse and patient first meet. A primary concern of the nurse is to find out why the patient sought help and if he did so voluntarily. Burgess and Burns[11] described six categories of reasons why people seek psychiatric help and an appropriate nursing approach for each (see Table 4-2). Determining the patient's reason will directly influence the establishment of mutuality between the nurse and the patient. It forms the basis of the nursing assessment and helps the nurse focus on the patient's presenting problem and determine his motivation.

TABLE 4-2

ANALYSIS OF WHY PATIENTS SEEK PSYCHIATRIC HELP

Reasons for patients' seeking psychiatric care	Appropriate nursing approach	Sample response
Environmental change from home to hospital: They desire protection, comfort, rest, and freedom from demands of their usual home and work environments.	Emphasis should be placed on ability of environment to provide protection and comfort while healing process of mind occurs.	"Tell me what it was at home/on the job that made you feel so overwhelmed."
Nurturance: They wish for someone to care for them, cure their illnesses, and make them feel better.	Respond by acknowledging their nurturance needs and assuring them that help and caring are available to them.	"We're here to help you feel better."
Control: They are aware of their destructive impulses to themselves or others but lack internal control.	Offer person sources of internal control such as medication, if prescribed, and reinforce external controls available through services of staff.	"We're not going to let you hurt yourself. Tell us when these thoughts come to mind and someone will stay with you."
Psychiatric symptoms: They describe symptoms of depression, nervousness, or crying spells. They know they need psychiatric help and actively want to help themselves.	Ask for clarification of symptom and strive to understand life experiences of patient.	"I can see that you're nervous and upset. Can you tell me about how things are at home/on the job so I can better understand?"
Problem solving: They identify a specific problem or area of conflict and express desire to reason it out and change.	Help patient look at problem objectively, and utilize problem-solving process with him.	"How has drinking affected your life?"
Advised to come to hospital: Family member, friend, or health professional has convinced them to come to hospital. They may feel angry, ambivalent, or indifferent about being there.	Confirm facts surrounding his seeking of help and set limits appropriate to agency, ward, etc.	"I see that you're angry about being here. Perhaps as you become part of the ward community, you'll feel differently."

Modified from Burgess, A., and Burns, J.: Am. J. Nurs. **73:**314, 1973.

■ **FORMULATING A CONTRACT.** As the nurse relates with the patient in this phase of the relationship, the tasks are to establish a climate of trust, understanding, acceptance, and open communication and formulate a contract with the patient. The accompanying box lists the elements of a nurse-patient contract. The contract begins with the introduction of the nurse and patient, exchange of names, and explanation of roles. This is often omitted by the nurse who has determined the patient's name from another source, such as a chart, family member, or other clinician, and fails to introduce herself because of her anxiety, discomfort, or lack of recognition of the patient as an individual worthy of respect. An explanation of roles includes the responsibilities and expectations of the patient and nurse with a description of what the nurse can and cannot do. This is followed by a discussion of the purpose of the relationship in which the nurse emphasizes that the focus of it will be the patient, his life experiences, and areas of conflict. Because the establishment of the contract is a mutual process, it is a good opportunity to clarify misperceptions held by either the nurse or patient.

With the "who" and the "why" determined, the "where, when, and how long" are discussed. Where will the meetings be held? When and how often will they occur? How long will each be and how long will the series of meetings be? The conditions for termination should be reviewed and may include a specified length of time, attainment of mutual goals, or the discharge of the patient if he is hospitalized. The issue of confidentiality is an important one to discuss with the patient at this time. Confidentiality does not imply secrecy or the exclusive possession of information. Rather, it involves the disclosure of certain information to another specifically authorized person. This means that information about the patient will be shared with people who are directly involved in his care in the form of verbal reports and written notes. This is important in providing for the continuity and comprehensiveness of patient care and should be clearly explained to the patient.

Establishing a contract is a mutual process in which the patient participates as fully as possible. In some cases, such as with the psychotic or severely withdrawn patient, the patient may be unable to fully participate, and the nurse must take the initiative in establishing the contract. As the patient's contact with reality increases, the nurse should review the elements of the contract when appropriate and strive to attain mutuality.

It is also possible to use a written contracting model to work therapeutically with patients and groups. Loomis describes a formal treatment contract as an openly negotiated, clearly stated set of mutual expectations that indicate what the nurse and patient expect of each other regarding the patient's health care.[44] Such a contract establishes a set of shared objectives as well as an understanding of the structure and process of arriving at mutually determined outcomes. This model identifies four levels of change contracts (see Table 4-3). Each higher level implies the inclusion of all lower level contracts.

The first level or care contracts involve the provision of physical and emotional safety. Level II or social contracts deal primarily with behaviors and situations that can be brought under the conscious control of the patient. Level III or relationship contracts focus on the repetitive or cyclical nature of patient problems as demonstrated in their day-to-day relationships. Level IV contracts involve structural change and require intensive psychotherapy. The emphasis here is on reworking the entire pathological structure as well as the here-and-now relationship process. Nurse therapists entering into Level IV contracts require master's degree preparation and perhaps even specialized training in the theory and application of structural change treatment approaches. Since the level of contract can change over time, this contracting model allows the nurse and patient to evaluate their progress over time, renegotiate their work together, and determine the termination of a treatment relationship.

■ **EXPLORING FEELINGS.** Both the nurse and patient may experience some degree of discomfort and nervousness in this phase of the relationship because of its newness and the future expectations each person brings to it. The nurse may be well aware of personal anxieties and fears, but the difficulty inherent in the patient's role is often overlooked. Receiving help can be difficult from the patient's point of view for the following reasons:

Elements of a Nurse-Patient Contract

- Names of individuals
- Roles of nurse and patient
- Responsibilities of nurse and patient
- Expectations of nurse and patient
- Purpose of the relationship
- Meeting location
- Time of meetings
- Conditions for termination
- Confidentiality

TABLE 4-3

LEVELS OF CHANGE CONTRACTS

Level and type of contract	Focus of care	Nursing action
I. Care contracts	Physical safety Emotional safety Avoid predictable negative outcomes	Provide physical care Protect from loss of functional abilities
II. Social control contracts	Increase self-care activities Increase problem-solving ability Alteration in time structuring Alteration in reinforcement patterns	Crisis intervention Brief therapy
III. Relationship contracts	Relationship patterns Life-script decisions Traumatic early scenes	Insight work Cognitive restructuring Marital, family, or relationship counseling
IV. Structural change contracts	Parental modeling Persistent early injunctions	Script analysis Reparenting work Psychotherapy

From Loomis, M.: J. Psychosoc. Nurs. **23**(3):10, 1985.

1. It may be hard to admit one's difficulties, first to oneself and then to another, and to see them clearly.
2. It is not easy to trust strangers and be open with them.
3. Sometimes problems seem too large, too overwhelming, or too unique to share them easily.
4. Sharing one's problems with another person can pose a threat to one's sense of independence, autonomy, and self-esteem. Some may view this sharing as a sign of weakness or failure.
5. It is very difficult to commit oneself to change. Solving a problem involves thinking about some things that may be unpleasant, viewing life realistically, deciding on a plan of action, and then, most important, carrying out whatever it takes to actually bring about a change. These activities will place great demands on the energy and commitment of the patient.

If this is the first psychiatric experience for the nursing student, she may feel particularly stressed. Stacklum[67] identified a process that all such new students go through in the beginning of their relationships. In the first stage, they experience a moderate to severe level of anxiety characterized by selective inattention to instructions, obsession with detail, dissociation of theory from practice, and avoidance behavior.

Stage two is characterized by the students' use of the defense mechanisms of denial of the patients' problems and strong identification with them. Social conversation with the patients predominates, and nursing actions tend to be concrete and simple. In the next stage, the students question their own ability and experience feelings of anger and omnipotence. Hostility is often projected onto the staff.

From these early reactions, students hopefully progress to a beginning adjustment stage, which marks the transition into the working phase of the relationship. Students are now truly able to hear what the patient is saying, their anxiety is decreased, their interactions show more depth and insight, and their nursing actions become more realistic. A therapeutic process has begun.

The tasks of the nurse in the orientation phase of the relationship are to explore the patient's perceptions, thoughts, feelings, actions; identify pertinent patient problems; and mutually define specific goals to pursue. It is not uncommon for patients to display manipulative or testing behavior during this phase as they explore the nurse's consistency and intent. They may also evidence temporary regressions during the sessions as reactions to a large amount of self-disclosure in a previous meeting or to the anxiety created by a particular topic.

■ Working phase

During the working phase the major part of the therapeutic work is carried out. The nurse and patient explore relevant stressors and promote the development of insight in the patient by linking together his perceptions, thoughts, feelings, and actions. These insights should be translated into action and integrated into the life experiences of the individual. The nurse helps the patient to master his anxieties, increase his independence and self-responsibility, and develop constructive coping mechanisms. Actual behavioral change is the focus of this phase of the relationship.

Resistance behaviors are usually displayed by patients during this phase of the relationship because it contains the greater part of the problem-solving process. As the relationship develops, the patient panics when he recognizes his beginning feelings of closeness to the nurse and fears impending disintegration. His response is to cling to his defensive structures, and he resists all attempts of the nurse to move forward. An impasse or plateau in the relationship results. Since overcoming resistance behaviors is crucial to the progress of the therapeutic relationship, they will be discussed in greater detail later in this chapter.

■ Termination phase

Termination is one of the most difficult, but most critically important, phases of the therapeutic nurse-patient relationship. However, little has been researched or written regarding the process and outcome of termination:

Of all the phases of the psychotherapeutic process, the one which can produce the greatest amount of difficulty and create substantial problems for patient and therapist alike is the phase of termination. It is at this time when the impact of the meaning, in affective terms, of the course of therapy and the nature of the therapist-patient relationship is experienced most keenly, not only by the patient but also by the therapist.[61:77]

During this phase, learning is maximized for both the patient and nurse. It is a time to mutually exchange feelings and memories and to evaluate the patient's progress and goal attainment. Levels of trust and intimacy are heightened, which reflects on both the quality of the relationship and the sense of loss that is experienced by both. The accompanying box lists criteria identified by Campaniello that can be used to decide if the patient is ready to terminate.

Although mutuality between the patient and therapist is most often desired in deciding when to terminate, this is not always possible. Sometimes the reason is beyond the control of either person, such as when it is due to an institutional rule, the end of a clinical ro-

---

Criteria for Determining Patient Readiness for Termination[12]

1. The patient experiences relief from the presenting problem.
2. The patient's social function has improved, and his isolation has decreased.
3. The patient has strengthened his own ego functions and attained a sense of identity.
4. The patient employs more effective and productive defense mechanisms.
5. The patient has achieved the planned treatment goals.
6. An impasse has been reached in the therapist-patient relationship because of resistance or countertransference that cannot be worked through.

---

tation, or the eventual move of the therapist.

Regardless of the reason, the tasks of the nurse during this phase revolve around establishing the reality of the separation. Together the nurse and patient review the progress made in therapy and the attainment of specified goals. Feelings of rejection, loss, sadness, and anger are expressed and explored. The patient's dependency on the nurse should decrease, and there should be an increase in the interdependence of the patient with his environment and with significant others. It may be helpful to prepare the patient for termination by decreasing the number of visits, incorporating others in the meetings, or changing the location of the meetings. If this is done, the reasons behind the change should be clarified with the patient, so he does not interpret it as rejection by the nurse. It may also be appropriate to make referrals at this time for continued care or treatment.

One's understanding of the feelings that accompany termination can be enhanced by examining Fox, Nelson, and Bolman's comparison[22] of the phases in the termination process to the phases of grief work:

The first phase is a period of denial in which the person attempts to ward off either recognition of the loss or important feelings associated with it. The second, a phase that begins when the denial breaks down, is one of considerable emotional expression, usually of grief and sadness but often including anger and expressions of narcissistic hurt. The third phase is a prolonged period in which the reality of loss and the associated feelings of grief and anger are bit by bit worked through in the multitude of current life experiences that bring up memories of the lost person. To the extent that the mourner is able to perform this grief work successfully, he is gradually able to detach or free the emotional ties that are essential for finding new people or interests.*

In light of this comparison, it becomes evident that successful termination requires that the patient work through those feelings related to separation from emotionally significant persons. The nurse can help the patient to accomplish this by allowing him to experience and feel the effects of the anticipated loss, express those feelings generated by the impending separation, and relate his feelings to former symbolic or real losses.

■ **REACTIONS TO TERMINATION.** Patients may react to termination in a variety of ways. They may deny the separation or deny the significance of the relationship and impending separation. The inexperienced nurse might not see the reasons behind this denial and might feel rejected by the patient or believe she has failed him. Patients may express anger and hostility either overtly and verbally or covertly through lateness, missed meetings, or superficial talk. These patients may view the termination as personal rejection, which reinforces their negative self-concept. Patients who feel rejected by the nurse may terminate prematurely. By abruptly ending the relationship, they experience a sense of power and control and assert themselves by rejecting the nurse before she rejects them. It is also common to see the onset of symptoms and maladaptive behavior when termination approaches. In this way the patient regresses to his earlier behavior pattern and hopes to convince the nurse not to terminate because he still needs help.

If the nurse is aware of these possible reactions, she can anticipate them and discuss them with the patient should they occur. For some patients, termination is a critical therapeutic experience because many of their past relationships were terminated in a negative way that left them with unresolved feelings of abandonment, rejection, hurt, and anger. All these patient reactions have a similar goal—to cope with the anxiety about the separation and to delay the termination process.

Levinson[43] has identified five factors that can influence the reaction of the patient to termination:

1. The greater the degree of involvement the patient has had in the treatment and with the therapist, the more intense will be the nature of the reaction to termination.
2. Reaction to termination will vary with the degree of success and satisfaction the patient feels with the treatment.

3. The greater the degree of transference involvement and wished-for gratification or fulfillment of childlike wishes, the more intense will be the nature of the patient's reaction to termination.
4. Patients who have sustained earlier losses of significant persons in their lives will reexperience, as termination approaches, the arousal of affects and conflicts from those earlier periods.
5. Whether the patient has experienced key losses or not, his reaction to termination will be influenced by the level at which he has achieved mastery of the early separation–individuation crisis.

In addition to these, the patient's response will be significantly affected by the knowledge, skill, experience, and willingness of the nurse to remain open, sensitive, empathic, and responsive to the patient's changing needs. Helping the patient to work through and grow through the termination process is an essential goal of each nurse-patient relationship. It is important therefore that the nurse does not deny the reality of it to herself, nor allow herself to be manipulated by the patient into repeated delays or postponements. Particularly in this phase of the relationship, as in the orientation phase, the patient will be testing the nurse's judgment, and the issues of trust and acceptance will again predominate.

During the course of the relationship and with the attainment of nursing goals, the nurse and patient come to realize a growing sense of equality. The nurse perceives a similarity between herself and the patient, and the impending termination can be as difficult for the nurse as it is for the patient. It is necessary for the nurse to deal with her reaction to the various aspects of termination if she expects to make this a positive learning experience for herself and the patient. If the nurse can take the initiative and begin reviewing her thoughts, feelings, and experiences, she will be more aware of her own motivation, as well as more responsive to the needs of her patient. Schultz states the following:

When the student shares her own feelings and explains how she, too, feels the pain and separation, the patient can learn it is not he alone who needs to be dependent on others and to cling to successful relationships, but that life is a series of making and breaking relationships. The student and the patient learn that to be involved with other human beings is part of living, often a very satisfying part, but there is a time to love and a time to leave.... That allowing another to mourn with you, to share the agony of separation unashamedly, could be an answer to bridging some of the gulf between human beings in need of one another.[63:41-42]

Learning to bear the sorrow of the loss while incorporating positive aspects of the relationship into one's

---

*Copyright 1969, National Association of Social Workers, Inc. Reprinted with permission from Social Work, vol. 14, no. 4 (October 1969), p. 53.

life is the goal of termination for both the nurse and the patient in the therapeutic relationship.

The major tasks of the nurse during each phase of the nurse-patient relationship are summarized in Table 4-4.

Facilitative communication

Communication can facilitate the development of a therapeutic relationship or serve as a barrier to block its development. Nurses should understand the elements of the communication process and utilize specific skills or techniques that help the patient in working through the problem-solving process. According to Carkhoff and Truax, "The central ingredient of the psychotherapeutic process appears to be the therapist's ability to *perceive and communicate,* accurately and with sensitivity, the feelings of the patient and the meaning of those feelings."[16:285]

Every individual communicates constantly from birth until death. As Watzlawick and co-workers[73] have stated, all behavior is communication and all communication affects behavior. This reciprocity is central to the communication process. One of the most widely respected of the communication theorists is Ruesch. He has defined communication as "all those processes by which people influence one another."[59] Spitz is in agreement with the preceding theorists when he defines communication as "any perceivable behavioral change, intentional or not, directed or not, which helps one or more persons influence the perception, feelings, emotions, thoughts or actions of one or more persons, whether that influence is intentional or not."[66] The most prominent similarity among these three definitions is the focus on behavioral change and interpersonal influence.

The relevance of communication theory to nursing practice is quite apparent. First, communication is the vehicle for establishing a therapeutic relationship, since it involves conveying information and exchanging thoughts and feelings. Second, communication is the means by which people influence the behavior of another. Thus, it is critical to the successful outcome of nursing intervention, since the nursing process is directed toward promoting behavioral change in the direction of achieving a maximum level of wellness for the individual. Finally, communication is the relationship itself, since without it, a therapeutic nurse-patient relationship is not possible.

TABLE 4-4

NURSE'S TASKS IN EACH PHASE OF THE RELATIONSHIP PROCESS

Phase	Task
Preinteraction	Explore own feelings, fantasies, and fears Analyze own professional strengths and limitations Gather data about patient when possible Plan for first meeting with patient
Introductory or Orientation	Determine why patient sought help Establish trust, acceptance, and open communication Mutually formulate a contract Explore patient's thoughts, feelings, and actions Identify patient's problems Define goals with patient
Working	Explore relevant stressors Promote patient's development of insight and use of constructive coping mechanisms Overcome resistance behaviors
Termination	Establish reality of separation Review progress of therapy and attainment of goals Mutually explore feelings of rejection, loss, sadness, and anger and related behaviors

■ Verbal communication

Communication takes place on two levels: verbal and nonverbal. Verbal communication occurs through the medium of words, spoken or written. Taken alone, verbal communication can convey factual information accurately and efficiently. It is a less effective means of communicating feelings or nuances of meaning, and it represents only a small segment of total human communication.

Another limitation of verbal communication is that words can change meanings with different cultural groups or subgroups in a society. This is because words have both denotative and connotative meanings. The denotative meaning of a word is the concrete representation of it or its specific meaning. For example, the denotative meaning of the word "bread" is "a food made of a flour or grain dough which is kneaded, shaped, allowed to rise and baked." The connotative meaning of a word, in contrast, is its implied or suggested meaning. Thus the word "bread" can conjure up many different connotative or personalized meanings. Depending on a person's past experiences, preferences, and present frame of reference, he may be thinking of French bread, rye bread, a sesame seed roll, or perhaps pita bread. The phrase, "Give me some bread" can even have another meaning. When used as slang, it may be commonly understood to mean "give me some money." Once again, the characteristics of the speaker and the context in which the phrase is said influence the specific meaning of verbal language.

When communicating verbally, many people assume that they are both "on the same wavelength." But since words are only symbols, they seldom mean precisely the same thing to two people and, if the word represents an abstract idea such as "depressed" or "hurt," the chance of misunderstanding or misinterpretation may be quite great. In addition, many feeling states or personal thoughts cannot be put into words easily. A nurse who wishes to communicate effectively must be aware of the limitations and possible problems inherent with verbal language. She should strive to overcome them by validating her interpretation and incorporating information from the nonverbal level as well.

■ Nonverbal communication

Nonverbal communication includes everything that does not involve the spoken or written word, and it involves all of the five senses. It has been estimated that about 7% of meaning is transmitted by words; 38% is transmitted by paralinguistic cues, such as voice; and 55% is transmitted by body cues.[47] Nonverbal communication serves many functions in relating to another: supplementing, substituting, reinforcing, contradicting, and emphasizing verbal language; displaying affect; and regulating the flow of information. This level of communication is often unconsciously motivated and may more accurately indicate a person's meaning than the words he is saying. This is because people tend to verbalize what they think the receiver wants to hear, whereas less acceptable or more honest messages may be communicated simultaneously by the nonverbal route.

■ **TYPES OF NONVERBAL BEHAVIORS.** Various types of nonverbal behaviors have been identified in the literature. Of these, five categories of nonverbal communication will be briefly described. **Vocal cues,** or paralinguistic cues, include all the noises and sounds that are extraspeech sounds. Some examples include pitch, tone of voice, quality of voice, loudness or intensity, rate and rhythm of talking, and unrelated nonverbal sounds, such as laughing, groaning, nervous coughing, and sounds of hesitation ("um," "uh"). These are particularly vital cues of emotion and can be powerful conveyors of information.

Action cues are body movements that are sometimes referred to as kinetics. They include automatic reflexes, posture, facial expression, gestures, mannerisms, and actions of any kind. Facial movements and posture can be particularly significant in interpreting the mood of the speaker.

Object cues are the speaker's intentional and nonintentional use of all objects. Dress, furnishings, and possessions all communicate something to the observer about the speaker's sense of self. They are often consciously selected by the individual, however, and therefore may be chosen to convey a certain "look" or message. Thus, they can be less accurate than other types of nonverbal communication.

Space provides another clue to the nature of the relationship between two people. Hall[27] extensively researched proxemics, the use of space between communicators. He identified the following four zones of space that are demonstrated interpersonally in North America:

1. Intimate space—up to 45.5 cm (18 inches). This allows for maximum interpersonal sensory stimulation.
2. Personal space—45.5 to 120 cm (18 inches to 4 feet). This is used for close relationships and touching distance. Visual sensation is improved over the intimate range.
3. Social-consultative space—270 to 360 cm (9 to 12 feet). This is less personal and less dependent. Speech must be louder.
4. Public space—360 cm (12 feet) and over. This is used in speech giving and other public occasions.

Observation of seating arrangements and use of space by patients can yield valuable information to the nurse that has implications for both her assessment of the patient and the way in which her nursing intervention should be implemented.

Touch involves both personal space and action. It is possibly the most personal of the nonverbal messages and one's response to it is influenced by the setting, cultural background, type of relationship, sex of communicators, ages, and expectations. Touch can have many meanings.[71] It can express a striving to connect with another person as a way of meeting them or relating to them. It can be a way of expressing or conveying something to another, such as concern, empathy, or caring. Touch can also be used receptively as a way of sensing, perceiving, or allowing someone else to leave their imprint on another. Finally, Krieger[38] has developed the concept of "therapeutic touch," or the nurse's laying hands on or close to the body of an ill person for the purpose of helping or healing. She believes touch to be the imprimatur of nursing and contends that the therapeutic, comforting effects of touch have been often overlooked in nursing.

Touch is a universal and basic aspect of all nurse-patient relationships and has been described as the first and most fundamental means of communication.[4] Nevertheless, relatively little is really known about touch as it relates to health.[75] This is clearly one area in which many questions exist and many aspects remain unexplored. The therapeutic value of touch truly merits further examination through nursing research.

■ **INTERPRETING NONVERBAL BEHAVIOR.** All of these types of nonverbal messages are important, but interpreting them correctly can present numerous problems to the nurse. Body messages are rapid, often imprecise, and extremely complex. It is impossible to examine nonverbal messages out of context, and there are times when one's body reveals a number of different and perhaps conflicting feelings simultaneously. Cultural background is also a major influence on the meaning of nonverbal behavior. In America, with its diverse ethnic communities, such messages between people of different upbringing can easily be misinterpreted. Certain people may have been taught to suppress hands and facial expressions, whereas others may not show emotional response. For instance, Arabs tend to stand closer together when speaking, and Orientals tend to touch more; touching in America is often minimized because of perceived sexual overtones or one's puritan heritage. Because the meaning attached to nonverbal behavior is so subjective, it is essential that the nurse validate its meaning.

Nurses should respond to the variety of nonverbal behaviors displayed by the patient, particularly voice inflections, body movements, gestures, facial expression, posture and physical energy levels. Incongruent behavior or contradictory messages are especially significant. The nurse should refer to the specific behavior observed and attempt to validate its meaning and significance with the patient. If the nurse's words and tone of voice indicate that she is truly clarifying, suggesting, or validating, she will usually not create a defensive reaction in the patient. Three kinds of responses may be used by the nurse:

1. Questions or statements intended to increase the patient's awareness
2. Content reflections
3. Statements reflecting the responsiveness of the nurse

These possible responses are illustrated in the following interaction.

PATIENT: (**Shifting nervously in her chair, eyes scanning the room and avoiding the nurse) What . . . what do you want to talk about today?**

NURSE: **I sense that you are uncomfortable talking to me. Could you describe to me how you are feeling?**

NURSE: **You're not sure what we should be talking about and you want me to start us off?**

NURSE: **You look very nervous to me and I can feel those same feelings in me as I sit here with you.**

The nurse's first possible response is a reflection and attempt to validate the feelings of the patient. The purpose is to communicate to the patient the nurse's awareness of his feelings, to show acceptance of those feelings, and to request that he focus on them and elaborate on them. The nurse's second possible response deals with the content of the patient's message. The nurse here is clarifying what the patient is trying to say. The third possible response shares both the nurse's perception of her patient's feelings and the personal disclosure that she too has some of those same feelings. This type of response may help the patient feel accepted and understood by the nurse.

■ **IMPLICATIONS FOR NURSING CARE.** In addition to responding to the patient's nonverbal behavior, the nurse should incorporate aspects of it in implementing care. This may be most evident in the use of space in the nurse-patient relationship. A patient who is resistant to closeness will most certainly recoil from entry into his intimate space. The close distance area of personal space may also be intolerable to a patient who fears closeness. The nurse can assess the patient's level of spatial tolerance by observing the distance the patient maintains with other people. The nurse can also be alert to the patient's response when she interacts with him.

If she sits next to him on the sofa, does he get up and move to a chair? If she pulls her chair closer to him, does he move his chair away to reestablish the original space? Sometimes increasing the space between the nurse and an anxious patient can alleviate the anxiety enough to allow the interaction to continue. A decrease in the distance that the patient chooses to maintain from others may indicate a decrease in interpersonal anxiety.

A related concept to those of personal distance and personal space is that of territoriality. It can be defined as the drive to acquire and defend territory in order to assure species' survival. In analyzing territorial behavior among the chronic institutionalized mentally ill, Cooper believes that it can be measured by determining the prevalence and degree of the following behaviors:

- Attempting to consistently sit in the same area or chair
- Arranging concrete boundaries around one's body
- Rearranging body position to face away from others
- Avoiding eye contact
- Sitting side-by-side rather than face-to-face
- Increased sleeping or retreat into drugs, fantasies, etc.
- Various adornments of the body[18]

She believes that whenever possible, an attempt should be made to allow the hospitalized individual control and enjoyment of personal possessions and private living space, no matter how small or seemingly insignificant. Specifically, residents should be allowed free access to their personal living quarters and, as soon as possible, free access out of doors, or at least, off the ward itself. Residents can also be encouraged to wear personal clothing and keep personal items. In summary, hospitalized patients' territorial behavior should be recognized and its free expression allowed, while simultaneously attempting to decrease the crowding and high density that threatens it.

Argyle[3] enumerates other spatial parameters that are interpersonally significant. Height may communicate dominance and submission. Communication is facilitated when both participants are at similar levels. Orientation of the participants' body positions is also significant. Face-to-face confrontation is more threatening than oblique body positions. The physical setting also has spatial meaning. Ownership of a space affects the communication context. A patient may be more comfortable in his own room than in the therapist's office, unless the patient's room is also defined as bedroom. Conrol issues are minimized when communication takes place in a neutral area that belongs to neither partici-

pant. However, people rather quickly identify their own turf, even in unfamiliar settings, and then begin to exert ownership rights over this area. A common example of this can be observed in most college classes. At the beginning of the semester, people seat themselves somewhat randomly, but the arrangement usually solidifies after a couple of classes. Students then feel vaguely annoyed if they arrive in class to find another person in "their seat." They are experiencing an invasion of personal space. Awareness of a patient's use of space can add a further dimension to the nurse's ability to understand the patient.

Touch also should be used judiciously. It is a powerful communicative tool. Patients who are sensitive to issues of closeness may experience a casual touch as an invasion or as an invitation to intimacy, which may be even more frightening. Physical contact with a person of the same sex may be experienced by the patient as a homosexual advance and may precipitate a panic reaction. If procedures requiring physical contact must be carried out, careful explanations should be given both before and during the procedure. An efficient, impersonal, but caring, approach to physical nursing care may be least threatening to a patient experiencing interpersonal anxiety.

The last point to be made here regarding nonverbal communication is that the nurse must not only be aware of the patient's nonverbal cues, but she must also be aware of her own. Nonverbal cues of the nurse can communicate interest, respect, and genuineness or disinterest, lack of respect, and an impersonal facade. La Crosse[40] did a study of nonverbal behaviors to determine which ones promoted relating to someone else and which ones prohibited it. He concluded that affiliative nonverbal behavior included smiles, positive head nods, gestures, 80% eye contact, and a 20% forward body lean. Unaffiliative nonverbal behavior included 40% eye contact, a 20% reclining body lean, and none of the other categories. Furthermore, affiliative counselors were perceived to be more attractive and persuasive than unaffiliative ones. The implication of this type of research is that nurses, as therapeutic helpers, need to be aware of a spectrum of nonverbal behaviors in their patients and themselves and then incorporate them judiciously in their care.

■ The communication process

Human communication is a dynamic process that is influenced by the psychological and physiological conditions of the participants. Ruesch[60] has identified the elements of the process as perception, evaluation, and transmission. Perception occurs by activation of the sensory end organs of the receiver. The impulse is then

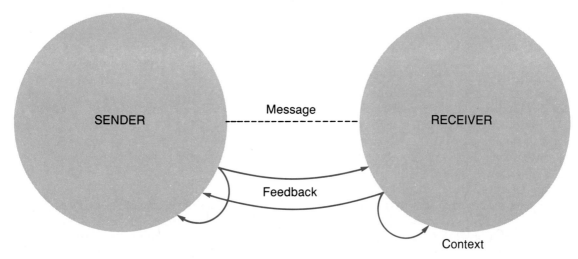

Fig. 4-4. Components of communication.

transmitted to the brain. Human beings are most reliant on visual and auditory stimuli for communications. Vision is the primary means of perceiving nonverbal communication, and hearing primarily responds to verbal stimuli. However, if one of the primary senses is dysfunctional, the other functional senses accommodate to improve the individual's perception. For instance, the deaf person can learn sign language and lip-reading, which rely on vision, to compensate for not being able to hear the verbal component of communication.

When the sensory impulse reaches the brain, evaluation takes place. The message is analyzed and categorized by the individual in terms of its meaning. Past personal experience is the matrix within which new experience is evaluated. If the individual encounters an entirely new experience for which there is no frame of reference, a feeling of confusion results. Evaluation results in a cognitive response that relates to the informational aspect of the message and an affective response that relates to the relationship aspect of the message. Most messages stimulate both types of responses.

When the evaluation of the message is complete, transmission takes place. This is perceived by the sender as feedback, thereby influencing the continued course of the communication cycle. Transmission must take place once communication has been initiated. It is impossible not to transmit some kind of feedback. Even lack of any visible response is feedback to the sender that the message did not get through, was considered unimportant, was an undesirable interruption, or any of a number of other possible interpretations, depending on the context. Feedback stimulates perception, evaluation, and transmission on the part of the original sender, and so the cycle continues until the participants

mutually agree to terminate it or one participant physically leaves the setting.

Theoretical models of the communication process help one to visualize its dynamic nature. They show visual relationships more clearly and thus can aid in finding and correcting communication breakdowns or problems. Two models, the structural and transactional analysis models, will be presented, since each gives a valuable, but different, perspective on the communication process.

■ **STRUCTURAL MODEL.** The structural model has five functional components in communication: the sender, message, receiver, feedback, and context[69] (Fig. 4-4). The **sender** is the originator of the message, which is then transmitted to the receiver. The **message** is a unit of information that is transmitted from the sender to the receiver. The **receiver,** then, is the perceiver of the message, which influences his behavior in some way. The verbal or behavioral response of the receiver is **feedback** to the sender. Feedback, as defined here, functions as described in general systems theory. Positive feedback promotes change within the system, and negative feedback promotes stability. An example of positive feedback might be the receiver unexpectedly telling the sender that the message made him angry, whereas negative feedback might be to respond exactly as the sender anticipated. When viewed structurally, communication is a circular process. The designation of sender and message and receiver and feedback is somewhat arbitrary once the cycle has begun, since feedback is also a new message initiated by the receiver, who then becomes the sender.

The fifth structural element of communication is the **context.** This is the setting in which the communication takes place. Knowledge of context is necessary to understand the meaning of the communication. For example, the phrase "I don't understand what you mean" may have different meanings in the context of a classroom or a courtroom. Context involves more than the physical setting for communication, however. It also includes the psychosocial setting, which encompasses the relationship between the sender and receiver, their past experiences with each other, and past experiences with similar situations, as well as cultural values and norms. Consider again the meaning of "I don't understand what you mean" in the following contexts: two college students discussing a philosophy assignment, a wife responding to her husband's accusation of infidelity, and a Japanese tourist asking directions in San Francisco. Although the content of the message is the same, its meaning is different, depending on the context in which the communication takes place.

Related problems. If one evaluates the communication process with regard to these five structural elements, specific problems or potential errors become evident. These are summarized in Table 4-5. First, the sender must be communicating the same message on both the verbal and nonverbal levels. If so, the sender's communication is termed **congruent.** If, however, the

levels are not in agreement, the communication is termed **incongruent,** which can be problematic.

CONGRUENT COMMUNICATION
VERBAL LEVEL: **I'm pleased to see you.**
NONVERBAL LEVEL: **Voice sounds warm, continuous eye contact, smiling.**

INCONGRUENT COMMUNICATION
VERBAL LEVEL: **I'm pleased to see you.**
NONVERBAL LEVEL: **Voice sounds cold and distant, avoids eye contact, neutral facial expression.**

Incongruent, or double-level, messages produce a dilemma for the listener because he does not know to which level he should respond, the verbal or nonverbal. Since he cannot respond to both, he is likely to feel frustrated, angry, or confused. This is a double-bind situation in which one is "damned if you do, and damned if you don't." Obviously, both patients and nurses can display incongruent communication, if they are not aware of their internal feeling states and the nature of their communication.

Another problem initiated by the sender is that of inflexible communication. This is communication that is either too rigid or too permissive. A rigid approach

TABLE 4-5

SPECIFIC PROBLEMS ASSOCIATED WITH THE STRUCTURAL ELEMENTS OF THE COMMUNICATION PROCESS

Structural element	Communication problem	Definition
Sender	Incongruent communication	Lack of agreement between the verbal and nonverbal levels of communication
	Inflexible communication	Exaggerated control or permissiveness by the sender
Message	Ineffective messages	Messages that are not goal-directed or purposeful
	Inappropriate messages	Messages not relevant to the progress of the relationship
	Inadequate messages	Messages that lack a sufficient amount of information
	Inefficient messages	Messages that lack clarity, simplicity, and directness
Receiver	Errors of perception	Various forms of listening problems
	Errors of evaluation	Misinterpretation due to personal beliefs and values
Feedback	Misinformation	Communication of incorrect information
	Lack of validation	Failure to clarify and ratify understanding of the message
Context	Constraints of physical setting	Noise, temperature, or various distractions
	Constraints of psychosocial setting	Impaired previous relationship between the communicators

is one of exaggerated control by the nurse and may be evident in the overuse of a standardized history or assessment form. It does not allow the patient to spontaneously express himself, nor does it allow him to contribute to the flow or direction of the interaction. Exaggerated permissiveness, on the other hand, refers to a nurse who does not share personal thoughts or impressions with the patient and thus the interaction lacks direction and mutuality. The patient may interpret the nurse's behavior as lack of interest or incompetency.

The next element of the communication process, the message, can also pose problems. Basically, these problems are messages that are ineffective, inappropriate, inadequate, or inefficient. Ineffective messages are not goal-directed or purposeful. They serve at least to distract, and at most to prevent the objectives of the nurse-patient relationship from being met. Inappropriate messages are those which are not relevant to the progress of the relationship. They may include failures in timing, stereotyping the receiver, or overlooking important information. Inadequate messages are basically those which lack a sufficient amount of information. The sender assumes the receiver knows more than he actually does. Inefficient messages lack clarity, simplicity, and directness. They use more energy than is necessary to confuse or complicate the message. This can be consciously or unconsciously done by the sender. It may reflect disease in the organ of communication, such as stuttering, or it can be due to lack of knowledge or poor use of language.

The third element, the receiver, is subject to the same problems as the sender but also some additional ones. He may experience errors of perception in which he might miss nonverbal cues, respond only to content and ignore messages of affect, be selectively inattentive to the speaker's message because of his own physical or psychological discomfort, be preoccupied with other thoughts, or have a physiological impairment of hearing organs. All of these errors are fundamentally problems of listening. The receiver may also experience problems in evaluating the message. He may misinterpret the meaning of the message because he is viewing it in terms of his own value system, rather than that of the speakers. In this case, he is not being open to the speaker but is judging him based on his own personal experiences and beliefs. He might also interpret a symbolic message literally or a literal one symbolically.

Errors in the feedback element include all of those which apply to the message. Feedback can also convey incorrect information to the sender about the message. Another serious error exists when the receiver fails to use feedback to validate his understanding of the message. Although feedback is the last step in the cyclical communication process, it has the potential for correcting previous errors and clarifying the nature of the communication.

The fifth element of context can also contribute to communication problems. The setting may be physically noisy, cold, or distracting to one or both parties. So, too, the psychosocial context, or past relationship between the communicators, may be one of mistrust or harbored resentment. From this analysis, the complexity of the communication process is evident, and it may even seem surprising that successful communication can occur, given all of these vulnerable areas. However, it can and does occur among those people who understand the process, have analyzed the elements of it, and use appropriate techniques.

■ **TRANSACTIONAL ANALYSIS MODEL.** Transactional analysis (TA) is the study of the communication or transactions that take place between people and of the sometimes unconscious and destructive ways ("games") that people relate to each other. This approach to personality was developed by Berne, a psychiatrist who made transactional analysis a popular theory through his book, *Games People Play: The Psychology of Human Relationships*.[5] It is a method of therapy as well as a model of communication.

The cornerstone of Berne's theory is that each person's personality is made up of three distinct components called **ego states.** An ego state is a consistent pattern of feeling, experiencing, and behaving. The three ego states that make up one's personality are the parent ego state (parent); adult ego state (adult), and child ego state (child) (Fig. 4-5). It is as though there are three "people" inside you: the parent-you, which incorporates all the attitudes and behavior you were taught (directly or indirectly) by your parents; the child-you, which contains all the feelings you had as a child; and the adult-you, which deals with reality in a logical, rational, computer-like manner. These three ego states are distinct, each having a consistent pattern of feeling, experiencing, and behaving.

The parent and child ego states are made up of the feelings, attitudes, and behaviors that are remnants of the past but can be reexperienced under certain conditions. The parent ego state consists of all the nurturing, critical, and prejudicial attitudes, behaviors, and experiences learned from other people, especially parents and teachers. The adult ego state is the reality-oriented part of the personality. It gathers and processes information about the world and is objective, emotionless, and intelligent in its approach to problem solving. The child ego state is the feeling part of the personality. In it resides feelings of happiness, joy, sadness, depression, and anxiety.

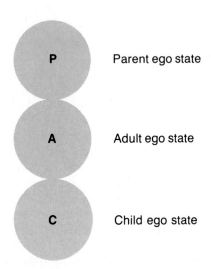

Fig. 4-5. Three ego states as described by Berne's theory of transactional analysis.

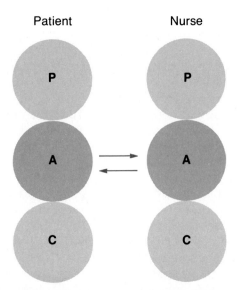

Fig. 4-6. Diagram of complementary transaction.

Berne's model of communication allows one to diagram transactions using these ego states. Transactional analysis then focuses on the communication between people. A transaction or communication between two people can be complementary, crossed, or ulterior. In a **complementary transaction** (Fig. 4-6), the arrows in the ego state diagram are parallel, and the communication flows smoothly.

COMPLEMENTARY TRANSACTION

PATIENT: **I know that when I get mad at my boss, I take it out on my wife and kids.**

NURSE: **Are you ready to think about some other ways you can handle your anger?**

If the arrows in the ego state diagram **cross**, however, communication breaks down (Fig. 4-7).

CROSSED TRANSACTION

PATIENT: **I know that when I get mad at my boss, I take it out on my wife and kids.**

NURSE: **Men always think that's okay, but the women have to suffer for it.**

The third type of transaction is termed **ulterior** (Fig. 4-8). It takes place on two levels: the social, or overt, level and the psychological, or covert, level. These transactions tend to be destructive because the communicators conceal their true motivations. One of the best known examples of this is the "Why Don't You . . . Yes But" (WDYYB) game. This game involves one person asking for a solution to a problem; however, every suggested solution is negated, until the helper is silenced. On the surface, the interaction is two adults problem solving, but in reality, one person is using his child to show what a bad parent the other person is.

ULTERIOR TRANSACTION

PATIENT: **I know that when I get mad at my boss, I take it out on my wife and kids but I don't know what else to do.**

NURSE: **Do you think you could let your boss know how you're feeling?**

PATIENT: **He'll fire me for sure.**

NURSE: **Perhaps you could talk it over with someone you work with.**

PATIENT: **I don't have time to chat on the job like that. Besides, no one cares about someone else's beefs.**

NURSE: **Sometimes physical exercise helps people get rid of their anger. Have you ever tried it?**

PATIENT: **Sure. I work out a lot, but it doesn't help.**

NURSE: **Perhaps you can explain all this to your family.**

PATIENT: **My wife's tired of "all my talk" as she puts it. She says she wants some action.**

The value of the transactional analysis model of communication is that it provides a framework for the nurse to use in exploring the patient's recurrent behaviors, identifying patterns, postulating causes, and planning alternative ways to respond. Thus nonproductive communication patterns can be stopped and new, more healthy, ones learned.

■ Therapeutic communication techniques

Ginott[26] believes that the two basic requirements for effective communication are that all communication be aimed at preserving the self-respect of both the helper and helpee and that the communication of understanding precede any suggestions of information or advice giving. These lay the groundwork for therapeutic com-

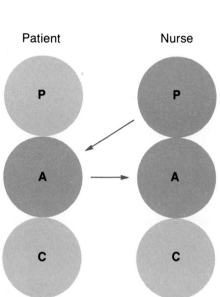

Fig. 4-7. Diagram of a crossed transaction.

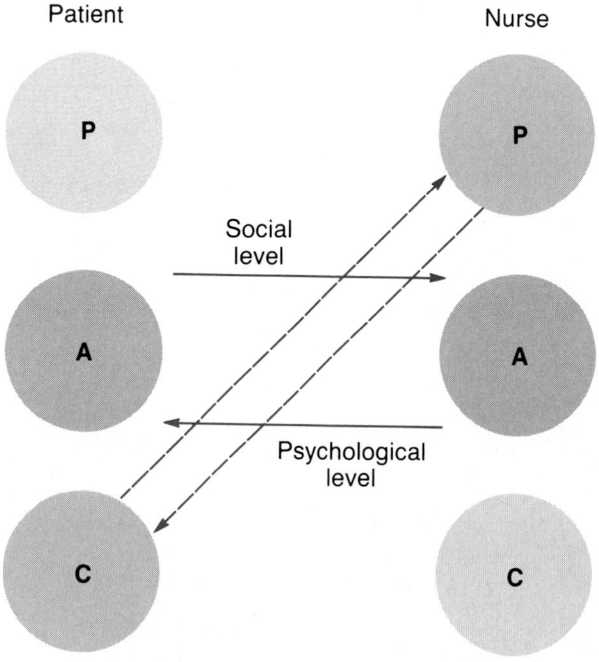

Fig. 4-8. Diagram of an ulterior transaction.

munication, which makes possible the formation of the nurse-patient relationship and the implementation of the nursing process. The collection of data and the planning, implementation, and evaluation activities are carried out *with* the patient, not *for* the patient, when the nurse uses therapeutic communication skills.

Some nurses reject the notion of therapeutic communication techniques because they view them as unnatural, ineffective, or stereotypical. Like all learned skills, they can be abused, used too frequently, or incorrectly applied, and knowledge of these skills does not ensure successful therapeutic communication. These techniques, although simple on the surface, are, in fact, difficult and require practice and conscious thought for mastery. Because they are techniques, they are only as effective as the person utilizing them. If they are incorporated into the nurse's existing interpersonal skills, they can enhance her effectiveness. If they are used as automatic responses and are inappropriate to the nurse's manner of personal expression, they will negate both the nurse's and the patient's individuality and divest them of their dignity.

To ensure that the nurse is using these skills appropriately and effectively, it will be necessary for the nurse to record interactions with the patient in some way and then analyze them. The nurse should also seek feedback from others. Many tools are available to help in this area. The nurse can benefit from maintaining a diary of her thoughts, feelings, and impressions in relation to her clinical work. This can prove to be valuable in working through difficult aspects of termination or countertransference reactions.

The nurse may decide to tape record or videotape interactions with the patient. These are two of the most informative recording methods, and they also allow the nurse the freedom to concentrate on the patient. They do, however, present problems. There is sometimes the need for another person to operate the equipment, there is always the possibility of failure, they can be expensive to obtain and operate, they may be prohibited by the agency, and they can raise questions concerning confidentiality.

Handwritten recordings are less expensive and do not require mechanical devices. They also allow the nurse to record her thoughts and feelings along with the verbal and nonverbal behavior. However, they require more physical time and energy. If they are written in the presence of the patient, they can be very distracting. If they are written afterward, some aspects of the interaction may be unconsciously forgotten or consciously ignored. Often, these are most significant omissions.

The advantages and disadvantages of the various methods of recording nurse-patient interactions are summarized in Table 4-6. These must be considered, along with the nurse's and patient's preferences before deciding on a particular method. Some form of recording that is as objective and comprehensive as possible is necessary. Only by analyzing the interaction will the nurse be able to evaluate the degree of success in utilizing therapeutic communication techniques.

Some of the most helpful of these techniques will now be described. Other sources present detailed information on the communication process and therapeutic and nontherapeutic communication techniques.[69,70] In addition, common errors in communication made by

TABLE 4-6

ADVANTAGES AND DISADVANTAGES OF VARIOUS METHODS OF RECORDING NURSE-PATIENT INTERACTIONS

Advantages	Disadvantages
Videotape	
Provides excellent opportunity to see, record, and analyze both nonverbal and verbal levels of communication	Mechanical devices are necessary
Participants are not distracted by writing	Mechanical failure can occur
Can be preserved for comparison with future interactions	At least one other person is necessary to operate equipment
Can provide participants with audiovisual feedback of their responses	Often distracting to participants, at least initially
Possible to see and hear entire interaction for review and supervision	Transcriptions are time consuming
Possible to replay segments for comparison, analysis, and supervision	Unless more than one monitor is available, comparison is time consuming
Tape recording	
Complete verbatim conversation is available	Mechanical devices are necessary
Participants are not distracted by writing	Mechanical failure can occur
Can be preserved for comparison with future interactions	Often distracting to participants, at least initially
Can provide participants with audio feedback of their responses	Transcriptions are time consuming
Possible to hear entire interaction for review and supervision	Unless more than one tape recorder is available, comparison is time consuming
Possible to replay segments for comparison, analysis, and supervision	Nonverbal communication is not available
	With cassette tape recorder, often necessary to disrupt interaction to turn tape over
Verbatim notes	
Possible to record thoughts and feelings during interaction	Difficult to concentrate on interaction until technique of writing without looking is mastered
Messages recorded as said rather than as what was intended	Often distracting to participants, at least initially
Possible to quickly review specific areas for comparison, analysis, and supervision	Requires greater skill in recording
Both verbal and nonverbal levels can be recorded	Segments of the interaction are usually missing or incomplete
No mechanical devices to distract participants	
General outline notes	
Possible to record thoughts and feelings during the interaction	Often distracting to participants, at least initially
Possible to quickly review specific areas for comparison, analysis, and supervision	Necessary to fill in general outline with specific data at a later time
Both verbal and nonverbal levels can be recorded	Often actual messages are distorted by intended messages
No mechanical devices to distract	
Requires less skill than verbatim notes	
Decreases amount of energy needed for writing during interaction, hence increases energy available for communication with client	
Postinteraction notes	
No distractions during interaction	Relies entirely on memory
Possible to focus attention entirely on communication process	Often actual messages are distorted by intended messages
Possible to record information at one's convenience	Often tends to be a more haphazard notation and analysis unless one is well organized

From Sundeen, S.J., et al.: Nurse-client interaction: implementing the nursing process, ed. 3, St. Louis, 1985, The C.V. Mosby Co.

students in psychiatric nursing are analyzed in an article by Sayre listed in the annotated suggested readings at the end of this chapter. Nontherapeutic techniques will not be discussed separately because basically they represent a failure to use an appropriate therapeutic skill. Rather, problems will be discussed relative to some of the therapeutic techniques, and it is hoped that the emphasis of learning will be on a theoretical understanding of therapeutic communication and its appropriate application in a facilitative nurse-patient relationship.

■ **LISTENING.** Listening is essential if the nurse is to reach any understanding of the patient. Only the patient can tell the nurse how he feels, what he thinks, and how he sees himself and the world. Only by listening to the patient can the nurse enter his world and see things as he does. Therefore the first rule of a therapeutic relationship is to listen to the patient. It is the foundation on which all other therapeutic skills are built.

Obviously one cannot listen if one is talking, yet inexperienced nurses often find it difficult not to talk. This may be due to their anxiety, need to prove themselves, or habitual manner of social interaction. It is helpful to remember that the patient should be talking more than the nurse during the interaction; the task of the nurse is to listen.

Real listening is difficult. It is an active, not a passive, process. The nurse's complete attention must be given to the patient, and she should not be preoccupied with herself. She should suspend her thinking of her own experiences and problems and her personal judgments of the patient. Listening is a sign of respect for the patient and is a powerful reinforcer. It reinforces verbalization by the patient, without which the relationship could not progress.

■ **BROAD OPENINGS.** Broad openings such as "What are you thinking about?" "Can you tell me more about that?" and "What shall we discuss today?" confirm the presence of the patient and encourage him to select topics to discuss. They can also indicate that the nurse is there, listening to him and following him. Also serving in this way are acceptance responses such as "I understand," "And then what happened?" "Uh huh," or "I follow you."

■ **RESTATING.** Restating is the nurse's repeating to the patient the main thought he has expressed. It, too, indicates that the nurse is listening. Sometimes only a part of the patient's statement is repeated. This technique can serve as a reinforcer or bring attention to something important that might otherwise have been passed over.

■ **CLARIFICATION.** Clarification occurs when the nurse attempts to put into words vague ideas or thoughts that are implicit or explicit in the patient's talking. It is necessary because statements about emotions and behaviors are rarely straightforward. The patient's verbalizations, especially when he is disturbed or feeling deeply, are not always clear and obvious. They may be confused, jumbled, hesitant, incomplete, disordered, or fragmentary. The nurse should not allow anything to go by that she does not hear or understand. Because of this uncertainty, clarification responses are often tentative or phrased as questions such as "I'm not sure what you mean. Are you saying that . . . ?" or "Could you go over that again?" This technique is important because one of the functions of the nurse-patient relationship is to help clarify feelings, ideas, and perceptions and to provide an explicit correlation between them and the patient's actions.

■ **REFLECTION.** Reflection goes beyond simple acceptance or restating responses. *Reflection of content* is also called validation, and it lets the patient know that the nurse has heard what he said and understands the content. It consists of repeating in fewer and fresher words the essential ideas of the patient and is like paraphrasing. Sometimes it helps to repeat a patient's statement, emphasizing a key word. Reflecting content is used to clarify the ideas that the patient is expressing and validate that the nurse's understanding is consistent with the patient's meaning.

PATIENT: **When I walked into the room, I felt like I was going to faint. I knew I had tried to do too much, too quickly, and I just wasn't ready for it.**
NURSE: **You thought you were ready to put yourself to the test but when you got there, you realized it was too much, too soon.**

Reflection of feelings consists of responses to the feelings that the patient has about the content. They let the patient know that the nurse is aware of what he is feeling. Broad openings, restatements, clarifications, and reflections of content need not represent empathic understanding. But reflection of feeling signifies understanding, empathy, interest, and respect for the patient. It increases the level of involvement between the nurse and patient.

The purpose of reflecting feelings is to focus on feeling rather than content to bring the patient's vaguely expressed feelings into clear awareness and to help him accept or "own" those feelings as a part of himself. Skillful use of this technique depends on the nurse's ability to identify feelings and cues for feelings from the patient's nonverbal and verbal behaviors. The steps in reflection of feelings are to determine what feelings the patient is expressing, describe these feelings clearly, observe the effect, and judge by the reaction of the patient whether the reflection was correct or not. Sometimes even inaccurate reflections can be facilitative because the patient may correct the nurse and state his feeling more clearly.

Although reflecting techniques are some of the most useful, they can also be used incorrectly by the nurse. One common error is stereotyping one's responses. This means that the nurse begins her reflections in the same monotonous way, such as "You think" or "You feel." A second error is in timing. Some nurses reflect back almost everything the patient says, which provokes feelings of irritation, anger, and frustration in the patient. The nurse appears to be insincere and, in fact, fails to be therapeutic with him. Other nurses may have trouble interrupting patients who continue talking in long monologues. Not only is it difficult to capture a feeling after it has passed, but in this case, the nurse is failing to be a responsible active partner in the relationship. Interruptions may, at times, be productive and necessary. Another error is the inappropriate depth of feeling. The nurse fails by either being too superficial in assessment of the patient's feelings or too deep. The final error is in the use of language that is inappropriate to the cultural experience and educational level of the patient. Effective language is language that is natural to the nurse and readily understood by the patient.

■ **FOCUSING.** Focusing helps the patient expand on a topic of importance. It allows him to discuss central issues related to his problem and keeps the communication process goal-directed. Intense focusing on an anxiety-producing topic can be detrimental to the relationship if it is not evaluated and balanced with other therapeutic techniques. Effectively used, it can help the patient become more specific, move from vagueness to clarity, and focus on reality.

By avoiding abstractions and generalizations, focusing helps the patient face his problems and analyze them in detail. It helps a patient talk about his situation or problem areas and accept the responsibility for improving them. If a patient is going to change his thoughts, feelings, or beliefs, he must first identify them as his own. If he fails to "own" them, he has lost control over a part of his life and becomes powerless to change it.

PATIENT: **Women always get put down. It's as if we don't count at all.**
NURSE: **Tell me how *you* feel as a woman.**

Encouraging a description of the patient's perceptions, encouraging comparisons, and placing events in time sequence are focusing techniques that promote specificity and problem analysis.

■ **SHARING PERCEPTIONS.** Sharing perceptions involves asking the patient to verify the nurse's understanding of what he is thinking or feeling. It is a way for the nurse to ask for feedback from the patient, while also possibly providing him with new information. Perception checking can consist of paraphrasing what the patient is saying or doing, asking the patient to confirm your understanding, and allowing him to correct your perception if it was incorrect. "You seem to be very irritated with me. Am I right about that?" It can also note the implied feelings of nonverbal language. When used in this way, it is best to describe the observed behavior first and then reflect on its meaning. "You say you really care about her, but everytime you talk about her, you clench your fists. I wonder if you don't feel betrayed by her?" It is also a way to explore incongruent or double-bind communication. "You're smiling, but I sense that you're really angry with me." Its value as a therapeutic technique lies in the understanding it conveys to the patient and its potential for clearing up confusing communication.

■ **THEME IDENTIFICATION.** Themes are underlying issues or problems experienced by the patient that emerge repeatedly during the course of the nurse-patient relationship. Once the nurse has identified the patient's basic themes, she can better decide which of the patient's many feelings, thoughts, and beliefs she should respond to and pursue. In this way the nurse can best promote the patient's exploration and understanding. Themes that are important will tend to be repeated throughout the relationship. They can relate to feelings (depression or anxiety), behavior (rebelling against authority or withdrawal), experiences (being loved, hurt, or raped), or combinations of all three.

■ **SILENCE.** Silence on the part of the nurse has varying effects, depending on how it is perceived by the patient. To a vocal patient, silence on the part of the nurse may be welcome, as long as he knows the nurse is listening. When the patient pauses in his talk, he often expects and desires a response from the nurse. Not to receive one may be perceived as rejection, hostility, or disinterest by the patient. The nurse's silence with a depressed or withdrawn patient may convey support, understanding, and acceptance. In this case, verbalization by the nurse may be perceived as pressure or frustration. Sharing a patient's silence can be a most difficult task for the nurse but an essential one to furthering the therapeutic relationship.

Silence has several beneficial values.[7] It can make the patient talk. Some introverted people find out that they can be quiet but still be liked. Silence allows the patient time to think and gain insights. And finally, silence can slow the pace of the interaction. In general, the nurse should allow the patient to break a silence, particularly when it has been introduced by the patient. Obviously, sensitivity is called for in this regard, and silence should not develop into a contest. However, if the nurse is unsure how to respond to a patient's comments, a safe approach is to maintain silence. If the nurse's nonverbal behavior communicates interest and involvement, the patient will often elaborate on his statement or discuss a related issue.

An ineffective technique would be to begin questioning the patient. As a general technique, direct questioning has limited usefulness in the therapeutic relationship. Repetitive questioning takes on the tone of an interrogation and negates the element of mutuality. "Why" questions are particularly ineffective and are to be avoided, as are questions that can be answered simply by yes or no responses. Excessive questioning tends to be characteristic of inexperienced helpers,[53] and one consequence of it is that patients do not take the initiative and are discouraged or prevented from engaging in the process of exploration.

■ **HUMOR.** Humor is a basic part of the personality and has a place within the therapeutic relationship. It resolves paradoxes, tempers aggression, and is a socially acceptable form of sublimation. It is a part of interpersonal relationships and is a constructive coping behavior, and, by learning to express humor, a patient may be able to learn to express other affects. Hutchinson[32] believes that humor can be used in three ways: (1) as an index to the developmental level of the patient, (2) as a planned approach for nursing intervention, and (3) as an indicator of change. As a planned approach to nursing intervention, humor can promote insight by making conscious repressed material, and a change in the expression of humor and the quality of interpersonal relationships may be indicators of significant change in the patient.

Another important feature of humor as described by Heuscher is that it can produce a sudden change or widening in the patient's experiential horizon. He believes that humor is an initial uncomplicated attempt at revealing new and wider visions of one's world and, as such, it can further the growth of the person who is able to integrate some of the new vistas in his world design. "At worst, joking in psychotherapy is a 'playing at change' that allows the therapist and patient to retain their uneasy security in their unchanging individual existences. At best, it is a helpful revelation of new options."[30]

There are no rules, however, for determining how, when, or where humor should be used in the therapeutic relationship. Rather, this depends on the nature and quality of the relationship, the patient's receptivity to such themes, and the relevance of the tale or witticism. Furthermore, the nurse must have insight into why she is using this technique and the dangerous ways it can be used to hide conflicts, ward off anxiety, manipulate the patient, and serve her own need to be liked and admired. Humor must be used cautiously. If it is indiscriminate, it meets only the nurse's needs, may be destructive to the relationship, and frightening to the patient.

■ **INFORMING.** Informing, or the skill of information giving, needs little elaboration. It is an essential nursing technique in which the nurse shares simple facts with the patient. It is a skill used by nurses in health teaching or patient education, such as in teaching a patient when to take medication and informing him about necessary precautions and side effects. Giving information, however, must be distinguished from giving suggestions or advice.

■ **SUGGESTING.** Suggesting is the presentation of alternative ideas relative to problem solving. It is an appropriate therapeutic technique if used at the proper time and in a constructive way. As a therapeutic technique, it is a useful intervention in the working phase of the relationship when the patient has analyzed the problem area and is exploring alternative coping mechanisms. At that time, suggestions by the nurse will increase his perceived options and choices.

Suggestion, or giving advice, can also be nontherapeutic. Some patients who seek help do not really expect to work out their own problems, but expect some pronouncement or sound advice on what to do from the health care professional. So too, nursing students often perceive their function as giving "common sense" advice. In these instances, giving advice shifts responsibility to the nurse and reinforces the patient's dependence on her.

Another limitation is that the patient may take the nurse's advice and still not have things work out. The patient then returns to blame the nurse for failure. Most commonly, though, patients do not follow the advice offered by others, as in the transactional analysis model. The request for advice is often a child's expression of dependency, and the patient really knows what to do. If the nurse falls into the trap and responds with advice, she will incur the patient's wrath and contempt. A more productive strategy is for the nurse to deal with the patient's feelings first—feelings of indecision, depen-

TABLE 4-7

THERAPEUTIC COMMUNICATION TECHNIQUES

Technique: **LISTENING**
Definition: An active process of receiving information and examining one's reaction to the messages received
Example: Maintaining eye contact and receptive nonverbal communication
Therapeutic value: Nonverbally communicates to the patient the nurse's interest and acceptance
Nontherapeutic threat: Failure to listen

Technique: **BROAD OPENINGS**
Definition: Encouraging the patient to select topics for discussion
Example: "What are you thinking about?"
Therapeutic value: Indicates acceptance by the nurse and the value of the patient's initiative
Nontherapeutic threat: Domination of the interaction by the nurse; rejecting responses

Technique: **RESTATING**
Definition: Repeating to the patient the main thought he has expressed
Example: "You say that your mother left you when you were five years old."
Therapeutic value: Indicates that the nurse is listening and validates, reinforces, or calls attention to something important that has been said
Nontherapeutic threat: Lack of validation of the nurse's interpretation of the message; being judgmental; reassuring; defending

Technique: **CLARIFICATION**
Definition: Attempting to put into words vague ideas or unclear thoughts of the patient to enhance the nurse's understanding or asking the patient to explain what he means
Example: "I'm not sure what you mean. Could you tell me about that again?"
Therapeutic value: Helps to clarify feelings, ideas, and perceptions of the patient and provide an explicit correlation between them and the patient's actions
Nontherapeutic threat: Failure to probe; assumed understanding

Technique: **REFLECTION**
Definition: Directing back to the patient his ideas, feelings, questions, and content
Example: "You're feeling tense and anxious and it's related to a conversation you had with your husband last night?"
Therapeutic value: Validates the nurse's understanding of what the patient is saying and signifies empathy, interest, and respect for the patient
Nontherapeutic threat: Stereotyping the patient's responses; inappropriate timing of reflections; inappropriate depth of feeling of the reflections; inappropriate to the cultural experience and educational level of the patient

Technique: **FOCUSING**
Definition: Questions or statements that help the patient expand on a topic of importance
Example: "I think that we should talk more about your relationship with your father."
Therapeutic value: Allows the patient to discuss central issues related to his problem and keeps the communication process goal-directed
Nontherapeutic threat: Allowing abstractions and generalizations; changing topics

Technique: **SHARING PERCEPTIONS**
Definition: Asking the patient to verify the nurse's understanding of what he is thinking or feeling
Example: "You're smiling but I sense that you are really very angry with me."
Therapeutic value: Conveys the nurse's understanding to the patient and has the potential for clearing up confusing communication
Nontherapeutic threat: Challenging the patient; accepting literal responses; reassuring; testing; defending

TABLE 4-7—cont'd

THERAPEUTIC COMMUNICATION TECHNIQUES

Technique: **THEME IDENTIFICATION**
Definition: Underlying issues or problems experienced by the patient that emerge repeatedly during the course of the nurse-patient relationship
Example: "I've noticed that in all of the relationships that you have described, you've been hurt or rejected by the man. Do you think this is an underlying issue?"
Therapeutic value: Allows the nurse to best promote the patient's exploration and understanding of important problems
Nontherapeutic threat: Giving advice; reassuring; disapproving

Technique: **SILENCE**
Definition: Lack of verbal communication for a therapeutic reason
Example: Sitting with a patient and nonverbally communicating interest and involvement
Therapeutic value: Allows the patient time to think and gain insights, slows the pace of the interaction and encourages the patient to initiate conversation, while conveying the nurse's support, understanding, and acceptance
Therapeutic threat: Questioning the patient; asking for "why" responses; failure to break a nontherapeutic silence

Technique: **HUMOR**
Definition: The discharge of energy through the comic enjoyment of the imperfect
Example: "That gives a whole new meaning to the word 'nervous,'" said with shared kidding between the nurse and patient
Therapeutic value: Can promote insight by making conscious repressed material, resolve paradoxes, temper aggression, reveal new options, and is a socially acceptable form of sublimation
Nontherapeutic threat: Indiscrimate use; belittling patient; screen to avoid therapeutic intimacy

Technique: **INFORMING**
Definition: The skill of information giving
Example: "I think you need to know more about how your medication works."
Therapeutic value: Helpful in health teaching or patient education about relevant aspects of patient's well-being and self-care
Nontherapeutic threat: Giving advice

Technique: **SUGGESTING**
Definition: Presentation of alternative ideas for the patient's consideration relative to his problem solving
Example: "Have you thought about responding to your boss in a different way when he raises that issue with you? For example, you could ask him if a specific problem has occurred."
Therapeutic value: Increases the patient's perceived options or choices
Nontherapeutic threat: Giving advice; inappropriate timing; being judgmental

dence, and perhaps fear. Then the request for advice can be looked at and responded to in its proper perspective.

Suggestion is also nontherapeutic if it occurs early in the relationship before the patient has analyzed his conflicts or if it is a technique used frequently by the nurse. Then it negates the possibility of mutuality and implies that the patient is not capable of assuming responsibility for his own thoughts and actions. This assumption is also present when suggestion by the nurse is really covert coercion as the nurse tells the patient how he *ought* to live his life.

The nurse's intent in using this technique thera-

peutically is to provide feasible alternatives and allow the patient to explore their potential value for himself. The nurse can then focus on facilitating the patient's exploration of the advantages and disadvantages and the meaning and implications of the potential alternatives. In this way suggestions can be offered in a nonauthoritarian manner with such phrases as "Some people have tried. . . . Do you think that would work for you?" When using the technique of suggesting, nurses must be careful about the timing of their intervention as well as their underlying motivation.

The therapeutic communication techniques presented in this chapter are summarized in Table 4-7.

Some Illness-Maintaining Responses of Nurses with Patients

1. The nurse using a patient (who was similarly exploited at home) to do errands for her (bring coffee, clean office, carry messages).
2. The nurse burdening the patient with tales of her exciting social life—putting the patient in the position of "audience" and at the same time having little interest, if any, in his concerns; to cheer him up by "one-upping" him!
3. The nurse making "pets" of a few patients and thereby reinforcing previous "pet" status for those patients and reinforcing "unfavorable comparison" for other patients. Giving gifts to some but not all patients.
4. Arbitrating siblinglike disputes among two patients, so that one loses and one wins, as in sibling disputes at home.
5. Responding to dependency bids in ways that confirm and reconfirm the patient's self-view: "I am helpless, dependent, etc."
6. Responding to patient bids for derogation or punishment by giving it, thereby confirming and reconfirming these patient self-views.

7. Permitting, inviting, and responding to "tale bearing" in which one patient "tattles" on another, thereby reinforcing the patient's "informer role," which further isolates the patient from constructive interaction with other patients as peers.
8. Allowing or permitting "coalitions across generations"; i.e., participating in nurse/patient discussion to the detriment of some other staff member. This replicates the patient's previous pattern of "pitting one against another," which may have effectively disunited mother and father, who are then reunited in concern for the now "identified patient."
9. Entering into pseudochum relationships with patients.
10. Nonuseful channeling of anxiety into overmedication, seclusion, EST, or work, rather than into investigation of circumstances that evoked the anxiety in a given situation.
11. Using various problematic verbal inputs such as "mixed messages," "double-binds," etc.

From Peplau, H.: Int. Nurs. Rev. **25**(2):44, 1978.

Responsive dimensions

Certain skills or qualities must be achieved by the nurse to initiate and continue a therapeutic relationship. They incorporate verbal and nonverbal behavior and the attitudes and feelings behind communication. Truax, Carkhoff, and Berenson[14-16] have identified specific core conditions for facilitative interpersonal relationships. They broadly divided them into responsive dimensions and action dimensions. The responsive dimensions include genuineness, respect, empathic understanding, and concreteness.

Many nurses believe that they already demonstrate these qualities with their patients. However, a number of studies have reported that nurses are low in the qualities traditionally associated with therapeutic effectiveness in counseling—genuineness, nonpossessive warmth, and empathy.[54] Furthermore, the helping process can impede the patient's growth rather than enhance it, depending on the level of the nurse's responsive and facilitative skills. Some of the ways in which nurses may consciously or unconsciously do this are given in the box on illness-maintaining responses.

The responsive dimensions are crucial in the orientation phase of a relationship to establish trust and open communication between the nurse and patient. The nurse's goal at this time is to gain an understanding of the patient and assist him to understand himself or gain insight. These responsive conditions then continue to be useful throughout the working and termination phases. All of the conditions are interrelated and contribute to each other in the therapeutic process, and some degree of all the responsive dimensions is necessary when one is initiating a relationship.

■ Genuineness

Genuineness implies that the nurse is an open, honest, sincere person who is actively involved in the relationship. She is a "real" person in a "real" encounter who is self-congruent, authentic, or "transparent."[35] Genuineness is the opposite of self-alienation, which occurs when many of one's real, spontaneous reactions to life are repressed or suppressed. Genuineness means that the nurse's response is sincere rather than phony. She is not thinking and feeling one thing and saying something different. The nurse expresses real feelings rather than presenting a defensive facade. "Being herself" simply means that at the moment the nurse is really whatever her response denotes. It is an essential quality because the nurse cannot expect openness, self-acceptance, and personal freedom in the patient if she lacks these qualities in the relationship.

Genuineness does not mean that the nurse must disclose her total self, but only that whatever she does show is a real aspect of herself and not merely a "professional" response that has been learned and repeated. It does not imply that the nurse will behave as she does with her family at home, neighborhood friends, or colleagues at a professional meeting. As she focuses on the patient, she puts aside much of her own need system and some of her usual ways of relating to others. Genuineness does not require that the nurse always express all her feelings; it requires only that whatever she does express is congruent. Neither does it imply impulsiveness or "anything goes." Carried to this extreme, genuineness can be destructive and work against the goals of a therapeutic relationship.

Following is an example of genuineness.

PATIENT: **I'd like my parents to give me my freedom and let me do my own thing. If I need them or want their advice, I'll ask them. Why don't they trust what they taught me? Why do parents have to make it so hard— like it's all or nothing?**

NURSE: **I know what you mean. My parents acted the same way. They offered advice, but what they expected was obedience. When they saw I could handle things on my own and used good judgment, they began to accept me as an individual. There are still times when they slip back into their old ways, but we understand each other better now. Do you think you and your parents need to share more openly and honestly your feelings and ideas?**

■ Respect

The quality of respect has also been called "nonpossessive warmth" or "unconditional positive regard."[15] Positive regard is unconditional in that it does not depend on the patient's behavior. Caring, liking, and valuing are other terms for respect. The patient is regarded as a person of worth; he is respected. The nurse's attitude is nonjudgmental, without criticism, ridicule, depreciation, or reservation. This does not mean that the nurse accepts all aspects of the patient's behavior as desirable or likeable or that she condones it. Yet the patient is accepted for what he is, as he is. She does not demand that he change to be accepted or that he be perfect. Imperfections are accepted along with mistakes and weaknesses as part of the human condition.

The inexperienced nurse may have difficulty accepting the patient without transferring her feelings about his thoughts or actions. However, acceptance means viewing his actions as coping behaviors that will change as the patient becomes less threatened and learns more adaptive mechanisms. It involves viewing his behavior as natural, normal, and expected, given his circumstances and perceptions.

Although there should be a basic respect for the patient simply as a person, respect is increased with understanding his uniqueness. Respect can be communicated in many different ways: by sitting silently with a patient who is crying, by genuine laughter with the patient over a particular event, by accepting the patient's request not to share a certain experience, by apologizing for the hurt unintentionally caused by a particular phrase, and by being open enough to communicate one's own anger or hurt caused by the patient. Being genuine with the patient and listening to him are also manifestations of respect for him. The nurse's ability to experience warmth for the patient depends in part on her ability to feel an unconditional positive regard for herself and an acceptance of both her own strengths and liabilities.

When the nurse communicates conditional warmth, she fosters feelings of dependency in the patient because she becomes the evaluator and superior in the relationship, making mutuality impossible. This might occur because of the nurse's need to be in control and dominant, or it might be fostered by the dependent, clinging patient. If dependency feelings should arise in the patient, the nurse can effectively deal with them by acknowledging them and exploring them with the patient.

■ Empathic understanding

Empathy has been defined by Kalisch as "the ability to enter into the life of another person, to accurately perceive his current feelings and their meanings. It is an essential element of the interpersonal process. When communicated, it forms the basis for a helping relationship between nurse and patient."[36:1548] Without it there is no basis for practice. It is understanding the patient's world from his internal frame of reference rather than from the nurse's own external frame of reference. Rogers described it as "to sense the client's private world as if it were your own, but without losing the 'as if' quality."[56:284] He believes that a high degree of empathy is one of the most potent factors in bringing about change and learning, and it is "one of the most delicate and powerful ways we have of using ourselves."[57:2]

Accurate empathy involves more than knowing

what the patient means. It also involves the nurse's sensitivity to the patient's current feelings and the verbal ability to communicate this understanding in a language attuned to the patient. It means frequently checking out with the patient the accuracy of one's perceptions and being guided by the patient's responses. It requires that the nurse lay aside personal views and values to enter another's world without prejudice. This can only be done by a nurse who is secure enough in herself that she knows she will not get lost in what may possibly be the strange or bizarre world of the patient and who can comfortably return to her own world when she wishes.

■   **DEVELOPMENT OF EMPATHY.** Empathic understanding consists of a number of stages. If the patient allows the nurse to enter his private world and attempts to communicate his perceptions and feelings, the nurse must be receptive to this communication. Next, the nurse must understand the communication of the patient. To do this, she must be able to put herself in the place of the patient and assume his role. She must then be able to step back into her own role and communicate her understanding to the patient. It is not necessary or desirable for the nurse to feel the same emotion as the patient. Empathy does not involve identification with the patient, and it should not be confused with sympathy. It is, instead, an appreciation and awareness of the patient's feelings. At deeper levels, empathy also involves enough understanding of human feelings and experiences to sense feelings that the patient only partially reveals.

A good deal of research has been conducted on empathy. The following discussion of the findings underscores its importance in counseling:

■   Empathy is clearly related to positive outcome.
■   Low empathy is related to a worsening in adjustment or pathologic conditions.
□   The ideal therapist is first of all empathic.
□   Empathy is correlated with self-exploration and process movement.
□   Empathy early in the relationship predicts later success.
□   The patient comes to perceive more empathy in successful cases.
□   Understanding is provided by the therapist, not drawn from her.
□   The more experienced the therapist, the more likely she is to be empathic.
□   Empathy is a special quality in a relationship, and therapists offer definitely more of it than even helpful friends.
■   The better integrated the therapist is within herself, the higher the degree of empathy she will be able to exhibit.

□   Experienced therapists often fall far short of being empathic.
□   Brilliance and diagnostic perceptiveness are unrelated to empathy.
■   An empathic way of being can be learned from empathic persons.

The findings highlighted with solid blocks are particularly relevant to improving nursing practice. The last statement indicates that the ability to be accurately empathic is something which can be learned; it is not something one is "born with." This is especially likely to occur if one's nursing educators and supervisors are themselves individuals of sensitive understanding and establish an empathic climate for learning.

The first two findings indicate that, depending on the empathic level of the therapist, therapeutic relationships can be "for better or worse." This is also true among nurses as evident in Williams' study,[76] which found that high and low levels of empathic communication were factors in changing the self-concept of institutionalized aged patients during group therapy.

Rogers[57] expands on the profound consequences empathy can have in promoting constructive learning and change. In the first place, it dissolves the patient's sense of alienation by connecting him on some level to a part of the human race. He can perceive that "I make sense to another human being . . . so I must not be so strange or alien. . . . And if I am in touch with someone else, I am not so all alone." On the other hand, if the patient is not responded to empathically, he may believe "If no one understands me, if no one can see what I'm experiencing, then I must be very bad off. . . . I'm sicker than even I thought." Another consequence of empathy for the patient is that he can see that someone values him, cares for him, and accepts him for the person he is. Then perhaps he can come to think "If this other person thinks I'm worthwhile, maybe I could value and care for myself. . . . Maybe I am worthwhile after all."

■   **EMPATHIC RESPONSES.** It is essential that the nurse first provides the contextual base for the relationship by her self-congruence or genuineness and her respect or unconditional positive regard for the patient. Then, the understanding conveyed to the patient through empathy gives him his personhood or identity. Each of us has the need to have our existence confirmed by another. Empathy gives the needed confirmation that one exists as a separate, valued, and unique person. The patient, as he perceives these new aspects of himself, incorporates them into his changing self-concept. And once his self-concept changes, his behavior changes, thus producing the positive outcome of therapy.

Gazda and co-workers[25] have described the following guidelines for responding with empathy:

1. Verbal and nonverbal behavior should be focused on by the helper.
2. The helper should formulate responses of empathy in a language and manner that is most easily understood by the helpee.
3. The tone of the helper's response should be similar to that of the helpee.
4. In addition to concentrating on what the helpee is expressing, the helper should also be aware of what is not being expressed.
5. The helper must accurately interpret responses to the helpee and use them as a guide in developing future responses.

A nursing study conducted by Mansfield[46] identified specific verbal and nonverbal behaviors that conveyed high levels of empathy to the patient:

- Having the nurse introduce herself to the patient
- Head and body positions turned toward the patient and occasionally leaning forward
- Verbal responses to the patient's previous comments, responses that focus on his strengths and resources
- Consistent eye contact and response to the patient's nonverbal cues, such as sighs, tone of voice, restlessness, and facial expressions
- Conveyance of interest, concern, and warmth by the nurse's own facial expressions
- A tone of voice consistent with facial expression and verbal response
- Mirror imaging of body position and gestures between the nurse and patient

Another study of nonverbal communication and empathy of patients and nurses showed that, in comparison to patients, nurses spent approximately twice as much interview time with direct eye gaze; three times longer with head nodding; and virtually the entire interview with legs crossed. Although nurses tended to smile more and laugh less than patients, these findings were not significant. The researchers then compared the behaviors of high- and low-empathy nurses. They reported that high-empathy nurses kept their legs still and in a crossed position, whereas low-empathy nurses had more extraneous leg movements and laughed twice as much as high-empathy nurses.[29]

Additional studies are needed in nursing to more precisely identify the behavioral indicators and outcomes of this important dimension of nursing care. The various methodologies utilized in empathic studies were reviewed by Gagan, who calls for additional studies to determine the precise nature and characteristics of the empathic process within the confines of the nurse-patient relationship.[23] Such research endeavors offer nursing the opportunity for scientific discovery and further advancement of its discipline.

■ **EMPATHIC FUNCTIONING SCALE.** Kalisch[36] devised a "Nurse-Patient Empathic Functioning Scale," which describes five levels or categories of empathy (Table 4-8). High levels of empathy (categories 3 and 4) communicate "I am with you," and the nurse's responses fit perfectly with the patient's conspicuous current feelings and content. Her responses also serve to expand the patient's awareness of his hidden feelings through the use of clarification and reflection. Such empathy is communicated by the language used, voice qualities, and nonverbal behavior, all of which reflect the nurse's seriousness and depth of feeling.

At low levels of empathy (categories 0 and 1), the nurse ignores the patient's feelings, goes off on a tangent of her own, or misinterprets what the patient is feeling. The nurse, at this low level, may be uninterested in the patient or concentrating on the "facts" of what the patient says rather than his current feelings and experiences. The nurse is doing other than listening; she may be evaluating the patient, giving advice, sermonizing, or thinking about her own problems or needs.

Empathic responses need to be properly timed within the nurse-patient relationship. Responses from category 4 in the orientation phase may be viewed as too intense and intrusive. Usually a number of category 2 responses are required initially to build an atmosphere of trust and openness. In the later stages of the orientation phase and, most particularly, in the working phase, categories 3 and 4 responses are appropriate and most effective. Responses from categories 0 and 1 are nontherapeutic at all times and block the development of the relationship.

The various levels of empathy are evident in the following example:

PATIENT: **I'm really jittery today, and I hope I can get things out right. It started when I saw Bob on Friday, and it's been building up since then.**

NURSE: **You're feeling tense and anxious, and it's related to a talk you had with Bob on Friday. (Category 2.)**

PATIENT: **Yes. He began putting pressure on me to have sex with him again.**

NURSE: **It sounds like you resent it when he pressures you for sex. (Category 3.)**

PATIENT: **I do. Why does he think things always have to be his way? I guess he knows I'm a pushover.**

NURSE: **It makes you angry when he wants his way even though he knows you feel differently. But you usually give in and then you wind up disappointed in yourself and feeling like a failure. (Category 4.)**

TABLE 4-8

NURSE-PATIENT EMPATHIC FUNCTIONING SCALE

Categories of nurse empathic functioning	Level of patient's feelings	
	Conspicuous current feelings	Hidden current feelings
Category 0	Ignores	Ignores
Category 1	Communicates awareness that is accurate at times and inaccurate at other times	Ignores
Category 2	Communicates complete and accurate awareness of essence and strength of feelings	Communicates an awareness of presence of hidden feelings but is not accurate in defining their essence or strength; effort being made to understand
Category 3	Same as category 2	Communicates an accurate awareness of hidden feelings slightly beyond what patient expresses himself
Category 4	Same as category 2	Communicates without uncertainty an accurate awareness of deepest, most hidden feelings

From Kalisch, B.: Am. J. Nurs. **73:**1548, 1973. Copyright © 1973, American Journal of Nursing Company. Reproduced, with permission, from American Journal of Nursing, September, vol. 73, no. 9.

PATIENT: **It happens just like that over and over. It's as if I never learn.**
NURSE: **So when the incident's all over, you're left blaming yourself and wallowing in self-pity. (Category 4.)**
PATIENT: **I guess that's right.**

Differences between nurses and patients are barriers to empathy. Differences in sex, age, religion, socioeconomic status, education, and culture can block the development of empathic understanding. Because everyone is unique, no one can completely understand another person. However, the wider a person's background and the more varied one's experiences, the greater will be the potential for understanding people.

Identical or similar experiences are not essential for empathy. No man can really experience what it is like to be a woman; no white can experience what it is like to be black. It is not necessary to be exactly like another, but it is desirable for nurses to prepare themselves in any way they can to understand potential patients. It is also important for nurses to realize that empathy can be learned and enhanced, and staff development programs have been documented as effective in raising a nurse's ability to perceive and respond with empathy.[41]

■ **Concreteness**

Concreteness involves the use of specific terminology rather than abstractions in the discussion of the patient's feelings, experiences, and behavior. It avoids vagueness and ambiguity and is the opposite of generalizing, categorizing, classifying, and labeling the patient's experiences. It has three functions: (1) to keep the nurse's responses close to the patient's feelings and experiences, (2) to foster accuracy of understanding by the nurse, and (3) to encourage the patient to attend to specific problem areas.[15] By focusing the patient in specific and concrete terms to his vague ramblings, the nurse helps the patient identify significant aspects of his problems.

The level of concreteness should vary during the various phases of the nurse-patient relationship. In the orientation phase, concreteness should be high and, at this time, it can contribute to empathic understanding. It is essential for the formulation of specific goals and plans. As the patient explores various feelings and perceptions related to his problems in the working phase of the relationship, concreteness should be at a relatively low level to facilitate a thorough self-exploration. At the end of the working phase when the patient is engaging in action and during the termination phase, high levels of concreteness are again desirable.

Concreteness is evident in the following examples:

EXAMPLE 1

PATIENT: **I wouldn't have any problems if people would**

quit bothering me. They like to upset me because they knew I'm high strung.

NURSE: **What people try to upset you?**

PATIENT: **My family. People think being from a large family is a blessing. I think it's a curse.**

NURSE: **Could you give me an example of something someone in your family did that upset you?**

EXAMPLE 2

PATIENT: **I don't know what the problem is between us. My wife and I just don't get along anymore. We seem to disagree about everything. I think I love her, but she isn't affectionate or caring—hasn't been for a long time.**

NURSE: **You say you're not sure what the problem is, and you think you love your wife. But the two of you argue often and she hasn't given you any sign of love or affection. Have you felt affectionate toward her, and when was the last time you let her know how you felt?**

These four responsive dimensions or conditions facilitate the formation of a therapeutic relationship. Few research instruments, however, have been developed in nursing to objectively evaluate nurse-patient interactions. Aiken and Aiken[1] have adapted the scales developed by Carkhoff and Truax relative to the core dimensions of empathic understanding, positive regard, genuineness, concreteness, and self-exploration. They divided each dimension into facilitative levels that would allow a practitioner to score herself on them. Methven and Schlotfeldt[49] developed an instrument designed to determine the nature of verbal responses nurses tend to give in emotion-laden situations typically encountered in nursing practice. Stetler[68] analyzed the relationship between empathy as perceived by a helpee and the communication of a helper in a therapeutic interaction. She reported on verbal, nonverbal, and vocal levels of communication. The therapeutic level at which nurses function is unknown at present. Additional research is greatly needed on nurse-patient interactions because there is little empirical evidence on which to base scientific practice in this area.

Action dimensions

Carkhoff identified the action-oriented or initiative conditions for facilitative interpersonal relationships to be those of confrontation, immediacy, and therapist self-disclosure. To these will be added the dimensions of catharsis and role playing. The separation of these therapeutic conditions into two groups, the understanding or responsive conditions and the initiating or action conditions, is not a distinct separation. To some extent all the dimensions are present throughout the therapeutic relationship. The action dimensions must have a context of warmth and understanding. This is important for the inexperienced nurse to recall because she may be tempted to move into high levels of action dimensions without having established adequate understanding, empathy, warmth, or respect. The responsive dimensions allow the patient to achieve insight, but this is not enough. With the action dimensions, the nurse moves the therapeutic relationship upward and outward by identifying obstacles to the patient's progress and the need for both internal understanding and external action.

■ Confrontation

Confrontation is an expression by the nurse of perceived discrepancies in the patient's behavior. Carkhoff[14] identifies three categories of confrontation:

1. Discrepancy between the patient's expression of what he is (self-concept) and what he wants to be (self-ideal)
2. Discrepancies between the patient's verbal expressions about himself and his behavior
3. Discrepancies between the patient's expressed experience of himself and the nurse's experience of him

Confrontation is an attempt by the nurse to bring to the patient's awareness the incongruence in his feelings, attitudes, beliefs, and behaviors. It may also lead to the discovery of ambivalent feelings in the patient. Confrontation is not limited to negative aspects of the patient. It also includes pointing out discrepancies involving his resources and strengths that are unrecognized and unused. It requires that the nurse collect sufficient data about the patient's history, perceptions, and observations of his verbal and nonverbal communication, so that validation of reality is possible.

Confrontation usually implies venting anger and aggressive behavior. This has the effect of belittling, blaming, and embarrassing the receiver—all of which are harmful and destructive in both social and therapeutic relationships. However, confrontation as a therapeutic action dimension is an assertive, rather than aggressive, action. It requires that the nurse take some risks, avoid venting her own feelings, and help the patient bring his discrepancies into his awareness.

The nurse must have developed an understanding of the patient to perceive discrepancies, inconsistencies in word and deed, distortions, defenses, and evasions. The relationship must also contain a bond that will weather the mild or severe crises which confrontation precipitates. The nurse must be willing and capable of working through this crisis after she confronts her patient. Without this commitment, the confrontation lacks therapeutic potential and can be quite damaging to both the nurse and patient. Without question, the effects of confrontation are challenge, exposure, risk, and the possibility for growth. When the nurse uses confrontation, she is modeling an active role to her patient in which she is using insight and understanding to remove ambiguity and inconsistency and thus seek deeper understanding.

■ **TIMING IN RELATIONSHIP.** Bromley[8] suggests that prior to confrontation, the nurse assess the following factors: the trust level in the relationship, the timing, the patient's stress level, the strength of his defense mechanisms, his perceived need for personal space or closeness, and his level of rage and tolerance for hearing another perception. The patient has the capacity to deny or accept the nurse's observations, and his response to the confrontation can serve as a measure of its success or failure. Acceptance indicates appropriate timing and patient readiness. Denial by the patient serves to allay the threat that the confrontation posed to the patient. It provides additional information to the nurse, since it tells her that the patient is resisting change and is unwilling to enlarge his view of reality at this time.

Confrontation must be appropriately timed to be effective. In the orientation phase of the relationship, the nurse should use confrontation infrequently and pose it as an observation of incongruent behavior. A simple "mirroring" of the discrepancy between a patient's actions and words is the most nonthreatening type of confrontation. The nurse might say, "You seem to be saying two different things." This type of confrontation closely resembles clarification at this time. She might also identify discrepancies between how she and her patient are experiencing their relationship, point out unnoticed strengths or untapped resources of the patient, or provide him with objective, but perhaps different, information about his world. According to Carkhoff, "Premature direct confrontations may have a demoralizing and demobilizing effect upon an inadequately prepared helpee.[14:93] This is because confrontation requires high levels of empathy and respect to be effective.

In the working phase of the relationship, more direct confrontations may focus on specific patient discrepancies. The nurse may confront the patient with areas of weaknesses or shortcomings or focus on the discrepancy between her experience of the patient and his own. This expands the awareness of the patient and helps him move to higher levels of functioning. As Carkhoff says, "Confrontation of self and others is prerequisite to the healthy individual's encounter with life."[14:93] Confrontation is especially important to point out when the patient has developed insight but his behavior has not changed. This enables him to see the

need to effect actual behavior change. This type of confrontation encourages the patient to act on his world in a reasonable and constructive manner, rather than assuming a dependent and passive stance toward life.

Research indicates that effective counselors use confrontation frequently, confronting patients with their assets more often in earlier interviews and with their limitations in later interviews.[2] Furthermore, Mitchell and Berenson[50] found that therapists who rated significantly higher on empathy, genuineness, respect, and concreteness confronted their patients significantly more often than those therapists who were less facilitative. In the initial interview, these confrontations were based on attempts to clarify the relationship, eliminate misconceptions, provide the patient more objective information about himself and his world, and emphasize the patient's strengths and resources.

Inexperienced nurses frequently avoid confrontation. Certainly it does involve a risk. It can be nontherapeutic when it is not associated with empathy or warmth or when it is used to vent the nurse's negative feelings of anger, frustration, and aggressiveness. However, carefully monitored confrontation can be viewed as an extension of genuineness and concreteness and is a useful therapeutic intervention that can further the patient's growth and progress.

Confrontation is evident in the following examples:

EXAMPLE 1

NURSE: **I see you as someone who has a lot of strength. You've been able to give a tremendous amount of emotional support to your children at a time when they needed it very much.**

EXAMPLE 2

NURSE: **It was my understanding that we were meeting together to talk about the problems that brought you to the hospital. But everytime I come, you ask me to play cards with you, share a game of table tennis, or toss around a basketball. It seems to me that we're not in agreement on what these meetings are all about.**

EXAMPLE 3

NURSE: **The fact that Sue didn't accept your date for Friday night doesn't necessarily mean she never wants to go out with you. She could have had another date or other plans with her family or girl friends. But if you don't ask her, you'll never find out why she refused you or if she'll accept in the future.**

EXAMPLE 4

NURSE: **We've talked three different times now and you've told me how you really don't have a problem or that other people make trouble for you. But I've noticed that on the ward you seldom talk to the other patients and little accidents like the spilled coffee at lunch really seem to upset you.**

EXAMPLE 5

NURSE: **You tell me how your parents don't trust you and never give you any responsibility, but each week you also tell me how you stayed out beyond your curfew or had friends over when your parents weren't home. Do you see a connection between the two?**

EXAMPLE 6

NURSE: **You say you want to feel better and go back to work, but you're not taking your medicine, which will help you to do that.**

EXAMPLE 7

NURSE: **We've been talking for 3 weeks now on how you need to get out and try to meet some people. We even talked of different ways to do that. But so far you haven't made any effort to join aerobics, take a class, or do any of the other ideas we had.**

■ Immediacy

Immediacy involves focusing on the current interaction of the nurse and the patient in the relationship. It is a significant dimension because the patient's behavior and functioning in the relationship are indicative of functioning in other interpersonal relationships. Most patients experience difficulty in interpersonal relationships; so the patient's functioning in the nurse-patient relationship must be evaluated. As Carkhoff states, "The way he relates to the counselor is a snapshot of the way he relates to others. . . . If the counselor does not focus on trying to understand these things, growth possibilities for clients can be missed."[14:192] The nurse has the opportunity to intervene directly with the patient's problem behavior, and the patient has the opportunity to learn and change his behavior. Immediacy may be viewed as empathy, genuineness, or confrontation that involves a particular content—the relationship between the nurse and the patient.

Immediacy connotes sensitivity by the nurse to the feelings of the patient and a willingness to deal with them rather than ignore them. This is particularly difficult when the nurse must recognize and respond to negative feelings expressed by the patient toward her. It is compounded by the fact that patients often express these messages indirectly and conceal them in references to other persons.

It is not appropriate or possible for the nurse to focus continually on the immediacy of the relationship. It is most appropriate to do so when the relationship seems to be stalled or is not progressing. Frequently this is due to factors in the immediate nurse-patient relationship, and focusing on them may help. It is also helpful to look at immediacy when the relationship is progressing particularly well. In both instances the patient is actively involved in describing what he feels is helping or hindering the relationship.

As with the other dimensions, high-level immediacy responses should not be suddenly presented to the patient. The nurse must first know and understand him and have developed a good, open relationship. The nurse's initial expressions of immediacy should be tentatively phrased, for example, "Are you trying to tell me how you feel about our relationship?" As the relationship progresses, observations related to immediacy can be made more directly, and, as communication improves, the need for immediacy responses may decrease.

Following are two examples of immediacy:

EXAMPLE 1

PATIENT: **I've been thinking about our meetings, and I'm really pretty busy now to keep coming. Besides, I don't see the point in them, and we don't seem to be getting anywhere.**

NURSE: **Are you trying to say you're feeling discouraged and you feel our meetings aren't helping you?**

EXAMPLE 2

PATIENT: **The staff here could care less about us patients. They treat us like children instead of adults.**

NURSE: **I'm wondering if you feel that I don't care about you or perhaps I don't value your opinion?**

■ Nurse self-disclosure

Self-disclosures have three characteristics. They are (1) subjectively true, (2) personal statements about the self, and (3) intentionally revealed to another person. In self-disclosure the nurse reveals information about herself, her ideas, values, feelings, and attitudes. She may share that she has had experiences or feelings similar to those of the patient and may emphasize both the similarities and differences. This kind of self-disclosure is an index of the closeness of the relationship and involves a particular kind of respect for the patient. It is an expression of genuineness and honesty by the nurse and is an aspect of empathy.

The rationale for nurse self-disclosure comes from the theoretical and research literature, which provides significant evidence that therapist self-disclosure increases the likelihood of patient self-disclosure. Patient self-disclosure is necessary for a successful therapeutic outcome. It must be emphasized, however, that self-disclosure by the nurse must be used judiciously, and this is determined by the quality, quantity, and appropriateness of her disclosures.

The number of self-disclosures appears to be crucial to the success of the therapy. Although too few nurse self-disclosures may fail to produce patient self-disclosures, too many may decrease the time available for patient disclosure or alienate him. There thus appears to be a nonlinear relationship between nurse genuineness and patient disclosure. The problem for the nurse is knowing where the middle ground is. Clinical experience is necessary to determine the optimal therapeutic level.

The appropriateness or relevancy of the nurse's self-disclosure is also important. The nurse should self-disclose in response to statements made by the patient. If her disclosure is far from what the patient is experiencing, it can serve to distract the patient from his problem or make him feel alienated from the nurse. A patient who is experiencing severe or panic levels of anxiety may feel threatened or frightened by the nurse's self-disclosure. She must be careful, in these cases, not to burden a patient with her own self-disclosures. Above all, disclosure by the nurse is always for the patient's benefit. The nurse does not disclose herself to meet her own needs or make herself feel better. She does not impose herself on the patient. When the nurse does self-disclose, she should have a particular therapeutic goal in mind.

Weiner has proposed guidelines that nurses can use to evaluate the potential usefulness of their self-disclosure.[74] These include:

1. Cooperation—Will the disclosure enhance the patient's cooperation, which is necessary to the development of a therapeutic alliance?
2. Learning—Will the disclosure assist the patient's ability to learn about himself, to set short- and long-term goals, and to deal more effectively with life's problems?
3. Catharsis—Will the disclosure assist the patient to express formerly held or suppressed feelings, important to the relief of emotional symptoms?
4. Support—Will the disclosure provide the patient with support or reinforcement for the goals that he is trying to accomplish in his life?

If so, then the nurse needs to consider the judicious use of nurse self-disclosure given the type and goal of treatment, the context of the nurse-patient relationship, the patient's ego strength, the patient's feelings about the nurse, and the nurse's feelings about the patient. These guidelines govern the "dosage and timing" of self-disclosures and help the nurse assess the appropriateness, effectiveness, and anticipated response of the patient to the disclosure.

Self-disclosure by the nurse is evident in the following example:

PATIENT: **When he told me he didn't want to see me again, I felt like slapping him and hugging him at the same time. But then I knew the problem was really me and no one could ever love me.**
NURSE: **When I broke off with a man I had been seeing, I felt the anger, hurt, and bitterness you just described. I remember thinking I would never date another man.**

In this example the nurse self-disclosed to emphasize that the patient's feelings were natural. She also reinforced the external cause for the separation (boyfriend's decision to leave versus the patient's inadequacy) and implied that, with time, the patient will be able to resolve the loss.

Even though research has indicated the importance of this dimension for patient growth, it appears to be an area of some discomfort for nurses. Johnson[33, 34] studied the level of reciprocal disclosure occurring between nurses and patients on four clinical units—medical, surgical, psychiatric, and critical care. She found that there was a tendency for both state and trait anxiety levels to be lower among nurses and patients as their levels of self-disclosure increased. In addition, she reported low reciprocal self-disclosure occurring in the psychiatric unit despite the verbal nature of psychiatric therapy and the lack of restrictions placed on talking about oneself. She concluded from her study that nurses and patients need to be assisted in learning to be open and authentic in their interactions with each other.

■ Emotional catharsis

Emotional catharsis occurs when the patient is encouraged to talk about things that bother him most. Fears, feelings, and experiences are brought out into the open and discussed with the nurse. The expression of feelings can be very therapeutic in itself, even if behavioral change does not ensue. The previously described responsive dimensions create an atmosphere within the nurse-patient relationship in which emotional catharsis is possible. The patient's responsiveness will depend on the confidence and trust he has in the nurse.

The nurse must be able to recognize cues from the patient that he is ready to discuss his problems. It is important that the nurse proceed with the patient at the rate he chooses and support him as he discusses difficult areas. If emotional catharsis is forced on the patient, it could precipitate a panic episode as his defenses are attacked, but sufficient alternative coping mechanisms are not available to him.

Patients are often uncomfortable about expressing feelings because of prohibitive social norms. Nurses may be equally uncomfortable with them, particularly with expressing feelings of sadness or anger. Frequently nurses assume they know the patient's feelings and do not attempt to specifically validate them. The dimensions of empathy and immediacy require the attendance to and expression of emotions. Unresolved feelings and feelings that are avoided can cause stalls or barriers in the nurse-patient relationship. Specific examples of this are transference and countertransference phenomena, which will be discussed later in the chapter.

If the patient is having difficulty expressing feelings, the nurse may help by suggesting how she might feel in the patient's place or how others might feel in that situation. She might validate with the patient the feeling he seems to be describing in a general way. Some patients respond directly to the question "How did that make you feel?" whereas others intellectualize and avoid the emotional element in their answer. When patients realize they can express their feelings within an accepting relationship, they expand their awareness and potential acceptance of themselves.

The following example illustrates emotional catharsis:

NURSE: **How did you feel when your boss corrected you in front of all those customers?**

PATIENT: **Well, I understood that he needed to set me straight, and he's the type that flies off the handle pretty easily anyhow.**

NURSE: **It sounds like you're defending his behavior. I was wondering how you felt at that moment.**

PATIENT: **Awkward . . . uh . . . upset, I guess (pause).**

NURSE: **That would have made me pretty angry if it happened to me.**

PATIENT: **Well, I was. But you can't let it show, you know. You have to keep it all in because of the customers. But he can let it out. Oh *sure* (emphatically)! He can tell *me* anything he wants. Just *once* I'd like him to know how *I* feel.**

■ Role playing

Role playing involves the acting out of a particular situation. It functions to increase the patient's insight into human relations and can deepen his ability to see the situation from another person's point of view. Sedgwick[64] identifies the intent of role playing to be a close representation of real life behavior that involves the individual holistically, to focus attention on a problem, and to permit the individual to see himself in action in a neutral situation. It provides a bridge between thought and action in a "safe" environment in which the patient can feel free to experiment with new behavior. It is a method of learning that makes actual behavior the focus of study, is action oriented, and provides immediately available information. Role playing consists of the following steps: defining the problem, creating a readiness for role playing, establishing the situation, casting the characters, briefing and warming up, considering the training design, acting, stopping, involving the audience, analysis and discussion, and evaluation.

When role play is used for attitude change, it relies heavily on role reversal. The patient may be asked to play the role of a certain person in a specific situation or to play the role of someone with opposing beliefs. Research indicates that role reversal can help a person reevaluate the other person's intentions and become more understanding of the other person's position.[6] After role reversal, patients may be more receptive to modifying their own attitudes.

As a method of self-awareness and conflict resolution, role playing may help the patient "experience" a situation, rather than just "talk about it." Role playing can elicit feelings in the patient that are similar in nature and intensity to those experienced in the actual situation. It provides an opportunity for insight and for the expression of affect. For these reasons, it is a useful method for heightening a patient's awareness of his feelings about a situation.

One of the specific ways in which role playing can be used to resolve conflicts and increase self-awareness is through a "dialogue" that requires the patient to take the part of each person or each side of an argument. He is then asked to "play out" the conflict through an imaginary dialogue. If the conflict is internal, the dialogue occurs in the present tense between his conflicting selves until one part of the conflict outweighs the other. If the conflict involves a second person, the patient is instructed to "imagine that the other person is sitting in the chair across from you." The patient is told to begin the dialogue by expressing wants and resentments about the other person. Then the patient changes chairs, assumes the role of the other person, and responds to what was just said. The patient assumes the first role again and responds to the other person. Dialoguing in this way not only serves as practice for the patient in expressing feelings and opinions, but also gives a reality base for the probable response from the other party involved in the conflict. This can often remove the barrier that is keeping the patient from making a decision and implementing the necessary action steps.

Role playing is included as an action dimension because it can facilitate the patient's development of insight. Nurses need a variety of intervention skills. Role playing can be effective when an impasse has been reached in the patient's progress, or when he is having difficulty translating insight into action. In these instances it can reduce tension and allow the patient the opportunity to practice or test out new behaviors for future use.

Table 4-9 summarizes the responsive and action dimensions for therapeutic nurse-patient relationships. In concluding this section of therapeutic dimensions, it must be emphasized that the nurse's effectiveness will be based on her openness to learn what works best with particular kinds of patients. Both the use of communication techniques and the therapeutic conditions must

TABLE 4-9

RESPONSIVE AND ACTION DIMENSIONS FOR THERAPEUTIC NURSE-PATIENT RELATIONSHIPS

Dimension	Characteristics
Responsive dimensions	
Genuineness	Implies that the nurse is an open person who is self-congruent, authentic, and transparent
Respect	Suggests that the patient is regarded as a person of worth who is valued and accepted without qualification
Empathic understanding	Viewing the patient's world from his internal frame of reference, with sensitivity to the patient's current feelings and the verbal ability to communicate this understanding in a language attuned to the patient
Concreteness	Involves the use of specific terminology rather than abstractions in the discussion of the patient's feelings, experiences, and behavior
Action dimensions	
Confrontation	The expression by the nurse of perceived discrepancies in the patient's behavior to expand his self-awareness
Immediacy	Occurs when the current interaction of the nurse and patient in the relationship is focused on and is used to learn about the patient's functioning in other interpersonal relationships
Nurse self-disclosure	Evident when the nurse reveals information about herself, her ideas, values, feelings, and attitudes to facilitate the patient's cooperation, learning, catharsis, or support
Emotional catharsis	Takes place when the patient is encouraged to talk about things that bother him most for its therapeutic effect
Role playing	The acting-out of a particular situation to increase the patient's insight into human relations and deepen his ability to see a situation from another point of view. It also allows the patient to experiment with new behavior in a safe environment

be individualized to the nurse's personality and the needs of her patients. Rote application can be destructive. The nurse must be willing to try other approaches and techniques that seem potentially helpful when the present approach seems ineffective at a given time with the patient.

Therapeutic impasses

Therapeutic impasses are blocks in the progress of the nurse-patient relationship. They arise for a variety of reasons and may take many different forms, but they all create stalls in the therapeutic relationship. These impasses provoke intense feelings in both the nurse and patient that may range from anxiety and apprehension to frustration, love, or intense anger. Four specific therapeutic impasses and ways to overcome them will now be discussed: resistance, transference, countertransference, and gift giving.

■ Resistance

Resistance is the patient's attempt to remain unaware of anxiety-producing aspects within himself. It is a natural reluctance or learned avoidance of verbalizing or even experiencing troubled aspects of self. The term *resistance* was initially introduced by Freud to mean the patient's unconscious opposition to exploring or recognizing unconscious or even preconscious material. The patient's ambivalent attitudes toward self-exploration, in which he both appreciates and avoids anxiety-producing experiences, are a normal part of the therapeutic process. Primary resistance is often caused by the patient's unwillingness to change when the need for change is recognized. Resistance behaviors are usually displayed by patients during the working phase of the relationship because it contains the greater part of the problem-solving process.

Resistance may also be a reaction by the patient to

Forms of Resistance Displayed by Patients

- Suppression and repression of pertinent information
- Intensification of symptoms
- Self-devaluation and a hopeless outlook on the future
- Forced flight into health where there is a sudden, but short-lived recovery by the patient
- Intellectual inhibitions, which may be evident when the patient says he has "nothing on his mind" or that he is "unable to think about his problems" or when he breaks appointments, is late for sessions, or is forgetful, silent, or sleepy

- Acting out or irrational behavior
- Superficial talk
- Intellectual insight in which the patient verbalizes self-understanding with correct use of terminology yet continues destructive behavior, or use of the defense of intellectualization where there is no insight
- Contempt for normality, which is evident when the patient has developed insight but refuses to assume the responsibility for change on the grounds that normality "isn't so great"
- Transference reactions

the nurse who has moved too rapidly or too deeply into the patient's feelings or who has intentionally or nonintentionally communicated a lack of respect. It may also simply be the result of a patient who has a nurse working with him who is an inappropriate role model for therapeutic behavior.

Secondary gain is another cause of resistance. It can become a powerful force in the perpetuation and propagation of an illness, since it makes the environment more comfortable. Favorable environmental, interpersonal, and situational changes occur, and material advantages may be secured as a result of the illness. Types of secondary gain include financial compensation, avoidance of unpleasant situations, the securing of increased sympathy or attention, escape from responsibility, attempted control of people, and lessening of social pressures.

Resistance may take many forms. The accompanying box lists some of the forms of resistance displayed by patients as identified by Wolberg.[77]

■ Transference

Transference is an unconscious response of the patient in which he experiences feelings and attitudes toward the nurse that were originally associated with significant figures in his early life. Such responses utilize the defense mechanism of displacement and may be triggered by some superficial similarity, such as a facial feature or manner of speech or by the patient's perceived similarity of the relationship. The term transference refers to a group of reactions that attempt to reduce or alleviate anxiety. The outstanding trait defining trans-

ference is the inappropriateness of the patient's response in terms of intensity.

Transference reduces the patient's self-awareness by helping him maintain a generalized view of the world in which all people are seen in similar terms. Thus the nurse may be viewed as an authority figure from the past, such as a parent figure, or as a lost loved object, such as a former spouse. Transference reactions are harmful to the therapeutic process only if they remain ignored and unexamined.

Two types of transference present particular resistances in the nurse-patient relationship. The first is the **hostile transference.** If the patient internalizes his anger and hostility, he may express this resistance as depression and discouragement. He may ask to terminate the relationship on the grounds that he has no chance of getting well. If the patient usually externalizes his hostility, he may become critical, defiant, and irritable. He may express doubts about the nurse's training, experience, or personal adjustment. He may attempt to compete with her by reading books on psychology and challenging her.

Hostility may also be expressed by the patient in detachment, forgetfulness, irrelevant chatter, or preoccupation with childhood experiences. An extreme form of uncooperativeness and negativism is evident in prolonged silences. Some of the most frustrating moments for the nurse are those spent in total silence with a patient. This is not the therapeutic silence that communicates mutuality and understanding. Rather, it is the silence that seems to be hostile, eternal, and oppressive. It is particularly disturbing for the nurse in the orientation phase before a relationship has been established. Generally, silences are more uncomfortable for the patient than they are for the nurse, but in this case the reverse may be true. The nurse's task is to understand the meaning of the patient's silence, and decide how to deal with it despite feeling somewhat awkward and useless.

A second difficult type of transference is the **dependent reaction transference.** This resistance is characterized by patients who are submissive, subordinate, and ingratiating and who regard the nurse as a "godlike" figure. The patient overvalues the characteristics and qualities of the nurse, and their relationship is in jeopardy because the patient views it as magical. In this reaction the nurse must live up to the overwhelming expectations of the patient, which is impossible because they are completely unrealistic. The patient continues to demand more of the nurse, and when she does not meet his needs, he is filled with hostility and contempt.

■ Overcoming resistance and transference

Resistances and transferences can pose difficult problems for the nurse. The psychiatric nurse must be prepared to be exposed to powerful negative and positive emotional feelings coming from the patient, often on a highly irrational basis. The relationship can become stalled and nonbeneficial if the nurse is not prepared for the patient's expression of feelings, is not prepared to deal with them, or is so preoccupied by her own needs and problems that she cannot clearly perceive what is happening.

Sometimes resistances occur because the nurse and patient have not arrived at mutually acceptable goals or plans of action. Perhaps the patient expected the nurse to give him advice or solve his problems for him. This may occur if the contract was not clearly defined in the orientation stage of the relationship. The appropriate action here is to return to the goals, purpose, and roles of the nurse and patient in the relationship.

Whatever the patient's motivations, the analysis of the resistance or transference is geared toward his gaining awareness of them and the development of his knowledge that he controls his behavior and ultimately he is responsible for all he does and experiences. The first thing the nurse must do in handling resistance or transference is to listen. When she recognizes the resistance, she then uses clarification and reflection of feeling. Clarification helps give the nurse a more focused idea of what is happening. Reflection of content may help the patient to become aware of what has been going on in his own mind. Reflection of feeling acknowledges the resistance and mirrors it back to the patient. The nurse may say, "I sense that you're struggling with yourself. Part of you wants to explore the issue of your marriage and another part says 'No—I'm not ready yet.'"

It is not sufficient, however, to merely identify that resistance is occurring. The behavior must be explored and possible reasons for its occurrence analyzed. The

Forms of Countertransference Displayed by Nurses

- Inability to empathize with the patient in certain problem areas
- Depressed feelings during or after the session
- Carelessness about implementing the contract by being late, running overtime, etc.
- Drowsiness during the sessions
- Feelings of anger or impatience because of the patient's unwillingness to change
- Encouragement of the patient's dependency, praise, or affection
- Arguing with the patient or a tendency to push the patient before he is ready
- Trying to help the patient in matters not related to the identified nursing goals

- Involvement with the patient on a personal or social level
- Dreaming about or preoccupation with the patient
- Sexual or aggressive fantasies toward the patient
- Recurrent anxiety, unease, or guilt feelings about the patient
- A tendency to focus repetitively on only one aspect or way of looking at the information presented by the patient
- A need to defend nursing interventions with the patient to others

depth of exploration and analysis engaged in by nurse and patient is related to her experience and knowledge base. The nurse prepared on the master's degree level has the background to review the material of resistance and work through the transference reaction with the patient. The process of supervision will aid her in this endeavor and minimize the effect of any negative reactions she may experience within herself.

■ Countertransference

Countertransference is a therapeutic impasse created by the nurse. It refers to her specific emotional response generated by the qualities of her patient that is inappropriate to the content and context of the therapeutic relationship or inappropriate in the degree of intensity of emotion. It is transference applied to the nurse. Inappropriateness is the crucial element, as it is with transference, because it is natural that the nurse will have a warmth toward or liking for some patients more than others for realistic reasons. She will also be genuinely angry with the actions of certain patients. But in countertransference her responses are not justified by reality. She will be identifying the patient with individuals from her past, and her own needs will be interfering with her effectiveness. Her unresolved conflicts about authority, sex, assertiveness, and independence will tend to create, rather than solve, problems.

Countertransference reactions are usually one of three types: reactions of intense love or caring, reactions of intense hostility or hatred, and reactions of intense anxiety often in response to resistance by the patient. Through the use of immediacy the nurse can identify countertransference in one of its various forms. The accompanying box lists some forms of countertransference displayed by nurses as described by Langs and Menninger.[42,48]

Forms of countertransference occur because the nurse is involved with the patient as a participant observer and is not a detached bystander. They can be powerful tools in exploration and potent instruments for uncovering inner states. They are destructive only if they are brushed aside, ignored, or not taken seriously.

These reactions, if studied objectively, can lead to further information and data about the patient. The analysis of countertransference can bring to light new material of which the nurse was not previously aware. The ability to remain objective does not mean that the nurse may not at times dislike what the patient says or may become irritated. The resistance of the patient to acquire insight and transform insight into action and the refusal of the patient to change maladaptive and destructive coping mechanisms can be frustrating. But

the capacity of the nurse to understand her feelings will help her to maintain a working relationship with the patient.

Countertransference may also be manifested as a group phenomenon. Psychiatric staff members can become involved in countertransference reactions when they overreact to a patient's aggressive behavior, ignore available patient data that would promote understanding, or become locked in a power struggle with a patient. Other types of countertransference might include ignoring patient behavior that doesn't fit the staff's diagnosis, minimizing the behavior of a patient, joking about or criticizing a patient, or becoming caught up in intimidation. Although these have been reported as phenomena of group countertransference, they can also be illustrative of individual countertransference reactions.

One difference between an inexperienced and an experienced psychiatric nurse is that the experienced nurse is constantly on the lookout for countertransference, becomes aware of it when it occurs, and holds it in abeyance or utilizes it to promote the therapeutic goals. In attempting to identify a countertransference the nurse must apply the same standards of honest self-appraisal to herself that she expects of the patient. She should subject herself to self-examination throughout the course of the relationship and particularly when the patient attacks or criticizes her. The following questions may be helpful:

- How do I feel about the patient?
- Do I look forward to seeing him?
- Do I feel sorry for or sympathetic toward him?
- Am I bored with him and believe that we are not progressing?
- Am I afraid of him?
- Do I get extreme pleasure out of seeing him?
- Do I want to protect, reject, or punish him?
- Do I dread meeting him and feel nervous during the sessions?
- Am I impressed by him or do I try to impress him?
- Does he make me very angry or frustrated?

If any of these questions suggest a problem, the nurse should pursue it. What is the patient doing to provoke these feelings? Who does the patient remind me of? The nurse must discover the source of the problem. Because countertransference can be detrimental to the relationship, it should be dealt with as soon as possible. When recognized, the nurse can exercise control over it. Frequently the nurse needs help in dealing with countertransference. Individual or group supervision can be most beneficial. Weekly clinical seminars, peer consultation, and professional meetings can also offer emotional support.

■ **PROBLEM PATIENTS.** Countertransference problems are most clearly evident when someone is labeled a "problem patient." Usually such a patient engenders strong negative feelings, such as anger, fear, and helplessness and is often described by nurses as "manipulative, a pain, dependent, inappropriate, and demanding." The label of "problem patient" implies that the patient should change his behavior for the sake of the helper rather than for his own benefit. A common consequence of this labeling is that the patient and nurse become adversaries, and the nurse avoids contact with him.

A study of the treatment records of "difficult patients" revealed some interesting findings. As compared to controls, difficult patients were simultaneously involved in or referred to two or more treatment programs, had no one person primarily responsible for coordinating their treatment programs, had incomplete documentation of treatment contacts, and lacked a comprehensive diagnosis and treatment plan.[52] A more recent study of therapist actions that address initially poor therapeutic alliances between the patient and therapist found that improved alliances and good outcomes were associated with (1) addressing the patient's defenses; (2) addressing the patient's guilt and expectations of punishment; (3) addressing the patient's problematic feelings in relation to the therapist; and (4) linking the problematic feelings in relation to the therapist with the patient's defenses.[21]

Rather than viewing him as a "problem patient," therefore, it is more productive for a nurse to view him as a patient who poses problems for herself. This turns the responsibility for action away from the patient and back onto the nurse. It forces the nurse to explore her responses to the patient and the behavior she displays that reinforces his unproductive behavior. In this way the nurse also makes the patient responsible for his own behavior. By stepping back and reviewing again the patient's needs and problems, the nurse becomes aware that she is failing to use the responsive dimensions of genuineness, respect, empathic understanding, and concreteness. And, without this therapeutic groundwork, a therapeutic outcome is impossible.

■ **Gift giving**

Gift giving is included in this discussion of therapeutic impasses, not because it necessarily precipitates an impasse, but because many nurses perceive it this way. This is partly because there has been a long-accepted taboo in nursing of accepting gifts from patients. Like many traditional taboos, it lacks a sound theoretical

rationale, inhibits the independent decision making of the nurse, and creates a feeling of anxiety or guilt.

Gifts can take many forms. They can be tangible or intangible, lasting or temporary. Tangible gifts may include such items as a box of candy, bouquet of flowers, hand-knit scarf, or a hand-painted picture. Intangible gifts can be the expression of thanks to a nurse by a patient who is about to be discharged or a family member's sense of relief and gratitude at being able to share an emotional burden with another caring person. The underlying element among all of these gifts is that something of value is voluntarily offered to another person usually to convey gratitude.

Because gifts can be so varied, it is inappropriate to lump them all together and uniformly arrive at an appropriate nursing action. Rather, the nurse's response to gift giving and the role it plays in the therapeutic relationship depends on the timing of the particular situation, intent of the giver, and contextual meaning of the giving of the gift. Occasionally, it may be most appropriate and therapeutic for the nurse to accept a patient's gift, although on other occasions it may be quite inappropriate and detrimental to the relationship.

■ **TIMING IN THE RELATIONSHIP.** The timing of the gift giving is an important consideration. In the introductory, or orientation, phase of the relationship, nurses may be asked, "Do you have a cigarette I can borrow?" or "Will you buy me a cup of coffee?" These seemingly minor requests may make the nurse feel uncomfortable refusing them. She may even rationalize her compliance by thinking that it indicates her interest in the patient and may help him to trust her. But these reponses by the nurse indicate her failure to examine the covert, or underlying, need of the patient who is making the request and her own needs in complying with it. Also, in this early phase of the relationship, the nurse may be the one to initiate gift giving by giving the patient a book, plant, or some other item that she believes expresses her interest.

In the orientation phase of the relationship, gift giving can be detrimental because it often meets personal needs rather than therapeutic goals. The patient, for example, may be trying to manipulate the nurse as his way of controlling the relationship and setting interpersonal limits on the level of intimacy he will allow. As such, it can be a form of resistance and act as a therapeutic impasse. The nurse as the gift giver may also be distorting the nature and purpose of the therapeutic relationship by her behavior. By giving gifts to the patient, she is attempting to relate through objects instead of the therapeutic use of self. She is avoiding exploring her own possible feelings of inadequacy of frustration. If the patient accepts the gifts, she may worry that he is relating to her out of a sense of obligation, and this aura of doubt may overshadow the course of the relationship. On the other hand, it may enhance the patient's sense of self to bring to his attention a magazine that has been on the ward and has an article on a topic of interest to him. The distinction lies in the meaning behind the gift and the sense of obligation it implies.

As the relationship progresses, gift giving may take on a different significance. In the working phase, for example, the patient may one day offer to buy the nurse a cup of coffee. This can be an indication of the patient's respect for the nurse and his belief in the mutuality of their work together. As an isolated incident, the nurse's acceptance of it can enhance the patient's confidence, self-esteem, and sense of responsibility.

Gift giving most often arises in the termination phase of the relationship, and it is in this phase that the meaning behind it can be the most complex and difficult to determine. At this time, gift giving can be tangible or intangible and can reflect a patient's need to make the nurse feel guilty, delay the termination process, compensate for feelings of inadequacy, or attempt to transform the therapeutic nurse-patient relationship into a social one that can possibly go on indefinitely. The nurse can initiate gift giving for similar reasons. The feelings evoked during the termination process can be very powerful, and they must be acknowledged and explored if termination is to be a learning experience for both participants. If feelings are identified and clarified, then a small gift that reflects gratitude and remembrance can be exchanged, accepted, and valued. In this case, it becomes not a therapeutic impasse, but a memento of a treasured growth experience.

Effectiveness of the nurse

The nurse's effectiveness in working with psychiatric patients is related to her knowledge base, clinical skills, and capacity for introspection and self-evaluation. The nurse and patient, as participants in an interpersonal relationship, are entwined in a pattern of reciprocal emotions that directly affect the therapeutic outcome. The nurse conveys feelings to the patient. Some of these will be in response to the patient; others will arise from the nurse's personal life and will not necessarily be associated with the patient. For example, a nurse is feeling angry because of an administrative problem involving the nursing service. Her patient may sense these feelings and misconstrue their source as being himself. If he does not have the confidence to discuss this with the nurse, she may be unaware of his misconception.

Many painful feelings arise within the nurse because of the nature of the therapeutic process, which can be stressful. These "normal" stresses are due to a variety of factors. Although the nurse must be a skilled listener, it is inappropriate for her to discuss her own conflicts or personal responses, except when they may help the patient. This bottling up of emotions can be painful. She is expected to empathize with the emotions and feelings of the patient. At the same time, however, she is expected to retain her objectivity and not be caught up in a sympathetic response. This can create a kind of double bind.

Termination poses another stress when the nurse must separate from a patient she has come to know well and care for deeply. It is common to experience a grief reaction in response to the loss. Many nurses find it emotionally draining when a patient communicates a prolonged and intense expression of emotion, such as sadness, despair, or anger. Discomfort also arises when the nurse feels unable to help a patient who is in great distress. Suicide dramatizes this situation. Treating suicidal individuals can arouse intense and prolonged anxiety in the nurse.

The painful nature of these emotional responses makes the practice of psychiatric nursing challenging and stressful. The therapeutic use of self involves the nurse's total personality, and total involvement is not an easy task. It is essential that the nurse be aware of her feelings and responses and receive guidance and support in her work.

■ Supervision

According to Haller, supervision is a "process whereby a therapist, frequently but not always a relative beginner, is helped to become a more effective clinician. The goals of supervision are not only to guide the therapist in the successful handling of the supervised case, but to catalyze the therapist's creative and therapeutic use of self."[28:36] The supervisor serves as a provider of theoretical knowledge and therapeutic techniques, validates the use of the nursing process, and supports the working through of transference and countertransference reactions. Consultation is different from supervision in that it denotes a peer or collegial relationship; it is discussed in detail in Chapter 26.

Supervision also functions as a support system for those providing care and is an essential element in therapeutic relationships. One must care about oneself and experience being cared for before one can give care to others. All practicing psychiatric nurses experience some degree of clinical stress. There are stresses associated with such patient behaviors as hopelessness, self-destruction, and manipulation, as well as the stress inherent in the intimacy, openness, and responsiveness required of the nurse who has established a therapeutic relationship. Supervision provides the nurse with a system of clinical support and contributes greatly, if indirectly, to the quality of nursing care.

In many ways the process of supervision parallels the nurse-patient relationship. Both involve a learning process that takes place in the context of a deep and meaningful relationship which facilitates positive change. Self-exploration is a critical element of both. The supervisor should provide the same responsive and action dimensions present in the nurse-patient relationship to help the supervised nurse become a person who is able to live effectively with herself and others.

Hughes advocates the use of a nursing model to provide the foundation for clinical teaching and supervision for the purposes of

- Improving the nurse's therapeutic relationships with patients
- Improving therapeutic nursing interventions
- Increasing knowledge of the theories of human behavior
- Increasing the nurse's self-awareness of the motivation of one's own behavior
- Furthering the development of the nurse's personal endowments[31]

She further identified three phases of supervision that parallel those of the nurse-patient relationship—contracting or beginning phase, working phase, and termination phase.

The most common forms of supervision are the dyadic or one-to-one relationship, in which the supervisor meets the supervisee in a face-to-face encounter; the triadic relationship, in which a supervisor and two nurses of similar experience and training meet for supervision; and group supervision, in which several supervised nurses meet together for a shared session with the supervisory nurse. All three forms of supervision have a similar purpose of exploring the problem areas and maximizing the strengths of the supervisees.

■ **THE PROCESS OF SUPERVISION.** The process of supervision requires the nurse to record the interactions with her patient. Both written processed recordings and audio recordings have been utilized for this purpose, but neither yields as accurate and complete information as that provided by videotape recordings.[51] Videotaped sessions minimize distortion of data. The supervised nurse then analyzes her data, extracts themes, and identifies problems relevant to her nursing care. She reviews the literature, draws inferences, evaluates her effectiveness, and formulates plans for her next session. In the supervision conference, she shares this analysis and receives feedback from her supervisor and peers, if it is a group conference.

Supervision can be viewed as either a didactic process in which the theory, concepts, and practice of the individual therapeutic relationship are enunciated, or it can be a quasi-therapeutic process that explores countertransference problems, attitudes, values, and the nurse's emotional needs and personal biases. The more widely accepted view recognizes that the supervisor-therapist relationship is more important than a simple didactic adjunct to the treatment process and that it has a major, if somewhat intangible, bearing on the therapist-patient relationship and the therapeutic process.

Three methods of supervision have been described. The first is **patient centered,** in which the therapist brings her technical problems with the patient to the supervisor and is given advice. The second type is **therapist centered,** in which the focus is on the therapist's blind spots and countertransference reactions, which helps the therapist to see her influence on the therapeutic process. The danger with this method is that when it is used to the extreme, the patient gets lost from sight, and the supervision evolves into personal therapy for the supervisee. The third approach is **process centered,** in which emphasis is on what is happening between the therapist, patient, and supervisor. The supervisor makes use of the analogy between the therapist-patient relationship and the therapist-supervisor relationship to help the supervisee use her own experience of emotional difficulties in receiving help from her supervisor to facilitate her understanding of the patient's situation.

Ekstein and Wallerstein[20] have developed a process-centered model of supervision that is neither personal therapy nor simply a didactic process of conveying information on theory and technique. In their model, the supervisor is an active participant in an affectively charged learning process, the focus of which is learning and personal growth, rather than psychotherapy for the supervisee. They describe how and in what ways the problems between the therapist and supervisor can shed light on and, in fact, often stand for problems that exist between the therapist and patient. The very problems experienced in the one relationship effect and are reflected in the other relationship, so that a parallel process exists between the supervisor-therapist relationship and therapist-patient relationship.

The goal of supervision, however, is not to eliminate these problems, but to use them to achieve greater understanding of the ongoing dynamic processes at work in therapy. The problems become the vehicles through which therapeutic progress may be made. They propose that the most effective supervision depends on active insight into the interplay of forces in the parallel processes of therapy and supervision.

Little research on the supervisory process is reported in the literature. One of the few studies to explore the nature of the process was conducted by Doehrman.[19] The results of this study highlight an important aspect of supervision—tension in the supervisory relationship is inevitable but when understood and handled skillfully, it is instrumental to the therapist's growth. Learning to be therapeutic inspires fear and resistance in the learner related to change. These are expressed in the supervisee's characteristic way of resisting authority. The therapist's ways of resisting help in supervision are intimately related to her difficulties in giving help to patients. Insight into these resistances will provide the supervisee with insight into her problems as a therapist and particular problems she experiences in the nurse-patient relationship. Deprived of these insights, the supervisee cannot grow as a therapist. There will be no learning, no change, and the status quo will be preserved.

Doehrman's study gives support to the Ekstein and Wallerstein model of supervision, which entails the supervisor's addressing herself to the problems of the supervisee that block her functioning as an effective therapist. Doehrman concludes that the supervisor should deal with the supervisee's feelings toward her and toward the supervisory process when these feelings interfere with the therapist's effectiveness with her patients or her ability to learn from her supervisor. The clarification of these problems requires the supervisor's use of certain therapeutic skills, such as the exploration and expression of feelings and encouraging insight, and this may be intensely therapeutic for the supervisee.

■ **PURPOSE AND GOALS.** Despite the intensity, however, supervision is not therapy. The essential difference between the two is a difference of purpose. The aim of supervision is the teaching of psychotherapeutic skills, whereas the goal of therapy is to alter the patient's characteristic patterns of coping to function more effectively in all areas of life. In contrast, the supervisee's problems in the supervisory and therapeutic relationships are dealt with only to the extent that they are affecting the nurse's ability to learn from her supervisor and be effective with her patients. Therefore, the problems are limited in scope and depth and do not include all other aspects of the supervisee's life situation. With the resolution of the particular problem, the focus of supervision returns to the teaching of psychotherapeutic skills and their implementation by the nurse with her patients. The therapeutic implications for the supervisee are therefore derivatives of the primary goal of supervision—the teaching of psychotherapeutic skills.

Supervision or consultation is necessary for the practicing psychiatric nurse. Although it is crucial for

DIRECTIONS FOR FUTURE RESEARCH

The following are some of the nursing research problems raised in Chapter 4 that merit further study by psychiatric nurses:

1. The extent to which psychiatric nurses possess the personal qualities associated with being able to help others
2. The levels of openness, authenticity, and empathic understanding in student-teacher relationships in nursing
3. The validity of Burgess and Burns' description of reasons why patients seek psychiatric care and which nursing approaches would be effective with each
4. Clinical investigation into the process and outcome of termination
5. The therapeutic effectiveness of touch as a nursing intervention
6. The affective and behavioral patient outcomes associated with the nurse's use of personal space and spatial parameters
7. Theoretical models of the communication process used by psychiatric nurses in identifying and correcting communication problems among patients
8. Valid and reliable instruments to measure the responsive and action dimensions of a therapeutic nurse-patient relationship
9. The extent to which psychiatric nurses demonstrate the responsive dimensions of genuineness, respect, empathic understanding, and concreteness and resulting therapeutic outcomes
10. The extent to which psychiatric nurses demonstrate the action dimensions of confrontation, immediacy, nurse self-disclosure, catharsis, and role playing and resulting therapeutic outcomes
11. An exploration of the role of gift-giving within the context of a nurse-patient relationship
12. The awareness, analysis, and resolution of the therapeutic impasses of resistance, transference, and countertransference by psychiatric nurses
13. The process, methods, and outcomes of supervision used with and by psychiatric nurses
14. The degree to which nursing education programs are successful in teaching nurses the communication and interpersonal relationship skills described in this chapter
15. Different levels of therapeutic relationship skills possessed by psychiatric nurses with varying educational and experiential preparation

novices, it is equally as important for experienced practitioners. Personal limitations create a need for assistance in remaining objective throughout the therapeutic process and the "normal" stresses it presents. Obviously supervision is only as helpful as the skill of the supervisor, the openness of the supervised nurse, and the motivation of both to learn and grow.

■ SUGGESTED CROSS-REFERENCES ■

This chapter serves as a foundation for formulating principles of psychiatric nursing and implementing psychiatric nursing practice. As such, it is related to all other chapters of this text.

■ SUMMARY ■

1. The therapeutic nurse-patient relationship is a mutual learning experience and a corrective emotional experience for the patient. In this relationship the nurse uses personal attributes and specified clinical techniques in working with the patient to bring about behavioral change. General goals of the relationship were identified.

2. Self-awareness was described as the first step in providing quality nursing care through the therapeutic use of self. The following qualities needed by nurses to be effective helpers were analyzed: the awareness of self, the clarification of values, the exploration of feelings, the ability to serve as a role model, altruism, and a sense of ethics and responsibility.

3. The four phases of the relationship process were described and tasks of the nurse in each of the phases were identified.

4. Communication incorporates the ideas of interpersonal influence and behavioral change and, as such, can play a facilitative role in the therapeutic relationship. Both the verbal and nonverbal levels of it were described, with elaboration on the nonverbal behaviors categorized as vocal cues, action cues, object cues, space, and touch. The elements of the communication process were identified as perception, evaluation, and transmission. The structural and transactional analysis models were used to examine components of the communication process and identify common breakdowns or problems. Helpful therapeutic communication techniques were also discussed.

5. The responsive dimensions of genuineness, respect, empathic understanding, and concreteness were presented. They interrelate with each other and contribute to each other in the therapeutic process, and some degree of all of them is necessary when initiating a relationship. The therapeutic level at which nurses function is unknown at present. Additional research on nurse-patient interactions is greatly needed because there is little empirical evidence on which to base scientific practice in this area.

6. The action dimensions of confrontation, immediacy, nurse self-disclosure, catharsis, and role playing stimulate and contribute to patient insight.

7. Therapeutic impasses are roadblocks in the progress of the nurse-patient relationship. As such, they should be dealt with by the nurse as soon as possible. One of these, resistance, was defined as the patient's attempt to remain unaware of anxiety-producing aspects within himself. Transference is an unconscious response of the patient in which he experiences feelings and attitudes toward the nurse that were originally associated with significant figures in his early life. Countertransference is the specific emotional response of the nurse, generated by the qualities of her patient, that is inappropriate to the content and context of the therapeutic relationship or inappropriate in the degree of intensity of emotion. It is transference applied to the nurse. Gift giving is often perceived to be a therapeutic impasse but the actual role it plays in the relationship depends on the timing of the situation, the intent of the giver, and the contextual meaning of the giving of the gift.

8. Supervision is a process in which the supervised nurse is helped to become a more effective clinician. It may occur individually or in groups and is distinct from consultation, which implies a peer relationship. A process-centered model of supervision was described that views therapy and supervision as parallel processes. Although supervision is crucial for novices, it is equally important for experienced practitioners.

■ REFERENCES ■

1. Aiken, L., and Aiken, J.: A systematic approach to the evaluation of interpersonal relationships, Am. J. Nurs. **73**:863, 1973.
2. Anderson, S.: Effects of confrontation by high- and low-functioning therapists on high- and low-functioning clients, J. Counsel. Psychol. **16**:299, 1969.
3. Argyle, M.: Bodily communication, New York, 1975, International Universities Press, Inc.
4. Barnett, K.: A theoretical construct of the concepts of touch as they relate to nursing, Nurs. Res. **21**:102, March-April 1972.
5. Berne, E.: Games people play: the psychology of human relationships, New York, 1964, Grove Press, Inc.
6. Bohart, A.: Role playing and interpersonal conflict reduction, J. Counsel. Psych. **24**:15, 1977.
7. Brammer, L., and Shostrum, E.: Therapeutic psychology, Englewood Cliffs, N.J., 1977, Prentice-Hall, Inc.
8. Bromley, G: Confrontation in individual psychotherapy, J. Psychiatr. Nurs. **19**(5):15, 1981.
9. Buber, M.: I and thou, New York, 1958, Charles Scribner's Sons.
10. Bugenthal, J.: The search for existential identity, San Francisco, 1976, Jossey-Bass, Inc., Publishers.
11. Burgess, A., and Burns, J.: Why patients seek care. Am. J. Nurs. **73**:314, 1973.
12. Campaniello, J.: The process of termination, J. Psychiatr. Nurs. **18**(2):29, 1980.
13. Campbell, J.: The relationship of nursing and self-awareness, Adv. Nurs. Sci. **2**(4):15, 1980.
14. Carkhoff, R.: Helping and human relations, vols. 1 and 2, New York, 1969, Holt, Rinehart & Winston, Inc.
15. Carkhoff, R., and Berenson, B.: Beyond counseling and

therapy, New York, 1967, Holt, Rinehart & Winston, Inc.

16. Carkhoff, R., and Truax, C.: Toward effective counseling and psychotherapy, Chicago, 1967, Aldine Publishing Co.

17. Coad-Denton, A.: Therapeutic superficiality and intimacy. In Longo, D., and Williams, R., editors: Psychosocial nursing: assessment and intervention, New York, 1978, Appleton-Century-Crofts.

18. Cooper, K.: Territorial behavior among the institutionalized, J. Psychosoc. Nurs. Ment. Health Serv. 22(12):6, 1984.

19. Doehrman, M.: Parallel process in supervision and psychotherapy, Bull. Menninger Clin. 40:9, 1976.

20. Ekstein, R., and Wallerstein, R.: The teaching and learning of psychotherapy, New York, 1958, Basic Books, Inc., Publishers.

21. Foreman, S., and Marmar, C.: Therapist actions that address initially poor therapeutic alliances in psychotherapy, Am. J. Psychiatry 142(8):922, 1985.

22. Fox, E., Nelson, M., and Bolman, W.: The termination process: a neglected dimension in social work, Soc. Work 14:53, Oct. 1969.

23. Gagan, J.: Methodological notes on empathy, Adv. Nurs. Sci. 5(1):65, 1983.

24. Gaylin, W.: Feelings, New York, 1979, Harper & Row Publishers, Inc.

25. Gazda, G., et al: Human relations development: a manual for educators, Boston, 1971, Allyn & Bacon, Inc.

26. Ginott, H.: Between parent and child, New York, 1965, Macmillan Co., Publishers.

27. Hall, E.: The silent language, Garden City, N.Y., 1959, Doubleday & Co., Inc.

28. Haller, L.: Clinical psychiatric supervision. In Kneisl, C.R., and Wilson, H.S., editors: Current perspectives in psychiatric nursing, vol. 1, St. Louis, 1976, The C.V. Mosby Co.

29. Hardin, S., and Halaris, A.: Nonverbal communication of patients and high and low empathy nurses, J. Psychosoc. Nurs. Ment. Health Serv. 21(1):14, 1983.

30. Heuscher, J.: The role of humor and folklore themes in psychotherapy, Am. J. Psychiatry 137(12):1546, 1980.

31. Hughes, C.: Supervising clinical practice in psychosocial nursing, J. Psychosoc. Nurs. Ment. Health Serv. 23(2):27, 1985.

32. Hutchinson, S.: Humor: a link to life. In Kneisl, C.R., and Wilson, H.S., editors: Current perspectives in psychiatric nursing, vol. 1, St. Louis, 1976, The C.V. Mosby Co.

33. Johnson, M.: Self-disclosure and anxiety in nurses and patients, Issues Ment. Health Nurs. 2(1):41, 1979.

34. Johnson, M.: Self-disclosure: a variable in the nurse-client relationship, J. Psychiatr. Nurs. 18(1):17, 1980.

35. Jourard, S.: The transparent self, New York, 1971, Litton Educational Publishing, Inc.

36. Kalisch, B.: What is empathy? Am. J. Nurs. 73:1548, 1973.

37. Kirschenbaum, H., and Simon, S., editors: Readings in values clarification, Minneapolis, 1973, Winston Press, Inc.

38. Krieger, D.: The therapeutic touch: how to use your hands to help or to heal, New York, 1979, Prentice-Hall, Inc.

39. Krikorian, D., and Paulanka, B.: Self-awareness—the key to a successful nurse-patient relationship? J. Psychosoc. Nurs. Ment. Health Serv. 20(6):19, 1982.

40. La Crosse, M.: Nonverbal behavior and perceived counselor attractiveness and persuasiveness, J. Counsel. Psychol. 22:563, 1975.

41. La Monica, E., and Karshmer, J.: Empathy: educating nurses in professional practice, J. Nurs. Educ. 17(2):3, 1978.

42. Langs, R.: The technique of psychoanalytic psychotherapy. vol. 2, New York, Jason Aronson, 1974.

43. Levinson, H.: Termination of psychotherapy: some salient issues, paper presented at the Illinois Society for Clinical Social Work, Chicago, Oct. 1975.

44. Loomis, M.: Levels of contracting, J. Psychosoc. Nurs. Ment. Health Serv. 23(3):9, 1985.

45. Luft, J.: Of human interaction, Palo Alto, Calif., 1969, National Press Books.

46. Mansfield, E.: Empathy: concept and identified psychiatric nursing behavior, Nurs. Res. 22(6):525, 1973.

47. Mehrabian, A.: Nonverbal communication, Chicago, 1972, Aldine Publishing Co.

48. Menninger, K.: Theory of psychoanalytic techniques, New York, 1958, Basic Books, Inc.

49. Methven, D., and Schlotfeldt, R.: The social interaction inventory, Nurs. Res. 11:83, Spring, 1962.

50. Mitchell, K., and Berenson, B.: Differential use of confrontation by high and low facilitative therapists, J. Nerv. Ment. Dis. 151(5):303, 1970.

51. Muecke, M.: Video-tape recording, Perspect. Psychiatr. Care 8:200, Sept.-Oct. 1970.

52. Neill, J.: The difficult patient: identification and response, J. Clin. Psychiatry 40(5):209, 1979.

53. Ornston, P., Cuchetti, D., Levine, J., and Freiman, L.: Some parameters of verbal behavior that reliably differentiate novice from experienced psychotherapists, J. Abnorm. Psychol. 73:240, 1968.

54. Peitchinis, J.: Therapeutic effectiveness of counseling by nursing personnel, Nurs. Res. 21(2):138, 1972.

55. Raths, L., Harmin, M., and Simon, S.: Values and teaching, Columbus, Ohio, 1966, Charles E. Merrill Publishing Co.

56. Rogers, C.: On becoming a person, Boston, 1961, Houghton Mifflin Co.

57. Rogers, C.: Empathic: an unappreciated way of being, J. Counsel. Psychol. 5(2):2, 1975.

58. Rokeach, M.: The nature of human values, New York, 1973, Macmillan, Inc.

59. Ruesch, J.: Communication and human relations: an interdisciplinary approach. In Ruesch, J., and Bateson, G.: Communication: the social matrix of psychiatry, New York, 1968, W.W. Norton & Co., Inc.

60. Ruesch, J.: Disturbed communication, New York, 1972,

W.W. Norton & Co., Inc.

61. Schiff, S.: Termination of therapy, Arch. Gen. Psychiatry **6**(1):77, 1962.
62. Schoffstall, C.: Concerns of student nurses prior to psychiatric nursing experience: an assessment and intervention technique, J. Psychosoc. Nurs. Ment. Health Serv. **19**(11):11, 1981.
63. Schulz, F.: The mourning phase of relationships, J. Psychiatr. Nurs. **2**(1):37, 1964.
64. Sedgwick, R.: Role playing: a bridge between talk and action, J. Psychiatr. Nurs. **14**(11):16, 1976.
65. Sigman, P.: Ethical choice in nursing, Adv. Nurs. Sci. **1**(3):37, 1979.
66. Spitz, R.: No and yes on the genesis of human communication, New York, 1957, International Universities Press, Inc.
67. Stacklum, M.: New student in psychology, Am. J. Nurs. **81**:762, 1981.
68. Stetler, C.: Relationship of perceived empathy to nurses' communication, Nurs. Res. **26**:432, 1977.
69. Sundeen, S., et al.: Nurse-client interaction: implementing the nursing process, ed. 3, St. Louis, 1985, The C.V. Mosby Co.
70. Travelbee, J.: Intervention in psychiatric nursing, Philadelphia, 1969, F.A. Davis Co.
71. Ujhely, G.: Touch: reflections and perceptions, Nurs. Forum **18**(1):18, 1979.
72. Uustal, D.: Values clarification in nursing: application to practice, Am. J. Nurs. **78**:2058, 1978.
73. Watzlawick, P., Beavin, J., and Jackson, D.: Pragmatics of human communication: a study of interactional patterns, pathologies, and paradoxes, New York, 1967, W.W. Norton & Co., Inc.
74. Weiner, M.: Therapist disclosure: the use of self in psychotherapy, Boston, Mass., Butterworths, 1978.
75. Weiss, S.: The language of touch, Nurs. Res. **28**(2):76, 1979.
76. Williams, C.: Empathic communication and its effect on client outcome, Issues Ment. Health Nurs. **2**(1):16, 1979.
77. Wolberg, L.: The technique of psychotherapy, vol, 2, New York, 1967, Grune & Stratton, Inc.

■ ANNOTATED SUGGESTED READINGS ■

*Abraham, I.: Support groups for nursing students in psychiatric rotation, Issues Ment. Health Nurs. **4**:159, 1982.

The content and process of a support group for undergraduate nursing students in clinical rotation in an inpatient psychiatric setting is presented and analyzed. Faculty might find this helpful reading.

*Albiez, Sr. A.: Reflecting on the development of a relationship, J. Psychiatr. Nurs. **9**(6):25, Nov.-Dec. 1970.

A nursing student describes her first experience in psychiatric nursing. She shares her feelings, fears, and problems in a way that other beginners can relate to, and this article can reassure the inexperienced nurse.

*Auvil, C., and Silver, B.: Therapist self-disclosure: when is it appropriate? Perspect. Psychiatr. Care **22**(2):57, 1984.

This article reviews three theoretical frameworks, assesses the implications of nurse self-disclosure and offers guidelines and criteria for appropriate self-disclosure. It is one of the few nursing articles to explore this responsive dimension.

Berne, E.: Games people play, New York, 1967, Grove Press, Inc.

The founder of transactional analysis uses it in this text to explore a number of specific "games." This thought-provoking book gives a different slant on relationships and challenges the reader to find ways to terminate destructive "games."

*Burnard, P.: Self-awareness for nurses. Gaithersburg, Md., 1986, Aspen Publishers, Inc.

This text contains practical exercises, charts and diagrams, and concise, clear information in a step-by-step guide to developing self-awareness.

*Campbell, J.: The relationship of nursing and self-awareness, Adv. Nurs. Sci. **2**(4):15, 1980.

The contributions to self theory by four theorists are reviewed in this article which then describes a holistic model of self-awareness that is related to nursing care. It presents a theoretical and conceptual discussion which is useful to both practice and future research endeavors.

Carkhoff, R.: Helping and human relations, vols. 1 and 2, New York, 1969, Holt, Rinehart & Winston.

Elements of research and practice in helping relationships are explored in these two volumes. Scales used to rate the "core therapeutic dimensions" are presented.

*Claud, E.: The plateau in therapist-patient relationships, Perspect. Psychiatr. Care **10**:112, July-Sept. 1972.

The theoretical basis for resistance is presented, and the author describes her approach in overcoming resistance in a patient she had been working with. Her clinical experiences are clearly related.

*Cooper, K.: Territorial behavior among the institutionalized: a nursing perspective, J. Psychosoc. Nurs. Ment. Health Serv. **22**(12):6, 1984.

The crux of this paper is that nurses are an important part of the ward milieu and should attempt, whenever possible, to allow the institutionalized individual control and enjoyment of personal possessions and private living space. It draws attention to the needs of an often overlooked group of patients.

Fromm-Reichmann, F.: Principles of intensive psychotherapy, Chicago, 1950, The University of Chicago Press.

This book presents formulations of principles of intensive psychotherapy with psychoneurotics and psychotics. Written for psychiatrists, it has application to psychiatric nurses as well, and it is a recommended source for nurses with advanced education or experience.

*Gagan, J.: Methodological notes on empathy, Adv. Nurs. Sci. **5**(1):65, 1983.

The methodological issues related to the measurement of empathy by nurses are discussed in this article. It presents a good review and identifies areas of need for nursing research.

*Geach, B., and White, J.: Empathic resonance: a counter-

*Asterisk indicates nursing reference.

transference phenomenon, Am. J. Nurs. **74**:128, 1974.

The authors document a unique countertransference event— presenting characteristics, antecedents, and consequences. They identify a need for nurses to record similar experiences.

*Hayes, M., Drake, N., and Lindy, J.: The evening shift: an occasion for acting out transference phenomena, J. Psychosoc. Nurs. Ment. Health Serv. **23**(10):24, 1985.

This article focuses on an underexplored aspect of nursing— issues on the evening shift. The authors view the nurse-patient contacts in light of transference reactions, and suggest that the disruptive, anxiety-producing behavior of patients, if viewed in this way, might have diagnostic and therapeutic value rather than being the occasion for professional self-doubt.

*Hughes, C.: Supervising clinical practice in psychosocial nursing, J. Psychosoc. Nurs. Ment. Health Serv. **23**(2):27, 1985.

The author advocates a nursing model of clinical supervision and reviews phases of supervision, supervisory functions, relationship, and teaching methods.

Jourard, S.: The transparent self, New York, 1971, Litton Educational Publishing, Inc.

This book proposes that man can attain health only as he gains courage to be himself with others and finds goals that have meaning for him. The author develops the concept of self-disclosure and the implications of it for the therapeutic relationship. Three chapters are specifically addressed to nurses and are highly recommended.

*Kalisch, B.: Strategies for developing nurse empathy, Nurs. Outlook **19**:714, 1971.

The author describes her experiment in developing empathic functioning in nursing students. The training includes discussion of the concept, discrimination training, communication practice, role playing, role model of empathy, and an experimental component.

*Karns, P., and Schwab, T.: Therapeutic communication and clinical instruction, Nurs. Outlook **30**(1):39, 1982.

The premise of this article is that nurse educators rarely apply therapeutic communication in their interactions with students in the clinical area. The need for it is documented, and possible inhibitors are suggested.

*Kasch, C.: Interpersonal competence and communication in the delivery of nursing care, Adv. Nurs. Sci. **6**(1):71, 1984.

This article suggests that one particular model for guiding nursing communication research lies in the area of interpersonal competence—viewed as the social-cognitive and functional-behavioral communicative abilities of nurses interrelated with the sociocultural context in health care. This is advanced theoretical reading for the nurse researcher.

*Krieger, D.: The therapeutic touch: how to use your hands to help or to heal, New York, 1979, Prentice-Hall, Inc.

This text presents the techniques of therapeutic touch with detailed directions offered for the nurse who wants to expand her healing abilities in this way.

*La Monica, E., and Karshmer, J.: Empathy: educating nurses in professional practice, J. Nurs. Educ. **17**(2):3, 1978.

This paper describes in detail a staff development program that was effective in raising nurses' abilities to perceive and respond with empathy. Valuable reading for nurse educators

and administrators who wish to design or use programs in behavioral empathy.

*McCann, J.: Termination of the psychotherapeutic relationship, J. Psychiatr. Nurs. **17**(10):37, 1979.

This article discusses the psychodynamics and theories of termination. It also has a good bibliography.

*Mihordin, R.: The nunsuch handbook, Perspect. Psychiatr. Care **12**:126, July-Sept., 1974.

This lighthearted article presents "rules" for psychiatric staff. It pokes fun at some common myths and staff prejudices and is fun, enjoyable reading.

Mueller, W., and Kell, B.: Coping with conflict—supervising counselors and psychotherapists, New York, 1972, Appleton-Century-Crofts.

This book explores the goals, relationships, and processes that define supervision. It reviews conflict as the core of supervision and discusses in depth the concepts, principles, and guidelines that characterize supervision. It can be valuable reading to both supervisors and practitioners.

*Murphy, K.: Use of territoriality in psychotherapy, J. Psychiatr. Nurs. **19**(3):13, 1981.

This is a brief, but useful, article. The author describes a case report in which she used the concept of territoriality in the therapeutic process.

Raths, L., Harmin, M., and Simon, S.: Values and teaching, Columbus, Ohio, 1966, Charles E. Merrill Publishing Co.

This is the classic text on value clarification. This book includes a theory of values, the value-clarifying method, the use of value theory, and research findings. It is well worth reading and studying.

*Sayre, J.: Common errors in communication made by students in psychiatric nursing, Perspect. Psychiatr. Care **16**(4):175, 1978.

This article should be required reading for all students in psychiatric nursing. It identifies many of the communication errors made in each phase of the relationship and gives a clinical example of each. It is a very useful article to enhance student learning.

*Schoffstall, C.: Concerns of student nurses prior to psychiatric nursing experience: an assessment and intervention technique, J. Psychosoc. Nurs. Ment. Health Serv. **19**(11):11, 1981.

The authors describe a study they conducted to assess and reduce the anxiety of students who are about to begin their clinical experience in psychiatric nursing. Educators may find this useful.

*Schroder, P.: Transference and countertransference, J. Psychosoc. Nurs. Ment. Health Serv. **23**(2):21, 1985.

The phenomena of transference and countertransference are clarified and elaborated on in this article. It is good supplementary reading on these topics.

*Sedgwick, R.: Role playing: a bridge between talk and action, J. Psychiatr. Nurs. **14**(11):16, 1976.

The uses and steps of role playing are described in this article. The techniques with a brief description of how they are accomplished are also included.

*Sundeen, S., et al.: Nurse-client interaction: implementing the nursing process, ed. 3, St. Louis, The C.V. Mosby Co.

This text describes the nursing process, including concepts related to self, communication, phases of the nurse-client relationship, and stress and adaptation. It is a useful reference for normative elements of relationship skills.

*Taylor, S.: Rights and responsibilities: nurse-patient relationship, Image **17**(1):9, Winter, 1985.

Nurse-patient relationships are examined in terms of rights and responsibility models of moral judgment, leading to a definition and description of maternalism.

*Uustal, D.: Values clarification in nursing: application to practice, Am. J. Nurs. **78**:2058, 1978.

Value clarification applied to nursing is the focus of this article. Ten strategies in applying the process are described that are helpful in identifying one's own values.

*Vidoni, C.: The development of intense positive countertransference feelings in the therapist toward a patient, Am. J. Nurs. **75**:407, 1975.

Transference and countertransference feelings that influence the nurse-patient relationship are described. This is an excellent article that explores this important aspect of therapeutic work.

*Warner, S.: Humor and self-disclosure within the milieu, J. Psychosoc. Nurs. Ment. Health Serv. **22**(4):17, 1984.

Humor is discussed within a theoretical framework in this article which emphasizes the positive and growth-producing use of humor as facilitative of self-disclosure.

*Witherspoon, V.: Using Lakovic's system: countertransference classifications, J. Psychosoc. Nurs. Ment. Health Serv. **23**(4):30, 1985.

Six types of countertransference responses in the nurse are described with three case reports in this brief article.

Wolberg, L.: The technique of psychotherapy, vols. 1 and 2, New York, 1967, Grune & Stratton, Inc.

This is a good reference text for the nurse therapist. It describes general principles of psychotherapy and analyzes each phase of treatment in depth. It is clearly written and includes pertinent case examples.

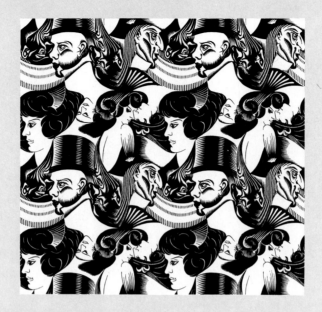

To be what we are, and to become what we are capable of becoming, is the only end of life.

Robert L. Stevenson, *Familiar Studies of Men and Books*

C H A P T E R   5

IMPLEMENTING THE NURSING PROCESS

After studying this chapter, the student should be able to:

- define nursing and its four characteristics as identified by the American Nurses' Association.

- define the nursing process and describe some of the unique challenges it presents when utilized with psychiatric patients.

- relate the need for a theoretical basis and conceptual framework for psychiatric nursing practice and its implications for the development and refinement of nursing theory.

- evaluate the role of culture in psychiatric care.

- describe the various psychiatric nursing activities in the phases of data collection, nursing diagnosis, planning, implementation, and evaluation.

- analyze the ways in which psychiatric nurses can be involved in organizational evaluation of patterns of care through quality assessment measures.

- discuss the ways in which psychiatric nurses demonstrate professional accountability.

- describe why participation in research is an essential part of psychiatric nursing practice.

- assess the need for documentation related to each phase of the nursing process and various tools that are used by nurses for this purpose.

- describe the three elements of the problem-oriented medical record and the format used for each.

- incorporate elements of the nursing therapeutic process in the student's work with psychiatric patients.

- identify directions for future nursing research.

- select appropriate readings for further study.

Nursing defined

The nurse-patient relationship is the vehicle for the application of the nursing process. The goal of nursing care is to maximize the person's positive interactions with his environment, promote his level of wellness, and enhance his degree of self-actualization. Through the establishment of a therapeutic nurse-patient relationship and the use of the nursing process, the nurse strives to promote and maintain patient behavior that contributes to integrated functioning. This is the essence of the nursing therapeutic process and the framework on which this text of psychiatric nursing is based.

The simplicity of this concept, however, should not override its significance. It is, rather, a complex process with many related components, and it requires a skilled nursing practitioner to utilize it successfully. **The American Nurses' Association defines nursing as "the diagnosis and treatment of human responses to actual or potential health problems."**[1:9] This definition suggests four defining characteristics of nursing*:

*American Nurses' Association: Nursing: a social policy statement, Kansas City, Mo., 1980. Reprinted with permission.

1. **Phenomena.** Nursing addresses itself to a wide range of health-related responses observed in sick and well people. The actual health problem is the focus of the practice of medicine, whereas a person's response to the problem is the focus of nursing diagnosis and treatment.

2. **Theory.** Nurses use theory in the form of concepts, principles, and processes to guide their observations and understand the phenomena that are the focus of their interventions. This understanding precedes and serves as a basis for determining nursing actions to be taken.

3. **Actions.** Nursing actions attempt to prevent illness and promote health. They are theoretically related to the observed phenomena and anticipated outcome of care.

4. **Effects.** The aim of nursing actions is to produce beneficial effects in relation to identified responses. The evaluation of outcomes of nursing actions suggests whether or not those actions have been effective in improving or resolving the conditions to which they were directed.

```
┌──────────┐                                                    ┌──────────┐
│          │                TABLE 5-1                            │          │
```

TABLE 5-1

COMPARISON OF THE STEPS IN PROBLEM SOLVING WITH THE PHASES OF THE NURSING PROCESS

Problem-solving steps	Phases of the nursing process
Observation and recognition of the problem	Data collection or assessment
Definition of the problem	Formulation of the nursing diagnosis
Formulation of the hypotheses or possible solutions	Planning of nursing care
Implementation of the hypotheses or possible solutions	Implementation of nursing interventions
Formulation of conclusions	Evaluation of the nursing assessment, care plan, and actions

These characteristics describe nursing as an applied science in which theory, investigation, and action are interrelated. They further suggest some essential components of the nursing therapeutic process that merit further exploration. The characteristic of *phenomena* suggests that psychiatric nurses need a model of health and illness so that they may more fully understand the range of actual and potential health problems which may arise and the possible responses to them. The characteristic of *theory* maintains that nurses need a theoretical basis and conceptual framework for psychiatric–mental health nursing practice. The characteristic of *action* requires the use of the nursing process as a problem-solving process, and the characteristic of *effects* relates to the need for standards of nursing practice to evaluate one's practice and the quality of care received by the patient. This chapter will discuss each of these components of the nursing therapeutic process. It will also relate them to the 1982 revised Standards of Psychiatric and Mental Health Nursing Practice* and the process criteria provided with each standard.

The nursing process

The nursing process is an interactive, problem-solving process used by the nurse as a systematic and individualized way to fulfill the goal of nursing care. It is a deliberate and organized approach requiring thought, knowledge, and experience. The nursing process acknowledges the autonomy of the individual and his freedom to make decisions regarding his own goals and be involved in his own care. Together the nurse and patient emerge as partners in a relationship built on trust and directed toward maximizing the patient's strengths,

*Reprinted with permission from the American Nurses' Association, Kansas City, Mo., 1982.

maintaining his integrity, and promoting his adaptive response to stress.

The problem-solving process is a scientific way of thinking and dealing with problems, and its principles are included in the nursing process. This is evident in Table 5-1 which compares the steps in problem solving with the phases of the nursing process.

When utilized with psychiatric patients, the nursing process presents some unique challenges.[8] Emotional problems are often vague and elusive and are not as tangible or visible as many physiological disruptions. Emotional problems vary in symptomatology or behavior and arise from multiple causes. Conversely, similar past events may be evident in widely differing present behaviors. Many psychiatric patients are initially not able to describe or identify their problems. They may be severely withdrawn, highly anxious, or out of touch with reality. Their ability to participate in the problem-solving process may be limited because of their perception of themselves as powerless victims who deny responsibility for their own behavior.

These factors make the use of the nursing process with psychiatric patients more difficult, but they do not negate it. Geach has identified the following three hallmarks of clinically valid problem solving for psychiatric patients:

1. That the nurse involve the patient in the process
2. That the problem to which the nurse and patient address themselves has immediate relevance to what is happening between them, at least initially
3. That there is some relatedness between the nurse and patient so that the solutions of the problems are experienced from within a relationship, not in isolation[8,12]

It is essential that the nurse and patient become partners in the problem-solving process. There is a great temptation for the nurse to exclude the participation of the patient, particularly if he resists becoming involved. This should be avoided for two reasons. First, learning is most effective when the patient directly participates in the learning experience. Second, the patient's isolation from others and self-alienation is part of his maladaptive life-style that needs to be modified. By including the patient as an active participant in the nursing process, the nurse will be helping to restore his sense of control over life and responsibility for action. It reinforces the message that the patient has been making decisions and continues to make them at present. His choice is between adaptive or maladaptive coping responses. Jourard states:

> If a person believes himself to be weak, helpless or doomed to some fate or other, he will tend to behave or suffer in the way expected. If, on the other hand, he has a concept of himself as a being with much untapped potential to cope with problems and contradictions in his life, then when these arise, he will persist in efforts to cope with them long after someone who sees himself as ineffective and impotent has given up.[17:34]

The phases of the nursing process as described by the *Standards of Psychiatric and Mental Health Nursing Practice* include data collection, formulation of the nursing diagnosis, planning, implementation, and evaluation (Fig. 5-1). Sometimes, the activities of data collection are also referred to as the assessment phase of the nursing process. Validation is part of each phase, and all phases may overlap or occur simultaneously.

Theoretical basis for practice
STANDARD I—THEORY
The nurse applies appropriate theory that is scientifically sound as a basis for decisions regarding nursing practice.
Process criteria
The nurse:

1. Examines basic assumptions on the nature of persons
2. Corrects erroneous beliefs
3. Utilizes theory and critical thinking to:
   a. Formulate generalizations, e.g., opinion, speculation, and assumption
   b. Generate and test hypotheses
4. Utilizes inferences, principles, and operational concepts
5. Applies relevant theories

All actions of the psychiatric nurse should arise from a theoretical base that includes an understanding of health-illness phenomena and a means for the evaluation of nursing care given. This theoretical basis is partially self-generated and partly drawn from other sciences but is integrated into a conception of nursing practice. The range of theories used by nurses includes intrapersonal, interpersonal, and systems theories. Intrapersonal theories explain within-person phenomena and are focused at the individual level of care. Interpersonal theories elaborate on interactions between two or more people. Systems theories aid the nurse in understanding complex networks or organizations, the dynamics of their parts, and processes in interaction. They are focused at the family, group, or community levels of care. Use of a range of theories is appropriate in nursing because of the great variance in the recipients of nursing care, types of health-illness responses, philosophical backgrounds of individual psychiatric nurses, and settings in which they work. No one theory is universally applicable; the appropriate theory should be selected for its relevance to the tasks at hand.

A conceptual framework is then formulated from relevant theoretical bases. It should reflect an integration of theory and nursing process and stimulate the evolution of a distinct body of nursing science by generating hypotheses, propositions, and relationships that can be empirically tested. In this way, conceptual frameworks provide a basis for the direction of nursing practice, research, and education and contribute to the development of nursing theory.

■ Nursing theory
A number of nursing theories are being developed at this time.[28] Some prominent nursing theorists who are developing conceptual models as a base for nursing practice include Roy,[35] Rogers,[34] Johnson,[16] Orem,[31] Neuman,[30] and King.[19] Flaskerud and Halloran have identified some areas of agreement in nursing theory development.[6] They believe that nurses generally agree on the following concepts in nursing: man-person, society-environment, health-illness, and nursing. As the nurse interacts with people in society to facilitate health, the nursing process occurs. Table 5-2 describes how various nurse theorists define these common concepts.

Some believe that psychiatric nursing has made little effort to apply the nursing models to its phenomena of concern. A notable exception to this is the work of Fitzpatrick, Whall, Johnson, and Floyd, which brings a unique perspective to psychiatric nursing theory.[5] Their text selects concepts and propositions from the larger body of knowledge in the behavioral sciences (such as Freudian theory, systems theory, and crisis theory) and relates them to the concepts of man, society, health-illness, and nursing. They believe there is a need to reformulate existing theories to achieve congruence with the world as nurses experience it. In such a way, psychiatric nurses would contribute to both theory refinement and the creation of clinically useful theory on which to base their practice.

 Data collection

STANDARD II—DATA COLLECTION
The nurse continuously collects data that are comprehensive, accurate, and systematic.
Process criteria
The nurse:

1. Informs the client of their mutual roles and responsibilities in the data-gathering process
2. Uses clinical judgments to determine what information is needed. Health data undergirding the nursing process for psychiatric and mental health clients are obtained through assessing the following:
   a. Biophysical, developmental, mental, and emotional status
   b. Spiritual or philosophical beliefs
   c. Family, social, cultural, and community systems
   d. Daily activities, interactions, and coping patterns
   e. Economic, environmental, and political factors affecting the client's health
   f. Personally significant support systems, as well as unutilized but available support systems
   g. Knowledge, satisfaction, and change motivation regarding current health status
   h. Strengths that can be used in reaching health goals
   i. Knowledge of pertinent legal rights
   j. Contributory data from the family, significant others, the health care team, and pertinent individuals in the community

Data collection may take place as a formal admission procedure outside of an established nurse-patient relationship. In this case, the information will be solicited from the patient in a direct and structured manner. Observing, interviewing, and examining are the basic methods of gathering information. An assessment tool or nursing history form can provide a systematic format that becomes part of the written record of a patient. It provides the facts on which the nurse can assess the patient's level of functioning and serves as a basis for the nursing diagnosis, planning, implementing, and evaluating of nursing care. The use of a specified data collection format helps to ensure that the necessary information will be obtained. It also reduces the patient's repetition of his history and provides a source of information available to all health team members. The mental status examination, as described in Chapter 6, may be included as part of the psychiatric nurse's evaluation.

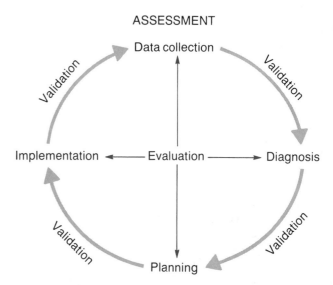

Fig. 5-1. Interrelated phases of the nursing process.

The assessment tool used by the nurse in collecting data about the patient should, ideally, be derived from a conceptual framework of psychiatric nursing. More frequently, however, it is determined by the setting or program in which the nurse works. Regardless of the format of the tool used, the nurse has the obligation to obtain as complete a picture as possible of the patient's life situation.

The process criteria of Standard II identify comprehensive areas in which data need to be collected. Each item listed (a–j) is important for a thorough and complete psychiatric nursing assessment. This list includes data relative to specific components of the nursing model of health-illness phenomena (see Chapter 3) utilized in this text—predisposing factors, precipitating stressors, primary appraisal of stressor, secondary appraisal of coping resources, and coping mechanisms as represented in Fig. 5-2. Together, these components represent the data needed to complete the **nursing assessment** phase of the nursing process. The process criteria also identify from whom the data are to be collected and represent various levels of the model of social hierarchy—individual, family, group, and community.

The baseline data should reflect both content and process, and the patient is the ideal source of validation. In collecting the data, the nurse should select a private place, free from noise and distraction, in which to interview the patient. Interviewing is a goal-directed method of communication that is required in a formal admission procedure. It should be focused, but as open ended as possible, progressing from general to specific, and allowing the patient the opportunity to express him-

---

TABLE 5-2

DEFINITION OF NURSING CONCEPTS BY NURSE THEORISTS

Nurse-theorist	Person	Environment	Health	Nursing
Roy[35]	"An adaptive system with cognator and regulator acting to maintain adaptation in regard to the four adaptive modes"	Conditions, circumstances, and influences surrounding, and affecting the development of an organism or group of organisms	The implied definition is that health exists if that person has adaptive responses that "promote the integrity of the person in terms of the goals of survival, growth, reproduction, and self-mastery"	Manipulating stimuli so that a person's coping mechanism can bring about adaptation
Rogers[34]	"Unitary man—a four-dimensional, negentropic energy field identified by pattern and organization and manifesting characteristics and behaviors that are different from those of the parts and which cannot be predicted from knowledge of the parts"	"A four-dimensional, negentropic energy field identified by pattern and organization and encompassing all that is outside any given human field"	Health not specifically defined; however, she does state that disease and pathology are value terms and since values change, phenomena perceived as disease such as hyperactivity may change over time and not be perceived as disease	Goal of nursing is that individuals achieve their maximum health potential through maintenance and promotion of health, prevention of disease, nursing diagnosis, intervention, and rehabilitation
Johnson[16]	Behavioral system composed of patterned, repetitive, and purposeful ways of behaving	Malfunctions in the behavioral systems are frequently due to "sudden internal or external environmental change"	It seems reasonable to assume that health would be considered behavior that is orderly, purposeful, predictable, and functionally efficient and effective	"External regulatory force which acts to preserve the organization and integration of the patient's behavior at an optimal level under those conditions in which the behavior constitutes a threat to physical or social health, or in which illness is found"

From Stanhope, M., and Lancaster, J.: Community health nursing, St. Louis, 1984, The C.V. Mosby Co.

---

self spontaneously. The tasks of the nurse are to maintain the flow of the interview, to listen to the verbal and nonverbal messages being conveyed by the patient, and to be aware of her own responses to the patient.

In an ongoing nurse-patient relationship, data collection may begin in the preinteraction or orientation phases of the relationship. Although the goal is to gather information, it is only one of many goals the nurse will be pursuing at this time. Other tasks of the nurse include establishing trust, acceptance, and open communication; formulating a contract; and exploring the patient's feelings and actions. The nurse's approach, therefore,

should be unstructured, flexible, and responsive to the cues of the patient. Rather than working from a formalized data collection tool, the nurse may attempt to focus the patient on observing and describing his present thoughts, feelings, and experiences. To supplement her knowledge of the patient, the nurse can use a variety of secondary sources of information, including the patient's medical record, nursing rounds, change-of-shift reports, nursing care plan, and the evaluation of other health professionals, such as psychologists, social workers, or psychiatrists. In using secondary sources of information, nurses should be cautioned against merely

TABLE 5-2—cont'd

DEFINITION OF NURSING CONCEPTS BY NURSE THEORISTS

Nurse-theorist	Person	Environment	Health	Nursing
Orem[31]	"A unity that can be viewed as functioning biologically, symbolically, and socially"	Although not explicitly defined, the role of the nurse in providing a developmental environment is discussed	"A term that has considerable general utility in describing the state of wholeness or integrity of human beings"	"A service, a mode of helping human beings" (Orem, 1980, p. 5); "nursing is contributed effort toward designing, providing, and managing systems of therapeutic self-care for individuals or multiperson units within their daily living environments"
Neuman[30]	"Man is a system capable of intake of extrapersonal and interpersonal factors from the external environment. He interacts with this environment by adjusting it to himself"	"Environment consists of the internal and external forces surrounding man at a point in time"	"Health or wellness is the condition in which all parts and subparts (variables) are in harmony with the whole man"	"Nursing can . . . assist individuals, families, groups to attain and maintain a maximum level of total wellness by purposeful interventions . . . aimed at reduction of stress factors and adverse conditions which affect optimal functioning"
King[19]	A social, sentient, rational, reacting, perceiving, controlling, purposeful, action-oriented, and time-oriented being	Refers to human being interacting with the environment but does not define it	Dynamic life experiences of a human being, which implies continuous adjustment to stressors in the internal and external environment through optimum use of one's resources to achieve maximum potential for daily living	"Nursing is perceiving, thinking, relating, judging, and acting vis-a-vis the behavior of individuals who come to a nursing situation"

accepting the assessment of another health team member. Rather, the nurse should apply the information she obtains to her nursing framework for data collection and formulate her own impressions and nursing diagnoses. This brings another perspective to the work of the health care team and an unbiased receptivity to the patient and his problems.

■ **CULTURAL CONSIDERATIONS.** Some aspects of the data collection phase merit additional discussion. One is the assessment of the patient's cultural, religious, and socioeconomic background. All too frequently these factors are assessed in a cursory way. Yet they exert a powerful influence on the success of the nursing process for two important reasons. The first is because sociocultural factors contribute to a patient's belief system of health and illness. One's religion, sex, race, culture, family ties, and economic status, for example, all have a formative influence on each component of the model of health-illness phenomena. Any one of a variety of sociocultural factors may play a dominant role in an individual's life. Therefore any attempt to promote the well-being of a patient must be based on an understanding of him as a unique individual who lives in a larger social, cultural, and religious community.

The second reason why sociocultural factors are important is that the response of the health care team is

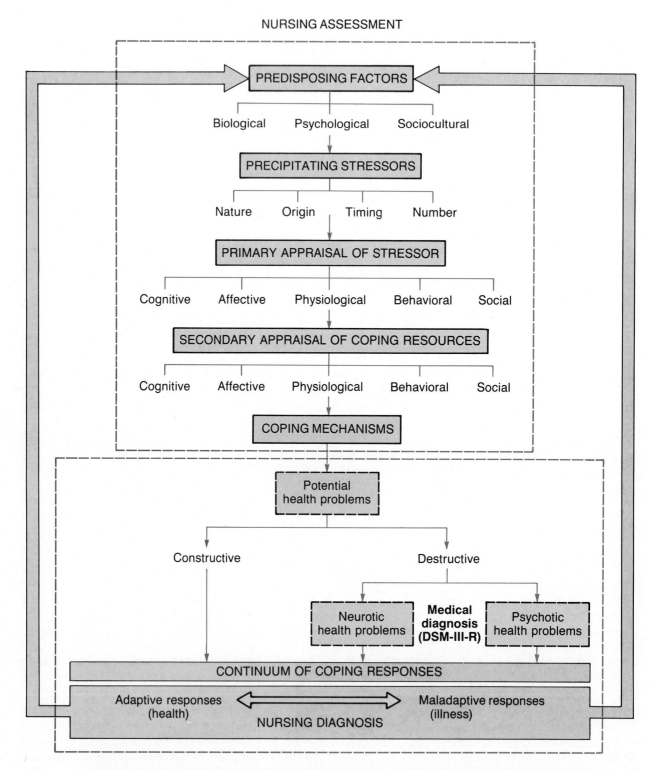

Fig. 5-2. Nursing model of health-illness phenomena and its relationship to nursing assessment and nursing diagnosis.

framed by the culture of which they are a part. The dominant psychotherapeutic approach of an era reflects the cultural attitudes of its time and place. This helps to explain why there are differences in observed symptoms, frequency, distribution, and outcome of psychiatric illness among countries and cultures throughout the world. For instance, in developing nations like Nigeria and India, the odds favor a fast and complete recovery from major psychoses. In the more technologically advanced countries, such as the United States, the prognosis is worse. This is due, in part, to the cultural stigma against mental illness that is prevalent in the West.

Cultural bias can also affect the process of psychotherapy. One study reported that minority group patients received the least intensive psychotherapy. They were discharged more often or seen for minimal supportive psychotherapy.[49] A study among public health nurses found that different judgments were made about patients as a function of their social class.[20] Still another aspect of this problem has been described as "institutional racism," which involves the notion that those who are not white are inferior.[11] Consequently, rather than viewing some patients as culturally different, they are viewed as disadvantaged, deprived, or underprivileged. Such prejudices do not form on the basis of race alone. They can also be based on a person's sex, religion, age, sexual preference, or ethnic background. However, the result is the same—prejudices influence the nurse's evaluation of the patient and limit the potential effectiveness of her care.

Psychiatry needs to embrace the idea of intercultural psychotherapy. Schlesinger[37] believes this occurs with the acknowledgment of the different cultural backgrounds between the patient and therapist and the resulting interaction of cultural variables. This has ramifications for self-awareness, communications, diagnosis, therapist-patient relations, therapeutic models, and treatment goals. It requires that the nurse have an awareness of her own sociocultural identity and values, an understanding of the roles social systems play in influencing behavior, and a willingness to learn from a patient with another cultural set.

■ **FAMILY SYSTEMS.** A final important aspect of data collection pertains to the significance of the patient as a family member. If the nurse views the patient as an interacting member of a family unit, it will be necessary for the data base to include the patient's view of the functional state of his family, as well as family resources and strengths. Sedgwick[38] describes the family as both a social organization and an emotional environment. As

a social organization, the purpose of the family is to develop within its members sets of skills necessary for productive membership in a larger social system. It is a focal point of interaction for the individual as he relates to other family members, other families, the community, and one's larger social network. So too, the broader social system makes demands, places expectations on the family, and requires it to process information, make decisions, attain financial and social productivity, and provide for the personal growth and development of its members.

The larger social context also influences the family's emotional environment. The family must create an atmosphere that is not only conducive to group living and cooperation, but individual development and disagreement as well. Although the emotional environment of the family is constantly changing, it is their mission to create an emotional climate that is trusting, warm, concerned, accepting of differences in opinions and abilities, and adaptable in light of the changes of individual members.

A healthy family unit is considered by Smilkstein[41] to be a nurturing unit that demonstrates integrity in five components: *a*daptability, *p*artnership, *g*rowth, *af*fection, and *r*esolve. The acronym APGAR was designed by him to refer to these components. To test these areas of family functioning, Smilkstein developed a brief screening questionnaire called the Family APGAR. Table 5-3 presents the functional components of the Family APGAR and relevant open-ended questions for family function information. This tool is useful in suggesting areas to be assessed relative to family functioning and potential areas of family strengths and resources.

Various types of family strengths may be noted. These include the ability to acquire resources, such as money or social support, and the productive use of them; the ability to communicate in depth with each other with openness and consensual decision making; the presence of encouragement, ego support, praise, recognition, respect for individuality, and flexibility of family functions and roles; and family unity, loyalty, and cooperation. All of these strengths serve as potential family resources. Other resources may be present in the family's cultural pride, religious affiliation, community ties, economic status, and educational background. The inclusion of these areas in the data collection phase of the nursing process not only gives depth to the nurse's assessment but also suggests the actions and resources that will assist in enhancing the patient's adaptation.

TABLE 5-3

DIMENSIONS OF THE FAMILY APGAR

Component	What is measured	Relevant open-ended questions
Adaptation	How resources are shared, or the degree to which a member is satisfied with the assistance received when family resources are needed	How have family members aided each other in time of need? In what way have family members received help or assistance from friends and community agencies?
Partnership	How decisions are shared, or the member's satisfaction with mutuality in family communication and problem solving	How do family members communicate with each other about such matters as vacations, finances, medical care, large purchases, and personal problems?
Growth	How nurturing is shared, or the member's satisfaction with the freedom available within the family to change roles and attain physical and emotional growth or maturation	How have family members changed during the past years? How has this change been accepted by family members? In what ways have family members aided each other in growing or developing independent life-styles? How have family members reacted to your desires for change?
Affection	How emotional experiences are shared, or the member's satisfaction with the intimacy and emotional interaction that exists in a family	How have members of your family responded to emotional expressions, such as affection, love, sorrow, or anger?
Resolve	How time (and space and money) is shared, or the member's satisfaction with the time commitment that has been made to the family by its members	How do members of your family share time, space, and money?

Modified from Smilkstein, G.: J. Fam. Pract. **6**:1231, 1978.

 Nursing diagnosis

STANDARD III—DIAGNOSIS

The nurse utilizes *nursing diagnoses* and standard classification of mental disorders to express conclusions supported by recorded assessment data and current scientific premises.

Process criteria

The nurse:

1. Identifies actual or potential health problems in regard to:
   a. Self-care limitation or impaired functioning whose general etiology is mental and emotional distress, deficits in the ways significant systems are functioning, and internal psychic and/or developmental issues
   b. Emotional stress or crisis components of illness, pain, self-concept changes, and life process changes
   c. Emotional problems related to daily experiences such as anxiety, aggression, loss, loneliness, and grief
   d. Physical symptoms that occur simultaneously with altered psychic functioning, such as altered intestinal functioning or anorexia
   e. Alterations in thinking, perceiving, symbolizing, communicating, and decision-making abilities
   f. Impaired abilities to relate to others
   g. Behaviors and mental states that indicate the client is a danger to self or others or is gravely disabled
2. Analyzes available information according to accepted theoretical frameworks
3. Makes inferences regarding data from phenomena

4. Formulates a nursing diagnosis subject to revision with subsequent data

On completion of the data collection, the nurse compares the information to documented norms of health and wellness. The psychosocial aspects of a patient's life present some special concerns for the nurse. It is important for her to remember that what is acceptable and appropriate behavior in one social group may be considered deviant and bizarre in another. Since normative standards of behavior are culturally determined, the nurse should make proper allowances for the patient's individual characteristics and the larger social group of which he is a member.

The nurse then must use logical decision making and independent judgment to analyze the collected data and derive a nursing diagnosis. **A nursing diagnosis is a statement of the patient's nursing problem that includes both the adaptive or maladaptive health response and contributing stressors.** These nursing problems concern aspects of the patient's health that may need to be promoted or with which the patient needs help in his biopsychosocial adaptation to stress. The subject of nursing diagnoses, therefore, is the patient's behavioral response to stress. This response, as represented in Fig. 5-2, may lie anywhere on the coping continuum from adaptive, healthy, to maladaptive, ill. Nursing diagnoses identify nursing problems that may be overt, covert, existing, or potential. The responsibility for therapeutic decisions regarding these patients' health responses is assumed by the professional nurse.

At the present time, the classification of nursing diagnoses is in its infancy. However, nurses must define and clarify what they do in the psychiatric setting, and this requires the formulation, dissemination, and use of nursing diagnoses. McClosky believes the following:

In today's world, unless nurses can name the health problems they treat, they are speechless before legislators, third party payors, administrators, other health professionals, and perhaps even nurses themselves. Nursing diagnosis pinpoints what nursing is and what it does.[17]

The North American Nursing Diagnoses Association has been working on identifying, defining, and describing a classification system of nursing diagnoses.[18] In addition, the Council on Psychiatric and Mental Health Nursing of the American Nurses' Association is developing a classification of phenomena of concern to psychiatric-mental health nurses (see Chapter 3). Additional work is needed both in defining the phenomena of concern to psychiatric nurses and in testing and validating the identified nursing diagnoses. If nurses use nursing diagnoses, record their observations and conclusions, and describe the health responses they treat,

the body of nursing knowledge will increase; and therefore, credibility and value placed on nursing care will also increase.

■ **RELATIONSHIP TO MEDICAL DIAGNOSES.** Nursing does not exist in a vacuum, however. Although nurses are the largest group of health care professionals, they must work with other groups, such as physicians, to maximize the health of patients. Each group of health care providers serves as a resource to the others as they collaborate for the improved health status of the patient.

The interrelationship between medicine and nursing includes the mutual exchange of data, the sharing of ideas and analyses, and the development of care plans that include all data pertinent to the individual patient. Interdependent and collaborative interventions are then based on the nursing assessment as well as the medical evaluation, and ensure a thorough and coordinated plan of treatment for the psychiatric patient. Nurses, therefore, while formulating nursing diagnoses and using the nursing process, should also be familiar with the medical diagnoses and treatment plans.

Medical diagnosis refers to the health problem or disease states of the patient. In the medical model of psychiatry, the health problems are mental disorders, which are classified in the Draft of the DSM-III-R in Development.[2] The Draft of the DSM-III-R in Development[2] comprehensively describes the manifestations of various mental disorders, but does not attempt to discuss cause or how the disturbances come about. Specific diagnostic criteria, however, are provided for each mental disorder. Chapters 2 and 3 of this text discuss the medical model and the Draft of the DSM-III-R in Development[2] in greater detail.

Nursing and medical diagnoses may complement each other, but one is not a component of another. A patient with one specific medical diagnosis may have a number of complementary nursing diagnoses related to his range of health responses. On the other hand, a patient may have a specific nursing diagnosis without any identified medical diagnosis.

Coler conducted a small study correlating identified nursing diagnoses specific to psychiatric—mental health nursing with the diagnostic categories of DSM-III.[3] The significance of the study is that it demonstrated the overlap of the diagnostic labels of nursing and psychiatry. For instance, the nursing diagnosis of ineffective individual coping was identified 37 out of 56 times and in all the DSM-III categories. The second most prevalent nursing diagnosis, potential for injury, appeared in all but two of the DSM-III categories. Additional research is needed to validate the phenomena represented in these diagnoses and to elaborate on their in-

```
┌─────────────────────────────────┐
│            TABLE 5-4            │
│                                 │
│   PRESENTATION OF MEDICAL AND  │
│     NURSING PSYCHIATRIC        │
│      DIAGNOSTIC CLASSES        │
└─────────────────────────────────┘
```

Medical diagnostic classes described in Draft of DSM-III-R in Development*	Psychiatric nursing diagnostic classes
Disorders usually first evident in infancy, childhood, or adolescence	Anxiety
Organic mental syndromes and disorders	Psychophysiological illness
Psychoactive substance use disorders	Alterations in self-concept
Sleep and arousal disorders	Disturbances of mood
Schizophrenic disorders	Self-destructive behavior
Delusional (Paranoid) disorders	Disruptions in relatedness
Psychotic disorders not elsewhere classified	Problems with expression of anger
Mood (Affective) disorders	Impaired cognition
Anxiety disorders	Substance abuse
Somatoform disorders	Variations in sexual response
Dissociative disorders	
Gender and sexual disorders	
Factitious disorders	
Impulse control disorders not elsewhere classified	
Adjustment disorder	
Other disorders associated with physical condition	
Personality disorders	

*American Psychiatric Association: Draft of the DSM-III-R in Development (subject to change), as proposed by the Work Group to Revise DSM-III. American Psychiatric Association, October 1985.

teraction with the accountable and requisite medical diagnostic categories.

The focus of this text is on psychiatric nursing and the identification and treatment of nursing problems. Chapters 9 to 21 are organized on this basis and are developed using a nursing process framework. Because quality nursing care requires an understanding of the patient's medical problems as well, each of these chapters will also incorporate a discussion of the medical diagnoses that may be relevant to the patient's health responses. In these chapters, a repeated format will be used to relate the nursing and medical diagnoses. Table 5-4 lists the 17 diagnostic classes identified by the Draft of the DSM-III-R in Development[2], along with the 10 psychiatric nursing diagnostic classes that are explored in this text. The purpose of including this content is to expand the nurse's understanding of the patient and provide a broader base for nursing actions.

Nursing diagnoses are usually formulated in the orientation phase of the relationship. Inexperienced nurses often feel pressured to identify nursing problems quickly and feel confused and frustrated by the withdrawn or noncommunicative patient who does not participate in the relationship and does not share his thoughts or feelings. In this case, the primary nursing problem may be the patient's social isolation related to feelings of inadequacy, or it may be lack of verbalization stemming from fear of interpersonal closeness. Nursing diagnoses describe current health responses of the patient. It is important for the nurse to begin with the behavior and coping responses displayed by the patient at the present time and to work from there. This requires both an acceptance of the patient and a setting of nursing priorities.

◆ Planning

STANDARD IV—PLANNING
The nurse develops a nursing care plan with specific goals and interventions delineating nursing actions unique to each client's needs.
Process criteria

1. The nurse collaborates with clients, their significant others, and team members in establishing nursing care plans
2. In the care plan the nurse:
   a. Identifies priorities of care
   b. States realistic goals in measurable terms with an expected date of accomplishment
   c. Uses identifiable psychotherapeutic principles
   d. Indicates which client needs will be a primary responsibility of the psychiatric and mental health nurse and which will be referred to others with the appropriate expertise
   e. Stresses mutual goal setting and shared responsibility for goal attainment at the level of the client's abilities
   f. Provides guidance for the client care activities performed by others under the nurse's supervision
3. The nurse revises the care plan as goals are achieved, changed, or updated

Careful planning builds on the data collection and nursing diagnosis phases of the nursing process and increases the probability of successful implementation and evaluation. The first step in planning is the development of clearly stated objectives, or goals, for nursing care. In developing methods for writing accurate goals, nursing has built on educational theory. The work of Mager[24] is highly recommended as a resource on this topic.

■ **GOAL CLARIFICATION.** There are four important aspects of goal setting: mutuality, congruency, realism, and timing. However, before goals can be adequately defined, the nurse must recognize that the patient frequently comes to therapy with goals of his own. Generally, they are expressions of the discomfort he feels and are related to symptom alleviation. Often the patient's goals are not directly stated and may be difficult to clarify. Taking nonspecific concerns and translating them into specific goal statements is no easy task for the nurse. He or she must understand the nature of the patient's coping responses and the predisposing and precipitating factors that influence them. Some of the difficulties in defining goals have been described as follows by Krumboltz and Thorensen[22]:

1. The patient may view his problem as someone else's behavior. This may be seen in the case of a parent who brings his adolescent son in for counseling. The parent may view the son as the problem, whereas the adolescent may feel his only problem is his father. An approach to handling this type of situation is to help the person who brings the problem into treatment, since he "owns" the problem at that moment. The nurse might suggest, "Let's talk about how I might help you deal with your son. A change in your response might lead to a change in his behavior also."
2. The patient may express his problem as a feeling, such as, "I'm lonely," or "I'm so unhappy." In addition to trying to help the patient clarify what exactly he is feeling, the nurse might ask him "What kinds of things could you do to make yourself feel less alone and more loved by others?" This helps the patient to see the connection between actions and feelings and increases his sense of responsibility for himself.
3. The patient's problem may be that he lacks a goal or an idea of what exactly he desires out of life. It might be helpful for the nurse, in this case, to point out that values and goals are not magically discovered but must be created by people for themselves. The patient can then be engaged in an active exploratory process to construct goals in his life or adopt the goals of a

social, service, religious, or political group with whom he identifies.
4. The patient's goals may be inappropriate, undesirable, or unclear. The solution here is not for the nurse to impose goals on the patient. Rather, even if the patient's goals seem to be against his best interests, the most the nurse can do is to reflect the patient's behavior and the consequences of it back to the patient. If he should then ask for help in setting new goals, the nurse can help him to do so.
5. The patient's problem may be a choice conflict. This is especially common if all of the choices are unpleasant, unacceptable, or unattainable. An example of this is a couple who wishes to divorce, but do not want to see their child hurt or suffer the financial hardship that would result. Although the nurse cannot make undesirable choices desirable, she can help patients use the problem-solving process and identify the full range of alternatives available to them.
6. The patient may have no real problem but may just want to talk. Nurses must then decide what role they can play with this person and carefully distinguish between a social and a therapeutic relationship.

It becomes obvious that the process of goal clarification is an essential step in the therapeutic process. Out of this clarification and the nursing diagnoses will emerge the mutually agreed on goals around which the therapeutic relationship will be based. There is often a tendency for the well-intentioned nurse to overlook the patient's goals and devise a care plan leading to an outcome that will be gratifying to herself. However, this imposition of supposedly beneficial goals by others may be one of the conflict-producing situations that the patient has experienced in the past. Therefore the experience of working cooperatively with the nurse to evolve mutually acceptable goals is an extremely beneficial experience. If a goal desired by the nurse cannot be shared by the patient, it may be best to defer it until he is able to share it.

■ **GOAL SPECIFICATION.** Once the goals are agreed on, the nurse must state them explicitly for herself and the patient. The more specifically one can state the goals of therapy, the more likely one is to achieve them. They also serve to guide later nursing actions and enhance the evaluation of care. It is therefore necessary that the objectives be written in behavioral terms. This means that the verb used in the statement of the objective should represent a behavior that may be observed. They should realistically describe what the nurse wishes to accomplish and within what time span. Often the requirement for explicit goals is avoided through the use of general statements that are applicable to all patients, such as the goals of forming a relationship or relieving depression. They may be valid in general terms, but they are not adequate in and of themselves.

Long- and short-term goals should be developed, with short-term goals contributing to the attainment of the long-term goals. Following are sample goals:

Long-term

> The patient will travel about the community independently within 2 months.

Short-term

1. At the end of 1 week the patient will sit on his front steps.
2. At the end of 2 weeks the patient will walk to the corner and back to his house.
3. At the end of 3 weeks the patient, accompanied by the nurse, will walk around the block.
4. At the end of 4 weeks the patient will walk around the block alone.

The hierarchy would continue until the desired goal is accomplished. It should be noted that the goal is stated in terms of observable behavior, includes a period of time in which it is to be accomplished, and incorporates any other conditions applicable to the goal, such as whether the patient is to be alone or accompanied by the nurse.

Most patients exhibit a number of nursing problems, each of which must be incorporated in the plan of care. Several goals may need to be written relative to each nursing diagnosis. As the nurse and patient work together to meet patient needs, new ones often arise. For this reason, it is necessary to make decisions concerning the relative importance or priority of meeting the various nurse-patient goals. Otherwise, care would become haphazard and fragmented, with the focus first on one goal and then on the next, based only on what happened to come up at the time. Important and immediate needs could get lost in the general chaos.

One of the most important tasks of the nurse and patient is to assign priorities to goals. Frequently, a number of goals can be pursued simultaneously. Goals related to the protection of the patient from self-destructive impulses always receive highest priority. With the identification of both long- and short-term goals, it is particularly important that the nurse keep the proposed time sequence firmly in mind.

Since the nursing care plan is dynamic and should ensure responsiveness to the patient's coping responses throughout his contact with the health care system, priorities are constantly changing. If the focus is always kept on the patient's behavioral responses, priorities can be set and modified as the patient changes. Nursing care is then personalized and the patient participates in its planning and implementation.

■ **GOAL ACHIEVEMENT.** Once the goals are formulated, the next task is to outline the plan or method for achieving these goals. The nursing care plan is based on application of theory from nursing and related physical and behavioral sciences to the unique responses of the individual patient. This presupposes that as the nurse identifies areas of patient need, appropriate theoretical resources will again be consulted. Failure to approach nursing care in this scientific manner is likely to result in illogical decision making and a plan based on tradition, intuition, or trial and error. Although use of any of these decision-making methods may result in a valid plan, consistency of depth and accuracy over time will suffer, as will the overall care of the patient. Skill in using the nursing process requires a commitment by the nurse to the ongoing pursuit of knowledge that will enhance professional growth.

Successful care planning is facilitated by the active involvement of the patient. If the nurse collects data, returns to the nurse's station, consults textbooks, and then writes up a plan of care, an important step has been missed. Once the nurse has formulated a tentative care plan, he or she must validate this plan with the patient. This saves time and effort for them both as they continue to work together and also communicates to the patient his responsibility in getting well. The patient can tell the nurse that a proposed plan is unrealistic regarding financial status, life-style, value system, or, perhaps, personal preference. There are usually several possible approaches to a patient problem. Utilizing the one that is most acceptable to the patient enhances the likelihood of goal accomplishment.

If the goal answers the question of "what," the plan of care answers the questions of "how" and "why." The plan chosen obviously will depend on the nursing diagnosis, the nurse's theoretical orientation, and the nature of the goals pursued. In general, the goals will influence the selection of therapeutic techniques. Failure to attain a goal by employing a particular plan can lead to the decision to adopt a new approach or to reevaluate the goal. Mutual planning and implementation activities commonly occur in the working phase of the relationship.

⟹ Implementation

STANDARD V—INTERVENTION

The nurse intervenes as guided by the nursing care plan to implement nursing actions that promote, maintain, or restore physical and mental health, prevent illness, and effect rehabilitation.

Process criteria

The nurse:

1. Acts to ensure that health care needs are met either by using nursing skills or by obtaining assistance from other health care providers when indicated
2. Acts as the client's advocate when necessary to facilitate the achievement of health
3. Reviews and modifies interventions based on patient progress

Implementation refers to the actual delivery of nursing care to the patient and his response to the care that is given. Good planning maximizes the probability of successful implementation. Such factors as available people, equipment, resources, time, and money must be considered as nursing actions are planned. Well-planned nursing care also takes into account the personalities and experiences of the nurse and the patient, and their interaction.

The most valid basis for nursing action is that which has been investigated by nursing researchers who have applied the scientific method to nursing practice. It is also acceptable to judiciously use theory from the physical and behavioral sciences to provide a rationale for nursing intervention. In most nurse-patient situations, there is more than one possible approach to accomplishing the stated objectives. It is helpful, when planning care, to identify alternative nursing actions that are appropriate to the goal. If this is done, the nurse is not left floundering should the only identified action fail. Consideration of several alternative nursing actions lends a great deal of flexibility to the implementation phase of the nursing process.

STANDARD V-A—PSYCHOTHERAPEUTIC INTERVENTIONS

The nurse (generalist) uses psychotherapeutic interventions to assist clients to regain or improve their previous coping abilities and prevent further disability.

Process criteria

The nurse:

1. Identifies the client's responses to health problems
2. Reinforces those responses to health problems that are functional and helps the client modify or eliminate those that are dysfunctional
3. Employs principles of communication, interviewing techniques, problem-solving, and crisis intervention when performing psychotherapeutic interventions
4. Uses knowledge of behavioral concepts such as anxiety, loss, conflict, grief, and anger to assist the client to cope, adapt, and constructively deal with feelings
5. Demonstrates knowledge about and skill in the use of psychotherapeutic interventions specifically useful in the modification of thought, perception, affect, behavior, and motivation
6. Utilizes health team members to help evaluate the outcome of interventions and to formulate modification of psychotherapeutic techniques
7. Reinforces useful patterns and themes in the client's interactions with others
8. Uses crisis intervention to promote growth and to aid the personal and social integration of clients in developmental, situational, or suicidal crisis

In implementing psychotherapeutic interventions, the nurse helps the psychiatric patient do two things: **develop insight** and resolve problems through **carrying out a plan of positive action**. These two areas for nursing intervention correspond with the responsive and action dimensions of the nurse-patient relationship described in Chapter 4. Insight refers to the development of new emotional and cognitive organizations by the patient. It frequently leads to an increase in anxiety as defense mechanisms are broken down. This is the time when resistances commonly occur. But knowing something on an intellectual level does *not* inevitably lead to a change in behavior. Nurses who terminate their interventions at this point are not fully carrying out the therapeutic process to the patient's benefit. An additional step is needed. The patient must decide if he will revert back to maladaptive coping mechanisms, remain in a resisting, immobilized state, or adopt new, adaptive, and constructive coping mechanisms.

The first step in helping a patient translate insight into action is to build adequate incentives to abandoning old patterns of behavior. The nurse should help the patient see that his old patterns do him more harm than good and inflict much suffering and pain on him. No new patterns can be learned unless the motivation to acquire them is greater than the motivation to retain old ones. Nursing activities therefore must include encouraging any desires the patient expresses for mental health, emotional growth, and freedom from suffering.

With sufficient motivation the patient must then be supported as he tests out new behaviors and coping mechanisms. Important in this regard will be the mobilization of the individual's social support system. This is relevant to all levels of nursing intervention—primary, secondary, and tertiary—and all patient populations.

STANDARD V-B—HEALTH TEACHING
The nurse assists clients, families, and groups to achieve satisfying and productive patterns of living through health teaching.
Process criteria
The nurse:

1. Identifies health education needs of clients
2. Employs principles of learning and appropriate teaching methods
3. Teaches the basic principles of physical and mental health
4. Teaches communication, interpersonal, and social skills
5. Provides opportunities for clients to learn experientially

Health education is an important nursing activity to help patients change maladaptive coping responses. It is incorporated in primary, secondary, and tertiary prevention activities. Specifically, it involves four steps.

1. Increasing a patient's awareness of issues and events related to one's mental health
2. Increasing a patient's understanding of the dimensions of potential stressors, possible outcomes, and alternative coping responses
3. Increasing a patient's knowledge of where and how to acquire the needed resources
4. Increasing the actual abilities of a patient

Therapeutic education can take place anywhere and with any group of individuals. For example, the effectiveness of a classroom course for psychiatric patients that focused on how to cope and regain control over their lives has been reported.[23] Similarly, patient education groups have been identified as having a positive effect on patient compliance to medication.[50]

There is also a movement to using an educational approach for working with families who have mentally ill relatives.[13] Such psychoeducational approaches give families an understanding of mental illness together with training in communication, problem solving, information giving, and behavioral management.

STANDARD V-C—SELF-CARE ACTIVITIES
The nurse uses the activities of daily living in a goal-directed way to foster adequate self-care and physical and mental well-being of clients.
Process criteria

The nurse:

1. Respects and protects the client's rights
2. Encourages the client to collaborate in the development of a self-care plan
3. Sets limits in a manner that is humane and the least restrictive necessary to assure safety of the client and others

STANDARD V-D—SOMATIC THERAPIES
The nurse uses knowledge of somatic therapies and applies related clinical skills in working with clients.
Process criteria
The nurse:

1. Utilizes knowledge of current psychopharmacology to guide nursing actions
2. Observes and interprets pertinent responses to somatic therapies in terms of the underlying principles of each therapy
3. Evaluates effectiveness of somatic therapies and recommends changes in the treatment plan as appropriate
4. Collaborates with other team members to provide for safe administration of therapies
5. Supervises the client's chemotherapeutic regimen in collaboration with the physician
6. Provides opportunities for clients and families to discuss, question, and explore their feelings and concerns about past, current, or projected use of somatic therapies
7. Reviews expected actions and side effects of somatic therapies with clients and their families
8. Uses prescribing authority for medications as congruent with the state nursing practice act

STANDARD V-E—THERAPEUTIC ENVIRONMENT
The nurse provides, structures, and maintains a therapeutic environment in collaboration with the client and other health care providers.
Process criteria
The nurse:

1. Assures that clients are adequately oriented to the milieu and are familiar with scheduled activities and rules that govern behavior and daily living
2. Observes, analyzes, interprets, and records the effects of environmental forces upon the client
3. Assesses and develops the therapeutic potential of the practice setting on behalf of clients through consideration of the physical environment, the social structure, and the culture of the setting
4. Fosters communications in the environment that are congruent with therapeutic goals
5. Collaborates with others in the development and institution of milieu activities specific to the client's physical and mental health needs
6. Articulates to the client and staff the justification

for use of limit setting, restraint, or seclusion and the conditions necessary for release from restriction to the client and staff

7. Participates in ongoing evaluation of the effectiveness of the therapeutic milieu
8. Assists clients living at home to achieve and maintain an environment that supports and maintains health

STANDARD V-F—PSYCHOTHERAPY

The nurse (specialist) utilizes advanced clinical expertise in individual, group, and family *psychotherapy*, child psychotherapy, and other treatment modalities to function as a psychotherapist and recognizes professional accountability for nursing practice.

Process criteria
The nurse:

1. Structures the therapeutic contract with the client in the beginning phase of the relationship, including such elements as purpose, time, place, fees, participants, confidentiality, available means of contact, and responsibilities of both client and therapist
2. Engages in interdisciplinary and intradisciplinary collaboration to achieve treatment goals
3. Engages clients in the process of determining the appropriate form of psychotherapy
4. Identifies the goals of psychotherapy
5. Uses knowledge of growth and development, psychopathology, psychosocial systems, small group and family dynamics, and knowledge of selected treatment modalities as indicated
6. Articulates a rationale for the goals chosen and interventions utilized
7. Fosters increasing personal and therapeutic responsibility on the part of the client
8. Provides for continuity of care for the client in the therapist's absence
9. Determines with the client, when possible, that goals have been achieved and facilitates the termination process
10. Refers clients to other professionals when indicated
11. Respects and protects the client's legal rights
12. Avails self of appropriate opportunities to increase knowledge and skill in the therapies utilized in nursing practice
13. Obtains recognized educational preparation and ongoing supervision for types of psychotherapy utilized, e.g., individual psychotherapy, group and family psychotherapy, child psychotherapy, psychoanalysis, or other forms of therapy
14. Uses clinical judgment in determining whether providing physical care (especially procedures prone to misinterpretation, e.g., injections, enemas) will enhance or impair the therapist-client relationship and delegates such care as needed

The standards of practice and related process criteria for the implementation of nursing care are quite detailed and explicit. The standards clearly identify the range of activities engaged in by psychiatric nurses as psychotherapeutic interventions, health teaching, self-care activities, somatic therapies, therapeutic milieu, and, if the nurse has advanced preparation, psychotherapy. The process criteria present a detailed description of the numerous specific activities psychiatric nurses employ in implementing nursing care.

Within the context of the nurse-patient relationship, adaptive goals can be actively pursued by the patient in a productive way. It is important for the nurse and patient to allow sufficient time for change. Many of the patient's maladaptive patterns have been building up over months and years and cannot be expected to change in a matter of days or weeks. Finally, the nurse must help the patient evaluate these new patterns, integrate them into his life experiences, and utilize the learning of problem solving as foresight for future experiences. In this way secondary prevention nursing interventions also fulfill primary and tertiary prevention goals. Chapters 9 and 11 describe primary and tertiary prevention nursing interventions in greater detail.

 # Evaluation

STANDARD VI—EVALUATION

The nurse evaluates client responses to nursing actions in order to revise the data base, nursing diagnoses, and nursing care plan.

Process criteria
The nurse:

1. Pursues validation, suggestions, and new information
2. Discusses observations, insights, and data with colleagues
3. Documents the results of evaluation of nursing care
4. Conducts a nursing audit

When evaluating nursing care, one should review all previous phases of the nursing process and determine the degree of goal achievement by the patient. The overall flow of the nursing process is evident in Fig. 5-3. From this representation, it is evident that many decisions are made by the nurse throughout the process. Evaluation of care requires that the nurse first consider if the conceptual framework was valid and appropriate to the particular patient situation. Next, was the data collection adequate and all relevant coping responses, objective signs, and subjective symptoms identified? The accuracy of the nursing diagnosis may be assessed with relation to the nature of normal parameters used, the

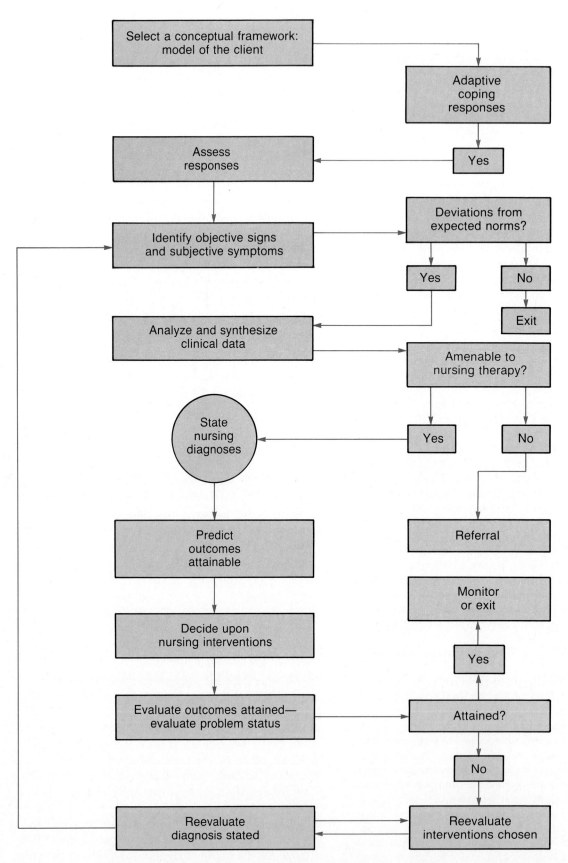

Fig. 5-3. Flowchart of the nursing process. (Modified from Gordon, M.: Nurs. Clin. North Am. **14**:492, 1979.)

analysis and synthesis of data, the application of theory, and its appropriateness for nursing therapy. The nursing goals and plan of care should be examined for their relevancy, priority, mutuality, and consideration of all realistic alternatives. In the area of implementation, the nurse needs to evaluate whether the nursing interventions were appropriate, efficient in use of time and energy and, most important, effective. The timing, relevance, communication, and outcome of the nursing interventions must all be critically analyzed. The achievement of goals is worth noting explicitly. Often progress with psychiatric patients is slow and occurs in imperceptible degrees rather than with dramatic suddenness. Realizing progress has been made can produce growth in itself and can evoke enthusiasm for further progress on the part of both the patient and the nurse.

One specific approach to evaluation in psychiatric nursing is the use of goal attainment scaling as described by Stanley.[45] This is a method for evaluating pre-established individual goals through the construction of a review plan. The steps involved in creating a review plan include

1. Identifying specific patient goals
2. Weighting the relative importance of each
3. Deciding on a way of measuring progress for each goal that is useful, relevant, and easily rated
4. Determining the expected patient outcome relative to each one
5. Creating a scale of levels of goal attainment
6. Setting a review date to assess a patient's overall progress towards the goals
7. Calculating a goal attainment score to provide an overall summary of patient progress

In using such an approach, evaluation becomes linked to planning, thereby strengthening the scientific basis of nursing practice by developing empirical methods. It could also be used by nurse administrators to assess the effectiveness of a service.

Flexibility is needed by the nurse to modify interventions on the basis of the patient's changing needs and the nurse's continuing evaluation. The need to modify a care plan does not connote failure of nursing care. Failure takes place if the plan of care is not relevant to the client's needs and is not revised as the needs change or are clarified. Thus, reassessment, reordering of priorities, new goal setting, and revision of the nursing care plan are all essential evaluation activities.

Evaluation is a mutual process based on the previously identified goals and level of satisfaction expressed by the patient. It is not a cumbersome task left for the termination phase of the relationship. Rather, it is a continuous, active process that begins with the initial phase of the relationship and is present throughout its development and completion. The key words for the evaluation phase of the nursing process can be summarized as mutual, continuous, adequate, effective, appropriate, efficient, and flexible.

■ **ORGANIZATIONAL EVALUATION.** There is another level of evaluation that nurses need to know about and actively participate in. This is the level of formal, systematic, organizational evaluation of overall patterns of care through *quality assessment measures.* In these activities, the focus is not on the nurse practitioner but on the patient and overall program of care. The present growth and commitment to critically reviewing and analyzing the quality of health care can be attributed to several sources: the demands of the consumer for quality, but reasonable, health care, third-party payees for controlled health care costs, the movement toward increased professional accountability, and regulatory and federal groups to monitor the quality of care given to providers. At this higher level of analysis, a comprehensive evaluation should theoretically include the following[40]:

- Systems evaluation of administration and management of treatment and allocation of resources
- Consumer evaluation of patient needs and satisfaction
- Clinical evaluation of treatment outcome and process

Of these three types of evaluation, clinical evaluation is the longest established and most common. Consumer evaluation is gaining attention and acceptance as the public is becoming more educated and assertive. Systems evaluation has primarily been limited to improving operations in private industry, and only recently has it been applied to health care.

Systems evaluation. Systems evaluation is the evaluation of the organization of the delivery system, which includes patient flow, paperwork, procedures for scheduling patients, staff-patient ratio, disciplinary mix, and the analysis of utilization of resources. It is intended to supplement clinical evaluation. Three components of systems evaluation have been identified: (1) systems analysis, (2) economic analysis, and (3) operations research. Systems analysis attempts to simplify and improve the organization. Economic analysis emphasizes monies spent and what, in turn, they produce. Operations research attempts to develop methods that will help hospital management plan for optimal allocation of the resources available. Together, these analyses bring a new dimension to the institution by evaluating the actual organization of treatment and have the potential

---

Functions of Quality Assurance

1. Tied to the philosophy of the hospital
2. Improves the performance of all professionals and protects the patients
3. Focuses on the quality of patient care
4. Sets the quality of care delivered against standards and measurable criteria
5. Prevents future losses or patient injuries by continuous monitoring of problem resolution areas
6. Searches for patterns of noncompliance with goals, objectives, and standards. The following steps of the quality assurance process are applied: problem identification, problem assessment, implementation of corrective action, follow-up, and reporting of findings.

From Orlikoff, J., and Lanham, G.: Hospitals **55**(15):55, 1981.

---

for improving the performance of the clinical operation.[40]

Consumer evaluation. Consumer evaluation of patient needs and satisfaction has not received as much attention in the psychiatric literature as it has in other areas of health care. One of the few studies to examine consumer satisfaction with nurse psychotherapy was reported by Hardin and Durham.[12] They found that 90% of the clients expressed satisfaction and 70% were extremely satisfied. Specific reasons for satisfaction were also reported by the authors. Assessing consumer satisfaction with nursing care is a difficult task because of the interdependent functioning of the health care team and the numerous variables that can explain the outcome measure of satisfaction. Nevertheless, additional studies are needed by nurses to both evaluate the services they provide, and document the cost-effectiveness of their activities.

Clinical evaluation. Clinical evaluation of ongoing programs is demonstrated in the form of various quality assurance activities that include both evaluation and corrective action.[32] Some of the functions of quality assurance are listed in the accompanying box. Zimmer[51] defines quality assurance as the estimation in degree of excellence in three areas: (1) patient health outcomes, (2) process or activity, and (3) resource cost outcomes. A common method reflecting two of these areas is the patient care audit, which, when restricted to nursing care, is also called the **nursing audit**. The topic of an audit may be a disease, nursing diagnosis, patient behavior, therapeutic measure, or nursing procedure. An audit that focuses on nursing actions is called a **process audit**. In a process audit, data are collected relative to a specific nursing activity, and they are then compared to a preset standard of nursing care, such as the American Nurses' Association *Standards of Nursing Practice*. If the audit focuses on the behavior of the patient in response to the care that has been provided, it is termed an **outcome audit**. This type of audit parallels the evaluation phase of the nursing process. Specific examples of nursing audits conducted in the psychiatric setting are described in some of the articles listed in the annotated suggested readings at the end of this chapter.

Both process and outcome audits have advantages, depending on the information desired. Zimmer[51] believes that in quality assurance efforts, nurses should first start with the determination of desired patient health outcomes and the degree to which they are attained. Next, nurses must proceed to the identification of the most powerful and cost-effective activities that cause these outcomes. Finally, when activities are identified and their relationship with specific outcomes is clear, nurses should proceed to the third step, determining the cost of the nursing activities and the related resources used to achieve specific outcomes.

Two important components of quality assurance should be emphasized. The first is the necessity for peer review, which should consist of expert nurse peers who are involved together in the delivery of care. They are the only persons who have the needed nursing knowledge to be able to make judgments about desired patient health outcomes, how patients should progress toward those outcomes, and nursing activities that cause the changes. They are also those people who will be most involved with the other component of quality assurance—the correction of deficiencies or problems of nursing care that the audit reveals. This idea of taking corrective action and actually making improvements is what differentiates quality assurance from simple program evaluation or evaluation research. The reports of quality assurance should reach the highest level of the organization, and it is expected that actions will be taken which will result in improvement. These may take the form of administrative changes in policies or procedures, continuing education programs, reallocation of personnel, changes in activities or procedures, or a need for further research.

Involvement in this level of clinical program evaluation is necessary for all nurses. Through such activities, nurses demonstrate professional accountability. As Zimmer has stated:

Members of the nursing profession will be able to take their place among the disciplines that function in patient health review when and only when they can identify the specific alterations in patient health status secured through nursing activities. The development and the use of nurses' capability to function in quality assurance thus deserves the highest priority in the nursing profession.[51:93]

Nurse accountability

STANDARD VII—PEER REVIEW

The nurse participates in peer review and other means of evaluation to assure quality of nursing care provided for clients.

Process criteria

The nurse:

1. Assumes responsibility for review of clinical practice with peers, supervisors, and/or consultants
2. Considers recommendations for change that may arise from review

STANDARD VIII—CONTINUING EDUCATION

The nurse assumes responsibility for continuing education and professional development and contributes to the professional growth of others.

Process criteria

The nurse:

1. Initiates independent learning activities to increase understanding and update skills
2. Participates in inservice meetings and educational programs either as an attendee or as a teacher
3. Attends conventions, institutions, workshops, symposia, and other professional meetings
4. Systematically increases understanding of theories related to psychiatric and mental health nursing
5. Assists others to identify areas of educational needs
6. Communicates formally and informally new knowledge regarding clinical observations and interpretations with professional colleagues and others

Implementing the nursing process is an ongoing activity that is the professional responsibility of every nurse. Inherent in this responsibility is the need for professional accountability requiring both peer review and continuing education on the part of each psychiatric nurse. Supervision by a peer, a group of peers, or a more experienced person is an important part of professional practice. Whether it is conducted formally or informally, peer review helps the nurse examine care planning and serves as an ongoing learning experience.

A nurse's need for continued growth can also be met through the more formalized process of continued education. This encompasses a variety of professional activities from reading journals to attending workshops to participating in psychiatric nursing organizations. A final important aspect of continued education involves the communication of new knowledge to one's professional colleagues in the mental health field.

STANDARD IX—INTERDISCIPLINARY COLLABORATION

The nurse collaborates with interdisciplinary teams in assessing, planning, implementing, and evaluating programs and other mental health activities.

Process criteria

The nurse:

1. Participates in the formulation of overall goals, plans, and decisions
2. Includes the client in the collaboration of the mental health team whenever possible and appropriate
3. Recognizes, respects, accepts, and demonstrates trust in colleagues and their contributions
4. Consults with colleagues as needed and is available to be consulted by them
5. Articulates knowledge and skills so that these may be coordinated with the contributions of others working with a client or program
6. Collaborates with other disciplines in teaching, supervision, and research

Planning and implementation of accountable nursing care do not take place in isolation from the patient's other experiences with the health care team and the health care system. The nurse has a responsibility to be sure that the nursing care plan is congruent with the plans of other health care professionals who are involved with the patient. Some degree of conflict can be avoided by personal contact with other professionals to discover how they define their roles and responsibilities. Knowledge of the distribution of responsibility within the health team enables the nurse to consult colleagues appropriately as indicated by the needs of the patient. Although the nurse may have information about these areas, it is a much more efficient and appropriate use of time and energy to refer the patient to team members who specialize in dealing with the patient's needs. Referral should be accompanied by adequate background information so that the assessment process is not duplicated.

STANDARD X—UTILIZATION OF COMMUNITY HEALTH SYSTEMS

The nurse (specialist) participates with other members of the community in assessing, planning, implementing, and evaluating mental health services and community systems that include the promotion of the broad continuum of primary, secondary, and tertiary prevention of mental illness.

Process criteria

The nurse:

1. Uses knowledge of community and group dynamics and systems theory to understand the structure and function of the community system
2. Recognizes current social and political issues that influence the nature of mental health problems in the community
3. Encourages active consumer participation in assessing and planning programs to meet the community's mental health needs
4. Brings the community's needs to the attention of appropriate individuals and groups, including legislative bodies and regional and state planning groups
5. Plans and participates in didactic and experiential educational programs related to the community's mental health
6. Uses consultative skills to facilitate the development and implementation of mental health services
7. Interprets mental health services to others in the community
8. Participates with other health care professionals and members of the community in the planning, implementation, and evaluation of mental health services
9. Participates in the delineation of high-risk population groups in the community and identifies gaps in community services
10. Assesses strengths and coping capacities of individuals, families, and the community in order to promote and increase their mental health
11. Uses knowledge of community resources to assist consumers' referral to and appropriate use of health care resources
12. Collaborates with staff at other agencies to facilitate continuity of service for individuals and families

Even when the focus of one's nursing care is at the level of the individual patient, the impact of the family and community must not be forgotten or overlooked. Interventions related to these other levels should be incorporated in each phase of the nursing process. The purpose of the psychiatric nurse generalist in working with these other levels, such as family and community, will be to enhance the resources of the patient and maximize adaptive health responses. The psychiatric nurse specialist can also function in implementing the nursing process with community health systems. At this level, the nurse uses consultative skills to impact on the health care needs of the larger community system.

Nursing research
STANDARD XI—RESEARCH
The nurse contributes to nursing and the mental health field through innovations in theory and practice and participation in research.

Process criteria

The nurse:

1. Approaches nursing practice with an inquiring and open mind
2. Utilizes research findings in practice
3. Develops, implements, and evaluates research studies as appropriate to level of education
4. Uses responsible standards of research in investigative endeavors
5. Ensures that a mechanism for the protection of human subjects exists
6. Obtains expert consultation and/or supervision as required

Nurses should realize that the relationship between theory, practice, and research is an interactive and reciprocal one.[46] For theory to be useful, it must have implications for practice, and for practice to be tested and validated, it must be theoretical. Theory that arises out of practice is validated by research, which returns to direct practice and has implications for clinical care. This cyclical relationship, as diagrammed by O'Toole,[33] is represented in Fig. 5-4. It shows how the casual, nonsystematic observation of a problem in practice leads to a more systematic observation and a definition of terms, including the nature of the problem and influencing factors. Descriptive, observational, and exploratory research designs are useful at this time in more precisely defining a problem or observation. Following this, hypotheses may be developed concerning relationships between identified variables. They may be tested in correlational or survey research designs. One might then propose causal relationships between the variables and test these predictions in experimental or quasiexperimental designs, in natural or controlled settings, with a specification of the predicted relationship. Only if a causal relationship has been established can one proceed to a prescriptive theoretical level and the testing of specific interventions aimed at changing the clinical problem. In this way, prescriptive studies feed knowledge back into practice to improve the quality of patient care.

This progressive process of observing from practice, theorizing, testing in research, and subsequently modifying practice must become an essential part of psychiatric nursing if it is to survive as a practice discipline.[33] Steps need to be taken to bridge the gap between research and practice. One way to do so would be to encourage closer collaboration between nurse researchers and nurse clinicians to ensure that the right questions are asked and the right variables are tested.[29]

Smoyak has noted that clinical practice in psychiatry

is "far more intuitive than it is scientific."[43:9] There are many reasons why research in this area is difficult to conduct. Problems such as sample size, outcome measurements, and the complexity of human behavior all compound the research difficulties. It is also difficult to balance the rights of the individual and the desire to accomplish sound research.[4,26] For example, consent to psychiatric research is complex. First, one needs to consider whether the subject is able to consent and the degree to which the consent constitutes an informed choice. Next is the issue of the experiment itself and whether it alters the subject's ability by changing his or her affect, perceptions, or ability to process information. The risks involved in psychiatric research must be carefully studied, and ethics must be maintained.

Research is sorely needed on the outcomes of nursing therapy to determine its effectiveness and to compare psychiatric nurses with other mental health care providers on relative effectiveness of services. Important data are being accumulated regarding the cost-effectiveness of nursing interventions in acute care, chronic care, primary care, and health promotion. Psychiatric nurses, in contrast, lag behind in documenting their practice. One controlled investigation conducted in England demonstrated that community psychiatric nurses' clinical and social care of neurotic patients was comparable with that provided by outpatient psychiatrists.[25]

In addition, the patients assigned to the nurses reported greater consumer satisfaction and had higher rates of discharge. Finally, over the whole study period, the care provided by the psychiatric nurses was less expensive. Research studies similar to this one need to be undertaken and reported by psychiatric nurses for the future survival and viability of this speciality area of practice.

Research about the practice of psychiatric nursing has increased in the past decade, and it is obvious that nurses have the ability to construct sophisticated designs with both theoretical and practical importance. The clinical problems are numerous, and as nurses gain the skills and experience to empirically validate their work, they have the potential of making a significant contribution to psychiatric theory and a substantial impact on practice.

Clinical case analysis

Clinical example 5-1 is a case study of a long-term relationship that demonstrates the use of the nursing process with a patient. It illustrates the interrelationship of the phases of the nurse-patient relationship, therapeutic dimensions, and various activities as the nurse works with the patient to bring about adaptive coping behavior and the more integrated functioning of the patient.

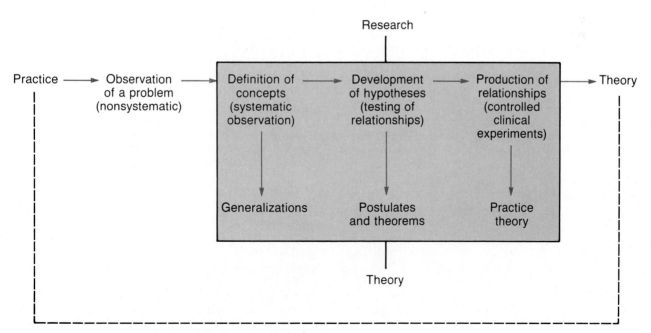

Fig. 5-4. Relationship between theory, practice, and research. (From O'Toole, A.: J. Psych. Nurs. Ment. Health Serv. **19**(2):11, 1981.)

CLINICAL EXAMPLE 5-1

Ms. G came to the psychiatric outpatient department of the local hospital requesting treatment with a female therapist. After consultation with a psychiatrist, the psychiatric nurse specialist agreed to perform the initial screening and evaluation and consider serving as her primary therapist.

ASSESSMENT

To collect the initial data, the nurse followed the admission format required by the department. A description of the presenting problem revealed that Ms. G was a 29-year-old single woman who was neat in appearance and markedly overweight. She reported feelings of "confusion and depression" and said that superficially she appeared "outgoing and friendly and played the role of a clown." In reality, however, she said she had few close friends, felt insecure about herself, felt unsuccessful in her job, and believed she "overanalyzed her problems."

Additional information was obtained in other significant areas of her life. Her psychosocial history revealed a disrupted family situation. Her mother died of tuberculosis when she was 11 years of age. Her father, age 73, was alive but had been an alcoholic "for as long as Mrs. G could remember." She had one sister, age 20, who married at age 16 and was now divorced. She also had one stepsister, age 45, who was married, had two adopted sons, and lived out of state. In exploring this family information, Ms. G revealed that her stepsister was her natural mother, but she had continued to call her father's wife "mother." After her "mother" died, her stepsister took over the house. Two years later, however, this stepsister married and moved out of state. Ms. G reported feeling closest to this stepsister and felt abandoned when she left. Ms. G then took charge of the house until age 14, when her father placed her and her sister in a group home where she had difficulty making friends.

She completed high school and college. In college she had four good friends who were all married now. Her only close heterosexual relationship was in high school, and this boyfriend eventually married her best friend. Since that time she had never dated and stated she had no desire to marry.

After college she obtained a job as a "girl Friday" for a law firm and expressed much pleasure with it. She then saw the opportunity to make more money as a waitress and switched jobs. She worked at a restaurant at present and her schedule involved day and night rotations as well as weekend shifts. She expressed dissatisfaction with many aspects of her job but an inability to identify alternatives. Her goal in life was to have a fulfilling career.

She lived alone. Her best friend was her immediate supervisor at work. She currently had no male friends and only two other female acquaintances.

Pertinent medical history revealed a major weight problem. She was 36 kg (80 pounds) overweight and extremely conscious of it. She viewed her body negatively and believed others were also "repulsed" by her weight. She was also recently recovered from infectious hepatitis. She drank an occasional beer when out with friends (once or twice a month), denied any drug use, and smoked three fourths of a pack of cigarettes a day.

NURSING DIAGNOSIS

After consultation the psychiatric nurse agreed to work with Ms. G as primary therapist. In the following session they established a contract for working together, and a fee was set by the agency's financial secretary. At this time they explored her expressed guilt over seeking help, the reason for her request for a female therapist, their mutual roles, and the confidential nature of the relationship. The nurse also shared with Ms. G. the maladaptive coping responses she had noted and the inferences she had made. They discussed these areas, and the following nursing diagnoses were identified from the psychiatric nursing diagnostic classes:

1. Self-concept, disturbance in self-esteem, related to childhood rejection and unrealistic self-ideals
2. Social isolation, related to ambivalence regarding male-female relationships and lack of socialization skills
3. Self-concept, disturbance in role performance, related to job dissatisfaction with working hours and nature of the work
4. Self-concept, disturbance in body-image, related to weight control problem
5. Anxiety, related to the possibility of change and the therapy process

PLANNING

In discussing these areas they agreed that problem 1 was a central one and problems 3 and 4 directly contributed to it. Her coping mechanisms included intellectualization and denial, and she compensated for her self-doubts by an outward appearance that was social, joking, and friendly, yet superficial. Prob-

CLINICAL EXAMPLE 5-1—cont'd

lem 5 presented an immediate demand on the therapeutic relationship. The strengths Ms. G brought to the therapy process included her introspective nature and ability to analyze events, her openness to new ideas, the resource people available to her in her immediate environment, and a genuine sense of humor. They mutually agreed to work on her problem areas in weekly therapy sessions. After 5 months they would evaluate the achievement of the following long-term goals:

1. Ms. G will describe her expectations of the therapeutic process and her commitment to it.
2. Aspects of Ms. G's self-ideal will be identified.
3. Factors influencing her self-concept and negative, stereotyped self-perceptions will be evaluated.
4. Interpersonal relationships will be analyzed to include her patterns of relating, her expectations of others, and specific areas of difficulty.
5. Alternative employment opportunities will be identified.
6. The advantages and disadvantages of a job change will be compared.

IMPLEMENTATION

Since they were in the introductory phase of the relationship, many of the goals involved areas needing further assessment. During this phase of treatment Ms. G displayed much anxiety, testing behavior, and ambivalence, and the nursing actions were focused on promoting respect, openness, and acceptance and minimizing her anxiety. Through the nurse's use of empathic understanding, Ms. G became less jovial and superficial and began to attain some intellectual insight into her behavior. With guidance she began to appraise her own abilities and became more open in expressing feelings.

She feared intimate personal involvement and could not tolerate physical closeness. The nurse incorporated this into nursing actions by initially minimizing confrontation, setting limits on anxiety-producing topics, and arranging the office seating to allow the patient to select her proximity to the nurse.

As they discussed the patient's relationships, the nurse confronted her with the dependent role Ms. G played in them and the unrealistic expectations she placed on others in the exclusiveness and amount of time she demanded from them. Her pattern of relating was also manipulative in that she elicited a sympathetic response and then used it to meet her own needs. She had great difficulty with mutuality and autonomy in relating to others. She was inexperienced in heterosexual relationships and missed many of the normal adolescent growth experiences in this area. Finally, she had much emotion and fear vested in her family of origin. The only trusting relationship Ms. G could recall was with her stepsister-mother. When this stepsister abruptly left home to marry, Ms. G perceived this as a personal rejection. She had since isolated herself from her family and continued to blame herself for her rejection by others, thus lowering her self-esteem and ability to trust others.

At the end of 4 months Ms. G was being considered for a promotion at work to hostess but on the basis of an evaluation by her best friend and supervisor was rejected for it. This precipitated a suicide attempt, which Ms. G revealed at her next regular session. At this point the issue of trust within the relationship became critical, as well as her inability to express anger because of fear of rejection. The nurse now began more actively confronting Ms. G in her areas of ambivalence and inconsistency, setting limits on her self-destructive behavior, and suggesting alternatives. Ms. G then revealed that her relationship with her friend-supervisor was also a sexual one, and she expressed fears of homosexuality and loss of identity.

In later sessions Ms. G's relationship with this friend would become a critical therapeutic issue because many of her conflicts were acted out in it. The therapy process presented a threat to the pathological nature of this relationship, and during the course of therapy Ms. G would need to choose between maladaptive behaviors and more growth-producing ones.

The relationship had now moved into the working phase where focus was placed on specifics, and problem-solving activities were begun. After 5 months the nursing diagnoses were reevaluated to include the following:

1. Violence, potential for self-directed, related to perceived rejection by friend
2. Self-concept, disturbance in personal identity, related to childhood rejection and unrealistic self-ideals
3. Social isolation, related to inability to trust, lack of socialization skills, and feelings of inadequacy
4. Powerlessness, related to fear of rejection by others

CLINICAL EXAMPLE 5-1—cont'd

5. Self-concept, disturbance in role performance, related to job dissatisfaction with working hours and nature of the work
6. Coping, ineffective individual, related to work and social stressors and lack of coping resources

At this time the nurse sought consultation as she further evolved her plan of care. Neither medication nor hospitalization were indicated. These formulations were shared with Ms. G, and together they collaborated about her future progress. They agreed to focus on changing Ms. G's maladaptive behavior by exploring past events and conflicts, and helping her learn more productive patterns of living. Ms. G was now ready to commit herself to the work of therapy and interpersonal change, and she began to assume increased responsibility for this therapeutic work.

Because her self-ideal was unrealistically high, specific short-term goals became essential. The nurse's theoretical orientation incorporated the dynamics of Sullivan's and Peplau's interpersonal theories, Beck's cognitive framework, and Glasser's reality therapy. The relationship was focused on frequently through the use of immediacy. It served as a model for examining many of her conflicts. This proved to be an excellent learning opportunity as Ms. G and the nurse dealt with resistance, transference, and countertransference reactions. During the next year Ms. G made much progress, including the following changes:

1. She moved into an apartment with another girl friend.
2. She left her previous job and resumed working in an office where she received more personal satisfaction and a work schedule that would allow her to increase her social activities.
3. She began a diet regimen.
4. She participated in additional activities, such as a dancing class and a health spa.
5. She learned to verbalize her anger more freely with the nurse, friends, and others at work. This included discussing the many relationships in her past that were terminated without her agreement and in which she had internalized the anger.
6. She contacted her stepsister-mother and visited her. This was an important therapeutic goal because it allowed her to review her early experiences and provided her with actual feedback from those involved. Consequently, many of her misperceptions became evident and open to exploration in therapy.
7. She was able to admit her ambivalent feeling about her friend-supervisor and discuss the negative aspects of the relationship. She stopped further sexual contact with her because she felt exploited in this area. Over time, the nature of this relationship changed, and it eventually became a casual acquaintance.
8. She learned about the variety of sexual feelings and responses and saw her needs in this area as appropriate developmental tasks.
9. Her perception of personal space changed, and her tolerance for physical closeness increased.
10. She developed new male and female friends and socialized frequently with them.

EVALUATION

The terminating phase of the relationship began after about 18 months. At this time Ms. G was independently solving problems and, in therapy, the nurse primarily validated and supported her thinking. She was now receiving and accepting much positive feedback from others, had lost 15 kg (40 pounds), was continuing to diet, was planning future career goals, and had achieved more satisfactory interpersonal relationships with both men and women. The mutual goals for therapy had been met.

Terminating was difficult because of the close, trusting bond that developed between them. The nurse had feelings of pleasure in Ms. G's growth, as well as personal satisfaction in her effectiveness as therapist. Ms. G openly described her feelings about terminating and raised the question of a possible social relationship between them. Over the course of 6 months she came to realize that the premise of the relationship was therapy and changing individual perceptions or patterns of relating would not be feasible or desirable. Most important, she had control for terminating this relationship and the opportunity to work it through in a positive way. The sessions were spaced to monthly intervals and considerable time was spent reviewing initial problem areas and the progress she had made in them. After 6 months, or 2 years of therapy, the nurse and patient mutually agreed to terminate regular sessions.

Documentation

The activities of each phase of the nursing process should be documented in writing. Written communication is essential to the successful planning and implementation of nursing care.

■ Assessment tools

Documentation by the nurse should begin with data collection activities. If information obtained from the nurse's data collection is not recorded, there is a tendency for other mental health clinicians to attempt to obtain the same information. This repetition for the patient is unnecessary and inappropriate. By entering all collected data on the patient record, omissions and areas of confusion can be easily identified and clarified with the patient.

An organized and systematic format should be used by the nurse in data collection activities. The tool used by the nurse for this purpose may be called a data collection tool, nursing assessment form, or nursing history. It may include elements of the psychiatric evaluation as described in Chapter 6 but goes beyond this evaluation to include subjective and objective data relative to a nursing diagnosis. A variety of such nursing assessment tools for the individual have appeared in the psychiatric nursing literature.* In addition, agencies, nursing departments, psychiatric units, educational programs, and individual nurse clinicians often use a tool that they have developed themselves. These tools may be adapted to the needs of a particular type of patient or institution.

At the present time, there is a need in psychiatric nursing for empirical testing of these tools for validity, reliability, and usefulness in nursing practice. One of the most complete data collection tools is the one developed by Francis and Munjas.[7] It consists of 315 questions divided into ten areas of assessment. The thoroughness of this tool, which is presented in its entirety in Appendix A, makes it a valuable basis for decisions regarding data collection. (See the box on page 176, which lists these and other areas to include in a complete nursing assessment.)

Three areas that are not specifically addressed by this tool, however, are the patient's social support network, medication and drug history, and physiological health status. Although a valuable and reliable assessment tool for measuring social support has not yet been developed, some elements that should be included in a clinical assessment of social support are listed in the box on nursing assessment.

---

*References 7, 9, 15, 42, 44.

Another critically important area of a psychiatric nursing assessment is the patient's medication and drug history. This assessment should be thorough and detailed, since it has major implications for efficacy of treatment and patient responsiveness to psychopharmocological agents. A detailed assessment form for medications and drugs is presented in Appendix B and it should include the aspects outlined in the box on nursing assessment.

An assessment of the patient's past and present physiological status should also be an essential part of the nurse's data collection, since maladaptive coping responses have physiological, as well as psychosocial, manifestations. Furthermore, physiological imbalances can cause or intensify symptoms indicative of emotional dysfunction. Other tools can be used to assess physiological functioning (Appendix C), and they should include the areas listed in the box on nursing assessment.

Finally although the data collection tool of Francis and Munjas does assess family information, there may be occasions when the nurse wishes to focus less on the individual and more on the quality of the family functioning, that is, the degree to which they are able to deal with problems successfully. To do this, the nurse may need to use an assessment tool for family analysis that examines the family as a unit, including its structure, relationships, and coping potential.[38, 48] Helm, at Yale University School of Nursing, developed a useful guide to family analysis (Appendix D). It assesses the aspects listed in the box on areas to include in a complete nursing assessment.

If the nurse were to undertake a complete biopsychosocial assessment of the patient based on these tools, it would require a number of hours to complete. At times, this might be necessary and appropriate. At other times, however, based on the patient's situation and the use of a team approach to care, the nurse may need to collect data relevant to only a few of these areas. A skilled practitioner, although possessing thorough knowledge of all areas of assessment, would then use judgment in determining the exact nature and extent of the data needed.

■ Nursing care plans

The next type of documentation used by nurses is the nursing care plan, which should reflect all of the remaining stages of the nursing process—nursing diagnosis, planning, implementation, and evaluation. Although the precise format of the care plan may differ somewhat among agencies, because it is based on the nursing process, the differences tend to be minor ones. A complete nursing care plan would include pertinent

Areas to Include in a Complete Nursing Assessment

Psychosocial

Demographic and vital data
  Name
  Address
  Birth
  Marital status
  Sex
  Race
Presenting data
  Nature of the problem
  Time of occurrence
  Reason for seeking care at this time
Family information
  Family system
  Communication patterns
  Interaction patterns
  Crisis response
Socioeconomic status
  Occupation
  Education
  Leisure time
  Residence
  Income
Life values
  Ethnicity
  Religious behavior
  Beliefs about illness
  Attitudes toward life
  Living standards
Social habits
  Eating
  Drinking
  Drug use
  Hygiene
Sexual behavior
  Preference
  Sex role
  Sex activity
Cognition
  Consciousness
  Orientation
  Attention
  Perception
  Apperception
  Thought content
  Thought form
  Thought progress
  Memory
  Self-concept
  Body image
Affect
  Depersonalization
  Continuum of despair to ecstasy
  Affective ambivalence
  Inadequate affect
  Inappropriate affect
  Anxiety
Conation (observed)
  Appearance
  Motor activity
  Communication

Social support

Size of social network
Intensity, durability, multidimensionality, dispersion, and frequency of social linkages
Normative context of the relationships
Social roles
Support available to meet role obligations during illness
Patterns of social affiliation
Need for social affiliation

Medications and Drugs

Psychiatric medications
Prescription (nonpsychiatric) medications
Over-the-counter (nonprescribed) medications
Alcohol and street drugs

Physiologic

Medical history
  Development
  Past illnesses and injuries
  Hospitalizations
  Family history
Physiological status
  Body systems
  Present illnesses
  Medications and ongoing treatments
Health maintenance
  Health goals

Family

Family's generational structure
Home environment
Physical and mental health
Financial status
Developmental stage in family life cycle
Family structure
Intrafamily relationships
Sociocultural family context
Strengths and weaknesses
Identified problem

Sample Nursing Care Format

Patient information
  Name _____
  Age _____
  Sex _____
  Marital status _____
  Race or ethnic group _____
  Religion _____
  Occupation _____
  Current living environment _____
  Immediate support system _____

Date of admission _____
Medical diagnosis _____
_____
_____

Medical treatment _____
_____
_____
_____
_____

Biopsychosocial behaviors		Nursing diagnosis	Priority	Goals		Nursing actions	Rationale	Evaluation
Objective data	Subjective data			Long-term	Short-term			
								Modification:

demographic data on the patient, objective and subjective behaviors of the patient, nursing diagnoses, priority of the diagnoses, nurse-patient goals, nursing actions, rationale, and evaluation with modifications of the plan. An example of a detailed and comprehensive nursing care plan format is given above.

There are a number of advantages to formulating a written record of the nursing care plan as it evolves. The nurse who initiates and writes the plan must think through the whole nursing process in a logical and structured manner. The likelihood of basing nursing care on sound rationale is greater, since nursing care plans are generally scrutinized by others, and the reasons for specific components of the plan may be questioned. Self-evaluation by the nurse is also facilitated. An up-to-date working care plan requires that application of the nursing process be consistently reviewed and revised.

Many agencies are aware that well-written nursing care plans reflect the course of the patient's contact with nursing personnel. It is frequently a practice to include the nursing care plan in the patient's permanent agency record. This can greatly enhance the quality of nursing care if the patient contacts the agency again in the future. Much data from the original assessment need not be collected again, thereby freeing the energy of both the patient and nurse to work on current concerns.

Detailed nursing care plans are useful learning tools.

However, the daily use of a care plan by the nursing staff and other personnel working with the patient may require an abbreviated form of the care plan. Recording care plan information in a concise manner can save both time and energy, but the dangers of vague generalities and routine analysis are great. The use of shortened care plans, such as Kardex forms, is prevalent in many institutions. A sample format for a psychiatric nursing Kardex form developed by Holden and Bedgio[14] is presented in Fig. 5-5. Nurses using such formats must ensure that patients are given clearly defined and individualized nursing care.

The documentation required in effective use of the nursing process sometimes poses problems for nurses. Transposing ideas into prose is often difficult, and usually the source of the difficulty is the fact that it is hard to crystallize one's thinking and be specific. Krall* suggests the following five guideline questions she found helpful in formulating written mental health treatment plans:

1. What is the exact behavior keeping the patient in the hospital?
2. Is the treatment plan written in behavioral terminology?

---

*From Krall, M.L.: Am. J. Nurs. **76:**236, 1976. Copyright by the American Journal of Nursing Co.

TREATMENT PLAN

Treatment goals
[ ] Decrease intensity of symptoms   [ ] Effective functioning
[ ] Reduction of conflicts   [ ] Improve personal relationships
[ ] Modify behavior   [ ] Improve grasp on reality

Precautions
[ ] Agitation   [ ] Emotional withdrawal   [ ] Drug use and withdrawal
[ ] Suicide   [ ] Agression   [ ] Acting out
[ ] Self-mutilation   [ ] Assault   [ ] Confusion
[ ] Elopement   [ ] Manipulation   [ ] Falling

Self-attitudes
Encourage socialization Yes [ ] No [ ]   Encourage dependence Yes [ ] No [ ]
Encourage verbalization Yes [ ] No [ ]   Allow withdrawal Yes [ ] No [ ]
Encourage responsibility Yes [ ] No [ ]   Matter of fact attitude Yes [ ] No [ ]

Socialization and visiting
[ ] Staff   [ ] Immediate family   [ ] Phone
[ ] Staff and patients   [ ] Family   [ ] Limited
    [ ] No restrictions   [ ] Unlimited

Recreation
[ ] Unit only   [ ] Off unit   [ ] Physical activities   [ ] Withhold activities
[ ] Recreational therapy   [ ] Accompanied   [ ] Moderate
    [ ] Unaccompanied   [ ] None

PSYCHIATRIC NURSING CARE PLAN

Background information: _____

Date	Problems and needs	Approach and evaluation

Room number	Patient's name	Age	Doctor	Admit date	Discharge date

Fig. 5-5. Psychiatric nursing Kardex form.

Date	Medications	Date	P.R.N. medications	Diagnostic & psychiatric tests	Req.	Done
		Date	Treatments	Special orders and concerns		

Allergies: Diagnosis: Diet:

Fig. 5-5—cont'd. Psychiatric nursing Kardex form. (From Holden, M., and Bedgio, R.: J. Psychiatr. Nurs. **19**(5):29, 1981.)

3. Is the stated behavior written in such a way that the patient can understand it?
4. Are the stated behaviors written in such a way that all nursing personnel can readily understand them?
5. How is the written treatment plan to be used?[21:236]

■ Charting

Santora and Willer[36] report on a study they conducted that examined the frequency, length, and content of staff's discussions and written reports about ninety hospitalized psychiatric patients. They found that nursing staff, as compared with psychiatrists, were more likely to record patient progress, but they were usually limited to behavioral descriptions; psychiatrists were more likely to focus on treatment goals or plans; and the overall quality of the records and reporting habits of the staff were low.

Partly as a response to such problems and the desire to avoid the duplication and dissatisfaction with traditional record keeping, Weed[47] developed the **problem-oriented medical record.** Traditional medical records have often been repetitive, confusing, and disorganized. Separation of nursing notes from the rest of the chart tended to block communication among various health team members. Nurses were often less motivated to write good notes, especially in settings where it was the

practice to destroy nursing notes a given period of time after the patient's discharge. Frequently, incidents that nurses thought were significant enough to record in detail were also recorded by other health team members. In the problem-oriented medical record, this duplication is avoided, because all notes are written chronologically. Therefore each person can concentrate on adding new observations to the chart. It is also convenient to read notes that are arranged sequentially, thus facilitating improved communication.

The problem-oriented medical record is used by many mental health facilities. It consists of three basic elements: (1) the data base, (2) the problem list and treatment plan, and (3) progress notes.[47] The data base is the sum total of information from which the patient's problems can be identified. Many mental health professionals, including nurses, psychiatrists, psychologists, and social workers, may contribute to its collection. The problem list and treatment plan are drawn up as soon after the patient is admitted as possible. Every significant problem of the patient and related treatment plan should be included. Problems may be active or inactive. They should be dated and appropriately labeled, and notation should be made when the problem is resolved.

Progress notes are usually written in SOAP format, and they are preceded by a date, problem number, and

TABLE 5-5

SAMPLE PROBLEM-ORIENTED MEDICAL RECORD

Problem list and treatment plan			
Date	Problem list	Treatment plan	Resolved
3-24-86	1. Agitated depression—loss of appetite, loss of interest in housework, difficulty sleeping	1. Amitriptyline (Elavil), 50 mg t.i.d. 2. Group therapy, Tuesdays 3. Explore patient's self-concept and perception of role performance 4. Encourage expression of emotion, particularly feelings of guilt, sadness, and hostility	
3-24-86	2. Marital conflict—states she and her husband are not compatible sexually and feels that he is not interested in her	1. Conjoint marital therapy, Fridays 2. Explore nature of sexual incompatibility 3. Confront patient with her inability to communicate her feelings and thoughts to her husband	

Treatment team progress notes		
Date and time	Problem list	Progress notes
3-29-86 4 PM	2. Marital difficulty	S Patient attended group therapy session today. Talked about difficulties with her husband, feels he doesn't love her. O Appears nervous in group, feigns eye contact, but does participate somewhat. A Still not comfortable with group members. Blames herself for problems at home, feels guilty. P Support her in group, encourage her to express her emotions freely. *F. Hawkins, R.N.*
4-20-86 2 PM	1. Depression	S Patient stated she was feeling better and liked participating in ward activities. O Appears more enthusiastic and motivated. Increase in appetite and better sleeping habits. A Adjusting to ward well. Appears antidepressants have taken effect. P Continue medication and encourage patient to become even more involved on the unit. *L. Wilson, M.D.*

problem name. The components of a SOAP note include the following:

S **Subjective data,** which include verbal comments, complaints, or information obtained from the patient or information obtained from a source other than the patient, such as the family

O **Objective data,** which may be a factual observation of a patient's behavior, such as his appearance or nonverbal behavior; a phys-

iological measurement, such as height, weight, or blood pressure; or a result of a test, such as an x-ray examination or laboratory data

A **Assessment,** which is the interpretation of the subjective and objective data

P **Plan,** which is the specific plan of action for the problem, including diagnostic studies, treatment approaches, and patient education plans.

The following is a sample SOAP note:

S "I'm scared to go for a job interview . . . scared of all the strange people looking at me."

O Patient's hand rubbed forehead, biting on fingernails, frequent changes in sitting positions, no eye contact. Patient smoked rapidly and continuously while discussing his employment status.

A Patient experiencing moderate anxiety over the thought of going for a job interview. Strangers continue to make him feel self-conscious and inferior.

P Encourage patient to verbalize his fears and anxiety. He must be approached by staff in a firm but caring manner, since he will not initiate social contacts. He requires persistent encouragement to verbalize feelings.

A sample of the two basic elements of the problem-oriented medical record, the problem list and treatment plan, and related progress notes are shown in Table 5-5.

Various methods of documentation have been presented. A more recent approach is the use of a computerized psychiatric treatment planning system used for writing, retrieving, and analyzing psychiatric treatment plans.[10] Such a system can provide rapid entry and retrieval of required treatment plans and produce a document that is clinically expressive and readable. It stores clinical data that may be used, additionally, for research, quality assurance, and management purposes.

The specific format used by the nurse may vary but the important issue is that information about the plan of care be disseminated, so that there can be consistency and continuity in the staff's approach to the psychiatric patient. Written records are subject to review by professional colleagues. Another dimension to the purpose and nature of documentation emerges when one realizes that in some states the identified patient also has access to documentation concerning his case. In one study,[39] patients on a psychiatric unit of a general hospital were given their complete medical records to read daily, and the practice was evaluated to determine its effect on patients and staff. Both medical and nursing staff along with patients found this practice to be an effective way to educate patients, help patients become more actively involved in their treatment, correct inaccuracies in the medical record, and promote thoughtful charting by the professional staff. Committing oneself in writing is a necessary part of implementing the nursing process. The implications of it should be seriously considered by all psychiatric nurses.

DIRECTIONS FOR FUTURE RESEARCH

The following are some of the nursing research problems raised in Chapter 5 that merit further study by psychiatric nurses:

1. The identification, classification, and validation of phenomena of concern to psychiatric nurses
2. The further refinement and empirical testing of nursing theories
3. The relationship of nursing theories to other theories from the behavioral sciences
4. The degree of mutuality present in the nurse-patient relationship at the various phases of the nursing process, particularly in a psychiatric care context
5. The extent to which the data collection process criteria are incorporated in psychiatric nursing assessments
6. The impact of cultural biases on the psychiatric care given to patients of different ethnic groups and social classes
7. Nursing diagnoses used by psychiatric nurses, including the extent and consistency of use, the format in which they are written, their validity and reliability, and their usefulness in suggesting nursing actions that will promote adaptive coping responses
8. The correlation and individuation of nursing and medical diagnoses
9. The degree to which nursing care plans are formulated, utilized, and evaluated by psychiatric nurses
10. The content, process, and structure of health teaching conducted by psychiatric nurses and related outcomes
11. The type of quality assessment measures utilized by psychiatric nurses
12. Outcomes of psychiatric nursing care including levels of patient satisfaction
13. The relative cost-effectiveness of psychiatric nurses compared with other mental health care providers
14. The quality assurance activities engaged in by psychiatric nurses and resulting patient outcomes, nursing activities, and costs
15. Models of interdisciplinary collaboration in psychiatric practice, research, and education
16. The validity, reliability, and usefulness of data collection tools in nursing practice
17. The nature and quality of documentation by psychiatric nurses

■ SUGGESTED CROSS-REFERENCES ■

This chapter serves as a foundation for formulating principles of psychiatric nursing and implementing psychiatric nursing practice. As such, it is related to all other chapters of this text.

■ SUMMARY ■

1. Through the establishment of a therapeutic nurse-patient relationship and the use of the nursing process, the nurse strives to promote and maintain the integrated functioning of the patient. This is the essence of the nursing therapeutic process and the framework for this psychiatric nursing text. The American Nurses' Association defines nursing as "the diagnosis and treatment of human responses to actual or potential health problems." It has four characteristics: phenomena, theory, actions, and effects.

2. The need for a theoretical basis and conceptual framework for psychiatric nursing practice was presented, along with its implication for the development and refinement of nursing theory.

3. The nursing process was defined as an interactive problem-solving process used by the nurse as a systematic and individualized way to fulfill the goal of nursing care. It is essential that the nurse and patient become partners in this process. The five phases of the nursing process—data collection, nursing diagnosis, planning, implementation, and evaluation—were described, with the American Nurses' Association's *Standards of Nursing Practice* used as the organizing framework.

   a. Data collection. Observing and interviewing are the basic methods of data collection. It may be facilitated by the use of a systematic assessment tool. Data should reflect both content and process, and information relative to the patient's biopsychosocial world. The patient is the ideal source of validation. The importance of cultural, religious, and socioeconomic data was emphasized, and the idea of intercultural psychiatry was introduced. The data base should also include the patient's view of the functional state of his family, as well as family strengths and resources.

   b. A nursing diagnosis is the independent judgment of a nurse through which the nursing problems of the patient are identified. These may be overt, covert, existing, or potential. The subject of nursing diagnoses is the patient's behavioral response to stress. The statement of a nursing diagnosis should include both the adaptive or maladaptive health response and contributing stressors.

   c. Planning involves setting goals that are mutual, congruent, realistic, and appropriately timed. Difficulties in defining and writing goals were described. The plan of nursing care also includes priorities and prescribed nursing approaches to achieve the goals derived from the nursing diagnoses.

   d. Implementation refers to the actual delivery of nursing care to the patient. With psychiatric patients, nursing interventions should be directed to helping them develop insight and resolve problems through carrying out a plan of positive action.

   e. Evaluation requires the review of all previous phases and the determination of the degree of goal achievement by the patient. It is a mutual continuous process that incorporates reassessment and modification of the care plan. Organizational evaluation of overall patterns of care through quality assessment measures was also discussed.

4. The need for nurse accountability was described in relation to peer review, continuing education, interdisciplinary collaboration, and utilization of community health systems.

5. The progressive process of observing from practice, theorizing, testing in research, and subsequently modifying practice must become an essential part of psychiatric nursing if it is to survive as a practice discipline. Research is also needed on the outcomes of nursing therapy to determine its effectiveness and to compare psychiatric nurses with other mental health care providers on relative cost-effectiveness of services.

6. A case analysis of a long-term relationship with a patient was used to illustrate the use of the nursing process, phases of the relationship, and various therapeutic dimensions.

7. Activities of each phase of the nursing process should be documented in writing. Examples of various tools that can be utilized by the nurse were presented. The problem-oriented medical record was described.

■ REFERENCES ■

1. American Nurses' Association: Nursing: a social policy statement, Kansas City, Mo., 1980, The Association.

2. American Psychological Association: Draft of DSM-III-R in Development (subject to change), as proposed by the Work Group to revise DSM-III. American Psychological Association, October 1985.

3. Coler, M.: I am nursing diagnosis: color me DSM-III green. In Kim, M., McFarland, G., and McLane, A., editors: Classification of nursing diagnoses, St. Louis, Mo., 1984, The C.V. Mosby Co.

4. Eichelman, B., Wikler, D., and Hartwig, A.: Ethics and psychiatric research: problems and justification, Am. J. Psych. **141**(3):400, 1984.

5. Fitzpatrick, J., Whall, A., Johnson, R., and Floyd, J.: Nursing models and their psychiatric mental health applications, Bowie, Md., 1982, Robert J. Brady Co.

6. Flaskerud, J., and Halloran, E.: Areas of agreement in nursing theory development, Adv. Nurs. Sci. **4**:1, 1980.

7. Francis, G., and Munjas, B.: Manual of social psychologic assessment, New York, 1976, Appleton-Century-Crofts.

8. Geach, B.: The problem-solving technique: as taught to psychiatric students, Perspect. Psychiatr. Care **12**:9, Jan.-March 1974.

9. Green, N.C.: A psychiatric assessment tool for staff and students, J. Psychiatr. Nurs. **17**(4):28, 1979.

10. Hammond, K., and Munnecke, T.: A computerized psychiatric treatment planning system, Hosp. and Community Psych. **35**(2):160, 1984.

11. Hankins-McNary, L.: The effect of institutional racism on the therapeutic relationship, Perspect. Psychiatr. Care **17**(1):25, 1979.

12. Hardin, S., and Durham, J.: First rate: exploring the structure, process, and effectiveness of nurse psychotherapy, J. Psychosoc. Nurs. Ment. Health Serv. **23**(5):8, 1985.

13. Hatfield, A.: Change in working with families: the need for a new theory, Paper presented to symposia: Our chronic patient's future in a changing world. 138th Annual Meeting of the American Psychiatric Association, May 1985.

14. Holden, M., and Bedgio, R.: Kardex forms for psychiatric nursing, J. Psychiatr. Nurs. **19**(5):29, 1981.

15. Joel, L., and Davis, S.: A proposal for baseline data collection for psychiatric care, Perspect. Psychiatr. Care **11**:48, April-June 1973.

16. Johnson, D.: The behavioral system model for nursing. In Riehl, J., and Roy, S.C., editors: Conceptual models for nursing practice, ed. 2, New York, 1980, Appleton-Century-Crofts.

17. Jourard, S.: Toward a psychology of transcendent behavior in explorations. In Otto, H., editor: Human potentialities, Springfield, Ill., 1966, Charles C Thomas, Publisher.

18. Kim, M., McFarland, G., and McLane, A., editors: Classification of nursing diagnoses, St. Louis, Mo., 1984, The C.V. Mosby Co.

19. King, I.: A theory for nursing: systems, concepts, process, New York, 1981, John Wiley and Sons.

20. Kini, J.: The effects of patient social class on the judgments of public health nurses, Nurs. Res. **17**(3):261, 1968.

21. Krall, M.L.: Guidelines for writing mental health treatment plans, Am. J. Nurs. **76**:236, 1976.

22. Krumboltz, J., and Thorensen, C.: Behavioral counseling, cases and techniques, New York, 1969, Holt, Rinehart & Winston.

23. Laffal, J., Brown, M., Pearlman, L., and Burns, G.: Therapeutic education of psychiatric inpatients in a classroom setting, QRB **9**:190, 1983.

24. Mager, R.: Preparing instructional objectives, Palo Alto, Calif., 1962, Fearon Publishers.

25. Mangen, S., Paykel, E., Griffith, J., Burchell, A., and Mancini, P.: Cost-effectiveness of community psychiatric nurse or out-patient psychiatrist care of neurotic patients, Psychol. Med. **13**:407, 1983.

26. Mann, L., and Whall, A.: Informed consent and the deinstitutionalized patient, J. Psychosoc. Nurs. Ment. Health Serv. **22**(1):22, 1984.

27. McClosky, J.: Nurses' orders: the next professional breakthrough, RN **431**(2):99, 1980.

28. Meleis, A.: Theoretical nursing: development and progress, Philadelphia, 1985, J.B. Lippincott.

29. Mercer, R.: Nursing research: the bridge to excellence in practice, Image **16**(2):47, 1984.

30. Neuman, B.: The Neuman systems model: application to nursing education and practice. Norwalk, Conn., 1982, Appleton-Century-Crofts.

31. Orem, D.: Nursing: concepts of practice, ed. 2, New York, 1980, McGraw-Hill Book Co.

32. Orlikoff, J., and Lanham, G.: Why risk management and quality assurance should be integrated, Hospitals **55**(15):55, 1981.

33. O'Toole, A.: When the practical becomes theoretical, J. Psychosoc. Nurs. Ment. Health Serv. **19**(2):11, 1981.

34. Rogers, M.: An introduction to the theoretical basis of nursing, Philadelphia, 1970, F.A. Davis.

35. Roy, S.C., and Roberts, S.: Theory construction in nursing: an adaptation model, Englewood Cliffs, N.J., 1976, Prentice-Hall.

36. Santora, E., and Willer, B.: The reporting habits of staff in a psychiatric hospital, Hosp. Community Psychiatry **26**:362, June 1975.

37. Schlesinger, R.: Cross-cultural psychiatry: the applicability of Western Anglo psychiatry to Asian-Americans of Chinese and Japanese ethnicity, J. Psychosoc. Nurs. Ment. Health Serv. **19**(9):26, 1981.

38. Sedgwick, R.: Family mental health: theory and practice, St. Louis, 1981, The C.V. Mosby Co.

39. Simonton, M., et al.: The open medical record: an educational tool, J. Psychiatr. Nurs. **15**:25, 1977.

40. Singh, A., May, P., and Messick, J.: The role of operations research and systems analysis in holding down the cost of hospitals and clinics, J. Psychiatr. Nurs. **16**(9):24, 1978.

41. Smilkstein, G.: The family APGAR: a proposal for a family function test and its use by physicians, J. Fam. Pract. **6**:1231, 1978.

42. Smith, L.: A nursing history and data sheet, Nurs. Times **77**:749, 1980.

43. Smoyak, S.: Clinical practice: intuitive or based on research? J. Psychosoc. Nurs. Ment. Health Serv. **20**(4):9, 1982.

44. Snyder, J., and Wilson, M.: Elements of a psychological assessment, Am. J. Nurs. **77**:235, 1977.

45. Stanley, B.: Evaluation of treatment goals: the use of goal attainment scaling, J. Adv. Nurs. **9**:351, 1984.

46. Stevens, B.: Nursing theory, Boston, 1979, Little, Brown & Co.

47. Weed, L.: Medical records, medical education and patient care, Cleveland, 1969, The Press of Case Western Reserve University.

48. Whall, A.: Nursing theory and the assessment of families, J. Psychiatr. Nurs. **19**(1):30, 1981.

49. Yamamoto, J., James, Q., and Palley, N.: Cultural problems in psychiatric therapy, Arch. Gen. Psychiatry **19**:45, July 1968.

50. Youssef, F.: Adherence to therapy in psychiatric patients: an empirical investigation, Int. J. Nurs. Stud. **21**(1):51, 1984.

51. Zimmer, M.: Quality assurance in the provision of hospital care. A model for evaluating nursing care, Hospitals **48**:91, 1974.

■ ANNOTATED SUGGESTED READINGS* ■

*American Nurses' Association: Affirmative action: toward quality nursing care for a multiracial society, Kansas City, Mo., 1976, The Association.

Unique needs of ethnic minority patients and suggestions for removing barriers to quality care in a multiracial society are explained in this collection of papers.

*American Nurses' Association: Issues in evaluation research, Kansas City, Mo., 1976, The Association.

This is a collection of papers by nursing leaders and researchers that presents a comprehensive view on the subject of evaluation research as it relates to quality assurance.

*Apostoles, F., Little, M., and Murphy, H.: Developing a psychiatric nursing audit, J. Psychiatr. Nurs. 15:9, May 1977.

This article describes the experience of developing the first nursing audit, primarily a process one, in one clinical division of a large psychiatric hospital. Eight specific steps are described in a way that makes it useful reading for nurses involved in a similar process.

*Babich, K., editor: A sourcebook: research in psychiatric mental health nursing. Boulder, Colo., 1983, Western Interstate Commission for Higher Education.

This monograph is a compilation of research studies that identifies and classifies psychiatric mental health nursing research. It both reflects the state of the field and serves as a useful reference source.

*Bevilacqua, J.: Voodoo—myth or mental illness? J. Psychiatr. Nurs. 18(2):17, 1980.

This is a fascinating clinical study of a 14-year-old Haitian girl's experience with what has been diagnosed as mental illness. The author raises many questions on etiology, interventions, and influence of voodoo and causes the reader to consider how the system that we work in perpetuates mental illness rather than relieves it.

*Boettcher, E.: Nurse-client collaboration: dynamic equilibrium in the nursing care system, J. Psychiatr. Nurs. 16:7, Dec. 1978.

This article explores the process of nurse-client collaboration, which parallels the nursing process. It is highly recommended for the clinical example it includes that describes a nursing care plan, including behaviors, nursing diagnosis, mutual goals, specific interventions, rationale, and evaluation.

*Carson, V., and Huss, K.: Prayer: an effective therapeutic and teaching tool, J. Psychiatr. Nurs. 17(3):34, 1979.

The authors contend that the spiritual components of nursing care are often neglected. The article provides a brief review of the literature on the importance of spirituality in psychiatry. It describes a project conducted at a state mental institution in which actions to meet spiritual needs of patients were implemented and evaluated.

*Erickson, H., Tomlin, E., and Swain, M.: Modeling and role-modeling, Englewood Cliffs, N.J., 1983, Prentice-Hall.

This easy-to-read text presents a practical approach to the study of a theory-based model for nursing. Its basis is that the nurse should understand the client's model of his world and then role model that world so that the client can grow healthier. Clinical examples are provided.

*Evans, C., and Lewis, S.: Nursing administration of psychiatric-mental health nursing. Rockville, Md., 1985, Aspen.

This is the only existing text that addresses psychiatric nursing administration. Relevant chapters discuss evaluation, continuing education, documentation, and research implementation.

*Fitzpatrick, J., Whall, A., Johnson, R., and Floyd, J.: Nursing models and their psychiatric mental health applications, Bowie, Md., 1982, Robert J. Brady Co.

This important text examines borrowed theories that psychiatric nurses frequently use and explores their congruence with nursing models. Highly recommended reading.

*Foreman, M.: Building a better nursing care plan, Am. J. Nurs. 79(6):1086, 1979.

This article presents a general semantics approach to formulation of a nursing care plan. The author believes that by asking oneself a series of questions, a more specific and more useful plan of care can be developed. This well-written article presents a concise and unique approach to care plan writing.

*Francis, G., and Munjas, B.: Manual of social psychologic assessment, New York, 1976, Appleton-Century-Crofts.

This text presents a systematic method for nurses to assess the sociological and psychological aspects of clients. A comprehensive analysis of variables is presented along with suggested questions. It is a valuable resource for nurse practitioners.

*Hankins-McNary, L.: The effect of institutional racism on the therapeutic relationship, Perspect. Psychiatr. Care 17(1):25, 1979.

The author explores the idea of racism and the many ways it influences the patient-therapist relationship. This is a topic that is not frequently discussed in the literature, and this article is thoughtful reading for all nurses.

*Hauser, M., and Feinberg, D.: Problem solving revisited, J. Psychiatr. Nurs. 15:13, Oct. 1977.

The authors present a framework consisting of a combination of the problem-solving process and the creative thinking process. The processes directed in a complementary manner are suggested as a means of solving problems creatively in situations that call for unique and novel solutions.

*Joel, L., and Davis, S.: A proposal for baseline data collection for psychiatric care, Perspect. Psychiatr. Care 11:48, April-June 1973.

The authors describe a data collection tool they developed for the psychiatric unit of a Veterans Administration general hospital. The article thoroughly discusses the pertinent data, sample questions, and data utilization in determining goals, problems, and approaches.

*Lucas, M., and Folstein, M.: Nursing assessment of mental disorders on a general medical unit, J. Psychiatr. Nurs. 18(5):31, 1980.

The authors of this study found that current nursing assessments on general medical units failed to identify cognitive dis-

---

orders and symptoms of emotional distress. To correct this omission, the authors suggest the use of two brief tools to quantitatively measure psychiatric disorders.

Mager, R.F.: Preparing instructional objectives, Palo Alto, Calif., 1962, Fearon Publishers.

This is a classic text on the art of writing behavioral objectives. It is written in a programmed learning format and is easy to read, but at the same time, it is very informative. This is highly recommended for inexperienced objective writers.

Mangen, S., Paykel, E., Griffith, J., Burchell, A., and Mancini, P.: Cost-effectiveness of community psychiatric nurse or out-patient psychiatrist care of neurotic patients, Psychol. Med. **13**:407, 1983.

A prospective, controlled investigation comparing psychiatric nurse and psychiatrist care is described in this article. This type of research is greatly needed in the psychiatric nursing field.

*Meleis, A.: Theoretical nursing: development and progress, Philadelphia, 1985, J.B. Lippincott.

This text delineates components of theory, identifies strategies used to develop theories, discusses existing nursing theories, and provides insights into nursing's theoretical past and future challenges.

*Mercer, R.: Nursing research: the bridge to excellence in practice, Image **16**(2):47, 1984.

The links between research and practice are explored in this article including problems and ways in which they may be overcome.

*Miller, T., and Lee, L.: Quality assurance: focus on environmental perceptions of psychiatric patients and nursing staff, J. Psychiatr. Nurs. **18**(2):9, 1980.

A unique application of quality assurance is described in this study, which assessed the ward atmosphere of an inpatient psychiatric service and utilized this information for the benefit of staff education and enrichment.

Olson, D., and McCubbin, H.: Families: what makes them work, Beverly Hills, Calif., 1983, Sage Publications.

"Normal" family life is described in this book that is based on a study of over 1000 families. Types of families, stresses they encounter, and coping resources are all explored.

*O'Toole, A.: When the practical becomes theoretical, J. Psychosoc. Nurs. Ment. Health Serv. **19**(12):11, 1981.

The relationship among practice, theory, and research is explored in this article, and studies in psychiatric nursing are reviewed with an assessment of the progress of the field in developing practice theory. Implications and suggestions for future direction highlight important areas that psychiatric nursing needs to address to survive.

*Rowan, F.: The chronically distressed client, St. Louis, 1980, The C.V. Mosby Co.

Eight in-depth psychiatric case studies are used by the author to illustrate the application of the nursing process methodology. It is highly recommended for its consistent and thorough analysis in a case-specific presentation.

*Schlesinger, R.R.: Cross-cultural psychiatry: the applicability of Western Anglo psychiatry to Asian-Americans of Chinese and Japanese ethnicity, J. Psychosoc. Nurs. Ment. Health Serv. **19**(9):26, 1981.

This excellent study focuses on Asian-Americans of the East Asian group and investigates the applicability of Western psychiatry to this particular cultural group. Stimulating and enlightening reading.

*Schmidt, C.: Withdrawal behavior of schizophrenics: application of Roy's model, J. Psychosoc. Nurs. Ment. Health Serv. **19**(11):26, 1981.

This article describes a study that tested the applicability of Roy's adaptation model to one problem identified by the nurse— withdrawn behavior of schizophrenic patients. It is an excellent example of the interrelatedness of theory, research, and clinical practice.

*Singh, A., May, P., and Messick, J.: The role of operations research and systems analysis in holding down the costs of hospitals and clinics, J. Psychiatr. Nurs. **16**(9):24, 1978.

In this article the applications of operations research and systems analysis techniques are explored to find ways to improve clinical operations and contain costs within medical care facilities.

*Stanley, B.: Evaluation of treatment goals: the use of goal attainment scaling, J. Adv. Nurs. **9**:351, 1984.

Goal attainment scaling is described in detail in this article. The authors argue that the key to successful evaluation lies in evaluation planning which strengthens the scientific basis of nursing practice by empirical methods.

*Whitley, M.: Administrative use of systems analysis to troubleshoot a problematic work situation, J. Psychosoc. Nurs. Ment. Health Serv. **21**(2):25, 1983.

This is a case study that offers some administrative tools for assessing and communicating to investors of a residential psychiatric care facility the adjustments necessary in order to promote a profit while meeting the needs of the residents.

*Zimmer, M.J., editor: Symposium on quality assurance, Nurs. Clin. North Am. **9**(2):305, 1974.

Quality assurance is the topic addressed in this group of articles. It is highly recommended reading for those nurses interested in further information on the subject.

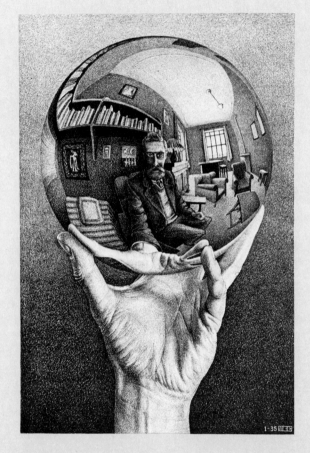

Information is of no value for its own sake, but only because of its personal significance.

Eric Berne

C H A P T E R   6

PSYCHIATRIC EVALUATION

E. SUSAN BATZER

LEARNING OBJECTIVES

After studying this chapter, the student should be able to:

- state the role of the nurse in the psychiatric evaluation of patients and the knowledge and skills needed by nurses to function in this area.

- identify the two basic elements of a psychiatric interview and appropriate interviewing skills.

- describe the stages of the psychiatric evaluation as they relate to the collection of data on the presenting problem, patient's history, mental status examination, formulation of a diagnostic impression, and case disposition.

- identify the major categories of data that should be collected by the nurse with regard to the patient's presenting problem, history, and mental status.

- analyze the specific aspects of the patient's behavior that should be assessed in each of the six major categories of the mental status examination.

- discuss additional resources the nurse can use to complete an assessment of the patient, including various psychological and physiological measurements.

- identify the potential usefulness of brain visual imaging for future psychiatric practice.

- relate the formulation of a medical diagnosis with that of a nursing diagnosis.

- describe the factors that need to be considered in making a decision about a case disposition.

- discuss future trends in the psychiatric evaluation of patients.

- identify directions for future nursing research.

- select appropriate readings for further study.

CLINICAL EXAMPLE 6-1

Late one night two police officers escort a young woman into the emergency room. The nurse observes her to be an attractive brunette, but her manner of dress is rather bizarre. She is wearing a bright purple satin shirt, cut-off jeans, white boots studded with rhinestones, and sunglasses. She is demanding to be released, stating that she has important business that must be taken care of immediately. The young woman approaches the nurse and states in a loud tone of voice that she is being held against her consent and that the authorities will be contacted about the matter. The police inform the nurse that the woman was picked up at the courthouse that evening after they received a phone call from the security guard. She had been walking around the state office building placing flyers on all the doors. She approached the security guard, demanding entrance to the courthouse for a scheduled private meeting with the chief judge.

This vignette, somewhat typical of a person with a manic episode, might also represent other conditions, such as substance-induced organic disorder or schizophrenic disorder. What information does the nurse need to assess this woman's current mental functioning and to determine whom to ask for further assistance?

CLINICAL EXAMPLE 6-2

A 57-year-old unemployed mailman who recently stopped drinking and is an avid member of Alcoholics Anonymous is admitted to the medical unit of a general hospital for a gastrointestinal workup because of bowel complaints, which he attributes to recent minor surgery he had for a rectal abscess. The results of the x-ray examinations and laboratory tests are all within normal limits. This man is to be discharged to his home, where he lives with his 90-year-old mother, who suffered a mild stroke 6 months ago. The nurse enters his room the evening before discharge and finds that he has stabbed himself in the abdomen with a pocket knife.

Was this man's depression so well masked that no clinical symptoms were evident during his hospital stay? Were there any clues recorded in the initial interview and assessment? Was a psychiatric evaluation done along with evaluation of the gastrointestinal, genitourinary, cardiopulmonary, and other systems medically scrutinized by all on admission?

These clinical examples demonstrate the importance of a psychiatric evaluation. They have several things in common: a psychiatric problem, nurse-patient interaction, and a lack of sufficient data to effectively assess and plan a treatment program. As vital members of the health care team, nurses must assume a role in the psychiatric evaluation of patients.

Role of the nurse

At one time the task of psychiatric evaluation was ascribed to the physician, usually a psychiatrist. However, Imboden[10] points out the need for a psychiatric evaluation as part of the routine physical examination of patients. If the patient's problem is psychologically based, a psychiatric evaluation might save the patient the time and expense of costly tests and procedures. The holistic approach to the study of humans implies assessment of psychological needs and potential. Nurses who are trained in caring for the patient as a total being will include the psychiatric evaluation as part of the assessment skills they acquired in nursing school.

A psychiatric evaluation is not something totally new to be learned. It is primarily a reorganization of knowledge and skills acquired by nurses. Basic knowledge of human behavior and psychodynamics, psychopathology, and psychotherapy, combined with interviewing and assessment skills are the tools nurses need to perform a psychiatric evaluation. Like most things, it is a skill easily learned with practice. What might often impede nurses in their performance is not a lack of knowledge but an uneasiness with psychiatric problems in their patients. It is important therefore that nurses be aware of their own negative reactions or feelings toward patients with psychiatric symptoms.

As in other areas of nursing, the role assumed by the nurse will depend on the level of nursing preparation achieved and the health care setting in which the nurse is employed. The general practitioner should include the psychiatric evaluation as part of the nursing history obtained to identify the nursing diagnoses and related plan of care. Clinical example 6-3 illustrates such an assessment.

This illustration presents the roles of two nurses. The staff nurse performed an assessment of the patient, including a brief psychiatric evaluation, and then called

---

CLINICAL EXAMPLE 6-3

An attractive 21-year-old woman is admitted to the gynecological service for a dilation and curettage. While orienting her to the unit, the nurse observes that she is chain smoking and continuously moving about the room. When asked some general questions about her illness, she begins to cry and tells the nurse about her boyfriend, who was recently killed in an automobile accident. The nurse pursues the conversation and from an assessment decides to call the psychiatric liaison nurse for assistance.

---

on the liaison nurse. This nurse consultant has advanced knowledge in the area of psychiatric nursing that will enable her to determine the nature of the patient's problem and assist the staff nurse in designing a plan of care to meet the patient's psychological and physiological needs.

Nurses working in a community mental health center may have advanced knowledge in psychiatric nursing through education at the master's degree level or through experience and in-service education in the mental health field. They often perform the initial evaluation of the patients seen in the center and call on other health team members such as the psychiatrist and psychologist for consultation to confirm the psychiatric diagnosis and treatment plan. Nurses in this setting may also be involved in certain aspects of the identified plan of care, such as arranging for hospitalization or engaging the patient in a form of psychotherapy, including crisis intervention, insight-oriented therapy, or other modes of therapy.

Nurses working in a psychiatric inpatient setting can perform a variety of functions based on the philosophy of the unit where they are employed. Whether this includes primary nursing, patient advocate, or other conceptually defined roles, nurses need to assess and continuously review their patient's mental functioning. This provides for a focus on the patient's problems and a vehicle for ongoing evaluation of the patient's needs.

The psychiatric interview

The basic elements of a psychiatric interview are the psychiatric history and the mental status examination. For the purpose of clarity these will be addressed separately in this chapter. However, this is not to imply a clear-cut demarcation in the clinical performance of the psychiatric evaluation. The interview provides the structure for assessment of the patient. Assessment denotes systematic collection of pertinent data about the patient. A data base on which nursing judgments can be made is collected through history taking and the mental status examination. Throughout the interview valuable data are obtained by observation of and communication with the patient.

There is no best way to perform a psychiatric evaluation. The nurse's approach and line of inquiry will vary depending on the nature of the presenting problem and the individual patient being assessed. There are many formats for performing and recording the psychiatric evaluation.[1, 10-12] This chapter presents one framework for organizing and systematically recording assessment data.

The purpose of the psychiatric interview is to establish rapport with the patient, gain knowledge of his characteristic patterns of living and coping behaviors, and assess how his mind is working. The interview is goal-directed communication that provides an opportunity for the nurse to experience who the patient is and to understand how he has developed through the course of life events. This attempt at fully acknowledging and understanding the patient as a unique human being enables the nurse to more effectively determine the patient's needs and an appropriate plan of care. How often does the plan of care fail or the problem reappear because of a lack of concern for the patient as an individual? Consider the patient with high blood pressure who is told to relax by the nurse who does not know he has six children to feed and bills to pay and is the only working member of his family. It is not surprising to find that this man has both uncontrolled blood pressure and is depressed when he next visits the hospital. The loss of appetite and inability to sleep, characteristic of an affective disorder, have compounded the original problem of high blood pressure.

Establishment of rapport is often taken for granted or viewed as an intuitive skill. However, it is a goal to be achieved by the nurse and should be thought about and planned for as any other nursing goal. A basic factor is respect for and awareness of the feelings of security in the patient. A threat to the individual's security produces anxiety, which, in turn, influences the nature of the data obtained in the interview. The nurse conveys a sensitivity to the patient's feelings by demonstrating a genuinely warm and concerned approach. This atmosphere of acceptance facilitates the expression of feelings and concerns by the patient.

Addressing the patient by name and introducing herself by name and title is a way the nurse conveys respect to the patient. Following this identification, a definition of purpose should be established so that a framework for the interview is set. This provides an opportunity for the sharing of expectations and the allaying of anxiety of the participants, since both individuals are clear about what is to follow. The nurse as interviewer is governed by the purpose of the interview, which is distinct and specific for each situation encountered. For example, with a patient who has had a thoracotomy as part of the treatment for Hodgkin's disease and is struggling with acceptance of this chronic condition and its effects on her current life-style, the psychiatric liaison nurse will provide consultation for the purpose of advising and perhaps facilitating the securing of competent psychiatric treatment elsewhere. A second type of interview is the initial meeting in brief psychotherapy or in a continued treatment situation. The nurse's purpose here is to establish both a diagnosis and a professional acquaintance with the intent of carrying on treatment herself. A third type of interview with a different purpose would be with the parents of a child who is handicapped or has a chronic disease. Although the focus of the interview might be a discussion of an identified problem the child is having, an assessment of the particular difficulties and needs of the parents must be considered in planning for the child's treatment.

Whenever the nurse conducts an interview the environment should be one that provides for an atmosphere of privacy. Ideally, this would include a comfortable room used solely by the interviewer and the person being interviewed. More often than not, this kind of privacy only occurs in settings where there are private offices in which the patient and nurse can meet. The nurse must often overcome environmental constraints, and her creativity is called on to convey an atmosphere of privacy to the patient. This can be accomplished by turning chairs in a crowded room away from others so that distractions are at a minimum or by leaving a message with other personnel that the interview is being conducted and should be interrupted only for identified reasons.

■ Interviewing skills

Thus far, understanding the patient through demonstrating respect, acceptance, and concern for him as an individual has been stressed. However, setting the stage for self-disclosure is not enough. The nurse must actively participate in the process by being what Sullivan[13] refers to as a participant observer. This implies both participation with and observation of the patient in an attempt to collect relevant data on which nursing care can be based.

Skill in the art of communication is a valuable tool of the participant observer. Maintenance of eye contact and the use of open-ended questions and reflection are familiar techniques used by the nurse in promoting communication. It should be noted, however, that active participation in the interview is not synonymous with increased verbalization by the nurse. A facial expression that reflects interest and concern is just as effective as a verbal message in denoting participation with the patient.

Two skills of utmost importance in conducting a psychiatric interview are listening and observation. Here they are specifically addressed because they are perhaps the most difficult skills to acquire. Attentive listening to and observing another involves transcending oneself and this is a difficult task. Being sure that what is spoken is what is heard as the sender of the message intended, and not as the receiver of the message had either expected or hoped for, requires continuous introspection on the part of the nurse who is the receiver of valuable information about the patient.

When communicating with the patient, the nurse must listen both to what is being said and what is not being said. A patient's verbal description of his mother is that she was "kind, loving, helpful, someone he could always turn to." However, as more information is shared, the patient describes his mother as "having been out of the house a lot working and leaving him with various babysitters throughout his childhood." From these limited data the nurse might begin to wonder how the mother was able to communicate the kind, helpful, loving attitude that her son describes. Or the nurse might question if this is more a description of what the patient as a child needed and wanted but did not receive from his mother. As a result of this conflict, the defense mechanisms of denial and fantasizing may be operating to protect the patient as he tells the nurse the story of his early childhood. Much more information is needed before an assumption such as this one can be made. What is implied in this description is that the nurse strives to understand what the patient is trying to communicate. Does she know what he means by his statements? Could it mean something other than what immediately occurs to her?

Throughout the interview the nurse must also listen for the themes that develop as the patient describes himself and his current and past history. In describing his life events a 22-year-old patient pointed out that his parents taught him at an early age to please other people. It also became evident to the nurse that his parents were consulted on most of the decisions he made throughout his life, such as the friends he had, the schools he attended, what his major was in college, and where he chose to live with his wife. He expressed trouble at work in placing limits on his co-workers who constantly asked him to do favors for them and join clubs, which he was not able to refuse. One of the themes inherent in this description is the patient's inability to assert himself. It is important to focus on this, since it may be one of the predisposing stressors related to his complaint of depression.

Observation also requires a special kind of attentiveness in the nurse. It is important to observe the verbal content as well as the nonverbal communication of the patient represented in the body language he uses. Does he look older or younger than his stated age? Is there a message in his style of dress or the gestures he uses in the interview? Does his manner of communicating reflect his educational level? Is his affective response to a particular topic congruent with the content he presents? In Clinical example 6-4 there are many nonverbal cues that the nurse should note.

These observations, along with others obtained in the mental status examination, form the data base on which nursing diagnosis and a treatment plan is made. Other observations will be addressed in more depth in the discussion of the mental status examination.

If the skills described are used by the nurse, an open atmosphere that encourages self-disclosure by the patient will be created. A tense, hurried, and anxious approach should be avoided. The nurse's awareness of her feelings, subjectivity, and misperceptions before meeting the patient should help her to avoid communicating her anxiety to the patient. If immobilized by her own insecurity and anxiety, the nurse will prevent the open atmosphere that allows for participation in the other individual's, her patient's, experience.

A vital concern of the beginning clinician is where to begin with the patient. Simply stated, it is best to start where the patient is. Yet few patients spontaneously begin on their own; rather, they will wait for the nurse to open the interview. A brief statement of what the nurse has learned about the patient, either from observation or from a referral, is usually enough to provide him with the opportunity to tell his story in his

---

CLINICAL EXAMPLE 6-4

Although Mrs. S is only 31 years of age, her torn clothing that fits loosely and her slumped posture and furrowed brow give an appearance of someone much older who has weathered many storms. She continuously wrings her hands as she talks about the death of her husband 6 years ago when her children were still infants. At one point she begins to tear while talking about her inability to give her children the things she would like them to have.

own way. The patient with Hodgkin's disease described earlier was approached by the nurse in the following way.

MS. J: **Good afternoon, Ms. X. My name is Ms. J and I am a psychiatric nurse.**

MS. X: **(Looks up) Hello.**

MS. J: **The head nurse, Ms. K, asked me to come and talk with you today. She is concerned about you because she has noticed that you had been crying on several occasions when she entered your room.**

MS. X: **(Beginning to tear) I'm tired of talking, I'm tired of tests, I just want to be left alone.**

MS. J: **It sounds like you are feeling frustrated.**

MS. X: **(Looking directly at the nurse) What would you know? All of this, and for what? Most people with cancer end up dead, so what's the use?**

The nurse had provided the patient a chance to ventilate and begin to disclose some of her feelings about her illness and her fear of death. From this point, considering the patient's emotional status and readiness, the nurse can proceed with the psychiatric evaluation.

With the hospitalized patient an account of the presenting problem and events leading up to the hospitalization as well as historical data about the patient may have previously been obtained and recorded in the chart by other health care professionals. If so, the nurse would modify her approach and discuss particular areas not included in the original evaluation or areas believed to be important to the patient's current mental functioning. The nurse can rely on collateral sources of information such as the medical history or social history and select the focus for the interview.

■ Presenting problem

A clear account of the presenting problem must be obtained. This consists of a detailed chronological reconstruction of the present illness. If it is not spontaneously offered by the patient or identified elsewhere, the nurse uses her skills in obtaining this information from the patient. How is the problem perceived by the patient? Is it interpersonal, somatic, or sociological? When was the problem first noticed (onset)? How long has it lasted (duration)? Does the patient have any ideas as to the possible causes of the problem? Has it become worse (progressed) or changed in degree? If so, when did the change occur? Has the patient found any solution or obtained any type of relief?

In eliciting this information from the patient, the nurse would look for other factors related to the current problem of which the patient may not be consciously aware, such as a change in personal relationships, job, financial condition, and other circumstances surrounding the initial occurrence. In the preceding dialogue it

was assumed, perhaps because of the nurse's own conflicts, that the patient's crying spells were related to her present condition—the thoracotomy for Hodgkin's disease. When specifically asked about the onset of her crying, the patient then proceeded to tell the nurse about her husband's recent loss of his job and inability to find another. Just this amount of information could change the entire assessment of this patient's needs. She may have already worked through acceptance of the chronic illness and currently be concerned with medical insurance for future treatment. Although the original statement she makes about cancer leading to death might reflect an ongoing conflict for her, without more specific inquiry by the nurse her immediate concerns could go unnoticed.

It is therefore necessary to strive for specificity. At times the nurse will need to guide the patient in an attempt to obtain an accurate account of events. Encouraging the patient to describe actual incidents and recording these in the patient's own words rather than making a general statement will be useful in achieving a correct assessment of the patient's conflicts and in the formulation of appropriate nursing diagnoses. Skill in discouraging trivia and repetitions will be needed in helping the patient to focus on the current problem.

After a clear concise statement is obtained about the presenting problem and the incidents that led to its occurrence, the patient's view of responsibility for the problem needs to be assessed. Does he see the problem as something he needs to change, something someone else is responsible for, or something that no one can control, as in the case of someone who believes the devil has entered his body and is controlling his actions?

Whom the patient views as being responsible for the problem directly relates to what changes are desired. The 22-year-old man previously described felt depressed and questioned what he could do to overcome these feelings. Although the relationship he had with his parents may have been a causative factor in his depression and a conflict he could work through in therapy, this was not his current focus. However, placing limits on expectations he had of himself and that others at work had of him was something he consciously desired to do. This allowed for a focus on an identified problem and a definition of goals. Agreement between the nurse and patient on problem identification is essential if resolution is to occur. Whether the nurse's task is to refer the patient for treatment or to personally undertake therapy with the patient, a mutually agreed on nursing diagnosis is essential.

In the initial stage of the psychiatric interview the nurse has created an open atmosphere by demonstrating a genuinely warm concerned approach to the patient and has also gathered information about his present illness. The major symptoms have been described by the patient in behavioral terms, such as a desire to be alone or frequent fighting with spouse, and in body disturbances, such as an inability to sleep, loss of weight, or palpitations of the heart. How the presenting problem is viewed by the nurse would depend on whether there were previous episodes, if the problem is an exaggeration of long-term trends, or something entirely new. To make an assumption about the characteristic patterns of living and coping behaviors of the patient, further data collection will be necessary.

■ History taking

A brief survey of the patient's past life in the second stage of the interview provides the nurse with a rough social sketch of the patient. Of particular significance are events in the patient's life that may contribute to a psychological disruption, which may be secondary to maladaptive coping behaviors or indicate resources and strengths to consider in treatment planning. To help the patient see the relevance of questions about the past, the nurse can summarize briefly what the patient has said of his problems and then make a transition to the past history, for example, "For me to understand you better and the events of your present situation, I will need to learn something about your past life."

There are significant variations in the methods and forms used in obtaining historical information about the patient.[10-12] However the history is obtained, information about medical and psychiatric history, family history, and a personal history are necessary. The historical information should also include a sexual history and a drug history (see Appendices A-D). The latter two areas are not usually covered spontaneously because of the anxiety-laden material. Starting with a survey of the patient's past life provides for an initial discussion of areas that are perceived by the patient as less threatening. In this way the nurse guides the patient without arousing undue anxiety by progressing from topics that promote the least anxiety to those which promote the most. The interview will have a smoother progression if the nurse asks questions in a logical sequence without abrupt changes from one topic to another.

■ **MEDICAL HISTORY.** The depth of information included in the medical history will depend on the age of the patient, the problems encountered in his life, and the resources available to the nurse. If the patient is a young woman who reports being in good physical health throughout her life, the amount of detail required would be less than from the middle-aged man who states that he has always had some physical ailment since childhood. Other family members or significant others in the

patient's life, such as mother or family physician, can be vital sources of data. This is true especially if the patient is uncertain about the events surrounding a particular illness or hospitalization.

Following are areas addressed in the general medical history of the patient:

1. Illnesses and operations, with a focus on when they occurred, the outcome, and the chronicity of the condition
2. Congenital, biological, chemical, or physical injury to the nervous system, specifically any head injuries sustained
3. Current medical treatments the patient is involved in or medication he is taking

When an account of these experiences is given, it is important to place emphasis on the patient's reaction to the illnesses, operations, or accidents he has had in his life.

■ **PSYCHIATRIC HISTORY.** Following the medical history, inquiry about any previous psychiatric illnesses or encounters with a psychiatrist, psychologist, or other mental health professional is made. Have there been any psychiatric problems in the past? Is the current episode similar to these or different as the patient perceives it? What were the frequency and duration of the past episodes? If the patient was involved in treatment, what kind was it and how did he feel about it?

The psychiatric history would also include related data about the patient's family. Relatives who have had psychiatric illnesses along with the prevalence of suicide in the family should be identified. The significance of this to the patient's present illness is twofold. In certain psychiatric disorders, such as the affective disorders, heredity is considered to be one of the predisposing factors.[3] The occurrence of a psychiatric illness or suicide in the patient's family may also give a perspective on how individuals in the patient's life coped with stress and whether this has influenced the patient's repertoire of coping behaviors. It is essential to point out, however, that the patient's reaction to mental illness in his family is of more significance than the isolated fact itself.

■ **FAMILY HISTORY.** Assessment of the patient's capacity to form interpersonal relationships begins with the family history. It is through the relationship the infant has with the significant adults in his life, usually the parents, that the basis of his security is formed. Sullivan[13] believes that the goal of life is interpersonal security. By assessing the patient's interpersonal relationships throughout his life, data can be obtained about his interpersonal needs and level of self-esteem. The family environment provides the first learning situation for the individual. Areas of dysfunction and support need to be determined, since the family can be considered one of the support systems available to the patient throughout his life.

Although the patient may not remember a lot about his early childhood, he has often been told of certain significant events. These may include when and where he was born, his place in the family structure, what the family circumstances were, including any financial stresses, and whether the patient's birth was planned. He may know of any problems his mother experienced during the pregnancy or labor and delivery, who besides the parents was frequently in the home, what the characteristics of discipline were, and what his parents' attitudes toward his development and life events seemed to be. The interactions the patient had with parents, siblings, and other family members during childhood with specific reference to brutality, rejection, deaths, or separations from significant others would be important factors influencing the patient's original development of his sense of self as being either "good" or "bad."

■ **PERSONAL HISTORY.** These data will give the nurse an impression of what the emotional climate was for this individual's beginning personality development from his point of view. When and how early developmental tasks were achieved, such as toilet training and entering school, leads into the personal history of the patient. A continuation of the chronological approach in pursuit of the individual's personal history incorporates important areas of life experiences. These areas include schooling, vocational pursuits, sexual experiences, and drug experimentation. These life experiences are more easily addressed if they are presented in a historical perspective of when they first occurred.

Starting school is a big event in childhood. It is also the first opportunity the individual has to compare himself to others. Socialization patterns have begun to develop. The age on entering school, type of school (private, parochial, public), grades repeated, level of academic performance, including special achievements, episodes of truancy, and disciplinary difficulties will portray the early attitudes developed about study and work. The relationships with teachers and fellow students, friendships formed, and special interests and activities, such as scouts, will portray the early social values established. If the individual developed close relationships during this time, he can usually remember the names of his closest friends and may know something about what they are doing now. Conflicts experienced during the early primary years are expressed in behaviors such as nail biting, nightmares, sleepwalking, and enuresis. Although most children exhibit some of these behaviors, the response of the parents and what the individual remembers about the behavior are important to elicit.

As the individual approaches adolescence, a time of rapid physical development and emotional turmoil, he begins the task of identification of self and the formation of intimate relationships. During this period of the individual's life, people outside the family structure become important sources for comparisons of values, attitudes, and experiences. Experimentation with drugs, including alcohol, and sex are likely to occur and should be addressed while information about this stage of development is being obtained.

On entering high school, what was the extent and type of participation in sports, parties, church, and political activities? What was the individual's experience with groups and leadership, especially during school? Was he a member of the "in group"? Did his level of academic performance change? What was his age and status on leaving school? Did he graduate or leave school to work? Did he have any special interests or hobbies? Were they solitary or group activities? When did he first drink alcohol, smoke marijuana, and experiment with other drugs, such as LSD, amphetamines, or barbiturates? What pattern was established at the time and how has it changed? Being asked questions about drug use can be intimidating to the individual. It is important to phrase the questions so that the individual feels free to answer without having a value judgment placed on him. Phrases such as "when" or "how often," rather than "do you," assume that the behavior has occurred and make it easier for the individual to answer than when he first must decide if he wants to admit to the behavior being addressed.

With the onset of puberty, sexual attitudes become important. How and from whom did the patient learn about sexual matters? With the woman, information surrounding the time of menarche is elicited. Who told her about menstruation? Her reaction to the first and subsequent periods should be ascertained. With both women and men it should be determined at what age pubic and axillary hair appeared. Did the individual experience an early or delayed onset of body development and what was the reaction to this in relation to peers? When did the man first experience an erection and orgasm and was it with or without ejaculation? When did the individual first masturbate? What were the experiences with necking, petting, and intercourse? How were these experiences viewed by family and friends? Friendship, dating, and early sexual experiences, including autosexual, homosexual and heterosexual activities are usually important issues for the adolescent. Were these experiences comfortable or pleasurable ones or associated with guilt?

The sex life of an individual can be viewed as a barometer of emotional health. It is therefore important to ascertain if there have been any changes in the individual's sexual habits. The nurse must feel comfortable discussing sexual matters with the patient to be able to talk about the patient's sexual habits in each stage of his life. This is an area that is sensitive to most people, and further information about what areas to address and how to discuss sexual material with patients can be obtained in the publication *Assessment of Sexual Function*.[9]

An individual's occupational and marriage history are included in the assessment of the period of maturity. What are his goals and ambitions, positions held, promotions, and relationships with bosses and peers? Are there any discrepancies between stated goals and the individual's efforts to achieve them? Continuing education and military experiences can be discussed as part of the occupational history of the patient when applicable.

The marriage history should include a history of dating and courtship, the circumstances of the marriage, sexual adjustment, frequency of relations, living conditions, financial difficulties experienced, and previous marriages. If there are any children in the family, what were the reactions to the pregnancies and births and are there any prominent problems in the family now? What is the patient's relationship with his parents? If they are deceased, what was the patient's reaction to the loss?

To complete the social sketch of the patient, it is essential to determine his talents, strengths, and assets to gain a total view of him as a person. Asking him to describe his daily activities can give a clue as to what the patient is trying to achieve. The richness or poverty of activities in his life-style may indicate the meaning of life for him. Church, community, and leisure activities are often sources of emotional support for an individual that can be used especially in times of stress.

The second stage of the evaluation has simply been an attempt to understand how the patient comes to be there in relation to the prominent landmarks that have characterized his course of life up until the present. This information depicts the development of the patient's self-concept. As with any assessment that the nurse would perform, the amount of detail required will depend on the individual patient, his presenting complaint, and the environmental constraints such as time. Hopefully, the areas just addressed will be included in some detail in each psychiatric evaluation completed by the nurse.

Clinical example 6-5 illustrates the type of data obtained in the first two stages of the psychiatric evaluation.

Mental status examination

The historical information obtained will give the nurse a perspective on areas with which the patient may have difficulty, such as forming interpersonal relationships, consistent job performance, and other significant life experience areas. Further supportive data for assessment of both the patient's limitations and strengths will be obtained in the mental status examination, which is the third stage of the psychiatric evaluation.

The mental status examination is a way of organizing observational data about all aspects of a patient's mental functioning. While obtaining information about the presenting problem and taking a history, the nurse is informally and indirectly accumulating information about the patient's mental functioning. However, formal questioning is usually needed at the end of the interview to complete an accurate and comprehensive mental status examination. Verbatim samples of the patient's speech and thought content are useful to present a precise picture of the patient. For clarity, the mental status examination should be recorded in a certain order and organized according to certain categories, that is, general observations, sensorium and intelligence, thought processes, affect, mood, and insight. Each item will be addressed with clinical examples for clarification followed by a continuation of the case history presented earlier.

■ General observations

Specific aspects of the patient's behavior are included in detail in the remainder of the mental status examination. It is useful, however, to record in the beginning the general observations of the patient, especially those characteristics which appear outstanding to the interviewer.

■ **APPEARANCE.** The patient's appearance should be described in terms of consistency with his age and station in life, his manner of dress (conservative, tasteful, meticulous, inappropriate), his personal habits (clean, unkempt, disorderly), his characteristic facial expression (alert, vacant, sad, bewildered, hostile, masklike), and his state of health and general nutrition.

■ **REACTION TO INTERVIEW.** The patient's reaction to the interview, with the circumstances surrounding it taken into account, is addressed. Has he been cooperative, friendly, evasive, ingratiating, indifferent, passive, dependent, or hostile in his responses to the interviewer? If he has been observed in various situations, does he respond differently to various types of people (physicians, nurses, other patients)? Each patient

CLINICAL EXAMPLE 6-5

Ms. T is a 22-year-old single, white, unemployed clerical worker who comes to the mental health clinic stating that she does not socialize any more and is becoming increasingly self-conscious about going out of the house for fear of "making a fool" of herself. She is currently living with her father, three siblings, and an aunt in the aunt's home. She states she would like to "make something" of herself but is afraid that people won't accept her.

Ms. T relates the onset of her feelings to the problems that occurred at work 18 months ago. She states she felt a lot of pressure at work, felt "extremely nervous" around her boss, was denied two promotions for "trivial reasons," and began to feel inferior to other workers, which made her depressed and led to her resignation.

During the time when problems were occurring at work, several incidents happened at home that also affected how Ms. T was feeling. Her younger sister was using drugs and the police had been called to the home several times. Ms. T was concerned about the effect this had on her aunt for whom she has a great deal of affection and gratitude. Her paternal grandmother had died in February and her twin brother had married and left the home in June. Both these individuals were a source of support to Ms. T. She wishes that her siblings and father would move out of the house, leaving only herself and the aunt because "none of them are decent people anyway and they only cause trouble for my aunt."

Her medical history includes hospitalization at age 6 for a tonsillectomy. Ms. T says she enjoyed being in the hospital and remembers playing in the play area. She had no major illnesses during childhood or adolescence that she could recall. She believes that she had the usual childhood illnesses, measles and mumps.

Ms. T's psychiatric history was negative for herself and her family. She was seen by Dr. X at the Community Health Facility 6 months ago for a questionable somatoform disorder. Her father has been seen by Dr. X for 10 years for multiple physical complaints.

Ms. T was born and raised in Baltimore. She is the eldest, along with a twin brother, of five children. She has two sisters, age 21 and 19, by her father's first marriage and one sister, age 15, by his second. Ms. T states she has little recollection of her biological mother. She remembers going to the movies with her at about age 4 and has heard from other family members that she was a "nice lady." Her father was described as a "very emotional" person who gets "very upset" easily. He drank heavily when the children were young and was taken out of the house several times by the police for disorderly conduct. Ms. T and her siblings were basically raised by her paternal aunt and grandmother. Even after the father's second marriage, she and her siblings lived with the aunt and the grandmother. Her father remarried when Ms. T was 6 years old and lived with his second wife in an apartment close to her aunt's home. She states that the family would celebrate holidays together and go on picnics but that she never felt close to any of her siblings or to her father.

Ms. T started school at age 5 and achieved "above average" grades. She was a safety in grade school and a cheerleader for 3 years in high school. She graduated from high school at age 17 without any failures. Ms. T says she was a "shy kid" most of her life but had several girl friends. However, she rarely brought them home because of her father's drinking.

She had dated one boy steadily from age 18 to 20. Her sexual experience included kissing and petting. Ms. T states she wants to be a virgin when and if she marries. She learned about menstruation from girl friends and a movie at school and her first period was at age 13. She states that she has never talked with family members about sexual matters.

Ms. T feels she has cut herself off from friends during the past 2 years. Several of them still call or drop by but she never goes out to socialize with them. She spends most of her day cleaning the house, making the meals, and listening to music in her room.

The only position Ms. T held was as a clerical worker at the bank. She acquired the job after graduation and believes that she did okay until 18 months ago. She gives a vague description of her boss, stating he just "didn't like me" and was "always on my back about something."

Ms. T denies any experimentation with drugs. She used to drink wine on social occasions when dating but stopped after she broke up with her boyfriend.

The patient was interviewed in her room on the fourth day of hospitalization. She was a white woman slightly overweight, neatly dressed in jeans and a sweater and appeared younger than her 36 years of age. Although she was cooperative, her guarded responses to all questions seemed excessively self-centered. She gave the interviewer the feeling that she didn't trust anyone and was preoccupied during the interview. When asked how other people treated her, she refused to answer with an angry "I'd rather not say!"

will react to the situation whether he is hospitalized, referred for psychiatric evaluation by the court, or voluntarily seeking counseling.

■ **CONSISTENCY OF BEHAVIOR.** As previously discussed, throughout the interview, communication is both verbally and nonverbally expressed. Examples of the patient's verbal and nonverbal behavior are included and the consistency of both is noted. Characteristics of the patient's speech, such as speed, vocabulary, and goal directedness are observed. Any overt motor behaviors, such as finger tapping, hair twirling, hand wringing, pacing, posturing, gait, and bizarre movements are described.

■ **RESPONSE TO PATIENT.** It is important that the nurse also become aware of the response she has to each of the patients she interviews. The response can contain diagnostic information about the patient. A depressed patient may elicit a sense of sadness and hopelessness in the nurse. In contrast, the nurse might experience anger toward a patient who is angry and hostile. The principal feeling elicited should be identified and the behaviors observed that are associated with the feeling should be clearly stated, as in Clinical example 6-6.

■ **Sensorium and intelligence**

This section describes the patient's state of consciousness and his ability to accurately perceive the environment. The patient's state of consciousness, orientation, memory, intellectual function, judgment, and comprehension are assessed. Impairment in more than one area may relate to a diagnosis of an organic mental disorder.[11] Since the disorder can vary from mild transient alterations to a permanent disruption of all areas, it is important to carefully document each area.

■ **LEVEL OF CONSCIOUSNESS.** A variety of terms can be used to identify the patient's level of consciousness. Is the patient alert and awake or stuporous and sleepy? Is he easily distracted or hyperalert? Can he sustain attention to both external and internal stimuli? A clouded state of consciousness is an essential feature in delirium and is therefore essential to assessment for accurate diagnosis and treatment.

■ **ORIENTATION.** The patient is questioned regarding his orientation to time, place, person, and situation. Does the patient know who he is, where he is, who the people around him are, and the date? Does he seem to understand the rationale for the interview and his role in it? Patients with organic disruptions may give grossly inaccurate answers, especially for time relationships.[3] In contrast, the schizophrenic disorders may cause the patient to say he is someone else or somewhere else or in some way reveal his personalized orientation to the world.

■ **MEMORY.** Memory impairment is a prominent behavior observed in dementia that can range from forgetfulness to a total lack of understanding of significant persons and events in the individual's life. There are three areas to be tested under memory: immediate recall, recent memory, and remote memory. Immediate recall involves attention and concentration as well as an ability to retain material just learned. The digits-span test requires that the patient repeat digits either forward or backward within a 10-second interval. The nurse recites a series of randomly selected digits to the patient, beginning with three digits and progressing until the patient is unable to repeat the digits in proper sequence. The same procedure is then repeated, but the patient is asked to say the number with the order reversed. An example may need to be given so that the procedure is understood. An approximate comparison to educational level can be made: five digits forward and four digits backward equals an eighth-grade education, and seven digits forward and five digits backward indicates a twelfth-grade education. However, high anxiety may interfere with the patient's ability to concentrate and should be considered if the performance is poor.

Recent memory can be tested by asking the patient when he came to the hospital and to recall the events of the past 24 hours. A reliable informant may be needed to verify the statements made by the patient. A test of recent memory can be performed by asking the patient to remember three words (an object, a color, an address) and then having him repeat them back 15 minutes later in the interview.

The patient's ability to give a consistent account of his past history requires an intact remote memory. Available records or reliable informants are needed to verify information, such as date of birth, age, when started and finished school, date of marriage, birth dates of children, and other significant life events.

■ **INTELLECTUAL FUNCTION.** A patient's intellectual functioning is assessed in relation to his educational, occupational, and attainment levels. Testing the patient's vocabulary, counting and calculating ability, abstract ability, and fund of general knowledge provides some information about the patient's intelligence. Vocabulary can be assessed by asking for word definitions or synonyms. Counting and calculating involve doing simple arithmetic problems ($9 \times 6, 21 + 7$) and asking the patient to serially subtract 7 from 100. If he has difficulty subtracting 7 from 100, he can be asked to subtract 3 from 20 in the same manner. This task also involves the ability to concentrate and complete a task.

The ability to conceptualize and abstract can be tested by having the patient explain a series of proverbs. The patient is given an example of a proverb with its interpretation and then asked to tell what several proverbs mean to him. Following are frequently used proverbs: "When it rains, it pours," "A stitch in time saves nine," "A rolling stone gathers no moss," and "The proof of the pudding is in the eating." Most adults are able to interpret proverbs as a representation or symbolization of human behavior or events. Cultural background is a set factor that should be considered when the patient is not able to complete the task. If the patient's educational level is less than ninth grade, asking him to list similarities between a series of paired objects will assess his ability to abstract. The following series of paired objects are frequently used: bicycle, bus; apple, pear; television, newspaper. A good reply would be in terms of function, whereas an answer in terms of structure may indicate a tendency toward concrete thinking.

To determine the patient's fund of general knowledge, he can be asked to name the last five presidents, the mayor, five large cities, the capital of France, or other similar questions congruent with his educational background. With all these tests it is essential to keep in mind the patient's educational and vocational background so that he is given tasks he is able to perform. If the patient cannot read or does not work, he may not be able to state recent events or local news but could relate plots of television shows or local neighborhood information. On completion of some general tests of intelligence, if the nurse has doubts about the patient's intelligence level or suspects deterioration from a history of changes at work, home, or school, a referral for psychological testing should be considered.[6]

■ **JUDGMENT.** The patient's judgment can best be assessed from an account of past decisions and how they were reached and from the patient's responses to the interview situation. Judgment involves the ability to understand facts and draw conclusions from relationships. In discussion of recent events does he appear to exercise sound judgment? The young teenage boy referred for counseling after repeated arrests for car theft exhibits poor judgment. It is useful to determine if the judgments are deliberate, impulsive, or inappropriate. Several hypothetical situations can be presented for the patient to evaluate: What would he do if he found a stamped, addressed envelope lying on the ground? How would he find his way out of a forest in the daytime? What would he do if he entered his house and smelled gas?

■ **COMPREHENSION.** Throughout the interview the patient's ability to understand the meaning of the questions is assessed, as well as his ability to comprehend incidents in his environment, such as local, political, and personal events that affect him and his community. Does he understand his role as a patient, and, if hospitalized, does he understand the hospital routine? An organic brain syndrome could interfere with the patient's level of comprehension.[11]

The assessment data obtained in the area of sensorium and intelligence is of particular importance in determining disorders classified as organic mental disorders. The acute picture presented to the clinician is often easy to identify, whereas the more subtle changes that can occur as a result of a degenerative disease or brain lesion require attentive observation by the nurse and, as previously mentioned, carefully documented behaviors, as shown in Clinical example 6-7.

CLINICAL EXAMPLE 6-7

It was apparent that the patient was alert and awake but almost totally distracted by something within himself. Questions and directions were repeated frequently so that they were understood. He was oriented to person, place, and situation. He performed six digits forward and three digits backward and remembered two of three objects after 15 minutes. He remembered the third with help. He listed presidents to Truman and performed serial sevens with relative ease, making two mistakes. He could not identify any recent events or discuss television shows and seemed limited in his fund of general knowledge. This may relate to his social isolation since quitting school at age 16, as described by his mother.

■ Thought processes

■ **FORM OF THOUGHT.** Observation of thought process is made through the patient's speech. The patterns or forms of verbalization, rather than the content of speech, are assessed. What is the rate or flow of speech? Is it overly fast or retarded? Does the patient's speech proceed in a clear, logical, goal-directed manner? As he talks about topics relating to himself, the nurse should note if the patient is able to express himself in an understandable manner or if his ideas are vague, leaving her uncertain about their meaning. Is he able to move freely from one topic to another with relative ease and flexibility? Is there continuity of thought or are his associations disconnected (loose), constantly changing (flight of ideas), wide of the point (tangential), interrupted suddenly (blocked), or distorted and bizarre, as when new words are made up to express ideas symbolically (neologisms).

■ **CONTENT OF THOUGHT.** Recurring patterns of content, such as delusions, hallucinations, or illusions may be observed and reflect a disruption in perception. Misperceptions include a variety of thoughts, feelings, or fears the patient may have that interfere in some way with his reality testing.

Hallucinations refer to sensory perceptions for which there are no external stimuli. Sometimes the patient's behavior will indicate that he is hallucinating; he may adopt a listening attitude, mumble, pick at unseen objects, or stop suddenly as if he is guarding himself. Asking if he has heard noises or voices when no one was around or had any unusual experiences will provide an opportunity for the patient to describe any such experiences to the nurse. Characteristics such as the source, manner of reception, content, and time of the experience should be described.

Delusions are recurring false beliefs that are not congruent with the patient's culture or background. Again, tactful questioning will be useful in helping him to focus on delusional material. Does he misinterpret what happens to him, giving it special or false meaning? Does he feel that he has been singled out or watched? Does he experience his thoughts or actions as being controlled by an external force? Can people read his mind or does he have psychic powers? These concerns may be complicated and will be concealed by the patient and require extensive questioning.

Illusions refer to misperceptions that have an external stimulus. The hospitalized patient may believe his room is a jail cell and the staff members are security guards. A schoolteacher with an organic mental disorder may perceive her family as pupils and the bedside table as her desk.

The patient's thoughts can be focused on obsessions, compulsions, or phobias that also interrupt the normal thought process. Repetitive thoughts, impulses, or behaviors unwanted by the individual are defined as obsessions or compulsions. These can be assessed by asking the patient if there are any intrusive recurring thoughts or actions that he feels unable to control and that occupy an extensive amount of his time. Objects and/or situations irrationally feared by the patient in a persistent manner are identified as phobias. The individual can exert great energy avoiding certain situations or thinking about the feared object.

Disruptions in both the form and content of thought are seen in the schizophrenias, affective disorders, anxiety disorders, organic mental disorders, and paranoid disorders in varying degrees of intensity and varying combinations. In the following example, the nurse includes a detailed description of the patient's form and content of thought in an assessment of his thought processes:

The patient's speech was rapid and he acknowledged feeling as if his thoughts were coming too fast, "My mind is racing ahead." The rapidity of his speech compounded the difficulty understanding him as he quickly moved from one topic to another in what appeared to be an unrelated manner. He denied any visual or auditory hallucinations; however, he believed that he could talk with God if he needed a consultant on his life situation. He felt this was a special blessing given to him over other men.

■ Affect

Observations of the range, appropriateness, and intensity of the patient's emotional expressions (affect) in relation to the circumstances of the interview and the ideas expressed are documented. Does the patient demonstrate variability in the expression of feeling or does his affectual response appear blunted or restricted in some way? Does he report significant life events without any emotional component (flat)? Is the patient's affectual response congruent with the content of his speech? Does he report that he is being persecuted by the police and laugh? Does he rapidly shift from one affectual response to another (labile)? The patient's statements of emotion and the nurse's empathic responses to the patient may provide clues to the appropriateness of the affect or character of the prevailing mood.

■ Mood

The pervasive, relatively enduring, emotional state of the patient reflects his mood and can influence his perception of his life situation. Does the patient's appearance reflect his mood? Does he look "down in the dumps"? A description of the patient's appearance, as well as his verbalizations about his mood, are recorded.

How would he describe his mood? Does it remain the same or change during the day or from day to day? Asking the patient to rate his mood on a scale of 0 to 10 can be useful for an immediate rating of his mood and valuable for comparison of changes that occur during treatment. When the clinical picture is highlighted by a continuous intensification or change in the patient's mood, an affective disorder is suspected.

While eliciting the patient's feelings, if the nurse perceives a potential for suicide, she should attempt to bring out the patient's thoughts about self-destruction. Information about suicidal or homicidal thoughts should be directly addressed. Has he had the desire to harm himself or someone else? Has he made any previous attempts, and, if so, what events surrounded the attempts? To make a judgment about the suicidal or homicidal risk present, the nurse assesses the details of the plans, ability for implementation (availability of guns), patient's attitude about death, and support systems available to him as shown in the following example:

The patient responded to most of the questions asked in a flat dull manner. Although he stated he felt sad about the recent changes in his life, his lifeless posture and tone of voice did not convey any emotional response. He denied any suicidal or homicidal ideation or plans. He related having made two previous suicidal gestures in the past year by "taking pills."

■ Insight

The degree of insight the patient has about the nature of his problem and how it affects his feelings, thoughts, and behavior may be assessed informally as he talks about his problems. It is important to determine if he sees the problem as something brought on by external factors or from within himself. Whether he can see his treatment needs realistically would affect the treatment plan and the setting of mutual goals to meet the patient's needs. Several questions may be helpful to ascertain the patient's degree of insight. What does he think about all he has told the nurse? What does he want to do about it? What does he want others, including the nurse, to do about it? The following example illustrates a patient's level of insight:

The patient enumerated several problems he encountered at work. He reluctantly stated that he might have to change, but really thought that his difficulties were because of his wife's drinking. He believed he could do nothing until she changed.

This third stage of the psychiatric interview completes the assessment of the patient. The mental status examination describes comprehensive data about the patient's mental functioning in an organized manner. Clinical example 6-8 finishes the clinical portrayal of Ms. T.

CLINICAL EXAMPLE 6-8

Ms. T was a stylishly dressed, neatly groomed, slender female, in apparent good physical health who appeared her stated 22 years of age. She was cooperative during the interview but had difficulty expressing herself in specific terms. Her vague responses at times left the interviewer feeling perplexed about the difficulties she was describing.

The patient was alert and awake and oriented to person, place, and situation. Immediate recall and recent memory were intact, demonstrated in her ability to recall three unrelated objects immediately and again in 15 minutes. Some of the historical information given was inconsistent with historical factors reported by her father. Although the vocabulary used by Ms. T and her knowledge of general information was congruent with her twelfth-grade education and past employment, she had difficulty completing the serial sevens but performed serial threes with relative ease. She stated she was "nervous," which may be a factor related to performance. She was able to abstract two of three proverbs presented.

Proverb	Interpretation
Don't cry over spilled milk.	"If something happens, then forget about it. Maybe things will get better."
A rolling stone gathers no moss.	"A good person gathers no enemies. If a person stays active, he won't get depressed."
People who live in glass houses shouldn't throw stones.	"The glass will break."

Her responses to hypothetical situations were appropriate; however, the manner in which she coped with difficulties at work and home showed impairment in judgment about personal issues.

Ms. T's speech was clear, coherent, and of normal rate and tone. Except for the vague tangential manner in which she discussed her concern for her aunt, her communication was goal directed. There were no apparent delusions, hallucinations, or illusions. She denied any obsessions, compulsions, or phobias.

The central theme during the interview was her fear of being irresponsible and hurting her aunt. Her sadness and concern about her behavior in relation to the aunt pervaded the interview. She appeared nervous (looking away, fidgeting) and cried whenever she talked about her aunt. She described her mood as "low" and rated it as a four. She denied any suicidal or homicidal ideation or plan previously or at the present time.

Her insight is questionable, since she questioned her need for treatment, although she agreed to return. She knew a problem existed but was unaware of the causative factors related to her behavior.

Elements of Psychiatric Evaluation

A. Data collection
1. Presenting problem
   a. Onset, duration, symptoms noted, and progression
   b. Solutions attempted
   c. Significant changes in the patient's life
   d. How responsibility for the problem is viewed
2. Characteristic patterns of living and coping behaviors
   a. Medical history and current problems
   b. Psychiatric history for self and family
   c. Family history and personal history: Chronological approach with emphasis on interpersonal relationships and major areas of life experiences
3. Mental status examination
   a. General observations: Appearance, reaction to the interview, consistency of behavior, and response to the patient
   b. Sensorium and intelligence: Level of consciousness, orientation, memory, intellectual functioning, judgment, and comprehension
   c. Thought processes: Characteristics of speech, patterns of verbalizations, manner of communication of thoughts, organization of ideas, coherence of associations, recurring patterns of thoughts, and misperceptions described
   d. Affect: Range, appropriateness, and intensity of affect
   e. Mood: behavioral manifestations and description of mood; and suicidal/homicidal ideation or plan
   f. Insight: Understanding of current situation and solutions
B. Organization and interpretation of data
1. Problem identification: Medical and nursing diagnoses
2. Identification of patient resources
C. Treatment plan

The nurse has assembled a comprehensive data base through history taking and the mental status examination. She has collected objective facts based on observation of the patient's behavior during the interview. In the final stage of the psychiatric evaluation the nurse critically examines the information she has organized in the preceding stages and interprets these data to formulate a treatment plan based on identified patient problems and nursing diagnoses. The elements of a psychiatric evaluation are summarized in the accompanying box.

Additional resources

The psychiatric interview provides the structure to obtain pertinent information about the patient. Additional resources are often utilized to complete a comprehensive assessment of the patient. The medical chart is one resource the nurse can use to collect information about the patient's medical and social histories. This information is recorded in designated sections of the patient's chart by various health team members.

Significant others in the patient's life, including family, friends, a minister, or the family physician can participate in the interview and share valuable perceptions about the patient and his current situation. Family theorists, such as Bowen,[4] stress the importance of the patient's social system in both diagnosis and treatment of psychiatric problems.

The expressive therapies are essential resources for the assessment and treatment of children. Children are often brought for psychiatric evaluation by the family or referred by the school system for behavioral disruptions. Art, dance, or play therapy can provide the means for establishing an initial relationship with the child. These therapies are especially important when the individual is unable to express his ideas verbally or does not want to talk. The family is, again, a vital resource to the clinician working with children.

■ Psychological measurements

Research in recent years has provided a variety of formalized questionnaires and standardized tests as adjunctive methods for assessment. Computers are now utilized for the collection and collation of data, the diagnosis of symptom clusters, and the evaluation of specific treatment modalities.[7] Rating scales can be used to gather information from the patient and significant others. The common rating scales given in the box on page 201 lists those most frequently used (also see Appendix E). Self-report questionnaires filled out by the patient give an account of the subjective distress experienced by the patient. This description can be a more accurate account of the emotional state of the patient than that inferred or elicited in the interview. Questionnaires directed to family members or friends can relate specific characteristics of the patient's social or family life. Some of the circumstances in which psychological testing may be useful are given in the situations testing box on page 202.

Psychological tests are of two types: those designed to evaluate intellectual and cognitive abilities and those designed to describe personality functioning. Some of these are briefly described in Table 6-1. Commonly used intelligence tests are the Wechsler Adult Intelligence Scale (WAIS) and the Wechsler Intelligence Scale for Children (WISC). Although intelligence tests are often criticized for being culturally biased, their ability to determine an individual's strengths and weaknesses within the culture provides essential therapeutic information.

Material obtained from projective tests reflects aspects of an individual's personality functioning, including reality testing ability, impulse control, major defenses, interpersonal conflicts, and self-concept. A battery of tests are usually administered to provide comprehensive information. The Rorschach Test, Thematic Apperception Test (TAT), Bender Gestalt Test, and Minnesota Multiphasic Personality Inventory (MMPI) are commonly used by the clinical psychologist for assessment.

A more detailed discussion of the types of psychological tests available and their clinical applicability can be found elsewhere.[6] It is important for the clinician to be aware of the resources available and the general information that can be obtained from standardized scales and tests. These tests may be administered by the nurse or may require the knowledge and skill of the psychologist for administration and interpretation. Collaboration with the psychologist to review the assessment data obtained and to plan treatment is a responsibility of the nurse as a member of the health team.

■ **Physiological measurements**

Special diagnostic procedures are especially important when the patient or his family describes abrupt changes in his manner of behaving or incidents of loss of consciousness for even brief periods of time. These are the electroencephalogram (EEG), CT scan, lumbar puncture, and blood chemistry values. A listing of normal laboratory values is presented in Table 6-2. Electroencephalography provides a mechanism for recording any changes in the electrical activity in various areas of the brain. The test is useful in diagnosis of epilepsy, brain lesions, and other diseases of, or injury to, the brain. According to the area of the lesion in the brain,

---

Common Rating Scales

Beck Depression Inventory
Hamilton Depression Scale (HAM-D)
Manic-State Scale
Nurses' Observation Scale (NOSIE)
Brief Psychiatric Rating Scale (BPRS)
Clinical Global Impressions Scale (CGI)
Hamilton Anxiety Scale (HAM-A)
Self-Report Symptom Check List (SCL-90).

---

specific symptoms would be demonstrated. The symptom complex would reflect the disruption in the function of the area of the brain involved. Distortion of the senses of taste, smell, sight, or hearing could occur. The patient's ability to speak clearly or understand what is being said to him could affect his pattern of communication. Changes in his personality or mental ability could be displayed in lapses of memory, absentmindedness, or loss of initiative. All these behaviors would be ascertained in the mental status examination. However, if the symptoms are treated from a psychopathological frame of reference, a brain tumor or seizure disorder could be overlooked and the appropriate treatment denied. The EEG, CT scan, and lumbar puncture are essential procedures for the detection of specific brain dysfunctions.

Chemical analysis of various substances in the blood can provide the clinician with diagnostic information. This is especially valuable when a drug-induced delirium is suspected. Many drugs and poisons can cause an organic mental disorder. The most commonly implicated are the opiates, barbiturates, amphetamines, and hallucinogens. The patient may display behaviors ranging from mild confusion and drowsiness to overwhelming anxiety and hallucinations. The blood level and toxic level of the particular drug involved would be important, possibly life-saving, information needed to determine a plan of care.

Symptoms of cerebral dysfunction, including mental confusion, hallucinations, and convulsions, might also occur in certain hypoglycemic states. In this instance the patient's behavior reflects a variation in the normal amount of glucose found in the blood. The etiological factors that might be involved are numerous. It is of particular importance in the organic mental disorders to differentiate these factors so that the appropriate treatment can be instituted.

Situations Where Testing Is Frequently Indicated

Children

1. *Presence of a learning disorder*
   Psychological testing can help delineate the probable etiology and appropriate course of treatment in learning disabilities which may involve central nervous system dysfunction, intellectual deficiency, and/or personality and emotional factors. Tests often provide clues to family and/or school influences in the situation.

2. *Emotional-social disturbances*
   Psychological testing can be useful in gaining understanding of such problems as hyperactivity; antisocial behavior; excessive withdrawal; difficulty adapting to peers, home, and/or school; and language disorders.

3. *Developmental deviations*
   Testing gives information relative to the age-appropriateness of the child's functioning in a wide variety of areas (intellectual, personal-social, perceptual-motor coordination).

Adults

1. *Mental retardation/intellectual deficiency*
   Testing can throw light on the factors interfering with an adult's use of intelligence, as well as provide an assessment of the degree of mental ability in the case of mental retardation. State laws may require an IQ score as part of the diagnosis of mental deficiency in certain situations, such as for custodial care, and support for children with learning disabilities.

2. *Psychotherapy*
   A psychological evaluation can help determine the most appropriate therapeutic mode and goals and is often useful in deciding when to terminate therapy, or understand changes that are occurring during therapy.

3. *Differential diagnosis*
   Psychological evaluations provide measures of a person's functioning ranging from perceptual-cognitive and ego level factors to personality structure, dynamics, and unconscious factors. The analysis of strength and weakness contributes to an understanding of the patterns of the whole person that can be used to derive a differential diagnosis. For adults, testing is often helpful in detecting borderline psychosis, early signs of organicity, and early signs of schizophrenia before symptoms become clearly manifest in clinically observable symptomatology.

4. *Forensic psychiatry*
   A psychological evaluation is often a helpful adjunct in cases involving mental illness or central nervous system impairments following injury. Psychological testing also has many applications in the criminal justice system.

From DeCato, C.M., and Wicks, R.J.: J. Psychiatr. Nurs. **14:**25, June 1976

■ Brain visual imaging in psychiatry

Although techniques of brain visual imaging have not yet affected the clinical practice of psychiatry in a profound way, they show great promise for increasing knowledge of the pathophysiology of mental illness, enhancing diagnostic assessment, and choosing more specific treatments for individual patients. Psychiatric research studies using these five new imaging techniques attempt to identify structural and physiological brain abnormalities underlying the functional impairments in psychiatric illnesses. The following descriptions, from Brown[5] and Friedel,[8] provide a brief explanation of each technique:

1. Computed tomography (**CT scan**) is a radiologic technique which takes cross-sectional x-rays of the brain. Structural changes, like ventricular enlargement, can be identified. These changes have been found in psychiatric patients with a variety of diagnoses and after chronic ingestion of substances like alcohol, but the research concentration to date has been focused on schizophrenia. CT scanning is an expensive

TABLE 6-1

COMMONLY USED PSYCHOLOGICAL TESTS

Name	General classification	Description	Special features
Bellak Children's Apperception Test	Projective technique	Drawings of animals for children	Designed specifically for children
Bender (Visual-Motor) Gestalt Test	Graphomotor technique; may be used as projective technique	Geometric designs that the patient is asked to draw or copy, with design in view	Useful for detecting psychomotor difficulties correlated with brain damage
California Personality Inventory	Objective personality test	Seventeen scales developed presumably for normal populations for use in guidance and selection	Less emphasis on mental illness than MMPI scales, such as, dominance, responsibility, socialization
Cattell 16 Personality Factor Questionnaire (16 PF)	Objective personality test	Questionnaire covering 16 personality factors derived from factor-analytical studies	Bipolar variables allow for interpretation of scores varying either above or below the norm, such as reserved vs. outgoing; trusting vs. suspicious, timid vs. venturesome
Draw-a-Person Test	Graphomotor projective technique	Patient asked to draw a person and then one of the sex opposite to the first drawing	Projects body image, how the body is conceived and perceived; sometimes useful for detecting brain damage; modifications include: draw an animal; draw a house, a tree, and a person (H-T-P); draw your family; draw the most unpleasant concept you can think of
Minnesota Multiphasic Personality Inventory (MMPI) (Forms: Individual, Group, and Shortened R)	Objective personality test	Questionnaire yielding scores for 9 clinical scales in addition to other scales	Includes scales related to test-taking attitudes; empirically constructed on basis of clinical criteria; computer interpretation services available
Rorschach Technique	Projective technique	Ten inkblots used as basis for eliciting associations	Especially revealing of personality structure; most widely used projective technique
Rosenzweig Picture Frustration Test	Projective technique	Cartoon situations, dialogue to be completed by subject	Designed specifically to assess patterns of reaction to typical stress situations; child, adolescent, and adult forms
Sentence Completion Test (SCT)	Varies from direct-response questionnaire to projective technique	Incomplete sentence stems that vary as to their ambiguity	Highly flexible; may be used to tap specific conflict areas; reveals generally more conscious, overt attitudes and feelings
Symonds Picture Story Test	Projective technique	Pictures of adolescents	Designed specifically for adolescents
Thematic Apperception Test (TAT)	Projective technique	Ambiguous pictures used as stimuli for making up a story	Especially useful for revealing personality dynamics; some pictures are designed specifically for women, men, adolescent girls, and adolescent boys

Continued.

TABLE 6-1—cont'd

COMMONLY USED PSYCHOLOGICAL TESTS

Name	General classification	Description	Special features
Wechsler Adult Intelligence Scale (WAIS)	Intelligence test	Eleven subtests: vocabulary, comprehension, information, similarities, digit span, arithmetic, picture arrangement, picture completion, object assembly, block design, and digit symbol	Most commonly used intelligence scale that yields a measure of intelligence expressed as IQ scores; differences in subtests can also be useful clinically
Wechsler Intelligence Scale for Children (WISC)	Intelligence test	Similar to the WAIS	Standardized for children ages 5 to 15
Wechsler Preschool and Primary Scale of Intelligence (WPPSI)	Intelligence test	Similar to the WAIS and WISC	Standardized for children ages 4 to 6½
Word-Association Technique	Projective technique	Stimulus words to which patient responds with first association that comes to mind	Flexible; may be used to tap associations to different conflict areas; generally not as revealing as SCT responses

Modified from Freedman, A.M., Kaplan, H.I., and Sadock, B.J., editors: Comprehensive textbook of psychiatry, ed. 3, Baltimore, 1980, The Williams & Wilkins Co.

TABLE 6-2

BOEHRINGER MANNGEIM 8700
Normal values for blood chemistry. *

BUN	6–22	mg/dl	Creatinine	0.5–1.5	mg/dl	Alkaline phosphatase	29–74	μ/l
Na	131–146	mEq/l	Ldh	112–217	μ/l	Bilirubin	0.1–1.2	mg/dl
K	3.5–5.0	mEq/l	SGOT	6–36	μ/l	Uric acid	2.5–7.7	mg/dl
Cl	95–108	mEq/l	SGPT	9–54	μ/l	Total protein	5.8–7.7	gm/dl
CO_2	23–31	mEq/l	Ca	8.5–10.5	mg/dl	Albumin	3.0–4.5	gm/dl
Glucose	70–110	mg/dl	Phosphorus	2.4–4.2	mg/dl	Cholesterol	0–170	mg/dl

*The range may vary slightly depending on the laboratory where the analysis was done.

procedure with some risk of x-ray overexposure to the patient. It is not indicated if a patient does not show gross neurological deficits on careful mental status or physical examination or on an EEG. Newer imaging techniques are likely to yield more information with less risk.

2. Brain electrical activity mapping (**BEAM**) uses computer analysis to topographically display EEG (electroencephalography) rhythms and evoked response (external electrical and sensory stimulation, i.e., flashes of light, noise, muscle stimulation, etc.) data. The BEAM uses color maps of condensed and summarized data on electrophysiologic activity in the brain. It involves easy and relatively inexpensive modifications of equipment that are familiar and accessible. It seems likely that this technique will be useful for patients who do not fit Draft of the DSM-III-R in Development[2] diagnostic categories and who may be suspected to have subtle organic impairments that are not fully characterized after initial neurologic screening. Thus far, results implicate the frontal lobes as a pathologic site of dysfunction in schizophrenia.

3. Regional cerebral blood flow techniques (**CBF**) utilize probes applied to the scalp to measure decreasing activity of a chemically inert and diffusable gas that emits gamma activity. CBF provides information on blood flow in gray matter and white matter and on relative tissue weights. The gas inhalation technique is used more often than injection into the internal carotid artery. CBF techniques have been used for research purposes to study a variety of psychiatric disorders, are less expensive than PET scanning, and may prove useful in the study of transient mental states. Single photon emission computed tomography (SPECT) is one method used to study CBF, and offers a means of assessing presumed neuronal activity in resting states and with tasks and pharmacological challenges.

4. Positron emission tomography (**PET**) scanning is a tool that quantitatively measures physiological and biochemical functions occurring in live tissue. A compound tagged with a positron-emitting nuclide is given to the patient either by inhalation or by injection. As the positrons are annihilated, these events are measured, and a computer generates color-coded displays. The PET scanner has provided measures of cerebral glucose use which are directly related to functional activity in regions of the brain. These results have shown glucose use to be abnormal in

a variety of psychiatric disorders. PET scanning is an extremely expensive procedure requiring sophisticated equipment, and it entails exposing a patient to a dose of radiation. Although PET scanning is in an early stage of development, it is likely to have a major effect on theory and knowledge of the pathophysiology of mental illness. We can now look at the sites of action of drugs by imaging the drug receptor molecules on the surface of cells in living humans.

5. Nuclear magnetic resonance (**NMR**) imaging is a new technique for obtaining cross-sectional pictures of the entire body. It can provide information on the metabolic and biochemical status of live organs. Simply stated, certain nuclei possess magnetlike behaviors. NMR images are formed by placing the appropriate part of the patient's body within a stationary magnetic field, which causes the nuclei to align in the direction of the field. This direction is then changed or deflected by the application of a radio-frequency pulse, generating an electrical signal which produces a cross-sectional image. After the pulse is turned off, nuclei return to their original direction. The time it takes for this to occur is called "relaxation time." Each atom has specific relaxation times depending on its biological surroundings. Computer-coded visual displays of these relaxation times can be generated. NMR imaging can detect lesions resulting from tumors, metastases, strokes, and abscesses, and can detect abnormalities in some psychiatric disorders in addition to drug effects. This technique does not expose the patient to x-rays or to any apparent health risks, thereby allowing for studies of children and repeated studies of patients over many years. Several potential uses are to study cell energy metabolism and to determine specific sites of action of drugs in the brain.

Diagnostic impression

At this point in the psychiatric evaluation a diagnostic impression is formulated from an integration of significant historical data, observations of the mental status examination, and results of specific tests that have been assembled. Formulating a diagnosis implies an awareness of identified problems, which can be overt, covert, existing, or potential. When an identification of the patient's problems and needs has occurred, it is important to validate these with the patient so that a plan of care can be implemented.

Organization and interpretation of the data collected involve formulating a diagnostic impression. The presenting problem has been identified in terms of the nature of onset, duration, and course. The nurse has clarified the relationship of the patient's behavior to stressors, or the precipitating factors that resulted in his seeking help at this time. These behaviors, along with those assembled in the interview, are compared to documented norms to identify deviations. One's theoretical base may include personality development theory, behavior theory, or systems theory. Each provides a framework for comparing behaviors and identifying deviations. Personality development involves the completion of identified tasks and incorporation of certain skills at various points in an individual's life. Behavior theory encompasses the broad spectrum of human behavior and incorporates individual set factors, such as culture and nationality, in determining the function of certain behavior for an individual in terms of its usefulness. Systems theory can also be used to provide a framework for evaluating factors in the patient's environment (family, community, nation) that influence his behavior.

The patient's behavior is the critical evidence used in formulating a diagnostic impression, regardless of the theoretical framework of the observer. The difficulty that arises in psychiatric diagnosis is in part due to the lack of specificity and simple, valid criteria for the classification of human behavior. Thus psychiatric diagnosis is a complex and controversial issue.

DSM-III and its current revision, Draft of the DSM-III-R in Development,[2] have attempted to increase the reliability of symptomatic diagnosis through the inclusion of specific diagnostic criteria to define each diagnosis. These criteria were utilized in clinical facilities throughout the United States during the development process to identify and solve problems in the classification of disorders. The predecessors to the Draft of the DSM-III-R in Development,[2] DSM-I and DSM-II, lacked sufficient detail in the classification for either clinical or research purposes.

In the DSM-III and Draft of the DSM-III-R in Development,[2] clinically significant behavioral or psychological syndromes that include symptom clusters of patient behaviors are classified as mental disorders (Chapters 2 and 3). A descriptive approach is utilized in the discussion of each disorder and in the division of each disorder into diagnostic classes. This results in the grouping together of syndromes that have common clinical features.

The DSM-III points out that the classification categorizes disorders, not individuals, and that each disorder is not an entity unto itself. Thus the need for an individualized approach to diagnosis is warranted. The approach of the DSM-III and the Draft of the DSM-

III-R in Development,[2] are atheoretical in relation to etiology unless a specific pathophysiological process is known to be causative, and then it is included in the definition of the disorder.

The nurse should possess a working knowledge of the DSM-III and the Draft of the DSM-III-R in Development,[2] so that effective communication can occur through the sharing of a common terminology among health team members. The nurse's knowledge can also be beneficial in helping her to ascertain other behavioral characteristics present in the patient who displays some behaviors suggestive of a particular syndrome. With certain disorders, especially the schizophrenic and affective disorders, effective treatments can be considered according to the similarity of problems exhibited within each category.

Although the DSM-III and the Draft of the DSM-III-R in Development,[2] follows a medical model in its description of symptoms of illness, the identification of specific observable behaviors of the clinical syndromes makes correlation with the nursing process model possible. The nurse, knowledgeable of the clinical syndrome involved, would focus on the nursing diagnosis identified from the assessment data obtained in the evaluation. The nursing diagnosis is a statement that reflects a discrepancy between the patient's behavior and the expected behaviors for a person with similar set factors as related to the stressors involved. For example, alteration in self-concept might be inferred from certain patient behaviors: shabby clothing, unkempt hair, preoccupation with physical concerns, refusal to participate in social activities. Specific nursing actions are then correlated with the nursing problem identified. The patient exhibiting an alteration in self-concept might benefit from specific information on grooming and self-care.

The organization and interpretation of the assessment data depend on the purpose of the interview and the background of the interviewer. As previously discussed, the nurse is guided by the purpose of the interview in determining the assessment data to be collected. A complete psychiatric evaluation is not always warranted, as in an emergency situation, but could be conducted over several interviews with the patient. The nurse may perform the mental status examination along with clarification of the presenting problem and rely on other resources, such as the medical chart, to obtain the pertinent historical data needed in an emergency situation.

The woman described in the beginning of this chapter may not be able to give an accurate account of historical factors when seen by the nurse. However, her mental status at the time needs to be assessed to determine the degree of incapacitation present and the immediate ramifications of it, if any. She was disturbing the peace, but should she be kept in jail overnight or allowed to leave the hospital in her current state of functioning? These are examples of the type of judgment in which the nurse will be involved when assessing patients in an emergency room or crisis clinic.

The educational background and experience of the nurse will also determine the comprehensiveness of the psychiatric evaluation and interpretations made. Nurses employed in mental health facilities will have more opportunity to practice skills in psychiatric evaluation. However, it should be stressed that all nurses need to be knowledgeable about the psychiatric evaluation process and be able to identify deviations from the norm in the patients they assess. The nurse may need to call on someone more knowledgeable in the area of psychiatry, such as the clinical specialist, for assistance in identifying particular disorders and determining a plan of care. The importance is in assessing the patient as a total being, including his state of mental health. This involves a basic knowledge about psychological behaviors as well as the sociological and biological behaviors.

■ Case disposition

A brief summary of factors to consider in making a decision about a case disposition will be presented. The three general areas to consider are the identified problem, the limitations and strengths of the individual, and the treatment resources available. Each area will be discussed separately and followed by a continuation of the case study of Ms. T.

The problem areas identified in the psychiatric evaluation are addressed in order of priority. The symptoms described by the patient in the presenting problem should be addressed first, since they are usually those causing most discomfort to the patient at the time he seeks treatment. However, as in other areas, the patient may not always be aware of or admit to problems that are of importance. Priority is always given to those which, if not treated, will threaten the life of the individual or the life of another. An individual's suicidal or homicidal potential must be considered first and an appropriate treatment plan provided. Another factor to consider in deciding priorities is whether the behavior observed is an expression of a failure of the individual's coping mechanisms, as in a crisis, or an expression of lifelong maladaptive behavior. The limitations of the individual in coping with the identified problems, especially in self-protection, are considered. In certain instances of psychotic behavior the individual may not be aware of his inability to care for himself and therefore may need brief hospitalization. The depressed individual is also a candidate for hospitalization, and his suicidal

risk must be evaluated at all times. The support system available to the patient is considered in determining what modality of treatment is used. A number of factors should be considered in determining whether the patient should be hospitalized or referred for outpatient treatment. These include the family and significant others available to the patient; his strengths, including past coping abilities; the values and beliefs he has regarding his life; and his ability to meet the demands of the situation.

The nature of the problem will indicate the treatment modality and related goals. For example, the patient who complains of an inability to form intimate relationships may benefit from both individual and group therapy. The man who complains of impotence with his spouse may be best able to work on this problem and related issues in couples therapy.

If the nurse is involved in the implementation of therapy, the problem should be defined in measurable terms so that both the nurse and the patient can evaluate if change is occurring in the therapeutic process. It is useful to ascertain what change the patient wants, since this allows for a focus on a particular issue and the definition of goals for therapy.

Whatever the nurse's goal might entail, on completion of the psychiatric evaluation she should be able to make a recommendation to the patient. This involves being knowledgeable about the community agencies available to the patient and what services they can and cannot provide.

Clinical example 6-9 (on page 208) illustrates how the data obtained in a psychiatric evaluation are used in a final disposition with identified problem areas and a formulated treatment plan. The techniques of interviewing, differentiating symptoms, establishing a diagnosis, and formulating a treatment plan are skills the inexperienced nurse will develop with experience and a sound theoretical base.

As in other areas of nursing, it is essential that the nurse become aware of the health team members working with the patient in the health care system. The treatment plan identified must be congruent with the plans of the other health care professionals working with the patient. Communication among those involved in the patient's care, such as the physician, social worker, and psychologist, should occur throughout all stages of the nursing process if a successful outcome is to be achieved.

The psychiatric evaluation is similar to the nursing process model in that it is a systematic problem-solving approach to patient care. Assessment data are obtained during the initial stages of the evaluation, and a treatment plan with identified goals is formalized in the final stage of the psychiatric evaluation. Whether the nurse

---

CLINICAL EXAMPLE 6-9

Ms. T stated she does not socialize any more, as evidenced by her leaving her job and withdrawal from family and friends. She spends her day at home cleaning, cooking, and listening to the radio alone in her room, which are solitary activities. She stated she felt inferior to her peers at work and was denied two promotions. She feels fearful about going out because she might make a fool of herself.

Ms. T's history reveals a lack of consistent nurturing in the home and an unstable family structure. The grandmother seemed to be a source of support and nurturance to Ms. T and has recently died. There was no evidence of role models for the development of intimate relationships in the home. Ms. T described herself as a "shy kid" who had few friends in childhood. She expressed feelings of hatred for most of her siblings. The aunt has provided for her, and the overwhelming concern Ms. T has about hurting the aunt may relate to fear of rejection, thereby losing the one stable relationship she believes she has left.

Ms. T presented an attractive appearance. She appeared to have difficulty relating to the interviewer, which was evidenced in her vague responses. She seemed to hide behind the sunglasses that she wore throughout the interview. She stated a concern about her decreasing ability to relate to others and a fear of attempting to do so.

The developmental tasks of the young adult include an increase in socialization and intimacy. It is a time when an individual's involvement in relationships and special interests provide for a sense of self-satisfaction. A pursuit of career goals occurs. The relationships formed and goals attained related to work or school become a source of positive feelings about oneself. In comparing the data obtained in the interview with developmental norms, a discrepancy exists. Two problem areas are evident: a decrease in socialization and a decrease in self-esteem.

The related nursing diagnoses would include (1) social isolation related to increased stress at work and home evidenced in withdrawal and (2) disturbance in self-concept related to feelings of guilt evidenced by statements of self-blame.

The treatment modality selected is long-term individual psychotherapy with the following goals. The patient will (1) establish a relationship with the therapist, (2) reestablish contact with friends, (3) resume vocational activities (school or work), and (4) experience activities within her capabilities to increase self-esteem. Conjunctive therapies considered are group and family therapy. Group therapy would provide the patient with the opportunity to develop and test socialization skills. Family therapy would focus on the interrelationship of the patient's problem with the family process. The selection of the type of therapy depends on the framework of the therapist and the availability of other modalities.

---

is involved only in the initial contact with the patient or participates in the treatment plan identified, she has completed the stages of the nursing process. Through interaction with the patient the nurse has been involved in assessment, planning, intervention, and evaluation even though the actual time spent in the last two stages may be minimal if a referral is made.

Future trends

It is difficult to project what might occur in the future. The experience and wisdom developed in the past century have brought changes no one could have foreseen. The study of the psyche is something that has historically perplexed human beings. Various schools of thought have emerged in an attempt to understand the development of the uniqueness of the human species. Theories of personality were developed by Freud, Sullivan, Erikson, and others as they observed and recorded the behavior of their patients over extended periods of time. Objective evaluation of behavior as an expression of the inner self remains a difficult task for the practitioner. Psychiatric evaluation still takes place in the subjective experience which evolves in the relationship that develops between the individuals involved. As advancement in technology has influenced the efficiency and effectiveness of the care a patient receives in the health care field, in the future the evaluation of the subjective side of humans will become increasingly more objective.

Psychological testing is being used more by practitioners in an attempt to expand or validate their objective impressions, as described earlier in the discussion of the resources available to the practitioner. Research has produced a variety of assessment tools, such as questionnaires, that aim to elicit certain information about the patient which can be compared to standardized results. A method for computerized psychiatric evaluation has been developed.

The role of the nurse in the health care system is being redefined as nurses continue to increase their independent functions and identify their unique contribution to the health care team. Nurses with advanced knowledge and experience in psychiatry are becoming private practitioners to meet the psychosocial demands of the population. Nurses in private practice often utilize other nurses, as well as psychiatrists, as consultants to their practice.

In considering the future trends in psychiatric evaluations, the legal implications increase as the population becomes more health oriented and adept at pursuing the right to health care. Diagnosis and treatment of health problems are scrutinized by the population and by the courts. Reported cases of negligence and malpractice are on the rise. This trend makes objective evaluation essential for the future practitioner. The integration of research and clinical practice is crucial for optimum care of human psychosocial needs. Care implies prevention and maintenance in the realm of mental health, and it should complement the established goal, cure.

◼ SUGGESTED CROSS-REFERENCES ◼

The Draft of the DSM-III-R in Development,[2] and the medical model are discussed in Chapters 2 and 3. Therapeutic relationship skills are discussed in Chapter 4. Impaired cognition is discussed in Chapter 19.

◼ SUMMARY ◼

1. As vital members of the health care team, nurses must assume a role in the psychiatric evaluation of patients. Basic knowledge of the concepts of psychodynamics, psychopathology, and psychotherapy combined with interviewing and assessment skills are the tools nurses need to perform a psychiatric evaluation. The role assumed by the nurse will depend on the level of nursing preparation obtained and the health care system in which the nurse is employed.

2. The basic elements of a psychiatric evaluation are the psychiatric interview and the mental status examination. The interview provides the structure for systematic collection of pertinent data about the patient through history taking and the mental status examination. The purpose of the psychiatric interview is to establish rapport with the patient, gain knowledge of his characteristic patterns of living and coping behaviors, and assess his mental functioning. Listening and observation skills are used by the nurse to create an open atmosphere that encourages self-disclosure by the patient.

3. A clear account of the presenting problem and the events that led up to the occurrence, or history of the pre-

---

DIRECTIONS FOR FUTURE RESEARCH

The following are some of the nursing research problems raised in Chapter 6 that merit further study by psychiatric nurses:

1. Investigation of the role of the psychiatric nurse as the primary evaluator
2. Reformulation and standardization of the psychiatric interview format leading to specific nursing diagnoses
3. Use of the psychiatric interview factors as predictors of outcome in patient response to treatment
4. A study of the Draft of the DSM-III-R in Development[2] diagnoses and their correlation with the formulation of nursing diagnoses
5. Exploration of the effect of medical status on the mental status of hospitalized, psychiatric patients
6. Exploration of the establishment of rapport and the effective collection of data
7. Measurement of the reliability of subjective patient history through the use of the mental status exam as an objective tool—pre- and post-examination
8. Early identification of patients at risk for expression of depression through self-destructive behaviors
9. A study of the assessment of specific factors of organicity which affect nursing care plan expectations in the psychiatric, inpatient setting
10. Exploration of comparisons between patient and interviewer perceptions of the presenting problem and its effect on the formulation of nursing diagnoses

---

senting problem, is obtained in the initial stage of a psychiatric evaluation.

4. Data collection through history taking involves obtaining information about the patient's medical and psychiatric history, family history, and personal history, including a sexual and drug history. These data are collected in the second stage of the psychiatric evaluation.

5. The mental status examination organizes observational data about a patient's mental functioning in six categories: general observations, sensorium and intelligence, thought processes, affect, mood, and insight. These data represent the third stage of a psychiatric evaluation.

6. Additional resources for data collection include the medical chart, significant others in the patient's life, formalized questionnaires, and standardized tests.

7. Brain imaging techniques may be helpful in completing a thorough assessment.

8. A diagnostic impression is formulated from an integration of significant historical data, observations of the mental status examination, and the results of special tests and diagnostic procedures. The nurse critically examines the comprehensive data obtained and interprets her findings on the basis of the comparison of patient behaviors to documented norms. Formulating a diagnostic impression entails the identification of the clinical syndrome displayed and the nursing diagnoses identified.

9. The organization and interpretation of the collected data and identification of a case disposition complete the final stage of a psychiatric evaluation. Making a case disposition involves awareness of the identified problems and related nursing diagnoses, the limitations and strengths of the individual, and the treatment resources available. Communication with other health professionals involved in a patient's care is imperative to ensure goal achievement.

10. Psychiatric evaluation is similar to the nursing process model in that it is a systematic, problem-solving approach to patient care. The assessment data obtained and their organization and interpretation depend on the purpose of the interview and background of the interviewer, the nurse.

11. Future trends in the psychiatric evaluation of patients include the development of more objective tests and measurements in computerized form. A practical consideration in obtaining skill in the psychiatric evaluation of patients is the legal implication of an undiagnosed psychiatric problem.

■ REFERENCES ■

1. Alston, J.F., and Levet, J.M.: What's happening: practical application of the mental status exam, Nurs. Pract. **2:**37, July-Aug. 1977.
2. American Psychiatric Association: Draft of the DSM-III-R in Development (subject to change), as proposed by the Work Group to Revise DSM-III. Washington, D.C., 1985, The Association.
3. Balis, G.U., Wurmser, L., and McDaniel, E.: Clinical psychopathology, Woburn, Mass., 1978, Butterworth Publishers, Inc.
4. Bowen, M.: Family therapy in clinical practice, New York, 1978, Jason Aronson, Inc.
5. Brown, R.P., and Kneeland, B.: Visual imaging in psychiatry. Hosp. Community Psychiatry **36**(5):489-495, May 1985.
6. DeCato, C.M., and Wicks, R.J.: Psychological testing referrals: a guide for psychiatrists, psychiatric nurses, physicians in general practice, and allied health personnel, J. Psychiatr. Nurs. **14:**24, June 1976.
7. Freedman, A.M., Kaplan, H.I., and Sadock, B.J., editors: Comprehensive textbook of psychiatry, ed. 3, Baltimore, 1980, The Williams & Wilkins Co.
8. Friedel, R.O., Cormack, MacL. A., Kuhar, M.J., et al.: Changing colors in psychiatry, Proceedings of a Symposium: Changing colors in psychiatry: Advances in brain imaging techniques, p. 1-51, 1984.
9. Group for the Advancement of Psychiatry: Assessment of sexual function: a guide to interviewing, New York, 1973, Mental Health Materials Center, Inc.
10. Imboden, J.B.: Practical psychiatry in medicine. Part 16. Psychiatric evaluation of the medical patient, J. Fam. Pract. **10:**4, April 1980.
11. Nyman, G.: The mental status examination. In Balis, G.U., Wurmser, L., and Grenell, R.: Psychiatric foundations of medicine, Woburn, Mass., 1978, Butterworth Publishers, Inc.
12. Snyder, J.C., and Wilson, M.F.: Elements of a psychological assessment, Am. J. Nurs. **77:**235, 1977.
13. Sullivan, H.S.: The psychiatric interview, New York, 1954, W.W. Norton & Co., Inc.

■ ANNOTATED SUGGESTED READINGS ■

American Psychiatric Association: Diagnostic and statistical manual of mental disorders, Draft of the DSM-III-R in Development (subject to change) as proposed by the Work Group to Revise DSM-III. Washington, D.C., 1985, The Association.

This book presents the most recent classifications of mental disorders with a comprehensive description of each diagnostic category.

*Cihlar, CR.: Mental status assessment for the ET nurse: psychologic impact of physical trauma, J. Enterostomal Ther. **13**(2):49-53, Mar.-Apr. 1986.

The author discusses characteristic reactions to physical trauma in the emergency trauma patient and the specific assessment of mental status particularly in reference to nursing care approaches.

*Critchley, D.L.: Mental status examination with children and adolescents: a developmental approach, Nurs. Clin. North Am. **14:**3, Sept. 1979.

The author describes the developmental framework she utilizes for organization of the mental status examination with children and adolescents. Suggestions for age-appropriate activities, such as play and art, are included in a discussion of the structure of the interview.

*Cunningham, R.: Nursing assessment of depression in the aged adult, Home Health Nurse **2**(4):9-16, July-Aug. 1984.

The author explores the differentiation of depression in the elderly through assessment of characteristics specific to the geriatric patient.

*DeCato, C.M., and Wicks, R.J.: Psychological testing referrals: a guide for psychiatrists, psychiatric nurses, physicians in general practice and allied health personnel, J. Psychiatr. Nurs. **14:**24, June 1976.

---

*Asterisk indicates nursing reference.

This article describes the nature of psychological evaluation and gives general guidelines for making referrals for psychological testing.

Freedman, A.M., Kaplan, H.I., and Sadock, B.J., editors: Comprehensive textbook of psychiatry, ed. 3, Baltimore, 1980, The Williams & Wilkins Co.

An in-depth discussion of the diagnosis and classification of symptoms observed in the psychiatric patient is presented in the chapters that address psychiatric evaluation. Specific guidelines are provided to the clinician in a well-organized, easily understood format for obtaining pertinent information in the psychiatric interview, taking a history, and performing the mental status examination.

Friedman, S., Feinsilver, D., Davis, G., et al.: Decision to admit in an inner-city psychiatric emergency room: beyond diagnosis—the psychosocial factors, Psychiatr. Q. **53**:259-274, 1981.

This article addresses historical factors in the assessment of patients, which influence psychiatric admission.

Group for the Advancement of Psychiatry: Assessment of sexual function: a guide to interviewing, New York, 1973, Mental Health Materials Center, Inc.

The publication gives a straightforward approach to the assessment of sexual function of the individual. Specific questions are included with the discussion of various age groups and particular problems that might occur at the stages of development.

Groves, J.E.: Taking care of the hateful patient, N. Engl. J. Community Ment. Health **6**:313-318, 1970.

The article explores the specific dynamics related to a behavioral diagnosis and its assessment.

Hankoff, L.D., Mischorr, M., et al.: A program of crisis intervention in the medical setting, Am. J. Psychiatry **131**(1):47-50, 1974.

This article deals with interventions associated with the assessment of problems affecting general medical patients.

*Hays, R.: The set test to screen mental status quickly, Geriatric Nurse **5**(2):96-7, Mar.-Apr. 1984.

The author introduces a tool for brief assessment of mental status in the elderly inpatient.

Hoehn, S.R., Hatcher, M., and Weiskopf, C.: Disposition of psychiatric emergency patients: patient characteristics associated with hospitalizations, Ann. Emerg. Med. **9**:605-609, 1980.

The author identifies a patient population who exhibit symptomatology which most often requires further psychiatric intervention and treatment.

Imboden, J.B.: Practical psychiatry in medicine. Part 16. Psychiatric evaluation of the medical patient, J. Fam. Pract. **10**:4, April 1980.

The importance of a psychiatric evaluation of the medical patient is conveyed in the discussion of the relationships between biological and psychosocial factors in illness. A general review of the broad classification of psychiatric illness, elements of a psychiatric diagnosis, factors to consider in a psychiatric interview, and the format for a psychiatric evaluation are clearly and concisely described.

*Johnson, M.N.: Theoretical basis for nursing diagnosis in mental health nursing, Issues Ment. Health Nurs. **6**(1-2):53-71, 1984.

The author describes the dynamic theorems that represent the formulation of nursing diagnoses in the psychiatric setting.

*Lancaster, J.: Adult psychiatric nursing, New York, 1980, Medical Examination Publishing Co., Inc.

Chapter 6 presents an assessment tool for the psychiatric setting. The tool outlines the areas included in a psychiatric evaluation and incorporates specific questions that address each area.

Lesser, A.L.: Problem-based interviewing in general practice: a model, Med. Educ. **19**(4):299-304, July 1985.

This article integrates mental health and evaluation principles into the general assessment of medical patients, presenting to the general practitioner a systems approach to diagnosis.

McIntyre, J.S.: Mania: the common symptoms of several illnesses, Postgrad. Med. **66**:1, July 1979.

Case histories of patients coming to the emergency room with mania are utilized for discussion of the assessment data necessary for evaluation and appropriate treatment.

*Ninns, M., and Makohon, R.: Alzheimer's disease functional assessment of the patient, Geriatric Nursing **6**(3):139-42, May 1985.

A timely article about early detection of Alzhiemer's disease related to observations of behavioral levels of function.

Nyman, G.: The mental status examination. In Balis, G.U., Wurmser, L., McDaniel, E., and Grenell, R.: Psychiatric foundations of medicine, Woburn, Mass., 1978, Butterworth Publishers, Inc.

A comprehensive discussion of the mental status examination is presented here. Case histories are included and compared as each section of the mental status examination is discussed. This is an excellent reference for a more thorough examination of the psychiatric patient.

Paykel, E.S.: The clinical interview for depression: development, reliability and validity, J. Affective Disord. **9**(1):85-96, July 1985.

The author explores specific characteristics of depression and the mechanism of interview technique to formulate the diagnostic impression. Statistical validity of the methodology is reviewed.

Rapp, M.S.: Re-examination of the clinical mental status examination, Can. J. Psychiatry **24**:8, Dec. 1979.

The author questions the objectivity of the data obtained in the mental status examination, especially in the areas of insight, memory, judgment, and intelligence. He implies that individual differences in the examiner and patient could distort the judgments made.

*Rector, C.S., and Foster, M.E.: Assessment and care of the patient experiencing alcohol withdrawal syndrome, Crit. Care Nurse **4**(4):64-8, July-Aug. 1984.

This article defines characteristics of alcohol withdrawal syndrome and the subsequent nursing care involved as a result of individual assessment techniques.

*Robitaille-Tremblay, M.: A data collection tool for the psychiatric nurse, Can. Nurse. **81**(7):26-31, Aug. 1984.

The author has developed a structured brief assessment tool for systematic collection and analysis of psychiatric patient data.

Spitzer, R.L., Skodol, A.E., Gibbon, M., and Williams, J.B.W.: DSM-III case book, Washington, D.C., 1981, The American Psychiatric Association.

This collection of case vignettes is helpful in its descriptive correlation of clinical material to the principles of the DSM-III. The discussion following each vignette includes the rationale for the diagnosis according to the diagnostic criteria outlined in the DSM-III.

Sullivan, H.S.: The psychiatric interview, New York, 1954, W.W. Norton & Co., Inc.

In this book Sullivan describes both the patient and therapist as they interact during the psychiatric interview. He stresses the importance of the patient-therapist relationship in understanding the patient as a unique person. Assessment of the patient is incorporated throughout the book as the stages of the interview are presented.

Taylor, M.A., Abrams, R., Faber, R., and Almy, G.: Cognitive tasks in the mental status examination, J. Nerv. Ment. Dis. **168**:3, March 1980.

A neuropsychological approach to the mental status examination is presented. The article outlines cognitive tasks, dysfunctions, abnormal responses, and suggested localization of cortical dysfunction.

Taylor, M.: The neuropsychiatric mental status examination, New York, 1982, Spectrum.

An update of the mental status examination which includes the exploration of organicity factors in cognitive function.

Winslow, G.S., Ballinger, B.R., and McHarg, A.M.: Standardized psychiatric interview in elderly demented patients, Br. J. Psychiatry **147**:545-6, Nov. 1985.

This article presents a specific interview for dementia which yields statistical data for reliability and validity.

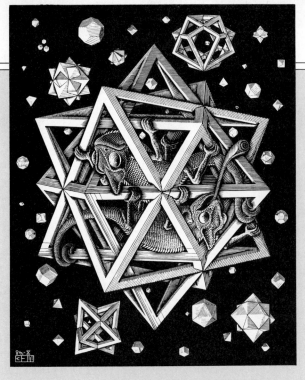

Pinel immediately led Couthon to the section for the deranged, where the sight of the cells made a painful impression on him. Couthon asked to interrogate all the patients. From most, he received only insults and obscene apostrophes. It was useless to prolong the interview. Turning to Pinel, Couthon said: "Now, citizen, are you mad yourself to seek to unchain such beasts?" Pinel replied calmly: "Citizen, I am convinced that these madmen are so intractable only because they have been deprived of air and liberty."

Philippe Pinel, Traité Complet du Régime Sanitaire des Alienes 56 (1836)

C H A P T E R 7

LEGAL AND ETHICAL ASPECTS OF PSYCHIATRIC CARE

LEARNING OBJECTIVES

After studying this chapter, the student should be able to:

- state the admission, discharge, and status of civil rights as they pertain to informal, voluntary, and involuntary admission to a psychiatric hospital.

- describe the legal justification for commitment, the commitment process, and the three types of resulting hospitalization.

- analyze the moral, legal, and psychiatric implications of involuntary commitment, including the issues of assessing dangerousness and freedom of choice.

- identify the common civil and personal rights retained by psychiatric patients.

- define the following terms: testamentary capacity, incompetency, confidentiality, privileged communication, and malpractice.

- evaluate the potential benefits and problems that may arise from the right to treatment, the right to refuse treatment, and the right to treatment in the least restrictive setting.

- discuss the rights, responsibilities, and potential conflict of interest attendant in the three legal roles of the nurse: as provider, employee, and citizen.

- compare and contrast the four sets of criteria commonly used in the United States to determine the criminal responsibility of a person believed to be mentally ill.

- assess the role of ethics in psychiatric nursing.

- define an ethical dilemma and relate one that arises in psychiatric nursing practice.

- apply the model for ethical decision making to a personally encountered ethical dilemma.

- critique the five forces currently affecting the mental health delivery system and the mechanisms and resources needed to improve the quality of mental health care in this country.

- identify directions for future nursing research.

- select appropriate readings for further study.

To assess the awareness of psychiatric professionals of the legal rights of their patients, Trancredi and Clark[40] conducted a study that included psychiatrists, psychiatric residents, nurses, and social workers. The results indicated that they were generally unaware of a patient's legal rights at the time of admission and during hospitalization. Yet the relationship between psychiatry and law reflects the tension between individual rights and social needs, and the two areas have many similarities. Both psychiatry and law deal with human behavior, interrelationships between people, and responsibilities people assume based on these relationships. Both also have a role in society's desire for control of undesirable behavior. Together they mutually analyze when psychiatric treatment is therapeutic, custodial, or incarceration.

There are also discrete differences between the two disciplines. Psychiatry is concerned with the meaning of behavior and personal life satisfaction. Law addresses the outcome of behavior and has developed a system of rules and regulations to facilitate orderly social functioning. These differences are evident in terminology when it is recognized that "insane" and "legal commitment" are predominantly legal, not psychiatric, terms. Lawyers, judges, and juries determine whether a person was insane when he acted and whether a psychotic individual should be legally committed for a period of treatment.

The practice of psychiatric nursing is influenced by the law, particularly in concern for the rights of patients and the quality of care they are receiving. In the past 20 years, civil, criminal, and consumer rights have been established and expanded through judicial decision. Previously powerless and neglected groups such as the mentally ill are now using the legal system as both a forum for the expression of legitimate grievances and as a vehicle for social change. Many of the laws vary from state to state, and professionals are required to become familiar with the legal provisions of their own states because knowledge of the law enhances the freedom of both the nurse and patient.

Hospitalizing the patient

One out of every eight Americans needs some form of mental health services, and a fourth of the people receiving psychiatric care are hospitalized. Not everyone

TABLE 7-1

DISTINGUISHING CHARACTERISTICS OF THE THREE TYPES OF ADMISSION TO PSYCHIATRIC HOSPITALS

	Informal admission	Voluntary admission	Involuntary admission
Admission	No formal application needed	Formal application must be completed by patient	Application did not originate with patient
Discharge	Initiated by patient	Initiated by patient	Initiated by hospital or court but not by patient
Status of civil rights	Retained in full by patient	Retained in full by patient	Patient may retain none, some, or all, depending on state law
Justification	Voluntarily seeks help	Voluntarily seeks help	Mentally ill and one or more of the following: 1. Dangerous to others 2. Dangerous to self 3. Need for treatment

who requires psychiatric care receives it, but the population statistics of mental hospitals are still imposing. Ten of every 10,000 Americans are patients in public mental hospitals, and state hospitals provide a major portion of long-term care for those patients with chronic illness. More than 25% of all hospital beds in the country are occupied by psychiatric patients, and there are three times as many patients on record at psychiatric hospitals as there are criminals in prison.[30] The process of hospitalization can be traumatic or supportive for the individual, depending on the institution, attitude of family and friends, response of the staff, and type of admission. Three major types are used at present: informal, voluntary, and involuntary. Characteristics that distinguish the three major types of hospitalization are summarized in Table 7-1.

■ Informal admission

This type of admission to a psychiatric hospital occurs in the same way a person is admitted to a general medical hospital, that is, without formal or written application. The individual is then free to leave at any time, as he would be in a general medical hospital. The patient is often requested to sign himself out "against medical advice," but he is not required to do so.

■ Voluntary admission

Under this procedure any citizen of lawful age may apply in writing (usually by use of a standard admission form) for admission to a public or private psychiatric hospital. He agrees to receive treatment and abide by the hospital rules. His reason for seeking help may be his own personal decision or may be based on the advice of family or a health professional. If a person is too ill to complete the admission process but voluntarily seeks help, a parent or legal guardian may request admission for him. In most states a child under the age of 16 may be admitted if his parents sign the required application form.

This is a preferred type of admission because it is similar to that of any medical hospitalization. It indicates that the individual acknowledges problems in living, is seeking help in coping with them, and will probably actively participate in finding solutions. The majority of patients who enter private psychiatric units of general hospitals are voluntary.

When admitted in this manner, the patient retains all his civil rights. These include such privileges as the right to vote, possess a driver's license, buy and sell property, manage personal affairs, hold office, practice a profession, and engage in a business. It is a common misconception of the public that all admissions to a mental hospital involve the loss of civil rights.

If the voluntary patient wishes to be discharged from the hospital, most states require that he give written notice to the hospital. In some states he can be released immediately; in others he can be detained from 48 hours to 15 days before being discharged. This allows the hospital staff time to confer with the patient and family members and decide if additional inpatient treatment is necessary. If it is and the patient will not withdraw his request for discharge, the family may initiate involuntary commitment proceedings and thereby change the status of the patient.

Although voluntary admission is most desirable, it is not always possible. Sometimes a patient may be acutely disturbed, suicidal, or dangerous to self or others and yet rejecting of any therapeutic intervention. In these cases involuntary commitments are then initiated.

■ Involuntary admission (commitment)

In the late 1940s the World Health Organization reported that almost 90% of admissions to state mental hospitals in the United States were involuntary commitments. Conversely, only little more than 10% were voluntary. The trend has definitely shifted to more voluntary admissions. In 1963, 30% were voluntary, and by 1971 nearly half of all admissions to psychiatric hospitals were initiated by the patient himself.[5] This trend is due to the greater variety of admission statuses and more stringent limitations placed on the use of involuntary commitment. This is still in striking contrast to England, however, where over 80% of the patients are admitted voluntarily.

Although involuntary commitment has come under more intense scrutiny, the United States Supreme Court continues to recognize it based on two legal theories: first, under its "police power," the state has the authority to protect the community from the dangerous acts of the mentally ill; second, under its *parens patriae* powers, the state has an interest in providing care for citizens who cannot care for themselves, such as some mentally ill persons. In the past 20 years, and particularly over the most recent ones, the police power rationale for civil commitment has been supplanting the *parens patriae* doctrine by means of statutory changes. In addition, there has been a related trend toward increasing the requirements for standards of proof and procedural due process for such commitments.

Involuntary commitment does not always imply compulsion. It means that the request for hospitalization did not originate with the patient and may signify that either it was actively opposed by him or he was indecisive and did not resist. The criteria for commitment vary among states and reflect the confusion present in the medical, social, and legal arenas of society. Most laws justify commitment of the mentally ill on three grounds: (1) dangerous to others, (2) dangerous to self, or (3) need for treatment. The important element appears to be whether the person can function in a reasonable manner in the outside world without becoming an undue burden on his family or the community. The vagueness of these criteria is reflected in the patients committed to psychiatric hospitals. Those suffering from psychoses account for less than half of all admissions, and the aged, the neurotic, and others account for the majority.[23]

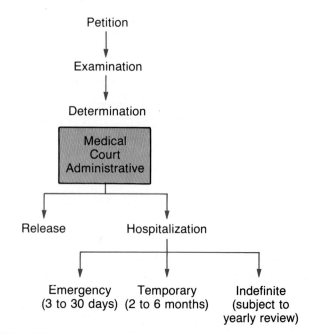

Fig. 7-1 Diagrammatical model of the involuntary committment process.

■ THE COMMITMENT PROCESS.

State laws on commitment vary, but they attempt to protect the individual who is not mentally ill from being detained in a psychiatric hospital against his will for political, economic, family, or other nonmedical reasons. Certain procedural elements of the commitment process are common. Action is begun with a sworn petition by a relative, friend, public official, physician, or any interested citizen stating the person is mentally ill and is in need of treatment. Some states allow only specific individuals to file such a petition. An examination of the patient's mental status is then completed by one or two physicians. Some states require at least one of the physicians be a psychiatrist.

The decision as to whether the patient requires hospitalization is then made. Precisely who makes this decision determines the nature of the commitment. **Medical** certification means a specified number of appointed physicians make the decision. This power to certify is given to all physicians and not limited to psychiatrists. **Court or judicial** commitment is decided on by a judge or jury in a formal hearing. In this case the court is required to notify the patient so that he can retain legal counsel to prepare for the hearing if he desires to contest it. A jury trial is not mandatory in most states but can be requested by the patient. Most states recognize the right of the patient to have legal counsel, but only about half actually appoint a lawyer for the patient if he does not have one. **Administrative** commitment is deter-

TABLE 7-2

DISTINGUISHING CHARACTERISTICS OF THE THREE TYPES OF INVOLUNTARY HOSPITALIZATION

	Emergency	Temporary	Indefinite
Goals	Controlling an immediate threat to self or others	Diagnosis and short-term therapy	Treatment until determined ready for discharge
Time limit	3 to 30 days	2 to 6 months	Indeterminate

mined by a special tribunal of hearing officers. The Fourteenth Amendment to the United States Constitution protects citizens against infringements on liberty without "due process of the law." Because of this, medical certification is used infrequently and primarily in emergency situations, and administrative commitment is subject to judicial review.

If the individual is determined to be in need of treatment, the final step of the commitment process then occurs and he is hospitalized. This may be for varying lengths of time, depending on the needs of the patient. Fig. 7-1 presents a diagrammatical model of the involuntary commitment process. It identifies three types of hospitalization: emergency, temporary, and indefinite. Characteristics that distinguish these types of hospitalization are described in Table 7-2.

Emergency hospitalization. Almost all states have provisions for emergency commitment for patients who are acutely ill. The goals for the commitment are short term, and it is primarily intended as a means of controlling an immediate threat to self or others. In those states lacking such a law the acutely ill individual is often taken into custody by the police and kept in jail on a disorderly conduct charge, which is a criminal charge. Such a practice is inappropriate and frequently detrimental to the mental status of the patient.

To obtain an emergency commitment, the patient's family, a physician, or someone designated by the state must file a petition that includes a supporting report by a psychiatrist. It is then reviewed by a judge or hospital official, and hospitalization is provided. Most state laws limit the time the person can be detained under emergency commitment to from 3 to 30 days. Emergency hospitalization allows for detainment in a psychiatric hospital only until proper legal steps are taken to provide for additional hospitalization.

Temporary or observational hospitalization. This type of commitment is primarily used for the pur-

pose of diagnosis and short-term therapy and does not require an emergency situation, as does the emergency hospitalization. Again, the commitment is for a specified period of time, but in this case it ranges from 2 to 6 months. The commitment process is similar to that just described. Some states require a court order for all temporary commitments, whereas others require one only if the person protests the hospitalization. If at the end of the stipulated period of time the patient is still not ready for discharge, a petition can be filed for an indefinite commitment.

Indefinite hospitalization (formal commitment). A formal commitment provides for the hospitalization of a patient for an indeterminate amount of time or until he is ready for discharge. The process is usually that of a court commitment. Patients in public or state hospitals more frequently have indefinite commitments than patients in private hospitals. Even when committed, these patients maintain their right to consult a lawyer at any time and to request a court hearing to determine if additional hospitalization is necessary. The hospital ultimately discharges the patient, however, and a court order is not necessary to do this.

■ Commitment dilemma

In nine states involuntary commitment assumes incompetency and is accompanied by the patient's loss of his civil rights. He is restricted in his ability to make contracts, vote, drive, obtain a professional license, serve on a jury, marry, or enter into civil litigation. In addition, the patient must suffer the stigma attached to the label "committed" in all his future activities. Because of the large number of people affected by involuntary commitment and the loss of personal rights that it entails, it becomes a matter of great legal, moral, social, and psychiatric significance. In the practice of general medicine there is no equivalent divestment of individual rights except for rare cases of mandated quarantine for carriers of some potentially epidemic diseases.

The question may be asked "How disturbed or ill does one need to be to merit commitment as insane?" A psychotic state is not a necessary or sufficient cause for commitment, as evident in the number of elderly, addicted, and neurotic patients hospitalized, as well as the many psychotic individuals who remain at liberty. Perhaps a person's dangerousness to himself or others is a more pertinent consideration. Certainly psychiatric professionals consider hospitalization in this instance as a humanitarian gesture and as a protection of the individual and society. "Dangerousness," however, is an undefined, unspecified term.

Dangerousness. It is interesting to note that people who are mentally healthy and dangerous have their freedom guarded by the courts so that after a prison sentence is served, the individual is automatically released and can no longer be retained. However, someone who is mentally ill and dangerous can be confined indefinitely. Ennis makes the following observation:

Of all the identifiably dangerous groups in society, only the mentally ill are singled out for preventive detention and . . . they are probably the least dangerous as a group. Why should society confine a person if he is dangerous and mentally ill but not if he is dangerous and sane?[12:101]

To support his suggestion that the mentally ill are probably less dangerous than the mentally healthy, he cites a 5-year study of 5000 patients discharged from a state mental hospital in New York. The results showed that their arrest rate was one twelfth that of the general population.

Similar findings were reported in a major study by Steadman and Cocozza.[37] Following the transfer of nearly a thousand patients from maximum-security "prison" mental hospitals to civil psychiatric hospitals, they reported that 97.3% of the allegedly dangerous mental patients had remained free of assaultive behavior 4½ years after transfer. Of 98 patients released and followed up in the community, approximately 98% had been nonassaultive. The idea of preventive detention does not exist in most areas of the law where the ability to predict an action does not confer the right to control the action in advance. Only illegal acts result in a prolonged loss of liberty for most citizens, except the mentally ill.

Another aspect of this dilemma also revolves around this idea of dangerousness. Extensive reviews of the literature have concluded that there are no reliable indicators of dangerousness.[38] Furthermore, even if some mentally ill individuals are potentially dangerous, it has not been proved that psychiatrists are good predictors of future violence. Frequently psychiatrists overpredict the patient's potential for dangerous acts and the extent of his illness.

Oran[27] believes this is because of the medical training of the psychiatrist, which has taught him that underdiagnosis is more harmful than overdiagnosis. It is compounded by his conflicting roles as agents of both the patient and community, which require him to be therapist, warden, and judge. If he underpredicts a psychiatric illness and the patient later causes harm, the community's anger is directed at him. If he overpredicts illness, however, a patient is subjected to treatment against his will. It has been suggested, therefore, that multidisciplinary teams rather than psychiatrists alone should be involved in determining dangerousness.[20] The input of those with knowledge of the patient's home setting and sociocultural background might also improve evaluations.

Szasz[39] states that whether a person is dangerous is not the real issue, but it is rather who he is and how he is dangerous. He believes society condones danger in some ways but not others. For example, drunken drivers are very dangerous and kill many more people than people with paranoid ideation. But drunken drivers are not committed, and people labeled paranoid are. In fact, some kinds of dangerous behaviors required in certain roles, such as race car driver, trapeze artist, and astronaut are admired and valued. It has been suggested that the assessment of danger involves four separate questions[9]:

1. What type of harmful act is to be considered dangerous: physical or psychological harm, harm to persons, or harm to property?
2. What degree of injury constitutes harm: verbal abuse, assault, or assault with a weapon?
3. How likely is it that the harmful act will occur? Do actuarial tables or clinical judgment give us predictive ability?
4. How frequently will the harmful act recur? Do the compulsively repeated acts of the exhibitionist make him more dangerous than a man whose only violent act was the murder of both his parents?

The answers to these questions can be very subjective, which suggests that the underlying issue is one of noncomformity in ways that offend others. In this context social role becomes important.

Before the law all men and women are equal, but it is also true that the majority of committed patients are members of the lower classes. Scheff has observed the following:

There is a large portion of the patient population, 43 percent, whose presence in the hospital cannot readily be explained in terms of their psychiatric condition. Their presence suggests the punitive character of the societal reaction to deviance.[34:168]

The behavioral criterion of dangerousness for commitment can be said to change the function of the psychiatric hospital from a place of therapy for mental illness to a place of confinement for certain offensive behavior. It suggests that the covert function of the psychiatric hospital is that of social control. This idea is supported by the various behavioral disorders that justify commitment, including drug addiction, alcoholism, and sexual offenses. In addition, epileptics are vulnerable to commitment in almost 40% of the states despite the fact that epilepsy is not a mental illness but a controllable physical abnormality.

Freedom of choice. The legal and psychiatric question being raised is one of freedom of choice. Some professionals believe that at certain times the individual cannot be responsible for himself. For his own protection and the protection of society it is necessary to confine him and to make decisions for him. An example is the suicidal patient. In most states it is against the law to kill oneself. Law and psychiatry join therefore to protect the person and help him resolve his conflict.

How does this compare with the cancer or cardiac patient who may reject medical advice and his identified therapeutic regimen? Should society, through law and medicine, attempt to cure him by involuntary methods? Some physicians, like Chodoff,[7] view civil commitment as basically a benevolent system that can make bona fide treatment available. He disagrees with the assumption that the mentally ill are competent to exercise free will and make decisions in their own best interest, such as decisions about whether to take medications or whether to be out in the streets instead of in a hospital. He contends that there are mentally ill people who may not be physically dangerous but nevertheless endanger their own prospects for a normal life. Chodoff believes institutions can at least protect them and in many cases help them. Thus he views the abolition of involuntary civil commitment as gravely immoral.

Other individuals, such as Szasz, oppose intervention. Szasz argues for responsibility for self and the right to choose or reject treatment. Should one's actions violate criminal law, he suggests the individual be punished for those actions through the penal system:

For some time now I have maintained that commitment—that is, the detention of persons in mental institutions against their will—is a form of imprisonment; that such deprivation of liberty is contrary to the moral principles embodied in the Declaration of Independence and the Constitution of the United States; and that it is a gross violation of contemporary concepts of fundamental human rights. The practice of "sane" men incarcerating their "insane" fellow men in "mental hospitals" can be compared to that of white men enslaving black men. In short, I consider commitment a crime against humanity.[39:113*]

There is currently a trend toward due process and evidentiary procedures and standards that approach or adopt the rigor of procedures and standards used in the criminal process. These changes are reflected in the Massachusetts Mental Health Act of 1970, which recoded the statutes governing the admission, treatment, and discharge of the mentally ill and mentally retarded. The changes in the Massachusetts statute were both substantive and procedural. The most significant substantive change was the elimination of very broad and vague criteria for commitment. These vague criteria were replaced by ones which required that the likelihood of serious harm to self or others be proven prior to involuntary hospitalization.

There were also two important procedural changes made in this act. One was the abolition of an indefinite period of involuntary hospitalization. The commitment was required to be for limited periods. The second important change was the requirement of fact evidence, rather than just expert opinions, as to whether the prospective patient met the legal criteria for commitment. The significance of these changes is indicated by the fact that nine other states (Maine, Nebraska, New Mexico, Ohio, Rhode Island, South Carolina, Tennessee, Washington, and Wisconsin) have statutorily adopted either the identical or substantially the same language as the Massachusetts standard for civil commitment.

■ **ETHICAL CONSIDERATIONS.** Whether to take a stand for or against commitment is an issue each nurse must resolve for herself. What should be done if the nonconformist does not wish to change his behavior? Does he maintain his freedom to choose even if his thinking appears to be irrational or divergent from the norm? Does the concept of mutuality exclude coercion? Can social interests be served by a means less restrictive than total confinement, such as outpatient therapy? Every nurse should assume the responsibility for reviewing the commitment procedures in her state and work for legislative amendments that would facilitate the necessary reforms.

The commitment dilemma therefore exposes present practices and opens areas of controversy for the future. The present mental hospital has been described as a jail, hospital, poorhouse, and home for the elderly. It protects, treats, feeds, maintains, and houses socially

---

*Excerpt from *Ideology and Insanity* by Thomas Szasz. Copyright © 1970 by Thomas S. Szasz. used by permission of Doubleday & Co., Inc.

incompetent individuals who are often feared by society. When they are discharged from the hospital, they are frequently left without alternatives and come to the attention of law enforcement agencies or welfare offices.

It has been estimated that approximately one third to one half of the homeless in the United States are believed to be mentally ill.[13] Robert Jones, the president of the Philadelphia Committee for the Homeless, blamed deinstitutionalization as the major cause, but he also mentioned as significant contributors economic recession, high unemployment rates, and cutbacks in federal programs.[15] In addition to blaming cutbacks in aid to individuals, he also noted the cutbacks in programs for medical care, aging studies, alcoholism and drug abuse, families and children, and employment training. Finally, he mentioned urban renewal for severely cutting into the number of available low-cost housing units and for increasing the number of evictions.

Local communities deny the problem by resisting the establishment of halfway houses or sheltered homes in their neighborhood. Third-party insurance seldom covers extended outpatient psychiatric care. In today's mobile and impersonal society, family and friends are often unwilling or unable to care for the newly released patient, who may end up in a dismal run-down hotel or boarding house with nothing to do but watch television and wander the streets.

These issues need to be addressed by psychiatric nurses, patients, and citizens across the country. The value of commitment, goals of hospitalization, quality of life, and rights of patients must be closely aligned and resolved through the judicial, legislative, and health care systems.

Discharge

A patient who voluntarily admits himself into the hospital can be discharged by the staff when he has received "maximum benefit" from the treatment, or he may initiate his own discharge request. Most states require that he give written notice of his desire for discharge, and some hospitals will also request he sign a form that states he is leaving "against medical advice." These forms then become part of his permanent record. He is usually released 24 to 72 hours after submitting a discharge request. In the event that a voluntarily admitted patient elopes from the hospital, he can be brought back only if he again voluntarily agrees. Staff frequently attempt to contact such a patient and discuss alternatives with him. If he refuses to return to the hospital, he must either be discharged or involuntary commitment procedures must be initiated.

An involuntarily admitted or committed patient has lost the right to leave the hospital when he wishes. Temporary and emergency commitments specify the maximal length of detainment. Indefinite commitments do not, although periodic reviews of the patient's status should be held, and the patient may apply for another commitment hearing to determine if additional hospitalization is necessary. If a committed patient elopes, the staff has the legal obligation to notify the police and committing courts. Frequently these patients return home or visit family or friends and can be easily located. The legal authorities then return the patient to the hospital, and additional steps are not necessary, since the original commitment is still effective.

There are three specific kinds of discharges. These include the conditional discharge, absolute discharge, and judicial discharge.

■ Conditional discharge

Many committed patients are assisted in the transition from the hospital into the community by specified leaves of absence or liberties. These are known as conditional discharges because certain things are expected of the patient. Most frequently he is required to attend outpatient therapy through the hospital or community mental health center. If he is progressing well, his leaves may be extended for 30 to 90 days or more. During this time the commitment order is still in effect, and, should he relapse while in the community, he can be brought back to the hospital and treatment continued.

This type of discharge planning allows for a gradual integration into the community, and many patients have benefited from it. If at the end of the conditional period the patient demonstrates a good adjustment, the hospital can issue an absolute discharge of the patient.

■ Absolute discharge

As the name implies, absolute discharge is the termination of the patient's relationship with the hospital. It is a final discharge, and if the patient needs to return to the hospital at some future time, new admission proceedings must be initiated. Usually the hospital is required to notify the court when a committed patient is given an absolute discharge.

This type of discharge is employed most often when substantial progress has been made by the patient and he is able to function well in the community. However, there are also instances when patients who have not improved and are unlikely to improve in the future are granted absolute discharges. In these instances arrangements are made with the families or guardians to provide satisfactory care for the patient. In addition, some laws require that other state officials be notified by the hospital.

■ Judicial discharge

Nearly 40 states now have laws that allow a patient or his family the right to appeal to the court for a discharge even though the hospital does not agree with the discharge request. The process and requirements for such cases vary from state to state, but they allow the patient an additional recourse for grievance if he believes hospitalization is no longer apppropriate. Such legislation may be instrumental in further defining patients' rights in future years.

Patients' rights

In 1973 the American Hospital Association issued a Patient's Bill of Rights, which many general hospitals throughout the country have adopted. Psychiatric hospitals, however, continue to struggle with the issue of the basic civil rights of the individual. In recent years the civil and personal rights of the mentally ill have been supported in legislative acts throughout the country. In retrospect the new laws also reflect the restrictions and discriminations suffered by the mentally ill in the past. Some states are now allowing the committed patient to retain all his civil rights, similar to the voluntary patient, except the right to leave the hospital and to terminate treatment.

Allowing for great variation among states, patients presently have the following rights[21]:

- Right to communicate with people outside the hospital through correspondence, telephone, and personal visits
- Right to keep clothing and personal effects with them in the hospital
- Right to religious freedom
- Right to be employed if possible
- Right to manage and dispose of property
- Right to execute wills
- Right to enter into contractual relationships
- Right to make purchases
- Right to education
- Right to habeas corpus
- Right to independent psychiatric examination
- Right to civil service status
- Right to retain licenses, privileges, or permits established by law, such as a driver's or professional license
- Right to sue or be sued
- Right to marry and divorce
- Right not to be subject to unnecessary mechanical restraints
- Right to periodic review of status
- Right to legal representation
- Right to privacy

- Right of informed consent
- Right to treatment
- Right to refuse treatment
- Right to treatment in the least restrictive setting

Some of these rights merit exploration in greater detail.

■ Right to communicate with people outside the hospital

This right entails the freedom of the patient to visit and hold telephone conversations in privacy and send unopened letters to anyone of his choice, including judges, lawyers, families, and staff. Although the patient has the right to communicate in an uncensored manner, the staff may place limits on the patient's access to the telephone or visitors when such access is detrimental to the patient's welfare or a source of harrassment for the staff. The hospital can also place limits on the times when telephone calls can be made and received and when visitors can enter the facility. On occasions hospital staff have intercepted letters presumed to be threatening or abusive and disposed of them. In states where this is not illegal, such activity raises the moral question of individual freedom vs. the good of the community.

■ Right to keep personal effects

This establishes the right of the patient to bring clothing and personal items with him to the hospital, taking into consideration the amount of space available for storage of them. It does not make the hospital responsible for their safety. Valuable items should preferably be left at home. If the patient brings something of value to the hospital, the staff should place it in the hospital safe or make other appropriate provisions for its safekeeping. This right does not relieve the hospital staff from ensuring a safe environment by removing dangerous objects from the patient's possession if necessary.

■ Right to be employed if possible

This includes the right to work whenever possible and the right to be compensated for it, including payment for work-therapy programs within the hospital. Involuntary servitude or work without pay within institutions is on the decline because courts have held that the Thirteenth Amendment, which abolished slavery, also applies to psychiatric patients. The consequence of these decisions is that mental institutions cannot force patients to work, either by punishing them or by making privileges or discharge dependent on work. If patients choose to work, they must be assigned jobs on documented therapeutic grounds and they must be paid the minimum wage.

The Department of Labor is notifying all institutions that if they fail to pay patient workers, they are violating the law. The ultimate effect of this move is not yet known. Some professionals fear that the money to pay patients will come out of treatment funds and that the patients will fare worse in the end. Others fear that hospitals will hire regular labor and leave the patients with nothing to do. Some argue that institutions will charge patients for room and board and recover much of the money. A further fear raised is that if the Department of Labor enforces the law and if institutions comply, they may be forced to close because of lack of funds.

■ Right to execute wills

A person's competency to make a will is known as *testamentary capacity*. He can make a valid will if he (1) knows that he is making a will; (2) knows the nature and extent of his property, and (3) knows who his friends and relatives are and what the relationships mean. Each of these criteria must be met and documented for the will to be considered valid. This means he must not be mentally confused at the time he signed his will. It does not imply that he must have the exact details of his property holdings or specific bank account figures. But he cannot attempt to give away more than he possesses. Furthermore, the law requires that he know who his relatives are but does not require him to bequeath anything to them.

The fact that a patient is committed or is diagnosed as psychotic does not immediately invalidate his will. The will is valid if it was made during a lucid period and the patient met the three criteria. The problem most debated in determining testamentary capacity is the delusional patient, particularly if the delusional thinking could alter the outcome of the will. The important question in this regard is whether the false belief or delusion caused the person to dispose of his property in a different way than he would have otherwise.

Two or three persons must witness the will by watching the person as he signs it and each other as they sign it. It is necessary therefore that they all be together at this time. At a later time a nurse may be summoned into court to give testimony on the condition of the person at the time he drew up his will. The nurse should testify relative to the three criteria, as well as report pertinent observations, recall information as accurately as possible, and express herself concisely and objectively. Hospital charts may also be used in the court proceedings, and the nurse's notes relative to the patient's behavior and mental status may provide additional information.

■ Right to enter into contractual relationships

Contracts are considered valid by the court if the person understands the circumstances involved in the contract and the natural consequences of it. Once again, a psychiatric illness does not invalidate a contract, although the nature of the contract and degree of judgment needed to understand it would be influencing factors.

■ **INCOMPETENCY.** An issue related to this right is the one of mental incompetency. Every adult is assumed to be mentally competent and possess the mental ability to carry out his affairs. To prove otherwise requires a special court hearing to declare him "incompetent." This is a legal term without a precise medical meaning. To prove that an individual is incompetent it must be shown that (1) he has a mental disorder, (2) this disorder causes a defect in judgment, and (3) this defect makes him incapable of handling his own affairs. All three elements must be present, and the exact diagnostic label is not as important in this regard. If a person is declared incompetent, a legal guardian will be appointed by the court to manage the patient's estate. This frequently is a family member, friend, or bank executive. Incompetency rulings are most often filed for persons with senile dementia, cerebral arteriosclerosis, chronic schizophrenia, and mental retardation.

The trend in legislation is to separate the concepts of incompetency and involuntary commitment, since the reasons for each are essentially different. Incompetency arises from society's desire to safeguard a person's assets from his own inability to understand and transact business. Involuntary commitments are usually initiated to protect the patient from himself (in the case of suicide), protect others from the patient (in the case of homicide), and administer treatment. However, many states still consider the two equivalent, and the policies and procedures of the hospital may impose the incompetent status on the patient.

As a result of an incompetency ruling, the person cannot vote, marry, drive, or make contracts. A release from the hospital is not necessarily an automatic restoration to competency. Rather, another court hearing is required to reverse the previous ruling and declare the individual competent and allow him to once again manage his own affairs.

■ Right to education

This right is being exercised by many parents on behalf of their emotionally ill or mentally retarded children. Everyone is guaranteed this right under the constitution, although many states have not made provisions for the adequate education of all groups of citizens and are now being required to do so.

Right to habeas corpus

Habeas corpus is an important right the person retains in all states even if he has been involuntarily admitted to the hospital. It originated in English Common Law and is provided for in the Constitution of the United States. The object of the writ is the speedy release of any individual who claims he is being deprived of his liberty and detained illegally. A committed patient may file such a writ at any time on the grounds that he is sane and eligible for release. The hearing takes place in a court of law where those people who serve to restrain the patient must defend their actions. A jury is sometimes impaneled to determine the sanity of the patient. A determination is then made, and if the court finds the patient to be sane, he is discharged from the hospital.

Right to independent psychiatric examination

Under the Emergency Admission Statute the patient has the right to demand a psychiatric examination by a physician of his own choice. If this physician determines that he is not mentally ill, the patient must be released.

Right to marry and divorce

Since marriage is a formal contract, the same general criteria for validity apply; that is, the marriage is considered valid if the individual understands the nature of the marriage relationship and the duties and obligations it entails. The crucial element is his mental capacity at the time of the marriage, not before it or after it. In general, courts are reluctant to declare a marriage void. Many states have laws forbidding the marriage of mentally ill persons. This is based on the notion that mental illness, whether genetically or environmentally induced, often runs in families. Thus the primary objective of such laws is to prevent the procreation of children who might be mentally ill. In these cases the law is not based on any scientific evidence of the inheritability of mental illness.

In most states psychiatric illness is not in itself grounds for divorce. However, some states will grant divorces if the mentally ill spouse has been committed to a hospital for a certain number of years (usually 3 to 5). It is sometimes also necessary to specify that the spouse is "incurably insane." Many psychiatric professionals are understandably hesitant to make such a determination.

Right to privacy

The right to privacy implies the right of the individual to keep some information about himself completely secret from others. *Confidentiality* involves the disclosure of certain information to another person, but this is limited to specifically authorized individuals. It is the responsibility of every psychiatric professional to safeguard a patient's right to confidentiality in all aspects of psychiatric treatment, including even the knowledge that a person is in therapy or in a hospital. Revealing such information might damage a person's reputation or hamper his ability to obtain a job. This was most dramatically evident when Senator Eagleton was running as a vice-presidential candidate in the 1972 presidential election. Unfortunately, as with most rights, the protection of the law cannot be applied in a discriminative manner, and thus potential ethical and professional dilemmas can be created, such as the one experienced by the nurse in the following true case,[19] Clinical example 7-1.

The issue of confidentiality is becoming increasingly important, since various agencies demand information about a patient's history, diagnosis, treatment, and prognosis and sophisticated methods for obtaining information (such as wiretapping and computer banks) have been developed. These threaten the individual's right to privacy. The clinician is free from legal respon-

---

CLINICAL EXAMPLE 7-1

On a Wednesday morning in 1981 in Springfield, Illinois, a man walked into Lauterbach's Cottage Hardware Store, grabbed an ax and began swinging. When he left, one person was dead and two others were critically injured. Ten days later, police received a call from Mr. K who was a patient in the 49-bed psychiatric unit at St. John's Hospital. Mr. K told the police that his roommate at the hospital confessed the crime. However, he didn't know his roommate's name. He asked Nurse M to identify him but she refused to do so, since she believed his name was shielded by a state law guaranteeing the privacy of mental health records. Hospital administrators supported her decision even after she was fined $250 by a county judge for refusing to give the man's name to a grand jury. Nurse M did tell the police that the suspect was not a patient in St. John's at the time of the murder and that he resembled their composite sketch.

sibility if information is released with the patient's written and signed request. As a rule it is best to reveal as little information as possible and discuss with the patient what the material will be.

The view of patients on this important issue has been subjected to very little research. A recent study that examined the views of psychiatric inpatients on issues related to confidentiality found that they valued confidentiality highly and were concerned about the possibility of unauthorized disclosures, particularly to employers.[35] They had little knowledge, however, of their legal rights or recourses should breaches in confidentiality occur. These data support contentions about the importance of confidentiality and suggest the need for additional research and patient education in this area.

The concept of confidentiality builds on the element of trust necessary in a patient-therapist relationship. The patient places himself in the care of others and reveals vulnerable aspects of his personal life. In return he expects high-quality care and the safeguard of his interests. Thus the patient-therapist relationship is an intimate one and demands trust, loyalty, and the maintenance of privacy.

■ **PRIVILEGED COMMUNICATION.** The phrase *privileged communication* is a legal one and applies only in court-related proceedings. It includes communications between husband and wife, attorney and client, and clergy and church member. The right to reveal information belongs to the person who spoke, and the listener cannot disclose the information unless the speaker gives permission. This privilege exists for the protection of the patient who could sue the listener for the disclosure of privileged information. Another purpose of it is to inspire confidence in the patient to encourage making a full account of symptoms and conditions so that they may be properly cared for and treated.

Privileged communication between health professionals and a patient exists only if a law specifically establishes it. Thirty-three states currently recognize privileged communication between physicians and patients; twelve do not. Five states have laws providing for privileged communication between nurses and patients, including Arkansas, New York, Oregon, Vermont, and Wisconsin.[28] In these states the nurse is exempt from giving information obtained in a professional capacity if the information was necessary to implement nursing care. All the other states do not, and a nurse would be required to reveal what the patient said to her in a court of law. In general, however, it is rare that a nurse is called into court to divulge information of this kind.

In 1975 the Federal Rules of Evidence were revised to extend physician-patient privilege only to psychotherapist-patient privilege. Acknowledging, however, that sometimes it was necessary to obtain information for the good of the public interest or to avoid fraud, the following exceptions were noted[43]:

1. Communications *not* made for purposes of diagnosis and treatment
2. Commitment and restoration proceedings
3. Issues as to wills or otherwise between parties claiming by succession from the patient
4. Actions on insurance policies
5. Required reports (venereal diseases, gunshot wounds, child abuse)
6. Communications in furtherance of the crime of fraud; mental or physical condition put in issue by the patient (personal injury cases)
7. Malpractice actions
8. Some or all criminal prosecutions, depending on the state

■ **PATIENT RECORDS.** Most hospitals keep psychiatric records separately and provide that they are less accessible than medical records. They are viewed by the law and psychiatric profession to be more sensitive than general medical records. Psychiatrists, for the most part, retain the right to decide if they should release medical information to the patient, and in some states patients are barred from viewing them at all. A hospital chart can be summoned into court, however, and anything that is written in it can be used in a lawsuit. Privileged communication does not apply to hospital charts, and nursing notes should be written carefully in all cases. Furthermore, it is a general rule that only those persons involved in a patient's care may read his chart. This includes physicians, nurses, aides, students, and others directly involved in the treatment process.

■ **PROTECTING A THIRD PARTY.** An added dimension to the concept of confidentiality and privileged communication has emerged from the case of *Tarasoff v. Regents of the University of California et al.*[41] In this case, the psychotherapist failed to warn Tatiana Tarasoff or her parents that his client had stated that he intended to kill her when she returned from her summer vacation. In the lawsuit that followed the death of Tatiana Tarasoff, California's Supreme Court determined that the treating therapist has a duty to warn the intended victim of a patient's violence. That means that when a therapist is reasonably certain that a patient is going to harm a particular third person, the therapist has the responsibility to breach the confidentiality of the relationship and warn or protect the third party. This obligation may be carried out in a number of ways, including alerting the proper authorities or having the patient hospitalized to prevent violent behavior.

■ Right to informed consent

Informed consent includes the disclosure by a physician of a certain amount of information to the patient about the proposed treatment and the attainment of the patient's consent, which must be competent, understanding, and voluntary. The physician must explain the special treatment, its possible complications, and its risks. The patient must be capable of giving consent and not be a minor or judged incompetent or insane by the court. Failure to obtain consent may be the basis for lawsuits of "assault and battery" or negligence.

Psychiatric outpatients usually express their consent by their willingness to come for treatment, and only unusual treatments, such as experimental drugs or ECT require specific written consent. Informally admitted and voluntary patients usually sign a paper on admission consenting to psychiatric treatment, which includes milieu therapy, chemotherapy, psychotherapy, and occupational therapy. Unusual treatments again need special permission. In the care of the involuntarily admitted patient, the commitment procedure gives the hospital the right to treat the patient.

Consent forms usually require the signature of the patient, a family member, and two persons who witnessed their signing it. Nurses are frequently called on in this regard. It then becomes a part of the patient's permanent hospital record.

■ Right to treatment

The concept of the right to treatment is a relatively recent development. In 1960 Birnbaum, a graduate student in both medicine and law, wrote, "there does not appear to have been any significant and realistic consideration given, from a legal viewpoint, to the problem of whether or not the institutionalized mentally ill person receives adequate medical treatment so that he may regain his health, and therefore his liberty, as soon as possible."[4] This cause received its impetus with a 1966 case in the District of Columbia *(Rouse v. Cameron)*. The court held that mental patients committed by criminal courts had the right to adequate treatment. Furthermore, it said that confinement without treatment was tantamount to incarceration and thus transformed the hospital into a penitentiary. It affirmed that the purpose of involuntary hospitalization was treatment, not punishment, and if this treatment was not provided, the patient could be transferred, released, or even awarded damages for his period of confinement. The court clarified that the hospital did not need to show that the treatment would improve or cure the patient but only that there was a true attempt to do so.

This right to treatment was extended in 1972 to all mentally ill and mentally retarded persons who were involuntarily hospitalized in a case in Alabama *(Wyatt v. Stickney)*. The court stated:

To deprive any citizen of his or her liberty upon the altruistic theory that the confinement is for humane therapeutic reasons and then fail to provide adequate treatment violates the very fundamentals of due process.[46]

It further defined criteria for adequate treatment in three areas:

1. A humane psychological and physical environment
2. A qualified staff with a sufficient number of members to administer adequate treatment
3. Individualized treatment plans

The keystone of the Wyatt decision is the requirement that an individualized treatment plan be formulated. Failure to provide it means the patient must be discharged unless he agrees to remain voluntarily.

This case is presently being appealed to a higher court, and if this decision is upheld, it will be an important one because it goes beyond the earlier right-to-treatment case and states that judicially enforceable standards of care in mental hospitals are required. It will also have economic implications, since meeting the three criteria of a humane environment, qualified staff in sufficient numbers, and individualized treatment plans will clearly cost more money. Upholding the court's decision might very well force states to reconsider the economic resource allocation presently allotted to mental health.

A landmark court decision in this area was given in June 1975 by the Supreme Court in the case of *Donaldson v. O'Connor* in which a Florida State psychiatric patient was freed after 15 years of confinement. The court ruled that he was not dangerous and was not receiving treatment and therefore to continue to confine him would be in violation of his right to liberty.

The constitutional basis for the right to treatment is found in the Eighth and Fourteenth Amendments. The Eighth Amendment deals with the issue of cruel and unusual punishment and the Fourteenth deals with due process and equal protection under the law. Various right-to-treatment cases have been introduced in the state courts throughout the country, and the outcome of them will greatly affect the care of the mentally ill.

This new right, however, also poses several questions. One involves the appropriateness of treatment and whether confinement itself can be considered therapeutic. A second problem raises the question of what to do with the patient who is untreatable. Should a length of time be set after which the patient is released?

Another problem is the unwilling patient. Might a person refuse treatment and then seek his release, claiming he was denied his right to adequate treatment? A more pressing question is whether the public is willing to pay the magnitude of the costs required to provide adequate treatment to the mentally ill in public institutions? In current times of high inflation and reduction in government funds, programs are often struggling for survival at existing funding levels, let alone expansion. Thus fiscal constraints may play an even greater role than judicial decisions in affecting the care of the mentally ill.

■ Right to refuse treatment

The relationship between the right to treatment and the right to refuse treatment is a complex one. The right to refuse treatment includes the right to refuse involuntary hospitalization and has been called the "right to be left alone." Some people believe that therapy has the power to control a person's mind, regulate his thoughts, and change his personality, and the patient should be protected against this by the right to refuse treatment. This argument states that involuntary therapy conflicts with two basic human and legal rights. The first is freedom of thought and the second is the right to control one's own life and actions as long as they do not interfere with the rights of others. An issue related to this is the right to refuse experimentation. A minimum requirement for any experimental treatment is the written consent of the patient. But evidence exists that in certain institutions inadequate consent had been obtained and in others no attempt at all was made to obtain consent.[36]

The landmark case in establishing this right for psychiatric patients was decided in 1979 in *Rogers v. Okin*. In this case the court went farther than in any previous case in establishing the rights of hospitalized psychiatric patients to refuse medication by reinforcing the standard that restraint may be used only in cases of emergency, such as the occurrence of, or serious threat of, extreme violence, personal injury, or attempted suicide. In writing the opinion for the court, Judge Tauro held that:

The committed patient has a right to be wrong in his analysis of that information (regarding a particular treatment program)—as long as the consequences of such error do not pose a danger of physical harm to himself, fellow patients or hospital staff. And so, while the state may have an obligation to make treatment available, and a legitimate interest in providing such treatment, a competent patient has a fundamental right to decide to be left alone, absent an emergency.[33]

Thus the fundamental premise of the court's decision in this case was that committed psychiatric patients were presumed competent to make decisions with respect to treatment in nonemergencies.

On the other hand, the 1982 Supreme Court decision in *Youngberg v. Romeo* supported the exercise of professional judgment in the use of seclusion or restraint.[47] The standard to be applied is that of usual and customary professional practice.

The questions raised by the right-to-refuse-treatment concept are many. Does the right apply to all treatment techniques, including medications, or only to those which are hazardous, intrusive, or severe, such as psychosurgery? How can staff meet the obligation to implement the right to treatment when a patient refuses to be treated? How does one differentiate between refusal, resisting treatment, and noncompliance and does each of these interpretations require a different course of action? There are no existing solutions to these complex issues, but they are of concern to nurses, who are frequently responsible for delivering prescribed treatment modalities such as medications.

An additional perspective is provided by Rhoden, who suggests that if refusals are too easily overridden by means of a generalized presumption of doing "what is best for the patient," the opportunity for increased patient-staff communication and cooperation might be lost.[31] She believes that this area is seriously complicated by the dilemma that although drug treatment is more likely to restore a patient's autonomy, taking his views seriously by not forcing the medication shows respect for the patient and may, in itself, be therapeutic.

A mental health staff faced with the patient who is refusing medication has a number of options. First, they can consider offering the patient a lower dosage of medication—or no medication at all. A second option would be to discharge the patient against medical advice if no other staff action would help to relieve the symptoms of the illness and the patient does not meet the criteria for commitment. Another option would be to have the patient declared incompetent and seek a court order permitting the use of the medication. Similarly, a guardian can consent to medication when the patient's refusal can be shown to be a result of his incompetence and resultant inability to make a rational decision.

At this time nurses should make their judgments on a case-by-case basis. The Task Force on Behavior Therapy has examined the issue of coerced treatment and suggested three criteria that may justify it[2]:

1. The patient must be judged to be dangerous to himself or others.
2. It must be believed by those administering treatment that it has a reasonable chance to benefit the patient and those related to him.

3. The patient must be judged to be incompetent to evaluate the necessity of the treatment.

They stress that even if these three conditions are met, the patient should not be deceived. He should be informed as to what will be done to him, the reasons for it, and its probable effects.

Future court decisions will certainly explore the many aspects of this issue. Peck indicates possible outcomes:

> The right-to-treatment movement . . . will undoubtedly do away with some of the injustices and deplorable conditions that have resulted in support for the right to refuse treatment and involuntary hospitalization. The end result might be more humane hospitals and treatment, which would lessen the impact of this movement. On the other hand, the right to treatment will probably also tend to make hospitals force their treatment, out of fear of being sued, on persons who were previously ignored. This in turn might result in an increase in cases maintaining the right to refuse treatment.[29:315]

■ **Right to treatment in the least restrictive setting**

The right to treatment in the least restrictive setting is closely related to the right to adequate treatment. It refers to the goal of evaluating the specific needs of each patient and maintaining the greatest amount of personal freedom, autonomy, dignity, and integrity in determining the treatment or services he is to receive. Six clinical dimensions of the concept of restrictiveness in psychosocial nursing are presented in Table 7-3. This right applies to both community- and noncommunity-based programs. Greater consideration of this right might well limit some of the controversy surrounding the commitment dilemma and the right to refuse treatment.

The cases behind this right assert that if patients can function in some setting other than a mental hospital, the court has the responsibility of placing them in that setting. This was the ruling in the case of *Dixon v. Weinberger* in 1973 when the judge ruled that patients in Washington, D.C., have a statutory right to confinement in the least restrictive facility.[11] Responsibility was placed on Washington, D.C., and the federal government to develop a plan to identify those who should be transferred to community-based facilities and the means for achieving this transfer, including the creation of alternative facilities if necessary.

Even though the right to the least restrictive alternative tends to support patient's needs for normalization in a much more effective way than the right to treatment cases, they are complicated by the fact that new models, more facilities, and increased financial resources must be applied to the concept of aftercare, so that discharged

TABLE 7-3

SIX CLINICAL DIMENSIONS OF THE CONCEPT OF RESTRICTIVENESS IN PSYCHOSOCIAL NURSING

Dimension	Component
Structural	Type of treatment setting and objective means of physical restraint or limitations on physical freedoms
Institutional policy	Rules, procedures, routines, and regulations for operating the institution and degree of patient involvement in planning
Enforcement	Staff-determined consequences of rule-breaking or inability of the patient to leave the setting
Treatment	Use and level of antipsychotic medications and the use of other somatic treatments such as electroconvulsive therapy or psychosurgery
Psychosocial atmosphere	Status difference between patients and staff and degrees of staff authoritarianism
Patient characteristics	Patient's ability to manage his own care and level of functioning as influenced by the severity of his disorder

From Garritson, S.: J. of Psychosoc. Nurs. **21**(12):9, 1983.

and chronically ill patients can be supported in the community.

For example, despite the growing emphasis on treatment in the least restrictive setting, it has been noted that states rarely use commitment to outpatient treatment as an alternative to involuntary hospitalization. One study examined the effects of changes in North Carolina commitment laws designed to facilitate the appropriate use of outpatient commitment.[24] The changes resulted in some increase in the appropriate use of outpatient commitment. But the clinicians who worked at hospitals continued to doubt its efficacy and remained reluctant to use outpatient commitment.

This right to treatment in the least restrictive setting raises a number of difficult questions. How do mental health professionals balance human rights versus the human needs of patients? Will sufficient funds be allocated to provide adequate supportive care in the community? What will happen to the remaining chronically ill patients who are not discharged into less restrictive alternatives? Will the community centers be able to provide a quality of care that is better than that provided by institutions? How can one stem the antipathy that exists in the larger community toward local placement of mentally ill patients? And most important, given the present economic constraints, will the limited resources allotted to mental health be given to community centers at the expense of large hospitals?

■ Nursing's role in patients' rights

The National League for Nursing in 1977 issued a statement on the nurse's role in patients' rights.[26] Respect and concern for patients and assurance of competent care were identified as basic rights, along with patients receiving the information they need to understand their illness and make decisions about their care. The League urged nurses to directly involve themselves in assuring the human and legal rights of patients.

Many of the patients' rights identified by the League include those previously mentioned. They also list the following rights*:

- Right to health care that is accessible and that meets professional standards, regardless of the setting
- Right to courteous and individualized health care that is equitable, humane, and given without discrimination as to race, color, creed, sex, national origin, source of payment, or ethical or political beliefs
- Right to information about their diagnosis, prognosis, and treatment, including alternatives to care and risks involved
- Right to information about the qualifications, names, and titles of personnel responsible for providing their health care
- Right to refuse observation by those not directly involved in their care
- Right to coordination and continuity of health care
- Right to information on the charges for services, including the right to challenge these
- Above all, the right to be fully informed as to all their rights in all health care settings

Perhaps the single most important factor in the implementation of the rights of patients is the attitude of psychiatric professionals. A sensitivity to patients' rights

---

*National League for Nursing: Nursing's role in patients' rights, New York, 1977, The League. Used with permission.

cannot be imposed by the court, the legislature, administrative agencies, or professional groups. If nurses show disdain for those rights, implement them perfunctorily, or are outwardly hostile about honoring them, patient's rights remain an empty legal concept. But if they are sensitive to the rights in all aspects of their relationships with patients, they will secure these human and legal rights.

■ Summary

The 1978 report from the President's Commission on Mental Health[30] recommends that each state have a "Bill of Rights" for all mentally disabled people which should be incorporated in educational programs directed to patients, staff, families, and the general public. It proposes that a copy of the rights be prominently displayed in all mental health settings, be given to each patient using the services, and be explained in an easily understandable manner.

The Mental Health Systems Act of 1980 supported the recommendations of the President's Commission on Mental Health and included within the act itself is a Bill of Mental Health Rights.[22] (See accompanying box on the 1980 Mental Health Systems Act's Rights and Advocacy.) Unfortunately, presidential commissions, mental health legislation, and litigation have primarily brought abstract victories to patients. Efforts to implement these decisions have been marked by confusing requirements, inadequate resources, and insufficient knowledge.

Clearly the reforms mandated by the law will cost money, yet public willingness to pay for both more and better psychiatric care is questionable at present. The limitations on resources will continue to be a major factor, regardless of how well organized, numerous, and well intentioned are the advocates of better mental health care. Thus the protection of the rights of the mentally ill will be greatly dependent on evaluating the effectiveness of any new programs arising from executive, judicial, or legislative orders.

Legal role of the nurse

Professional nursing practice is not determined by a simplistic adherence to patients' rights. Rather, it emerges from an interplay between the rights of patients, the legal role of the nurse, and concern for quality psychiatric care (Fig. 7-2). There are three roles that the psychiatric nurse moves in and out of in the process of completing professional and personal responsibilities. These are the roles of provider of services, employee or contractor of services, and private citizen. These roles are played simultaneously, and each role has attendant rights and responsibilities.

1980 Mental Health Systems Act's Rights and Advocacy

1. Right to appropriate treatment supportive of a person's personal liberty
2. Right to an individualized, written treatment plan and its appropriate periodic review and reassessment
3. Right to ongoing participation in the treatment plan and a reasonable explanation of it
4. Right not to receive treatment, except in an emergency situation
5. Right not to participate in experimentation without informed, voluntary, written consent
6. Right to freedom from restraint or seclusion
7. Right to a humane treatment environment
8. Right to confidentiality of records
9. Right to access of one's mental health care records
10. Right to access of telephone, mail and visitors
11. Right to be informed of these rights
12. Right to assert grievances based on the infringement of these rights
13. Right of access to a qualified advocate to protect these rights
14. Right to exercise these rights without reprisal
15. Right to referral to other mental health services upon discharge

■ Nurse as provider

■ **MALPRACTICE.** All psychiatric professionals have legally defined duties of care and are responsible for their own work. If these duties are violated, malpractice exists. Malpractice involves the failure of a professional person to give the kind of proper and competent care that is given by members of his profession in the community, resulting in harm to the patient. Most malpractice claims are filed under the law of negligent tort. A *tort* is a civil wrong for which the injured party is entitled to compensation. Because, under the law, everyone is responsible for his own torts, each nurse can be held responsible in malpractice claims. Under the law of negligent tort the plaintiff must prove the following:

1. A legal duty of care existed
2. The nurse performed the duty negligently
3. Damages were suffered by the plaintiff as a result
4. The damages were substantial

When patients are admitted to a psychiatric hospital for treatment, the problems of litigation in connection with their care are many and varied. The Bill of Rights in the Mental Health Systems Act helps to clarify the sometimes conflicting role of mental health professionals when it asserts the following[22]: a health professional is not obligated to administer treatment contrary to her clinical judgment, prevent the discharge of any person for whom appropriate treatment is or has become impossible as a result of the person's refusal to consent, admit any person who has repeatedly frustrated treatments in the past by withholding consent to the proposed treatment, or provide treatment to any person admitted solely for diagnostic or evaluative purposes.

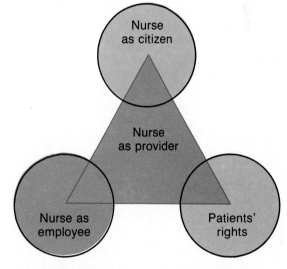

Fig. 7-2. Model of interactive influences of psychiatric nursing practices.

Such legislation helps to shed some light on the role of nurses and other health providers in such issues as right to treatment and right to refuse treatment.

Litigation. Lawsuits alleging malpractice in psychiatric diagnosis or treatment were once rather rare, but now appear to be growing in number. The American Psychiatric Association has identified the following as the most frequent sources of claims, in order of decreasing frequency:

- Patient suicide
- Improper treatment
- Ineffective or improper medication
- Breach of confidentiality

- Wrongful commitment
- Injuries resulting from electroshock therapy
- Sexual abuse of patients
- Failure to obtain informed consent[42]

Similarly, lawsuits against nurses were relatively uncommon. However, they can occur when errors are made by the nurse in either dependent or independent functioning. The accompanying box describes three recent cases involving psychiatric nurses. A study of nursing malpractice litigation between 1967 and 1977 indicated that approximately 14 cases occurred in psychiatric hospitals.[6] Of the total incidents the majority involved administration of treatments, communications, supervision of patients, and administration of medications.

The most common causes of malpractice suits against psychiatric nurses are negligence in the areas of suicide precautions and assisting in ECT. When a patient is believed to be suicidal, the psychiatrist writes an order for suicide precautions. The nurse then has the responsibility to implement that order in a way that assures the patient's safety. The exact procedure varies from hospital to hospital, but it should include close observation of him, limiting his activity to the ward only, and removing from him any objects that may possibly be used to injure himself. Another potential problem area concerns the patient receiving ECT. Proper precautions must be taken by the nurse to prepare him before the treatment and to monitor his status when he returns until he is fully conscious and alert.

■ **LEGAL RESPONSIBILITIES.** Creighton[8] stresses that the nurse is responsible for reporting pertinent information about the patient to co-workers involved in caring for him. The degree of nursing care she must use with patients must be dependent on the patient's condition, with the seriously ill demanding a higher degree of care to protect them from injury and self-destruction.

Reporting information includes written as well as oral communication, and the importance of accurate records cannot be overemphasized. Many potential problems can be avoided with clear, concise nursing notes. For example, notes that record the specific suicidal precautions that were implemented with a patient clarify the nurse's functioning. The nurse should also record the occasion when she explained to a patient and his family the food precautions he needed to observe when taking his MAO inhibitor medication. Such a note would prevent a possible lawsuit should the patient violate his dietary restrictions and become ill while on a leave of absence from the hospital. Accurate reporting is an element of good nursing care and should be completed promptly and with diligence.

The exact legal responsibilities of nonphysician therapists have not yet been well defined. It would be valuable for the nurse to practice the following preventive measures to avoid possible lawsuits:

1. Implement nursing care that meets the *Standards of Psychiatric–Mental Health Nursing Practice* as described by the American Nurses' Association.
2. Know the laws of the state in which one practices, including the rights and duties of the nurse as well as the rights of the patients.
3. Keep accurate and concise nursing records.
4. Maintain the confidentiality of patient information.
5. Consult a lawyer should any questions arise.

■ Nurse as employee

The role of employee, or contractor of service, is much less known and less frequently scrutinized, but is also very important. This is the role that mandates the practitioner's rights and responsibilities in relation to one's employers, partners, consultants, and other professional colleagues. The rights and responsibilities of employees and contractors of service are not widely known by professionals. But it is here that one's economic security, professional future, and peer relationships are based.

As an employee, a nurse has the responsibility to provide adequate supervision and evaluation of those under her authority for the quality of care given, to observe her employer's rights and responsibilities to clients and other employees, to fulfill the obligations of the contracted service adequately, to adequately apprise the employer of circumstances and conditions that impair the quality of care given, and to report observations of negligent care by others when and where appropriate. This includes the legal duty to communicate concerns about other mental health professionals who may be errant through nursing administration channels.

In return for fulfilling these responsibilities, a nurse can expect certain things from her employer, including the right to consideration for service, the right to provision of an adequate working environment and conditions, the right to adequate and qualified assistance where necessary, and the right to respect all of her other rights and responsibilities.

■ Nurse as citizen

The third role that the nurse plays is that of citizen. This role is particularly significant because all other roles, rights, responsibilities, and privileges are awarded because of the inherent rights of citizenship. Our form of democratic government grants these rights as inher-

Selected Litigation Involving Psychiatric Nurses

Case 1: Valentine v. Strange (597 F. Supp. 1316 VA)

Problem: Nurses sued when psychiatric patient set self on fire

Facts: Despite two previous attempts to burn herself, the health care providers permitted the patient to keep her cigarettes and lighter. Patient subsequently set fire to her clothing and suffered third-degree burns.

Legal Lesson: The failure of health care professionals to take precaution in the face of imminent danger to the life of an involuntarily committed patient constitutes a violation of liberty interests protected by the due process clause of the Fourteenth Amendment.

Case 2: Vattimo v. Lower Bucks Hospital (428 A. 2nd 765—Pa.)

Problem: Need for restraint and supervision of patients by psychiatric nurses

Facts: A patient with a psychotic fascination with fire set fire to his hospital room resulting in the death of the other occupant. The patient had been diagnosed as a paranoid schizophrenic, and staff had been warned of his preoccupation with fire.

Legal Lesson: The hospital was required to exercise reasonable care under the circumstances to restrain, supervise, and protect mentally deficient patients.

Case 3: Delicata v. Bourlesses (404 N.E. 2nd 667—Mass.)

Problem: Nursing psychiatric assessment versus the psychologist's

Facts: A nursing assessment indicated that a depressed patient should be closely supervised as potentially suicidal. An evaluation by the staff psychologist advised that suicidal precautions were *not* necessary. The patient subsequently killed herself in a locked bathroom.

Legal Lesson: Medical orders by a staff psychiatrist or an evaluation by a staff psychologist must be questioned when there is a change or deterioration in a patient's condition. Nursing assessments should include the evaluation of such changes in the patient's apparent physical and psychological condition. The responsibility of assessment includes the necessity for making appropriate nursing judgments and implementing nursing actions based on these assessments.

---

ent: civil rights, property rights, right to protection from harm, right to a good name, and right to due process. These rights form the foundation for the extension of other legal relationships of the nurse.

■ **CONFLICT OF INTEREST.** Unfortunately, the best interests of the patient, the nurse, and the employer do not always merge, and conflict can occur when, for example, the nurse's right to live and work without threat to personal security is violated by a patient who causes the nurse physical or emotional harm. The many dimensions of this potential conflict are illustrated in the case of a psychotic patient who has hallucinations that are adequately controlled with psychotropic medications but who refuses to take them. Intervention with this patient needs to take into consideration the following possibilities:

■ Failing to medicate the patient may be a denial of his right to treatment.

■ Failing to medicate the patient could have harmful side effects, such as the unnecessary and possibly irreversible continuation of his illness.

■ Failing to medicate the patient may lead to a psychotic episode and result in violence and injury to himself, other patients, or the staff.

■ Failing to medicate the patient may lead to a psychotic episode but no violence.

Maryland Nurses' Association
The Bill of Rights for Registered Nurses

We, the Council on Human Rights of the Maryland Nurses' Association, in order to promote increased knowledge and understanding of the rights and responsibilities of all registered nurses, have developed The Bill of Rights for Registered Nurses. We propose that this Bill will aid in educating consumers and health care professionals about the rights of registered nurses, as well as their corresponding reponsibilities. Therefore, we submit the Bill of Rights for Registered Nurses as a position statement of the Maryland Nurses' Association.

The nurse has a right:

The nurse has a responsibility:

Individual

to practice according to the Maryland Nurse Practice Act.

to make independent nursing judgments.

to question any delegated medical order or any plan of care that may cause possible harm to the patient/client or others.

to refuse to carry out any delegated medical order or any plan of care that may cause possible harm to the patient/client or others.

to pursue quality continuing education.

to teach individuals and groups health care practices that facilitate treatment, prevent illness, and provide optimal wellness.

to assume personal accountability for individual nursing judgments and actions which consider the individual value systems and the uniqueness of each patient/client.

to implement the nursing process in providing individualized nursing care.

to safeguard the patient/client and the public from incompetent, unethical, or illegal health care practices.

to refuse to perform any nursing action which will jeopardize the patient/client or the public, and the obligation to communicate the rationale to the proper authority.

to avail one's self of opportunities which will broaden knowledge and refine and increase skills.

to educate the patient/client and the public.

Employment

to competitive hiring and promotion which is based on knowledge and experience and which is unrestricted by consideration of sex, race, age, creed, or national origin.

to realistic assignments that can assure the patient/client quality care that includes safety, dignity, and comfort.

to negotiate salary and individual conditions of employment.

to work in a safe and adequately equipped environment.

to work with qualified, competent nursing personnel.

to periodic, fair, objective evaluations by peers.

to pay increases based on demonstrated performance.

to due process whenever accused of unethical, incompetent, illegal, or unqualified practice or of prejudicial or inappropriate conduct.

to be an advocate for the patient/client and the public when health care and safety may be affected by incompetent, unethical, or illegal practices.

to representation by a negotiator in labor matters.

to maintain competence and prepare one's self adequately for promotion.

to evaluate one's own work environment and to communicate and document unrealistic work loads through appropriate channels.

to make known individual convictions and preferences prior to hiring.

to assess, evaluate, document, and correct unsafe conditions and to communicate such information to the appropriate authority promptly.

to objectively document and report to appropriate authority evidence of competent, as well as incompetent performance and to evaluate, inform, counsel, and teach nursing personnel when indicated.

to participate in the development of reliable and valid evaluation criteria for peer review.

to maintain competence, incorporate new techniques and knowledge, and continuously upgrade the quality of health care.

to participate in the planning, establishment, and implementation of procedures to ensure due process.

to be alert to any instances of incompetent, unethical, or illegal practices by any member of the health care system and to take appropriate action regarding these practices.

to select and utilize a knowledgeable and impartial negotiator.

Maryland Nurses' Association
The Bill of Rights for Registered Nurses—cont'd

The nurse has a right:	The nurse has a responsibility:
Professional	
to receive support from the nursing profession at all levels.	to participate in activities that contribute to the ongoing development of the profession's body of knowledge.
to belong to an autonomous nursing organization.	to be an active member and to participate in the nursing organization's effort to implement and improve standards of nursing.
to have expert testimony supplied by the nursing organization for both legal and legislative issues.	to provide knowledgeable, objective, articulate expert testimony.
to full and equal representation on all decision-making bodies concerned with health care.	to provide knowledgeable, active, and effective collaborating with members of the health professions.
to be involved actively in the political decision-making process at all levels of the government.	to be knowledgeable, active, and effective in the legislative process by direct involvement, effective education and selection of representative legislators, lobbying, and creating citizen awareness in promoting local, state, and national efforts to meet the health needs of the public.

■ Medicating the patient in the absence of an emergency situation and without a clear threat of violence is in violation of his right to refuse treatment.

In this case, the staff decided not to medicate the patient. When the night nurse went to check on the patient in his room that evening the patient struck the nurse in the face, which resulted in severe bruises and the loss of some teeth. This development leads to a host of new questions.

■ Was the patient competent and legally liable for his actions?

■ What were the circumstances of the incident?

■ Was the nurse sufficiently aware of the potential hazard and, if so, was she responsible for assuming the risk?

■ Was the staffing pattern adequate to discourage, respond to, and control a potentially violent situation?

■ Was there a provision in the environment of the unit for potentially violent patients and, if so, why wasn't it used for this patient?

Obviously, there are no simple or perhaps even equitable resolutions to such dilemmas; yet they are real and ever present. It would appear that prevention needs

to be the focus of concern by mental health professionals. This requires a knowledge of legislation, rights, and responsibilities with a serious appreciation of the potential conflicts that might emerge.

Nurses in one state, Maryland, have demonstrated an awareness of these issues and have developed the bill of rights for registered nurses shown on the opposite page and above. This document is commendable in that it serves to educate nurses and the public and also to clarify rights and responsibilities. In addition, professional nursing judgment requires a careful examination of the context of nursing care, the possible consequences of one's actions, and the feasible alternatives one might employ. Only then do rights and responsibilities take on any real meaning.

Psychiatry and criminal responsibility

The determination of criminal responsibility concerns the accused person's condition at the time of the alleged offense. It has received much public attention when used in the "insanity defense." This defense proposes that a person who has committed an act that in a usual situation would be criminal is held not guilty by reason of "insanity." This is a difficult decision to make; usually the defense attorneys and prosecutors offer many arguments pro and con and frequently psychiatrists are called on to testify. Nurses are seldom directly involved in the legislative process, but they should have an understanding of the law in this area both as citizens and psychiatric professionals.

The idea behind this type of defense is an essentially humanitarian one. The rationale for it is that a person should not be blamed if he "did not know what he was doing" or "could not help himself." With the complexity of today's society and the judicial system, however, many believe this defense is being abused, and it has created great controversy in the legal and psychiatric professions.[45] Much of this controversy has been stimulated by the attempt on President Reagan's life. The conflict among citizens, legal authorities, mental health professionals, and in the news media has been heightened by the "not guilty by reason of insanity" verdict by the John Hinckley, Jr., case in 1982. This might precipitate changes in the present law. One such change is the movement away from the use of the defense of "not guilty by reason of insanity" (NGBI) to the more recent of "guilty but mentally ill" (GBMI).

At the present time there are four sets of criteria used in the United States to determine the criminal responsibility of an offender who is suffering from a mental illness: the M'Naghten Rule, the Irresistible Impulse Test, the Durham Test, or "Product Rule," and the American Law Institute's Test, or the ALI Test, the most frequently used criteria (see Table 7-4).

■ M'Naghten Rule

This law originated with the trial of Daniel M'Naghten in London in 1832 when he was tried for the murder of Edward Drummond, the private secretary of Sir Robert Peele. M'Naghten had suffered from delusions of persecution, and on numerous occasions had complained to public authorities. Receiving no help, however, he decided to resolve the situation himself. He began watching the house of Sir Robert Peele and one evening, under the belief he was shooting Peele, shot Edward Drummond as he emerged from the house. When he came to trial, his attorney entered an appeal of "partial insanity" and M'Naghten was declared of unsound mind and was committed to an institution for the criminally insane. In deciding the case, the judges identified two rules to use in determining the criminal responsibility of a person who pleads insanity. The first rule states that the individual at the time of the crime did not "know the nature and quality of the act." The second states that if he did know what he was doing, he did not know that what he was doing "was wrong." These two rules are simply referred to as the "nature and quality" rule and "right from wrong" test.

This case was the first major test for determining criminal responsibility, and it is still used in most states and criminal courts. It has become less popular in recent years, however, because of the narrow wording, which some people believe ignores aspects of the whole personality such as emotions and will.

■ Irresistible Impulse Test

About 15 states have adopted this test along with the M'Naghten Rule. It is never used in isolation. According to this test, a person may know the difference between right and wrong but finds himself impulsively driven to commit the criminal act. It is usually necessary to show a lack of premeditation and that the strength of the urge was so great that it would have been carried out regardless of the circumstances. This test is frequently used as a defense for sudden, violent behavior displayed under stress.

■ Durham Test, or "Product Rule"

This test is based on a 1954 decision that took place in the District of Columbia. The rule states that the accused is not criminally responsible if his act was the "product of mental disease." Thus it is sometimes called the "Product Rule," although this phrase and "mental disease" have been difficult to define. Many people object to the use of this test because it greatly expands the number and scope of individuals who may use the insanity defense. At this time it is only used in New Hampshire, Maine, and the Virgin Islands.

■ American Law Institute's Test

This test is similar to the combination of the M'Naghten Rule and Irresistible Impulse Test. It states that a person is not responsible for his criminal act if he lacks the capacity to "appreciate" the wrongfulness of it or to "conform" his conduct to the requirements of the law. It also excludes "an abnormality manifested only by repeated criminal or otherwise antisocial conduct." This last condition thereby excludes the psychopath who has repeated criminal conduct. This test has become popular over the years, and it is now used by all the federal circuit courts and at least ten states' courts.

■ Disposition of mentally ill offenders

If a person is found not guilty by reason of insanity (NGBI), he is not often set free. In some states he may be committed at the discretion of the court, and in almost a third of the states he is automatically hospitalized. Some offenders are treated in special hospitals, others are sent to state mental hospitals, and still others are sent to treatment facilities provided in the penal institution. If a person is found guilty but mentally ill

---

TABLE 7-4

FOUR SETS OF CRITERIA COMMONLY USED TO DETERMINE THE CRIMINAL RESPONSIBILITY OF A MENTALLY ILL OFFENDER

Name of test	Criteria
M'Naghten Rule	1. The individual did not know the nature and quality of the act. 2. The individual did not know that what he was doing was wrong.
Irresistible Impulse Test	An individual is impulsively driven to commit the criminal act with lack of premeditation and a strong urge to do so. This test is seldom used in isolation.
Durham Test, or Product Rule	An individual's act was the "product of mental disease." This test is only used in three states.
American Law Institute's Test	An individual lacks the capacity to "appreciate" the wrongfulness of his act or to "conform" his conduct to the requirements of the law. It excludes the psychopath and is a popular criteria for determining criminal responsibility.

(GBMI), he is never set free. Since the insanity defense is used most often in capital offenses, it is usually desirable to make security provisions available and penal institutions lend themselves best to this.

After hospitalization and on recovery, the patient may be discharged by the court that ordered his commitment. In other states he may be discharged by the governor. Still others allow the mental institution to make that decision. The major criteria for discharge of the patient are that he is not likely to repeat his offense and that it is relatively safe to release him to the community.

Ethics in psychiatric nursing

Ethical considerations combine with legal issues to impact on all the elements of the psychiatric nursing process. The concept of ethics has different meanings to each individual. It implies what is right and wrong and becomes intermingled with one's ideas on values and morality.

■ Ethical standards

An ethic is a standard of valued behavior or beliefs adhered to by an individual or group. It describes what ought to be, rather than what is. It is a goal to which one aspires. These standards of behavior are learned through socialization, growth, and experience. As such, they are not static entities; they evolve and change concurrent with social change. Ethical standards can only be implemented in conjunction with personal value systems.

Groups, such as professions, can also hold a code of ethics that reflects the profession's desire to protect its clients. It functions to define behavior that is viewed to be desirable by the profession in its service to consumers, not in service to itself, and it serves as a framework for decision making for members of the profession. Moore[25] has defined two major purposes for a code of ethics as that of "structuring" and "sensitizing." This first purpose of structuring has a basically preventive value and aims to hold back impulsive and unethical behavior. The second purpose of sensitizing has an essentially educative value and aims to raise one's ethical consciousness.

The American Nurses' Association published a code of ethics for nurses (see the box on page 236).[1] It places heavy emphasis on the accountability of the nurse for the quality of patient care and the nurse's duty to act as a patient advocate in ensuring the quality of care rendered by others.

These professional standards are intended to be used by nurses in the daily conduct of health care delivery. Knowledge of one's own personal values and implementation of them within the framework of the nursing ethical code can shape the quality of the nursing care one gives patients and increase the satisfaction the nurse receives from her practice.

■ Power and paternalism

A discussion of ethics and nursing must take into consideration the crucial element of power. In the psychiatric setting, the nurse can function in many roles,

American Nurses' Association Code for Nurses

1. The nurse provides services with respect for human dignity and the uniqueness of the client unrestricted by considerations of social or economic status, personal attributes, or the nature of health problems.
2. The nurse safeguards the client's right to privacy by judiciously protecting information of a confidential nature.
3. The nurse acts to safeguard the client and the public when health care and safety are affected by the incompetent, unethical, or illegal practice of any person.
4. The nurse assumes responsibility and accountability for individual nursing judgments and actions.
5. The nurse maintains competence in nursing.

From American Nurses' Association: Code for nurses with interpretive statements, Kansas City, Mo., 1976, The Association. Reprinted with permission.

6. The nurse exercises informed judgment and uses individual competence and qualification as criteria in seeking consultation, accepting responsibilities, and delegating nursing activities to others.
7. The nurse participates in activities that contribute to the ongoing development of the profession's body of knowledge.
8. The nurse participates in the profession's efforts to implement and improve standards of nursing.
9. The nurse participates in the profession's efforts to establish and maintain conditions of employment conducive to high-quality nursing care.
10. The nurse participates in the profession's effort to protect the public from misinformation and misrepresentation and to maintain the integrity of nursing.
11. The nurse collaborates with members of the health professions and other citizens in promoting community and national efforts to meet public health needs.

from a custodial keeper of the keys to a skilled therapist. Each of these roles, however, has a certain amount of power inherent in it, since all nurses have the ability to influence the patient's course of treatment. Nurses serve as the major source of information regarding a patient's behavior. This is particularly true in inpatient settings, where longer contacts can occur between a nurse and patient and the nursing staff is the only group to work a 24-hour day. Nurses also participate in team meetings, individual and group psychotherapy, and behavior modification programs. Finally, nurses can greatly influence decisions about patient medications, such as the type, dosage, and frequency of the prescribed drugs.

The literature describes the ethical dilemmas that arise from health care professionals' "paternalistic" attitude toward their patients. Paternalism can be defined as acting on one's own idea of what is best for another person, without asking the involved individual. It occurs when something is done "for the patient's own good" even though the patient would likely disagree with the action. This attitude tends to reduce the adult patient to the status of a child and interferes with a patient's freedom of action.

Gert and Culver present five criteria to evaluate whether a particular action is truly paternalistic.[14] They suggest that a nurse is acting paternalistically if, and

only if, the nurse's behavior indicates that the nurse believes that

1. One's action is for the patient's good
2. One is qualified to act on the patient's behalf
3. One's action involves violating a moral rule (such as deceiving, breaking a promise, causing pain)
4. One is justified in acting on the patient's behalf whether or not the patient has ever given or will ever give consent
5. The patient thinks (perhaps falsely) that he knows what is for his own good

Paternalism, defined by these criteria therefore, involves acting on one's own beliefs, as well as violating a commonly held moral rule.

To avoid this potential danger, the nurse should realize that her ethical obligations span a wide range of individuals, including the patient, the patient's family or support system, herself, her own family, other health care professionals, the health care institution or organization in which she works, and the larger social community. Furthermore, her ethical obligations arise within a context of laws and government regulations that may, at times, create ethical dilemmas which involve and affect the nurse. To the extent that she is aware of them, she can examine these problems not only from a clinical perspective, but also from an ethical one.

■ Ethical dilemmas

An ethical dilemma exists when moral claims conflict with one another. It can be defined as (1) a difficult problem that seems to have no satisfactory solution or (2) a choice between equally unsatisfactory alternatives. Ethical dilemmas pose such questions as "What should I do?" and "What is the right thing to do?" They can occur both at the nurse-patient-family level of daily nursing care and at the policy-making level of institutions and communities. Although ethical dilemmas arise in all areas of nursing practice, some problems are unique to psychiatric and mental health nursing. Many of these dilemmas come together under the umbrella issue of behavior control.

On first analysis, behavior control may seem like a simple concrete issue—behavior is a personal choice, and any behavior that does not impose on the rights of others is acceptable. Unfortunately, this simple proposition does not help one address complex situations. For example, a severely depressed person may choose suicide as an alternative to an intolerable existence. This is, on one level, an individual choice not directly harming others, yet suicide is strongly prohibited in American society. In many states, suicide is a crime that can be prosecuted. So too, in some states, it is illegal for consenting adults of the same sex to have sexual relations, although it is not illegal for a man to rape his wife. These examples raise some difficult questions: When is it appropriate for society to regulate personal behavior? Who will regulate this behavior? Is the aim of this regulation personal adjustment, personal growth, or adaptation to social norms? And finally, how do we measure the costs and benefits of attempting to control personal freedom in a free society?

One of the most fundamental problems is that psychiatry lacks definitions for mental health, normalcy, mental illness, and insanity. These terms have been debated for hundreds of years, yet society lacks consensus on universally accepted definitions. This is evidence of the blurring boundaries between science and ethics in the field of psychiatry. Theoretically, science and ethics are viewed as two separate entities. Science is descriptive, deals with "what is," and rests on validation; ethics is predictive, deals with "what ought to be," and relies on judgment. However, psychiatry is neither purely scientific nor value free.

The fact that psychiatry is not a predictable science is reflected in the existence of over 100 schools of psychotherapy, each with its own theory of causation, treatment goals, and therapeutic practices, which range from screaming cures (Janov's primal therapy), to reasoning cures (Ellis' rational therapy), to realism cures (Glasser's reality therapy), to orgasm cures (Reich's orgone therapy), to profound-rest cures (transcendental meditation), and even to chemical cures (megavitamin therapy).[16] What emerges is the sense that psychiatry represents neither pure science nor pure ethics, but a branch of the healing professions that resides somewhere in between and that often may be affected by culture, chance, and faith.

Despite these ambiguities, each mental health professional must identify the nature of one's professional commitment. Is one committed to the happiness of the individual or the smooth functioning of society? Ideally, these values should not conflict, but in reality they sometimes do. The patient's rights to treatment, to refuse treatment, and to informed consent highlight this conflict-of-interest question. As a nurse, one must consider if one is reinforcing an individual's personal unhappiness to force him to be socially or politically acceptable to society. As such, the nurse may not actually be working for either the patient's best interests or her own; she may be acting as an agent of society and not be really aware of it.

All nurses participate in some therapeutic regimens in psychiatry whose scientific and ethical bases are ambiguous. Any health professional who has witnessed electroconvulsive therapy, for example, has probably questioned the effectiveness, coerciveness, precision, or humaneness of psychiatry. Yet the American health care system continues to apply a medical model of wellness and illness to human behavior. Wellness is socially acceptable behavior, and illness is socially unacceptable behavior. Within this context, it becomes critically important for each nurse to analyze such ethical dilemmas as freedom of choice versus coercion, defining adequate treatment, deciding on resource allocations, helping versus imposing values, and focusing on cure versus prevention.

■ Ethical decision making

Ethical decision making involves trying to determine right from wrong in situations where clear guidelines are not evident.

Everything is neither right nor wrong. The right or wrong is the choosing, the keeping, the losing. All paths are light and shadow, and every path is a different thing to each man. The right and the wrong, the good and the evil lie not upon the silent pathway, but in the man that walks it.[32:198]

There are three dimensions to ethical decision making. Each of these dimensions influences one's analysis of the dilemma and decisions related to it:

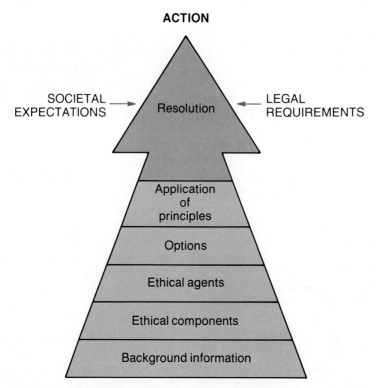

Fig. 7-3. Model for ethical decision making. Societal expectations and legal requirements may sway the resolution of the conflict one way or another. But one must not confuse the notions of what is legal (or expected) with what is good, right, or proper—they may or may not coincide. (From Curtin, L.: Nurs. Forum **17**(1):12, 1978.)

1. The existence of a code of value judgments or ethics that is known to the individual
2. The awareness of one's personal moral beliefs and values
3. A complex social context with normative and legal implications

It is necessary for the nurse to correlate the code of nursing ethics with her own personal value system and to identify areas of harmony and incongruence. This will allow the nurse to base ethical decisions on behavior that involves responsibility, accountability, risk, and commitment. Responsibility requires the capacity for rational, moral decision making. Accountability signifies action. Risk involves the undertaking of peril, jeopardy, or chance of loss, and commitment implies loyalty, trust, and a pledge of self. In addition, the nurse's ethical choice must take into consideration the circumstances of the specific situation, social mores, and legal ramifications arising from it.

■ **MODEL FOR ETHICAL DECISION MAKING.** A decision-making model can be a useful tool in identifying factors that impinge on the decision and principles which need to be clarified. Curtin[10] proposed a model

for critical ethical analysis (Fig. 7-3). It describes steps or factors that the nurse needs to consider between encountering an ethical dilemma and resolving it. The first step is **gathering background information** to get as clear a picture as possible of what precisely is the problem. This includes finding out what information is available and what information is needed to clarify one's understanding of the underlying issues. The next factor is **identifying the ethical components** or the nature of the dilemma, such as freedom versus coercion or treating versus accepting the right to refuse treatment. The next step is the **clarification of the rights and responsibilities of all ethical agents,** or those involved in the decision making. This involves the patient, the nurse, and possibly many others, including the patient's family, physician, health care institution, clergy, social worker, and perhaps even the courts. All involved ethical agents may not agree on how the situation should be handled, but the scope of their rights and duties can be clarified. **All possible options must then be explored** in light of the rights and responsibilities of everyone involved, as well as the purpose and potential result of each option. This step serves to eliminate those alternatives that violate rights or can be certain to produce harm.

The nurse then engages in the **application of principles,** which are derived from her philosophy of life and nursing, her store of scientific knowledge, and the ethical theory to which she subscribes. Ethical theories suggest ways of structuring or clarifying ethical dilemmas and help one to judge potential solutions. Following are four such positions[3]:

1. **Utilitarianism** focuses on the consequences of actions and on the greatest amount of happiness or the least amount of harm for the greatest number. It is embodied in the idea of "the greatest good for the greatest number."
2. **Egoism** is a position in which one seeks the solution that is best for oneself. The self is of paramount importance, and others are viewed secondarily, if at all.
3. **Formalism** requires the consideration of the nature of the act itself and the principles or rules involved. It involves the universal application of a basic principle, such as "do unto others as you would have them do unto you."
4. **Fairness** is based on the concept of justice, and benefit to the least advantaged in society becomes the norm for decision making.

The final step is the **resolution into action.** Within the context of social expectations and legal requirements, the nurse decides on the goals and methods of implementation. Table 7-5 summarizes the steps the nurse takes in ethical decision making and suggests questions she can ask herself as she deals with the challenge and complexity of ethical choice in psychiatric nursing practice.

Future challenges

The interface between psychiatry and the law is becoming increasingly complex. Historically, the mental health delivery system had only two components—mental health professionals and the patient. Now, however, the system has grown to include five forces, each of which must be taken into account when dealing with any mental health problem. This pentagonal relationship (Fig. 7-4) has been described by Kopolow[17] to be composed of consumers, providers of services, governmental regulators and lawmakers, the judiciary, and third-party insurers. Members of each of these groups have related, but slightly different, interests. The consumer is concerned that services be available when and where he wishes them, that they are appropriate to his needs, and that he is involved in establishing the priorities of the program. The provider has clinical and professional biases. If outside controls must exist, the provider wants them equitably applied and with one's

TABLE 7-5	
STEPS AND QUESTIONS IN ETHICAL DECISION MAKING	
Steps	**Relevant questions**
Gathering background information	Does an ethical dilemma exist? What information is known? What information is needed? What is the context of the dilemma?
Identifying ethical components	What is the underlying issue? Who is affected by this dilemma?
Clarification of agents	What are the rights of each involved party? What are the obligations of each involved party? Who should be involved in the decision making? For whom is the decision being made? What degree of consent is needed by the patient?
Exploration of options	What alternatives exist? What is the purpose or intent of each alternative? What are the potential consequences of each alternative?
Application of principles	What criteria should be used? What ethical theories are subscribed to? What scientific facts are relevant? What is one's philosophy of life and nursing?
Resolution into action	What are the social and legal constraints and ramifications? What is the goal of one's decision? How can the resulting ethical choice be implemented? How can the resulting ethical choice be evaluated?

responsibilities and liabilities clearly defined. The government wants citizens to have access to quality care at the least cost and wants the providers to be accountable for the care they provide. The courts, after years of neglect, have recently assumed the role of guardian of patients' constitutional rights and have begun to scru-

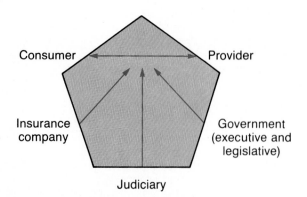

Fig. 7-4. Pentagonal relationship that characterizes the mental health delivery system. (From Kopolow, L.: Patient's rights and psychiatric practice. In Barton, W., and Sanborn, C., editors: Law and the mental health professions, New York, 1978, International Universities Press, Inc.)

tinize patient care and treatment. Finally, insurance companies are concerned with either making a profit, or remaining solvent while seeking assurances that they are paying for covered services by appropriately licensed and credentialed professionals. The changing priorities and interactions of these five forces affect the quality, availability, and responsiveness of mental health services in this country.

At present there is a simultaneous urge to adequate treatment of the psychiatrically ill and protection of their constitutional rights. Both of these trends are emerging at a time of fiscal restraint. It would appear as if one's choice is between abandoning former patients to their rights in the community or warehousing them in large institutions, whether these be hospitals or jails.[44]

Mental health professionals are concerned about the quantity and quality of care received by psychiatric patients. Legal reformers are indignant about the lack of rights experienced by these patients and object to a law that justifies commitment under the uncertain prediction by a single professional of some unproven and unknowable harm. Criminal court judges are angry that in the day-to-day implementation of the commitment law, the only option left to them is to prosecute the mentally ill defendant. Psychiatric hospitals are understaffed and underfunded and are attacked on all sides for their inability to "care" for and "cure" psychiatric patients. Community programs are few and poorly supported and have resulted in deinstitutionalized patients living without treatment in urban ghettos or finding their way into the criminal justice system. The public is frightened at the thought of having psychiatric patients in their neighborhoods, and concerned citizens demand that mental health programs exercise greater control over this population perceived to be dangerous.

Clearly, mechanisms are needed by which patients, mental health professionals, attorneys, and concerned citizens can work together to improve mental health care and advance the rights of all patients. The priorities of the mentally ill extend beyond protection of their legal rights to protection of their clinical needs and general welfare. No one profession or group unilaterally can fulfill all of these needs, but increased cooperation among the various mental health advocates can make this goal possible.

■ Advocacy and patient education

Mental health advocacy is evolving into one effective method for protecting and advocating the rights of all citizens to high-quality mental health care that is clinically and constitutionally appropriate. New Jersey, for example, has a Division of Mental Health Advocacy mandated by the state legislature that works to produce a better system of mental health care and delivery. It is staffed by lawyers, psychologists, psychiatric nurses, social workers, and others who work as advocates for those caught up in the psychiatric system. Other states, such as Minnesota, New York, Michigan, and California, have adopted similar programs. The purpose of mental health advocacy is to assure that both clinical and legal considerations of the patient are properly weighed, and it is increasingly being considered as part of the range of services to which patients are entitled.

Simultaneously, the advocacy for patients' rights movement has been criticized for lack of adequate definition of terms and selected irresponsible advocacy. "Advocate," "legal representative," and "ombudsman" often do not carry the same or even similar meanings in different programs or when used by different people. "Legal advocacy" and "legal services" are also confused, and "information and advice" are often equated with "advocacy." Lamb has also noted that the patients' rights activist has power without clinical responsibility.[18] He cautions that major problems can result when power is wielded by people who lack an appreciation of the clinical complexities of work with the severely mentally ill. There is a need for mental health professionals, therefore, to distinguish responsible advocacy from irresponsible advocacy. He suggests that advocates be required to have in-depth experience providing direct service to severely disturbed patients for 6 months to a year and that advocates be rigorously screened within bureaucracies.

It has been noted that the ratio of patients to prisoners is three to one and suggested that for every public defender there should be three mental health lawyers. Whether or not such an idea becomes a reality, it is still possible to safeguard the rights of patients by (1) pe-

---

DIRECTIONS FOR FUTURE RESEARCH

The following are some of the nursing research problems raised in Chapter 7 that merit further study by psychiatric nurses.

1. Awareness by psychiatric nurses of a patient's legal rights at the time of admission and during the psychiatric hospitalization.
2. Perceptions of psychiatric nurses of the dangerousness of patients, including criteria defining it, assessing it, predicting it, and its effect on nursing care.
3. Knowledge of psychiatric nurses of the statutes governing the admission, discharge, and rights of the mentally ill in the states in which they work.
4. Attitudes of psychiatric nurses toward various important legal and ethical issues, such as commitment, privileged communication, informed consent, right to treatment, and right to refuse treatment.
5. The ability of psychiatric nurses to evaluate the potential dangerousness of psychiatric patients.
6. The nature of nursing involvement in caring for the homeless mentally ill.
7. Patients' rights most commonly violated in psychiatric settings.
8. Nursing interventions implemented with patients who refuse medication.
9. Litigation involving psychiatric nurses, including the number of cases, basis of the lawsuit, other persons named in the suit, and outcome.
10. Knowledge of psychiatric nurses' rights and responsibilities as employees.
11. Resolution of conflict of interest relative to the legal roles of the psychiatric nurse as provider, employee, and citizen.
12. The ethical dilemmas arising from psychiatric nurses' paternalistic attitude toward their patients.
13. The dimensions of the ethical decision-making process used by psychiatric nurses in critically analyzing ethical issues.
14. The level of participation of psychiatric nurses in formal and informal mental health advocacy programs.
15. Mechanisms used by psychiatric nurses to impact on mental health issues at the local, state, and national levels and identification of issues in which they are involved.

riodic reviews of those involuntarily committed, (2) considering the least restrictive setting when determining treatment or services, and (3) greater use of alternatives to hospitalization, including foster home and day treatment programs. Impetus for change in this area is requiring that states reorder their priorities, yet it is occurring at a time when a number of states have been forced to cut their mental health budgets. One can only speculate on what the impact of all this activity will be in the future.

In the Sixteenth Century the deranged were expelled, shipped off, or executed; in the Seventeenth Century the insane were locked up in jails and houses of correction; in the Eighteenth Century madmen were confined in madhouses; in the Nineteenth Century lunatics were sent to asylums; in the Twentieth Century the mentally ill are committed to hospitals; in the Twenty-first Century . . . .
K. Jones, *Lunacy, Law, and Conscience*

■ SUGGESTED CROSS-REFERENCES ■

This chapter serves as a foundation for formulating principles of psychiatric nursing and implementing psychiatric nursing practice. As such, it is related to all other chapters of this text.

■ SUMMARY ■

1. Informal admission to a psychiatric hospital occurs without formal or written application. The patient admitted in this way is free to leave at any time.

2. Voluntary admission requires the individual to make written application to a psychiatric hospital and agree to receive treatment and abide by hospital rules. If he wishes to be discharged, it is usually required that he give written notice to the hospital.

3. Involuntary admission means that the request for hospitalization did not originate with the patient, and when he is committed, he loses the right to leave the hospital when he wishes. It is usually justified on the grounds of (a) dangerous to others, (b) dangerous to self, or (c) need for treatment. The procedure for commitment includes filing a petition, completing a mental status examination, and determination of the need for hospitalization, which can be a medical, court, or administrative decision.

    a. Emergency involuntary admission may be used for patients who are acutely ill, and most states limit the amount of time the person can be detained to from 3 to 30 days.

    b. Temporary or observation involuntary admission is used for the purpose of diagnosis and short-term therapy. The commitment is for a specific period of time ranging from 2 to 6 months.

c. Indefinite involuntary admission, or formal commitment, detains a person for an indeterminate length of time or until he is ready for discharge. It usually involves a court decision.

4. There are three types of discharges.

    a. A conditional discharge is a patient's specified leave of absence from the hospital. Certain expectations are placed on him, the most common being that he attend outpatient therapy.

    b. An absolute discharge is a final one and marks the patient's termination of his relationship with the hospital. New admission proceedings must be initiated if the patient wishes to return to the hospital after receiving an absolute discharge.

    c. A judicial discharge is one issued by the court. It is provided for by laws that allow a patient or his family to appeal for discharge even though the hospital may oppose this request.

5. The civil and personal rights of psychiatric patients are presently being supported in legislative acts throughout the country. The nature of these rights varies greatly from state to state.

    a. The person's competency to execute wills is called the testamentary capacity. To make a valid will, it is required that he (1) know he is making a will, (2) know the nature and extent of his property, and (3) know who his friends and relatives are and how he is related to them.

    b. "Incompetency" is a legal term that must be proved in a special court hearing. To determine incompetency, it must be shown that the person has a mental disorder that causes a defect in judgment, and this defect makes him incapable of handling his own affairs. As a result of this ruling he is deprived of many of his civil rights. This can be reversed only in another court hearing that declares him competent.

    c. Habeas corpus is an important right all patients retain. It provides for the speedy release of any individual who can show he is being deprived of his liberty and detained illegally.

    d. The right to privacy implies the right to keep some information about oneself completely secret from others. "Confidentiality" involves disclosure of certain information to another specifically authorized person. "Privileged communication" applies only in court-related proceedings and must be established by law. At present, most states do not provide for privileged communication between nurses and patients.

    e. The right to informed consent requires that a physician explain the treatment to the patient, including its possible complications and risks. The patient's consent to it must imply competency, understanding, and volition. All unusual and experimental treatments require special permission.

    f. The rights to treatment, refuse treatment, and receive treatment in the least restrictive setting are recent developments that are being delineated in various court decisions.

6. The psychiatric nurse has rights and responsibilities attendant to each of three legal roles: nurse as provider, nurse as employee, and nurse as citizen.

    a. As a provider, every nurse is responsible for the quality of care she gives to patients and can be held responsible in malpractice claims. For a nurse to be proved negligent it must be shown that (1) a legal duty of care existed, (2) the nurse performed the duty negligently, (3) the patient suffered damages, and (4) the damages were substantial.

    b. As an employee, the nurse has responsibilities to peers, employer, and colleagues.

    c. As a citizen, her rights form the foundation for the extension of the nurse's other legal relationships. It is possible for the nurse to experience a conflict of interest among these rights and responsibilities.

7. Criminal responsibility concerns the accused person's condition at the time of the alleged crime. The "insanity defense" has received much attention in this regard. At present, three tests are commonly used in the United States to determine criminal responsibility. These are the M'Naghten Rule, the Irresistible Impulse Test, and the American Law Institute's Test. A fourth test, the Durham Test, or "Product Rule," is seldom used.

8. An ethic is a standard of valued behavior or beliefs adhered to by an individual or group. It describes a goal to which one aspires. An ethical dilemma exists when moral claims conflict with one another. In psychiatric nursing, many of these dilemmas center on the issue of behavior control. Ethical decision making involves trying to determine right from wrong in situations where clear guidelines are not evident. A model for critical ethical analysis was presented and discussed.

9. Five forces currently affect the mental health delivery system—the consumer, the provider, the government, the judiciary, and the insurance companies. The future must provide for independent, responsible, and collaborative approaches to advocacy so that it can become an effective mechanism for the creation of a more responsive mental health system.

■ REFERENCES ■

1. American Nurses' Association: Code for nurses with interpretive statements, Kansas City, Mo., 1976, The Association.

2. Arkin, A., et al.: Behavior modification, N.Y. State J. Med. **76:**190, Feb. 1976.

3. Aroskar, M.: Anatomy of an ethical dilemma: the theory, Am. J. Nurs. **80:**658, 1980.

4. Birnbaum, M.: The right to treatment, Am. Bar Assoc. J., p. 499, 1960.

5. Brakel, S.J., and Kock, R.S.: The mentally disabled and the law, revised ed., Chicago, 1971, University of Chicago Press.

6. Campazzi, B.: Nurses, nursing and malpractice litigation: 1967-1977, Adv. Nurs. Sci. **4**(1):1, 1980.

7. Chodoff, P.: The case for involuntary hospitalization of the mentally ill, Am. J. Psychiatry **133**:496, 1976.

8. Creighton, H.: Law every nurse should know, Philadelphia, 1975, W.B. Saunders Co.

9. *Cross v. Harris,* 418 F 2d (D.C. Cir. 1969).

10. Curtin, L.: A proposed model for critical ethical analysis, Nurs. Forum **17**(1):12, 1978.

11. *Dixon v. Weinberger,* No. 74285 (C.D.D.C. Feb. 14, 1974).

12. Ennis, B.J.: Civil liberties and mental illness, Criminal Law Bull., p. 101, 1971.

13. Fustero, S.: Home on the street, Psych. Today **18**(2):56, 1984.

14. Gert, B., and Culver, M.: Paternalistic behavior, Philos. Pub. Affairs. **6**:45, 1976.

15. Jones, R.: Street people and psychiatry: an introduction, Hosp. Community Psychiatry **34**(9):807, 1983 Suppl.

16. Karasu, T.: Psychotherapies: an overview, Am. J. Psychiatry **134**:851, 1977.

17. Kopolow, L.: Patients' rights and psychiatric practice. In Barton, W., and Sanborn, C., editors: Law and the mental health professions, New York, 1978, International Universities Press, Inc.

18. Lamb, R.: Securing patients' rights—responsibly, Hosp. Community Psychiatry **32**(6):393, 1981.

19. Law briefs, Time, p. 44, July 6, 1981.

20. Levinson, R., and Ramsay, G.: Dangerousness, stress and mental health evaluations, J. Health Soc. Behav. **20**:178, 1979.

21. McGarry, L., and Kaplan, H.: Overview: current trends in mental law, Am. J. Psychiatry **130**:627, 1973.

22. Mental Health Systems Act, Report No. 96-980, Amendment to Senate Bill 1177, Sept. 23, 1980.

23. Merton, R.K., and Nisbet, R.A., editors: Contemporary social problems, New York, 1961, Harcourt, Brace & World.

24. Miller, R., and Fiddleman, P.: Outpatient commitment: treatment in the least restrictive environment? Hosp. Community Psychiatry **35**(2):147, 1984.

25. Moore, R.: Ethics in the practice of psychiatry: origins, functions, models and enforcement, Am. J. Psychiatry **135**:157, 1978.

26. National League for Nursing: Nursing's role in patient's rights, Pub. No. 11-1671, New York, 1977, The League.

27. Oran, D.: Judges and psychiatrists lock up too many people, Psychol. Today **7**:27, Aug. 1973.

28. O'Sullivan, A.: Privileged communication, Am. J. Nurs. **80**:947, 1980.

29. Peck, C.: Current legislative issues concerning the right to refuse versus the right to choose hospitalization and treatment, Psychiatry **38**:303, Nov. 1975.

30. President's Commission on Mental Health: Report to the president, vol. I, Washington, D.C., 1978.

31. Rhoden, N.: The presumption for treatment: has it been justified? Law, Med. Health Care **13**(2):65, 1985.

32. Rogers, C.: Nakao: Blackfoot philosophy, New York, 1972, Warner Books, Inc.

33. *Rogers v. Okin,* 478, Fed. Supp. 1342, 1979.

34. Scheff, T.: Being mentally ill: a sociological theory, Chicago, 1966, Aldine Publishing Co.

35. Schmid, D., Applebaum, P., Roth, L., and Lidz, C.: Confidentiality in psychiatry: a study of the patient's view, Hosp. Community Psychiatry **34**(4):353, 1983.

36. Spece, R.: Conditioning and other techniques used to 'treat'? 'rehabilitate'? 'demolish'? prisoners and mental patients, South Calif. Law Rev., p. 616, 1972.

37. Steadman, H., and Cocozza, J.: Careers of the criminally insane, Lexington, Mass., 1974, D.C. Heath.

38. Stone, A.: Mental health and law: a system in transition, Rockville, Md., 1975, National Institute of Mental Health, U.S., Department of Health, Education, and Welfare.

39. Szasz, T.: Ideology and insanity, New York, 1970, Doubleday & Co., Inc.

40. Tancredi, L., and Clark, D.: Psychiatry and the legal rights of patients, Am. J. Psychiatry **129**:328, 1972.

41. *Tarasoff v. Regents of the University of California et al.,* 529 p. 2d 553.

42. Taub, S.: Psychiatric malpractice in the 1980s: a look at some areas of concern, Law, Med. Health Care **11**(3):97, 1983.

43. 28 USCS Appendix 476, 1975.

44. Whitmer, G.: From hospitals to jails: the fate of California's deinstitutionalized mentally ill, Am. J. Orthopsychiatry **50**(1):65, 1980.

45. Williams, R., and Robitscher, J.: Should psychiatrists get out of the courtroom? Psychol. Today, **11**:85, Dec. 1977.

46. *Wyatt v. Stickney:* 344, Fed. Supp. 373, 375, 1972.

47. *Youngberg v. Romeo:* 102 Supreme Ct. 2452, 1982.

■ ANNOTATED SUGGESTED READINGS ■

*Aroskar, M.: Anatomy of an ethical dilemma: the theory, the practice, Am. J. Nurs. **80**:658, 1980.

In these articles, the author first describes the theory related to ethical dilemmas and decision making and then uses the theory to analyze a specific clinical dilemma. The application to practice makes this reading particularly useful.

Barton, W., and Sanborn, C., editors: Law and the mental health professions, New York, 1978, International Universities Press, Inc.

This is a compilation of papers by recognized authorities in both the legal and mental health professions. They examine the implications of recent judicial decisions that have affected psychiatric practice and suggest possible routes toward a smoother interface between law and psychiatry. Topics covered include informed consent, malpractice, confidentiality, competence, patient rights, involuntary admissions, and dangerousness.

Chodoff, P.: The case for involuntary hospitalization of the mentally ill, Am. J. Psychiatry **133**:496, 1976.

---

*Asterisk indicates nursing reference.

The author examines three points of view on the question of involuntary hospitalization. He believes that there is an over-reliance on the dangerousness standard, and he favors a return to the use of medical criteria by psychiatrists.

Ennis, B.: Prisoners of psychiatry, New York, 1972, Harcourt, Brace, Jovanovich, Inc.

This book contains specific case histories of men and women whose lives were changed by the label "mental illness." It is written by a lawyer who represented mental patients, and it makes interesting reading on a more personal level.

Ennis, B., and Siegel, L.: The rights of mental patients, New York, 1973, Avon Books.

This guide was published in cooperation with the American Civil Liberties Union and presents a brief description of the various rights of psychiatric patients. It also suggests how these rights can be protected.

Feileger, D.: The battle over children's rights, Psychol. Today **11**:89, July 1977.

Thirty-eight states have laws allowing parents or guardians to commit their children as voluntary patients to mental institutions. This article questions if children should have the right to be heard independently. It describes the federal court decision of Kremens v. Bartley, *which decided that children are entitled to protection against abuses in the commitment process. The issue is a complex one because the child's right to liberty is pitted against the parent's authority and claim to control of the child.*

*Fenner, K.: Ethics and law in nursing, New York, 1980, Van Nostrand Reinhold Co.

The purpose of this book is to help nurses distinguish ethical from unethical practice and be alert to potential problems in exceeding the legal parameters of health care. Theory and case studies are combined to stimulate much needed discussion on ethics and nursing.

*Fromer, M.: Paternalism in health care, Nurs. Outlook **29**(5):284, 1981.

The author contends that nurses, physicians, and administrators exhibit paternalism—the tendency to limit the patient's autonomy. One reason for this is the socialization process of nurses. This is a studious and analytical discussion of an important problem in psychiatric practice.

*Garritson, S.: Degrees of restrictiveness in psychosocial nursing, J. Psychosoc. Nurs. **21**(12):9, 1983.

Six dimensions of the concept of restrictiveness are explored in this important article: structural, institutional policy, enforcement, treatment, psychosocial atmosphere, and patient characteristics. Highly recommended reading for the analysis it presents.

*Garritson, S., and Davis, A.: Least restrictive alternative: ethical considerations, J. Psychosoc. Nurs. **21**(12):17, 1983.

This is an excellent article that critically evaluates how the principles and assumptions underlying the least restrictive alternative concept relate to the human rights versus human needs dilemma that confronts practitioners. Specifically, four issues are addressed: rights, paternalism, autonomy, and needs.

Golann, S., and Fremouw, W., editors: The right to treatment for mental patients, New York, 1976, Irvington Publishers, Inc.

This book is a result of the Amherst Conference on the Right to Treatment, which focused attention on the rights of institutionalized persons and the professional and political issues involved in implementing these rights.

*Gonzalez, H.: The consumer movement: the implications for psychiatric care, Perspect. Psychiatr. Care, **14**:186, Oct.-Dec. 1976.

This worthwhile article briefly examines the consumer movement and its two major components: the consumer as consumer and the consumer as a provider of health care. The author then analyzes the implications of the consumer movement for health care providers in the delivery of psychiatric care. It is a thought-provoking article.

Jones, R.: Street people and psychiatry: an introduction, Hosp. Community Psychiatry **34**(9):807, 1983.

This is an excellent review article on the problem of the homeless in the United States today. It provides a historical perspective as well as the work of advocacy organizations in dealing with this contemporary concern.

Karasu, T.: The ethics of psychotherapy, Am. J. Psychiatry **137**(12):1502, 1980.

The ethics of psychotherapy are addressed in terms of the interface between science and ethics, the goals of treatment, the therapeutic relationship, and special issues of confidentiality and therapist-patient sex. It is thought-provoking reading.

Kesey, K.: One flew over the cuckoo's nest, New York, 1962, Viking Press.

This is a popular novel that has also been adapted for the theater and movies. It describes the plight of the central character, MacMurphy, who has been committed to a state mental hospital. The story records his attempt to fight the hospital system and obtain a release. Many of the elements of institutionalization are dramatized in this powerful and enjoyable tale.

Kittrie, N.: The right to be different, Baltimore, 1971, Johns Hopkins University Press.

The author describes the conflict between the humanitarian ideals of the therapeutic state and the practical results of the administration of criminal law. He examines the problems of mental illness, commitment, and due process and the future implications of implementing a therapeutic state. Particular attention is devoted to delinquent youths, psychopaths, addicts, alcoholics, and methods of dealing with the population explosion. This book provides advanced reading in this controversial area.

Kopolow, L., and Bloom, H., editors: Mental health advocacy: an emerging force in consumers' rights, Rockville, Md., 1977, U.S. Department of Health, Education, and Welfare.

This publication seeks to stimulate interest in patient advocacy. The first part reviews major concepts in advocacy; the second part describes statewide mental health–advocacy programs. The third part describes a unique judicial decision, and the appendix includes a model state advocacy statute and an excellent bibliography.

*Laben, J., and MacLean, C.: Legal issues and guidelines for nurses who care for the mentally ill, Thorofare, N.J., 1984, Charles B. Slack.

This essential book explores and clarifies basic legal concepts in clear, concise language. It is a well-researched and author-

itative reference that includes both discussion of issues and case decisions.

McGarry, L., Schwitzgebel, K., Lipsitt, P., and Lelos, D.: Civil commitment and social policy, Rockville, Md., 1981, U.S. Department of Health and Human Services, National Institute of Mental Health.

This monograph is the final report from a research project that documented the impact and consequences of the new mental health law in Massachusetts on the civil commitment of the mentally ill. This is one of the few studies to actually examine the consequences of such legal changes.

Means, H.: Criminal case number 16836: *the State of Maryland vs. Sherry Windt*, The Washingtonian **38**:102, Feb. 1978.

This article describes the interplay between psychiatry and the law in a true case presentation of 16-year-old Sherry Windt, who killed her mother. The reporter has access to both legal and psychiatric records, and he presents the complex sequence of events relative to her trial and psychiatric assessment. It is a stimulating article that provokes numerous questions regarding psychiatry and the law.

*Nations, W.: Nurse-lawyer is patient advocate, Am. J. Nurs. **73**:1039, 1973.

This article describes the innovative role of a nurse who has both nursing and legal qualifications as she acts as an ombudsman for psychiatric patients in a Veterans Administration Hospital. The functions she performs are identified as responding to requests for help from patients and families, serving as consultant and advisor about patient problems to administration, and helping the director see the operation of the institution through the eyes of the patient.

Rubin, J.: Economics, mental health and the law, Lexington, Mass., 1978, D.C. Heath & Co.

This is an exploration of the economic bases and implications of recent mental health litigation. Important issues of the book are the need to consider what is being demanded and supplied in regard to mental health care, at what cost is it produced, and the willingness of people to pay for it.

*Saunders, J., and Du Plessis, D.: An historical view of right to treatment, J. Psychosoc. Nurs. **23**(9):12, 1985.

This article analyzes the responsibilities of the professional nurse in the right to treatment issue. This is described as providing active psychiatric treatment on an individualized basis and monitoring the patient's environment, thus safeguarding the legal rights of the mentally ill.

Szasz, T.: Law, liberty, and psychiatry, New York, 1963, The Macmillan Co., Publishers.

This classic text presents a critical inquiry into the social and legal uses of psychiatry. The author's aim is to show that psychiatry today in the United States is often used to subvert tra-

ditional political guarantees of individual liberty. He describes many of the faults committed in the name of mental illness and proposes solutions for them. The 20 chapters cover more of the pertinent issues that arise between law and psychiatry and this text is considered to be a classic in its field.

Szasz, T.: Psychiatric slavery, New York, 1977, The Macmillan Co., Publishers.

The author supports the concepts of freedom and personal responsibility and in this text he examines the problem of involuntary mental hospitalization. He parallels it to involuntary servitude and illustrates his thesis through the use of the Donaldson case.

Tancredi, L., Lieb, J., and Slaby, A.: Legal issues in psychiatric care, New York, 1975, Harper & Row, Publishers, Inc.

This text is written for students in all areas of mental health. It explores the many complex legal issues that confront the psychiatric professional in a thorough and concise manner and clearly understood language. Illustrative case examples are used to provoke discussion and apply pertinent theory. It can serve as a valuable and ready reference for psychiatric nurses.

*Thorner, N.: Nurses violate their patients' rights, J. Psychiatr. Nurs. **14**:7, Jan. 1976.

The author reports on a study she conducted on the refusal of medication by patients. Her findings revealed that medication refusals do not occur with a high frequency in the psychiatric setting, and nurses deal with refusals by first using psychological methods. She also reported that nurses in the study did not have an adequate knowledge of the patients' right to refuse medication and the legal responsibility in medication administration.

Williams, R., and Robitscher, J.: Should psychiatrists get out of the courtroom? Psychol. Today **11**:85, Dec. 1977.

Psychiatrists have become increasingly active in pretrial screenings for mental competence, courtroom debates about sanity and responsibility, and posttrial decisions on the probability of rehabilitation. In this article the author debates the role of the psychiatrist in the courtroom. His final recommendation is to make forensic psychiatrists more responsible and to refine the theory of criminal responsibility so that judges and juries get less confusing advice.

*Winkler, L., and Fennell, K.: Values and nursing ethics: a bibliography, J. Psychiatr. Nurs. **19**(4):19, 1981.

The authors present a complete bibliography of journal articles on values and nursing ethics. They have done a literature review for us all!

*Witt, P.: Notes of a whistleblower, Am. J. Nurs. **1983**:1649, 1983.

This is the personal story of a psychiatric nurse who saw abuse in her work setting and tried to stop it. It is a chronology of one nurse's attempt to resolve a legal and ethical dilemma she experienced in her psychiatric nursing practice.

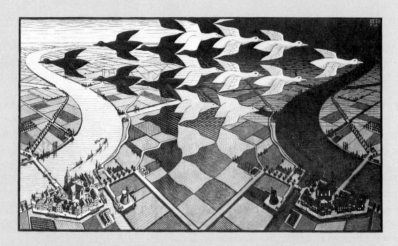

'What can't be cured must be endured,' is the very worst
and most dangerous maxim for a nurse which was ever
made. Patience and resignation in her are but other
words for carelessness or indifference—contemptible, if in
regard to herself; culpable, if in regard to her sick.

Florence Nightingale, Notes on Nursing

C H A P T E R   8

FUTURE CHALLENGES IN PSYCHIATRIC
NURSING

LEARNING OBJECTIVES

After studying this chapter, the student should be able to:

- describe the nursing practice issues that are of concern to psychiatric–mental health nurses.

- discuss the actions necessary to influence current trends in psychiatric nursing education.

- identify the importance of the development of a consistent and generally accepted psychiatric nursing diagnostic nomenclature.

- describe the need for psychiatric nursing research.

- discuss current trends in the mental health care delivery system.

- compare and contrast the role of the nurse in various community-based mental health care settings.

- analyze the psychiatric nursing services needed by special populations of patients.

- discuss the role of the nurse in client advocacy and political action.

- select appropriate readings for further study.

If there is truth in the saying, "There is opportunity in a time of crisis," then the 1980s are a time of great opportunity for psychiatric nursing. Within nursing, movement is underway to confront issues that have been brewing for many years. These include education for practice, credentialing, control of professional practice, scope of practice, and reimbursement. All of these in one way or another affect the professional life of the psychiatric nurse.

At the same time, the mental health care system has been undergoing a profound change. The almost exclusively hospital-based system of the past has moved very rapidly toward a community focus. Populations in need of service have been redefined based on recognition of past deficiencies and changing demographics. Attention has been drawn to the issue of the rights of patients and, more recently, the rights of staff. Awareness of the need for cost containment has brought attention to efficient and effective delivery of mental health services.

Nurses who work in mental health settings must be familiar with these issues and aware of the potential effect they may have on their own practice. Passive acceptance of decisions made by legislators, bureaucrats, and other health care providers will lead to the decline of psychiatric nursing as an important influence on the future of the mental health care system. Senator Daniel Inouye of Hawaii has said, "You nurses, you can have whatever you want, you can control the health care system, you have more power than any other group, including all the oil lobbyists, but you will go to your graves with 'docile' written on your tombstones."[1] This challenge by one of our staunchest supporters must be met.

Psychiatric nursing practice challenges

■ Education for practice of psychiatric–mental health nursing

Twenty years ago, psychiatric nursing educators were in the vanguard of nursing education. Graduate education for psychiatric nursing practice was well established. Federal funding of nursing programs and student traineeships was readily available. As a result of this progressive educational system, nurses were actively involved in the changes in the mental health care system that occurred in the 1960s and 1970s. However, since 1980, drastic changes have taken place. Funding for nursing education programs of all types has been drastically reduced. For psychiatric nursing, it is now necessary to compete for limited funds with other disciplines. Unfortunately, psychiatric nurses have never been able to mobilize their potential political clout sufficiently to compete effectively with the other mental health care disciplines. As a result, the graduate psychiatric nursing education system is in a precarious position.

Another trend with serious implications for psychiatric nursing in the future is the declining enrollment of students in schools of nursing. As more job opportunities are becoming open to women, fewer are choosing the traditionally female occupations, such as nursing. The image of the nurse as subservient to the physician, overworked, and underpaid does little to encourage young women to enter the field. At the same time, the identification of nursing as a "woman's profession" discourages men from entering schools of nursing in large numbers. Recently, the American Nurses' Association has recognized this problem and has launched a nationwide campaign to update the image of nursing. However, individual nurses must become more active in promoting a positive image to the public.

Although recruitment to nursing in general has declined, the percentage of nursing graduates who select psychiatric nursing as their area of practice has declined even more rapidly. A study conducted by Lowery, Banchik, and Miller[2] in 1982 revealed that only 4.9% of senior baccalaureate nursing students planned to seek employment in psychiatric nursing. A similar study conducted by Mitsunaga, Bloch, and Burckhardt[5] found only 5% stating a preference for psychiatric nursing. In recent years, enrollments in graduate programs in psychiatric–mental health nursing have decreased steadily. This specialty used to attract nurses who looked forward to independent practice and greater autonomy, but other nursing specialties, such as nurse midwifery and nurse practitioners of various types, now offer those same benefits and have done a better job of marketing their opportunities.

Nurse educators and administrators have proposed explanations for the waning interest in psychiatric nursing. One theory is that the integrated nursing curriculum separated psychiatric nursing out as a unique area of practice.[6] Some students completed their nursing education program with no experience in an inpatient psychiatric setting and were therefore not attracted to that as a place of employment. Stereotypical images of mental hospitals remained unchallenged by personal experience. In addition, graduating students were routinely advised by faculty to "get basic medical-surgical nursing experience before you go into a specialty area like psych." This message is reinforced by nurse administrators who require medical-surgical nursing experience before employment in psychiatric settings. Although probably well meant, this advice is discouraging to new graduates who would otherwise consider exploring mental health nursing as a career option. It is time for psychiatric nursing leaders to reevaluate the integrated curriculum and approaches to career counseling so that sufficient numbers of nurses may be attracted to psychiatric nursing careers and to graduate education for advanced practice. Options such as concentrated clinical study in psychiatric settings and internships for new graduates should be expanded.

In order to be viable as a mental health care discipline, graduate education must be focused on theory and practice skills that are valued in the marketplace. Mansfield and colleagues[3] reported a study that compared objectives for graduate education that were prioritized by consumers, educators, and practitioners. Table 8-1 illustrates the five highest priorities for each group. It should be noted that the set of objectives for consumers was developed by a group of consumers for all mental health disciplines. The educator and practitioner set was developed by a group of mental health nursing educators. Clearly, there is a great need for communication and collaboration among these groups.

■ Delineation of psychiatric nursing practice

The nature of mental health care delivery has created problems for psychiatric nursing in delineating the scope and characteristics of practice. Just as psychiatry has been less well defined than other areas of medical specialty practice, the phenomena of concern to psychiatric nurses have also proved to be difficult to define. However, efforts are underway to correct this problem. A committee of the ANA Council of Psychiatric and Mental Health Nursing is in the process of developing a set of psychiatric nursing phenomena which will then serve as the foundation for formulation of a set of psychiatric nursing diagnoses. It is hoped that the resulting psychiatric nursing classification system will then be merged into the NANDA nursing diagnostic nomenclature (see Chapter 3) to create a unified set of nursing diagnoses and correct a current deficiency in the NANDA structure.

A real benefit of the new nomenclature will be its potential impact on reimbursement for psychiatric nursing practice. In order to be paid for providing a service, the supplier must be able to clearly describe the nature of the service. Until now, nurses have been limited to trying to describe nursing services in medical terms. This has curtailed nursing's ability to receive reimbursement for the delivery of nursing services. This has also limited the ability to demonstrate the cost-effectiveness of psychiatric nursing intervention, thus handicapping nurse executives in their efforts to justify the employment of clinical nurse specialists. The present focus on cost containment in all health care settings mandates the documentation of cost-benefit data relative to psychiatric nursing practice.

Issues related to competition in the mental health care marketplace must also be addressed by mental health nurses. Free competition requires that equal reimbursement for services be available to all providers. At this time, this is not the case in most states. Psychiatric nurses, through their professional organization, must continue to lobby federal and state legislators to extend full reimbursement to psychiatric nurse specialists. In addition, vigilance is required to be sure that the Federal Trade Commission retains its jurisdiction over professional practice in order to prevent attempts

TABLE 8-1

COMPARISON OF PSYCHIATRIC–MENTAL HEALTH NURSING EDUCATIONAL OBJECTIVES

Consumer	Educator	Practitioner
Respect client dignity	Select and apply appropriate theory	Concept of stress
Patient rights	Skill in crisis intervention	Assess client's needs, goals, and motivation
Early intervention and recognition of symptoms	Articulate conceptual framework for own psychiatric nursing practice	Termination of relationship
Women, stress, and changing roles	Clinical specialist role: theory and practice	Skill in eliciting client's perceptions
Awareness of own value conflicts	Assess family interaction problems	Capacity to form therapeutic relationships

Adapted from Mansfield, E. et al.: Comparison of psychiatric–mental health nursing education objectives, J. Psychosoc. Nurs. **20**:29, May 1982.

to restrain or limit practice of some disciplines. In recent sessions of Congress, the American Medical Association has promoted legislation to revoke this FTC power. A coalition of the other health care disciplines has been successful thus far in blocking this effort.

Consumers must also be assured that the providers of psychiatric nursing care are well qualified. The profession has a responsibility to set and maintain standards of practice. In addition, certification for specialty practice and peer review for quality assurance are responsibilities of all nurse specialists. There has been a steady increase in the number of mental health nurses who are certified at the specialist and generalist levels. This trend must continue in order to elicit public confidence in nurses as mental health care providers.

■ Psychiatric nursing research

Psychiatric nurses must become more active in research. Delineation of the scope of practice, the effectiveness of specific nursing interventions, and approaches to changing the image of the psychiatric nurse are but a few of the topics that need investigation. Since competition for research funding is keen and since nurses must compete with members of the other mental health care disciplines for scarce funds, it is critical that doctorally prepared nurses provide leadership in this area. The Council of Directors of Graduate Programs in Psychiatric Nursing has recently confronted the National Institutes of Mental Health regarding the underrepresentation of nursing in membership on grant review panels and in receipt of grant awards. However, the success of this effort will be compromised if nurses do not submit high-quality grant applications. It is important that nurse researchers find out about NIMH priorities and funding initiatives. Research theory and the development of research skills should form a thread through all levels of nursing education. Staff nurses should be given an opportunity for involvement in research projects that are taking place in the workplace. Without paying adequate attention to nursing research, the future of psychiatric nursing practice will be severely compromised.

Mental health care system challenges

■ Evolution of new services

Mechanic[4] notes, "Although nursing has a long tradition in inpatient psychiatric settings, the potentials for nursing in the mental health arena remain undeveloped." He goes on to note that in 1955, 50% of the episodes of mental health care took place in public hospitals. In contrast, in 1980, less than 10% of mental health care episodes were in these settings. At the same time, total episodes of mental health care increased from 1.7 million in 1955 to 6.4 million in 1980. These massive shifts in locus of service delivery and amount of service delivered have led to enormous demands on providers of mental health services. Nurses must be able to meet the challenges presented by the system.

As more mental health services are provided in community settings, innovative approaches to service delivery are developed. It has become apparent that for seriously mentally ill people, the traditional private office or clinic appointment is not effective in providing mental health care. These patients need services that are tailored to their needs and provided when and where they need them. Because of their long tradition of providing services in community settings, nurses are well prepared to take a leading role in initiating creative service systems.

Community residential services are required for deinstitutionalized people. The publicity in most large cities about the large numbers of former mental hospital patients in the homeless population underscores the need for these services. Nurses would seem to be uniquely well qualified to run community residential programs.

Other former hospital patients will be found in home settings. Nurses from home health agencies could provide a valuable service to families who frequently have difficulty managing the disturbed behavior of the mentally ill member. However, reimbursement restrictions have slowed the extension of home health services to this population. Nurses need to publicize the potential availability of this service and to demonstrate its cost-effectiveness in keeping people out of hospitals. Clinical nurse specialists in psychiatric–mental health nursing who work in home health settings could also provide crisis intervention services. In addition, they could assist families to provide care to homebound patients with organic brain syndromes. Some home health agencies do provide these services, but there is potential for enormous growth. Nurses should not wait for health care administrators or physicians to establish mental health home care agencies. There is no reason why nurses should not seize this opportunity to initiate nurse-owned and -operated services.

Many mental health care systems are shifting to a rehabilitative rather than a medical focus. More specific information about this approach will be found in Chapter 11. Slavinsky[7] has proposed that nurses need to develop case management skills in order to work in a rehabilitation-oriented system. The components of case management are

1. Continuity of care
2. Client advocacy
3. Coordination of care
4. Preventive education
5. Resource development
6. Accountability

None of these should be unfamiliar to the psychiatric nurse. They have always been an important part of nursing practice. However, it is another example of an area of functioning that has not been well enough defined or communicated by psychiatric nurses to other disciplines and to consumers. Therefore, it is now being hailed in nonnursing literature as a new approach to mental health care. Despite the confusion as to its "newness," there is no doubt that this particular complex of services, while valued by nurses, has not been adequately delivered to consumers. Nurses must propose service delivery models that assure case management for all who need it.

■ Service delivery to special populations

Increased public attention to social problems emanating from specific populations of mentally ill people has resulted in the development of programs targeted to the needs of those groups of patients. Recently, the spotlight has been particularly directed toward the young and the old. Federal funding initiatives for research and for education have been directed toward programs for children and adolescents and for the elderly. Emphasis in both areas has been on both prevention and intervention.

Increases in delinquent behavior and in substance abuse which frequently leads to crime has created interest in developing mental health programs for young people. Other areas that have received a great deal of publicity recently are adolescent suicide and eating disorders. In particular, there is a great need for research to increase the understanding of the origins of these problems, in order to develop approaches to prevention. The need for nurses prepared as specialists in child and adolescent psychiatric–mental health nursing will continue to grow in the near future. There is an urgent need for these nurses to take a leadership role in modeling innovative and effective intervention and preventive strategies for this population.

Demographics have led to the interest in providing mental health services to the elderly. Psychogeriatric nursing is the newest mental health nursing specialty. Historically, the elderly have been the most neglected group of the mentally ill. The work was considered to be unrewarding, and providers of these services received little glory. However, the services that were provided were provided by nurses. This has resulted in a wealth of practical knowledge regarding psychogeriatrics, which needs to be validated through research. In addition, nurses need to translate past experiences into new approaches to providing care to the mentally disabled elderly. Ideally, every nursing home and every home care agency should employ a psychiatric nurse consultant to assist nursing staff to intervene with disturbed psychosocial behavior. This also requires a massive effort to prepare at the graduate level the future leaders in this specialty.

More work also needs to be done in providing acceptable and accessible services to members of minority groups. The volume and quality of available mental health services still remain focused on the needs of middle class and higher socioeconomic groups. The number of psychiatric nurses who are members of minority groups continues to be very low. Efforts must be continued to interest members of racial and ethnic minorities to pursue careers in psychiatric nursing. Their input is essential to enable the development of services that are appropriate to the needs of minority groups.

■ Advocacy and patient rights

Mental health system consumers historically have been a silent and forgotten minority. This is changing. Groups of primary consumers and their families are coming forth as a new voice in the care delivery system. Nurses need to recognize this as a healthy development and an opportunity to forge partnerships with consumers. The political system is particularly sensitive to the concerns of the average person, once these concerns are articulated in the context of an organized group. The lack of involvement of consumers in the past has had a negative effect on the amount of money available for service delivery. As a poster caption beneath a blank square says, "Mental illness has no poster child." The stigma attached to mental illness has compounded the handicap by fostering an environment of secrecy. Nurses can assist consumers in developing their political clout by providing information about needed services, participating in public education about mental illness, volunteering time for community mental health projects, and joining advocacy groups.

As patients have become more vocal about their needs, they have also become more assertive in demanding their civil rights. The new involvement of the legal system in the mental health system is threatening to some providers. Nurses need to be involved in determining the boundaries of the two systems. When does legal concern encroach on the therapeutic relationship? This question will need to be answered in the near future, and the answer will affect the practice of every psychiatric nurse. There is no doubt that patient abuse must be eliminated. However, more nebulous

issues such as the right to treatment and the right to refuse treatment need clarification. Further discussion of legal and ethical issues related to psychiatric nursing may be found in Chapter 7.

■ Political action

In order for nurses to accomplish the level of influence that they need relative to all the issues and trends identified in this chapter, they absolutely must become a recognized force in the political system. The numbers are there. The question is, is the will there also? Political action and accountability is the only route to acquiring professional autonomy and leadership in mental health care. Nurses must become educated in the legislative and regulatory processes. They must be involved in political campaigns, and they must testify in legislative hearings. In coalition with other mental health care providers and consumers, they must lobby for government budgets that provide adequate funding for mental health service delivery, professional education, and research. Then, psychiatric nurses must assert their right to an equitable share of the resources, given the value of the services they provide. For psychiatric nurses, this means that the days of reaction are past. Proaction is the key to meeting the future challenges of psychiatric nursing.

■ SUGGESTED CROSS-REFERENCES ■

The roles and functions of psychiatric nurses are discussed in Chapter 1. A nursing model of health-illness phenomena is discussed in Chapter 3. Legal and ethical aspects of psychiatric care are discussed in Chapter 7.

■ SUMMARY ■

1. Challenges to psychiatric nursing practice and their relationships to education, practice, and research were discussed.

2. Attention needs to be paid to the recruitment of students into schools of nursing and of nurses into psychiatric nursing.

3. There needs to be a reassessment of the place of psychiatric nursing in the undergraduate nursing curriculum.

4. The development of a diagnostic nomenclature for psychiatric nursing was discussed, and the importance of this for definition of practice and reimbursement was addressed.

5. Issues of competition in the mental health care marketplace were explored.

6. There was discussion of the psychiatric nurse's responsibility for maintaining professional competency through certification and peer review.

7. The urgent need for psychiatric nursing research was emphasized.

8. Mental health system challenges were described.

9. Challenges were presented related to the increase in

community-based care and the need for innovative services.

10. Challenges were presented related to the needs of special populations of patients, including children, adolescents, the elderly, and minorities.

11. Challenges were presented related to the need for psychiatric nurses to establish collaborative relationships with consumer advocacy groups and become politically active.

■ REFERENCES ■

1. Lang, N.: Nurse-managed centers, will they survive? Am. J. Nurs. **83:**1290, 1983.
2. Lowery, B., Banchik, D., and Miller, J.: National survey of clinical and educational interests of nurses. In Proceedings: psychiatric mental health nursing recruitment to the specialty, Washington, D.C., 1982, U.S. Department of Health and Human Services.
3. Mansfield, E. et al.: Comparison of psychiatric–mental health nursing education objectives: consumers, educators and practitioners, J. Psychosoc. Nurs. Ment. Health Serv. **20:**29, May 1982.
4. Mechanic, D.: Nursing and mental health care: expanding future possibilities for nursing service. In Aiken, L.H., editor: Nursing in the 80s: crises, opportunities, challenges, Philadelphia, 1982, J.B. Lippincott Co.
5. Mitsunaga, B.K. et al.: Designing psychiatric/mental health nursing for the future: problems and prospects, J. Psychosoc. Nurs. Ment. Health Serv. **20:**15, Dec. 1982.
6. Pearlmutter, D.R.: Recent trends and issues in psychiatric–mental health nursing, Hosp. Community Psychiatry, **36:**56, Jan. 1985.
7. Slavinsky, A.T.: Psychiatric nursing in the year 2000: from a nonsystem of caring to a caring system, Image **16:**17, Winter 1984.

■ ANNOTATED SUGGESTED READINGS ■

*Dumas, R.G.: Social, economic and political factors and mental illness, J. Psychosoc. Nurs. Ment. Health Serv. **21:**31, March 1983.

This psychiatric nursing leader challenges nurses to become involved in the mental health care system. She advocates an activist role in social and political movements. She also emphasizes the need for nurses to become more involved in activities related to primary prevention.

*McBride, A.B.: Present issues and future perspectives of psychosocial nursing, J. Psychosoc. Nurs. Ment. Health Serv. **24:**9, Sept. 1986.

Developments in nursing theory and research are reviewed in this article. The author contends that psychosocial nursing has "come of age," and identifies tasks for future development.

Mechanic, D.: Nursing and mental health care: expanding future possibilities for nursing services. In Aiken, L.H., editor: Nursing in the 80s: Crises, opportunities, challenges, Philadelphia, 1982, J.B. Lippincott Co.

It is instructive for nurses to be aware of how they are viewed by members of other disciplines. This article is written by a sociologist who has studied nursing. His observations point out many areas where nursing may potentially contribute a great deal to the development of a progressive mental health care delivery system.

*Peplau, H.E.: Some reflections on earlier days in psychiatric nursing, J. Psychosoc. Nurs. Ment. Health Serv. **20:**17, Aug. 1982.

In order to gain perspective on the current status of psychiatric nursing, it is useful to consider the past. The author has provided psychiatric nurses with an instructive and entertaining description of some of the problems and concerns of the psychiatric nurses of earlier times.

*Stuart, G.: An organizational strategy for empowering nursing, Nurs. Econ. **4:**2, Apr. 1986.

A new approach for empowering nursing is described in this article. It advocates nurses acting as a united group and the impact they can then have on the organizations in which they work. It presents a challenging perspective on a familiar problem.

*Asterisk indicates nursing reference.

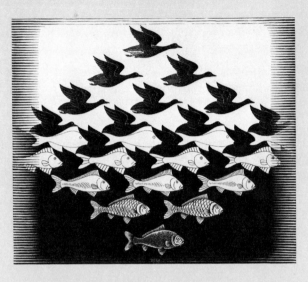

*What is this thing called health?
Simply a state in which the individual
happens transiently to be perfectly
adapted to his environment. Obviously,
such states cannot be common, for the
environment is in constant flux.*

H.L. Mencken, in the American Mercury, March 1930*

C H A P T E R   9

PREVENTIVE MENTAL HEALTH NURSING

*Reprinted with permission of Aspen Publishers, Inc.

LEARNING OBJECTIVES

After studying this chapter, the student should be able to:

- define primary, secondary, and tertiary prevention.

- compare and contrast the epidemiological, behavioral, and nursing paradigms of primary prevention.

- assess the vulnerability of the following groups to developing maladaptive coping responses: children and adolescents, new families, established families, women, mature adults, and the elderly.

- describe the levels of intervention and activities related to the following primary prevention nursing interventions: health education, en-

vironmental change, and supporting social systems.

- compare and contrast group psychotherapy, therapeutic groups, and self-help groups in relation to group goals, desired outcomes, and role of the nurse.

- assess the importance of evaluation of the nursing process when applied to primary prevention.

- identify directions for future nursing research.

- select appropriate readings for further study.

Prevention of mental disorders is regarded by many people, at least in principle, as a desirable goal that should be actively pursued. Although this may appear to be straightforward, in fact, the issues raised in a discussion of prevention are quite complex and even controversial. The basic concepts underlying preventive mental health endeavors were articulated by Caplan in his classic work, *Principles of Preventive Psychiatry.*[10] In it, he applies the three levels of preventive intervention from the public health model to mental illness and emotional disturbance. He defined **primary prevention** as lowering the *incidence* of mental disorders or reducing the rate at which new cases of a disorder develop. **Secondary prevention** involves reducing the *prevalence* of a disorder by reducing its duration. Techniques for the control of a disorder that focus on early case finding, screening, and prompt effective treatment can all be considered secondary prevention activities. **Tertiary prevention** activities attempt to reduce the *severity* of a disorder and the disability associated with it.

At the present time the major thrust in the United States is in secondary prevention activities or the treatment of mental disorders. This is evident in the allocation of economic resources, the nature of caregiving organizations and institutions, and the characteristic activities of psychiatric professionals. Similarly, much of this textbook is focused on the treatment of existing mental disorders. Tertiary prevention is evident in rehabilitative activities that often reflect a chronically ill patient group. This group is underserved and under-

valued and, although it represents a substantial number of the mentally ill, their needs appear to have a low priority within present American society. Chapter 11 examines the area of tertiary prevention in more depth.

Although primary prevention is often espoused with such slogans as "An ounce of prevention is worth a pound of cure" or "Curing is costly—prevention, priceless," it has yet to evolve as a substantial force in the mental health movement. This is partly because of the fuzziness of the concepts and definitions underlying the issues. For example, primary prevention programs may be aimed at an entire population or only at persons believed to be at high risk for developing a disorder. This depends on how one views primary prevention in general—is it disease prevention or health promotion? There also needs to be agreement on what one is promoting or preventing to best determine what action should be taken.

Conceptualizing primary prevention

The idea of promoting mental health in general is a very attractive one. Promotion sounds optimistic and positive. It is consistent with the idea of self-help and taking responsibility for one's own health. It implies changing human behavior and draws on a holistic approach to health. A continuing problem, however, with the strategy of promoting mental health is the vastness and vagueness of its goals. As Kessler and Albee note,

"Nearly everything, it appears, has implications for primary prevention, for reducing emotional disturbance, for strengthening and fostering mental health."[51:355] Thus goals are frequently ill defined, and evaluation of promotion activities is difficult at best. Even if goals of a project can be identified and measured, their relation to long-term goals and behavior remains questionable. For example, successfully teaching coping skills to schoolchildren may attain one's short-term goals, but what this precisely means for their mental health as adults is unclear and unsupported by empirical evidence.

■ Epidemiological prevention paradigm

Another problem is that there is basic disagreement on what is most important in understanding and preventing mental disorders. One group of mental health professionals favors the genetic-biochemical explanation that each mental disease has a separate physical cause. The prevention model they favor focuses narrowly on genetic counseling and on biochemical and brain research to discover the specific separate causes of each mental illness. They argue that there is no real proof that social stresses cause mental illness, and that the high rate of mental illness among the poor may be because disturbed people tend to "drift downward" from the upper and middle classes into poverty.

Lamb and Zusman, in a critique of primary prevention, state this view boldly:

The cause and effect relationship between social conditions and mental illness is extremely questionable. In the area of mental health, most—if not all—successful primary preventive activities have been aimed at specific diseases. In contrast to the situation in large areas of physical illness, there is no evidence that it is possible to strengthen "mental health" and thereby increase resistance to mental illness by general preventive activities. Despite massive efforts to combat poverty (at least partly in the name of mental health), to increase social welfare and Social Security benefits, and to change the educational systems and methods of child rearing, there is no indication of a decrease in frequency of any of the functional mental illnesses. Nor is there obvious evidence that other countries with stronger social welfare systems and different child-rearing practices have different rates of mental illness. Thus, as far as we can see, the major functional mental illnesses (as well as the very frequent diagnosable minor illnesses) remain untouched by primary prevention in the sense of trying to strengthen mental health.[55:13]

This suggests that primary prevention activities are perhaps best focused on illness prevention. Viewing mental illness as a disease in the medical model perspective allows one to use the classic, epidemiological paradigm in primary prevention. This paradigm consists of the following steps:

1. **Identify a disease of sufficient importance to justify the development of a preventive intervention program. Develop reliable methods for its diagnosis so that people can be divided with confidence into groups according to whether they do or do not have the disease.**
2. **By a series of epidemiological and laboratory studies identify the most likely theory of that disease's path of development.**
3. **Mount and evaluate an experimental preventive intervention program based on the results of those research studies.**[2:182]

Unquestionably this paradigm has been effective for a broad array of communicable diseases, such as smallpox, typhus, malaria, diphtheria, tuberculosis, rubella, and polio, and nutritional diseases, such as scurvy, pellagra, rickets, kwashiorkor, and endemic goiter. It has also proved useful in a variety of mental disorders caused by poisons, chemicals, licit or illicit drugs, electrolyte imbalances, and nutritional deficiencies. All these diseases have one thing in common. For each, there is a known necessary, although not always sufficient, causative agent.

■ Behavioral prevention paradigm

A contrasting view of the causes and prevention of mental illness is presented by those mental health professionals who support a social-learning model in which mental disorders are believed to result from faulty early learning of social coping skills, from low levels of competence, from low self-esteem, and from poor support systems interacting with high levels of stress. This viewpoint emphasizes that mental disorders do not appear to have a single identified precondition and that mental illnesses in particular may have causative factors that are multiple, interactive, situational, and sociocultural in nature. They thus require that prevention of mental illness be conceptualized in a more behavioral way as the prevention of problems or maladaptive responses. Hollister supports this view. He calls for prevention of the following:

1. **Specific behaviors** that are self-defeating or harmful to others, such as poor or unhealthy habits, overeating, procrastinating, evasiveness, blaming others, and "setting the stage" to fail
2. **Role failures,** as a student, a parent, or an employee
3. **Relationship breakdowns** between husband and wife, parent and child, boss and employee, including detection and control of interpersonal "games" that are destructive
4. **Feeling overreactions,** such as panics, new situation anxiety, flights, and temper tantrums

5. **Psychological disabilities,** such as the social deterioration of a confined ill person, decompensation, "going to pieces," or falling into melancholia instead of experiencing normal grieving.

With such a conceptualization, many of the commonsense services already given in the community by mental health and other helping agencies can be identified and publicly acknowledged as prevention efforts.[44:41-48]

By defining problems in this way they can include both single-episode events, such as a divorce, or a long-standing condition, such as marital conflict. They can also reflect either an acute health problem or a chronic health problem. For example, Room[76] has identified the following categories of problems that can arise from the abuse of alcohol:

1. Acute health problems, such as overdose or delirium tremens
2. Chronic health problems, such as cirrhosis or head or neck cancer
3. Casualties, such as accidents on the road, in the home or elsewhere, and suicide
4. Violent crime and family abuse
5. Problems of demeanor, such as public drunkenness and use of alcohol by teenagers
6. Default of major social roles—work or school and family roles
7. Problems of feeling state—demoralization and depression and experienced loss of control

This conceptualization requires the use of a new paradigm for primary prevention, which has been developed by Bloom.[5] It assumes that problems are multicausal, that everyone is vulnerable to stressful life events, and that any disability or problem may arise as a consequence of them. For example, four vulnerable persons can face a stressful life event—perhaps the collapse of their marriage, or the loss of their job. One person may become severely depressed, the second may be involved in an automobile accident, the third may head down the road to alcoholism, and the fourth may develop a psychotic thought disorder or coronary artery disease. This behavioral paradigm does not search for a cause for each problem. Rather, it attempts to reduce the incidence of stressful life events as outlined in the following steps:

1. **Identify a stressful life event that appears to have undesirable consequences in a significant proportion of the population. Develop procedures for reliably identifying persons who have undergone or who are undergoing that stressful experience.**

2. **By traditional epidemiological and laboratory methods, study the consequences of that event and develop hypotheses related to how one might go about reducing or eliminating the negative consequences of the event.**

3. **Mount and evaluate experimental preventive intervention programs based on these hypotheses.[5:183]**

This paradigm shifts attention from nonspecific predisposing factors of mental illness to more discrete and identifiable precipitating stressors. These factors may be single-episode life events, such as loss of a job, or more long-term life event stressors, such as job dissatisfaction. By narrowing the focus of one's study in this way, one is able to limit the population at risk and allow for a more judicious use of one's financial and program resources.

■ Nursing prevention paradigm

It is possible to identify the specific dimensions needed for nurses to engage in primary prevention activities based on the nursing model of health-illness phenomena utilized in this text. Basically, it would involve the systematic application of the nursing process with a focus on the primary prevention of maladaptive health responses associated with an identified stressor. This would incorporate the following aspects:

1. *Assessment.* **Identification of a stressor that precipitates maladaptive responses and a target or vulnerable population group that is at high risk in relationship to it.**

2. *Planning.* **Elaboration of specific strategies of prevention and relevant social institutions and situations through which the strategies may be applied.**

3. *Implementation.* **Application of selected nursing interventions aimed at decreasing maladaptive responses to the identified stressor and enhancing adaptation.**

4. *Evaluation.* **Determining the effectiveness of the nursing interventions with regard to short- and long-term outcomes, use of resources, and comparison with other prevention strategies.**

The nursing process can thereby be used in a goal-directed way to decrease the incidence of mental illness and promote mental health among individuals, families, groups, and communities.

Assessment

Three types of primary prevention programs have been identified by Bloom: community-wide, milestone, and high-risk.[6] In a community-wide program, the target group is all individuals living within a specified geographic area. The people receiving intervention are not selected on a case-by-case basis but rather are included based on geographic considerations. In a milestone program, residents of a community become the target of an intervention at a particular point in the life cycle. Examples of such programs include those aimed at women who are pregnant for the first time, and preschool screening programs whose goals are to identify and provide effective intervention for children who are thought to be at risk for emotional or learning problems in later years. The third type of primary prevention program is a high-risk program in which specific individuals or groups are identified as being at increased risk for certain conditions and become the target of an intervention program.

While all people and all families face similar developmental tasks, not everyone adapts to them or copes with them in a positive way. This may be because certain individuals or groups in our society have additional stressors placed on them, inadequate coping resources, and fewer positive experiences to balance out their perceived stress. These people and groups are thus particularly vulnerable or at high risk for developing maladaptive responses. It is extremely helpful if the nurse has an awareness of these vulnerable people. The increased sensitivity that results from this awareness will affect the nurse's assessment of both existing and potential problems and actual work with people from these high-risk groups. Nurses, as the largest group of health care providers, can make a significant impact in promoting mental health if they would anticipate problems and commit their time and skill to preventing their occurrence.

Assessment in primary prevention therefore involves identifying groups of people who are vulnerable to developing mental disorders or maladaptive coping responses to specific stressors or risk factors. To complete such an assessment, the nurse needs to draw on information generated from theory, research, and clinical practice. Some of these vulnerable groups will now be briefly described. Each group could merit, in itself, a separate chapter or perhaps a textbook. The intent of this discussion, however, is to highlight the unique ways in which some people are particularly vulnerable to maladaptive responses.

It should also be noted that these are not the only high-risk groups for developing mental disorders. The actual identification of vulnerable groups is greatly dependent on one's geography and life experiences. And not all individuals within these groups are at equal risk. What these groups do share, however, is the experience

of a life event, stressor, or risk factor that represents a loss of some kind or places an excessive demand on one's ability to cope. These broad categories are intended to help one conceptualize common stressful experiences. Utilizing them in clinical research or practice would necessitate a further specification of a particular subgroup within these broad categories based on a particular stressor or risk factor. The more clearly the subgroup can be defined, the more specific the prevention strategies can be researched, identified, and implemented.

■ Children and adolescents

The mental health needs of children are noteworthy. It has been estimated that approximately 2 million children have severe mental disorders that require immediate help, and another 8 to 10 million need help but less urgently. At present, only 500,000 of these children receive any kind of treatment through the mental health care system. In contrast, about 74% of the 7.6 million physically handicapped children in this country receive some sort of service.[1]

Many adult problems have their origins in childhood. Childhood and adolescence are periods for learning coping skills, and the success in achieving such skills can have profound effects throughout life. Childhood conditions that merit a primary prevention effort are presented in the box on page 258. Some of these problems probably result from a dysfunction in the biological development and organization of the brain. Others may be the result of major stressors beyond the child's control. Regardless, they must be viewed from the most holistic nursing perspective because they occur in the context of the fragile relationships of a child's genetic endowment, mental development, physical health, and family and social environment.

Adolescence is an accepted time of tremendous biological, psychological, and social change. The demands placed on the young person are great, and not all adolescents have sufficient resources to cope with them. One usual resource of the adolescent, the peer group, can actually become a stressor by pressuring the young person to participate in experiences, such as drugs or sex, that may not be in his or her best interests. Concerns about sex typing and homosexuality may develop at this time, as do questions about contraception, pregnancy, abortion, and venereal disease.

Late adolescence may be a time of moving away from home, making an initial career choice, or becoming involved in advanced schooling. All of these occurrences may lead to questions about independence, motivation, competence, control, and capacity for intimacy. The need to develop intimate psychosocial relationships with

Childhood Conditions Meriting Primary Prevention Intervention

1. Antisocial behavior
   a. Physical aggressiveness (e.g., fighting, wanton destructiveness, robbery)
   b. Other antisocial behaviors (e.g., truancy, running away, petty theft)
2. Learning disorders
3. Mental retardation
4. Childhood schizophrenia
5. Suicide
6. School failure
7. Child abuse and neglect (including sexual abuse)
8. Severe neurotic disorders
9. Psychiatric sequelae of chronic medical illness

others may be a major source of stress even though it is considered to be a normal developmental task. Many questions and insecurities may surround the issues of marriage, selecting a mate, conjoint living, and shared decision making. Each of these demands placed on adolescents may come together and compound their level of stress. If this occurs and their coping resources are not adequate, this group will be highly vulnerable to the development of maladaptive responses.

There is a tremendous amount of documentation related to the adolescent's potential for developing maladaptive responses. Reporting the many studies and statistics pertaining to this high-risk group is beyond the scope of this chapter but the problems are self-evident in the large numbers of adolescent suicides, runaways, drug abusers, and school failures, and the tremendous problems posed by juvenile prostitution, unwanted pregnancies, delinquency, and crime. These problems are discussed in Chapter 31. Certainly not all adolescents develop problems, but in the face of additional stressors from peers or family, this is one population group that is particularly vulnerable to a range of social, psychological, and behavioral problems.[77]

■ New families

The whole arena of family life poses opportunities for primary prevention. In a society beset with stress and rapid change, the stability and smooth functioning of the family can no longer be taken for granted. Issues such as working mothers, divorce, and single-parent families have ramifications for nursing as does the broader area of parenting.

The stress involved in decisions regarding children, conception, birth, and assuming the parental role has been well documented in both the professional literature and popular press. The decision whether or not to have children has become increasingly complex with recent changes in American society. Women now may have more extensive career options, less geographical proximity to their own families of origin, more earning potential, greater medical technology available, changing sex-role perceptions, and a more frequently used option to have children later in their adult years. However, these changes may be at odds with the cultural norms or personal beliefs of the couple, and, rather than serving to increase one's options, they may instead create conflict and dissonance. How the couple copes with this stress has far-reaching implications for their own health and that of their children.

Clearly new parents are at high risk for developing maladaptive responses. Bieber and Bieber[4] describe a psychiatric syndrome that appears not uncommonly in the first year after the birth of a child in both men and women. The signs and symptoms include combinations of acute anxiety, depression, psychosomatic disorders, changes in affectional responses toward the spouse, changes in sexual behavior, the onset of various types of frigidity in the woman, potency difficulties in the man, an apparent loss of interest in the marriage, and the first involvement in extramarital relations, often leading to divorce. Pregnancy thus sets in motion a series of changes and stressors that challenge the coping resources of the man and the woman and can result in either adaptive or maladaptive responses.

■ MOTHERS.

The transition to motherhood is accepted as a stressful period for women of all ages. Pregnancy and the postpartum period are generally regarded as maturational crises for women equal in importance to those of adolescence and midlife. Stressors undergone during this period include the following:

1. Endocrine changes
2. Changes in body image
3. Activation of psychological conflicts pertaining to pregnancy
4. Intrapsychic reorganization of becoming a mother

The result of these stressors is often the experience of a postpartum depression of varying intensity, or with some women, a postpartum psychosis. Studies indicate that from 20% to 40% of women report emotional disturbance or cognitive dysfunction or both in the early postpartum period.[46] Another study found 65% of mothers describing depression postpartum, with 25% of the women reporting symptoms continuing longer than a week.[72] Disturbances of psychotic proportions occur much less frequently but obviously with greater impairment.

■ **FATHERS.** The response of men to pregnancy and fatherhood has most often been described in the literature in terms of the benefits of parental involvement to father, mother, and infant. Little attention has been given to their more problematic responses, despite the fact that minor emotional reactions are common, and severe reactions are not rare.[24] Lacoursiere[54] reported that about 2% of hospitalized patients with a diagnosis of paranoid psychosis developed symptoms in relation to fatherhood. An interesting study found that one of the most important factors in female maladjustment to pregnancy was rejection of the pregnancy by the husband or father of the child.[38]

Yet, if one views childbirth as a maturational crisis, it must serve as a stressor for the man as well as the woman. For both, it is a time to recapitulate some of the developmental problems of earlier phases. The following variables have been suggested as significant instigators of psychopathological reactions in men: increased financial responsibility, triggering of latent homosexual conflicts by restriction of heterosexual opportunities during the prenatal period, rearousal of unacceptable childhood anger toward parents or siblings, reactivation of unresolved oedipal conflict, and frustration of dependency demands as the wife's attention is diverted to the baby's needs.[52] Fishbein[24] suggests that the essential determinant of what happens to the man psychodynamically appears to be how satisfactorily the man has resolved his own developmental attachment-individuation-separation processes.

■ **INFANTS.** The mental health of the parents also directly affects the health of the infant. This is demonstrated in a study by Nuckolls, Cassel, and Kaplan,[70] which found that the proportion of women having pregnancy and birth complications was significantly higher among those women who had experienced a high frequency of life changes accompanied by a low degree of social–emotional support during their pregnancies, and that when social support was high, there was no increase in complications. Conflict over the acceptance of pregnancy has been associated with increased length of the labor process, as well as increased levels of maternal anxiety,[57] and the degree of wantedness of the pregnancy has been associated with increased risk of low birth weight. Cobb[13] cites several studies which show that wanted children tend to adapt to or cope with the

stresses of growing up better than do those who began life under circumstances where the parental preference had been for abortion. Wanted children fared better in terms of the decreased incidence of juvenile delinquency and need for psychiatric treatment and were better able to adapt to the school socialization and educational achievement processes.[25]

Another dimension of stress in this high-risk group is related to the bonding and attachment process and the development of parent-child relationships. Stressors related to childbirth can place the family at risk for child maltreatment. A number of circumstances, including a medically abnormal pregnancy, difficult labor or delivery, neonatal separation, other separations in the first 6 months, illnesses in the infant during the first year of life, and maternal illness during the first year of life all place a family at risk for child maltreatment. Threats to the parent-infant bond are particularly dangerous. In one study,[62] 66% of the abused children were found to have experienced 48-hour separations from their parents in the first week of life, whereas only 3% of those same children's siblings had been separated. Medically high-risk infants are particularly in danger. In a study[50] of 146 infants who had been in an intensive care nursery, it was found that a lack of parental visits was associated with the likelihood of later maltreatment.

Although these results are not in and of themselves definitive, when combined with other research findings they are persuasive. Disruption in parent-infant bonding predicts greater risk for maltreatment.[29] Where the mother has an active role and high status in the childbirth process, there are fewer medical complications, less resort to medications that suppress infant functioning, fewer cesarean section deliveries, and fewer induced labors.[21] These, in turn, have a positive influence on the child and may serve to reduce the risk of child maltreatment.

■ **ROLE TRANSITIONS.** The abuse and neglect of children are evidence of parental difficulty in assuming the maternal or paternal role. Both roles are assumed through a complex social and cognitive learning process. They are not intuitive, nor are they universally present in couples who have given birth. Many variables have been identified as having an impact on the maternal role. Mercer[64] identifies these as age, perceptions of the birth experience, early maternal-infant separation, support system, self-concept and personality traits, maternal illness, child-rearing attitudes, infant temperament, infant illness, and socioeconomic status. Although all of these variables have been described in the literature, there is no evidence that one variable is most predictive or how they interact to account for variance in the maternal role. The nursing framework proposed by Mercer for studying these variables is necessary to guide research projects that can identify stressors and suggest prevention strategies.

A similar nursing research paradigm has been developed by Cronenwett and Kunst-Wilson[17] for the transition to fatherhood. They believe that a separate paradigm for fathers is necessary because the experience of becoming a parent differs for men and women, and the stress associated with becoming a parent is least understood for men. The framework they propose for understanding the processes involved in a man's transition to fatherhood incorporates many pertinent variables and can help stimulate the formulation of theoretical questions for further research. More precise knowledge of the nature of the stress and the intervening variables that promote adaptation will be necessary for the nurse to actively work to prevent potential problems.

Three other subgroups of new parents may also be particularly vulnerable in their role transitions. These include teenage parents, unwed parents, and the parents of adopted children. Pregnancy in adolescence brings together two maturational crises, each of which compounds the problems of the other. At this time, the adolescent has not yet achieved his or her own sense of identity and independence and yet must assume the role of parent for an infant who is totally dependent. The unwed mother of any age experiences to some degree a lack of coping resources that may include social support, financial assistance, and shared care-taking responsibilities. The stressor of parenthood thus makes excessive demands on one's coping ability.

Stress is also experienced by parents throughout the process of adoption. The parents who are not able to conceive their own child have undergone an extensive period of testing, waiting, hoping, and accepting one's physiological limitations. Once the decision to adopt has been made, a long waiting period usually follows. The actual arrival of an adopted child of any age requires a readjustment of roles and family dynamics. In addition, the relatively recent phenomena of surrogate mothers may initiate changes and problems that are new to the couple and society at large.

■ Established families

In American society the family unit is of critical importance. It continues to be a primary personal and cultural institution that has undergone some major and minor changes in structure in response to the larger social environment. The majority of Americans continue to seek and contract marriages, desire and have children, and live in households independent of the nuclear family. Important changes have also occurred. Because of increased longevity and fertility control, the "shape" of the family life cycle has changed, so that parenting no longer dominates most of the family's life cycle. Raising a family may only occupy half or a third of a couple's married life. In addition, today over 50% of American mothers work outside the home. This statistic is expected to increase to 75% by 1990. Of all married women with children under the age of 6, 45% are employed.[87] The employment of married women thus appears to be an accepted and perhaps even expected social pattern because of economic and personal fulfillment needs. Of those women who work, two thirds are single, widowed, divorced, or separated, or have husbands who earn less than $10,000.[87] A final important change is the increasing divorce rate, which has given rise to single-parent families. It is estimated that one out of five children lives in a single-parent home. Remarriage is also increasing, with the result that families may have stepparents, stepchildren, and multiple sets of grandparents.

Although it can be argued that these changes are not necessarily destructive in themselves, they all do place demands on the family's functioning and create a more complex set of needs. For example, all parents need some relief from their child and home care responsibilities. Often these needs can be met through an evening out or an informal arrangement with families and friends. However, in families in which both parents work, child care that is consistent, dependable, and of high quality becomes a necessity.

Another type of family at high risk for developing problems is the one in which there is lack of knowledge of effective parenting. Because parenting is not an established course in educational curriculum and families are more geographically mobile, it is not surprising that this need has emerged. Yet one's child-rearing practices do have a significant effect on one's children and even future generations.

Pratt[73] has observed that the use of the developmental style of child rearing (reasons, information, rewards, and autonomy) tends to be more effective than disciplinary methods in assisting children to develop resources and capacities for coping, learning, and taking care of themselves. Maladaptive behaviors associated with the strongly disciplinary style of child rearing have been identified as social aggressiveness, hostility, and dependency in boys and regressiveness, fearfulness, and social withdrawal in girls. Studies have shown that, when parents have tended to be lax or inconsistent in the use of appropriate rules or controls, their children's failure to develop adequate coping mechanisms in early life can cause subsequent maladjustment in their neurophysical development and lead to lifelong patterns of psychosomatic as well as social complications.[47]

It becomes apparent that there are numerous subgroups of families under stress. Many of these high-risk family groups have been researched, analyzed, and reported on in both the popular literature and that of the psychiatric community. Although the potential problems are significant, there is a major deficit in programs to either prevent them or alleviate them once they develop. The lack of quality day care programs, the government's cancellation of the 1981 White House Conference on Children, and federal reductions in programs aiding children and families all reveal the low priority given to families under stress.

■ **DIVORCE.*** The divorce rate in the United States has risen sharply in the past few years, provoking a crisis situation in many families and necessitating immediate intervention directed toward stress reduction. Although the increasing divorce rate is startling, attention is also directed toward the number of marriages that do not dissolve but rather maintain themselves in a constant state of disequilibrium.

Divorce, one of the most traumatic crises a family faces, confronts each member with the task of examining and often changing his role in the family system. Although divorce is often a healthy step toward reestablishing family homeostasis, stress is involved. A body of knowledge is being accumulated regarding the reactions of both spouses and children to the experience. The first year after the divorce is particularly difficult. During this time money constitutes a major source of stress as one household divides into two, each needing financial support. Women complain of feeling helpless and physically unattractive and of experiencing an acute loss of identity. On the other hand, men describe not knowing who they are, feeling as though they have no roots, structure, or predictable home life. Many divorced men buy sports cars and flashy clothes and plunge into a wide range of social activities to offset the loneliness of apartment living.[41]

Divorce therapy is gaining attention as a tool for primary prevention. The ultimate goal of divorce counseling or therapy is to help the couple disengage from their former relationship with a minimum amount of destructive and malicious behavior toward each other or their children. Divorce is dealt with as a family systems problem, which includes not only the immediate family but also the extended family. Each person in the family has an opinion about the situation and may need to lay blame on someone; each is affected by the family disruption.

*This section was contributed by Jeanette and Wade Lancaster.

One framework for understanding the dynamics associated with divorce moves through the stages of grief to explain reactions to the separation and loss.[40] Regardless of how fraught a marriage is with frustration and conflict, it is never easy to terminate. Even painful relationships have meaning for the participants. Denial serves to shield the marriage partners from the reality of the separation and their subsequent loss, since it "buys" time for individuals to reconstruct coping abilities. In nursing intervention, denial is supported by the nurse's listening to and helping the person describe his fear and dismay at the situation. Denial is transitory and is not supported when it becomes disproportionate to the actual situation.

Anger often follows denial and may be directed outwardly toward the ex-spouse or inwardly when it is manifested as depression. As the former partners are forced into new roles, they may feel helpless. Since helplessness causes a person to feel vulnerable, a common coping mechanism is to become angry and attempt to impose control on the situation. Just as in the stages of grief, bargaining often follows anger. One or both spouses wonder if the marriage could have been saved "if I had just. . . ." Depression typically occurs when one or both parties realize that the emotional investment they once had in a marriage no longer exists. The final stage, acceptance, is seen when the individual can move beyond regret and begin to make plans. Throughout the counseling, but particularly once acceptance begins, the primary nursing approach is problem solving, or application of the nursing process to assess, plan, and implement coping strategies.

A major issue in relation to divorce counseling is that of family roles. Traditional family roles are often disrupted as each spouse assumes responsibilities previously carried out or shared with the other partner. Men may assume responsibility for household maintenance when previously their wives handled this task. Women may be forced to support themselves and their children; for some, employment may constitute a major alteration in role.

Specific interventions are either child centered, relationship focused, or adult centered.[49] Child-centered interventions assist the parents to understand and deal with age-related responses to divorce. Children are particularly at risk for mental health disruption during a divorce in that they are often caught in the middle of bitter parental battles, and visitation rights, custody, and child support can become bargaining issues. Children from divorced families also tend to constitute a major portion of the case loads in psychiatric facilities with common problems being depression, aggressive outbursts, or behavioral problems at school or in social

TABLE 9-1

RESPONSES TO DIVORCE AND RELATED NURSING INTERVENTIONS

Behavior observed	Nursing intervention
Preschool	
Regression, confusion, irritability	Provide guidance to custodial parent who serves as child's best support person
Difficulty understanding what is happening	
Repeatedly asks same questions (e.g., "Where is Daddy?" "When is Daddy coming home?")	Teach communication skills related to interpreting meaning of divorce
	Examine alternatives for intervening in the child's regressive behavior
Early latency	
Often immobilized by parental separation	Open discussion may be too threatening; nurse might use a "divorce monologue" to talk about how other children react to divorce
Developmentally denial does not serve these children well, yet open confrontation with reality is traumatic	
Nearly insatiable need to maintain contact with both parents	Focus on helping both parents support child's need for contact
Anger (common reaction)	"Divorce monologue" may give child permission to express anger
Later latency	
Torn in loyalty toward parents	Encourage child to express fears and worries to parents
Worries a great deal	Support child as he deals with pain and anger
Can both express their feelings verbally and channel them into organized activities	Encourage parents to be consistent and firm in approach
Superego controls may be threatened as external controls decrease because of stress	
Adolescence	
Intense feelings of pain (anger, sadness, loss, and betrayal)	Provide an opportunity for open discussion of feelings, including helping them plan ways to express feelings directly and constructively
Strong feelings of shame and embarrassment	
Concern about their own future as a marital partner	Discuss feelings of shame, embarrassment, and fear of the future
Concern about adequacy as a sexual partner in their current dating, as well as for future married life	
Often unrealistic concern about finances	Use communication strategies, such as role playing or psychodrama to help adolescents learn to deal with feelings
Shortened disengagement from and shift in perceptions of parents	Practice improved, honest, open communication
Accelerated individuation from parents	
Heightened awareness of parents as sexual objects	
Loyalty conflicts	
Strategic withdrawal as a defense against pain	

Modified from Kelley, J., and Wallerstein, J.: Am. J. Orthopsychiatry **47:**23, 1977.

groups. Of the children, 7 to 16 years old, that Shanok and Lewis studied,[80] 48% of those referred to a juvenile court clinic were from broken homes, and children of divorce constituted 49% of those referred to a child guidance clinic. Similarly, Kalter[48] reported that 41% of the children receiving services at a large university department of psychiatry were from homes in which the parents were separated, divorced, or remarried.

Some frequently observed age-specific responses to divorce and pertinent nursing interventions are given in Table 9-1.[49]

Relationship-centered interventions are used when knowledge of growth and development is less an issue than is the ability to cope with the stress of divorce. Many parents become immobilized with their increased responsibility and the pressing need to make decisions and deal with the daily reactions of family members to the divorce. Frequently children get caught up in the parental conflict. Nursing intervention helps the family members remain open and honest with one another and not use each other for harmful purposes.

Adult-centered counseling focuses on helping the partner who seeks counseling adapt to his new role and cope with the stresses implicit in a major life change. Even the most desperate marriage provides some security and division of labor. Women particularly need to examine their alternatives in advance of major decisions to make the most advantageous choice as they assume expanded roles, which often include financial support of self or family.

■ **ILLNESS.** Another major source of stress for all families is illness in any form. The illness of one family member affects all other members and can result in maladaptive responses and a variety of pathological states. The premature birth of a child, the child born with a genetic defect, and the handicapped child all place great and unanticipated demands on the family. Parents of such children, and the children themselves, have special individualized needs. Studies show that parental attitudes about having produced handicapped children vary quite widely (regret, denial, anger, and rejection), since these children may represent parental incompetence both to the parents themselves and to others.[53] Voysey[88] reported that parental coping patterns include the projection of false reports of progress, statements of grief, and the development of cynical acceptance of the disabilities.

Nurses are particularly aware that major and minor illnesses of family members take a significant toll. Illnesses requiring hospitalization and surgery precipitate multiple threats to the family unit. Adapting to a hyperactive child, an alcoholic parent, a psychotic sibling, or an arthritic spouse may be impossible without the extended use of outside resources.

A final well-documented stressor for the individual and family is the death of a member. Bereavement and its sequelae have been studied in various forms—widows, widowers, stillborn death, death of a parent, death of a child, sudden death, sudden infant death, and death after a protracted illness. Research in this area has led to the elaboration of the normal mourning or grieving process and the identification of strategies for anticipatory guidance, support systems, and preventive intervention. These are described in Chapter 15. Perhaps of all the vulnerable groups discussed in this chapter, the bereaved have been the focus of the most research and the most clearly articulated prevention strategies. The task of adequately implementing these strategies remains to be done.

■ Women

In a descriptive nursing research study, Griffith analyzed broad areas of stress, common stress responses, and usual coping patterns of women according to their age group.[31, 32] The stress categories and factors included in the study are presented in Table 9-2. One fourth of all women in the study reported that their physical health was a major stressor. Women between 25 and 34 years old indicated that personal time and personal success were also major stressors, while for women over 35, physical health was the primary stressor, followed by personal time. Younger women were more likely to report physical and emotional symptoms of stress than older women. The physical symptoms most frequently reported included restlessness, sinus problems, frequent backaches and headaches, and trouble sleeping. Emotional responses to stress included feeling overweight, depression, nervousness, anxiety, sudden mood shifts, and irritability.

Women's usual coping patterns also vary with age. Younger women were more likely to talk with friends or associates about their problems, while older women relied on work or religion. Almost one third of the women in the study used consumption of food as a means of coping with their problems. These are significant findings because they document both the physical and mental health care needs of women in present American society. Additional research is necessary to identify effective ways to assist women in reducing their stress symptoms and developing more adaptive coping responses. Nursing, as a predominantly female profession, has the potential of making a significant impact in health promotion and illness prevention with this high-risk population.

■ **MENTAL HEALTH NEEDS.** The mental health of women is intimately connected to the idea of equality: "The equal right to participate in all areas of the life of society and to pursue one's unique psychological potential in all of its aspects."[11:1320] Unfortunately American society is one of structured social inequality based on gender, race, and class differences to name a few. Women have a disadvantaged status in this society, which increases their vulnerability to stress and their potential for developing maladaptive responses. The status of women is summarized in the 1978 President's Commission on Mental Health:

1. **Salary.** More than half of all women are now employed outside of the home, but they are clustered in the lowest paying occupations and at the bottom of the achievement ladder. One woman in four compared to one man in 18 lives on an annual income of less than $4000.
2. **Dual roles.** Whether or not a woman is employed

TABLE 9-2

CATEGORIES AND FACTORS OF POTENTIAL STRESSORS EXPERIENCED BY WOMEN

Category	Factors
Love relationships	Being in love Satisfactory sex life Relationship with loved one
Personal success	Success in life Success in occupation/role Degree of recognition Personal growth and development
Physical health	Nutrition and eating patterns Physical attractiveness General health and physical condition Exercise and physical activity
Parent-child relationships	Being a parent Relationship with children
Personal time	Time to oneself Balance between work, family, leisure, home, and self
Social relationships	Relationships with close friends Relationships with co-workers Social life with significant others

From Griffith, J.: Women's stressors according to age group: part I, Issues in Health Care of Women, 6:311, 1983.

outside the home, housework remains largely "women's work." Thus many American women have two full workdays in every 24 hours.

3. **Politics.** Only about 3.5% of the House and 2% of the Senate of the United States and about 9% of the state legislators are women. This greatly reduces the political capacity of women to improve their status.
4. **Business.** It is still unusual to see women in the bastions of financial power and in high corporate echelons.
5. **Law.** In many states when a woman marries, she trades the rights of a person for the duties of a wife. A husband who deserts his wife and takes a temporary job in another state can seriously affect his wife's credit rating, right to vote, serve on juries, run for office, and so on.[74:1027]

The Subpanel on the Mental Health of Women of this commission reported that circumstances and conditions which society accepts as normal and ordinary often lead to despair, anguish, and mental illness in women.[74] The subpanel documented the ways in which inequality creates dilemmas and conflicts for women in the contexts of marriage, family relationships, reproduction, child rearing, divorce, aging, education, and

work. These same conditions encourage the frequency of incest, rape, and marital violence, which also heighten women's vulnerability to mental illness. Finally, the epidemiological data that establish conditions associated with mental illness are particularly relevant to women. These include poverty, alienation, and powerlessness. The convergence, therefore, of multiple stressful events with the chronic stressful conditions in which women frequently live, produces a high susceptibility to mental disorders among women.

This susceptibility is substantiated by a high incidence and prevalence of mental illness among women. One of the most consistent findings is that depression is closely associated with being female. The ratio of depressed women to men is about two to one. The data also show that young poor women who head single-parent families and young married women who work at dead-end jobs have shown the greatest rise in the rate of both treated and untreated depression.[33] The most recent research data suggest, however, that the excess of psychological symptoms in women is not intrinsic to femaleness but to the conditions of subordination, stress, and powerlessness that characterize traditional female roles.

■ **POWERLESSNESS.** Families are usually viewed as providing support networks for people, yet Carmen, Russo, and Miller[11] believe that it is in the traditional construct of marriage that the subjugation of women is the most apparent and destructive. For example, it is in rigidly traditional families that female adults and children are at highest risk for violence and sexual abuse.[74] Violence is said to occur in 50% of American families,[42] and it has been estimated that 1% of all girls have been sexually abused by their fathers.[39] The problem of family abuse and violence is discussed in detail in Chapter 32.

These destructive patterns of family roles and relationships are reinforced by society's pervasive pattern of sex discrimination. Women who leave unhappy or violent homes are denied equal educational, vocational, and economic opportunities; quality and supportive child care facilities, and a legitimate self-supporting role in society. Women are clustered in "female" jobs that are characterized by low pay. In the same occupation, they earn less than men. They are not equally compensated with men for work involving similar education or experience. In 1979, the median annual income of women who worked full time was 60% that of men. The earnings gap is greatest for minority women.[87] Of divorced women, only 14% are awarded alimony, and only 44% are awarded child support. Less than half of these, or only 21% of divorced mothers, collect child support regularly, and even then the payments are generally insufficient.[85] It would appear then, that the alternative to depression in an unhappy marriage can be a life of poverty with a dead-end job and great difficulty in attempting to provide adequate care for one's children.

The idea of powerlessness in the development of psychological distress and mental disorders among women is evident in one study, which reported that women who became depressed had previously made many attempts to cope. Those with the highest rates of depression were continuously faced with multiple and chronic stresses affecting themselves and their children. Efforts to deal with these stresses led to repeated frustration in employment possibilities, housing conditions, protection against violence and crime, child care assistance, and the unhelpful responses of social service and mental health agencies.[30]

■ **RESPONSE OF THE MENTAL HEALTH SYSTEM.** If one's goal is illness prevention and health promotion, one cannot overlook this last concern—the responsiveness of the health community. New knowledge about women, men, and sex roles has not generally been incorporated in mental health education or clinical practice. This is evident in the following criticisms:

1. There is a double standard for mental health based on sex-role stereotyping and adjustment to one's environment. Broverman's now classic study[8] of mental health clinicians' attitudes indicates that healthy women are viewed differently from men and adults of unspecified gender in being more submissive, less independent, less adventurous, more suggestible, less competitive, more excitable in minor crises, more likely to have their feelings hurt, more emotional, more conceited about appearance, less objective, and more illogical. Although this study was conducted in 1970, Sherman[82] in 1980 concluded that there is still sex-role stereotyping in mental health standards and that sex role–discrepant behaviors are viewed as more of a maladjustment. Although nurses were not included in Broverman's study, Davis[19] believes that as a group, they are not very different from others practicing in the mental health field. She notes that despite nurses' perceptions to the contrary, research seems to indicate that as an occupational group, nurses have a traditional view of sex roles.

2. Sexual abuse and exploitation in the male therapist–female patient relationship is more common than has previously been realized. This includes such erotic activities as kissing, hugging, touching, and therapist-patient sex. Some studies have indicated that as many as 10% of men psychiatrists and psychologists in practice report having sexual contact with women patients.[18]

3. A related danger in the male–female therapeutic relationship is that the dyad may replicate rather than remedy the "one-down" position in which women frequently find themselves in life. This may encourage the fantasy that an idealized relationship with a more powerful other is a better solution to life problems than is taking autonomous action. This possibility is strengthened by the predominance of male therapists.[12]

4. Therapeutic theories have often supported stereotypes about sex roles, including the assumption that dependency, masochism, and passivity are normal for women and that assertiveness and aggression should be treated differently for women than for men.[8] Women are also subjected to the theories based on a "blame-the-mother" tradition, particularly in reference to schizophrenic children and a general "antifeminine Freudian" position.

5. A pervasive sex bias has been documented in the therapeutic relationship. There is evidence that therapists' knowledge about issues affecting the lives of women is inadequate.[82] Adjustment to traditional roles is stressed, yet there has been a lack of realistic appraisals of the occupational hazards of the housewife role. Anger in women is often labeled pathological and inappropriate.[58] Thus many women experience conflict about anger and have difficulty expressing it adaptively.

The consequences of these practices affect both the

quality and quantity of mental health care available to women. Carmen notes:

> Women can be considered *both* overserved and underserved by mental health delivery systems. For disorders congruent with sex-role stereotypes, such as depression, conversion hysteria, and phobias, women show higher rates of service utilization than do men. In contrast, problems of women that are congruent with societal views of male authority and female devaluation, such as rape, incest, and wife beating, have been ignored. Thus, services for female victims of male aggression have been provided largely through the coordinated efforts of women themselves at a time when mental health professionals were often either blaming the victims or not noticing them. Similarly, for disorders that are incongruent with society's idealized view of women, such as alcoholism and illicit drug abuse, women's service needs have usually been hidden and ignored.[11:1327]

Yet the incidence of alcoholism among women is high, and in the United States more than two thirds of all tranquilizers, stimulants, and antidepressants are used by women.[22] Homemakers over age 35 have been identified as the largest single group of tranquilizer users.[16] What one can conclude from this discussion is that women at high risk for psychiatric illness are often separated or divorced, nonwhite, poorly educated, of low socioeconomic status, and coping with the stress of raising small children and being a breadwinner on a low income.[34]

■ **WORKING MOTHERS.*** An increasing number of women are in the labor force because of personal career choice or financial need. Within the United States, because of the increasing divorce rate, more women are becoming the primary financial support for themselves and their children. It is often difficult to juggle three roles—wife, mother, employee. Employment outside the home can engender positive, growth-producing feelings, resulting in an increased self-esteem and heightened sense of independence, as well as negative, often immobilizing feelings of guilt and anxiety about "abandoning" one's family. It is not uncommon for a working mother to assume responsibility for everything that goes askew with the family in her absence. Many women are socialized to accept the belief that a woman's place is in the home; hence, when a woman seeks employment, she thinks she is functioning in opposition to societal norms.

Although the new freedom of emergent feminism has expanded some opportunities for women, it has also created new dilemmas. Four new syndromes have been identified as a result of these changes: (1) reentry anxiety

when a long homebound woman returns to work in the outer world, (2) performance anxiety and fear that career success may be viewed as social failure, (3) conflict between social expectations of accommodation and compliance and the need to assert herself and fight for her rights when they have been imposed on, and (4) conflict between a woman's sense of personal identity and her professional identity, in which marriage or family may be viewed as a threat to autonomy.[65]

Three defense mechanisms seem symptomatic of underlying guilt: rationalization, projection, and overcompensation. In rationalization the mother thinks up a socially approved reason for her behavior, such as "I would just play bridge or do volunteer work if I stayed at home." Projection involves blaming someone or something else for one's need to work, and overcompensation is evidenced by trying to repay the child with gifts.[56]

There are a number of ways in which nurses can help the working mother cope with her myriad of roles. First, they can encourage and provide a medium in which the mother can come to grips with her conflicting feelings. The mother needs to be aware that it is the quality rather than the quantity of mother-child interactions that has the greatest impact on growth and development. Moreover, children often benefit from their mother's feelings of self-satisfaction related to job success.

The nurse can also support working mothers as they make or change child care arrangements. Few situations have as profound an effect on the working mother as disruptions in child care. Essentially, selecting the best arrangement for each family is a problem-solving strategy whereby the family examines each available alternative and selects the one that seemingly will bring more comfort.

Another problem-solving area relates to assignment of responsibility for household chores. It is estimated that it takes 105 hours a week to carry out full-time employment and meet the domestic responsibilities of the family. A variety of household management alternatives exist, and the nurse can help the mother select the one that suits the needs of her family. Five guidelines have been developed for nurses working with mothers who are experiencing role conflict[56]:

1. Help the mother examine and accept her reasons for working.
2. Encourage the woman to choose a job carefully. Working mothers cannot afford the luxury of displacing accumulated hostility from the job onto the family.
3. Communicate honestly with family members to

---

*This section was contributed by Jeanette and Wade Lancaster.

determine their response to employment. Discussion of differences cannot occur without honest expression.

4. Assist the mother in finding a suitable surrogate whose attitudes are consistent with hers.
5. Explore ways in which help can be provided by others, the family, or the housekeeper.

■ Mature adults

The issues of midlife and advancing age are problematic for some, but not all, adults. As people approach midlife they reflect on the choices they have made and their progress in attaining the goals they had set for themselves. Marriage, life-style, children, career, and quality of life all are subject to scrutiny. Certain types of stressors, including career changes (promotion, change of job, demotion, or being fired), changes in the family unit (death, divorce, or departure of the last child), and the aging process, may precipitate anxiety, depression, or psychosomatic illnesses. In essence, midlife is the time when previous choices in important life areas and one's related success, failure, satisfaction, and disappointment are reviewed and reworked in light of one's previous goals, currently perceived limitations, finiteness of opportunities, and time itself. It combines the sense of "another chance" with that of a "final chance."[84]

Midlife has traditionally been given very little attention in theory, research, or practice. Recent works by Neugarten,[66] Sheehy,[81] Levenson,[59] and Gould[28] have explored it as a time of development and change, rather than a period merely focused on impending aging and death. The middle years range in the 30s to 40s, although precisely defining it by chronological age has been more recently criticized. Neither can it any longer be defined as the time of menopause for the woman. Rather, it relates to a combination of biological, psychological, and sociological events. Notman compares it to the period of adolescence:

This importance of separation, the change in relationship to family, and the potential for further development of one's own interests, are common to both periods. However, the differences are highly significant. At adolescence the separation is from parents, who are incestuous object choices. At midlife the separation is from children, and the experience often revives some sense of loss. The adolescent perspective of infinite time and choices to be made differs from the midlife sense of the finite and the reassessment of choices that have been made. The reality is that time is limited and that although choices do exist or even increase, there is also a limited range and variety of careers, new physical pursuits, and new relationships.[69:1273]

Important in a discussion of midlife is the fact that it is viewed differently by men and women. According to Levenson's work,[59] men give central importance to the role of work in establishing oneself in the world. Work, not family, appears to be the organizing theme of men's lives. Thus, at midlife, men focus heavily on evaluating their work and their career goals. Women, on the other hand, focus on the world in relation to their family or potential to have one, as well as their work or career goals. Women who have not had children feel a last chance to consider motherhood. Women with children experience a decrease in their absorption in the burdens of child care. One's children may either be launched into the world or functioning quite independently at home. Consequently, these women may feel relieved, renewed, and ready to return to the work world.

Although this can be an exciting time, it can also be viewed negatively if one feels displaced, unprepared, or unaccepted. Extramarital affairs, divorces, and major life changes can result from a midlife crisis and can pose problems for the individual, as well as the family.

■ The elderly

Another time of increased stress for the individual has, in the past, been largely ignored by researchers and clinicians in the mental health field who focus heavily on the early developmental stages. This is the period of later adulthood and old age. One of the most obvious reasons for this may be evident in the changing distribution of the population. In 1900, only 28% of the American population exceeded the age of 35 and only 3% had reached the age of 65. In contrast, in 1981, 45% exceeded age 35, and 11% of the population were 65 or older. During the same period of time, life expectancy in America has increased from an average of 51 years to 76 years for men.[79] Furthermore, the United States census in 1970 identified more than 106,000 Americans 100 years of age or older.

Elderly people are at high risk for mental health disruption for several reasons, including their susceptibility to the effects of rapid social and environmental change. Since the 1950s social and technological changes have occurred at an unprecedented pace. This poses problems for elderly people who are physiologically less able to adapt to rapidly changing events in their lives.

A number of barriers exist for the elderly, which interfere with their ability to meet their mental health needs. First, a far greater share of national resources are devoted to children than to the elderly. Also, elderly people who live on fixed incomes are especially susceptible to the effects of inflation. People are at high risk for lowered self-esteem during inflationary periods when their expectations for either social mobility or maintenance of at least an adequate standard of living are destroyed by the high cost of living. Elderly people are susceptible to lowered self-esteem and resignation when they have spent a lifetime of saving for retirement only to find that they are not able to make ends meet. In addition, transportation often presents a major barrier for the elderly who do not have ready access to services. Retirement also can deal a serious blow to self-esteem, since so much of contemporary society revolves around what people do for a living.

Although the majority of the present elderly population is not poor (only 14% of those over 65 are under the poverty line) and 95% of those over 65 remain community, rather than institutional, residents,[79] there are noticeable changes that begin to impose constraints on the aging adult. In reviewing the literature, Hefferin[37] identified three life stages of people living beyond age 65. The first stage is between ages 65 and 75, in which most people continue with normal activities unless there is a specific illness. In the second stage, from age 75 to 85, normal activities can also be carried out, although the effects of aging are evident. The final stage occurs after 85, in which most people need some help to maintain normal activities, and some may even require institutionalization.

As these stages reflect, the period of the life course extending from middle age into early old age is often characterized at the outset by the height of social and economic success as well as physical well-being. But slowly changes occur that for most people are simply a somewhat lower level of physical and psychological energy, accompanied by society's subtle and open pressures to make room for the next generation. It has been shown that the documentable quantitative changes in learning ability, intellectual competence, and other contextual behavior are relatively small and often within the realm of individual and environmental compensatory interventions. The evidence is strong, also, that individual differences in the maintenance of behavioral competence are related primarily to the person's state of health and the opportunities and tendencies to be fully involved in a stimulating environment.

Despite this evidence, society still holds many myths and stereotypes about the elderly that mitigate against the maintenance of feelings of worth. Language and humor are replete with examples of clichés that cast elderly people in a negative light. Phrases like the "old goat," "silly old biddy," or "dirty old man" do not reflect a positive image of the elderly. The very word elderly tends to call forth a set of images, including graying and thinning hair, a slow stooped gait, and a tendency toward forgetfulness. In a major study by the National Council on Aging[3] it was found that older people were almost as negative in their attitudes about aging as were their younger counterparts. Few people in a sample of 4000 chose the years between 60 and 80 as "the best of my life" and about one third considered this period as the least desirable time of their life.[9]

■ **LIFE STRESSORS.** The extension of the normative life span into a long period of postparental and postvocational behavior is creating new life stressors and resulting maladaptive responses. For example, certain life events, such as enforced retirement, and loss of friends and family become more likely with increasing age, and loss of a spouse is often perceived as the single greatest loss that an individual can experience in the life cycle. The combined physical, social, financial, and psychological changes that result from the loss of a spouse severely tax the coping ability of the bereaved.

Although death of a spouse may be perceived as the greatest stressor, multiple other stressors that are social, psychological, and biological in origin overlap, interact, and enhance the vulnerability of aging adults. These are described in detail by Goodstein.[26] He notes that the social sphere presents a major source of stress, including family-cultural, employment, commercial, logistical, financial, and discriminatory stresses as described in Table 9-3. He observes that the elderly's social status and physical function have decreased at the same time this population has increased.

The elderly also have a bombardment of emotional pressures as they struggle with the issues of integrity and independence. Stressors involving mastery, coping style, generation gap, fears, love cues, self-image, loss, death of family and friends, relocation, money, retirement, deteriorating body functions, attractiveness, visual and auditory acuity, prestige, sex, and cognition (Table 9-3) all pose emotional hardship to the elderly. Goodstein believes that no matter what the specific psychological stress, the commonalities of sequelae to loss are reduced self-esteem and dignity, plus the implication that life and personal usefulness are slipping away.

Finally, without question, biological stress takes a toll on the elderly. Consider these statistics:

The elderly represent one third of the nation's health bill, one third of the family physician's practice time, two times the number of outpatient visits of other age populations, twice the number of days in the hospital of other age populations, three and a half times the cost of health care in other age populations, and 45% of the elderly have some physical limitations.[26:226]

Major sources of biological stress for the elderly include illness and accidents, physiological aging, medications, other ingested substances, and iatrogenic biological stresses (Table 9-3).

TABLE 9-3

SUMMARY OF STRESSES FACING THE ELDERLY

Category of stress	Influencing factors	Outcomes
Social Stresses		
Family-cultural	Smaller family size	Weakened traditional nuclear family unit
	Increased mobility	Less opportunity for role modeling by elderly
	One fourth of elderly have no children	Shift from family to public responsibility for
	One half of elderly have only distant relatives	care of the aged
Employment	Security not based on ability to work but on government and union pensions	Retirement represents a major change that may be responded to adaptively or maladaptively
	Elderly capable of work function beyond age 65	Some models of part-time work have been developed
	In 1900, 66% of those over 65 still worked	
	Now less than 33% work	
	Retirement age is now 70 by new federal law	
Commercial	Society values youth and views older people and objects as obsolescent	Aging is devalued
	Commercial advertising is aimed at youth and deplores aging in principle	
Logistical	Physical disabilities, costs, fears, access, distances, and weather are all problems affecting the mobility of the elderly	Transportation is difficult for many of the elderly
		Access to activities and health care is often limited
		The elderly are easy targets for robbery and assault
Financial	Pensions are outstripped by the cost of living	Inflation has a severe impact on the elderly
	Health insurance is often inadequate with rising premiums and poor psychiatric coverage	
	Statistics for physical and psychiatric illness demonstrate the elderly's great need for services	
Discriminatory	Negative stereotypes of the elderly are commonly accepted	Ageism, or prejudice toward the elderly, exists in American society
	Providing health care to the elderly lacks prestige and is often avoided by caregivers	Health problems of the elderly often receive inadequate treatment
	Courses in aging and care of the aged are seldom part of the educational curricula of health care professionals	
Psychological Stresses		
Mastery	The elderly experience decreasing influence over their outer life and preoccupation with their inner life	Through denial and projection the elderly evolve a "magical mastery" of their external environment
Coping style	The elderly tend to use coping styles that were effective earlier in life	If previously used and trusted coping styles fail, the elderly may display maladaptive responses
	Denial, somatization, projection, and constructed affect may occur	

Continued.

Despite these multiple stresses, most elderly persons are able to live in the community reasonably secure financially and in social contact with family and friends. However, those older persons experiencing multiple stresses and inadequate coping resources are at greater risk to require some form of institutional support.

Access to and use of social support systems are important determinants of an older person's response to stress along with previous life experiences, premorbid coping styles, physical and emotional status, and the approach health professionals provide to the elderly from both a practical and an attitudinal standpoint.

TABLE 9-3—cont'd

SUMMARY OF STRESSES FACING THE ELDERLY

Category of stress	Influencing factors	Outcomes
Generation gap	At the time of the elderly's need, younger relatives may be at crucial points in their own lives and lack the time and insight to help	Younger relatives have difficulty understanding the aging process
Fears	Common fears include the following: 1. Maintaining control over their lives and environment 2. Maintaining physical functioning 3. Retaining a sense of purpose and productivity 4. Maintaining independence while acknowledging the possible need of a dependent status for survival 5. Failing cognition and senility 6. Death 7. Losing the interest of others	Predictable fears are common among the elderly and may cause significant psychological stress
Love cues	The elderly have acquired skills in interpreting nonverbal communication. They easily detect and respond to cues of lack of interest or respect	If the elderly perceive lack of interest or honesty, they believe they are unliked and respond by withdrawing
Self-image	The elderly may dislike their dependent status or interpret it as a sign of their own failures	The elderly may have an aversion to youth or an acceptance of the stereotypes of the aged
Loss	Losses are predictable, steady, numerous, and often arrive in bunches	Losses for the elderly represent the most basic psychological stress
Death of family and friends	Loss of family and friends suggests impending loss of self	Results in loss of security and companionship and depletion of the pool of caregivers
Relocation	Relocation can involve loss of privacy, accustomed diet, favorite belongings, and familiar faces. It may be accompanied by a feeling of aloneness or abandonment	Stress is a function of losing the familiar and facing the unsure new environment
Money	Loss of money affects the availability of goods, care, identity, and status	This compounds any other stressor experienced by the elderly
Retirement	Some external sources of gratification may be lost, and the couple may have to deal with changes in privacy and daily routine	Results in changes in income, identity, and life-style
Deteriorating body function	This decreases a person's skills	Loss of body functioning may affect one's identity and sense of productivity and usefulness
Attractiveness	Aging produces physical changes. The effect of aging on one's physical appearance is subject to personal evaluation	One potential outcome is negative self-image and withdrawal from others
Visual and auditory acuity	Acuity in sensory cues is important for orientation, processing information, and maintaining daily activities	Diminution in sight or hearing can create inaccurate interpretation of the environment and may lead to paranoid or avoiding behavior

■ **BARRIERS TO MENTAL HEALTH CARE.*** Attitude barriers on the part of both the elderly and health care providers interfere with effective service utilization.

*This section was contributed by Jeanette and Wade Lancaster.

Hagebak and Hagebak[35] described psychological barriers held by both therapists and the elderly. They found six major attitude barriers commonly held by therapists: (1) the "you can't teach an old dog new tricks" attitude, which discounts the elderly person's ability to learn, adapt, or change; (2) the "my God, I'm mortal too"

TABLE 9-3—cont'd

SUMMARY OF STRESSES FACING THE ELDERLY

Category of stress	Influencing factors	Outcomes
Prestige	The elderly often are retired from membership in decision-making bodies or are given an "honorary" membership without voting privileges	They perceive that their opinions are not valued and that their experience does not count
Sex	Sexual ability is determined by availability of a partner, past sexual activity, physical health, and support from family and health professionals The elderly may be embarrassed to discuss their sexual needs or experience side effects from medications One's ability to enjoy sex can be maintained throughout the life cycle	Natural physiological changes, if explained to the elderly and understood by them, can result in increased closeness, satisfaction, and communication
Cognition	Subtle changes in cognitive ability are detected first by the elderly Cognitive changes can be compounded by other life stresses	Resulting changes and perceptions can affect practical coping abilities and be psychologically disturbing
Biological Stresses		
Illness and accidents	Result in decreased function and pain	Can erode activity, appearance, finances, employability, and self-esteem
Physiological aging	Aging inevitably occurs in body organs, biochemical and metabolic pathways, musculoskeletal systems, and central nervous system It occurs at different rates in different people and among different organs in the same person	Requires specific and sensitive guidelines for treatments, medications, education, and compliance
Medications	The elderly tend to collect large numbers of medications from multiple sources, using an average of 13 prescriptions a year They often take higher than prescribed doses and for longer periods of time Of psychogeriatric admissions, 20% are precipitated by adverse effects of psychotropic drugs	Prescribing medications must be accompanied by proper discussion, written instructions, and careful monitoring
Other ingested substances	Changes in appetite, decreased activity, and poor physical function interfere with proper food intake among the elderly Assessment of caffeine, nicotine, and alcohol is often overlooked in the elderly	Nutrition is often a problem for the elderly Drugs and alcohol may be used as tranquilizers or to allay loneliness
Iatrogenic biological stresses	The negative stereotypes of aging may block the reality of medication side effects and infection sequelae	Major iatrogenic problems arise from failing to diagnose and treat the causes of illness because of stereotyped thinking and an inappropriate prescription of medications to "keep the patient happy"

Modified from Goodstein, R.: Am. J. Orthopsychiatry **51**(2):219, 1981.

syndrome, which forces therapists to acknowledge their own aging process; (3) the "why bother?" attitude, which holds that since elderly people have a shortened life span it is hardly worth the effort to work with them; (4) the "I'm a child" belief, which is seen when role reversal occurs and the therapist responds to the older person as though to a parent; (5) the "patient is a child" approach, which discounts the elderly people's abilities by treating them like children; or (6) "senility is natural," which expects the elderly person to be forgetful, slow, etc. Often the elderly respond to these attitudes like a self-fulfilling prophecy and thus behave accordingly.

Nurses can overcome these attitude hurdles by first

Potential Primary Prevention Measures

Education and information measures

- Increasing the public's awareness, through planned campaigns utilizing the appropriate media, that stress can be an antecedent of illness and that stress management can be an important component of health
- Creating new educational pathways for developing enhanced professional skills in bio-behavioral fields of medicine and public health
- Developing the capacities of health care professionals in stress diagnosis and management
- Helping parents recognize and deal with stress
- Training secondary, elementary, and preschool teachers to include discussion of stress recognition and management in school health curricula
- Training of police in handling calls involving domestic and interpersonal disputes which would potentially lead to violent behavior
- Public education, especially for high risk groups, on steps to take to reduce risks of rape
- Training all "helping" professionals regarding signs which indicate high risk for suicide
- Helping the public be aware of indicators of possible suicide

Service measures

- Hotlines for people under acute stress (suicide, child abuse prevention)
- Stress management programs in work places
- Stress management programs targeted to adolescents, parents, and the elderly
- Stress appraisal analysis (self-administered or performed by a legitimate objective outside source)
- Professional and social support systems to assist in resolution of stressful life events, including mutual aid and self-help groups such as Reach for Recovery, child abusing parents, bereavement groups, single parent groups

- Information and counseling with regard to individually appropriate leisure and stress-reducing activities including exercise
- A variety of self-help relaxation and biofeedback techniques, which can be individualized in concert with a diversity of life-styles and work requirements
- Psycho-physiologic tests to aid in assisting employees who are having difficulty adjusting to their work and to their co-workers
- Support services for inevitable or necessary life change events—especially in relation to death, separation, job changes, and geographic relocation
- Domestic crisis teams to defuse domestic disputes
- Targeting the above measures to high risk populations and individuals with low coping abilities
- Evaluating intervention efforts
- Follow-up services for persons who have attempted suicide
- Shelters for abused wives (and husbands)
- Training all health (and other human services—including educational) personnel to be alert to evidence of child abuse

Technological measures

- Actions by employers, labor, and government to reduce stress-creating work environments
- Reducing stressful aspects of the environment such as noise pollution and overcrowding

Legislative and regulatory measures

- Activities to create employment opportunities for youth
- Action to limit the availability of handguns, to reduce homicides and suicides that occur during stressful periods
- Strengthening mandatory child abuse reporting laws

Modified from U.S. Department of Health and Human Services: Promoting health, preventing disease: objectives for the nation, Washington, D.C., 1984, Public Health Service.

recognizing that the older person is a person who just happened to grow older but is not basically different from other people. The next step is introspection or conscious examination of one's feelings toward aging and death. Attitudes, beliefs, and feelings are generally clearly transmitted to others, hence, personal awareness is extremely important.

Like nurses and other health care providers, elderly people often hold attitudes that are barriers to obtaining mental health services. They often believe that "senility is natural" and expect to evidence psychological changes. Thus they view any mental health changes as inevitable and often fail to seek assistance for problems that could be treated or reversed. Elderly people often question their value by asking "who/why am I?" They believe that since they no longer work and their children are grown they have lost their value to society. A third attitude held by the elderly is one of fierce independence, or "do for yourself," whereby they hesitate to seek the assistance of others. The counterpart to this attitude is "I'm distrustful and afraid," in which the elderly fear the services provided by anyone associated with the mental health system. Last, elderly people may evidence a "doing what's expected" syndrome in which they support stereotypes or their perceptions of what others expect of them.[35] These barriers tend to arise because both nurses and the elderly are unfamiliar with the aging process.

Severe psychological decline is not an inevitable part of aging. Although some physiological changes do occur with aging, many others can be prevented by modification of the environment, such as overcoming attitudes that expect the elderly to respond in less than functional ways, reducing stress, and simple techniques, such as speaking clearly and audibly. As with all age groups, stress interferes with accurate perception of environmental cues as well as problem-solving ability. Stimuli that tend to set off a stress response are those which are novel, rapidly changing, or unexpected.

The most common psychiatric problem among the elderly is depression. Old age is a time of numerous losses. For many, retirement, while eagerly anticipated, reflects a loss of meaningful involvement with the larger society. Also, friends and family members begin to die, skills and abilities may diminish, and even homes and familiar possessions are lost. The effects of several drugs commonly consumed by elderly people contribute to depression, including digitalis; antihypertensives, especially reserpine; antiparkinsonism drugs; corticosteroids; antianxiety drugs; and even some antidepressants.[22]

The interaction of drugs is a particular problem for the elderly who often mix medications. Comfort[14] says that the first operation in geriatric psychiatry is the "plastic bag test," which means to collect all the medication the patient is taking. Often some were prescribed, others were purchased over the counter, and still other medication was provided by friends or family. Not only do the elderly inadvertently mix medications but many use drugs and alcohol to cope with stress, loneliness, or feelings of fear, anxiety, or loss.

The elderly are not a homogeneous group. Each one is a unique person with needs, desires, assets, and

support networks. In providing mental health services it is important to remember that most elderly people do not live in institutions but rather are able to maintain their own home or live with friends or family members. Often a primary mental health goal is that of helping the family identify and use its own strengths to support and respond effectively to elderly members.

Hamrick and Blazer[36] describe a program that helps family members identify and use their own strengths to help elderly relatives. They assess areas such as recent events that may have been stressful, the developmental history of both the patient and the family, impairments in the older adult, family conflicts, and support (both tangible and intangible). Once the assessment is completed, one or more of five major approaches is generally used: (1) explain the patient's impairment and capabilities to the family, (2) inform the family about community resources and how to use them, (3) evaluate respite activities of the family, (4) allow members to express and work through their feelings, and (5) provide opportunities for the family to make decisions about the care of the older adult.

To respond effectively to the mental health needs of the elderly, nurses must use an integrated approach that takes into account the multiple stressors as well as the resources available for effective coping. Schaie believes that "the quality of life in developed societies can be readily sensed from the manner in which transition from midlife to old age is accomplished with a minimum of stress and the preservation of maximum personal freedom and opportunities."[79:216] If this is true, primary prevention activities directed toward the elderly must command the attention of psychiatric nurses and other health professionals.

♣ Planning and implementation

Under the sponsorship of the Public Health Service, a national incentive has been undertaken to promote health and prevent disease in this country. A number of potential measures have been identified to meet one of the 1990 objectives for the control of stress and violent behavior. These include education, service, technological, and legislative measures as identified in the box on the opposite page.[86] This list provides the nurse with a good overview of the many areas appropriate for nursing intervention.

In addition, the nursing model of health-illness phenomena presented in Chapter 3 and represented in Fig. 9-1 is useful for the nurse in planning strategies for primary prevention. It suggests both target areas and types of activities that might be useful. If one's overall nursing goal is to promote constructive coping mech-

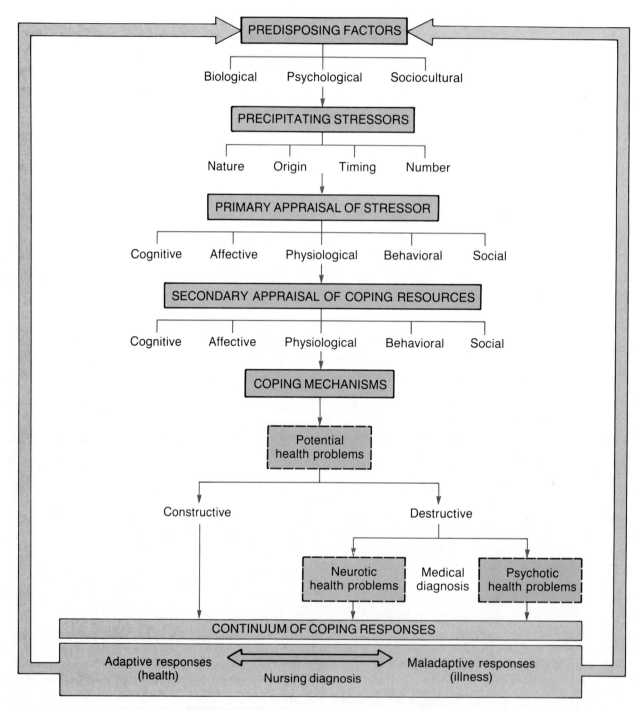

Fig. 9-1. Nursing model of health-illness phenomena.

anisms and maximize adaptive coping responses, then the model suggests that prevention strategies should be directed toward influencing predisposing factors, precipitating stressors, appraisal of stressors, and coping resources and mechanisms through the following interventions: (1) health education, (2) environmental change, and (3) supporting social systems. Because the

process depicted in the model is a dynamic one, it is not possible to discretely link a particular strategy with a particular component of the model. Rather, the strategies can affect multiple aspects of a person's life. For example, an environmental change, such as changing jobs, can affect one's predisposition to stress, decrease the amount of stress, change one's appraisal of the threat, and perhaps increase one's financial or social coping resources. This interactive effect can thus serve to justify the use of these prevention strategies for vulnerable groups.

■ Health education

This strategy of primary prevention in mental health involves the strengthening of individuals and groups through **competence building.** It is based on the assumption that many maladaptive responses are the result of a lack of competence, that is, a lack of perceived control over one's own life, of effective coping strategies, and the lowered self-esteem that results. Bloom[5] believes that competence building is perhaps the single, most persuasive preventive strategy for dealing with individual and social issues in most communities. A competent community is one that is aware of resources and alternatives, can make reasoned decisions about issues facing them, and can cope adaptively with problems. In this sense the concept of a competent community parallels the concept of positive mental health.[45]

■ **LEVELS OF INTERVENTION.** Health education or competence building can be viewed as having four aspects. The first is increasing the individual's or group's awareness of issues and events related to health and illness. Awareness of normal developmental tasks and potential problems must be a foundational element. The second aspect is increasing one's understanding of the dimensions of potential stressors, possible outcomes (both adaptive and maladaptive), and alternative coping responses. A third element is increasing one's knowledge of where and how to acquire the needed resources. Many health professionals assume this is common knowledge, although for many groups of individuals it is not. The fourth and final aspect of health education focuses on increasing the actual abilities of the individual or group. This means improving or maximizing one's coping skills, such as problem-solving skills or interpersonal skills, tolerance of stress and frustration, motivation, hope, self-esteem, and power. Ryan contends the following:

Self-esteem is to some extent an essential requirement to the very survival of the human organism . . . and is partially dependent on the inclusion of a sense of power within the self-concept. . . . A mentally healthy person must be able to perceive himself as at least minimally powerful, capable of influencing his environment to his own benefit, and further . . . this sense of minimal power has to be based on the actual experience and exercise of power.[78:50]

■ **PROGRAMS AND ACTIVITIES.** Health education has long been regarded by nurses as an essential part of nursing practice, yet it is difficult to quantify the degree or quality of mental health education actually implemented by nurses. It can take place in any setting, can assume a formal or informal structure, can be directed toward individuals or groups, and can be related to predisposing factors or potential stressors. Health education directed toward strengthening an individual's predisposition to stress can take various forms. Growth groups may be formed for parents that focus on parent-child relations, normal growth and development, or effective methods of child rearing. Groups of children or adolescents can discuss peer relationships, sexuality, or potential problem areas, such as drug abuse or promiscuity. Employee groups can be formed to discuss career burnout and related issues. Or a more activity-centered educational program can be initiated, such as Outward Bound, which helps the individual discover that step by step one can expand competence in mastering new, unexpected, and potentially stressful situations in an adaptive way.

Probably the most common type of health education program implemented at present is one that aids the individual in coping with a specific potential stressor. Consider, for example, the impending stressor or risk factor of marital separation. Families about to experience marital separation are vulnerable to emotional problems, physical complaints, and increased utilization of health care f 'lities.[7,89] Children and adults about to experience ι vent may be offered educational and supportive group intervention aimed at enhancing their ability to cope. Education groups can similarly be offered to those experiencing retirement, bereavement, or any other stressful event.

Parent education classes are a well-known example of the type of anticipatory guidance that can be offered to high-risk groups. Although raising children is considered a serious aspect of American life, until recently little attention has been directed to the belief that effective parenting is not an innate ability. Whether nurses subscribe to a specific set of beliefs and strategies for parenting or choose an eclectic approach, the opportunities for promoting mental health abound. Possibly one of the most beneficial results of parent education is the acknowledgment that all parents become frustrated, angry, and ambivalent toward their children. Parent education goes beyond acknowledging feelings and includes learning and practicing alternative ways of interacting with children. During these classes, situations are anticipated and discussions focus on identifying potential crisis situations and dealing with them through simulated encounters such as role playing. Education for mental health can thus address the needs of both children and parents as family roles shift and respond to societal change.

Finally, health education activities can be directed to the larger community. One way to do this is by changing the attitudes and behavior of health care providers and consumers. This may involve activities related to dispelling myths and stereotypes associated with vulnerable groups, providing knowledge of normal parameters, increasing sensitivity to psychosocial factors affecting health and illness, and enhancing the ability to give sensitive, supportive, humanistic health care.

An example of one such activity is an educational pamphlet published by the Parental Stress Center of Pittsburgh.[2] The Center serves families in which one or both parents abuse or neglect their children, many of whom are infants when the pattern of abuse begins. The pamphlet was conceptualized as a resource for new mothers to help them understand and prepare for the special stresses inherent in mothering their infants during the first 3 months of life. In providing this mental health information, the Center considered the issues of the social stigma of mental illness, the cognitive ability of the patient, educational background, legitimacy of popular psychotherapy fads, and the use of an appropriate communication medium.

Another community-level strategy requires public education on mental health issues and community resources. Misconceptions regarding vulnerable subgroups of the population need to be corrected. The stigma, misunderstanding, and fear surrounding mental illness is related to both the agencies providing mental health services and the people receiving these services who are often elderly, poor, or members of social minority groups. Unlike physical illness, which tends to evoke sympathy and the desire to help, mental disorders tend to disturb and repel people. Yet everyone encounters stress, and all people are subject to maladaptive coping responses. Mental health professionals can educate the public in the idea that health is a continuum, and illness is caused by a complex combination of factors. "In this way we may begin to understand that none of us is immune from mental illness or emotional problems, and that the fear, the anxiety, and even the anger we feel about people who suffer these problems may merely reflect some of our own deepest fears and anxieties."[74:57]

■ **Environmental change**

Activities in primary prevention involving environmental change have a social setting focus. They require the modification of an individual's or group's immediate environment or the larger social system. They are particularly appropriate actions when the environment has placed new demands on the person, when it is not responding to his developmental needs, and when it pro-

vides a diminished level of positive reinforcement for the individual. The nursing literature gives evidence that this is not an area of primary prevention in which nurses have been actively involved.

For the individual, various types of environmental changes may prove to promote one's mental health, including changes in one's economic, work, housing, or family situations. **Economically,** there may be the location of resources for financial aid or assistance obtained in the budgeting and managing of income. **Work** changes may include vocational testing, guidance, education, or retraining that can result in a change of jobs or careers. It may also mean that an adolescent, a homemaker, or an older adult may be placed in a new career option. Changes in one's **housing** situation can involve moving to new quarters, which may mean leaving family and friends or returning to them, improvements in existing housing, or the addition or subtraction of co-inhabitants, whether they are family, friends, or roommates. Environmental changes that may benefit the **family** include attaining child care facilities, enrollment in a nursery school, grade school, or camp, or obtaining access to recreational, social, religious, or community facilities.

The potential benefit of all of these changes should not be minimized or overlooked by mental health practitioners. They can promote mental health by increasing one's coping resources, modifying the nature of one's stressors, and possibly increasing one's positive, rewarding, and self-enhancing experiences.

■ **ORGANIZATIONS AND POLITICS.** Nurses can also effect environmental changes at a larger organizational and political level. One way is by influencing health care structures and procedures. Given the vulnerability of new parents, for example, nurses can work to implement birthing rooms and family suites in obstetrical settings. One might also become involved in the training of community, nonprofessional caregivers as one way of increasing the social supports available to vulnerable groups. Another approach would be to stimulate support for women's issues related to mental health, such as through studying the psychology of women; dispelling sex-role stereotypes; promoting feminist therapy[75]; sponsoring programs, conferences, and workshops on women's issues; and recruiting more women professionals into the mental health field.

Obviously, if nurses believe that their profession makes a valuable contribution in promoting health, they should document the cost-effectiveness and quality of nursing care, lobby for greater patient access by nurses, and seek adequate compensation and reimbursement for nursing services. Many of these goals can be obtained if nursing has greater participation in the decision-making structures of health care institutions, such as hospital boards, advisory groups, health system agencies, and legislative bodies.

Within organizations, environmental change can be achieved through program consultation. Such consultation with a large corporation, for example, may lead to the formulation of more flexible retirement plans or a preretirement counseling program. Involvement in community planning and development can have an impact in many different areas. For instance, a community may be helped to meet the needs of the elderly for educational opportunities, recreational programs, and access to social support networks through telephone tielines or special transportation services. So too, the stress associated with environmental pollutants, such as chemicals and radiation, can be addressed.

Some environmental changes require involvement at the national level. It may be directed toward the media's portrayal of violence, laws on drunk driving, gun control legislation, access to family planning services, federal funding of abortion, the advocation of changes in child-rearing practices, including the provision of day-care centers, flex time and paternity leave, or the passage of equal rights legislation.

Of course many attitudes in and areas of the social system are in need of change, including racism, sexism, ageism, inadequate housing, poverty, and problems with the educational system. The dilemma is that global problems such as these are too broad, too pervasive, and too diffuse to be adequately addressed, let alone resolved. Furthermore, the changes under Reagan's program of the "New Federalism" clearly mean that fewer governmental resources are available to aid such primary prevention efforts. For any prevention strategies to be successful in the future, it will be necessary to document the ways in which a particular group is vulnerable to a specific stressor, how the proposed prevention program will be beneficial and cost-effective, and the degree to which it succeeded or failed.

■ Supporting social systems

As a primary prevention strategy, supporting social systems is not an approach that attempts to remove or minimize the stressor or risk factor. Rather, its rationale is that of strengthening social supports as a way of buffering or cushioning the effects of a potentially stressful event. It is such an important concept for all levels of prevention—primary, secondary, and tertiary—that an entire section of the President's Commission on Mental Health was devoted to exploring ways to expand personal and social networks of families, neighbors, and community organizations to which people naturally turn to help them cope. It has implications for pro-

moting health, helping people seek help earlier, supporting them in times of stress, and aiding the situation of the chronically mentally ill. Social support systems can be helpful in emphasizing the strengths of individuals and families and focusing on health rather than illness. For these reasons the commission recommended that "a major effort be developed in the area of personal and community supports which will":

1. Recognize and strengthen the natural networks to which people belong and on which they depend
2. Identify the potential social support that formal institutions within communities can provide
3. Improve the linkages between community support networks and formal mental health services
4. Initiate research to increase our knowledge of informal and formal community support systems and networks[74:15]

Given the goal that social support systems should be maximized, how does one go about achieving it? First, one needs to determine how much social support a high-risk group will need and then compare it to the amount of social support that is available. Although the question is straightforward, it is complicated by the fact that there are multiple determinants of each element. One's need for social support will be influenced by one's predisposing factors, the nature of the stressors, and the availability of other coping resources, such as economic assets, individual abilities and skills, and defensive techniques. The availability of social supports will similarly be influenced by one's predisposing factors, such as age, sex, or socioeconomic status, the nature of the stressor, and the characteristics of the environment. Acute episodic stressors tend to elicit more intense support, whereas in chronic problems, support resources tend to not persist. So too, changes or stressors viewed in a positive way by one's social network, such as the birth of a baby or a promotion, may elicit a great deal of support, whereas a negative event, such as a sudden death, may generate little support.

In addition, the quantity and type of social support that meets one need may not meet another. Research suggests that different characteristics of social support may be needed for different stresses. For example, in one study, family cohesiveness, family expressiveness, and spouse support were significant sources of support for the patient receiving dialysis, but the presence of a confidant was not.[20] However, Brown's study[9] found that an important factor in preventing depression in women was an intimate confiding relationship with a husband or boyfriend. Support from other relationships was not shown to be a specific factor. In Hirsch's study[43] of major life changes, he found that low-density, multidimensional support systems were more adaptive to the women he studied. Yet high-density support systems have commonly been regarded as the socially desirable, cultural ideal. Thus the match between the type and level of social support and the nature of the stressor is an important, but not entirely understood, one.

■ **TYPES OF INTERVENTIONS.** Even though many variables related to social support need further study, one can still use social support in designing and implementing interventions in primary prevention. Four particular types of interventions are possible. First, social support patterns can be used to assess communities and neighborhoods to identify problem areas and high-risk groups. Not only will this give information as to the quality of life, but the social isolation of a particular group might become apparent as well as central individuals whose aid may then be enlisted in developing community-based programs.

A second preventive intervention would be to improve linkages between community support systems and formal mental health services. Frequently mental health professionals are not aware of or comfortable with the existence or functioning of community support systems. To correct this, they should be taught the skills involved in utilizing and mobilizing community resources and social support systems. All types of health care providers need to be able to recognize when patients need social support and to provide them with access to appropriate community support systems.

The third type of intervention is to strengthen natural, existing caregiving networks. Health professionals can provide information and support to the variety of informal caregivers in the community who serve a very important and somewhat different function from more formalized and organized support systems. Gottlieb[27] notes that informal support systems provide (1) a natural training ground for the development of problem-solving skills, (2) a medium in which personal growth and development is based on repeated episodes of people learning to direct the process of change for themselves, and (3) a supportive milieu that capitalizes on the strength of existing ties among people in our communities, rather than fragmenting intact social units on the basis of diagnosed needs or specialized services.

Numerous such informal support groups exist. They may include church groups, civic organizations, clubs, women's groups, or work and neighborhood supports. Self-help groups are becoming more common as members organize themselves to solve their own problems. The members all share a common experience, work together toward a common goal, and use their own strengths to gain control over their lives. The processes involved in self-help groups are social affiliation, learning self-control, modeling methods to cope with

stress, and acting to change the social environment.[60]

Self-help groups are familiar to the public through such groups as Alcoholics Anonymous, Weight Watchers, Parents Without Partners, and Parents Anonymous. They have also demonstrated their ability to help those people experiencing grief reactions, such as widows[15] and parents of children who died from the sudden infant death syndrome. Since self-help groups utilize a variety of methods and membership criteria, each group should be assessed individually for its general effectiveness and appropriateness for particular individuals and families. Newton has identified some areas for the nurse to assess before recommending involvement in a self-help group.[67] These are presented in Table 9-4.

Working with natural, informal support systems should be done cautiously, however, to minimize undesirable consequences. One should attempt to create the least amount of disruption possible. Gottlieb[27] warns against the potentially damaging effects of well-intentioned consultation with informal caregivers by inadvertently suppressing their natural repertoire of helping behaviors. This might be an important point to remember in relation to all primary prevention strategies.

Finally, if an individual's social support is inadequate, interventions may need to be more direct. To determine what interventions are possible, Norbeck suggests that the following questions be asked:

1. What is the capacity of the network to change?
   a. *Network structure.* Are there persons who can be brought into (or back into) the network?
   b. *Network functioning.* Can existing network members be assisted to provide the kind of support that is needed (e.g., allow talk about the pregnancy or about a loss)?
   c. *Network disruption.* Can policies be changed or resources employed to minimize network disruption (e.g., due to hospitalization at a distant tertiary care facility)?
2. Does the individual have the interpersonal skills and attitudes required to establish and maintain contact with network members?
3. Is the individual receptive to using existing self-help or support groups or to having contact with a person who has coped with a similar experience?
4. If help from the indigenous social support system cannot be made available or acceptable, exactly what support does this individual require to cope with the current stressors or illness?
5. What long-term help would be required to assist the individual to establish and maintain an adequate social support network?[68:54]

A fourth possible intervention may be to help the person or group develop, maintain, and use their net-

---

TABLE 9-4

ASSESSMENT GUIDELINES FOR SELF-HELP GROUPS

Questions for the group	Questions for the potential member
1. What is its purpose? 2. Who are the group members and leaders? 3. What are the beneficial aspects of the group? 4. For whom would the group not be suitable? 5. What problems are inherent in the group? 6. Is the group effective in preventing further emotional distress?	1. How does the person feel about attending a self-help group? 2. How compatible is the group and the individual's approach to the problem? 3. How accessible is the group to the potential member?

From Newton G.: J. Psychosoc. Nurs. Ment. Health Serv. **22**(7):27, July 1984.

---

work. The person may also be encouraged to consider expanding his network. This might require health education strategies with the goal of competence building. Alternatively, one can influence the network more directly. Network therapy involves assembling and mobilizing all the important members of the family's kin and friendship network. The focus is then on tightening social bonds within the network and breaking dysfunctional patterns.[83] For families who are isolated and whose networks are depleted, network members may not be available for such a strategy. In this case, arranging for the use of mutual support groups may be effective.

Finally, it should be noted that although supporting social supports is an effective intervention, it is not one that is limited to primary prevention activities. Rather, all nurses in all settings can utilize this strategy as a way of providing holistic care to maximize the health of individuals, families, and groups.

■ Working with groups

The nurse who is working in the area of primary prevention in mental health may be working with any level of the social hierarchy—individuals, families, communities, or even the larger society (Fig. 9-2). At this time she is likely to be working with groups of people as a way of maximizing the impact she can make and mobilizing the environment's potential to be supportive. A group approach, however, may not always be the most effective or efficient one. To decide if a group approach is indicated for a particular intervention, Loomis suggests that the nurse ask herself the following questions:

1. What are the client needs I am attempting to meet?
2. Can these needs be met in a group?

3. What are my own objectives for the proposed group?
4. What are the expectations of the system relative to the proposed group?
5. Is there any discrepancy or conflict between the answers to questions 1 through 4?[61:18-20]

Assuming that a group approach has been decided on, the next task of the nurse is to decide what type of group would be most appropriate. This may be accomplished by considering one's group goals, desired outcomes, and role of the nurse. It is particularly important to examine the role of the nurse, because different types of groups often have similar goals and even outcomes. For example, providing emotional support to members is usually a function of many groups—formal, informal, natural, and professional. So too, the imparting of new information to members can be a common outcome. A distinguishing characteristic, however, can be found in how the nurse functions in the group.

■ TYPES OF GROUPS. Marram describes three types of groups that the psychiatric nurse is particularly likely to be involved in.[63] The first is **group psychotherapy,** which uses the group process to treat people with existing mental disorders. They may vary in intensity and in the underlying theoretical framework used by the leaders. These groups can be distinguished by their overall emphasis on (1) personality reconstruction, (2) insight without reconstruction, (3) remotivation, (4) problem solving, (5) reeducation, or (6) support.[63] Nurses who lead such groups are actively and formally engaging patients in a therapeutic endeavor. However, the context is changed from that of a one-to-one relationship to that of a group relationship. Regardless, the responsibility for group psychotherapy resides with the nurse, and, for her to function in this role, she needs to have advanced education or extensive supervised ex-

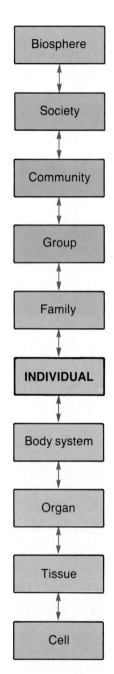

Fig. 9-2. Levels of organization that make up the social hierarchy.

perience. This type of group is associated with secondary and tertiary levels of prevention, and examples of it include inpatient groups, outpatient groups, special problem groups, family groups, therapy groups, and married couples groups.

The second type of group is commonly implemented in primary prevention strategies. This is the **therapeutic group,** which may be differentiated from group psychotherapy according to (1) how large a role

emotional stress has played in the person's current level of health and (2) the primary goal or central objective of the group experience.[63] In group psychotherapy the emotional stress of the patient is of primary importance, and the group goal is one of treatment. In therapeutic groups, stress is the result of some change or life event that has the potential of producing a maladaptive response. One's goal, therefore, is that of prevention, education, and providing support. The individual in this group is on the healthy end of the health-illness continuum, although he may be experiencing a situational crisis of some type. The nurse still maintains responsibility for these groups, although her role may now be that of a health educator and facilitator. Examples of these groups can be found in general hospitals, clinics, nursing homes, industrial settings, business, schools, and penal institutions.

The third type of group is the **self-help, or mutual support, group,** which has been described under the strategy of supporting social systems. Their primary aims are to (1) control member behavior, (2) ameliorate stress due to common problems, and (3) maintain member self-esteem and social integration.[63] They do not focus on personality reconstruction or insight analysis. Although the goals of these groups may not necessarily differentiate them from other types of groups, they do differ in one very important criterion; they are led by the group members themselves. If a nurse is the leader with primary responsibility for the group, then it is not a self-help, or mutual support, group. In these groups, if professionals participate at all, they do so by invitation and usually only in an ancillary role.

Finally, the nurse who is utilizing a group approach should have an understanding of the development and processes that occur in groups to increase the therapeutic potential of the group for its members. These are described in Chapter 28.

 Evaluation

Throughout this chapter on primary prevention in mental health, mention has been made of the lack of clarity of concepts and assumptions, the lack of empirical studies identifying causal or predictive relationships, and the lack of understanding of the essential processes underlying preventive interventions. All of these problems are serious, and perhaps they all contribute to the lack of support for primary prevention as a public priority. Until we know more about an optimum fit between an individual and his social environment, it will be difficult to be able to help people define, select, create, and use environments that are growth producing for them.

There is a tendency when talking about primary

prevention to think in terms of the total elimination of mental illness and stress. Yet these are not realistic goals, and maintaining them can only discourage any possible action. Perhaps it is possible to set goals of the reduction in suffering and the enhancement of the capacity to cope. But even these may be unattainable, given that the environment is constantly changing and adaptation to it is an ongoing challenge. Rather, if one focuses on the specific problems of a vulnerable group in our society, one's activity becomes more directed, and the chance of success increases.

Clearly there is a need for the evaluation of programs in primary prevention. In a world of shrinking resources, only those programs with proven effectiveness are likely to be supported in the future. It needs to be demonstrated that the prevention strategy used had both short-term and long-term effects which benefited the individual and society. One also needs to determine if the specific strategy implemented was the most effective, appropriate, and efficient one. Considering alternative approaches and comparing outcomes is an essential part of the evaluation process.

Offord believes that in the initial evaluation of primary prevention programs close attention must be given to two points: (1) the program or intervention must be described in reproducible terms; and (2) the target of the intervention program must be stated.[71] Given these two prerequisites, he has identified the following points that should then be considered in evaluating particular primary prevention interventions or programs.

1. *Efficacy.* Does the program or intervention do more good than harm among those who agree to it?
2. *Effectiveness.* Does the intervention do more good than harm to those to whom it is offered?
3. *Efficiency.* Is the intervention being made available to those who could benefit from it with optimal use of resources?
4. *Length and timing of intervention.* Is there any evidence about the optimal length or timing of an intervention program?
5. *Harmful effects.* Are there data to suggest that the interventions may have harmful effects perhaps due to the unfavorable consequences of labeling?
6. *Screening programs.* Is there any evidence about the sensitivity, specificity, and predictive accuracy of the screening program?
7. *Possible high-risk groups.* Is there any evidence that the program would be more efficient if it were applied to those at increased risk for the disorder to be prevented?

DIRECTIONS FOR FUTURE RESEARCH

The following are some of the nursing research problems raised in Chapter 9 that merit further study by psychiatric nurses:

1. Mental health services available to women on a regional basis in relation to rape, family violence, and substance abuse
2. Study of psychiatric nurses' attitudes toward sex roles
3. Identification of specific stressors and intervening variables that precipitate maladaptive responses and a target or vulnerable population group that is at high risk in relationship to them
4. Responsiveness of the mental health community to specified vulnerable groups
5. Specific preventive strategies and relevant social institutions and situations through which the strategies may be applied
6. The degree, level, and type of environmental change implemented by psychiatric nurses
7. The extent of participation of nurses in mutual support groups
8. The degree, domain, and type of mental health education implemented by psychiatric nurses
9. The effectiveness of preventive nursing interventions with regard to short- and long-term outcomes, use of resources, and comparison with other prevention strategies
10. The degree and type of intervention used by psychiatric nurses in supporting social systems
11. Preventive programs implemented by nurses who work with the mental health needs of women
12. The extent to which nurses engage in the primary prevention measures identified to meet the national 1990 objectives for the control of stress and violent behavior

---

8. *Economic analysis.* What are the results of the cost-benefit and cost-effectiveness analyses?

Finally, when evaluating certain aspects of the interventions, Offord suggests that the quality of the evidence supporting the conclusion should be rated systematically in the following way:

Grade I: If evidence is obtained from at least one properly randomized control trial

Grade II-1: If evidence is obtained from well-designed cohort or case-controlled analytic studies

Grade II-2: If evidence is obtained from comparisons between times and places with or without the intervention

Grade III: If support is derived from the opinions of respected authorities, based on clinical experience, descriptive studies or reports of expert committees

He believes that when this grading system is applied to a particular primary prevention intervention or program, it will make explicit the strength of the scientific evidence supporting its possible implementation, and provide a framework from which research priorities can be readily identified.[71]

Although preventing all illness is not possible, preventing some particular problems is. But a number of barriers exist that make it difficult to expand primary prevention activities. When faced with a choice, the needs of the presently ill consistently take precedence over preventing problems in the future. This holds true for nurses, as well as for the larger society. Yet by being more farsighted both groups could benefit greatly. Nursing has long maintained its role in health education and supportive care. If it can document these actions and their effectiveness, it will demonstrate its value as a profession and its importance in promoting the well-being of society.

■ SUGGESTED CROSS-REFERENCES ■

The model of health-illness phenomena, including stressors, coping resources, social support systems, and family assessment, are discussed in Chapter 3. Chapter 25 describes prevention in relation to community mental health. Therapeutic aspects of groups are discussed in Chapter 28. Problems experienced by adolescents are discussed in Chapter 31, and problems of family violence and abuse are discussed in Chapter 32. Problems experienced by the elderly are discussed in Chapter 35.

■ SUMMARY ■

1. Caplan's three levels of preventive intervention were described. The major thrust in present psychiatric care is in secondary prevention, and primary prevention has yet to evolve as a major force in the mental health movement. Definitional problems related to primary prevention were identified.

2. The idea of promoting mental health was critiqued, and it was suggested that primary prevention activities focus on illness prevention to be effective. Mental illness was conceptualized as having causative factors that are multiple, interactive, situational, and sociocultural, all of which result in maladaptive behaviorial responses. A paradigm for primary prevention was presented that attempts to reduce the incidence of particular stressful life events for vulnerable groups. The

application of the nursing process with this view of primary prevention was described.

3. Assessment in primary prevention was presented as the identification of groups of people who are vulnerable to developing mental disorders or maladaptive coping responses to specific stressors or risk factors. The following vulnerable groups were described: children and adolescents, new families, established families, women, mature adults, and the elderly.

4. Prevention strategies should be directed toward influencing predisposing factors, precipitating stressors, appraisal of stressors, and coping resources through the following interventions: health education, environmental change, and supporting social systems.

  a. Health education involves the strengthening of individuals and groups through competence building.

  b. Environmental change involves the modification of an individual's or group's immediate environment or the larger social system.

  c. Supporting social systems is a way of buffering or cushioning the effects of a potentially stressful event. Four strategies for supporting social systems were described.

5. Working with groups is useful to maximize the preventive impact of the nurse's actions and the environment's potential to be supportive. Three types and groups, group psychotherapy, therapeutic groups, and self-help groups, were described in relation to group goals, desired outcomes, and role of the nurse.

6. Evaluation of primary prevention activities is impeded by the lack of clarity of assumptions, empirical studies in the area, and essential processes underlying preventive interventions. In evaluating preventive strategies, one needs to consider specific criteria and utilize a systematic rating scale of scientific evidence.

■ REFERENCES ■

1. American Journal of Psychiatry: Research on mental illness and addictive disorders: progress and prospects, **142**(7):25, July 1985.

2. Angier, J.: Issues in consumer mental health information, Bull. Med. Libr. Assoc. **72**(3):262, July 1984.

3. Beverly, E.: The beginning of wisdom about aging, Geriatrics **30**(7):117, 1975.

4. Bieber, T., and Bieber, T.: Postpartum reactions in men and women, J. Am. Acad. Psychoan. **6**(4):511, 1978.

5. Bloom, B.: Prevention of mental disorders: recent advances in theory and practice, Community Ment. Health J. **15**(3):179, 1979.

6. Bloom, B.: The evaluation of primary prevention programs. In Roberts, L., Greenfield, N., and Miller, N., editors: Comprehensive Mental Health, Madison, 1968, University of Wisconsin Press.

7. Bloom, B., Asher, S., and White, S.: Marital disruptions as a stressor: a review of analysis, Psychol. Bull. **85**:867, 1978.

8. Broverman, I., Broverman, D., and Clarkson, F.: Sex-role stereotypes and clinical judgments of mental health, J. Consult. Clin. Psychol. **34**:1, 1970.

9. Brown, F., and Harris, T.: Social origins of depression, London, 1978, Tavistock Publications, Ltd.

10. Caplan, G.: Principles of preventive psychiatry, New York, 1964, Basic Books, Inc., Publishers.

11. Carmen, E., Russo, N., and Miller, J.: Inequality and women's mental health: an overview, Am. J. Psychiatry, **138**:1319, 1981.

12. Chesler, P.: Women and madness, New York, 1972, Doubleday Publishing Co.

13. Cobb, S.: Social support as a moderator of life stress, Psychosom. Med. **38**(5):306, 1976.

14. Comfort, A.: Geriatric psychiatry: mental symptoms in old age, Ala. J. Med. Sci. **18**(2):177, 1981.

15. Conroy, R.C.: Widows and widowhood, N.Y. State J. Med. **77**(3):357, 1977.

16. Cooperstock, R.: Sex differences in psychotropic drug use, Soc. Sci. Med. **12B**:179, 1978.

17. Cronenwett, L., and Kunst-Wilson, W.: Stress, social support and the transition to fatherhood, Nurs. Res. **30**(4):196, 1981.

18. Davidson, V.: Psychiatry's problem with no name: therapist-patient sex, Am. J. Psychoanal. **37**:43, 1977.

19. Davis, A.: The woman as therapist and client, Nurs. Forum **16**(34):250, 1977.

20. Diamond, M.: Social support and adaptation to chronic illness: the case of maintenance hemodialysis, Res. Nurs. Health **2**:101, 1979.

21. Elkins, V.: The rights of the pregnant parent: two continents, New York, 1976, Schocken Books, Inc.

22. FDA Drug Bulletin, Feb. 1980, U.S. Government Printing Office.

23. Filner, B., and Williama, R.: Health promotion for the elderly: reducing functional dependency. In Healthy people: the surgeon general's report on health promotion and disease prevention, Washington, D.C., 1979, U.S. Department of Health, Education and Welfare.

24. Fishbein, E.: Fatherhood and disturbances of mental health: a review, J. Psychiatr. Nurs. **19**(7):24, 1981.

25. Forssman, H., and Thuwe, I.: One hundred and twenty children born after application for therapeutic abortion refused, Acta Psychiatr. Scand. **28**(1):21, 1974.

26. Goodstein, R.: Inextricable interaction: social, psychologic, and biologic stresses facing the elderly, Am. J. Orthopsychiatry **51**(2):219, 1981.

27. Gottlieb, B.: The primary group as supportive milieu: application to community psychology, Am. J. Community Psychol. **7**(5):469, 1979.

28. Gould, R.: The phases of adult life: a study in developmental psychology, Am. J. Psychiatry **129**:521, 1972.

29. Gray, J. et al.: Prediction and prevention of child abuse and neglect, Child Abuse Negl. **1**:45, 1977.

30. Greywold, E., Reese, M., and Belle, D.: Stressed mothers syndrome: how to short circuit the stress depression cycle, Behav. Med. **7**(11):12, 1980.

31. Griffith, J.: Women's stressors according to age groups: part I, Issues in Health Care of Women **6**:311, 1983.

32. Griffith, J.: Women's stress responses and coping patterns according to age groups: part II, Issues in Health Care of Women **6**:327, 1983.

33. Guttentag, M., Salasin, S., and Belle, D., editors: The mental health of women, New York, 1980, Academic Press, Inc.

34. Guttentag, M., Salasin, S., and Legge, W.: Women's utilization of mental health services studied, Evaluation **3**:30, 1976.

35. Hagebak, J., and Hagebak, B.: Serving the mental health needs of the elderly: the case for removing barriers and improving service integration, Community Ment. Health J. **16**:263, 1980.

36. Hamrick, K., and Blazer, D.: Older adults and their families in a community mental health center: strategies for intervention, Hosp. Community Psychiatry **31**:332, 1980.

37. Hefferin, E.: Life-cycle stressors: an overview of research, Fam. Community Health **2**(4):71, 1980.

38. Helper, M. et al.: Life-events and acceptance of pregnancy, J. Psychosom. Res. **12**:183, 1968.

39. Herman, J.: Father-daughter incest, Pro. Psychol. **12**(1):76, 1981.

40. Herman, S.: Divorce: a grief process, Perspect. Psychiatr. Care **12**:108, May 1974.

41. Hetherington, M., Cox, M., and Cox, R.: Divorced fathers, Psychology Today **10**:42, April 1977.

42. Hilberman, E.: Overview: the "wife-beater's wife" reconsidered, Am. J. Psychiatry **137**:1336, 1980.

43. Hirsch, B.: Natural support systems and coping with major life changes, Am. J. Community Psychol. **8**:159, 1980.

44. Hollister, W.: Basic strategies in designing primary prevention programs. In Klein, D., and Goldston, S., editors: Primary prevention: an idea whose time has come, Department of Health, Education, and Welfare No. (ADM)77-447, Rockville, Md., 1977, National Institute of Mental Health.

45. Iscoe, I.: Community psychology and the competent community, Am. Psychol. **29**:607, 1974.

46. Jarrahi-Zadeh, I. et al.: Emotional and cognitive changes in pregnancy and early puerperium, Br. J. Psychiatry **115**:797, 1969.

47. Jonas, A.D., and Jonas, D.F.: The influence of early training on the varieties of stress responses: an ethological approach, J. Psychosom, Res. **19**(5-6):325, 1975.

48. Kalter, N.: Children of divorce in an outpatient psychiatric population, Am. J. Orthopsychiatry **47**(1):40, 1977.

49. Kelley, J. and Wallerstein, J.: Brief interventions with children in divorcing families, Am. J. Orthopsychiatry, **47**:23, 1977.

50. Kennell, J., Voos, D., and Klaus, M.: Parent-infant bonding. In Heffer, R., and Kempe, C., editors: Child abuse and neglect: the family and the community, Cambridge, Mass., 1976, Ballinger Publishing Co.

51. Kessler, M., and Albee, G.: An overview of the literature of primary prevention. In Albee, G., and Jaffe, J., editors:

Primary prevention of psychopathology, Hanover, N.H., 1977, University Press of New England.

52. Ketai, R., and Brandwin, M.: Childbirth-related psychosis and familial symbiotic conflict, Am. J. Psychiatry **136**(2):190, 1979.

53. Klein, C.: Coping patterns of parents of deaf-blind children, Am. Ann. Deaf **122**(3):310, 1977.

54. Lacoursiere, R.: Fatherhood and mental illness: a review and new material, Psychiatr. Q. **46**:109, 1972.

55. Lamb, H., and Zusman, J.: Primary prevention in perspective, Am. J. Psychiatry **136**(1):12, 1979.

56. Lancaster, J.: Coping mechanisms of working mothers, Am. J. Nurs. **75**:1322, 1975.

57. Lederman, R.P. et al.: Relationship of psychological factors in pregnancy to progress in labor, Nurs. Res. **28**(2):94, 1979.

58. Lerner, H.: The taboo against female anger, Menninger Perspect. **5**:5, Winter, 1977.

59. Levenson, D., Darrow, C., and Kelin, E.: The seasons of a man's life, New York, 1978, Alfred A. Knopf, Inc.

60. Levy, L.: Self-help groups: types and psychological processes, J. Appl. Behav. Sci. **12**:310, 1976.

61. Loomis, M.E.: Group process for nurses, St. Louis, 1979, The C.V. Mosby Co.

62. Lynch, M.: Ill-health and child-abuse, Lancet, vol. 2, Aug. 16, 1975.

63. Marram, G.D.: The group approach in nursing practice, ed. 2, St. Louis, 1978, The C.V. Mosby Co.

64. Mercer, R.: A theoretical framework for studying factors that impact on the maternal role, Nurs. Res. **30**(2):73, 1981.

65. Moulton, R.: Some effects of the new feminism, Am. J. Psychiatry **134**(1):1, 1977.

66. Neugarten, B., editor: Middle age and aging, Chicago, 1968, University of Chicago Press.

67. Newton, G.: Self-help groups: can they help? J. Psychosoc. Nurs. Ment. Health Serv. **22**(7):27, July 1984.

68. Norbeck, J.: Social support: a model for clinical research and application, Adv. Nurs. Sci. **3**(4):42, 1981.

69. Notman, M.: Midlife concerns of women: implications of the menopause, Am. J. Psychiatry **136**:1270, 1979.

70. Nuckolls, K.B., Cassel, J., and Kaplan, B.H.: Psychosocial assets, life crisis and the prognosis of pregnancy, Am. J. Epidemiol. **95**:431, 1972.

71. Offord, D.: Primary prevention: aspects of program design and evaluation, J. Am. Acad. Child Psychiatry **21**(1):225, 1982.

72. Pitt, B.: Atypical depression following childbirth, Br. J. Psychiatry **114**:1325, 1968.

73. Pratt, L.: Child-rearing methods and children's health behavior, J. Health Soc. Behav. **14**(3):61, 1973.

74. President's Commission on Mental Health, vols. 1 to 4, Washington, D.C., 1978, U.S. Government Printing Office.

75. Rawlings, E., and Carter, D.: Psychotherapy for women, Springfield, Ill., 1977, Charles C Thomas, Publisher.

76. Room, R.: The case for a problem prevention approach to alcohol, drug and mental problems, Public Health Rep. **96**(1):26, 1981.

77. Rutter, M.: Changing youth in a changing society, Cambridge, Mass., 1980, Harvard University Press.

78. Ryan, W.: Preventive services in the social context: power, pathology and prevention. In Bloom, B., and Buch, D., editors: Preventive services in mental health programs, Boulder, Colo., 1967, Western Interstate Commission for Higher Education.

79. Schaie, K.: Psychological changes from midlife to early old age: implications for the maintenance of mental health, Am. J. Orthopsychiatry **51**(2):199, 1981.

80. Shanok, S., and Lewis, D.: Juvenile court versus child guidance referral: psychological and parental factors, Am. J. Psychiatry **134**:1130, 1977.

81. Sheehy, G.: Passages, New York, 1974, E.P. Dutton, Inc.

82. Sherman, J.: Therapist attitudes and sex-role stereotyping. In Brodsky, A., and Hare-Merstin, R., editors: Women and psychotherapy, New York, 1980, The Guilford Press.

83. Speck, R., and Rueveni, V.: Network therapy—a developing concept, Fam. Process **8**:182, 1969.

84. Sundeen, S., Stuart, G., et al.: Nurse-client interaction: implementing the nursing process, ed. 3, St. Louis, 1985, The C.V. Mosby Co.

85. "To . . . form a more perfect union . . .": Justice for American Women: Report of the National Commission of the Observance of International Women's Year, Washington, D.C., 1976, U.S. Government Printing Office.

86. U.S. Department of Health and Human Services: Promoting health, preventing disease: objectives for the nation, Washington D.C., 1984, Public Health Service.

87. U.S. Department of Labor: Twenty facts on women workers, Washington, D.C., 1980, Office of the Secretary, Women's Bureau.

88. Voysey, M.: Impression management by parents with disabled children, J. Health Soc. Behav. **13**(1):80, 1972.

89. Weiss, R.: Marital separation, New York, 1975, Basic Books, Inc., Publishers.

■ ANNOTATED SUGGESTED READINGS ■

*Boettcher, E.: Linking the aged to support systems, J. Gerontological Nurs. **11**(3):27, Mar. 1985.

A conceptual framework is presented based on socioeconomic factors, social exchange, power, and linkages that can help nurses formulate and implement more effective care plans for the elderly.

*Cronenwett, L., and Kunst-Wilson, W.: Stress, social support and the transition to fatherhood, Nurs. Res. **30**(4):196, 1981.

The authors present a paradigm of variables that are involved in the transition to fatherhood. Such a paradigm can be used

---

*Asterisk indicates nursing reference.

to generate theories, test hypotheses, and develop appropriate preventive interventions. Additional work of this type is greatly needed in nursing.

*Delgado, M.: A model for mental health education in Hispanic communities, J. Psychiatr. Nurs. **18**(8):16, 1980.

This article describes a mental health education program specifically targeted to reach Hispanics. It discusses methods, settings, logistics, and recommendations for similar projects.

Eisenberg, L.: A research framework for evaluating the promotion of mental health and prevention of mental illness, Public Health Rep. **96**(1):3, 1981.

This excellent review article addresses specific topics and ways in which health may be promoted. Broad in scope and important in content.

*Ellison, E.: Social networks and the mental health caregiving system: implications for psychiatric nursing practice, J. Psychosoc. Nurs. Ment. Health Serv. **21**(2):18, Feb. 1983.

This article examines the social network perspective as it relates to the design and delivery of mental health services for the chronically mentally ill. Assessment, diagnoses, and intervention strategies are described.

*Gammonley, J.: New directions for mental health education, J. Psychiatr. Nurs. **16**(12):40, 1978.

This is one of the few articles in the psychiatric nursing literature that focuses on mental health education. It is described in relation to both preventive and therapeutic programs.

Guttentag, M., Salasin, S., and Belle, D., editors: The mental health of women, New York, 1980, Academic Press, Inc.

This edited book is a very good overview of issues related to women—a high-risk group for mental health problems.

Harman, D., and Brim, O.: Learning to be parents: principles, programs and methods, Beverly Hills, Calif., 1980, Sage Publications, Inc.

This is a major assessment of the field of parent education that includes the rationale and issues behind parent education and the methods, curriculum, and evaluation of parent education programs. Timely, practical, and thorough.

Hefferin, E.: Life-cycle stressors: an overview of research, Fam. Community Health **2**(4):71, 1980.

This article is precisely what the title describes—a review of research on life-cycle stressors that is very extensive, thorough, and well-organized. A valuable reference article.

*Jacobson, A.: Melancholy in the 20th century: causes and prevention, J. Psychiatr. Nurs. **18**(7):11, 1980.

Depression among women is explored in this paper with a particular focus on primary prevention using support networks and anticipatory guidance for this high-risk population during critical developmental stages.

*Johnson, S.: High-risk parenting, Philadelphia, 1979, J.B. Lippincott Co.

The nurse-author describes families who are at risk because of a variety of social, psychological and physiological stressors. This is an important book, which is recommended for all nurses working with families under stress.

Journal of Family Issues

This quarterly journal focuses on the family in contemporary

society. It includes theoretical and applied research writing with special issues focusing on a particular topic in depth.

Kastenbaum, R.: Old age and the new scene, New York, 1981, Springer Publishing Co., Inc.

This is an anthology of psychosocial gerontology. The contributors are scholars and researchers whose viewpoints promote reevaluation of the elderly and greater awareness of the potential of later life.

Mace, D.: Prevention in family services, Beverly Hills, Calif., 1983, Sage Publications, Inc.

This text describes marriage and family enrichment programs used throughout the country that make the difference between strong families and broken families. It reflects a vital approach to family services and prevention.

*Marram, G.D.: The group approach in nursing practice, ed. 2, St. Louis, 1978, The C.V. Mosby Co.

This text treats the scope, nature, and process of group work in nursing. Since all nurses work with and in groups, the content of this book should be essential knowledge.

*Mercer, R.: A theoretical framework for studying factors that impact on the maternal role, Nurs. Res. **30**(2):73, 1981.

This article is recommended for its presentation of a theoretical framework useful in studying variables influencing the maternal role. This type of nursing theorizing and research can make a valuable contribution to the field.

*Newton, G.: Self-help groups: can they help? J. Psychosoc. Nurs. Ment. Health Serv. **22**(7):27, July 1984.

Assessment guidelines for evaluating self-help groups are described in detail. This article will help nurses to determine the therapeutic potential of such groups since not all of them are effective for all people.

*Nix, H.: Why parents anonymous? J. Psychiatr. Nurs. **18**(10):23, 1980.

This article describes the formation of Parents Anonymous, the self-help group aimed at preventing child abuse. The group's definition, structure, roles, and processes are well described.

*Norbeck, J.: Social support: a model for clinical research and application, Adv. Nurs. Sci. **3**(4):43, 1981.

In this substantive article the author outlines the concept of social support and discusses how it may be incorporated in nursing practice. An excellent bibliography on the subject is also included.

Norman, W., and Scaramella, T.: Midlife developmental and clinical issues, New York, 1980, Brunner/Mazel, Inc.

The authors focus beyond the losses and deprivations of midlife to the potential for active fulfilling growth. Addressed are social and intrapsychic factors that affect perceptions of self and adaptational patterns, developmental challenges, options, and potentially problematic areas that are critical in the clinical setting.

Peterman, P.: Parenting and environmental considerations, Am. J. Orthopsychiatry **51**(2):351, 1981.

The efficacy of establishing a self-help group in a poor urban area is described in this brief article. The effects of environmental factors and their use as intervention strategies to help promote positive parenting roles is discussed.

*Roberts, F.: A model for parent education, Image **13**:86, Oct. 1981.

This well-written article looks at why parent education is often ineffective and presents a new model for reconceptualizing its planning and delivery. The model has applicability for preventive health education in other areas as well.

*Robinson, K.: Working with a community action group, J. Psychiatr. Nurs. **16**(8):38, 1978.

This article describes the role of nurses working with a community action group. The stages of group development and related problems are analyzed.

Rutter, M.: Changing youth in a changing society, Cambridge, Mass., 1980, Harvard University Press.

This text is a review of the psychosocial problems of adolescents in society. It addresses whether there are definable problems specifically associated with the adolescent age period, whether the problems are increasing or changing in character, and how the health and social services should be geared to cope with them.

Satir, V.: Peoplemaking, Palo Alto, Calif., 1972, Science & Behavior Books.

According to the author, the family is the "factory" where human beings are made. This is a book written for families about family process. It analyzes self-worth, communication systems, and family rules in a most enjoyable way.

*Sedgwick, R.: Family mental health: theory and practice, St. Louis, 1981, The C.V. Mosby Co.

This excellent text on working with families is divided into three sections: an overview of concepts and principles, a discussion of the clinical process, and clinical application through case illustrations. This is one text that should be read by all nurses.

Smyer, M., and Gatz, M.: Mental health and aging. Beverly Hills, Calif. 1983, Sage Publications, Inc.

This book can familiarize nurses with a broad range of proven mental health interventions. Case studies of different programs, each of which has been rigorously evaluated, demonstrate how and why each program works.

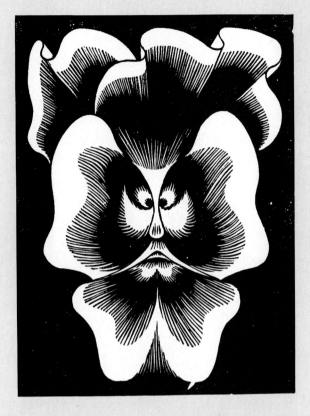

Our moulting season, like that of the fowls, must be a crisis in our lives.

Henry David Thoreau

C H A P T E R   1 0

CRISIS INTERVENTION

SANDRA E. BENTER

LEARNING OBJECTIVES

After studying this chapter, the student should be able to:

- describe the history of crisis theory, specifying the contributions of Lindemann and Caplan.

- define crisis and explain its potential for disorganization or personal growth.

- relate Caplan's four phases of a crisis and impinging "balancing factors."

- discuss the etiology of the three types of crises: maturational, situational, and adventitious.

- analyze the goal, scope, and phases of crisis intervention.

- assess the relationship between nursing diagnoses and medical diagnoses appropriate to crisis intervention.

- describe four levels of crisis intervention and eight therapeutic techniques.

- evaluate the various modalities of crisis intervention and the settings in which they may be employed.

- apply crisis intervention principles in the care of a patient

- discuss future trends in crisis therapy.

- identify directions for future nursing research.

- select appropriate readings for further study.

Historical perspective

Historically, crisis theory is an outgrowth of psychoanalytical theory. Analytical theory proposes that there are unconscious links to behavior and that dynamic formulations can be made to explain the causes of behavior. The causes are found in one's early experiences of infancy and childhood and affect one throughout his life span. There are many areas of conflict within the individual, and for those conflicts to be resolved constructively, they must be geared toward adaptation to the environment. For example, to be socially acceptable, one's aggressive impulses can be channeled into competitive business practices rather than the physical harm of a rival.

Those who studied and practiced preventive psychiatry used psychoanalytical concepts to develop crisis theory. They explored the feasibility of intervening briefly during stressful periods to resolve the problem in an adaptive or positive way. They observed a specific sequence of phases that individuals experienced when faced with stressful situations and studied the outcomes of the crises. Crisis intervention techniques were then determined for facilitating favorable outcomes.

Eric Lindemann,[26] in 1944, studied 101 patients in crisis. He included psychoneurotic patients who lost a relative during the course of treatment, relatives of patients who died in the hospital, bereaved disaster victims (Coconut Grove fire) and their relatives, and relatives of members of the armed forces. Lindemann observed the course of normal grief and the symptomatology of morbid grief reactions. Those bereaved individuals undergoing normal grief showed signs of somatic distress, preoccupation with the image of the deceased, hostile reactions, guilt, changes in patterns of activity, and sometimes the taking on of characteristics of the deceased. Those individuals undergoing morbid grief reactions demonstrated either delayed or distorted reactions. Distorted reactions included overactivity without a sense of loss, the acquisition of symptoms belonging to the last illness of the deceased, the development of a medical disease, an alteration in relationships to friends and relatives, the development of furious hostility against specific persons, and the development of a clinical agitated depression.

Lindemann saw the role of mental health workers to be that of helping the patient extricate himself from his ties to the deceased and find new patterns of rewarding interaction. He believed the concept of intervention during bereavement could be applied to intervention during other stressful situations such as marriage and the birth of a child. Thus the prevention of psychiatric disorders could be accomplished. He envisioned this accomplishment as taking place in the community and being patterned after a public health model so that many people could be reached. Lindemann, along with Gerald Caplan, actually set up a community mental health clinic in Massachussets where crisis intervention was practiced.

In 1964 Caplan formally introduced concepts of community mental health practice. In addressing himself to primary, secondary, and tertiary preventive aspects of practice, he clearly defined crisis theory and described crisis intervention as a formal therapy in itself.[6] He viewed **primary prevention** as the social and interpersonal actions that ensure the provision of basic supplies to a community to help it deal constructively with its crises. The prevention of mental disorder is the aim. Social action deals with efforts to work with political and social policies to help people cope with crises, whereas interpersonal action deals with helping individuals with their specific stresses.

Secondary prevention aims to decrease the number of existing cases through early diagnosis and effective treatment. Early referral, screening programs, and improvement in diagnostic tools are all examples of secondary prevention. This type of prevention is the more traditional treatment-oriented method of approaching mental illness. Caplan emphasizes that attention must be paid to effective use of mental health workers and knowledge so that the numbers treated successfully will be large enough to make a difference in community rates.

Tertiary prevention aims to reduce the rate of defective functioning caused by one's lowered capacity to contribute to the community after the mental disorder has ceased. Rehabilitation programs therefore focus on tertiary prevention. Secondary prevention includes primary prevention, and tertiary prevention includes both primary and secondary. Crisis therapy is a primary prevention concept and is seen as one of the most effective ways of preventing mental disorder.

In 1963 President Kennedy issued a message on mental illness and mental retardation. After the message, communities began to take on further the responsibility of caring for their own mental health needs. Although many clinicians believed that long-term psychoanalytical psychotherapy was still the preferred treatment, it was impractical in that it was expensive, required a lengthy time commitment, and generally did not meet the needs of all socioeconomic strata. It was believed that a method of treatment that was brief, direct, and here-and-now–oriented was necessary. Crisis therapy therefore became more widely used.

Definition of crisis

A crisis is an internal disturbance that results from a stressful event or a perceived threat to self. The individual's usual repertoire of coping mechanisms becomes ineffective in dealing with the threat, and the individual experiences a rise in anxiety. The threat, or precipitating event, can usually be identified. It may

have occurred weeks or days ago, and its significance may or may not be linked (in the individual's eyes) to the crisis state. Precipitating events are perceived losses, threats of losses, or challenges.[6] Losses may include the death of a spouse, divorce, or loss of a job. Threats of losses may include illness of a family member or an increase in arguments with a spouse. Challenges may include a change in responsibilities at work or a change to a different line of work. Additional threats or stresses are identified in the Social Readjustment Rating Scale (Chapter 3).

In response to the threat or precipitating event the individual's level of anxiety rises and Caplan's[6] four phases of a crisis emerge. In the first phase the anxiety stimulates one's usual methods of coping into action. If these do not bring relief and there is inadequate situational support, the individual progresses to the second phase in which he becomes even more anxious as a result of the failure of his coping mechanisms. In the third phase the individual tries out new coping mechanisms or redefines the threat so that old ones can work. Resolution of the problem therefore can occur in this phase. If resolution does not occur, however, the individual goes on to the fourth phase in which the continuation of severe or panic levels of anxiety may lead to psychological disorganization.

In describing the phases of a crisis, some important balancing factors need to be considered.[1] These balancing factors are one's perception of the event, situational supports, and coping mechanisms. Successful resolution of the crisis is more likely if the individual's perception of the event is realistic rather than distorted, if there are situational supports available to the individual so that others can help him solve the problem, and if the individual has coping mechanisms available to him that alleviate anxiety. These balancing factors are represented in the paradigm developed by Aguilera and Messick (Fig. 10-1).

The phases of a crisis and the impact of balancing factors parallel the components of the nursing model of health-illness phenomena described in Chapter 3 of this text. However, by definition, crises are self-limiting. Individuals in crisis are too emotionally uncomfortable to sustain such a high level of anxiety indefinitely. A period of 6 weeks has classically been considered the time span needed for resolution, whether it be a positive solution or a state of disorganization. However, that time span has recently been questioned by researchers who consider it unlikely that any specific time can be applicable to all individuals undergoing all crises.[3]

Symptoms of individuals in crisis are myriad. They can include helplessness, anxiety, confusion, depression, anger, withdrawal, psychosomatic symptoms, ineffi-

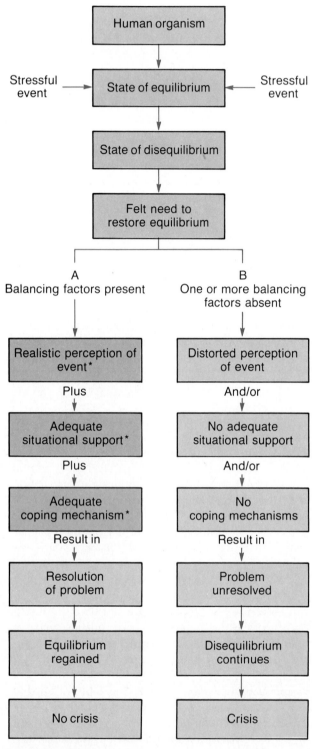

*Balancing factor

Fig. 10-1. Effect of balancing factors in a stressful event. (From Aguilera, D.C., and Messick, J.M.: Crisis intervention: theory and methodology, ed. 5, St. Louis, 1986, The C.V. Mosby Co.)

ciency, and hopelessness. Suicidal and homicidal thoughts may be present. Feelings of alienation from others occur frequently. Sometimes the formation of these symptoms can cause further hardships. For example, inefficiency at work may lead to the loss of a job, financial problems, and ultimately lowered self-esteem.[23] Crises can also be complicated by old internal conflicts. Previous conflicts can be reactivated by the present conflict and make crisis resolution more difficult to attain.

An important aspect of crisis theory is that the period of intense conflict is a time of increased vulnerability, and can produce increased growth. It is what one does with the crises that will determine whether growth or disorganization results. Growth comes from experiencing and learning in new situations. Individuals in crisis feel uncomfortable and often reach out for help. They are in turmoil and are ready to accept influence from others until they feel psychological equilibrium has returned. The fact that crises can stimulate personal growth is an important one for the nurse to consider when working with patients in crisis situations.

Types of crises

Crisis can be divided into three types: maturational, situational, and adventitious. Sometimes more than one type of crisis can occur at the same time. Thus an individual undergoing a maturational crisis can simultaneously have a situational stress that adds to his anxiety. For example, an adolescent who is having difficulty adjusting to his change of role and body image can, at the same time, experience the death of a parent.

■ Maturational crises

Developmental psychology describes a succession of steps one must take in the continuous task of growing toward maturity. As an individual passes from one stage to another, he goes through transitional periods during which his psychological equilibrium can be upset. These periods are developmental, or maturational, crises.

Erik Erikson[13,14] described eight stages of development from infancy to old age and the relationship of each stage to the ones before and after. Each stage presents a central problem or task that must be resolved by the individual for him to move on to the next developmental stage. Within his theory Erikson emphasizes that development is a continuum in which each stage has a part, and the tasks of each stage must be completed for the individual to grow further and move toward maturity. As the personality of the individual matures, he learns to cope with the stresses of life. Erikson points out that this mastery of tasks leads to successful solutions of maturational crises.

Havighurst[18] also identified specific developmental tasks for each major developmental period from infancy

CLINICAL EXAMPLE 10-1

Ms. J was a 19-year-old black, single, unemployed woman who came to the mental health clinic a month after the birth of her first child. Ms. J complained of feelings of depression. Her symptoms included difficulty falling asleep, early morning awakening, crying spells, a poor appetite, difficulty in caring for the baby because of fatigue and apathy, and thoughts of wanting to hurt the baby. The patient lived with her parents and siblings and had never lived on her own. She had always been dependent on her mother to take care of her and relieve her stresses. Her mother, however, worked and the patient was totally responsible for her daughter's care each day. Also, Ms. J's mother was angry that she had had a child and usually refused to care for the baby. The patient's boyfriend, who was the baby's father, had promised to marry her, but he had recently decided he was too young to handle the responsibility of a wife and child. In summary, a young woman who had unmet dependency needs of her own was now in a position of parenthood and had to meet the dependency needs of an infant. This precipitated a crisis state for her.

CLINICAL EXAMPLE 10-2

Mr. R was a 67-year-old white, married pharmacist who came to the mental health clinic complaining of anxiety, depression, and insomnia. His symptoms had begun 2 weeks previously and had steadily increased in intensity since that time. Two weeks ago the patient's wife had become insistent that they begin to make concrete plans to move to a retirement community in Florida. The patient described his wife as a strong willful woman who was also outgoing and charming and made friends easily. He considered himself a quiet nervous person who was comfortable only with old friends and his two sons and their families. Mr. R, although of retirement age, had continued to work as a pharmacist, doing relief work for a drugstore chain when the regular pharmacists were absent. In moving to Florida, the patient would lose his pharmacist's license, which was valid only for his present state of residence. He expressed difficulty in making the transition from a working person to a retired person. He had fears of becoming directionless and useless. He was anxious about leaving his sons and his friends. The possibility of both complete retirement and moving to another state precipitated his present distress.

through death. Table 10-1 compares Erikson's and Havighurst's developmental stages and tasks.[38] Together they present a comprehensive view of human development and its crises.

Maturational crises are periods requiring role changes. For example, when one grows from early childhood to middle childhood, he is expected to become socially involved with people outside the family rather than limiting his involvement to the family alone. When one advances from adolescence to adulthood, he is expected to be financially responsible for himself rather than being dependent on his parents. Both social and biological pressures to change can precipitate a crisis. The nature and extent of the maturational crisis can be influenced by the adequacy of role models, interpersonal resources, and the ease of others in accepting the new role.[41] Adequate role models provide the individual with an understanding of how to act in the new role. Interpersonal resources allow the individual the flexibility to try out many new interpersonal behaviors in his attempt to achieve role changes. The use of others in accepting the new role determines the strength or resistances one comes up against in making role changes. The greater the resistance of others, the more stress the individual faces in making the changes.

Transitional periods during adolescence, parent-

hood, marriage, midlife, and retirement are key times for maturational crises to occur. Some conflicts related to parenthood are in Clinical example 10-1.

Some of the conflicts related to retirement are presented in Clinical example 10-2.

■ Situational crises

Situational crises occur when a specific external event upsets an individual's psychological equilibrium or the equilibrium of a group of individuals such as members of a family. Examples of situational crises include the loss of a job, the loss of a loved one, an unwanted pregnancy, the onset or exacerbation of a medical illness, divorce, and school failure or other school problems. The loss of a job can result in financial stress, feelings of inadequacy as a breadwinner, and marital conflict caused by a spouse's anger over the lost job. The loss of a loved one results in bereavement and can also cause financial stress, change of roles of family members, and loss of emotional support. The onset or exacerbation of a medical illness causes fear of the loss of a loved one. Again, financial stress and change of roles of family members often occur. Divorce is similar to the stress of the loss of a loved one, and there is, in addition,

TABLE 10-1

COMPARISON OF ERIKSON'S AND HAVIGHURST'S DEVELOPMENTAL STAGES AND TASKS

Developmental stage	Erikson	Havighurst
Infancy	*Trust vs. mistrust* 1. Oral needs of primary importance 2. Adequate mothering necessary to meet infant's needs 3. Acquisition of hope	1. Learning to walk 2. Learning to take solid foods 3. Learning to talk 4. Learning to control elimination of body wastes 5. Learning sex differences and sexual modesty 6. Achieving physiological stability 7. Forming simple concepts of social and physical reality 8. Learning to relate oneself emotionally to parents, siblings, and other people 9. Learning to distinguish right and wrong and developing a conscience
Toddler years	*Autonomy vs. shame* 1. Anal needs of primary importance 2. Father emerges as important figure 3. Acquisition of will	
Early childhood	*Initiative vs. guilt* 1. Genital needs of primary importance 2. Family relationships contribute to early sense of responsibility and conscience 3. Acquisition of purpose	
Middle childhood	*Industry vs. inferiority* 1. Active period of socialization for child as he moves from family into society 2. Acquisition of competence	1. Learning physical skills necessary for ordinary games 2. Building wholesome attitudes toward oneself as a growing organism 3. Learning to get along with age mates 4. Learning an appropriate sex role 5. Developing fundamental skills in reading, writing, and calculating 6. Developing concepts necessary for everyday living 7. Developing conscience, morality, and scale of values 8. Developing attitudes toward social groups and institutions
Adolescence	*Identity vs. identity diffusion* 1. Search for self in which peers play important part 2. Psychosocial moratorium is provided by society 3. Acquisition of fidelity	1. Accepting one's physique and accepting a masculine or feminine role 2. New relations with age mates of both sexes 3. Emotional independence of parents and other adults 4. Achieving assurance of economic independence 5. Selecting and preparing for an occupation 6. Developing intellectual skills and concepts necessary for civic competence 7. Desiring and achieving socially responsible behavior 8. Preparing for marriage and family life 9. Building conscious values in harmony with adequate scientific world picture
Adulthood	*Intimacy vs. isolation* 1. Characterized by increasing importance of human closeness and sexual fulfillment 2. Acquisition of love	1. Selecting a mate 2. Learning to live with marriage partner 3. Starting family 4. Rearing children 5. Managing home 6. Getting started in occupation 7. Taking on civic responsibility 8. Finding congenial social group

TABLE 10-1—cont'd

COMPARISON OF ERIKSON'S AND HAVIGHURST'S DEVELOPMENTAL STAGES AND TASKS

Developmental stage	Erikson	Havighurst
Middle age	*Generativity vs. self-absorption* 1. Characterized by productivity, creativity, parental responsibility, and concern for new generation 2. Acquisition of care	1. Achieving adult civic and social responsibility 2. Establishing and maintaining economic standard of living 3. Assisting teenage children to become responsible and happy adults 4. Developing adult leisure activities 5. Relating oneself to one's spouse as a person 6. Accepting and adjusting to physiological changes of middle age 7. Adjusting to aging parents
Old age	*Integrity vs. despair* 1. Characterized by a unifying philosophy of life and a more profound love for mankind 2. Acquisition of wisdom	1. Adjusting to decreasing physical strength and health 2. Adjusting to retirement and reduced income 3. Adjusting to death of spouse 4. Establishing explicit affiliation with age group 5. Meeting social and civic obligations 6. Establishing satisfactory physical living arrangements

From Sundeen, S.J., et al.: Nurse-client interaction: implementing the nursing process, ed. 3, St. Louis, 1985, The C.V. Mosby Co.

the stress of dealing with the ex-spouse. An unwanted pregnancy is a stress in that it requires decisions to be made about whether to complete the pregnancy or to abort it, and whether to keep the baby or place it in adoption. If the baby is to be kept, changes in life-style will be required. School failure or other school problems stress the individual and can lead to serious feelings of inadequacy. Parents often blame themselves or each other, and total family disequilibrium can result.

Some of the stresses related to the exacerbation or onset of a medical illness can be seen in the situational crisis presented in Clinical example 10-3.

■ Adventitious crises

Adventitious crises are accidental, uncommon, and unexpected crises. Multiple losses with gross environmental changes result. For example, fires, earthquakes, or floods, which disrupt entire communities, are adventitous crises. Recent mass tragedies, which have become all too common, are also examples of adventitious crises and include group kidnappings (the taking of hostages), nuclear accidents, group killings in communities, and floods complicated by the deposit of industrial waste material along with water.

Unlike maturational and situational crises, adven-

CLINICAL EXAMPLE 10-3

Mrs. H is a 55-year-old white married woman whose husband was hospitalized for mitral stenosis. Heart surgery was scheduled for the following week. Mr. H appeared appropriately concerned, but the nursing staff noticed that the patient's wife was becoming increasingly anxious. She spent each day running from her husband's bedside to the nurses' station demanding constant attention. She moved and spoke rapidly and continuously, and at times her thoughts seemed confused. Mrs. H stated that once in the past she had had a "nervous breakdown" and she hoped the stress of her husband's surgery would not result in another one.

titious crises do not occur in the lives of everyone. When they do occur, however, they challenge every coping mechanism because of the severity of the stress state they impose. During adventitious crises mental health workers must reach larger numbers of people in crisis states. The multiple losses and gross environmental changes that result from adventitious crises can be seen

TABLE 10-2

FIVE PHASES OF HUMAN DISASTER RESPONSE

Phase	Response
Impact phase	Includes the event itself and is characterized by shock, panic, or extreme fear; the person's judgment and assessment of reality factors are very poor, and self-destructive behavior may be seen
Heroic phase	A cooperative spirit exists between friends, neighbors, and emergency teams; constructive activity at this time can help to overcome feelings of anxiety and depression but over-activity can lead to "burnout"
Honeymoon phase	Begins to appear 1 week to several months after the disaster; the need to help others is sustained, and the money, resources, and support received from various agencies causes life to begin again in the community; psychological and behavioral problems may be overlooked
Disillusionment phase	Lasts from about 2 months to 1 year; a time of disappointment, resentment, frustration, and anger; victims often begin to compare their neighbors' plights with their own and may start to resent, envy, or show hostility toward others
Reconstruction and reorganization phase	Individuals recognize that they must come to grips with their own problems; they begin to rebuild their homes, businesses, and lives in a constructive fashion; this period may last for years after the disaster

Data from Frederick, C., and Garrison, J.: Behav. Today **12**:32, Aug. 1981.

in the following situation described in a Department of Health, Education, and Welfare publication:

In West Virginia a river filled with coal sludge overflowed when a dam broke, and an entire community was damaged. There were many deaths and injuries, loss of homes and possessions, disruption or loss of employment, sudden relocation, and extreme demands on physical endurance. The solidarity of this isolated rural community was grossly disturbed. The residents suffered a high incidence of mental illness as a result.[9:5]

Disaster-precipitated emotional problems often surface weeks or even months after the disaster. The symptoms usually occur in roughly five phases, which are described in Table 10-2.[15] If the reconstruction phase does not begin within 6 months of the onset of the disaster, the likelihood of lasting psychological problems is greatly increased. The severe psychological stress resulting from adventitious crises can be further illustrated by the findings of Terr who studied 23 child kidnap victims:

In the town of Chowchilla, California, a school bus containing 26 children and a bus driver was stopped by three masked men and taken over at gunpoint. The captured chil-

dren were driven around in boarded-over vans for 11 hours and were then transferred to a buried truck trailer. After 16 additional hours, two of the oldest boys dug them out. The children suffered from initial misperceptions, fears of further trauma, and hallucinations. Later they experienced posttraumatic play reenactment, personality change, repeated dreams, fears of being kidnapped again, and a fear of common mundane experiences.[40:14]

Crisis intervention

Aguilera and Messick state:

Crisis intervention can offer the immediate help that a person in crisis needs in order to reestablish equilibrium. This is an inexpensive, short-term therapy that focuses on solving the immediate problem.[1:1]

Crisis intervention is frequently limited to a time period of 6 weeks. The goal of crisis intervention is for the patient to return to his previous precrisis level of functioning. Often the patient advances to a level of functioning that is higher than the precrisis level because he has learned new ways of problem solving. There are four phases of crisis intervention that are similar to those of the nursing process.[2] They are assessment, planning, implementation, and evaluation.

Assessment

The first step of crisis intervention is assessment. During this phase data regarding the nature of the crisis and its effect on the patient must be collected. It is from these data that a plan for intervention will be developed. It should be kept in mind that during this phase the nurse begins to establish a positive working relationship with the patient. A number of specific areas should be assessed by the nurse. These are the balancing factors that are important in the development and resolution of a crisis:

1. Identifying the precipitating event
2. Identifying the patient's perception of the event
3. Identifying the nature and strength of the patient's support systems
4. Identifying the patient's previous strengths and coping mechanisms

The components of the nursing model of health-illness phenomena that parallel the balancing factors in crisis intervention are highlighted in Figure 10-2.

■ **PRECIPITATING EVENT.** To help identify the precipitating event, the nurse should explore three areas during assessment. These areas are the patient's needs and the events that threaten those needs, the point at which symptoms appear, and the themes or memories that are verbalized by the patient. Four kinds of needs that have been identified are related to self-esteem, sexual role mastery, dependency, and biological function.[29,37] Self-esteem is achieved when the individual attains successful social role experience. Sexual role mastery is achieved when the individual attains vocational, sexual, and parental role successes. Dependency is achieved when a satisfying interdependent relationship with others is attained. Biological function is achieved when an individual is in a position of safety in which the continuation of his life is not threatened.

The nurse identifies which needs are not being met by questioning the patient about how he feels about himself, what areas of his life he considers to be successful, what kinds of relationships he has with others, and how safe and secure he feels in life. The nurse looks for obstacles that might interfere with meeting the patient's needs. What recent experiences have been upsetting? What areas of life have had changes?

■ **PERCEPTION OF THE EVENT.** The patient's perception of the precipitating event is of primary importance, because what may appear to the nurse as a trivial experience may have great meaning to the patient. An overweight adolescent girl may have recently been the only girl in the class not invited to a social event. This may have threatened her self-esteem. A man with two

unsuccessful marriages may have just been told by a girl friend that she wants to end their relationship. This may have threatened his need for sexual role mastery. An emotionally isolated, friendless woman may have had car trouble and been unable to find someone to give her a ride to work. This may have threatened her dependency needs. A chronically ill man who has had a recent exacerbation of his illness may have had his need for biological function threatened.

The point at which coping patterns become ineffective and symptoms appear is often after the stressful incident. When did the patient begin to feel anxious? When did his sleep disturbance begin? At what point in time did his suicidal thoughts start? If symptoms began last Tuesday, ask what took place in the patient's life on Tuesday or Monday. As the patient connects life events with the breakdown in coping mechanisms, an understanding of the precipitating event can materialize.

Themes and surfacing memories the patient verbalizes give further clues to the precipitating event. Present issues of concern are symbolically connected to past issues of concern. For example, a female patient who talks about the death of her father, which occurred 3 years ago, may, on questioning, reveal a recent loss of a relationship with a male. A patient who talks about feelings of inadequacy he had as a child because of poor school performance may, on questioning, reveal a recent experience in which his feelings of adequacy on his job were threatened. Since most crises involve losses or threats of losses, the theme of losses is a common one expressed. In assessment the nurse therefore looks for a recent occurrence that may be connected to an underlying theme.

■ **SUPPORT SYSTEMS.** The patient's living situation, with emphasis on supports in the environment, needs to be assessed. Information is sought concerning present and potential sources of support. Does the patient live alone or with family or friends? With whom is he close? Who does he think understands him and offers him strength? Is there a clergyman or church friend he thinks is supportive to him? Assessing the patient's support system is important in determining who should come for the crisis therapy sessions. It may be determined that certain family members should come with the patient so that the family members' support can be strengthened. It may be determined that since the patient has few supports in his life, he should be involved in a crisis therapy group so that the support of other group members can be elicited. Assessing the patient's support system is also vital in determining whether an inpatient hospitalization would be more appropriate than outpatient crisis therapy. If there is a

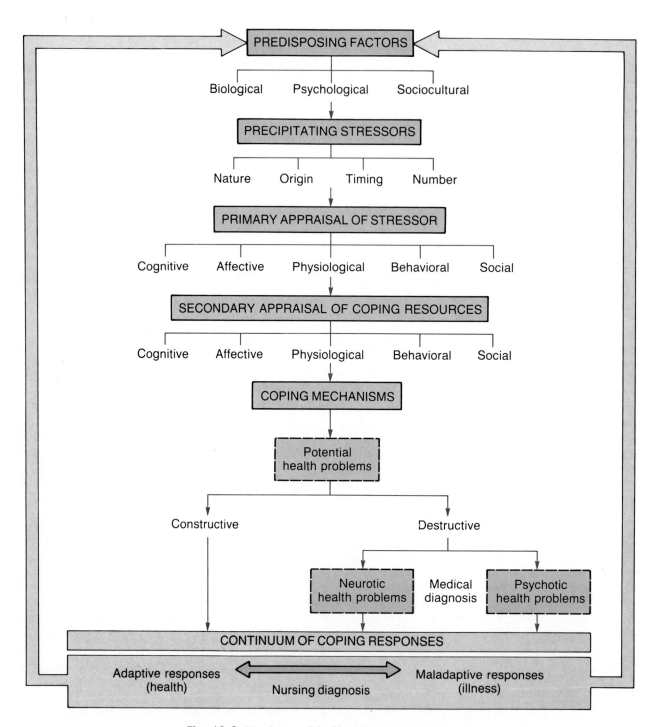

Fig. 10-2. Nursing model of health-illness phenomena.

high degree of suicidal and homicidal risk along with a weak outside support system, hospitalization may be a safer and more effective treatment.

■ **COPING MECHANISMS.** Next, the nurse assesses the patient's strengths and previous coping mechanisms. How has the patient handled other crises in his life? To whom has he turned? How did he relieve anxieties? Did the patient talk problems out with a relative? Did he leave his environment for a period of time to think things out from another perspective? Did he participate in physical activity to relieve tension? Did he find relief in crying? Besides exploring previous coping mechanisms, the nurse should also note the absence of other possible successful mechanisms.

■ **NURSING DIAGNOSES.** The final step in the assessment phase of crisis intervention is the formulation of nursing diagnoses. These diagnoses may be related to any aspect of the patient's life and can reflect the variety of nursing problems described in Chapters 12 to 21 of this text. The accompanying box presents the primary NANDA nursing diagnoses appropriate to crisis intervention and examples of complete nursing diagnoses. Nursing diagnoses related to the range of possible maladaptive responses of the patient are identified along with related medical diagnoses in Table 10-3.

■ **RELATED MEDICAL DIAGNOSES.** Relevant medical diagnoses may similarly pertain to a variety of psychiatric disorders. However many patients who require crisis intervention fall under the category of adjustment disorder. In addition, one type of anxiety disorder is particularly amenable to crisis intervention therapy. This is the posttraumatic stress disorder. If not treated early, posttraumatic stress disorder can become chronic.[5,10,16] For example, it is estimated that 20% to 60% of the 2.5 million Vietnam War veterans who saw combat have had or continue to have psychological adjustment problems at home. Their long-term adjustment should ideally follow four stages identified by Figley: (1) recovery, (2) avoidance, (3) reconsideration, and (4) adjustment.[5] In recovery, the veteran realizes that he is safe. In avoidance, he attempts not to think about his experiences so that he does not have to face overwhelming feelings. In reconsideration, the veteran reflects on his experiences and begins to deal with his thoughts and feelings. Finally, having successfully reflected, he enters the stage of adjustment. Immediate psychological assistance in following through these stages may prevent chronic disorder.[16] The medical diagnoses of adjustment disorder and posttraumatic stress disorder will now be briefly described.

Adjustment disorder. Adjustment disorder is a maladaptive reaction to an identifiable psychosocial stressor that occurs within 3 months of the onset of the stressor but has not persisted for more than 6 months. Behaviors include impairment in social or occupational functioning or symptoms of an excessive reaction to the stressor. There are various types of adjustment disorders, such as the following:

Adjustment disorder with depressed mood: The other essential feature is tearfulness or hopelessness.

Adjustment disorder with anxious mood: The other essential features are nervousness, worry, and jitteriness.

Adjustment disorder with mixed emotional features: The other essential feature is a combination of depression and anxiety and other disorders.

Nursing Diagnoses Related to Crisis Intervention

Primary NANDA Nursing Diagnoses

Coping ineffective, individual
Coping ineffective, family: compromised
Family process, alteration in

Examples of Complete Nursing Diagnoses

Ineffective individual coping related to child's illness evidenced by limited ability to concentrate and psychomotor agitation

Ineffective individual coping related to daughter's death evidenced by inability to recall events pertaining to the car accident

Ineffective family coping, compromised, related to separation from husband evidenced by excessive dependency on friends and preoccupation with having husband return home

Ineffective family coping, compromised, related to wife's cancer diagnosis evidenced by feelings of grief, fear, and guilt

Alteration in family process related to move to a new town evidenced by social withdrawal and rejection of help from others

Alteration in family process related to marriage of daughter evidenced by unclear family boundaries and distorted communication patterns

---

TABLE 10-3

MEDICAL AND NURSING DIAGNOSES RELATED TO CRISIS INTERVENTION

Related Medical Diagnoses (DSM-III-R)*	Related Nursing Diagnoses (NANDA)
Adjustment disorder with depressed mood	Altered growth and development
Adjustment disorder with anxious mood	Anxiety
Adjustment disorder with mixed emotional features	†Coping, ineffective family: compromise
Adjustment disorder with disturbances of conduct	†Coping, ineffective individual
Adjustment disorder with mixed disturbance of emotions and conduct	†Family process, alteration in
Adjustment disorder with work or academic inhibition	Fear
Adjustment disorder with withdrawal	Grieving, anticipatory
Adjustment disorder with physical complaints	Health maintenance, alteration in
Adjustment disorder NOS	Impaired adjustment
Posttraumatic stress disorder	Knowledge deficit
	Parenting, alteration in
	Post-trauma response
	Rape trauma syndrome
	Self-concept, disturbance in
	Social isolation
	Spiritual distress

*From American Psychiatric Association: Draft of the DSM-III-R in Development (subject to change), as proposed by the Work Group to Revise DSM-III. American Psychiatric Association, October 1985.
†Indicates primary nursing diagnoses for crisis intervention.

Adjustment disorder with disturbances of conduct: The other essential feature is the violation of the rights of others or of major age-appropriate societal norms and rules.

Adjustment disorder with mixed disturbance of emotions and conduct: The other essential features are both emotional features and a disturbance of conduct.

Adjustment disorder with work or academic inhibition: The other essential feature is a decrease in work or academic functioning.

Adjustment disorder with withdrawal: The other essential feature is social withdrawal without significant depressed or anxious mood.

Adjustment disorder with physical complaints: The other essential feature is the presence of physical symptoms such as headache, backache, or fatigue.

Adjustment disorder NOS: This is a residual category for disorders involving maladaptive reactions to psychosocial stressors that are not classifiable as specific types of adjustment disorder.

Posttraumatic stress disorder. The essential feature of posttraumatic stress disorder is the development of characteristic symptoms following a psychologically traumatic event that is generally outside the range of usual human experience. The characteristic symptoms involve reexperiencing the traumatic event; a numbing of responsiveness or reduced involvement with the external world; recurrent, distressing dreams of the event; and a variety of autonomic, depressed, or anxious symptoms.

■ Planning

The second step of crisis intervention is planning the intervention. During this phase the previously collected data are analyzed and specific interventions are proposed. Dynamics underlying the present crisis are formulated from the information regarding the precipitating event. Alternative solutions to the problem are explored, and steps for achieving the solutions are designated. The nurse decides which environmental supports to engage or strengthen and how to do this. He or she also decides which of the patient's coping mechanisms to develop and which ones to strengthen.

■ Intervention

The third step of crisis intervention is implementing the intervention itself. The intervention can take place on many levels with the use of a variety of techniques. Shields[33] has described four specific levels of crisis intervention, which represent a hierarchy from the most superficial to the most in-depth:

1. Environmental manipulation
2. General support
3. Generic approach
4. Individual approach

Each step includes the lower levels of intervention. The order of the steps also represents the degree of knowledge and skill needed by the nurse for application.

■ **ENVIRONMENTAL MANIPULATION.** Environmental manipulation includes those interventions that directly change the patient's physical or interpersonal situation for the purpose of providing situational support or removing stress. For example, a patient who is having difficulty coping with her six children may temporarily send several of the children to their grandparents' house. In this situation some stress is alleviated. Similarly, a patient having difficulty on his job may take a week of sick leave so he can be removed temporarily from that stress. A patient who lives alone may move in with his closest sibling for several days. In this situation some support is provided. Likewise, involving the patient in family or group crisis therapy provides environmental manipulation for the purpose of providing support.

■ **GENERAL SUPPORT.** General support includes those interventions which provide the patient with the feeling that the nurse is on his side and will be a helping person. The nurse's demonstration of the therapeutic elements of warmth, acceptance, empathy, and caring in addition to offering reassurance results in this type of support.

■ **GENERIC APPROACH.** The generic approach is a type of crisis intervention that is analogous to the public health model. It is designed to reach high-risk individuals and individuals of great numbers in as short a time as possible. It applies a specific method to all those individuals faced with a similar type of crisis. The course of the particular type of crisis is previously studied and mapped out. The intervention is then set up to ensure that the course of the crisis results in an adaptive resolution.

As described earlier in this chapter, grief is an example of a type of crisis with a known pattern that can be influenced toward a positive outcome. Lindemann's[26] study described the pattern of grief. He believed that helping the patient extricate himself from his ties to the deceased and find new patterns of rewarding interaction would influence the patient toward a positive or adaptive resolution of his grief. Applying this specific intervention to individuals experiencing grief, especially when a high-risk group is evident (e.g., families of local disaster victims) is an example of providing a generic approach. Use of the generic approach does not require the nurse to have a thorough understanding of the unique psychodynamics of the patient.[22]

■ **INDIVIDUAL APPROACH.** The individual approach is a type of crisis intervention analogous to the model of diagnosis and treatment of a specific problem in a specific patient. The nurse needs to have a thorough understanding of the patient's psychodynamics that led to the present crisis and must consequently use the intervention geared to aid the particular patient to achieve an adaptive resolution to his crisis. This type of crisis intervention can be effective with all types of crisis. It is of particular benefit in crises that are combined situational and maturational crises. The individual approach is also beneficial when symptoms include strong components of homicidal and suicidal risk. The individual approach should be applied to those crises for which a known course cannot be mapped. It also should be applied to those crises which have not responded to a trial of the generic approach. It is often helpful to consult with others when deciding which approach to use for a specific patient.

■ **TECHNIQUES.** The nurse's implementation of these levels of intervention is aided by the use of some techniques of crisis intervention that are active, focal, and explorative in nature. Since the focus of crisis intervention is on the present crisis, the intervention must be now oriented to achieve the goal of quick resolution. Furthermore, the nurse must be active in guiding the crisis intervention through its various steps. A more passive approach is inappropriate for this type of psychotherapy because of the time limitations of the crisis situation.

In her care the nurse is creative and flexible, trying whatever, within reason, may work. Some techniques might include abreaction, clarification, suggestion, manipulation, reinforcement of behavior, support of defenses, raising self-esteem, and exploration of solutions.[21, 32] The technique of interpretation is not emphasized in crisis intervention because a conscious solution to an immediate problem is the goal of crisis intervention. Interpretation deals with making unconscious elements of behavior conscious and is therefore not compatible with the goal. A brief description of these techniques will now be presented.

Abreaction is the ventilation of feelings that takes place as the patient verbally recounts emotionally charged areas. Awareness of affect is experienced, and tension reduction results. Usually abreaction is encouraged in crisis intervention. The nurse facilitates abreaction by asking the patient how he feels about his situation, recent events, and significant people involved in his crisis. The nurse asks open-ended questions and reflects the patient's words back to him so that he will further ventilate his feelings. The nurse does not discourage crying or angry outbursts but rather sees them as a positive release of feelings. Only when feelings seem out of control, such as in extreme rage or despondency, should the nurse discourage abreaction and help the patient concentrate on thinking rather than feeling. For example, if a patient angrily talks of wanting to kill a specific person, it is better to help him focus on thinking through the consequences of carrying out the act rather than encouraging free expression of the angry feelings.

Clarification is used when the nurse encourages the patient to express more clearly the relationship between certain events in his life, or the nurse herself may point out possible relationships. For example, helping a patient see that it was after he was passed over for a promotion that he began feeling too sick to go to work is clarification. Clarification enables the patient to gain a better intellectual understanding of his feelings and how they led to the development of a crisis. In crisis intervention the clarification of unconscious processes is minimal.

Suggestion is the process of influencing an individual so that he accepts an idea or belief. In crisis intervention the nurse influences the patient to see her as a confident, calm, hopeful, empathic leader who can help. By believing the nurse can help, the patient himself feels optimistic and in turn will feel less anxious. He also may want to please the nurse by fulfilling her expectations of getting better.

Manipulation is a technique in which the nurse uses the patient's emotions, wishes, or values to his benefit in the therapeutic process. Like suggestion, manipulation is a way of influencing the patient. For example, the nurse may want to point out to the patient who prides himself on his independence that he is capable of as well as responsible for much of the work of solving his problem.

Reinforcement behavior occurs when useful adaptive behavior of the patient is reinforced by the nurse. She strengthens positive responses made by the patient by agreeing with or complimenting those responses. For example, when a patient who has passively received berating from his boss states that he asserted himself in an interaction with his boss, the nurse can tell him she is pleased with his assertiveness.

Support of defenses occurs when the nurse encourages the use of defenses that result in adaptive gratification and discourages those which result in maladaptive gratification. Defense mechanisms are indirect behaviors used to cope with stressful situations. The purpose of defense mechanisms is to maintain self-esteem and ego integrity. When defenses deny, falsify, or distort reality to the point that the individual cannot deal effectively with reality, they are maladaptive. The nurse should encourage the patient to use defenses that result in adaptive gratification and discourage those which result in maladaptive gratification. For example, when a patient denies the fact that her husband wants to break up their marriage despite the fact that he has told her and demonstrated to her what he wishes, the nurse can point out to her that she is not facing facts and dealing realistically with the problem. This is an example of discouraging the use of the defense mechanism of denial. If a patient who is furious with an authority figure writes a letter to the authority's supervisor rather than assaulting the authority, the nurse should encourage his adaptive use of the defense mechanism of sublimation.

In crisis intervention, defenses are not attacked but rather are more gently encouraged or discouraged. When defenses are attacked, the patient cannot maintain his self-esteem and ego integrity. There is not enough time in crisis intervention to help replace the attacked defenses with new healthier defenses. Returning the patient to his previous level of functioning is the goal of crisis intervention, not the restructuring of defenses.

Raising self-esteem is a particularly important technique. The patient in a crisis feels helpless and may be overwhelmed with feelings of inadequacy. The fact that he has found it necessary to seek outside help for his problem may further increase his feelings of inadequacy. The nurse should help the patient regain his feelings of self-worth. She does this by communicating her confidence that the patient can participate actively in finding solutions to his problems. The nurse also communicates to the patient that he is a worthwhile person by listening to him, accepting his feelings, and relating to him with respect.

Exploration of solutions is essential because crisis intervention is geared toward solving the immediate crisis. The nurse and patient actively explore solutions to the crisis. Alternative solutions that the patient could not conceive of originally may become apparent as he talks to the nurse and his anxiety decreases. For example, a patient who has lost his job and has not been successful in finding a new one may become aware of the fact that he knows many people in his field of work whom he could contact to get information regarding the job market and possible openings.

These crisis intervention techniques are summarized in the accompanying box. In addition to using these techniques, Morley, Messick, and Aguilera[30] listed at-

Techniques of Crisis Intervention

Technique: **Abreaction**
Definition: The ventilation of feelings that takes place as the patient verbally recounts emotionally charged areas
Example: "Tell me about how you have been feeling since you lost your job."

Technique: **Clarification**
Definition: Encouraging the patient to express more clearly the relationship between certain events in his life
Example: "I've noticed that after you have an argument with your husband you become sick and can't leave your bed."

Technique: **Suggestion**
Definition: Influencing an individual so that he accepts an idea or belief, particularly the belief that the nurse can help and that he will feel better
Example: "Many other people have found it helpful to talk about this and I think you will too."

Technique: **Manipulation**
Definition: Using the patient's emotions, wishes, or values to his benefit in the therapeutic process
Example: "You seem to be very committed to your marriage and I think that you will work through these issues and have a stronger relationship in the end."

Technique: **Reinforcement of behavior**
Definition: Giving the patient positive responses to adaptive behavior
Example: "That's the first time you were able to defend yourself with your boss and it went very well. I'm so pleased that you were able to do it."

Technique: **Support of defenses**
Definition: Encouraging the use of defenses that result in adaptive gratification and discouraging those that result in maladaptive gratification
Example: "Going for a bicycle ride when you were so angry was very helpful since when you returned you and your wife were able to talk things through."

Technique: **Raising self-esteem**
Definition: Helping the patient to regain feelings of self-worth
Example: "You are a very strong person to be able to manage the family all this time. I think you will be able to handle this situation too."

Technique: **Exploration of solutions**
Definition: Examining alternative modes of action geared toward solving the immediate problem
Example: "You seem to know many people in the computer field. Couldn't you contact some of them to see if they might know of available jobs?"

titudes that are essential for the crisis worker to have. She should see her work as the treatment of choice with persons in crisis rather than as a second-best treatment. Assessment of the present problem should be viewed as necessary for treatment, but complete diagnostic assessment should be viewed as unnecessary. The goal and time limitations of crisis intervention should be kept in mind constantly, and unrelated material should not be explored. An active directive role must be taken, and flexibility of approach is mandatory.

■ Evaluation

The fourth step of crisis intervention is evaluation. During this phase the nurse and patient evaluate whether the intervention resulted in the desired effect, a positive resolution of the crisis. Has the patient returned to his precrisis level of functioning? Have the patient's original needs, which were threatened by the precipitating or stressful event, been met? Have the patient's symptoms, which demonstrated ineffective use

of coping mechanisms, subsided? Have the patient's useful coping mechanisms begun to function again? Does the patient have a strong support system to rely on now? The nurse reviews with the patient changes that have occurred and gives the credit for these changes to the patient so that he can see his own effectiveness. The nurse discusses with the patient how that which was learned from the experience of crisis intervention may help in coping with future crises. As in any evaluation process, if goals have not been met, the patient and nurse can go back to the first step, assessment, and continue through the four phases again. At the end of the evaluation process, if the nurse and patient believe referral for another type of professional help would be useful, the referral is made.

Clinical case analysis

The phases of crisis intervention just described can be seen in Clinical example 10-4.

CLINICAL EXAMPLE 10-4

ASSESSMENT

Mr. A was a 29-year-old, medium-built, casually dressed black man who was referred to the crisis clinic by another agency. The patient came to the clinic alone. The nurse working with Mr. A collected the following data.

The patient worked in a large steel-making company. The company was laying off many workers and reassigning others. One month before Mr. A was temporarily assigned to an area where he had had difficulty 2 years ago. The foreman, the patient believed, was now harrassing him as he had previously. Two weeks ago the patient got angry at the foreman and had thoughts of wanting to kill him. Instead of taking violent action, Mr. A became dizzy, and his head ached. He requested medical attention but was refused. He then "passed out" and was taken by ambulance to the dispensary.

Since that time Mr. A had a comprehensive physical examination and was found to be in excellent health. His physician prescribed diazepam (Valium) on an as-needed basis, but this was only slightly helpful. The patient returned to work for 2 days this week but felt "sick" again. The agency to which Mr. A registered a complaint against his foreman was the agency that referred him to the clinic.

Mr. A complained of being depressed, nervous, and tense. He was not sleeping well, was irritable with his wife and children, and was preoccupied with angry feelings toward his foreman. He had paranoid feelings about his foreman harassing him. Mr. A denied suicidal thoughts while admitting to homicidal thoughts. He felt the homicidal thoughts were under control. At one point during the initial interview the patient was tearful despite strong attempts at control. He demonstrated adequate comprehension, above-average intelligence, a good capacity for introspection, an adequate memory, an affect more of anxiety than depression, and paranoid ideation in regard to the foreman at work. His thought processes were organized, and there was no evidence of a perceptual disorder. Ego boundary disturbance was evident in the patient's paranoid thoughts. It seemed that the foreman was, in fact, a difficult man to get along with. However, the description of personal harassment seemed distorted. There were no depressive symptoms.

Mr. A was raised by his parents. His father was "boss" and beat him and his siblings often. His mother was quiet and always agreed with his father. Mr. A's parents were Jehovah's Witnesses, and he was Baptist. The patient had a younger brother, a younger sister, and an older sister. The patient and his brother had always been close. The two of them had stopped their father's beatings by ganging up on him and "psyching him out." As a child Mr. A hung around with a "tough crowd" and fought frequently. He stated he believed that he can physically overpower others, but tries to keep out of trouble by talking to people rather than fighting and by working hard.

Mr. A had never before sought aid from a mental health facility. His physical health, as stated, was excellent. He was taking no medication at the time of his first interview. Mr. A had a tenth-grade education and had always achieved above-average grades. His work record up until this time was good. His interests included bowling and other sports. He also periodically took courses at a local community college for his own personal growth rather than in preparation for a degree.

Mr. A had been married for 9 years. His wife was 2 years younger than he. They had three daughters ages 9, 7, and 9 months. Mr. A stated that his relationships with his wife and daughters were satisfactory. Both his wife and his brother were strong supports at this time.

Mr. A's usual means of coping were talking calmly with the threatening party and working hard on his job, in school, and in leisure activities. These coping mechanisms failed to work for him at this time but had been successful in the past. Other strengths the patient exhibited were a good work record under the other foreman and only mild impairment in spheres of his life outside work. He had no arrest record and showed the ability of not acting impulsively but rather of thinking through his actions. Mr. A showed strong motivation for working on his problem. He was reaching out for help, and the beginning of a therapeutic relationship was developing.

Environmental supports seemed strong. The patient's wife and brother were supportive, but the patient saw his problem as not involving them. It was therefore decided that the patient would be seen alone for the sessions. The patient felt no supports at work.

PLANNING

Mr. A was in a situational crisis, an internal disturbance that resulted from a perceived threat. The threat or precipitating stress in this case was the transfer to a new boss. The patient's need for sexual role mastery was not being met, since he was not

CLINICAL EXAMPLE 10-4—cont'd

attaining vocational role success. Soon after the transfer Mr. A's usual means of coping became ineffective and he experienced increased anxiety. Symptoms that appeared included attacks of dizziness, headache, passing out, and paranoid thinking. There was no suicidal intent, but feelings toward the foreman contained some homicidal ideation. The patient demonstrated enough control over his impulses that hospitalization was believed to be unnecessary. Memories and themes in the patient's verbalizations emphasized his feelings of being harassed. He had had difficulty with his new boss before. Difficulty with his boss was speculated to be a repetition of an earlier conflict, that is, the patient's feelings toward his father, another harassing boss.

The overall goal of treatment would be for the patient to return to at least his precrisis level of functioning. If possible, he could reach a level above, having learned new methods of problem solving. A crisis intervention approach was decided on that considered the patient's needs and desires, the presenting problem, and the limitations of the clinic. The patient demonstrated a good potential for problem solving and the nurse made a contract with him for crisis intervention on a weekly basis.

Possible solutions were mutually explored:

1. It was believed that the patient should remain away from work temporarily so that his rage would not be likely to explode.
2. The patient's intellectual understanding of the crisis would be sought. By understanding what had happened to cause his anxiety, the patient would be able to see more clearly ways of solving the problem. Intellectual understanding rather than affective understanding is sought because of the time limitations and goals of crisis intervention. Affective understanding involves long-term treatment with much emphasis on unconscious processes.
3. Old constructive ways of handling anger would be reinforced. These included submitting a formal complaint at work and ventilating his feelings both to the nurse during the sessions and to his family and friends at other appropriate times.
4. New ways of coping would be taught. These included seeking support at work and following several official avenues of protest.
5. Because of the strength of the patient's feelings toward his boss, it was possible that new ways of handling anger would not suffice and that a transfer to another department might be a better solution.

INTERVENTION

The level of intervention used by the nurse was the **individual approach,** which is the most sophisticated approach and includes the generic approach, general support, and environmental manipulation. The individual approach was chosen because the patient's crisis was not one for which a known course could be mapped. Also, since there was a homicidal component to the patient's symptoms, it was believed to be the safest approach. With a clear understanding of psychodynamics, the nurse geared the intervention to aid the patient to achieve an adaptive resolution to his crisis.

Environmental manipulation was achieved by having the patient remain home from work temporarily. Letters were written by the nurse to his employer explaining his absence in general terms. The patient was encouraged to talk to his wife about his difficulties so that she could understand his anxiety and be emotionally supportive.

General support was given by the nurse, who provided an atmosphere of reassurance, nonjudgmental caring, warmth, empathy, and optimism. The patient was encouraged to talk freely about the problem without having his feelings judged as good or bad. The nurse offered reassurance that the problem was one that could be solved and that the patient would be feeling better. The nurse let the patient know that she understood his feelings and would help him overcome his crisis.

The **generic approach** was used to decrease the patient's anxiety and guide him through the various steps of problem solving common to all crises. Levels of anxiety were assessed and means of reducing anxiety or helping the patient tolerate moderate anxiety were employed. The patient was encouraged to use his anxiety consciously and constructively to solve his problem and develop new coping mechanisms.

The **individual approach** was used in assessing the specific problems of Mr. A and treating those specific problems. An understanding of the patient's individual psychodynamics was sought and dealt with by the nurse and patient. The patient was reexperiencing harassment from a male authority figure as he had experienced with his father during his youth. Because of the repetition of harassing experiences, Mr. A perceived his treatment by his boss

Continued.

CLINICAL EXAMPLE 10-4—cont'd

in a personal and paranoid way. In other words, he was strongly sensitive to unfair treatment and overreacted as a result of early repetitive childhood experiences. His emotional response was to strike out physically, as his father had struck out at him. Intellectually, Mr. A knew this would be a disastrous action, and his conflict was solved by becoming sick and passing out so that he could not assault his boss. Mr. A's intense anger was recognized and a high priority was placed on channeling the anger in a positive direction.

The first two interviews were used for data gathering and establishing a positive therapeutic relationship. Through the use of **abreaction** the patient ventilated angry feelings but did not concentrate on wanting to kill his boss. The nurse used **clarification** to help the patient begin to attain an intellectual understanding of the precipitating event and its effect on him. **Suggestion** was used by influencing the patient to see the nurse as one who can help. The nurse told the patient the problem could be worked out by the two of them and that he would soon be feeling better. The patient decided to contact several people at work to obtain information about transferring to another department or being laid off. The patient and nurse therefore were **exploring solutions.** The nurse **reinforced** the patient's use of problem solving by telling him his ideas about alternative solutions were good ones well worth his looking into. Throughout these and other sessions the nurse **raised his self-esteem** by communicating her confidence that he could participate actively in finding solutions to his problems. She also listened to and accepted his feelings and treated him with respect. By contacting others at work in his pursuits, the patient found some supportive individuals at work.

During the third session the patient described an incident in which he became furious at a worker at an automobile repair shop. The repairs on the patient's car were never right, and the patient kept returning the car there. The patient shoved the worker but limited his physical assault to that. He then felt nervous and jittery. The patient had previously expressed pride in his ability to control his angry feelings and not physically strike out at others. **Manipulation** was used by telling the patient he showed control in stopping the assault before it had become a full-blown fight and it seemed apparent he could continue to exhibit this ability. During this session, also, the patient spoke of old angry feelings toward his father. Some of this ventilation was allowed, but soon thereafter the focus was guided back to the present crisis.

In the fourth session the patient reported no episode of uncontrollable anger. He still put much emphasis, however, on being harassed by others. The nurse questioned the fact that others were out to intentionally harass the patient. Mr. A's defenses were not attacked, but his gross use of projection was discouraged. In the fifth session the patient reported that a car tried to run him off the road. At a red traffic light the patient spoke calmly to the driver and the driver apologized. The nurse **reinforced this behavior** and **supported his use of sublimation as a defense.** Discussion of termination of the therapy was begun.

In the sixth session the patient told of his plans to return to work the following week. He would be going to a different department even though it seemed he would soon be laid off. He also talked about a course he had begun at a community college. He showed no evidence of anxiety or paranoia. Termination of the therapeutic relationship was further discussed. Only a few of the techniques of crisis intervention are described here. It should be kept in mind that the techniques, in actuality, are repetitively used in all sessions to be effective.

EVALUATION

The interventions resulted in the desired effect, an adaptive resolution of the crisis. The changes that occurred were discussed with the patient. The patient's need for sexual role mastery was being met. He was returning to work in a department in which he felt comfortable and successful. His symptoms of anxiety, paranoia, dizziness, headaches, passing out, and homicidal thoughts had ended. He no longer felt harassed. His original coping mechanisms were again effective. He was talking calmly to people he was having difficulty with, and he was again working hard in a goal-oriented way (i.e., a college course). He had learned new methods of coping, which included talking about his feelings to significant others, following administrative or official avenues of protest, and seeking support. The patient and nurse discussed how Mr. A could use the methods of problem solving he had learned from the experience to help cope with future problems. The goal, return to the precrisis level of functioning, had been attained.

It was also recommended to the patient that he engage in long-term psychotherapy so that he could deal with the old angers that interfered with his present life. The patient refused the recommendation at this time and stated he would contact the clinic if he changed his mind.

Modalities and settings for crisis therapy

Nurses are in the position to render crisis therapy frequently by virtue of the various settings in which they practice. The observant nurse will identify individuals in crisis and plan necessary action. Medical hospitalizations are stressful for patients and their families and are often precipitating causes of crises. The patient who becomes excessively demanding or withdrawn or the wife who becomes known as a "pest" to the nursing staff are possible candidates for crisis therapy. The loss of a limb, the limitations imposed on one's activities, and the changes in body image because of surgical intervention can all be viewed as losses or threats that may precipitate situational crisis. Simply the stress of being dependent on nurses for care can precipitate a crisis for the hospitalized patient. Strain and Grossman[35] identified the following categories of psychological stress in hospitalized patients:

1. Threat to narcissistic integrity
2. Fear of strangers
3. Separation anxiety
4. Fear of loss of love and approval
5. Fear of loss of control of developmentally achieved functions
6. Fear of loss or injury to body parts
7. Reactivation of feelings of guilt and shame and fear of retaliation

In addition, nurses who work in obstetric, pediatric, geriatric, or adolescent settings can readily observe patients or family members undergoing maturational crises. The anxious new mother, the acting-out adolescent, and the newly retired depressed patient are all possible candidates for crisis therapy. If physical illness is an added stress during maturational turning points, the patient is at an even greater risk.

Emergency room settings are flooded with crisis cases. People who attempt suicide, psychosomatic patients, and families of accident victims are all possible candidates for crisis therapy. If the nurse herself is not in a position to work with the patient on an ongoing basis, a referral for crisis therapy can be made. Community health nurses, having the advantage of observing patients in their own environments, can often spot and intervene in family crises. The child who refuses to go to school, the man who refuses to learn how to give himself the insulin injection, and the family with a member dying at home are, again, possible candidates for crisis therapy. Community health nurses are in a position to evaluate high-risk families for their need of crisis therapy. Families with new babies, ill members, recent deaths, and a history of difficulty coping are all possible high-risk families.

■ Family work

The family concept of crisis defines the crisis as a family problem, regardless of who is the identified patient.[7] The identified patient is the individual who is exhibiting symptoms. Since the crisis is seen as a family problem, responsibility for the patient's symptoms is placed on the family. It is assumed that a sequence of events occurring within the family led up to the decompensation of a member. The family is viewed as a system so that each member affects and is affected by each other member. For example, when a child refuses to go to school, it is believed not only that the child fears school and wishes to remain with mother but also that the mother is afraid to be alone and wants the child home with her. The crisis is a family one, not the child's crisis. It is also assumed that role problems cause disequilibrium in families, and new role assignments may be helpful. For example, if a mother appears to be the leader of the family and the father is discounted as ineffective, the nurse can assign certain tasks to the father, such as deciding on proper bedtimes for the children, so that the father will assume some leadership. At other times, tasks are given to the entire family so that emphasis is removed from the symptoms and conflicts. The family is given the responsibility of meeting each member's needs and of changing so that the present problem can be solved.[24]

One family crisis model developed by Hill[19] is based on family systems theory. It was formulated as a result of his research on induced separation and reunion during World War II. In the model, known as the ABCX model, the event (A) interacts with the family's coping resources (B) in combination with the family's definition of the event (C) and produces the crisis (X). If the crisis is not quickly resolved, the family eventually reorganizes into either an adaptive or maladaptive family structure. Another model adds postcrisis adaptation to Hill's model and is called the double ABCX model.[27] This model asserts that if the change in the family system continues over time, pile up results. Pile up is the addition of further hardships encountered by the family. New ways of perceiving the situation and new ways of coping occur and can result in new family organization.

Some practitioners initiate crisis intervention programs for families with specific problems. For example, programs have been implemented for families of servicemen missing in action,[39] families going through perinatal bereavement,[31] and families with children in the intensive care nursery.[11] One innovative program was established to help patients with chronic renal failure and their families adjust to the unique demands of home dialysis.[25]

Nurses in community mental health centers or departments of psychiatry, of course, see many patients in crisis. Patients and families have varied major complaints: depression, anxiety, marital conflict, suicidal thoughts, illicit drug taking, and psychotic symptoms. Crisis therapy modalities available in mental health centers include individual, family, and crisis groups.

■ Group work

Crisis groups function along the same sequential phases of resolution that individual intervention follows.[36] The nurse and group help the patient to attempt to solve his problem. Thereafter the group reinforces the patient's new problem-solving behavior. The nurse's role in the group is active, focal, and present oriented. The group follows the nurse's example and uses similar therapeutic techniques. The group acts as a support system for the patient and is therefore of particular benefit to socially isolated individuals. Often the way the patient functions in the group will highlight the faulty coping that is responsible for his present problem. For example, it may become apparent from a patient's interaction with group members that he does not appear to listen to anything said by others but continues verbalizing as though nothing were said. This same patient may be in a crisis because his girl friend left him because she thought he did not care about her thoughts and feelings. The nurse can comment on the faulty coping seen in the group and encourage group discussion about it.

Crisis groups can be open ended or time limited and can be geared toward a homogeneous or heterogeneous population. Donovan, Bennett, and McElroy[12] describe a limited crisis group in a health maintenance organization. They speculate that the group's success is attributable to cohesiveness of the group culture, the supportive and accepting attitude of the group, and the group's expectation that the patients will work out their problems. Chen[8] describes a successful open-ended crisis group in a community mental health center. She observes that process interventions can be creatively used to enhance the group interaction while maintaining the crisis-oriented focus. In her group, Chen uses an individual interpersonal focus and a mass group focus to help patients resolve their present crises. Homogeneous crisis groups have been initiated for groups with specific problems. For example, groups have been implemented for men accompanying women seeking abortion[17] and families in the waiting room for intensive care patients.[4]

There is a trend for psychiatric hospitalizations to be short term. Nurses practicing on these units can use crisis therapy in working with the patient and his family either individually or in groups so that the patient can return to the community as soon as possible. This can also prevent rehospitalization. The hospitalization itself may be viewed as an environmental manipulation and thus as part of the crisis intervention.

Crisis intervention is sometimes practiced by way of the telephone rather than in face-to-face contacts. Nurses working for hot lines or nurses who become involved in answering emergency telephone calls may find themselves practicing crisis intervention without the use of visual cues. Referrals for face-to-face contact should be made, but often, because of the patient's unwillingness or inability to cooperate, the telephone remains the only contact. Listening skills must therefore be emphasized in the nurse's role. Most emergency telephone services have extensive training programs to teach this specialized type of crisis intervention. Manuals are written for the crisis worker and include content such as suicide potential rating scales, community resources, drug information, guidelines for helping the caller discuss his concerns, and advice on understanding the limitations of one's role.[28]

■ Disaster work

As part of the community, nurses are called on when adventitious crises strike the community. Floods, earthquakes, airplane crashes, fires, nuclear accidents, and other natural and unnatural disasters precipitate large numbers of crises. Frederick and Garrison[15] have described a "service model" in which mental health workers in the immediate postdisaster period should go to places where victims are likely to congregate, such as morgues, hospitals, and shelters. Later, if Federal Disaster Assistance Centers are established, mental health workers may assist in the centers. Rather than waiting for people to publicly identify themselves as persons who are unable to cope with stress, it is suggested that the mental health workers work with the Red Cross, talk to people waiting in lines to apply for assistance, go door-to-door, or, at a relocation site, ask people how they are managing their affairs and explore their experiences to stress.

Nurses providing crisis therapy during large disasters would use the public health or generic approach so that as many individuals as possible can receive help in a short amount of time. Tragedies such as group kidnappings and group killings in communities may affect fewer people and may at times require the individual approach. The nurse may choose to work with families or groups rather than individuals during adventitious crises so that individuals can gain support from others in their family or community who are undergoing stresses similar to theirs.

A good example of mental health professionals helping victims of an adventitious crisis occurred in Kansas City, Missouri, in the days and weeks following the crash of the overhead walkways at the Hyatt Hotel in July 1981. Eight mental health centers in the Kansas City metropolitan area joined to help care for the emotional sufferings of the individuals involved.

The centers formed an unofficial coalition and prepared a joint press release describing the many aspects of the grieving process and publicizing the services that they would offer to the survivors of those killed at the hotel—the injured, the observers, and the rescue workers. The services were of three kinds. First, all the centers offered phone counseling and support groups free of charge. Second, special services were planned, such as a grief workshop that was attended by about 200 people who had been at the crash scene. Other related seminars were also held. Third, the centers and media worked together to let the general public know about other resources and services as these became available and to reassure people that their strong reactions to the tragedy were normal.

■ Preventive work

Crisis therapy is a major technique of preventive psychiatry. Maladaptive behavior can be prevented by identifying a crisis and intervening immediately. Crisis can actually be avoided by determining factors that can lead to a crisis and taking action to curtail the process. When the nurse sees a potentially stressful situation, she should watch the involved individual's level of anxiety. She should talk and listen to those under stress so that anxiety levels can be lessened before they reach severe or crisis proportions.

For example, an elderly patient with a known psychiatric illness was being seen in supportive long-term psychotherapy with his wife. The wife telephoned the nurse who was working with them to state that her husband had died 2 weeks ago and they therefore would not be coming back to the clinic. The nurse believed that the patient's death was most definitely a stress for his wife and that there was a potential for a crisis. The nurse asked the patient's wife to come into the clinic one more time so that they could evaluate how she was getting along. The wife was seen and the nurse encouraged her to talk about her husband's death and her future plans. The nurse assessed that the wife was going through the grieving process in a normal adaptive way and that as long as the wife continued talking about her feelings to family and friends, a crisis would be avoided.

It is also a preventive measure to intervene when a psychiatrically impaired individual undergoes a crisis so that further debilitation can be stopped. As Aguilera and Messick point out:

> All three levels of prevention are inherent and are practical in crisis intervention. It is possible that this may be a major reason why the concepts and techniques of this method of treatment have been so widely accepted.[1:140]

Nurses practice in primary, secondary, and tertiary prevention settings and can contribute greatly to prevention by case finding and treatment.

■ Patient education

Educating patients about crisis prevention and early adaptive response to stressful situations is important for reducing maladaptation. This education can be provided by the nurse to both individual patients and to society at large.

Although patient education takes place during the entire crisis intervention process, it is emphasized during the evaluation phase. At this time, the patient's anxiety has decreased, and he can better use his cognitive abilities. The nurse and patient recapitulate the course of the crisis and the intervention to teach the patient how to avoid other similar crises. For example, the nurse identifies, with the patient, the feelings, thoughts, and behaviors he experienced as his anxiety rose following the stressful event. She explains that if these feelings, thoughts, and behaviors are again experienced, the patient should immediately consider that he is stressed and needs to take action to stop the anxiety from escalating. She then teaches the patient ways in which he can use his newly learned coping mechanisms in future situations.

Nurses are also involved in identifying patients who are at high risk for developing crises and teaching coping strategies to avoid the development of the crises. For example, coping strategies which can be taught to potential patients (e.g., all hospitalized patients) are (1) how to obtain cognitive information, (2) how to elicit instrumental or concrete support, and (3) how to elicit emotional support.

The general public, as recipients or potential recipients of crisis therapy, are in need of education so that they can identify those in need of crisis services, be aware of available crisis services, change their attitudes so that people will feel free to seek crisis services, and obtain information about how others deal with potential crisis-producing problems. For example, a mother who learns about reactions to rape may identify her daughter as a rape victim. She then takes her daughter to the nearest crisis center which services rape victims. The mother, in encouraging her daughter to go to the crisis center, tells her daughter that rape is not the fault of the victim, thus enabling her daughter to change her attitude about the rape and feel positive about obtaining outside help. At the center, the mother is given a pamphlet, which describes how to help rape victims, and shares this pamphlet with friends so that they can cope quickly and effectively if their loved ones are raped.

The nurse provides education to society at large through participating in programs in the media (both publicly and privately funded), by leading or participating in educational groups in the community, and by taking every opportunity possible to advertise crisis services. For instance, if a nurse is a member of a church group that has developed crisis services, she should share the availability of these services with her child's parent-teacher association. Thus, the information is disseminated to the school's families, the teachers' families, and to other groups to which the parents and teachers belong. Crisis prevention and crisis therapy are necessary for improving the mental health of society. Nurses, as health care professionals, are in a position to provide much patient education about crisis on both a small and large scale.

Future trends

Crisis therapy is becoming more and more popular as the treatment of choice for primary, secondary, and tertiary preventive care of psychiatric problems. It is considered both practical and effective by mental health workers and patients. Because it is a short-term therapy, it is inexpensive in terms of time and money for patients and caregivers. In our mobile and fast-moving society crisis therapy is also practical because it requires a short-term commitment from the patient and caregiver. Many people can be reached in a limited period of time.

Persons other than mental health professionals are being educated to adequately do certain levels of crisis intervention. Neighborhood workers, police, clergy, bartenders, and lawyers are but a few of the many people who come in frequent contact with the target population. These non–mental health professionals who deal with people in crisis are being taught by professionals, including nurses, how to identify individuals in crisis, how to intervene on a generic level, and how to refer individuals needing professional treatment to mental health personnel.

There are some authors who believe that there is not one systematic model of crisis therapy, but many. Conceptualization of crisis work is vague rather than detailed and refined. More research is needed so that crisis theory can be better defined operationally.[34] The choice of crisis intervention modality for specific patients seems at times to be arbitrary and dependent on the practitioner's or agency's orientation rather than based on theory. Further research is needed to identify which crisis intervention modality—individual, group, or family—is most effective under which circumstances. At present the family modality is selected when the crisis directly involves other family members and when strong family support is essential for the individual. When the identified crisis patient is a child or adolescent, family crisis intervention is the preferred mode.[20]

At times, when family members are uncooperative and refuse to become involved in the treatment, an individual or group approach is selected. For those individuals in crisis who are isolated and have little family or friend support, a group is beneficial because the other group members form a support system. The individual approach is selected when the crisis does not seem to directly involve the family or when the patient believes he can best handle the crisis on his own. A patient whose crisis stems from his asserting his independence from his family may also want to be seen individually. Most recently, much attention in individual and family development study is being focused on normative rather than nonnormative developmental changes. For example, a new mother is described as going through a natural transition rather than a developmental crisis. But the differentiation between transition and crisis has not yet been clearly defined.

Nurses are more frequently being placed in the role of primary therapist and therefore are becoming more involved in the direct practice of crisis therapy. This trend seems to be continuing and will grow as certification procedures for nurses further develop. Nurses are also involved in indirect services in the field of crisis therapy. The theory and practice of crisis intervention is taught by nurses to other nurses in various settings and also to non–mental health professionals and paraprofessionals. Nurses are frequently in the role of consultant and advise others in their work with individuals in crisis. Additional nursing research is needed in the area of crisis therapy. What level of education and skill is needed to perform the different levels of crisis intervention? Which nursing interventions are most effective for whom? Follow-up studies are also needed so that the long-term effects of crisis therapy can be evaluated.

■ SUGGESTED CROSS-REFERENCES ■

Therapeutic relationship skills are discussed in Chapter 4. The phases of the nursing process are discussed in Chapter 5. Interventions in primary prevention are discussed in Chapter 9.

DIRECTIONS FOR FUTURE RESEARCH

The following are some of the nursing research problems raised in Chapter 10 that merit further study by psychiatric nurses:

1. The conditions under which natural developmental transitions become crises
2. The relationship between length of time for crisis resolution and individual personality factors
3. Appropriate outcome measures to utilize in evaluating the effectiveness of crisis theory
4. The relationship between the length of time for crisis resolution and type of crisis
5. Empirical validation of the course of grief
6. Useful content for nurses to include in anticipatory guidance of crisis patients
7. Family functioning characteristics associated with family vulnerability to crisis
8. The relationship between characteristics of role models and the incidence of developmental crises
9. Congruence between a patient's and nurse's perceptions of the seriousness of a precipitating event
10. Empirical validation of Caplan's four phases of crisis
11. Ability of nurses to utilize the four levels of crisis intervention
12. Early identification of individuals at risk for crisis
13. Knowledge of the long-term effects of crisis therapy
14. The level of nursing education and skill needed to perform the different levels of crisis intervention

■ SUMMARY ■

1. The theory and practice of crisis therapy developed as an outgrowth of analytical and preventive psychiatry. Eric Lindemann and Gerald Caplan were two of the first pioneers to define and practice crisis therapy.

2. A crisis is an internal disturbance that results from a perceived threat. An individual's usual repertoire of coping mechanisms becomes ineffective in solving problems and the individual experiences a rise in anxiety. Crises are a time of increased vulnerability and can stimulate personal growth.

3. Crises can be maturational, situational, or adventitious in etiology. Maturational crises develop from stress during transitional periods of the maturing process when psychological equilibrium is upset. Situational crises occur when a specific external event upsets one's psychological equilibrium. Adventitious crisis are accidental, uncommon, and unexpected crises with multiple losses and gross environmental changes.

4. Crisis intervention is a brief, here-and-now–oriented, active mode of psychotherapy with the goal of reestablishing psychological equilibrium. On completion of the process of crisis intervention, the patient is returned to at least his precrisis level of functioning.

5. The methodology of crisis intervention includes the steps of assessment, planning, intervention, and evaluation. Data are collected and analyzed, a plan of intervention is made and implemented, and results are evaluated. If goals have not been met, the patient and nurse can go back to the first step and continue through the four phases again.

6. In completing an assessment, the nurse attempts to identify the precipitating event, the patient's previous strengths and coping mechanisms, and the nature and strength of the patient's support systems. She further assesses the patient's needs and the events that threaten those needs, the point at which symptoms appear, and the themes or memories that are verbalized by the patient.

7. Levels of crisis intervention are environmental manipulation, general support, generic approach, and individual approach. Environmental manipulation includes those interventions which directly change the patient's physical or interpersonal situation for the purpose of providing situational support or removing stress. General support includes those interventions which provide the patient with the feeling that the nurse is on his side and will be a helping person. The generic approach includes those interventions which guide patients through a particular known course of a crisis so that an adaptive solution to the crisis will be the outcome. The individual approach includes those interventions which aid a particular patient to achieve an adaptive resolution to this crisis and requires a clear understanding of the patient's specific psychodynamics.

8. Techniques of crisis intervention include abreaction, clarification, suggestion, manipulation, reinforcement of behavior, support of defenses, raising self-esteem, and exploration of solutions.

9. Nurses are in the position to use crisis intervention techniques frequently by virtue of the various settings in which they practice. Settings include all areas of general hospitals, communities, mental health centers, psychiatric hospitals or units, emergency telephone services, and disaster areas. Modalities of crisis intervention used include the individual, family, and group approaches. Educating individuals and society about crises can reduce maladaptation. The nurse is in a position to provide this education on both a small and large scale.

10. Trends in crisis therapy seem to demonstrate continued use and sophistication of techniques. Nurses are involved with crisis therapy in both their direct and indirect services. Roles are growing for nurses as primary caregivers, teachers, consultants, and researchers. Further nursing research is needed so that theory can be better defined operationally. The use of specific techniques and modalities of crisis therapy need study.

▪ REFERENCES ▪

1. Aguilera, D.C., and Messick, J.M.: Crisis intervention: theory and methodology, ed. 5, St. Louis, 1986, The C.V. Mosby Co.
2. American Nurses' Association: Standards of nursing practice, Kansas City, Mo., 1973, The Association.
3. Auerbach, S.M.: Crisis intervention research: methodological considerations and some recent findings. In Cohen, W., Claiborn, W.L., and Specter, G.A., editors: Crisis intervention, New York, 1983, Human Sciences Press, Inc.
4. Bloom, N.D., and Lynch, J.G.: Group work in a hospital setting, Health Soc. Work 4:48, Aug. 1979.
5. Burgess, A.W., and Baldwin, B.A.: Crisis intervention theory and practice, Englewood Cliffs, N.J., 1981, Prentice-Hall.
6. Caplan, G.: Principles of preventive psychiatry, New York, 1964, Basic Books, Inc.
7. Chandler, H.H.: Family crisis intervention: point and counterpoint in the psychosocial revolution, J. Natl. Med. Assoc. 64:211, May 1972.
8. Chen, M.E.: Applying Yalom's principles to crisis work . . . some intriguing results, J. Psychiatr. Nurs. 16:15, June 1978.
9. Crisis intervention programs for disaster victims in smaller communities, Washington, D.C., 1979, Department of Health, Education, and Welfare Pub. No. (A.D.M.) 79-675, U.S. Government Printing Office.
10. Davidson, J., Swartz, M., Krishnan, P.R., and Hammett, E.: A diagnostic and family study of posttraumatic stress syndrome, Am. J. Psychiatry 142:1, Jan. 1985.
11. Dillard, R.G., Auerbach, K.G., and Showalter, A.H.: A parents' program in the intensive care nursery: its relationship to maternal attitudes and expectations, Soc. Work Health Care 5:245, Spring 1980.
12. Donovan, J.M., Bennett, M.J., and McElroy, C.M.: The crisis group—an outcome study, Am. J. Psychiatry 13:906, 1979.
13. Erikson, E.H.: Childhood and society, New York, 1963, W.W. Norton & Co., Inc., Publishers.
14. Erikson, E.H.: Identity, youth and crisis, New York, 1968, W.W. Norton & Co., Inc., Publishers.
15. Frederick, C., and Garrison, J.: Disaster and mental health: an overview, Behav. Today 12:32, Aug. 1981.
16. Friedman, M.J.: Post-Vietnam syndrome: recognition and management, Psychosomatics 22:54, 1981.
17. Gordon, R.H.: Efficacy of a group crisis—counseling program for men who accompany women seeking abortions, Am. J. Community Psychol. 6:239, June 1978.
18. Havighurst, R.J.: Human development and education, New York, 1953, Longman, Inc.
19. Hill, R.: Families under stress, New York, 1949, Harper.
20. Hoff, L.A.: People in crisis: understanding and helping, Menlo Park, Calif., 1984, Addison-Wesley.
21. Imboden, J.B., and Urbaitis, J.C.: Practical psychiatry in medicine, New York, 1978, Appleton-Century-Crofts.
22. Jacobson, G., Strickler, M., and Morley, W.E.: Generic and individual approaches to crisis intervention, Am. J. Public Health 58:339, 1968.
23. King, J.M.: The initial interview: basis for assessment in crisis intervention, Perspect. Psychiatr. Care 9:247, Nov.-Dec. 1971.
24. Langsley, D.G., and Kaplan, D.M.: The treatment of families in crisis, New York, 1968, Grune & Stratton, Inc.
25. Levenberg, S.B., Jenkins, C., and Wendorf, D.J.: Studies in family-oriented crisis intervention with hemodialysis patients, Int. J. Psychiatry Med. 9(1):83, 1978-1979.
26. Lindemann, E.: Symptomatology and management of acute grief, Am. J. Psychiatry 101:141, 1944.
27. McCubbin, H., and Patterson, J.: Family adaptation to crisis. In McCubbin, H., Cauble, A., and Patterson, J., editors: Family, stress, coping, and social support, Springfield, Ill., 1982, Charles C Thomas.
28. Mills, P.: Crisis intervention resource manual, Vermillion, S.D., 1973, Educational Research and Service Center.
29. Mitchell, C.E.: Identifying the hazard: the key to crisis intervention, Am. J. Nurs. 77:1194, 1977.
30. Morley, W.E., Messick, J.M., and Aguilera, D.C.: Crisis paradigms of intervention, J. Psychiatr. Nurs. 5:537, 1967.
31. Quirk, T.R., O'Donohue, S., and Middleton, J.: The perinatal bereavement crisis, J. Nurse Midwife. 24:13, Sept.-Oct. 1979.
32. Rusk, T.N.: Opportunity and technique in crisis psychiatry, Compr. Psychiatry 12:249, May 1971.
33. Shields, L.: Crisis intervention: implications for the nurse, J. Psychiatr. Nurs. 13:37, Sept.-Oct. 1975.
34. Smith, L.L.: Crisis intervention theory and practice, Community Men. Health Rev. 2:5, 1977.
35. Strain, J.J., and Grossman, S.: Psychological care of the mentally ill, New York, 1975, Appleton-Century-Crofts.
36. Strickler, M., and Allgeyer, J.: The crisis group: a new application of crisis theory, Social Work 12:28, 1967.
37. Strickler, M., and LaSor, B.: Concepts of loss in crisis intervention, Ment. Hygiene 54:302, 1970.
38. Sundeen, S.J., et al.: Nurse-client interaction: implementing the nursing process, ed. 3, St. Louis, 1985, The C.V. Mosby Co.
39. Teichman, Y., Spiegel, Y., and Teichman, M.: Crisis intervention with families of servicemen missing in action, Am. J. Community Psychol. 6:315, 1978.
40. Terr, L.C.: Psychic trauma in children: observations following the Chowchilla schoolbus kidnapping, Am. J. Psychiatry 138:14, Jan. 1981.
41. Williams, F.: Intervention in maturational crises, Perspect. Psychiatr. Care 9:240, Nov.-Dec. 1971.

■ ANNOTATED SUGGESTED READINGS ■

*Aguilera, D.C., and Messick, J.M.: Crisis intervention: Theory and methodology, ed. 5, St. Louis, 1986, The C.V. Mosby Co.

This book presents crisis theory and method in a detailed, comprehensive, and thorough manner. Content includes historical development, psychotherapeutic techniques, group therapy concepts, socioeconomic factors affecting intervention, the problem-solving approach, situational and maturational crises, and levels of prevention and trends as they relate to crisis intervention. Paradigms are included to facilitate understanding.

*Brownell, M.J.: The concept of crisis: its utility for nursing, Adv. Nurs. Sci. 6:4, July 1984.

The author explores the varying definitions and uses of the concept of crisis. She then presents a crisis continuum for conceptualizing crisis states. The article is scholarly and provides implications for nursing practice and research.

Burgess, A.W., and Baldwin, B.A.: Crisis intervention theory and practice, Englewood Cliffs, N.J., 1981, Prentice-Hall.

This clinical handbook provides guidance for practice by specifying a typology of six types of crises, and formats for intervention in each type. Many contemporary crisis-producing issues, such as sexual abuse, incest, divorce, mothers going to work, and combat stress are addressed in the typology.

*Burnside, I.M.: Crisis intervention with geriatric hospitalized patients, J. Psychiatr. Nurs. 8:17, March-April 1970.

The author describes her work with elderly hospitalized patients. She presents a guide for crisis intervention with this type of patient, emphasizing the need for grief work.

Caplan, G.: Principles of preventive psychiatry, New York, 1964, Basic Books, Inc.

A classic in psychiatry, this book places a historical perspective on the development of crisis intervention from preventive psychiatry. A public health model is used to explain the approaches of primary, secondary, and tertiary prevention of mental disorders.

*Chen, M.E.: Applying Yalom's principles to crisis work: some intriguing results, J. Psychiatr. Nurs. 16:15, June, 1978.

Written for the serious group therapist, this article translates some conventional group therapy principles into a crisis group theoretical framework. The literature on crisis groups is reviewed, followed by a description of an open-ended crisis group that uses Yalom's process-focused interventions. Theory is clearly defined and illustrated with clinical examples.

Cohen, L.H., Claiborn, W.L., and Specter, editors: Crisis intervention, New York, 1983, Human Sciences Press, Inc.

Written for the academician, researcher, or anyone interested in scientific information, this book presents material about crisis theory, technique, training, and research. It is written in a scholarly manner, presenting numerous citations on which its tenets are founded.

Crisis intervention programs for disaster victims in smaller communities, Washington, D.C., 1979, Department of Health, Education, and Welfare Pub. No. (A.D.M.) 79-675, U.S. Government Printing Office.

Although written for persons interested in the planning and delivery of disaster-related crisis intervention services, this monograph provides a wealth of information on the entire field of disasters and the use of crisis intervention to assist disaster victims.

Getz, W., et al.: Fundamentals of crisis counseling, Lexington, Mass., 1974, Lexington Books, D.C. Heath & Co.

This general text about crisis intervention includes historical development, definitions, goals, techniques, interviewing stages, telephone crisis, and crisis with minority groups. It is useful in that it includes many clinical examples and verbatim notes.

*Hall, J., and Weaver, B.: Nursing of families in crisis, Philadelphia, 1974, J.B. Lippincott Co.

This is a compilation of articles written by nurses dealing with families in crisis. The text attempts to increase the reader's understanding of crisis theory as it applies to nursing situations and provide examples of strategies and tactics that may be useful in helping families resolve crises. A variety of nursing practice settings are presented.

*Harrison, D.: Nurses and disasters, J. Psychosoc. Nurs. 19(2): 34, 1981.

This brief paper reviews some of the acute psychiatric problems that can result from disaster experiences. Effective use of nurses in these emergencies is also described.

Hoff, L.S.: People in crisis: understanding and helping, Menlo Park, Calif., 1984, Addison-Wesley.

In addition to presenting the theory and practice of crisis intervention, this book stresses the social and cultural contexts that influence that theory and practice. Crisis intervention approaches described include individual, group, family, and community networking.

Jacobson, G., Strickler, M., and Morley, W.E.: Generic and individual approaches to crisis intervention, Am. J. Public Health 58:339, 1968.

The authors describe the nature of crisis and present two possible approaches in crisis intervention, the general and individual approaches. Circumstances under which each approach is selected are identified, and clinical examples of each method are presented.

*Lancaster, J., and Berkovsky, D.: An ecological framework for crisis intervention, J. Psychiatr. Nurs. 16:17, Mar. 1978.

This article was written for the nurse educator. The authors describe how to help baccalaureate nursing students use an ecological framework for crisis intervention with children placed in an institution for dependent and neglected children. Both theory and clinical examples are presented, making this article a useful one for students too.

Lindemann, E.: Symptomatology and management of acute grief, Am. J. Psychiatry 101:141, 1944.

This article describes an early study of the grieving process. Stages of grief are identified and normal and morbid grief reactions are differentiated. The use of crisis intervention to guide grief toward a favorable outcome is explored.

McCubbin, H., and Figley, C., editors: Stress and the family, vol. 1 and 2, New York, 1983, Brunner/Mazel, Inc.

---

*Asterisk indicates nursing reference.

This book is written for those interested in understanding a family systems approach to stress, crisis, and adaptation. Its two volumes comprehensively describe how families cope with both time-limited and more prolonged stress such as in natural disasters, family transitions, and chronic illness in a child.

*Mitchell, C.E.: Identifying the hazard: the key to crisis intervention, Am. J. Nurs. 77:1194, 1977.

This article concentrates on identifying the precipitating or stressful event from which a crisis develops. The author tells in detail what clues to look for and how to use the clues to intervene effectively.

*Narayan, S.M., and Joslin, D.J.: Crisis theory and intervention: a critique of the medical model and proposal of a holistic nursing model, Adv. Nurs. Sci. 2:27, July 1980.

These authors provide an alternative to the disease prevention orientation of crisis intervention, in describing a holistic model that emphasizes the alteration of health potential as one strives for a high level of wellness. The medical and holistic nursing models of crisis are compared both theoretically and in implications for intervention.

National Institute of Mental Health: Crisis intervention programs for disaster victims in smaller communities, Rockville, Md., 1979, U.S. Department of Health, Education, and Welfare.

This government monograph provides both theoretical and practical knowledge that can help in the planning and implementing of disaster-related mental health programs that are efficiently and effectively organized. Although primarily focused on the rural area, its recommendations have a wider interest and applicability as crisis intervention programs for various disaster victims.

National Institute of Mental Health: Training manual for human service workers in major disasters, Rockville, Md., 1978, U.S. Department of Health, Education, and Welfare.

This highly recommended manual uses crisis intervention theory and is a training instrument to help people cope after a disaster strikes. Its excellent coverage includes phases of a disaster, key concepts, community relationships, selection and education of human service workers, special risk groups, self-awareness sessions, and identification of available resources.

Parad, H., editor: Crisis intervention: selected readings, New York, 1965, Family Service Association of America.

This compilation of readings presents a range of theoretical formulations of crisis theory, and shows the way crisis intervention is used in practice. It applies crisis theory to various practice settings and a number of commonly encountered stressful situations affecting the individual, group, and family. This is a highly recommended reading.

Strickler, M., and Allgeyer, J.: The crisis group: a new application of crisis theory, Soc. Work 12:28, 1967.

This article describes a study in which individuals in crisis were treated in group therapy. The authors claim most patients made progress in the crisis group modality and explain theoretically how the progress occurred. A clinical example is given to further illustrate the concepts.

*Wallace, M.A., and Morley, W.E.: Teaching crisis intervention, Am. J. Nurs. 70:1484, 1970.

Written for the nurse educator, this article describes problems that evolve in clinical supervision of graduate nursing students learning to practice crisis intervention. Both initial and advanced problem patterns are identified and solutions are described.

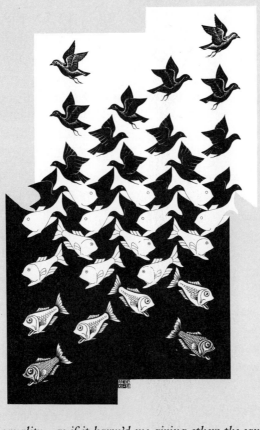

*Of equality—as if it harm'd me giving others the same
chances and rights as myself—as if it were not
indispensible to my own rights that others possess the same.*

Walt Whitman, Thought

CHAPTER 11

REHABILITATIVE PSYCHIATRIC NURSING

LEARNING OBJECTIVES

After studying this chapter, the student should be able to:

- define tertiary prevention and psychiatric rehabilitation.

- discuss concepts relative to an individual's rehabilitative nursing needs.

- identify four trends in the development of psychosocial treatment.

- describe stressors experienced by the chronically mentally ill.

- describe the concepts of primary and secondary gain as they pertain to psychiatric rehabilitation.

- analyze the readiness of a patient for discharge from a treatment program.

- identify and discuss five factors relative to assessment of the family's resources for assisting the patient.

- describe and evaluate community resources relative to the needs of the recovering psychiatric patient.

- analyze the concept of stigma as it operates in the community.

- discuss the role of the nurse in interaction with the needs of the recovering patient.

- identify and discuss eight principles of psychiatric rehabilitation.

- compare and contrast several models for the provision of rehabilitative psychiatric services.

- develop specific behavioral goals for rehabilitative psychiatric nursing care in conjunction with the patient and family.

- describe group interventions that are appropriate to tertiary prevention, including the nurse's role with self-help groups.

- discuss nursing interventions that are directed toward meeting the needs of families.

- develop a mental health education plan relevant to tertiary prevention.

- identify directions for future nursing research.

- select appropriate readings for further study.

- analyze the importance of nursing intervention at a community level, including mental health education, membership in advocacy groups, networking, and political action.

- describe the current status of tertiary prevention program evaluation.

- identify suggested readings for further study.

The public health model of prevention specifies three levels of preventive health care activity: primary, secondary, and tertiary. **Primary prevention,** as discussed in Chapter 9, is directed toward decreasing the incidence of a health problem by intervening before a potential disruption occurs. **Secondary prevention** is directed toward intervention to decrease the prevalence of a health problem by intervening promptly when illness occurs to limit its severity and duration. This is the traditional area of concentration for psychiatric nurses and is the subject of much of the content of this book. **Tertiary prevention** is the limitation of disability related to an episode of illness. It is the subject of this chapter.

Any episode of illness involves potential lasting change in the individual's level of functioning. The more serious the health problem, the greater is the possibility of a serious interference with the individual's ability to function productively in the community. Episodes of illness that involve hospitalization are generally more disruptive to the person's life-style and require a greater readjustment as part of the recovery process. Nurses who are providers of care at the secondary prevention level in institutional settings must maintain an awareness of the total range of present and potential patient care needs. Tertiary prevention usually begins prior to discharge from the hospital.

Caplan[15] defines the goal of tertiary prevention as one of reducing the rate in a community of defective functioning resulting from mental disorder. However this definition includes the other levels of prevention. He adds that common usage usually limits the meaning to reduction of the rate of residual defect.[15] This is the sense in which it will be used in this chapter.

Rehabilitation

Tertiary prevention is operationalized by the performance of activities identified as *rehabilitation*. Rehabilitation is the process of enabling the individual to return to his highest possible level of functioning. The goal is usually to match or exceed the pre-illness functional level. This may be achieved by capitalizing on strengths, relearning old skills, or learning new skills, depending on the effects of the health care problem and the person's response to it. Anthony identifies the goal of psychiatric rehabilitation as follows: "The goal of the psychiatrically disabled helpee is to perform the physical, intellectual and emotional skills needed to live, learn and work in her or his particular community, given the least amount of support necessary from agents of the helping professions."[2:30]

Like primary prevention, the tertiary level of prevention was largely ignored until the advent of community mental health programs in the 1960s. The development of effective treatment methodologies for psychosocial disruptions allowed mental health care providers to begin to think about the future of former patients who were able to reenter the community. Medication and psychotherapy, in particular, were instrumental in assisting patients to develop positive interpersonal relationships. Hospitalization was avoided for some patients who were able to continue to function in the community with the help of intensive intervention.

Psychiatric rehabilitation was given further impetus as attention turned to the civil rights of psychiatric patients. The right to treatment in the least restrictive setting was established in the courts and resulted in close scrutiny of people who had been hospitalized, in some cases for many years. As people were returned to communities, it became obvious that many of them lacked the skills they needed to function adequately. Scandals erupted in many areas as discharged psychiatric patients gravitated to shabby boarding houses, soup kitchens, and skid row. Unaccustomed to managing their daily affairs, many were victimized by people they encountered on the streets. Many returned to the hospital for brief admissions, creating a "revolving door" between the hospital and the community. Others became inmates of other kinds of institutions, especially jails and nursing homes, as they demonstrated their inability to cope.

The process of moving long-term hospital patients to the community is called **deinstitutionalization.** For this process to succeed, patients must be prepared to function at least minimally well in the community. This has become an important focus of psychiatric rehabilitation. However, all patients who have received treatment for a disruption in mental or emotional function-

ing are potentially in need of rehabilitative services. This chapter will focus on the nursing process as applied to psychiatric rehabilitation for any degree of residual impairment. The care of the chronically mentally ill person is discussed in greater depth in Chapter 34.

Psychiatric rehabilitation approaches have also been termed psychosocial treatments. Heinrichs[23] has identified four trends in the development of psychosocial treatment: (1) psychoeducation and the medical model, (2) working with families, (3) group therapy, and (4) social skills–social learning theory.

■ Psychoeducation and the medical model

The traditional medical approach to a patient with a physical illness includes identification of the problem by naming a diagnosis, telling the person what to expect from the illness, and discussing treatment alternatives. In the past, people with mental illnesses were discouraged from asking questions about their problems, leading to the development of misconceptions and fear. As more has been learned about the probable biological origin of the major illnesses, there has been more willingness on the part of mental health care providers to teach patients and families. Heinrichs[23:126] states,

An important function of psychoeducational work is to identify hitherto unspoken fears and to correct myths and prejudices by providing basic information in a context of respect and hope.

This is in contrast to the approach labeled "mystification" by Banes.[9] She relates this to a lack of education of patients about their illnesses, treatments, and medications.

■ Working with families

The professional has assumed the role of consultant to the family. This is in contrast to the suspicious and blaming stance that had characterized provider attitudes toward families in the past. Families can then be partners in providing care.

■ Group therapy

For many severely mentally disabled people, group treatment is more effective than individual therapy. Positive aspects of the group include an opportunity for ongoing contact with others, consensual validation of perceptions and an allowance for varying levels of activity and intensity of participation.

■ Social skills–social learning theory

This theoretical framework is based on a behavioral approach. It involves the teaching of specific living skills that the patient is expected to need in order to survive in a community setting. At the present time, research is needed to test the efficacy of this approach and the generalizability of skills learned outside of the real life setting.

Bennett[12] discusses the conflict between the needs of society and the needs of the mentally ill person. Closing hospital wards leads to loss of jobs for hospital staff. Community living expenses must be met through tax revenues. Taxpayers may object to this use of their funds. Families may have been relieved by the decision to hospitalize a troubled member. They may not be eager to take him back. He recommends that the resolution to this dilemma may rest in study of the needs of patients and of the characteristics of hospital and community environments.[12] Therapeutic and damaging elements in both settings should be identified and this information used to develop more helpful patient care settings.

Rehabilitative psychiatric nursing must be studied in the context of the person and his social system. This requires a focus by the nurse on each of three elements: the individual, the family, and the community. This chapter has been designed to discuss each of these elements of the social system relative to the phases of the nursing process. Relevant nursing interventions will be identified at each phase.

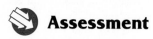 **Assessment**

■ **The individual**

Assessment of the person's need for rehabilitation begins at the time of the first contact between the nurse and the patient. A comprehensive psychiatric nursing assessment, as described in Chapters 5 and 6, is directed toward obtaining information that will enable the nurse to assist the patient to achieve his maximum possible level of functioning. This is, of course, the definition of rehabilitation. Nurses are expected to identify and reinforce the patient's strengths as one means of assisting him to cope with his weaknesses. This, too, is basic to the concept of rehabilitation. Thus good nursing care is really synonymous with rehabilitative nursing care.

The nursing model of health-illness phenomena (Fig. 11-1) may be applied within the context of rehabilitative nursing practice. It is particularly important for the nurse to identify stressors that may interfere with the patient's adjustment to a health-promoting life-style. The Holmes and Rahe[24] approach to rating life stressors has been presented in Chapter 3. Baker[8] and associates have questioned whether this list of stressors is appropriate for subpopulations, such as the chronically men-

tally ill. They conducted a study to identify life stressors that are relevant to this group. In order to evaluate the relative impact of stressors, they asked study participants to rate life events according to two sets of factors.

The first set of variables relates to the **valence** of the event. It may be either *positive* and growth-enhancing or *negative* and psychologically distressing. The other set focuses on the **source** of the event. A *pawn* event is not under the control of the individual. An *origin* event is initiated and therefore controlled by the person. If these parameters are paired, it is possible to hypothesize potentially more distressing events as one moves from a positive/origin combination to negative/pawn. Although the investigators did not report this type of analysis, they did find a concurrence between positive and origin and negative and pawn events. In other words, if an event was viewed as positive, it was more likely that the subject had initiated it. Pawn events were experienced as more distressing. Table 11-1 summarizes the major life events identified in this study, along with the source and valence ratings for each event. Nurses need to be aware of patients' perceptions of their experiences. Research provides guidelines for this. It is also essential to validate each individual's response to significant changes in his life.

When conducting the initial assessment of the patient, the nurse needs to think beyond the limits of her own patient care setting to try to anticipate the nature of the patient's other contacts with the health care system. In hospitals, this process is discharge planning and the need is obvious. However, nurses in community settings should also expect patients to progress to other levels of care. Although some people will need long-term maintenance outpatient care, many will be discharged from psychiatric care.

■ **PRIMARY AND SECONDARY GAIN.** To assess the patient's readiness to move from one level of care to another, the nurse must understand the concepts of primary and secondary gain. **Primary gain** refers to the individual's efforts to cope with the predisposing and precipitating stressors. For instance, a person who feels compelled to wash his hands repetitively experiences a reduction in anxiety as a result of the behavior. The decrease in anxiety is the primary gain. Nursing care at the secondary prevention level focuses on interventions to assist the patient to develop healthier ways of accomplishing the primary gain.

Secondary gain refers to the other advantages that are associated with the sick role. In the American culture, sick people are expected to be incapacitated with limited ability to meet their own needs. Therefore they expect to receive help and attention from others. In return, they are expected to cooperate with a plan of

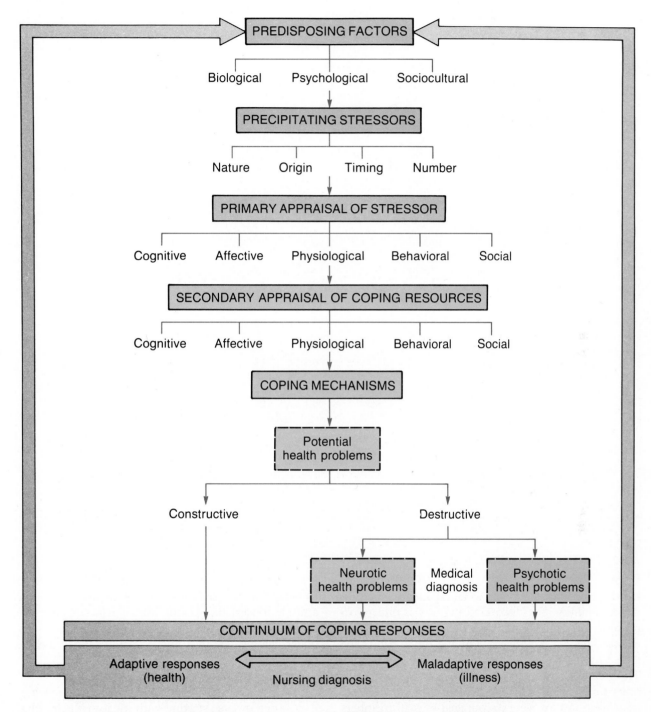

Fig. 11-1. Nursing model of health-illness phenomena.

care, indicating motivation to become well again. The extra attention and nurturing that is given to sick people can decrease the motivation to get better. Most people experience this even with a minor illness. A cold provides an excuse to stay home from school or work, sleep late, eat favorite foods, and indulge in relaxing activities. Even when one feels below par, there is pleasure asso-

ciated with the release from daily responsibilities and a reluctance to resume them. The problem is magnified for the person who requires health care because of difficulties in coping with the stresses of daily life. Patient status can protect the person from the need to confront anxiety-provoking situations.

Even when more effective coping mechanisms have

TABLE 11-1

OVERALL OCCURRENCE, SOURCE, AND VALENCE OF LIFE EVENTS REPORTED BY CLIENTS SURVEYED BY BAKER ET AL.

Major categories of life events	Overall occur-rence*	Source			Valence		
		Origin	Pawn	Un-known	Positive	Negative	Un-known
Changes in structured daily activities (N = 97)	19.8	77.3	21.6	1.0	37.1	8.2	54.7
Changes in residence (N = 64)	13.0	82.8	17.2	0	35.9	7.8	56.3
Changes in physical health (N = 50)	10.2	4.0	96.0	0	4.0	84.0	12.0
Changes in finances (N = 49)	10.0	20.4	73.5	6.1	22.4	34.7	42.9
Hospitalization (N = 47)	9.6	0	100	0	12.8	23.4	63.9
Changes in family relation-ships (N = 46)	9.4	50.0	43.5	6.5	23.9	21.7	54.3
Changes in interpersonal rela-tionships with nonrelatives (N = 46)	9.4	73.9	23.9	2.2	45.7	17.4	37.0
Changes in relationship with spouse (N = 19)	3.9	57.9	36.8	6.3	10.5	15.8	73.7
Other events (N = 73)†	14.9	35.6	61.6	2.7	27.4	35.6	37.0
Total	100.00	47.7	50.1	2.2	26.9	26.5	46.6

From Baker, F., et al.: Hosp. Community Psychiatry **36**:299, March 1985. Copyright 1985, The American Psychiatric Association. Reprinted with permission.
*Percent of 491 life events
†Comprises the nine categories containing the smallest number of events (changes in personal habits, operations, death of significant other, holiday or vacation, change in environmental conditions of current residence, notable personal achievement, legal problems, changes in transportation resources, and miscellaneous events)

been developed, it can be frightening to test them in a situation that was intolerable in the past. Bachmann[5] has described her experience as an expatient reentering the community. She discovered that it was difficult to relate to her old friends because of their difficulty understanding her experience. On the other hand, she lacked the self-confidence to reach out to new people. The greatest source of support for her was contact with other former patients. She comments that these significant relationships were discouraged by staff members who viewed them as a way of perpetuating illness. This emphasizes the need for the nurse to try to understand the patient's world and to respect his needs as he sees them. Bachmann also found the community boring compared to the hospital and began to develop a life pattern of working and sleeping. Nurses who are involved in busy community and family lives may fail to recognize the contrast that the patient experiences between the hospital and the community.

The resistance that is associated with secondary gain is sometimes thought to be a purposeful manipulation to avoid the resumption of responsibility. A punitive attitude toward the patient who is reluctant to move ahead is not helpful. The person needs support and understanding. Helpful nursing interventions include the following:

1. Planning with the patient to resume activities one by one, starting with the least threatening
2. Role playing difficult situations before attempting to confront them
3. Accompanying the patient into the community to offer support if needed
4. Providing honest and timely feedback about the patient's attempts to become reengaged in his environment
5. Advocating for the patient's needs with family members and community agencies

Over an extended period of time, the reluctance to reenter the community tends to grow gradually. When a person is hospitalized for months or years, the handicap that Wing[47] has referred to as "institutionalism" develops. This is characterized by social withdrawal and resistance to leaving the hospital, even when the surroundings are barely adequate. The institutional environment becomes comfortable because it is predictable and few demands are made. Some patients become angry or more symptomatic when they are being encouraged to move to the community. Some have hypothesized that this response of social withdrawal is a result of the lack of stimulation in the environment; others believe that it is a behavior related to severe mental illness, usually chronic schizophrenia. Although it is important that the cause be identified through research, in any case the nurse needs to work to assist the patient to develop trusting and caring relationships.

Discharge from an inpatient or partial hospitalization program should be based on careful interdisciplinary assessment of the patient's level of functioning. Gallagher[21] defines patient discharge as a process of social negotiation. He has reviewed the literature and identified other factors that frequently appear to determine readiness for discharge:

1. **Age.** Young patients are more likely to be discharged.
2. **Length of stay.** Potential for discharge decreases as the length of stay in the program increases.
3. **Life circumstances.** Housing and employment in the community increase the likelihood of discharge. Employment is a more important factor for men. Marriage, implying available housing, is more significant with women.
4. **Family wishes.** Family request facilitates release.
5. **Patient request for release.**

Although the success of the negotiation process and the influence of life factors may in reality determine discharge, nurses should strive to assess the patient's living skills and interpret this assessment to the patient, family, and interdisciplinary team. Anthony[2] has developed a matrix (Table 11-2) of the skills required for successful functioning in the community. He describes the physical, emotional, and intellectual components of the skills required for living, learning, and working. The nurse may use these examples in conjunction with the patient to identify the patient's strengths, establish goals, and set priorities for skill development. Use of such a model provides a rational basis for assessing the patient's readiness to function productively in the community. It also provides objective information that can be shared with the mental health care providers who will work with the patient in the agency to which he is transferred.

Nurses who work in community settings must also be concerned about the relevance of the given treatment to the needs of the patient. In a study of 99 long-term patients of a community mental health center, Spivack[41] and associates found that the patients' focus was on social interaction and health status rather than on work and task accomplishment. The investigators questioned whether the issues emphasized in the treatment setting would assist the patients to learn to function successfully in the community. They recommended the adoption of a skills development model to prepare patients for vocational settings.

■ The family

The image of the isolated chronically mentally ill person who returns to a community where he has no connections has been widely publicized in recent years. However, the majority of mentally ill people are involved with their families and will have frequent contact with family members while they are in the community.[30] Therefore family resources must be assessed when a rehabilitation plan is being developed. Unfortunately, an adversary relationship frequently evolves between the patient's family and health care providers. The family may be viewed as the cause of the problem or as resistant to the treatment plan. Family members have a right to provide input to the treatment plan. They can identify potential problem areas. If their support is enlisted, they can be helpful in enhancing the patient's compliance with the plan. Hatfield[22] describes the needs of family members. She encourages mental health care providers to build alliances with families. She conducted a survey of 89 families of schizophrenic patients. She was able to identify the following patient behaviors or results of behaviors that are most disturbing to families:

1. Tension related to unpredictable behavior
2. Irregular sleep patterns that keep other family members awake as well
3. Mealtime disruptions
4. Argumentativeness
5. Negative relationships with siblings
6. Marital discord between parents

Although one might expect families to be angry at the patient for creating a disrupted family life or guilty for possibly playing a role in the problems, Hatfield elicited more feelings of grief and depression. If anger was present, it was usually directed at fate or the system rather than the patient.[22]

TABLE 11-2

POTENTIAL SKILLED ACTIVITIES NEEDED TO ACHIEVE THE GOAL OF PSYCHIATRIC REHABILITATION

Physical	Emotional	Intellectual
Living skills		
Personal hygiene	Human relations	Money management
Physical fitness	Self-control	Use of community resources
Use of public transportation	Selective reward	Goal setting
Cooking	Stigma reduction	Problem development
Shopping	Problem solving	
Cleaning	Conversational skills	
Sports participation		
Using recreational facilities		
Learning skills		
Being quiet	Speech making	Reading
Paying attention	Question asking	Writing
Staying seated	Volunteering answers	Arithmetic
Observing	Following directions	Study skills
Punctuality	Asking for directions	Hobby activities
	Listening	Typing
Working skills		
Punctuality	Job interviewing	Job qualifying
Use of job tools	Job decision making	Job seeking
Job strength	Human relations	Specific job tasks
Job transportation	Self-control	
Specific job tasks	Job keeping	
	Specific job tasks	

From Anthony, W.A.: Principles of psychiatric rehabilitation, © 1980, University Park Press, Baltimore.

Doll[20] also conducted a survey of significant others of psychiatric patients. Whereas the Hatfield group was mostly upper middle class, the Doll group of 125 respondents was mostly lower middle and lower class. The findings of the two studies were quite consistent. The Doll group also denied shame or guilt connected to the patient's problem. These families were also able to accept some degree of deviant behavior, although there was a limit to their tolerance. High deviance did eventually lead to a decrease in acceptance of the patient. These families expressed the fear that there would be little or no change in the patient's condition. This was expressed as a feeling of being trapped.

Leavitt[31] interviewed the families of 16 patients who were being discharged from an inpatient psychiatric setting. They were all first-admission patients with an average length of stay of 1 month and 9 days. She found that the families were eager to discuss their responses to impending discharge with a receptive person. In general, the families were not prepared for the discharge of the hospitalized member. Leavitt identified several possible contributory factors relative to this response:

1. Pessimism about the future related to their opinion that the patient had not recovered
2. Lack of recognition of the hospital as a resource to the family
3. Lack of instruction and anticipatory guidance in how to respond to the patient's behavior
4. Failure to view themselves as a resource and as part of the treatment team
5. Limited communication with the staff concerning their perception of the patient's progress; inability to disagree with the staff's plan to discharge the patient

6. Absence of an empathic approach to the family by the staff

The nurse's assessment of the family should incorporate the growing body of knowledge about family responses to mental illness and about their needs. Supportive families need to be supported in turn so their resources are not depleted by the constant demands of the patient. Walsh[45] has identified factors that appear to be related to successful living at home for schizophrenic patients. These are summarized in Table 11-3.

For some patients the emotional climate of the family to which they return can have a significant effect on their adjustment. Wing[46] has noted that schizophrenic patients have more problems when they are members of a hostile, critical, or overinvolved family. Vaughn and Leff[44] have found that schizophrenics have recurrences of their illnesses more frequently when there is a high level of expressed emotion in the family. These families need help to understand that intense emotion, either positive or negative, raises the patient's anxiety level. The emotional climate influences nonschizophrenic patients as well. Oversolicitousness reflects family members' insecurity and their concern that they might inadvertently cause a relapse. Protectiveness can be stifling to a patient who is striving to be independent and resume control of his own life.

On the other hand, rejection of the patient may also be a problem. Families sometimes view mental illness as a characterological weakness that can be overcome by their exertion of moral effort. This type of familial attitude may result in guilt on the part of the patient who believes that he has disappointed his significant others. Guilt leads to increased anxiety and decreased self-esteem. These are conditions that interfere with the achievement of a high level of functioning.

Reintegration of a patient into the family requires a readjustment of roles, particularly if a family member has been hospitalized for several weeks or months. In the normal family structure, functions are distributed among family members. The combination of functions assigned to a family member constitutes his role in the family. When a member is absent, others must perform his essential functions. If the absence is brief, the family structure readily reverts to its usual pattern when the missing member returns. However, if the member is away for a prolonged time, the family reorganization assumes an aspect of permanence. The members become emotionally attached to the new structure and may be reluctant to return to the earlier organization. Clinical example 11-1 illustrates this problem.

The P family situation is not an unusual one. The structure of the health care system with the discontinuity

TABLE 11-3
FACTORS THAT HELP OR HINDER A SCHIZOPHRENIC PATIENT'S ADJUSTMENT TO LIFE IN A FAMILY SETTING

Factors conducive to success	Factors not conducive to success
Fairly high functional level; friends; social activities.	Disruptive to family routine
No younger siblings who are adversely affected	Siblings frightened; resentful
Accepting, noncritical family	Family critical, judgmental
Relaxed family milieu	Family life revolves around mentally ill member
Use of outside support group	No outside support group

between home and hospital leads to problems such as theirs. Transitional services such as predischarge family counseling and postdischarge home visiting would have detected the potential problem and assisted the family to cope with the role changes that occurred. Family counseling assisted them to understand the reasons for their behavior. It only took a few sessions to help them reach a state of family equilibrium because the family was basically sound. Longer term intensive family therapy is often needed when the family system is seriously disturbed.

The nurse who is assessing the family as part of a rehabilitation plan should include the following areas:

1. Family structure, including developmental stage, roles, responsibilities, norms, and values
2. Family attitudes toward the mentally ill member
3. The emotional climate of the family
4. The social supports that are available to the family, including extended family, friends, financial support, religious involvement, and community contacts
5. The family's understanding of the patient's problem and the plan of care

Some of this information may be obtained by collaboration with the social worker. However, it is still a

Ms. P was a 47-year-old woman who was hospitalized in the psychiatric ward of a general hospital following a suicide attempt. Her medical diagnosis was a major depressive episode. She gradually responded to interpersonal intervention and antidepressant medication and after 4 weeks felt well enough to return home.

The P family consisted of Mr. and Ms. P and their three children, a 16-year-old daughter and 12- and 10-year-old sons. The family was frightened and very concerned when Ms. P attempted suicide. The children worried about whether their behavior had caused their mother's depression. Mr. P spent a great deal of time reassuring them. He was more actively involved in the family than usual because he was the only available parent. He had to supervise the children's daily activities, assign chores, and referee their quarrels. He discovered that he liked getting to know his children better.

Lisa, the oldest child and only daughter, assumed many of her mother's household responsibilities. She cooked, organized the cleaning, and supervised her brothers when her father was away. She enjoyed her new adult relationship with her father as they discussed household plans and problems with the younger children. During visits to the hospital, she became reluctant to tell her mother very much about what was happening at home.

When Ms. P returned home, everyone seemed happy and relieved. However, when she went into the kitchen to start dinner, Mr. P and Lisa insisted that she rest. She accepted this and was glad to see that Lisa was so capable. She also felt a bit guilty that her daughter had been required to take on so many extra duties. As Ms. P began to take over her household responsibilities, she found that she was frequently in conflict with Lisa, who would criticize her or her work. In addition, she felt shut out of the new relationship between Mr. P and the children. Because of her recent illness, she questioned whether her feelings were based in reality or if she was again becoming depressed. Fortunately, Ms. P discussed her dilemma with her nurse-therapist in the outpatient clinic who arranged for family counseling.

nursing responsibility to be available and accessible to the family. This includes regular planned contacts with the family and inclusion of the family as part of the treatment team.

■ The community

The community at large exerts a significant influence on the rehabilitation of its mentally ill members. Mental health professionals have a unique role in the community because they are simultaneously community members and advocates of the mentally ill. It can be difficult for patients and their families to demand that the community provide adequate services. Care providers, including nurses, can and should assume a leadership role in assessing the adequacy and effectiveness of existing community resources and in recommending changes.

Nurses in all treatment settings need to become familiar with the agencies in the community that provide services to patients. Most communities have a directory of social and medical services that can be consulted for basic information, such as location, type, and cost of the services provided. Most agencies serve a population that comes primarily from a particular geographical area, such as one part of a city, or in a rural area, perhaps one or several counties. As the nurse works with that population, she will become more familiar with other agencies that are involved with the same people. Nurses should pay attention to patients' evaluations of the agencies from which they receive services. This information helps to identify agencies that are responsive and helpful as opposed to those which are difficult for patients to approach.

Personal contact with other community agencies can be very useful as part of a community assessment. This may be accomplished by arranging an appointment with an agency staff member. However, a more realistic picture of an agency's services can be obtained by accompanying a patient who is requesting services to the agency. This allows the nurse to see how the agency responds to the patient and how the patient handles his affairs in the community. The nurse can also provide emotional support to the patient if he is insecure about approaching a new situation. The nurse should identify herself to the staff of the agency and explain that she is accompanying the patient and also would like to learn more about the services that are offered. Collaborative relationships between mental health care providers and community agencies are absolutely essential if rehabilitation is to succeed.

There are a wide range of services that need to be provided to patients as part of the tertiary prevention system. Those which are directed toward basic needs include provisions for shelter; food, clothing, and household management; income and financial support;

TABLE 11-4

COMPREHENSIVE ARRAY OF SERVICES AND OPPORTUNITIES FOR CHRONICALLY MENTALLY ILL PERSONS

Basic needs/opportunities	Special needs/opportunities

Shelter

Protected (with health, rehabilitative, or social services provided on site)
Hospital
Nursing Home
Intermediate-care facility
Crisis facility
Semi-independent (linked to services)
Family home
Group home
Cooperative apartment
Foster care home
Emergency housing facility
Other board and care home
Independent apartment/home (access to services)

Food, clothing, and household management

Fully provided meals
Food purchase/preparation assistance
Access to food stamps
Homemaker service

Income/financial support

Access to entitlements
Employment

Meaningful activities

Work opportunities
Recreation
Education
Religious/spiritual
Human/social interaction

Mobility/transportation

General medical services

Physician assessment and care
Nursing assessment and care
Dentist assessment and care
Physical/occupational therapy
Speech hearing therapy
Nutrition counseling
Medication counseling
Home health services

Mental health services

Acute treatment services
Crisis stabilization
Diagnosis and assessment
Medication monitoring (psychoactive)
Self-medication training
Psychotherapies
Hospitalization: acute and long-term care

Habilitation and rehabilitation

Social/recreational skills development
Life skills development
Leisure time activities

Vocational

Prevocational assessment counseling
Sheltered work opportunities
Transitional employment
Job development and placement

Social services

Family support
Community support assistance
Housing and milieu management
Legal services
Entitlement assistance

Integrative services

Client identification and outreach
Individual assessment and service planning
Case service and resource management
Advocacy and community organization
Community information
Education and support

From Department of Health and Human Services Steering Committee on the Chronically Mentally Ill: Toward a national plan for the chronically mentally ill, Pub. No. (ADM)81-1077, Washington, D.C., 1981, U.S. Government Printing Office.

meaningful activities; and mobility and transportation.[19] Other services provide for special needs that may differ from one patient to the next, such as general medical services, mental health services, habilitation and rehabilitation programs, vocational services, and social services.[19] A third group of services are integrative, with the purpose of coordinating the system. These include patient identification and outreach, individual assessment and service planning, case service and resource management, advocacy and community organization, community information, and education and support.[19] This overview of a community service system was developed by the Steering Committee on the Chronically Mentally Ill of the United States Department of Health and Human Services. It is described in greater detail in Table 11-4. Although the plan was developed with a focus on the chronically mentally ill, it is comprehensive and may be used to assess the range of services available to patients with all types of mental health care needs.

These services may be provided in a variety of settings. Table 11-5 identifies the types of settings in which mental health care services might be provided according to the level of care that is needed.

■ **STIGMA.** It is important that an adequate number and type of services be available in the community. However, there is another aspect of community life that is more difficult to assess accurately and to deal with than that of service provision. This is the degree to which there is stigma attached to mental illness. According to Gallagher,[21] *stigma* was a term used by the Greeks to refer to body signs that indicated something negative about the person's worth. Today the stigma is attached to the behavior and does not relate to physical signs. A response to mental illness that is based on stigma is irrational and emotional. For this reason it is particularly difficult to change. Stigma is closely related to prejudice. Cumming and Cumming[17] found that student nurses tended to attribute mental illness to poor

TABLE 11-5

TYPICAL SETTINGS FOR PROVIDING SERVICE CLUSTERS

Acute treatment	Residential treatment	Rehabilitation	Psychosocial support
Housing setting			
Apartment/home (on site)	Public psychiatric hospital	Family	Family
Family (on site)	Nursing homes	Halfway house	Apartment
Foster family	Veterans hospital	Cooperative apartment (transitional)	Congregate housing (long term)
Crisis hostel	Forensic unit at public psychiatric hospital		Board and care home
Respite care home	Community forensic unit		Lodge
Emergency housing			Foster care home
General hospital			
Public psychiatric hospital			
Private psychiatric hospital			
Community mental health center inpatient unit			
Service setting			
Work		Social club	Social club
Telephone hotline		Psychosocial rehabilitation center	Psychosocial rehabilitation center
Other housing and hospital settings previously listed		Sheltered workshop	Sheltered workshop
		Industry setting	Community mental health center outpatient services
		Community college	Outpatient clinic
		Community mental health center outpatient services	Day treatment program
		Outpatient clinic	
		Day treatment program	

From Department of Health and Human Services Steering Committee on the Chronically Mentally Ill: Toward a national plan for the chronically mentally ill, Pub. No. (ADM)81-1077, Washington, D.C., 1981, U.S. Government Printing Office.

heredity or weak character. Although their landmark study of the effect of community education on attitudes toward the mentally ill was done in the 1950s, attitudes have changed little since then.

Gallagher[21] cites the contribution of the media to the perpetuation of stigma. Headlines always highlight the psychiatric history of a person who commits a crime. The positive achievements of rehabilitated formerly mentally ill people are seldom newsworthy. It would be rare, indeed, to see a headline stating "Child Saved from Burning House by Former Mental Patient." Television also contributes to the problem. Mental illness is portrayed as being a primary cause of violent behavior with the corollary that the mentally ill are always violent. This syllogistic message is destructive to the efforts of discharged patients to become productive community members. Banes[9] speaks of a process of "mentalism," in which a person's feelings are invalidated by labeling them as "sick." Patients are then viewed as "sick, incapable, and irresponsible—forever." This attitude allows the community to rationalize less than adequate care for the mentally ill.

Education is reported by Gallagher[21] to be the key factor in overcoming stigma. In general, more highly educated people have more realistic views of the range of behavior that may be associated with mental illness. However, this does not always correlate directly with complete acceptance. An individual might demonstrate intellectual understanding of mental illness and might be compassionate toward a friend or family member who receives psychiatric care. However, this same person might still oppose the establishment of a group home for the chronically mentally ill on his block or might refuse to ask a person with a history of psychiatric care to babysit for his children. These attitudes are as prevalent among nurses as they are among the general public. Consider this conversation between a head nurse and her supervisor:

NURSE: **Ms. T came back from sick leave today. She was in Riverview (a psychiatric hospital), you know.**
SUPERVISOR: **Yes, I know. How does she seem?**
NURSE: **All right, so far. I gave her a light assignment today, and I told her to come to me if she needs help.**
SUPERVISOR: **That's good. I hope she can handle things. She really *was* a good nurse.**
NURSE: **I do have one question for you. Should I let her have the medicine keys?**

On the surface, these two nurses seem concerned about the welfare of Ms. T and also seem to be appropriately planning for the care of the patients for whom they are responsible. However, they reflect some of the attitudes that can be most damaging toward people who are recovered from a mental illness. These include lack of confidence, an attitude of overprotectiveness and expectation of poor impulse control and unreliability.

Success in employment is a critical element of successful psychiatric rehabilitation. Prejudice toward mental illness can make it extremely difficult for an expatient to perform effectively in the work setting. Many employers are reluctant to hire people with a history of mental illness. For this reason mental illness, including alcoholism and drug abuse, is included in the federal law prohibiting job discrimination on the basis of handicap. This means that to reject a job applicant because of a history of mental illness, an employer must prove that the person's disability will make it impossible for him to perform the job. This law is helpful in terms of enabling more people to become employed. However, it does not prevent the more subtle manifestations of discrimination, such as social isolation and devaluation of ability to do a good job.

Many patients and their families try to avoid stigma by keeping the nature of the person's illness a secret. The need for secrecy places additional stress on the family system, because there is always the fear that the truth will be revealed. Secrecy is also destructive because the family is essentially buying into the prevailing prejudice and conveying that there is something shameful about the patient's need for psychiatric treatment. Families are a part of society and as such, share the prejudices of other community members. Caplan[15] discusses the importance of assessing the family's prejudices, so they can be given assistance in recognizing and overcoming them. Otherwise, the patient may return to a setting where he is not trusted. This attitude may extend to relationships outside of the family. The whole family may decide to avoid talking about the illness of one member, because they perceive that others will blame the family for the problem.

Nurses who are also community members are in a position to monitor community attitudes. They can be helpful in interpreting the community to patients and also in modeling a realistic attitude toward the mentally ill members of the community. This requires awareness of one's own attitudes toward mental illness and the involvement of the mentally ill in society.

 ## Planning and implementation

■ The individual

Treatment planning and intervention in rehabilitative psychiatric nursing focuses on fostering independence by maximizing the person's strengths. This is directly parallel to the nurse's role in physical rehabilitation. It differs from nursing care that is given to patients

TABLE 11-6

A COMPARISON OF STAFF ATTITUDES AT SOTERIA HOUSE TO THOSE IN A TRADITIONAL MENTAL HEALTH SETTING

Soteria House	Traditional setting
Psychosis a valid experience	Psychosis an illness, therefore not an intimate part of person
"Being with" the individual	Maintain objectivity and distance
Important event, should be taken seriously	Getting over it most important
Understanding the experience important	Putting the experience behind important
Allow individual to experience his psychosis	Shore up defenses to suppress, repress, and abort psychosis
Regression allowed	Regression prevented or interrupted when possible
Containing, holding environment	"Moving on" environment
Growth and learning from psychosis valued	Getting over psychosis quickly valued
Minimal pressure to "get going"	Length of stay seen as critical

From Mosher, L.R., and Menn, A.Z.: In Stein, L.A., and Test, M.A., editors: Alternatives to mental hospital treatment, New York, 1978, Plenum Press.

when they are acutely ill. During acute illness, whether physical or mental, people require a nurturing approach. The nurse must provide for all of the basic life functions that the person is unable to manage. However, the relationship gradually becomes less dependent as the patient grows stronger and better able to care for himself. Residual functional deficits may remain. The nurse and patient must then collaborate to devise ways for the patient to overcome any remaining impaired areas of functioning.

Peplau[37] described nursing roles relative to the patient's needs and ability to function. The unconditional mother-surrogate role related to the acutely ill phase and implied that the nurse would act in a maternal nurturing way. When the patient began to feel better, the nurse would assume a role characterized by some continuation of mother-surrogate functions with the addition of counseling, leadership, and resource person activities. The latter behaviors characterize the shift of responsibility from the nurse to the patient. People who choose nursing as a profession often have strong needs to nurture. It is important to be aware of this and not to let it interfere with the patient's need to develop self-care skills.

The close relationship between physical and psychiatric rehabilitation is demonstrated in the eight principles of psychiatric rehabilitation, as articulated by Anthony, Cohen, and Cohen.[4]

1. The primary focus of psychiatric rehabilitation is on improvement of capabilities and competencies.

2. The patient benefits by developing skills that will be useful in his own environment.
3. Psychiatric rehabilitation uses a variety of theories and therapeutic constructs. It is based on the philosophy and principles of rehabilitation.
4. Improvement of vocational outcome is a central focus.
5. Hope is essential for psychiatric rehabilitation.
6. Deliberately increasing independent behavior can ultimately lead to increased independent functioning.
7. The patient is encouraged to be actively involved in planning and implementing his own rehabilitation.
8. The fundamental psychiatric rehabilitation interventions are patient skill development and the development of environmental resources.

■ **ALTERNATIVE CARE SETTINGS.** It may be difficult to alter traditional nurse-patient roles in a hospital or clinic setting. In recent years, there have been efforts to develop alternative settings for the delivery of mental health care, such as foster homes, halfway houses, and psychosocial rehabilitation centers. One such alternative treatment program is Soteria House.[35] In Greek, *soteria* means deliverance. Soteria House was developed as an alternative for psychotic patients to treatment programs based on the medical model. This avoids many of the problems associated with the need to assume the role of patient, including the implied dependency and lack of personal responsibility for behavior. Mosher and Menn[35] have compared the attitudes typical of Soteria

House staff with those generally observed in a traditional mental health care setting (Table 11-6). Although it may appear that the Soteria approach fosters dependency, the ultimate objective is to help the person find meaning in his experience and to integrate it into his life. Staff acceptance of the patient and his right to experience is critical for the patient's ultimate ability to accept himself. In addition, decision making and responsibility are controlled by patients unless they are absolutely unable to do so.

Another alternative intervention program has as its goal the maintenance of patients in their own homes in the community. This is the Training in Community Living program designed by Stein and Test.[42] In this model, when a person is referred for hospital admission, the staff goes to the community with him rather than his going to the hospital to be with the staff. Nurses in this program accompany patients as they perform their usual activities, providing support and assistance when necessary. This real world experience with the patient enables the nurse to assess accurately the skills that the person needs to learn and to mutually agree on realistic goals. Staff contact is decreased as the patient demonstrates the ability to function independently. When the person is living with his family, they may also receive counseling and assistance in dealing with the patient's behaviors.

A third nonhospital intervention model is that developed by Polak and co-workers,[38] referred to as the Southwest Denver Model. They emphasize the need to consider and manipulate the social forces that influence the patient. This model also uses direct intervention in the social environment as the treatment approach. The major difference between this model and Training in Community Living is the focus. Whereas the latter model assists the patient to adjust to the environment, the Southwest Denver Model assists the environment to adjust to the needs of the patient. Intervention again takes place in the patient's social setting. If it is necessary for the patient to get away from his environment for a short time, foster care is arranged. Hospitalization is viewed as a last resort. If a patient is acutely psychotic or suicidal, an "intensive observation apartment" is available with close 24-hour supervision provided. A home day care program provides training in living skills in a home setting.

The programs described above generally maintain a clear distinction between the helpers and the helped. Chamberlin[16] has described three other models which profess to decrease or eliminate this differentiation. Her perspective is that of mental health services consumer.

- **Partnership model.** Recipients of the services of this type of program are told that they are partners. However, there is still a clear distinction between care givers and receivers. Chamberlin refers to these as "alternatives in name only." One example of a partnership model program is Fountain House. This program is described in detail in Chapter 34. It is run by professionals and according to Chamberlin, looks like and functions like an institution. She further criticizes the apparent assumption that all expatients are like the severely disabled people upon whom the program focuses.
- **Supportive model.** Membership is open to all who want mutual support. Expatients and those who have never been hospitalized are equal. It is believed that anyone is sometimes in need of help and sometimes able to provide help to others. Professionals are excluded except to generate community support or funding.
- **Separatist model.** Expatients support each other and run the service. All others are excluded. It is believed that anyone who has never experienced the psychiatric patient role will interfere with the consciousness-raising process and will have mentalist attitudes.

Chamberlin believes very strongly that alternative treatment programs should be run by patients. Successful programs also incorporate several other elements. They must be planned to address needs that have been identified by the clients, and participation must be voluntary. There should be options to participate in all or part of the total program. Help is either provided by clients to clients or by others whom the clients select. The service recipients are responsible for the administrative direction of the program. Criteria for participation are determined by the client group. Finally, the primary responsibility of the program is to the client and strict confidentiality is maintained, while making all information available to the client.

As experience with alternative treatment programs has become more extensive, it has also become apparent that there are subpopulations of patients who need modified or special programs. For instance, Setze and Bond[39] conducted a study of hospital readmission for 400 admissions to a psychosocial rehabilitation program. They found that women, whites, those under 21 years old, and those who had been hospitalized three or more times were more likely to be readmitted. This viewpoint is supported by Bachrach's[7] observation that there is an emerging recognition of the different service needs of men and women.

Bond[13] and associates have suggested three types of targeted interventions to be incorporated into psychosocial rehabilitation programs in order to prevent rehospitalization in high risk groups. They conducted a controlled study to test the three models. The add-on approach involves the creation of special programs for at-risk group members. These could include medication education classes or parents groups. The investigators question the usefulness of this method because it is not significantly different from the basic program model. The second intervention is program modification to reduce pressure on the patient by decreasing expectations of the patient. However, the usefulness of this approach was not supported by the study data. The third possibility is program substitution. When a totally new program was introduced to address the needs of the recidivists, the readmission rate was reduced. In addition to rehabilitation programming, housing needs of discharged patients must also be considered.

Foster home care is sometimes recommended for individuals who are discharged from the hospital, particularly those who have been hospitalized for a long time and have lost contact with relatives. There has been concern about foster home placement because lack of regulation of foster homes has resulted in situations where foster caregivers exploit the resident. However, well-run foster-care settings have been demonstrated to be effective.[32] Foster homes, of course, must be supplemented by treatment programs and provision for other psychosocial needs.

An example of an intervention designed specifically for a group of chronically mentally ill expatients is the "coffee group" described by Masnik, Olarte, and Rosen.[33] Nonstructured group sessions were used to assess the condition and progress of patients and to encourage socialization. The social aspect was reinforced by the provision of coffee and cookies at each session.

These program examples are not meant to be an exhaustive catalogue of approaches to psychiatric rehabilitation. They demonstrate the application of creativity to a complicated problem. Nurses have been involved in most of these programs. There is a risk involved in challenging the traditional mental health care structures, but also a potential reward as people who have been excluded from society are reintegrated as productive members. It should be noted that comprehensive psychosocial rehabilitation programs, exemplified by the Fountain House model, are widely recommended for intervention with chronically mentally ill patients. These programs are discussed in Chapter 34.

Rehabilitative psychiatric nursing is directed to-ward maximizing the person's strengths and minimizing his weaknesses. The nursing care plan should be organized around very specific behavioral goals that are derived from a comprehensive assessment of the patient's living skills. These goals should be an extension of those which are developed as part of the secondary prevention process. Examples of such goals may be found in Chapters 12 to 21. This part of the nursing care plan may be labeled the discharge plan in an inpatient treatment setting. Discharge plans should also be developed in community settings to remind both the nurse and the patient that the ultimate goal is for independent functioning. Even patients who need long-term medications can usually receive maintenance prescriptions from their family physician as part of their general health care program. This helps to put the mental illness into perspective as a chronic health problem that is not so different from other chronic problems the patient might have.

Determination of a desired level of functioning must be an interactive process between the patient and the nurse. If the patient resists taking on activities that the nurse believes would be helpful, it is important to try to understand why this is so. Sometimes nurses try to push a patient ahead too rapidly. Behavior that has developed gradually over time and that has served a useful function for the patient cannot be changed quickly. Learning new behavior patterns and giving up old ones is frightening and anxiety provoking.

Lamb[28] has suggested the following reasons that the homeless mentally ill may resist help:

1. Severe illness and disorganization
2. Low tolerance for intimacy and closeness
3. Rejection of the mentally ill identity
4. Desire to maintain an isolated life-style and anonymity
5. Fear of dependency

The nurse must be sure that the patient's coping skills are adequate to deal with the stress of growth. Feedback must be solicited from the patient to be sure that the rehabilitation plan continues to be responsive to his needs. Sometimes the plan assumes greater importance than the patient. The nurse needs to guard against this.

■ **PATIENT EDUCATION.** Several theorists have recommended educational approaches to assist with the rehabilitative process. Barter and associates[10] have described the Community Interaction Program in Sacramento, California. Three of the components of this program emphasize education. Transitional employment training teaches attitudes and behaviors consistent with success in the workforce. Adult basic education is offered to counteract deficits in basic academic education. Local teachers present these classes, thus fostering community involvement in the program as well. There are also weekly seminars on medications. These sessions are structured with a pretest followed by a lecture/discussion presentation and concluded with a posttest. At times, other topics such as health and nutrition have been added. This practical type of education is very useful in assisting people who have been institutionalized to survive in the community.

Bellack and associates[11] reported on a social skills training program. This is a structured learning experience that prepares the patient to initiate development of a social network and to decrease the stress of interpersonal conflict and failure. The content includes training on participating in brief conversations, assertiveness skills, and the expression of positive feelings. Special topics related to patient need such as dating or job interviewing may be added. A role modeling, role play, and feedback teaching method was used. It was concluded that the patients responded well to the high structure and goal orientation of the program.

Patient education should be an integral part of the nursing role. Buckwalter and Kerfoot[14] identified several topics that can assist the patient to avoid rehospitalization. These are presented in the format of a teaching plan in Table 11-7. A mental health education program such as this can be adapted for use in hospital or community settings. Specific content can be planned to meet the needs of individual patients or groups. Consumers are growing to expect health teaching as an integral part of professional services. Nurses are the health care providers who are best equipped to respond to this expectation.

Lamb et al.[29] have identified several guiding principles for the care of long-term psychiatric patients in the community. The first of these is that the patient must be given a sense of mastery over internal drives, symptoms, and environmental demands. To accomplish this, the care provider must use the second principle and work with the well part of the ego. "The goal is to expand the remaining well part of the person rather than to remove or cure pathology."[29:10] The third principle is that treatment should take place with the least possible envelopment of the patient and in a noninstitutional setting if possible. They advocate clear definition of goals as another principle. The next is that work therapy should be a cornerstone of the program. They state that the change of status from mental patient to normal community resident is a crucial principle. The final principle states that normalization of the person's environment should always be a goal. These last two principles can be carried out by giving socialization goals high priority and by encouraging social activities in the community with community members.[30]

The nurse can perform the important role of advocacy for the patient. Kohnke[27] has defined the two elements of the role of the nurse as advocate. They are to inform the patient about alternative approaches to his problem and to support his decision about how to respond. Significant others or community members may become impatient with the person as he struggles to regain control of his life. The nurse, with the patient's permission, can interpret the plan of care to others and enlist their support. She can also seek appropriate community services and assist the patient to make use of them. Human service systems are often not responsive to the needs of people who have problems dealing with stress. Role playing sometimes helps the patient practice the behaviors that he will need to use to find an apartment, obtain public assistance, or participate in a job interview. Group support may also be helpful. Small groups of people who are confronting similar challenges can provide a feeling of comradeship, as well as practical suggestions for handling specific situations. Nurses can organize and facilitate such groups.

■ **SOCIAL SUPPORT.** The role of nurses relative to social support groups has been described by Norbeck.[36] She relates the following theoretical assumptions underlying social support:

1. Supportive relationships are needed by people to manage everyday role demands and to cope with life transitions and unusual stressors.
2. A network of social relationships forms the context for the giving and receiving of social support.
3. Social network relationships are relatively stable over time, especially those that constitute the individual's primary ties.
4. In order to be supportive, a relationship should be basically healthy, not pathological.
5. The quantity and type of support that is needed is determined by the characteristics of the individual and the nature of the situation.
6. The quantity and type of support that is available is also determined by the characteristics of the situation and the individual.

Norbeck states that many psychotic patients have inadequate social supports characterized by a negative network orientation. Nursing interventions that she recommends for these patients are described in Table 11-8. The interventions are focused on the type of deficiency being experienced. Situational deficiencies are dealt with by the mobilization of coping skills or environmental supports. Pathological deficiencies require modification of the patient's behavior or of the network. The nurse may need to collaborate with other members

TABLE 11-7

MODEL OF AN EDUCATION PLAN FOR PSYCHIATRIC PATIENTS IN REHABILITATION PROGRAMS

Content	Instructional activities	Evaluation
Identify and describe common psychiatric diagnoses	Provide handouts outlining behaviors Discuss coping behaviors Assign homework from lay literature Compare mental illness to physical illness	Patient recognizes characteristics of the diagnosis he has been given Patient distinguishes between cure and coping
Describe the role of stress in contributing to psychiatric disorders	Sensitize the patient to signs of increased stress Define stress as a test of coping skills Teach relaxation exercises	Patient verbalizes level of stress Patient performs relaxation exercises and describes a reduction in perceived stress
Assist to gain a sense of control by recognizing personal pattern of signs and symptoms	Provide feedback when symptomatic behavior occurs Instruct patient to keep a diary of behavior and to identify symptoms	Patient consistently labels symptoms and seeks professional help when necessary
Development of social skills to enable participation in vocational and recreational activities	Role play social interaction in a variety of situations Field trips to community activities Supervised vocational training in real work settings	Patient participates in progressively more independent social and work activities
Identify and describe community support systems	Provide a list of community support programs, including self-help groups, mental health care agencies and social agencies Invite representatives of programs to speak to patient group Escort to first agency contact	Patient selects community programs that offer resources needed by him Patient becomes able to access agency independently
Describe and discuss psychoactive medications	Instruct about actions, side effects, and contraindications to common psychoactive medications Distribute handouts describing the patient's medications Suggest systems to help patient remember when to take medication and how much	Patient describes characteristics of prescribed medications Patient reports effects of prescribed medications Patient takes medication as prescribed

Modified from Buckwalter, K.C., and Kerfoot, K.M.: J. Psychosoc. Nurs. Ment. Health Serv. **20**:(5):15, May 1982.

of the health care team to assist the patient to overcome serious deficiencies.

Group support may also be found through involvement in self-help groups. These are groups of patients who meet to offer peer support and encouragement. Self-help groups do not solicit and frequently actively discourage involvement by mental health care providers. Providers may be viewed as representatives of an illness-focused system. Self-help groups emphasize the abilities of their members to serve as advocates for themselves and for others with similar problems. The nonthreatening experience of social support has been identified by Knight and co-workers[26] as the aspect of self-help groups that is most frequently described as helpful by members. Recovery, Inc., was the first self-help group formed by people with emotional problems. This group

TABLE 11-8

TYPOLOGY OF DEFICIENCIES IN SOCIAL SUPPORT AND RECOMMENDED INTERVENTIONS

Deficiencies	Nursing interventions
I. Situational	
1. Losses of network members	1. a. Assist client to deal with losses and provide temporary support
	b. Assist client to "repeople" the network
2. Crisis or problem exceeds network's capacity or experience	2. a. Influence key network member to provide support
	b. Volunteer linking
	c. Mutual aid groups
	d. Professional support
II. Pathological	
A. *Person deficiencies:*	
3. Inadequate social skills	3. a. Training in social skill development
	b. Environmental manipulation to facilitate interaction
4. Negative network orientation	4. a. Assist client to decrease over-generalization from pathological relationships to other relationships
B. *Network deficiencies:*	
5. Pathological relationships	5. a. Decrease face-to-face contact with key person
	b. Change attitudes and behavior of key person
6. Maladaptive network structure	6. a. Encourage non-kin contact
	b. Network therapy

From Norbeck, J.S.: J. Psychosoc. Nurs. Ment. Health Serv. **20:**(12):22, Dec. 1982.

was modeled after Alcoholics Anonymous. More recently, other groups have organized to bring together chronically mentally ill people or those with a specific medical diagnosis, such as schizophrenia. Some self-help groups draw their membership from the families of mentally ill people who often feel caught between the demands of the patient on one hand and the health care providers on the other. Nurses can make patients aware of these groups and encourage them to attend. They can also offer themselves as resources to the group if the members identify a need with which a nurse could be helpful. Membership in a self-help group can be an important step toward independence by a person who is recovering from a mental illness.

■ The family

The involvement of a supportive family is tremendously important to the successful rehabilitation of a mentally ill person. The mental illness of a member is often a shock and a source of great stress to the family. Nurses are in a good position to assist families to cope with the stress and to adapt to related changes in the family structure. Hatfield[22] has described several needs of families related to the mental illness of a member.

These are summarized in Table 11-9. One important need is for knowledge. Families want to be able to understand the patient's behavior and how to respond helpfully to disturbed behavior. They would like a clear nontechnical explanation of the illness, as well as a prognosis that is as accurate as possible. Nurses can provide information, refer families to other health team members for further information, and provide suggestions on how to respond to disruptive behavior. One particularly perplexing problem for families is to be involved enough and interested enough without being intrusive on the one hand or distant on the other.[47] Nurses can offer assistance in this area by providing feedback to families about interactions that they have observed and by modeling effective communication skills. In some families, interaction will be disturbed to the extent that family therapy is required. Unless she has advanced preparation in this therapeutic modality, the nurse should refer the family to a qualified family therapist. Families also need to know about behaviors that could indicate a recurrence of the illness, so they can encourage the patient to seek help before hospitalization is required. Group education sessions for family members can be productive because participants can share experiences while they learn. This approach combines group support and education. Zelitch[48] has described a workshop series that was developed to meet the needs of patients' families with the following goals:

1. To educate families about mental illness
2. To engage the family's active participation in the patient's treatment
3. To facilitate self-help and support among families with similar concerns
4. To help families identify resources in the community
5. To assist relatives to assign priorities to their concerns
6. To teach relatives basic behavioral techniques that can be applied in dealing with the patient

Families also identified the need to be informed about available resources.[22] This enables them to assist the patient to utilize resources.

The second major need identified by the families in Hatfield's study[22] was to have someone with whom they could talk. Most of the people surveyed were self-help group members and had found that this peer support was helpful to them. The National Alliance for the Mentally Ill (NAMI) has been actively engaged in promoting the development of peer support groups for families of mentally ill people. The third need was for respite care

resources. Respite care provides supervision for the patient in a community setting when the family needs relief from the demands of a mentally ill member. This service allows families to take a vacation or spend a short time away from the patient without feeling the guilt that they would if the patient was rehospitalized.

The final need expressed was for crisis services, including home visiting. It can be very difficult for a family to persuade a disturbed member to go to a treatment facility, particularly if the patient has been hospitalized in the past and suspects that he will be again. Families are sometimes forced to wait until the situation becomes so bad that they must call the police to take the patient into custody. Crisis intervention in the home could avert this distressing situation. Home visiting is an activity that is generally accepted by nurses, who are in turn usually well received in the community. Home health care is a service that needs to be made available to patients who are unwilling or unable to participate in other forms of outpatient care.

Walsh,[45] writing as a parent of a schizophrenic, has suggested several common trouble spots in family life. The first is disrupted communications. Another problem area has to do with the mechanics of everyday life. These include the need for privacy and control over one's own space, keeping a regular schedule, nutrition, television usage, money management, and grooming.

TABLE 11-9

NEEDS FREQUENTLY CITED BY FAMILIES OF PSYCHIATRIC PATIENTS AND SUGGESTED NURSING INTERVENTIONS

Needs	Nursing interventions
I. Knowledge	
A. Understand disturbed behavior and respond helpfully	Provide information
	Refer to other team members
	Suggest possible responses
B. Appropriate level of involvement	Provide feedback about interactions
	Role model effective communication
C. Signs and symptoms of recurrence	Arrange a group education program about the characteristics of mental illness
D. Community resources	Provide a list of available resources
II. Peer support	Refer to a self-help group
III. Respite services	Assist to find or create resources
IV. Crisis services	Refer to an emergency mental health service or alert community to the need for new services

Families are concerned about responding to hallucinations, delusions, and odd behavior. They are particularly in need of assistance in coping with threats of violence, whether directed toward others or the self in the form of suicidal behavior. Alcohol and drug use also cause disruptions in family life.

The last area of concern identified by Walsh is one that is frequently ignored by family members and professionals alike. That is the need for relatives to remember to take care of themselves. She recommends the following ways to accomplish this:

1. Accept the fact of a mentally ill family member.
2. Plan a self-care program.
3. Continue to pursue personal activities and interests.
4. Get involved with organizations such as self-help groups or churches.
5. Avoid the advice and opinions of those who have not lived with a schizophrenic.
6. Remember that happiness is possible.
7. Stop blaming yourself.

Reviewing this list gives the nurse some understanding of the pain and stress that is experienced by the family of a mentally ill person. Nurses can help alleviate that pain by providing advice such as that listed above.

■ **NURSE-FAMILY ALLIANCE.** Helpful attitudes for professionals working with families of mentally ill patients have been identified.[47] Instead of approaching the family as an expert, which can lead to feelings of impotence resulting in anger, Wing and Olsen recommend a relationship of mutual learning. The nurse can then concentrate on empathizing with the family and participating with them in problem solving.

Unfortunately, families and members of the mental health care treatment team, including nurses, sometimes become engaged in power struggles related to the care of the mentally ill family member. Spaniol, Zipple, and FitzGerald[40] suggest the following ways that professionals can share power with families to the ultimate benefit of the patient:

1. Clarify mutual goals.
2. Be knowledgeable about rehabilitative and educational methods.
3. Avoid imposing your model on families. Separate intervention from explanation of causation.
4. Acknowledge your limitations.
5. Develop a team relationship with the family and the community.
6. Recognize and identify the family's strengths.
7. Learn to accept criticism of the system.

8. Encourage family members to recognize and meet their own needs.
9. Keep up with current information about psychiatric illnesses and medications and share this knowledge with families.
10. Learn practical advice from families and incorporate it into health-teaching plans.
11. Seek knowledge about the availability and quality of community resources.
12. Establish a positive relationship with family support groups and refer families to them.
13. Demonstrate personal commitment through advocacy.
14. Learn to accept diverse beliefs.
15. Cultivate a personal support system.

Because nurses are usually viewed as supportive and helpful, they are in a good position to be sensitive to the stated needs of families and to address them in their practice.

■ **FAMILY INTERVENTION PROCESS.** Anderson, Hogarty, and Reiss[1] have described a four-phase process for intervention with the families of schizophrenic patients. This model is summarized in Table 11-10. Phase I focuses on establishing a connection with the family. At first the therapist "joins" the family by engaging in social conversation and information sharing. This decreases anxiety by creating an atmosphere that is familiar to the family. Next the therapist assumes the role of "family ombudsman." This implies an alliance with the family and the avoidance of assigning blame for the patient's problems. The therapist shares information with the family and solicits their input for the treatment plan. The clinician's role is established as the family's representative and link with other parts of the health care system. The family's reactions to the illness are elicited, and their concern is mobilized in the patient's behalf. Finally, a treatment contract is agreed on. This includes the establishment of mutual goals.

Phase II is directed toward teaching survival skills for living with schizophrenia. This is done in the context of a day-long workshop. It is also hoped that a support network will be formed among the families who attend. In Phase III, the content from the workshop is applied to the individual family. There are generally two main themes during this phase: reinforcing family boundaries and the patient's gradually resuming responsibility. Respect for boundaries is communicated by allowing individuals to speak for themselves, allowing members to engage in separate activities, and by recognizing each member's area of vulnerability and limitation. Responsibility is gradually assumed by the patient by first helping with simple tasks, then functioning more independently as readiness develops. The family is encouraged to be patient because this can be a long slow process. Expectations must be realistic with one change made at a time. Phase IV begins when goals have been attained to the greatest possible extent. At this point, the family chooses between traditional family therapy or decreased involvement focusing on maintenance.[1] Although the model was developed for work with the families of schizophrenic patients, many of the principles apply to other families as well. Intervention utilizing the model should not be attempted without advanced education at the graduate level. However, understanding of family needs can facilitate the nurse's approach to relatives in her contacts with them. Nurses are often the most accessible members of the health care team, especially in inpatient settings. They can be very helpful if they try to understand family needs and reinforce family coping mechanisms.

■ The community

There are several ways in which nurses may intervene in the community to encourage the establishment of tertiary prevention programs. Among these are health education, membership in advocacy groups, networking, and political action. It has been noted that stigma decreases with increased formal education. Cumming and Cumming[17] hypothesized that community-based health education programs on the topic of mental health might have the same effect. They conducted a study based on this hypothesis in an attempt to change negative community attitudes toward the mentally ill. They failed in their efforts, but had some interesting observations related to the study. They believed that they should have found a way to motivate the community members to want to learn. They also assumed that they were aware of community attitudes, but later discovered that this was not so. They had used a psychiatrist as the

TABLE 11-10

OVERVIEW OF THE FAMILY INTERVENTION PROCESS

Phases	Goals	Techniques
Phase I	Connect with the family and enlist cooperation with program Decrease guilt, emotionality, and negative reactions to the illness Reduction of family stress	Joining Establishing treatment contract Discussion of crisis history and feelings about the patient and the illness Empathy Specific practical suggestions that mobilize concerns into effective coping mechanisms
Phase II Survival skills workshop	Increased understanding of illness and patient's needs by family Continued reduction of family stress Deisolation—enhancement of social networks	Multiple family education and discussion Concrete data on schizophrenia Concrete management suggestions Basic communication skills
Phase III Reentry and application	Patient maintenance in community Strengthening of marital/parental coalition Increased family tolerance for low-level dysfunctional behaviors Decreased and gradual resumption of responsibility by patient	Reinforcement of boundaries (generational and interpersonal) Task assignments Low-key problem solving
Phase IV Maintenance	Reintegration into normal roles in community systems (work, school) Increased effectiveness of general family processes	Infrequent maintenance sessions Traditional or exploratory family therapy techniques

From Anderson, C.M., Hogarty, G.E., and Reiss, D.J.: Schizophr. Bull. **6:**495, 1980.

educator in the project. They later decided that it might have been more effective to use community members, provided they were well-informed about the subject. The psychiatrist was a good teacher, but this was not the role expected of him by the community members. Finally, they came to believe that they should have stimulated direct involvement between community members and patients by encouraging volunteer activity as a part of the program.

Most nurses have a strong background and a firm belief in health education. Mental health education at the community level provides a real opportunity to have an impact on the experience of patients as community members. Greater understanding of the realities of the usual behaviors and the needs of the mentally ill could increase community acceptance, leading to the development of better services. People who refuse to allow group homes in their neighborhoods usually have irrational fears fueled by the media's distorted portrayal of mentally ill people. Education combined with direct contact with members of rehabilitation programs can be helpful in overcoming negative attitudes. Nurses should take advantage of opportunities to speak to community groups about mental health.

Membership by nurses in community advocacy groups can also be helpful. By this means, nurses can join forces with other professional and lay people who share concerns about the care of the mentally ill. The National Mental Health Association is the largest advocacy group that addresses mental health issues. Members of this organization have been instrumental in drawing attention to the needs of the mentally ill and in supporting positive legislation at the federal and state levels. They monitor the effectiveness of the mental health care system. Nurses can provide useful input to this part of their activities.

At a broader level, nurses can stimulate the development of collaborative relationships among advocacy groups, professional organizations, self-help groups, and concerned citizens. As fewer funds are available for the care of the mentally ill, the formation of coalitions is essential to lobby for the allocation of resources to mental health care. Coalition formation is also referred to as networking. Mitchell and Trickett[34] have identified functions served by social networks. They include "emotional support; task-oriented assistance; communication of expectations, evaluation, and a shared world view; and access to new and diverse information and social contacts."[34:30] These functions are also the factors that capture members' commitment to united action.

The activities of community-wide networks are frequently directed toward the political system. Aside from allocation of money and other resources, the nature of mental health care in a community is strongly influenced by the political structure of that community. As has been seen in Chapter 7, legal issues have a profound effect on mental health care delivery. Nurses need to be aware of and involved in the political process. They should communicate directly with their legislators at all levels, sharing their interests and concerns. Politicians are well aware of the need to be responsive to the priorities of their constituents. The number of nurses in the United States makes them a potentially powerful political force, but that power has seldom been exerted. If nurses are committed to positive health care, particularly at the primary and tertiary prevention levels, they must become visibly involved.

Nurses can also become more directly involved in the political system. They can run for office and support other nurses who are legislators. Nurses are often invaluable members of appointed boards and commissions having to do with health care. Their knowledge can be shared with others who are planning community health care systems. These voluntary activities are time consuming, but they can have great impact on the health care system. Community-level policies can either inhibit or facilitate direct care efforts. Active involvement in professional organizations often leads to productive and rewarding community activities. There is a great sense of satisfaction to be found in selling a community on a new idea and seeing it become a reality.

Evaluation

■ Program evaluation

Many of the approaches to tertiary prevention that have been described are relatively new. Because of the long-term nature of many types of mental illness, the evaluation of these programs is in its early stages. Longitudinal studies will provide more valid and reliable measures of success or failure. Bachrach[6] has reviewed the literature on model programs for the care of chronically mentally ill people. She analyzed these programs at four levels. The first level is an evaluation of the success or failure of the individual program. The program may be measured according to a number of parameters. Externally determined criteria (e.g., cost-effectiveness or licensure standards), accomplishment of stated objectives, patient functioning, and patient or staff satisfaction are approaches to evaluation that have been used at the programmatic level. The second level is the assessment of commonalities among programs. Bachrach found the following eight common elements in successful programs[6]:

1. The targeting of a specific group of patients
2. Realistic linkages with other community resources
3. Provision of a full range of functions
4. Individualized treatment
5. Conformity with the local cultural system
6. Specialized training for staff
7. Liaison with a hospital for access to inpatient beds when needed
8. Presence of an internal evaluation system

The third level of evaluation relates to the reproducibility and generalizability of the program. This is identified as a problem by Bachrach for several reasons. One is that each program is developed in a cultural context that differs from others. Another is that model programs often have the advantage of special funding and other resources that are not available for duplicates. The very fact of being a model and therefore special can influence the outcome of a program. Another very important hindrance to reproducibility is the extent to which most successful programs depend on the leadership of one person or a small group of people who are extraordinarily committed to their program. There is frequently a charismatic leader associated with successful programs. Finally, the model programs are too new to tell whether they will stand the test of time.[6]

The fourth level of evaluation is that of relevance. This looks at the relationship of the program to the mental health care system. Bachrach[6] has named this impact evaluation. She questions whether model programs can really provide the answers to broader social problems. The model must be considered in the context of the system within which it exists.

■ Patient evaluation

Others have directed their efforts toward evaluating the effectiveness of rehabilitation programs by assessing the impact on the individual patient. Kelly and co-workers[25] looked for predictors of success in aftercare programs. They identified two, including involvement in occupational therapy and responsiveness to reinforcement in group therapy. Anthony and co-workers[3] have also recommended patient evaluation criteria. They settled on recidivism and posthospital employment as the most useful measures of community adjustment. However, they also recommend that evaluation efforts be extended and that rehabilitation programs take a closer look at their results.

Turkat and Buzzell[43] suggest an evaluation approach based on member movement within a psychosocial rehabilitation program. They found that as patients move from one program component to another,

---

DIRECTIONS FOR FUTURE RESEARCH

The following are some of the nursing research problems raised in Chapter 11 that merit further study by psychiatric nurses:

1. Nursing interventions that limit dependency by inpatients on the institution
2. Testing of the generalizability of social skills learned in a hospital or other institutional setting to a community environment
3. Exploration of various models of independent living skills training
4. Effective staffing patterns for psychosocial rehabilitation programs
5. Survey of the amount of classroom and clinical time allotted to content relative to rehabilitative psychiatric nursing in basic and graduate nursing programs
6. Nursing interventions that can increase public understanding of mental illness and the mentally ill with measurement of the effect on stigma
7. The relationship between contact with unrelated mentally ill people and attitudes toward mental illness
8. Constructive roles that nurses may perform relative to self-help groups
9. Evaluation of the helpfulness of self-help group membership as compared to participation in other types of treatment programs
10. Exploration of the impact of participation of family members in a self-help group on the recovery process of the patient
11. Description of community support groups planned to address the unique needs of subpopulations of the chronically mentally ill: women, young adults, the elderly
12. The extent to which nurses assume the role of patient advocate and their effectiveness in this role
13. Development of generalizable and reproducible evaluation criteria to be applied to tertiary prevention programs
14. The relationship of various tertiary prevention program elements to patient outcomes

---

there is not a consistent progression toward increased independence. Patients tend to move back and forth "alternating cycles of progression, regression and maintenance." Therefore, it is important not to base program evaluation on an expectation that most patients will progress in a stepwise fashion. A decrease in rehospitalization rates may be a more significant criterion of program success.

Cutler[18] identified clinical, programmatic, and administrative principles for psychosocial rehabilitation programs that may serve as evaluation guidelines. The clinical principles are continuity of care, availability of services, and the provision of services in the patient's natural environment. Programmatically, the services should be comprehensive. The administrative principles include integration of planning with all service providers and agencies, planned staff development, and a constant and ongoing evaluation program. Patients of the Living in the Community program in Oregon, on which these principles are based, experienced a 9% hospital recidivism rate in 6½ years.

It is becoming obvious that if tertiary prevention efforts are to be supported in the future, it is necessary to prove that they are effective in both human and economic terms. Therefore, evaluation criteria must be developed and utilized.

■ SUGGESTED CROSS-REFERENCES ■

The nursing process is discussed in Chapter 5. Intervention in social support systems is discussed in Chapter 9. Family assessment is discussed in Chapter 5, and identification of vulnerable families is discussed in Chapters 9 and 29. The care of the chronically mentally ill patient is discussed in Chapter 34.

■ SUMMARY ■

1. Tertiary prevention was defined as reduction of the rate of residual defect related to an episode of mental illness.

2. Psychiatric rehabilitation was identified as the process by which tertiary prevention is operationalized.

3. Four trends in the development of psychosocial treatment were identified as psychoeducation and the medical model, working with families, group therapy, and social skills–social learning theory.

4. Stressors were discussed in terms of the experience of the chronically mentally ill.

5. Concepts related to the assessment of the individual and rehabilitative nursing needs were described.

6. The concepts of primary and secondary gain were discussed as they relate to psychiatric rehabilitation.

7. Readiness for discharge from inpatient or partial hospitalization programs was analyzed in terms of patient characteristics and required skills.

8. Family assessment was discussed in the context of available resources for patient support. Important factors include family attitudes toward the patient, alterations in the roles of family members, the emotional climate of the family, the availability of social support, and the family's understanding of the patient's illness.

9. Community assessment was described in terms of the nurse's responsibility to identify and evaluate community resources.

10. The phenomenon of stigma was presented as a representation of the resistance encountered by patients who attempt to reenter the social system.

11. The role of the nurse in planning and intervening in rehabilitative psychiatric care was related to responsiveness to the patient's readiness for increased independence.

12. Eight principles of psychiatric rehabilitation were presented to demonstrate similarities to physical rehabilitation concepts.

13. Several model community programs for the provision of tertiary prevention services were described.

14. The development of specific mutual nurse-patient goals that are stated in behavioral terms was discussed relative to tertiary prevention.

15. Group intervention, including fostering self-help groups, was suggested as an appropriate activity for the nurse.

16. Strategies were presented for the support of the families of psychiatric patients. These included family education, involvement in a peer support group, provision for respite care, and crisis intervention, including home visiting.

17. A model mental health education plan for consumers of tertiary rehabilitation services was presented.

18. Community interventions were proposed to encourage and support the development of tertiary prevention services. These include mental health education, membership in advocacy groups, networking, and political action.

19. Program evaluation was discussed in terms of the state of the art. Some criteria were identified, as were levels of evaluation. However, there is a need for more work in this area.

■ REFERENCES ■

1. Anderson, C.M., Hogarty, G.E., and Reiss, D.J.: Family treatment of adult schizophrenic patients: a psychoeducational approach, Schizophr. Bull. **6**:490, 1980.

2. Anthony, W. A.: The principles of psychiatric rehabilitation, Baltimore, 1980, University Park Press.

3. Anthony, W. A., et al.: Efficacy of psychiatric rehabilitation, Psychol. Bull. **78**:447, 1972.

4. Anthony, W. A., Cohen, M.R., and Cohen, B.F.: Psychiatric rehabilitation. In Talbott, J.A., editor: The chronic mental patient: five years later, New York, 1984, Grune & Stratton, Inc.

5. Bachmann, B.J.: Reentering the community: a former patient's view, Hosp. Community Psychiatry **22**:19, April 1971.

6. Bachrach, L.L.: Overview: model programs for chronic mental patients, Am. J. Psychiatry **137**:1023, 1980.

7. Bachrach, L.L.: Chronic mentally ill women: emergence and legitimation of program issues, Hosp. Community Psychiatry **36**:1063, Oct. 1985.

8. Baker, F., et al.: The impact of life events on chronic mental patients, Hosp. Community Psychiatry **36**:299, Mar. 1985.

9. Banes, J.S.: An ex-patient's perspective of psychiatric treatment, J. Psychosoc. Nurs. Ment. Health Serv. **21**:(3):11, Mar. 1983.

10. Barter, J.T., Queirolo, J.F., and Ekstrom, S.P.: A psy-

choeducational approach to educating chronic mental patients for community living, Hosp. Community Psychiatry **35**:793, Aug. 1984.

11. Bellack, A.S., et al.: An examination of the efficacy of social skills training for chronic schizophrenic patients, Hosp. Community Psychiatry **35**:1023, Oct. 1984.

12. Bennett, D.: Deinstitutionalization in two cultures, Health Society **57**:516, 1979.

13. Bond, G.R., et al.: Preventing rehospitalization of clients in a psychosocial rehabilitation program. Hosp. Community Psychiatry **36**:993, Sept. 1985.

14. Buckwalter, K.C., and Kerfoot, K.M.: Teaching patients self care: a critical aspect of psychiatric discharge planning, J. Psychosoc. Nurs. Ment. Health Serv. **20**:(5):15, May 1982.

15. Caplan, G.: Principles of preventive psychiatry, New York, 1964, Basic Books, Inc., Publishers.

16. Chamberlin, J.: On our own, New York, 1978, McGraw-Hill Book Co.

17. Cumming, E., and Cumming, J.: Closed ranks: an experiment in mental health education, Cambridge, Mass., 1957, Harvard University Press.

18. Cutler, D.L., et al.: Disseminating the principles of a community support program, Hosp. Community Psychiatry, **35**:35, Jan. 1984.

19. Department of Health and Human Services Steering Committee on the Chronically Mentally Ill: Toward a national plan for the chronically mentally ill, Pub. No. (ADM)81-1077, Washington, D.C., 1981, U.S. Government Printing Office.

20. Doll, W.: Family coping with the mentally ill patient: an unanticipated result of deinstitutionalization, Hosp. Community Psychiatry **27**:183, Mar. 1976.

21. Gallagher, B.J., III: The sociology of mental illness, Englewood Cliffs, N.J., 1980, Prentice-Hall, Inc.

22. Hatfield, A.B.: The family as partner in the treatment of mental illness, Hosp. Community Psychiatry **30**:338, 1979.

23. Heinrichs, D.W.: Recent developments in the psychosocial treatment of chronic psychotic illnesses. In Talbott, J.A.: The chronic mental patient: five years later, New York, 1984, Grune & Stratton, Inc.

24. Holmes, T.H., and Rahe, R.H.: The social readjustment rating scale, J. Psychosom. Res. **11**:213, 1967.

25. Kelly, J.A., et al.: Objective evaluation and prediction of client improvement in mental health aftercare, Soc. Work Health Care **5**:187, Winter, 1979.

26. Knight, B., et al.: Self-help groups: the members' perspectives, Am. J. Community Psychol. **8**:53, Jan. 1980.

27. Kohnke, M.F.: Advocacy: what is it? Nurs. Health Care **3**:314, June 1982.

28. Lamb, H.R.: Deinstitutionalization and the homeless mentally ill, Hosp. Community Psychiatry **35**:899, Sept. 1984.

29. Lamb, H.R., et al.: Community survival for long-term patients, Washington, D.C., 1976, Jossey-Bass, Inc., Publishers.

30. Lamb, H.R., and Goertzel, V.: The long-term patient in the era of community treatment, Arch. Gen. Psychiatry **34**:679, 1977.

31. Leavitt, M.: The discharge crisis: the experience of families of psychiatric patients, Nurs. Res. **24**:33, Jan.-Feb. 1975.

32. Linn, M.W., et al.: Hospital vs. community (foster) care for psychiatric patients, Arch. Gen. Psychiatr. **34**:78, Jan. 1977.

33. Masnik, R., Olarte, S.W., and Rosen, A.: "Coffee groups": a nine-year follow-up study, Am. J. Psychiatry **137**:91, Jan. 1980.

34. Mitchell, R.E., and Trickett, E.J.: Task force report: social networks as mediators of social support, Community Ment. Health J. **16**:27, Spring 1980.

35. Mosher, L.R., and Menn, A.Z.: Lowered barriers in the community: the Soteria model. In Stein, L.I., and Test, M.A., editors: Alternatives to mental hospital treatment, New York, 1978, Plenum Press.

36. Norbeck, J.S.: The use of social support in clinical practice, J. Psychosoc. Nurs. Ment. Health Serv. **20**:(12):22, Dec. 1982.

37. Peplau, H.E.: Interpersonal relations in nursing, New York, 1952, G.P. Putnam's Sons.

38. Polak, P.R.: A comprehensive system of alternatives to psychiatric hospitalization. In Stein, L.I., and Test, M.A., editors: Alternatives to mental hospital treatment, New York, 1978, Plenum Press.

39. Setze, P.J., and Bond, G.R.: Psychiatric recidivism in a psychosocial rehabilitation setting: a survival analysis, **36**:521, May 1985.

40. Spaniol, L., Zipple, A., and FitzGerald, S.: How professionals can share power with families: Practical approaches working with families of the mentally ill, Psychosoc. Rehab. J. **8**:77, Oct. 1984.

41. Spivack, G., et al.: The long-term patient in the community: life style patterns and treatment implications, Hosp. Community Psychiatry **33**:291, April 1982.

42. Stein, L.I., and Test, M.A.: An alternative to mental hospital treatment. In Stein, L.I., and Test, M.A., editors: Alternatives to mental hospital treatment, New York, 1978, Plenum Press.

43. Turkat, D., and Buzzell, V.: Psychosocial rehabilitation: a process evaluation, Hosp. Community Psychiatry **33**:848, Oct. 1982.

44. Vaughn, C.E., and Leff, J.P.: The influence of family and social factors on the source of psychiatric illness, Br. J. Psychiatry **129**:125, 1976.

45. Walsh, M.: Schizophrenia: straight talk for families and friends, New York, 1985, William Morrow and Co., Inc.

46. Wing, J.K.: Social psychiatry in the United Kingdom: the approach to schizophrenia, Schizophr. Bull. **6**:556, 1980.

47. Wing, J.K., and Olsen, R.: Community care for the mentally disabled, New York, 1979, Oxford University Press.

48. Zelitch, S.R.: Helping the family cope: workshops for families of schizophrenics, Health Soc. Work **5**:47, Nov. 1980.

■ ANNOTATED SUGGESTED READINGS ■

Anderson, C.M., Hogarty, G.E., and Reiss, D.J.: Family treatment of adult schizophrenic patients: a psychoeducational approach, Schizophr. Bull. **6**:490, 1980.

The authors describe in detail an innovative approach to family intervention. Education is the focus until the family is ready to choose to deal with more psychodynamic issues. This article would be of interest to nurses with graduate level preparation who are involved in a family intervention program.

Anthony, W. A.: The principles of psychiatric rehabilitation, Baltimore, 1980, University Park Press.

This is an excellent book that describes a psychiatric rehabilitation program in great detail. It is clearly written and reflects the author's extensive experience in training mental health care providers to care for the seriously mentally ill.

Bachrach, L.L.: Deinstitutionalization: an analytical review and sociological perspective, Department of Health, Education, and Welfare Pub. No. (ADM)79-351, Washington, D.C., 1979.

In this work the author attempts to pull together the many theories and opinions related to deinstitutionalization. It provides a good overview of the issues and includes a sociological analysis by the author. It is recommended for the advanced student or the nurse who is interested in performing research.

*Banes, J.S.: An ex-patient's perspective of psychiatric treatment, J. Psychosoc. Nurs. Ment. Health Serv. **21**(3):11, March 1983.

Reflecting the perspective of a mental health professional who was a mental patient, the author writes eloquently about the mental health system. Her observations about the effects of institutionalization and the dilemmas of deinstitutionalization should be read by all nurses who work with troubled people. She challenges us to help our patients overcome the obstacles to a fulfilling life.

Bennett, D.: Deinstitutionalization in two cultures, Health Society **57**:516, 1979.

This article is an interesting exploration of the differences in the United States and United Kingdom approach to deinstitutionalization. The author conveys an understanding of the issues and events that have shaped these cultural differences. The contrast is fascinating.

Bogin, D.L., et al.: The effects of a referral coordinator on compliance with psychiatric discharge plans, Hosp. Community Psychiatry **35**:702, July 1984.

This report of a research project clearly demonstrates the importance of actively assisting patients to become involved in aftercare services. The researchers found that the intervention of a specific staff person who was responsible for discharge planning enhanced patient compliance with outpatient treatment.

Chamberlin, J.: On our own, New York, 1978, McGraw-Hill Book Co.

This book presents the viewpoint of a woman who was a client of the mental health system. She describes her experiences in a graphic manner. She also discusses in detail alternative approaches to mental health care that she believes to be more humane and helpful than those which she experienced. She presents a strong case for greater patient involvement in planning and carrying out treatment and rehabilitation.

Cooley, R.N., Jr.: Developing a sense of community in chronic inpatients through religious and social activities, Hosp. Community Psychiatry, **33**:486, June 1982.

The author, who is a chaplain, describes a group called Happy Travelers which used a religious base to assist chronic patients to experience supportive social interaction. The group shared both in and out of hospital experiences, including the establishment of ties to community churches.

Department of Health and Human Services, Steering Committee on the Chronically Mentally Ill: Toward a national plan for the chronically mentally ill, Pub. No. (ADM)81-1077, Washington, D.C., 1981, U.S. Government Printing Office.

This publication provides current and comprehensive information on the status of the care of the chronically mentally ill in the United States. Mental health nurses should be familiar with its content and will find that it is a useful reference.

Gudeman, J.E., and Shore, M.F.: Beyond deinstitutionalization: a new class of facilities for the mentally ill, N. Engl. J. Med. **311**:832, Sept. 1984.

The authors identify five groups of patients who do not function adequately in the community. These include: the elderly, demented, and behaviorally disturbed; the mentally retarded and psychotic; the brain-damaged and assaultive; the psychotic and assaultive; and the chronically schizophrenic, disruptive, and endangered. They suggest specialized inpatient units for these people to provide long-term treatment-oriented care.

*Hjorten, M.K.: A volunteer support system for the chronically ill, Persp. Psychiatr. Care **20**:17, Jan.-Mar. 1982.

A nursing student writes a personal account of her experience planning and later directing a community support program for the chronically mentally ill. She provides several suggestions for the organization of such programs. She demonstrates the value of volunteer services and community involvement.

Hospital and Community Psychiatry

This journal, published by the American Psychiatric Association, is a rich resource of information about psychosocial rehabilitation. Most current research in this field is reported here. The focus is multidisciplinary.

Keys, L.M.: Former patients as volunteers in community agencies: a model work rehabilitation program, Hosp. Community Psychiatry **33**:1017, Dec. 1982.

This article focuses on a vocational rehabilitation program that places patients in volunteer jobs in local community agencies. Advantages for the patients include increased self-esteem related to task accomplishment, learning social and work skills, and experiencing a normal environment.

*La Duke, D.L., et al.: Operation homeward bound—a military psychiatric transition program, J. Psychosoc. Nurs. Ment. Health Serv. **18**(7):22, July 1980.

The authors describe a psychiatric rehabilitation program that was implemented in a military setting. The primary interven-

---

*Asterisk indicates nursing reference.

tions were educational in nature and focused on adaptation to the community, interpersonal skills, and job survival skills.

Langsley, D.G., Barter, J.T., and Yarvis, R.M.: Deinstitutionalization—the Sacramento story, Compr. Psychiatry **19**:749, 1978.

These authors demonstrate the effect of legislation on the provision of mental health care. They describe the changes that took place in Sacramento, California, in response to the passage of the Lanterman-Petris-Short Act, which reorganized the mental health care system in the state.

*Leavitt, M.: The discharge crisis: the experience of families of psychiatric patients, Nurs. Res. **24**:33, Jan.-Feb. 1975.

This research report describes the results of interviews with the families of 16 psychiatric patients prior to discharge from the hospital. The investigator concluded that the families were not prepared to deal with the patient at home. She analyzes several reasons for this response.

*McMordie, W.R.: Helping patients control their own money: money management training, Persp. Psychiatr. Care **20**:33, Jan.-Mar. 1982.

The inability to manage money frequently prevents the mentally or neurologically disabled person from living successfully in the community. The author recommends a skills training approach to assist them to learn about transactions involving money.

*Norbeck, J.S.: The use of social support in clinical practice, J. Psychosoc. Nurs. Ment. Health Serv. **20**(12):22, Dec. 1982.

This is an excellent discussion of the concept of social support. Relevant research findings are presented. The author developed a typology of social support-related problems and suggests nursing interventions.

*Reid, L.: Approaches to the aftermath of schizophrenia, Perspect. Psychiatr. Care **17**:257, 1979.

The author discusses the reactions of the individual following hospitalization for psychotic behavior. A group approach focused on patient education is advocated, with encouragement of patients to ask questions and discuss their experiences. This is a good description of an effective nursing approach in a partial hospitalization setting.

Skirball, B.W., and Pavelsky, P.L.: The compeer program: volunteers as friends of the mentally ill, Hosp. Community Psychiatry **35**:938, Sept. 1984.

The authors describe a program in which trained volunteers provide support services to mentally ill people. This relationship is coordinated with the patient's therapist and provides the patient with an added dimension of a normal friendship.

*Sweeney, D., et al.: Mapping urban hotels: life space of the chronic mental patient, J. Psychosoc. Nurs. Ment. Health Serv. **20**(5):9, May 1982.

Community care providers should seek out patients on their own turf. Many live in urban hotels. Nurses need to visit these hotels and enlist proprietors and/or staff as community caregivers. The object is not to "professionalize" them, but to assist them to provide social support to the residents.

Talbott, J.A.: The chronic mental patient: five years later, New York, 1984, Grune & Stratton, Inc.

This important anthology includes chapters written by most of the recognized authorities in the care of the chronically mentally ill. The scope of the topics covered and the depth of the presentations make this an invaluable resource to the psychiatric nurse.

Walsh, M.: Schizophrenia: straight talk for families and friends, New York, 1985, William Morrow and Co., Inc.

This book is recommended to nurses as an excellent presentation of the impact of schizophrenia on the family. The author is very frank in describing her experiences with the mental health care system and those of other families. Nurses should also recommend this book to families of patients. It contains much information and advice, including a list of rehabilitation resources.

Whitmer, G.L.: From hospitals to jails: the fate of California's deinstitutionalized mentally ill, Am. J. Orthopsychiatry **50**:65, Jan. 1980.

This is a presentation of the darker side of the deinstitutionalization experience as mandated by law in California. The author maintains that people who were forced out of state hospitals are now being found in state prisons. He criticizes the law in terms of the actual effect on people. It is a good demonstration of the impact of a political decision on human services.

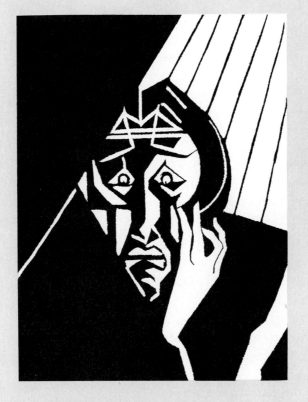

. . . . The fears we know
Are of not knowing . . . It is getting late.
Shall we ever be asked for? Are we simply
Not wanted at all?

W. H. Auden, The Age of Anxiety

C H A P T E R   1 2

ANXIETY

LEARNING OBJECTIVES

After studying this chapter, the student should be able to:

- describe the characteristics of the concept of anxiety.

- compare and contrast the four levels of anxiety with regard to one's perceptual field, potential for learning, and continuum of coping responses.

- discuss the predisposing factors that have been proposed for the origin of anxiety.

- analyze precipitating stressors that contribute to the development of anxiety.

- state the value of a unified multicausal model of anxiety.

- identify the physiological, behavioral, cognitive, and affective behaviors that are associated with anxiety.

- identify and describe the coping mechanisms associated with task-oriented and ego-oriented reactions.

- analyze the position of anxiety within the nursing model of health-illness phenomena.

- formulate individualized nursing diagnoses for patients with varying levels of anxiety.

- assess the relationship between nursing diagnoses and medical diagnoses associated with anxiety.

- develop long-term and short-term individualized nursing goals with patients who are experiencing anxiety.

- apply therapeutic nurse-patient relationship principles with appropriate rationale in planning the care of the patient who is experiencing anxiety.

- describe nursing interventions appropriate to the needs of the patient who is experiencing panic, severe, moderate, and mild levels of anxiety.

- analyze the indications for, techniques of, and problems associated with promoting the relaxation response.

- develop a mental health education plan to promote a patient's adaptive anxiety responses.

- assess the importance of the evaluation of the nursing process when working with patients who experience anxiety.

- identify directions for future nursing research.

- select appropriate readings for further study.

During the past 20 years over 500 articles or books have been published on the topic of anxiety, which appears to be a pervasive aspect of contemporary life. It is created within the environment by threats of war, monetary inflation, the energy crisis, and political kidnappings. Anxiety is also created within the individual as one experiences inner confusion, conflicting values, role diffusion, and personal disenchantment. The seventeenth century was known as the Age of Enlightenment, the eighteenth as the Age of Reason, the nineteenth as the Age of Progress, and the twentieth as the Age of Anxiety. But anxiety is as old as human existence and belongs to no particular era or culture. It derives from the greek root meaning "to press tight" or "to strangle"; the Latin term for "anxious" also denotes narrowness or constriction, usually with discomfort.

Although the concept of anxiety is timeless, its great impact on human life has been realized only in recent years. It is all-pervasive, and every corner of human endeavor is affected by anxiety. It is closely related to the terms "anger," when defined as "grief or trouble," and "anguish," which is described as "acute pain, suffering, or distress." Anxiety is a multidimensional concept, and it is manifested as a somatic, experiential, and interpersonal phenomenon. It therefore involves one's body, perceptions of self, and relationships with others. These elements make it a foundational concept in the study of psychiatric nursing and human behavior.

Continuum of anxiety responses

May defines anxiety as "diffuse apprehension that is vague in nature and associated with feelings of uncertainty and helplessness."[21:190] Feelings of isolation, alienation, and insecurity are also present as the person perceives that the core of his personality is being threatened. Experiences provoking anxiety begin in infancy and continue throughout life, concluding with the fear of the greatest unknown, death.

■ Defining characteristics

Understanding the concept of anxiety can be enhanced by exploring some of its characteristics. Anxiety is an emotion and a subjective experience of the individual. It is an energy, and as such cannot be observed directly. The perception of a nurse that a patient is anxious is an inference based on certain behaviors of the patient. As with all inferences, the nurse needs to validate this with the patient. Also, anxiety is an emotion without a specific object. It is provoked by the unknown and precedes all new experiences such as entering school, starting a new job, or giving birth to a child.

This characteristic of anxiety differentiates it from **fear,** which is an ideation of the individual that has a specific source or object which the person can identify and describe. Fear involves the intellectual appraisal of a threatening stimulus; anxiety involves the emotional response to that appraisal. When a person says he fears something, he is generally referring to a set of circumstances that are not present but that may occur at some point in the future. A fear is activated when a person is exposed, either physically or psychologically, to the stimulus situation he considers threatening. When the fear becomes activated, he experiences anxiety. Fear then, is the appraisal of danger; anxiety is the unpleasant feeling state evoked when fear is stimulated. This distinction is evident in the phrases used in speaking of the two emotions; one speaks of *having* a fear but of *being* anxious.

Another important characteristic of anxiety for the nurse is the fact that it is communicated interpersonally. This means that if a nurse is talking with a patient who is anxious, within a short time the nurse will also experience feelings of anxiety. Similarly, if a nurse is anxious in a particular situation, this will be readily communicated to the patient. The contagious nature of anxiety can therefore have positive and negative effects on the therapeutic relationship and must be diligently monitored by the nurse. It is also important to remember that anxiety is part of the fabric of everyday life. It is basic to the human condition and provides a valuable warning system to the individual. In fact, the capacity to be anxious is necessary for survival.

The balance between survival and death addresses the crux of anxiety—preservation of self. Anxiety occurs as a result of a threat to a person's selfhood, self-esteem, or identity. Tillich describes it as "the state in which a being is aware of its possible non-being."[31] It occurs when something central to one's personality, essential to one's existence and security, is being threatened. It may be connected with the fear of punishment and disapproval, withdrawal of love, disruption of a relationship, isolation, or loss of body functioning. Anxiety is experienced when the values a person identifies with his existence as a person are threatened. In this way culture is related to anxiety in that culture determines in part the values the individual holds as most important. These values include the physical, social, moral, and emotional elements of life. Underlying every fear is the anxiety of not being able to preserve one's own being, and this is the frightening element. However, a person can meet the anxiety and grow from it to the extent that his values are stronger than the threat.

All people therefore need a balance between courage and anxiety to preserve themselves, fulfill their beings, and affirm their existence. It is only by moving through anxiety-creating experiences that one achieves self-realization. Whenever a person moves through new possibilities, he enlarges his self-awareness, increases the scope of his activity, and expands his freedom. As May summarizes it, "the positive aspects of selfhood develop as the individual confronts, moves through and overcomes anxiety-creating experiences."[21:234]

■ Levels of anxiety

In defining the concept of anxiety, Peplau[27] identified four levels of anxiety and described the effects of each on the individual (Fig. 12-1). The first is **mild anxiety,** which is associated with the tension of day-to-day living. During this stage the person is alert and his perceptual field is increased as he sees, hears, and grasps more than previously. This kind of anxiety can motivate learning and can produce growth and creativity in the individual. The second level is **moderate anxiety,** in which the person focuses on immediate concerns and blocks out the periphery. His perceptual field is narrowed as he sees, hears, and grasps less. He thus experiences selective inattention but can attend to more if he is directed to do so. The third level is **severe anxiety,** in which the person's perceptual field is greatly reduced. He tends to focus on a specific detail and not think about anything else. All his behavior is aimed at getting relief, and he needs much direction to focus on another area. The final level is **panic,** which is associated with awe, dread, and terror. At this time details are blown out of proportion. Because the individual is experiencing a loss of control, he is unable to do things even with direction. Panic involves the disorganization of the personality. It is a state in which a person can no

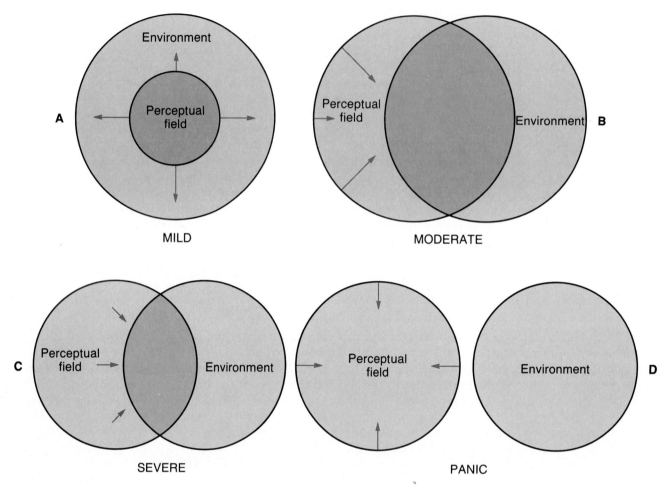

Fig. 12-1. Levels of anxiety.

longer function as an organized human being. With panic there is increased motor activity, decreased ability to relate to others, distorted perceptions, and loss of rational thought.[25] This is a frightening and paralyzing experience for the individual in which he is unable to communicate or function effectively. This level of anxiety cannot persist indefinitely. It is incompatible with life, and, if it continued over a prolonged period, exhaustion and death would result.

The nurse working with a patient will be able to identify which level of anxiety is present on the basis of the behaviors she observes. The anxiety response may then be conceptualized on the continuum of coping responses described in the nursing model of health-illness phenomena (Chapter 3). Fig. 12-2 characterizes the anxiety response as ranging from the most adaptive response of anticipation to the most maladaptive response of panic. The nurse's identification of the patient's level of anxiety and its position on the continuum of coping responses will be relevant to the nursing di-

agnosis and will subsequently affect the type of intervention she chooses to implement.

Assessment

■ Predisposing factors

Anxiety is a prime factor in the development of the personality and formation of individual character traits. It is natural, then, that various theories of the origin of anxiety would exist. However, the present core of definitely established facts to support these theories is small.

■ **PSYCHOANALYTIC VIEW.** Freud initiated the study of anxiety, and his position underwent a drastic change 30 years after he first formulated it. In the beginning Freud regarded anxiety as a purely physiological reaction to a person's chronic inability to reach an orgasm in sexual relations. He believed that if the sexual instincts were not allowed to express themselves directly, their energy would be converted into anxiety. Alleviation of anxiety therefore merely required the

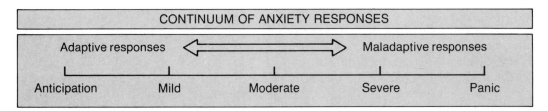

Fig. 12-2. Continuum of anxiety responses.

proper adjustments in the patient's sexual technique. Not until much later did he see the importance of anxiety for a theory of personality development.[14,15]

His change in viewpoint led him to describe two types of anxiety—primary and subsequent. The essence of primary anxiety is the "traumatic" state, which originates in the infant as a result of the sudden stimulation and trauma of the birth process. The process of birth is the first experience attended by anxiety, and experiences of anxiety continue with the possibility that one's physical needs of hunger and thirst might not be met. Primary anxiety therefore was viewed as a state of tension or a drive produced originally by external causes. The environment was seen as being capable of threatening as well as satisfying, and this implicit threat predisposed the individual to anxiety in later life.

With increased age and ego development, a new kind of anxiety arises. Freud viewed this subsequent anxiety as the emotional conflict that takes place between two elements of the personality—the id and the superego. The id represents one's instinctual drives and primitive impulses, whereas the superego reflects one's conscience and culturally acquired restrictions. The ego, or I, serves as the battleground as it tries to mediate the demands of these two clashing elements. Freud therefore suggested that one major function of anxiety was to warn the person of impending danger. It was a signal to the ego that it was in danger of being overtaken.

■ **INTERPERSONAL VIEW.** Sullivan[30] disagreed with Freud in that he believed that anxiety could not arise until the ego reached a minimum stage of development in which the organism had some awareness of its environment. Sullivan viewed the fear of disapproval as central to his theory of anxiety. He looked to the origin of anxiety in the early bond between the infant and mothering one. Through this close emotional bond, anxiety is first conveyed by the mother to the infant, who responds as if he and his mothering person were one unit. As the child grows older, he sees this discomfort as related to what he himself does and conceives of his mother as approving or disapproving of his behavior. In addition, developmental traumas such as separations and losses can lead to specific vulnerabilities.

Sullivan believed that anxiety in later life arises in interpersonal situations in which a person perceives he will be viewed unfavorably or will lose the love of another person whose opinion he values.

Sullivan identified two other aspects of anxiety that will be important in the nurse-patient relationship. The first is that a mild or moderate level of anxiety is frequently expressed as anger by the individual. The second is that areas in the personality marked by anxiety often become the areas of significant growth when, as in a therapeutic relationship, the individual can learn to deal with his anxiety constructively.

Will[33] believes that an individual's level of self-esteem is an important factor related to anxiety. A person with a high predisposition to anxiety is one who is easily threatened, has a low level of self-esteem, or has a poor opinion of himself. This is evident in a person with test anxiety. His anxiety is high because he doubts his ability to succeed. This may have nothing to do with his actual abilities, how prepared he is, or how much he studied; the anxiety is due only to his perception of his ability, which reflects his self-concept. He may, for instance, be well prepared for the examination, but his severe level of anxiety will reduce his perceptual field significantly and he may omit, misinterpret, or distort the meaning of the test items. He may even block out all his previous studying when handed the examination. The result will be a poor grade, and this will in turn reinforce his poor perception of self. Research supports the theory that individuals with high anxiety appear to have a greater discrepancy between their perceived self and ideal self.[29] Thus low self-esteem can be a cause of proneness to high anxiety.

■ **BEHAVIORAL VIEW.** Some behavioral theorists propose that anxiety is a product of frustration, which is anything that interferes with one's ability to attain a desired goal. The actual precipitating factor may be any of a number of internal or external stressors, but it acts to block the individual's attempt to obtain satisfaction and security. An example of an external frustration for a young man might be his factory's decision to lay off a certain number of employees, including himself. In this instance, many of his goals may be potentially blocked, such as financial security, pride in work, and perception of self as family provider. An internal frustration is evidenced by the young college graduate who sets unrealistically high personal career goals and continues to be frustrated by job offers of a clerical or apprentice nature. In this case his view of self is being threatened by his unrealistic goals, and he is likely to experience feelings of failure, insignificance, and mounting anxiety.

Other experimental psychologists regard anxiety as a learned drive based on an innate desire to avoid pain. They believe that anxiety begins with the attachment of pain to a particular stimulus, and, if the reaction is strong enough, it may become extended or generalized to similar objects and situations. Learning theorists believe that individuals who have been exposed in early life to intense fears are more likely to demonstrate a high predisposition to anxiety in later life. In this respect, parental influences are important. The child who sees his parents respond with anxiety to every minor stress soon develops a similar pattern. This can also occur if the child's parents are completely unmoved by potentially stressful situations. In this case the child feels alone and lacks emotional support in family stress situations. It is the appropriate emotional response of parents that gives the child security and helps him learn constructive coping methods of his own.

Another way in which anxiety is theorized to arise is through conflict, which is defined as the clashing of two opposing interests. The person experiences two competing drives and must choose between them. A reciprocal relationship exists between conflict and anxiety; conflict produces anxiety and yet anxiety produces feelings of helplessness, which in turn increases one's perceived conflict. Dollard and Miller[11] conceptualize conflict as deriving from two tendencies: approach and avoidance. Approach is the tendency to do something or move toward something, whereas avoidance is the opposite tendency—not to do something or not to move toward something. The authors identify four kinds of conflict (Fig. 12-3). The first is the **approach-approach** conflict in which the individual is motivated to pursue two equally desirable but incompatible goals. This type of conflict seldom produces anxiety, which is more prevalent in conflicts involving avoidance. **Approach-avoidance** conflict occurs when the individual wishes both to obtain and avoid a goal at the same time. This can be evident in the patient who desires to express his anger but feels great anxiety and fear in doing so or in the business executive who wishes to be advanced

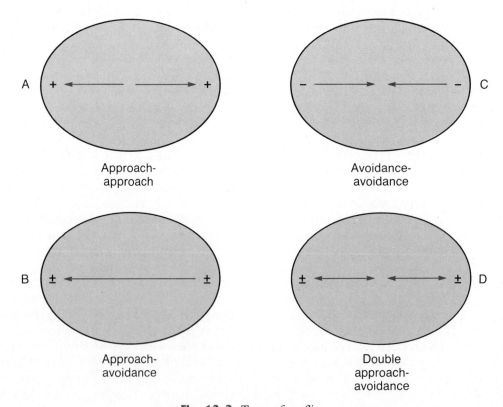

Approach-
approach

Avoidance-
avoidance

Approach-
avoidance

Double
approach-
avoidance

Fig. 12-3. Types of conflict.

within his company but to be promoted must compromise his values of honesty and loyalty. **Avoidance-avoidance** is a third kind of conflict in which the person must choose between two undesirable goals. This is a difficult choice, since neither alternative seems beneficial, and it is usually accompanied by much anxiety. The most common type of conflict situation is the **double approach-avoidance.** In this case the person can see both desirable and undesirable aspects of both alternatives. Frequently this is the kind of conflict experienced by a person who must choose between continuing to live with the pain of his social and emotional life and destructive coping patterns or expose himself to the threat and potential pain of the therapy process, should he seek psychiatric help. These kinds of double approach-avoidance conflict feelings are frequently described as ambivalence. In summarizing their theory, Dollard and Miller stress the importance of conditioning early in life but assert that still little is known about how most complex learned drives are acquired or about those factors which permit one person to easily resolve a conflict while another is plunged into a tumultuous emotional state.

■ **FAMILY STUDIES.** Epidemiological and family studies show that anxiety disorders clearly run in families and that they are common and heterogeneous.[32] There is an overlap within the anxiety disorders and between anxiety disorders and depression. In addition, there is an increased probability that a person with one anxiety disorder will have another or will have a major depression within his or her lifetime.

It has been estimated that the prevalence of all anxiety disorders is about 4% to 8% of the general population and only about a quarter of persons with anxiety disorders receive treatment for these problems. However, these persons are high users of health care facilities for reasons other than emotional problems.[32]

■ **BIOLOGICAL BASIS.** Basic science advances in understanding anxiety have been considerable in recent years. Investigators have learned that the brain contains specific receptors for benzodiazepines, and that these receptors probably help to regulate anxiety. The discovery of benzodiazepine receptors has prompted a search for naturally occurring brain substances that bond to them. The inhibitory neuroregulator gamma-aminobutyric acid (GABA) also may play a major role in biological mechanisms relating to anxiety, as may the endorphins. Although the theory is still controversial, some investigators believe that an area deep in the brain called the locus ceruleus, which is known to be important in a number of behaviors, may have a key role in certain forms of anxiety. Rigorous studies of drugs that relieve and produce anxiety should help provide additional information regarding the biological basis for anxiety disorders.

In addition, it has been shown that an individual's general health has a marked effect on his predisposition to anxiety. Anxiety may accompany some physical disorders, and growing evidence suggests that it can worsen such dangerous illnesses as hypertension, heart disease, and peptic ulcer. Hyperthyroidism, hypoglycemia, and severe pulmonary disease are other illnesses associated with high levels of anxiety. One's coping mechanisms may be impaired by toxic influences, dietary deficiencies, reduced blood supply, hormonal changes, and other physical causes. In the presence of physical illness, there is input from somatic sources that may reduce one's capacity to cope with additional stressful inputs. One study that examined the relationship between selected health-related stressful life events and anxiety levels found that anxiety was strongly related to the number of days the individual had been sick during the last month, as well as the incidences of hospitalization, involvement in an accident, and four out of five medical conditions.[12] In addition, symptoms from some physical disorders, including hyperthyroidism, may mimic or exacerbate anxiety.

Similarly, fatigue increases irritability and feelings of anxiety. It appears that fatigue produced as a result of nervous factors predisposes the individual to a greater degree of anxiety than does fatigue that has resulted from purely physical causes. Thus fatigue may actually be an early symptom of anxiety, and patients complaining of nervous fatigue may already be suffering from a moderate anxiety state and be more susceptible to future stress situations.

■ **Precipitating stressors**

Given these numerous theories about the origin of anxiety, what kinds of events might precipitate feelings of anxiety within the individual? It is possible to group precipitating stressors into two categories: threats to one's physical integrity and threats to one's self-system.

■ **THREATS TO PHYSICAL INTEGRITY.** This category suggests impending physiological disability or decreased capacity to perform the activities of daily living. They may include exposure to viral and bacterial infection or to environmental pollutants or safety hazards (external source); failure of one's own physiological mechanisms, such as the heart, immune system, or temperature regulator (internal source); lack of adequate housing, food, or clothing (external source); normal biological changes that might occur with pregnancy or aging (internal source); traumatic injury (external source); or failure to participate in preventive health practices in such areas as dental care, exercise, rest, or routine physical examinations (internal source). Pain is often the first indication that one's physical integrity is being threatened. It creates anxiety that often motivates the person to seek health care. Thus some preventive health programs try to generate mild anxiety. Because threats to one's physical integrity do produce anxiety, many of the patients nurses work with will experience these feelings.

■ **THREATS TO SELF-SYSTEM.** Threats derived from this second category are quite pervasive. Basically, they imply harm to one's identify, self-esteem, and integrated social functioning. They may include a variety of losses, such as a spouse, parent, or close friend through death, divorce, or relocation (external source); interpersonal difficulties at home, at work, or in the community (internal sources); change in job status (external source); assumption of a new role, such as parent, student, employee, or group leader (internal source); ethical dilemmas arising from one's religious, family, or work situation (external source); social or cultural group pressures (external source); and many of the threats to physical integrity previously mentioned, since the mind-body relationship is an intimate and overlapping one.

This distinction of categories is only theoretical, since the person responds to all stressors, whatever their nature and origin, as an integrated whole. Nor will any specific event be as equally stressful to all individuals or even to the same individual at different times.

■ **AN INTEGRATIVE MODEL.** A true understanding of anxiety requires integration of knowledge from all of the various points of view. Akiskal has proposed an integrative model that accommodates data generated from psychoanalytic, interpersonal, behavioral, genetic, and biological perspectives.[1] This multicausal model provides a useful frame of reference for the nurse because it is holistic in nature and encourages the assessment of behaviors and perceptions in developing appropriate nursing interventions. It also suggests a variety of causative factors and stresses the interrelationship of them in explaining present behavior. It proposes that anxiety disorders can best be understood as an integration of the following factors:

1. There is a built-in neurobiological substance that prepares the individual to cope with danger.
2. Evolution has affected this substance in such a way that certain stimuli that are threatening to survival are selectively avoided.
3. Certain individuals may be born with a central autonomous nervous system that is overly sensitive to stimuli that are generally harmless.
4. Childhood and adult learning experiences may ultimately determine the extent, severity, and nature of the situations that will evoke anxiety.

5. Chronic inability to cope with dangerous situations adaptively could create a high tendency to respond with anxiety.
6. The cognitive functions of humans might permit continual focusing on anxiety reactions, such that the mere anticipation of aversive stimuli would provoke anxiety.
7. Such a person would perhaps be more vulnerable to insecurities, especially if intelligent and inclined toward introspection.

Thus, the person's response will depend on the number and timing of the stressor and the predisposing factors previously described, as well as on the person's perception of the event and the resources he has available. By observing specific behaviors, the nurse will be able to assess the individual's level of anxiety, identify his coping responses, and then formulate an appropriate nursing diagnosis.

■ **Behaviors**

Anxiety can be expressed directly through physiological and behavioral changes. It can also be indirectly manifested through the formation of symptoms or coping mechanisms that attempt to defend one against anxiety. The nature of the behaviors displayed by the patient depends on his level of anxiety. The intensity of the behaviors will increase with increasing anxiety.

In describing anxiety's effects on **physiological responses,** it can be seen that mild and moderate anxiety heighten one's capacities, whereas severe and panic levels paralyze or overwork capacities and structures. The physiological responses associated with anxiety are primarily mediated through the autonomic nervous system. This involves the internal adjustment of the body without a conscious or voluntary effort by the individual. There are two kinds of autonomic responses: the sympathetic, which serve to activate body processes, and the parasympathetic, which act to conserve body responses.

Experimental studies support the predominance of the sympathetic reaction, which prepares the body to deal with an emergency situation by either a "fight" or "flight" reaction. When the cortex of the brain perceives a threat, it sends a stimulus down the sympathetic branch of the autonomic nervous system to the adrenal glands. Because of a release of epinephrine, respiration deepens, the heart beats more rapidly, and arterial pressure rises. Blood is shifted away from the stomach and intestines to the heart, central nervous system, and muscle. Glycogenolysis is accelerated, and the blood glucose level rises. For some individuals, however, the parasympathetic reaction may coexist or predominate and produce somewhat opposite effects. Other physiological reactions may also be evident. The variety of physiological responses to anxiety that the nurse may observe in patients are summarized in Table 12-1.

Psychomotor manifestations, or **behavioral responses,** will also be evident by the patient in the anxious state. Its effects have both personal and interpersonal aspects. High levels of anxiety affect one's coordination, involuntary movements, and responsiveness. They also act as disjunctive forces in human relationships. In an interpersonal situation, anxiety can be a warning that discomfort is to be anticipated and the person had best withdraw from the threatening situation. It is therefore common to see signs of withdrawal and decreased personal involvement with others displayed by the anxious patient. The possible behavioral responses the nurse might observe are presented in Table 12-2.

Mental, or intellectual, functioning is also affected by anxiety. **Cognitive responses** the patient might display when experiencing moderate, severe, or panic levels of anxiety are described in Table 12-2.

Finally, the nurse will be able to assess a patient's emotional reactions, or **affective responses,** to anxiety by his subjective description of his personal experience. Frequently patients describe themselves as "tense, jittery, on edge, jumpy, worried, or restless." One patient attempted to describe his feelings in the following way: "I'm expecting something terribly bad to happen, but I don't know what. I'm afraid, but I don't know why. I guess you can call it a generalized bad feeling." All these phrases are expressions of a person's apprehension and overalertness. They convey the impression that all is not well, and it seems clear that the person interprets his anxiety as a kind of warning sign. Additional affective responses are listed in Table 12-2.

Anxiety is an unpleasant and uncomfortable experience that no one wants or will seek out. Most people will go to extremes to avoid it and frequently try to replace its awareness by some other feeling that is more tolerable. Pure anxiety is rarely seen, but it is usually observed in combination with other emotions. Patients might describe feelings of anger, boredom, contempt, depression, irritation, worthlessness, jealousy, self-depreciation, suspiciousness, sadness, or helplessness, which may be viewed as defenses to shield them from the distress of anxiety. This may present problems for the nurse who is trying to discriminate between anxiety and depression, for instance, because the content expressed by the patient may be similar.[23]

In fact, there are close ties between anxiety, depression, guilt, and hostility, and these emotions often function in a reciprocal manner—one feeling acts to generate and reinforce the others. The relationship between anx-

---

TABLE 12-1

PHYSIOLOGICAL RESPONSES TO ANXIETY*

Cardiovascular

Palpitations
Heart racing
Increased blood pressure
Faintness (p)
Actual fainting (p)
Decreased blood pressure (p)
Decreased pulse rate (p)

Respiratory

Rapid breathing
Shortness of breath
Pressure on chest
Shallow breathing
Lump in throat
Choking sensation
Gasping

Neuromuscular

Increased reflexes
Startle reaction
Eyelid twitching
Insomnia
Tremors
Rigidity
Fidgeting
Pacing
Strained face
Generalized weakness
Wobbly legs
Clumsy movement

Gastrointestinal

Loss of appetite
Revulsion toward food
Abdominal discomfort
Abdominal pain (p)
Nausea (p)
Heartburn (p)
Diarrhea (p)

Urinary Tract

Pressure to urinate (p)
Frequency of urination (p)

Skin

Face flushed
Localized sweating (palms)
Itching
Hot and cold spells
Face pale
Generalized sweating

*(p) indicates parasympathetic response

---

iety and hostility is particularly close, since the pain one experiences with anxiety frequently gives rise to anger and resentment toward those perceived to be responsible, and these feelings of hostility then serve to increase one's level of anxiety.

This cycle is evident in the case of a dependent and insecure wife who was very attached to her husband and who expressed numerous vague fears. In exploring her feelings, she also expressed great hostility toward him and their relationship, which symbolized her helplessness and increased her feelings of weakness. Verbalizing these angry feelings, however, served to further increase her anxiety and her unresolved conflict.

Thus it is evident that anxiety frequently finds

TABLE 12-2

BEHAVIORAL, COGNITIVE, AND AFFECTIVE RESPONSES TO ANXIETY

Behavioral	Cognitive	Affective
Restlessness	Impaired attention	Edgy
Physical tension	Poor concentration	Impatient
Tremors	Forgetfulness	Uneasy
Startle reaction	Errors in judgment	Tense
Rapid speech	Preoccupation	Nervous
Lack of coordination	Blocking of thoughts	Fearful
Accident proneness	Decreased perceptual field	Scared
Interpersonal withdrawal	Reduced creativity	Frightened
Inhibition	Diminished productivity	Alarmed
Flight	Confusion	Terrified
Avoidance	Hypervigilant	Jittery
Hyperventilation	Self-conscious	Jumpy
	Loss of objectivity	
	Fear of losing control	
	Frightening visual images	
	Fear of injury or death	

---

expression in anger, and a tense and anxious person is more likely to become angry.

■ Coping mechanisms

As the level of anxiety increases to the severe and panic levels, the behaviors displayed become more intense and injurious to the individual. It is obvious that these behaviors may be painful, uncomfortable, and unpleasant. It is also understandable, then, that people seek to avoid anxiety and the circumstances in which it arises. When experiencing anxiety, the individual uses various coping mechanisms to try to allay it, and the inability to cope with anxiety constructively is a primary causative factor in the creation of pathological behavior. In an attempt to neutralize, deny, or counteract anxiety the individual develops patterns of coping, and the pattern he uses to cope with mild anxiety tends to remain dominant when anxiety becomes more intense. It can be said that anxiety plays a major role in the psychogenesis of emotional illness, since many symptoms of illness develop as attempted defenses against anxiety. These symptoms also provide the outward but disguised symbolical expression of elements of the conflict.

It is beneficial for the nurse to be familiar with the coping mechanisms people use when experiencing the various levels of anxiety. The **mild level of anxiety** is the anxiety one experiences as the tension of day-to-day living. Menninger[24] identified a number of coping mechanisms people use to relieve this kind of tension.

These include crying, sleeping, eating, yawning, laughing, cursing, physical exercise, daydreaming, and oral behavior, such as smoking and drinking. In interpersonal situations the individual copes with low levels of anxiety through superficiality, lack of eye contact, use of clichés, and limited self-disclosure. The person can also protect himself from anxiety by assuming roles he is comfortable in and limiting his close relationships to those with people having values similar to his own. Mild levels of anxiety are often handled without conscious thought and their effects can be easily minimized.

Moderate, severe, and panic levels of anxiety, however, pose greater threats to the ego and require the use of more energy to cope with the threat. It is possible to categorize these coping mechanisms as task-oriented reactions and ego-oriented reactions.

■ TASK-ORIENTED REACTIONS.
Task-oriented reactions involve one's cognitive abilities in an attempt to solve problems, resolve conflicts, and gratify one's needs. They are aimed at realistically meeting the demands of the stress situation, which has been objectively appraised. These are consciously directed and action oriented. These types of reactions can include attack, withdrawal, and compromise.

In **attack behavior** a person attempts to remove or overcome obstacles to satisfy a need. There are many possible ways of attacking problems, and this type of reaction may be destructive or constructive. Destructive patterns are usually accompanied by great feelings of anger and hostility, which may be discharged in negative or aggressive behavior that violates the rights, property, and well-being of others. Constructive patterns reflect a problem-solving approach and are evident in self-assertive behaviors that affirm one's own rights while also respecting the rights of others.

Withdrawal behavior may be expressed physically or psychologically. Physically, withdrawal involves removing oneself from the source of the threat. This can apply to biological stressors, such as smoke-filled rooms, exposure to irradiation, or contact with contagious diseases. An individual can also withdraw in various psychological ways, such as by admitting defeat, becoming apathetic, or lowering aspirations. As with attack, this type of reaction may be constructive or destructive. When it is used in a way that isolates the individual from others and interferes with his ability to work, the reaction begins to create additional problems for the individual and is often accompanied by the emotional states of fear, hostility, and guilt.

Because some situations cannot be resolved through either attack or withdrawal, **compromise** is frequently necessary. This involves changing one's usual way of operating, substituting goals, or sacrificing aspects of one's personal needs. Compromise reactions are usually constructive and are frequently employed in approach-approach and avoidance-avoidance situations. When the decision resolves the problem, the individual can then move on to other activities. Occasionally, however, the person realizes with time that the compromise is not acceptable, and he must then renegotiate a solution or adopt a different coping mechanism.

A person's capacity for task-oriented reactions and effective problem solving is greatly influenced by his expectation that he is likely to succeed in achieving at least a part of his goals. This, in turn, will depend on his remembering that he was successful in the past in situations of similar difficulty and that he was able to overcome the presenting obstacles. On this basis, he can go forward and attempt to do something about the stressful situation. Perseverance in problem solving also depends on the person's expectation that a certain level of pain and discomfort is likely to be involved and his belief that people like himself are capable of tolerating this. Here lies the balance between courage and anxiety.

■ **EGO-ORIENTED REACTIONS.** Task-oriented reactions are not always successful in coping with stressful situations. Consequently, ego-oriented reactions are often used to protect the self. These reactions, also called **ego defense mechanisms,** serve as one's first line of psychic defense. Everyone uses defense mechanisms, and they frequently help one cope successfully with mild and moderate levels of anxiety. They function to protect the person from feelings of inadequacy and worthlessness and prevent awareness of anxiety. They can be used to such an extreme degree, however, that they distort reality, interfere with interpersonal relationships, limit one's ability to work productively, and promote ego disintegration instead of self-integrity.

As coping mechanisms they have certain drawbacks. First, they operate on relatively unconscious levels so that the person has little awareness of what is happening and little control over events. Second, they involve a degree of self-deception and reality distortion. Therefore they are usually not adaptive in helping the individual to realistically cope with the problem. Many defense mechanisms have been identified in the literature. Some of the more common ones are identified in Table 12-3.

It is important to conclude a discussion of ego-oriented reactions, or defense mechanisms, with the observation that individuals frequently monitor their own level of emotional tolerance and consequent need for the employment of ego defenses. Caplan notes:

> I have learned to wait patiently, while exercising appropriate, direct and indirect surveillance, to see whether the person will feel strong enough after a while to begin to confront the loss, disappointment or threat and little by little to relax his defenses. This may sometimes take quite a long time.[9:416]

This idea is supported by Elliott,[13] who believes that one defense mechanism in particular, denial, may be used as an effective mechanism to actually allay anxiety immediately following a stressful event. She believes that if denial is gradually eliminated as the stress begins to subside, the person may better adapt to the new situation.

The evaluation of whether the patient's use of certain defense mechanisms is adaptive or maladaptive revolves around the consideration of four issues:

1. The accurate recognition of the patient's use of the defense mechanism by the nurse.
2. The degree to which the defense mechanism is used. Does it imply a high degree of personality disorganization? Is the person unresponsive to facts about his life situation?
3. The degree to which use of the defense mechanism impedes the patient's progress toward regained health.
4. The need underlying the patient's use of the ego defense mechanism.

A consideration of these areas by the nurse will enhance understanding of the patient and the plan for his nursing care.

If the ego defense mechanisms are not successful and the person's level of anxiety remains high, he is forced to use exaggerated and inappropriate coping

TABLE 12-3

EGO DEFENSE MECHANISMS

Defense mechanism	Example	Defense mechanism	Example
Compensation: Process by which a person makes up for a deficiency in his image of himself by strongly emphasizing some other feature that he regards as an asset.	Mr. L, a 42-year-old businessman, perceives his small physical stature negatively. He tries to overcome this by being aggressive, forceful, and controlling in his business dealings.	**Projection:** Attributing one's own thoughts or impulses to another person. Through this process one can attribute his own intolerable wishes, emotional feelings, or motivations to another person.	A young woman who denies she has sexual feelings about a co-worker accuses him without basis of being a "flirt" and says he is trying to seduce her.
Denial: Avoidance of disagreeable realities by ignoring or refusing to recognize them; probably simplest and most primitive of all defense mechanisms.	Mrs. P has just been told that her breast biopsy indicates a malignancy. When her husband visits her that evening, she tells him that no one has discussed the laboratory results with her.	**Rationalization:** Offering a socially acceptable or apparently logical explanation to justify or make acceptable otherwise unacceptable impulses, feelings, behaviors, and motives.	John fails an examination and complains that the lectures were not well organized or clearly presented.
Displacement: Shift of emotion from a person or object toward which it was originally directed to another usually neutral or less dangerous person or object.	Timmy, a 4-year-old boy, is angry because he has just been punished by his mother for drawing on his bedroom walls. He begins to play "war" with his soldier toys and has them battle and fight with each other.	**Reaction formation:** Development of conscious attitudes and behavior patterns that are opposite to what one really feels or would like to do.	A married woman who feels attracted to one of her husband's friends treats him rudely.
Dissociation: The separation of any group of mental or behavioral processes from the rest of the person's consciousness or identity.	A man is brought to the emergency room by the police and is unable to explain who he is and where he lives or works.	**Regression:** Retreat in face of stress to behavior characteristic of any earlier level of development.	Four-year-old Nicole who has been toilet trained for over a year begins to wet her pants again when her new baby brother is brought home from the hospital.
Identification: Process by which a person tries to become like someone he admires by taking on thoughts, mannerisms, or tastes of that individual.	Sally, 15 years old, has her hair styled similarly to her young English teacher whom she admires.	**Repression:** Involuntary exclusion of a painful or conflictual thought, impulse, or memory from awareness. It is the primary ego defense, and other mechanisms tend to reinforce it.	Mr. R does not recall hitting his wife when she was pregnant.
Intellectualization: Excessive reasoning or logic is used to avoid experiencing disturbing feelings.	A woman avoids dealing with her anxiety in shopping malls by explaining that she is saving the frivolous waste of time and money by not going into them.		
Introjection: Intense type of identification in which a person incorporates qualities or values of another person or group into his own ego structure. It is one of the earliest mechanisms of the child; important in formation of conscience.	Eight-year-old Jimmy tells his 3-year-old sister, "Don't scribble in your book of nursery rhymes. Just look at the pretty pictures."	**Splitting:** Viewing people and situations as either all good or all bad. Failure to integrate the positive and negative qualities of oneself.	A friend tells you that you are the most wonderful person in the world one day, and how much she hates you the next day.
		Sublimation: Acceptance of a socially approved substitute goal for a drive whose normal channel of expression is blocked.	Ed has an impulsive and physically aggressive nature. He tries out for the football team and becomes a star tackle.
		Suppression: A process often listed as a defense mechanism, but it is really a conscious analogue of repression. It is intentional exclusion of material from consciousness. At times, it may lead to subsequent repression.	A young man at work finds he is thinking so much about his date that evening that it is interfering with his work. He decides to put it out of his mind until he leaves the office for the day.
Isolation: Splitting off of emotional components of a thought, which may be temporary or long term.	A second-year medical student dissects a cadaver for her anatomy course without being disturbed by thoughts of death.	**Undoing:** Act or communication that partially negates a previous one; primitive defense mechanism.	Larry makes a passionate declaration of love to Sue on a date. On their next meeting he treats her formally and distantly.

mechanisms that may appear deviant or abnormal to others. These coping patterns are maladaptive responses and include the many hidden, unconscious, and devious pathways in which the effects of anxiety are converted psychologically.

Obviously, many coping mechanisms are available to the individual to use in minimizing anxiety. The use of some of these defense mechanisms appears to be essential for all human beings if they are to maintain emotional stability. The exact nature and number of the defenses used by the individual strongly influence his personality pattern. When these defenses are overused or used unsuccessfully, they are responsible for many physiological and psychological symptoms commonly associated with emotional illness. As Freud has said, "One thing is certain, that the problem of anxiety is a nodal point linking up all kinds of most important questions; a riddle, of which the solution must cast a flood of light upon our whole mental life."[14:118]

Nursing diagnosis

Formulating a nursing diagnosis depends on a clear understanding of the position of anxiety within the larger perspective of the nursing model of health-illness phenomena (Fig. 12-4). First, it emerges as a "generalized anxiety reaction" to a person's primary appraisal of a stressor that is perceived to be threatening or harmful. Three aspects of anxiety are activated at this time:

1. The central nervous system is aroused.
2. Anxiety is felt and is evident in various cognitive, affective, physiological, behavioral, and social changes.
3. Ways of coping with anxiety are brought into play.

These coping mechanisms may be constructive or destructive in nature and may represent neurotic or psychotic health problems.

■ Differentiating anxiety responses

Most of the behaviors and coping mechanisms described in this chapter in relation to anxiety could be classified as neurotic disorders or health problems. A **neurosis** is a mental disorder characterized by anxiety but in which there is no distortion of reality. Neurotic disorders are maladaptive anxiety responses associated with moderate and severe levels of anxiety (Fig. 12-4).

Psychosis, however, can emerge with the panic level of anxiety as the individual feels he is "breaking into pieces."[3] Unlike neurosis, the anxiety of psychosis is not just fear of failure or fear of being unable to cope with the threatening situation. It is the fear that the failure will reveal defeat in the "process of living" and failure in the "process of being." This can be seen in the woman who has just given birth to a baby and experiences a postpartum psychosis. In this case the fear manifests itself in connection with being a mother as the woman identifies with her own mother and with the child and experiences feelings of unfulfilled needs and personal inadequacies.

In addition to differentiating between neurotic and psychotic anxiety responses, the nurse will need to be able to discriminate between anxiety and depression.[4] There is frequently an overlap in this area because anxious patients are often depressed and depressed patients are often anxious. Specific differences between the two groups, and these are described in Table 12-4.

■ Identifying nursing problems

The nurse who has adequately assessed a patient and uses a conceptual model for understanding anxiety will be able to formulate a nursing diagnosis based on the patient's position on the continuum of anxiety responses. In doing so, the nurse will review the objective data collected, as well as the subjective responses of the patient to questions and statements. The patient's history will be important, as will be the nurse's personal response to the patient, since anxiety is one experience that is readily communicated interpersonally.

In formulating the nursing diagnosis in relation to anxiety, the research of Lagina[18] shows that nurses tend to refer more frequently to subjective observations than to objective behaviors. They appear to rely heavily on the patient's medical diagnosis of health problems, prognosis, and the therapy indicated. Lagina stresses the need for nurses to go beyond the patient's medical diagnosis to find out what behavior the patient is displaying and his pattern of responding to anxiety. She also suggests that nurses, in diagnosing their patients' anxiety, may be projecting their own anxiety, and she underscores the need to distinguish between the two.

The formulation of a nursing diagnosis requires that the nurse determine the quality and quantity of the anxiety experienced by the patient and the constructive or destructive nature of the coping mechanism mobilized. In considering the quality of the anxiety, the nurse might question the appropriateness of the patient's response to the perceived threat. Is it warranted, sensible, and adaptive or absurd and irrational? A problem may exist if the response is out of proportion to the threat. This would indicate that the patient's cognitive appraisal of the threat is unrealistic. The quantity of the reaction is the next consideration as the nurse attempts to determine the degree or level of anxiety present. The escalation of the anxiety to the severe and panic levels indicates that the conflict is increasingly problematic and incapacitating for the patient.

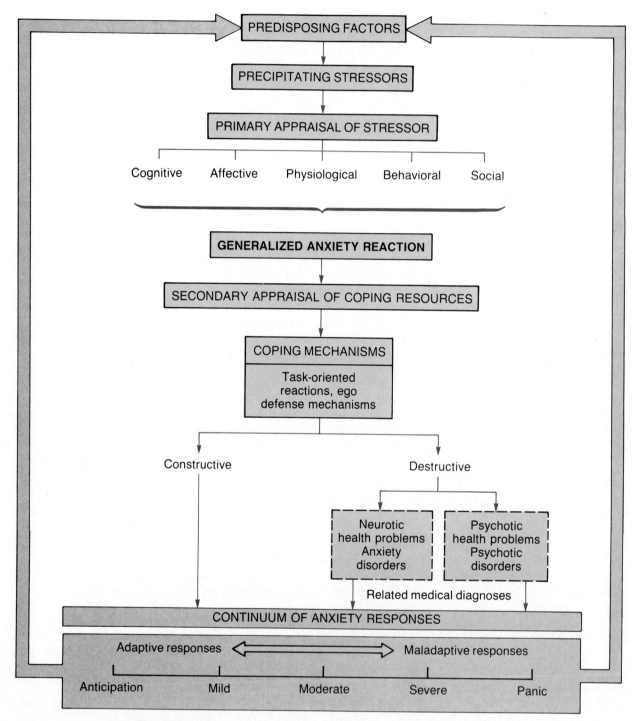

Fig. 12-4. Nursing model of health-illness phenomena related to anxiety.

The nurse also needs to explore how the anxiety is being met or coped with. Constructive coping mechanisms are protective responses that confront the threat on the level of conscious awareness. Destructive coping mechanisms involve repression into the unconscious and tend to be ineffective, inadequate, disorganized,

inappropriate, and exaggerated. They may be evident in bizarre behavior or symptom formation.

Finally, the question may be posed as to the overall effect of the anxiety on the individual. Is it stimulating growth? Or is it interfering with effective living and life satisfaction? Is it enhancing one's sense of self? Or is it

TABLE 12-4

DIFFERENCES BETWEEN ANXIETY AND DEPRESSION

Anxiety	Depression
Negative appraisals are selective and specific and do not encompass all areas of functioning.	Negative appraisals are pervasive, global, and exclusive.
Sees some prospects for the future.	Sees the future as blank and has given up all hope.
Does not regard defects or mistakes as irrevocable.	Regards mistakes as beyond redemption.
Uncertain in his negative evaluations.	Absolute in his negative evaluations.
Anticipates possible damage to his health, satisfaction, and survival.	Regrets he has lost sources of gratification but believes he is incapable of change.
Predicts that only certain specific events may go badly.	Global view that nothing will turn out right for him.

depersonalizing and despiritizing? Whenever possible, the patient should be included in identifying problem areas. This may not always be feasible, however, particularly if the patient's anxiety level is at the severe or panic level.

An appropriate nursing diagnosis would reflect these criteria. It should include the nursing problem, the related stressor, and maladaptive health response. Primary NANDA nursing diagnoses and examples of complete nursing diagnoses related to anxiety are presented in the accompanying box. Obviously, a complete nursing assessment would include all maladaptive responses of the patient, and many additional nursing problems would be identified from the way the patient's anxiety reciprocally influences his interpersonal relationships, self-concept, cognitive functioning, physiological status, and other aspects of his life. The identification of nursing problems should be as complete as possible to ensure an adequate plan of care and intervention. Nursing diagnoses related to the range of possible maladaptive responses of the patient are identified in Table 12-5.

Nursing diagnoses can be formulated for any patient experiencing anxiety. It may be a coping response to a physical illness, a psychological illness, or a perceived threat to one's physical integrity or self-system. The patient may or may not also have been medically diagnosed.

■ Related medical diagnoses

Many patients experiencing anxiety of a transient or less severe nature have no medically diagnosed health problem. However, patients experiencing more severe levels of anxiety most commonly have neurotic disorders that fall under the category of anxiety disorders in the Draft of the DSM-III-R in Development.[2] The eight

Nursing Diagnoses Related to Anxiety

Primary NANDA Nursing Diagnoses

Anxiety
Coping, ineffective: individual
Fear

Examples of Complete Nursing Diagnoses

Panic level of anxiety related to family rejection evidenced by confusion and impaired judgment
Severe anxiety related to sexual conflict evidenced by repetitive handwashing and recurrent thoughts of dirt and germs
Severe anxiety related to marital conflict evidenced by inability to leave the house
Moderate anxiety related to financial pressures evidenced by recurring episodes of abdominal pain and heartburn
Moderate anxiety related to assumption of motherhood role evidenced by inhibition and avoidance
Moderate anxiety related to poor school performance evidenced by excessive use of denial and rationalization
Ineffective individual coping related to daughter's death evidenced by inability to recall events pertaining to the car accident
Ineffective individual coping related to child's illness evidenced by limited ability to concentrate and psychomotor agitation
Fear related to impending surgery evidenced by generalized hostility to staff and restlessness

TABLE 12-5

MEDICAL AND NURSING DIAGNOSES RELATED TO ANXIETY

Medical Diagnostic Class	Psychiatric Nursing Diagnostic Class
Anxiety disorders	Anxiety
Related Medical Diagnoses (DSM-III-R)*	**Related Nursing Diagnoses (NANDA)**
Panic disorder	†Anxiety
Agoraphobia without panic attacks	Bowel elimination, alteration in
Social phobia	Breathing pattern, ineffective
Simple phobia	Communication, impaired: verbal
Obsessive-compulsive disorder	†Coping, ineffective: individual
Post-traumatic stress disorder	†Fear
Generalized anxiety disorder	Health maintenance, alteration in
Anxiety disorder NOS	Impaired adjustment
	Impaired social interaction
	Injury, potential for
	Nutrition, alteration in
	Post-trauma response
	Powerlessness
	Self-concept, disturbance in
	Sensory-perceptual alteration
	Sleep pattern disturbance
	Social isolation
	Stress incontinence
	Thought process, alteration in
	Urinary elimination, alteration in

*From American Psychiatric Association: Draft of the DSM-III-R in Development (subject to change), as proposed by the Work Group to Revise DSM-III. American Psychiatric Association, October 1985.
†Indicates primary nursing diagnoses for anxiety

major disorders included in this category are listed in Table 12-5. Each one will now be briefly described.

■ **PANIC DISORDER.** The essential features of this disorder are recurrent panic (anxiety) attacks that occur at times unpredictably, though certain situations, such as driving a car, may become associated with a panic attack. They are manifested by the sudden onset of intense apprehension, fear, or terror, and are often associated with feelings of impending doom. The most common symptoms experienced during an attack are: shortness of breath, choking, palpitations, chest pain, sweating, faintness, dizziness, nausea, depersonalization, numbness, hot flashes, trembling, fear of dying, and fear of going crazy or doing something uncontrolled. Attacks usually last minutes; more rarely, hours. The individual often develops varying degrees of nervousness and apprehension between attacks.

■ **AGORAPHOBIA WITHOUT PANIC ATTACKS.** The essential features are a fear of being away from a safe place or person, especially in situations where incapacitation may occur. The individual experiences gen-

eralized travel restrictions, often needs a companion away from home, and has a markedly altered life-style. Agoraphobia has been classically described as "fear of the market place" but more recently is viewed as a fear of experiencing panic or anxiety away from a safe place or person and thus a "fear of fear." Agoraphobia is one of the most complex and disabling of the anxiety disorders.

■ **SOCIAL PHOBIA.** The essential feature is a persistent, irrational fear of, and compelling desire to avoid, situations in which the individual may be exposed to scrutiny by others. There is also the fear that the person may behave in a manner that will be embarrassing. Anticipatory anxiety occurs if the individual is confronted with entering such a situation and therefore attempts to avoid it. The avoidant behavior causes marked distress and is recognized by the individual as excessive or unreasonable. Examples include fear of speaking or performing in public, using public lavatories, eating in public, or writing in the presence of others.

■ **SIMPLE PHOBIA.** The essential feature of simple

phobia is a persistent, irrational fear of, and a desire to avoid, an object or situation, other than having a panic attack or humiliation in social situations. The fear interferes with functioning and is recognized by the individual as unreasonable. The most common simple phobias involve that of animals, particularly of dogs, snakes, insects, and mice. Other phobias include: acrophobia—fear of heights; claustrophobia—fear of closed spaces; monophobia—fear of being alone; pyrophobia—fear of fire.

■ **OBSESSIVE-COMPULSIVE DISORDER.** These reactions may be experienced singularly or in combination, and the presence of either one of the two is sufficient to warrant the diagnosis. The essential feature of an obsessive-compulsive disorder is an incessant preoccupation with impulses and anxieties which the individual believes are groundless, senseless, and impossible. An *obsession* is a recurring thought that is unwanted but which cannot be voluntarily excluded from consciousness. They are intrusive, repetitive, and unwanted thoughts, images, or impulses that generate resistance. The content of such thoughts is typically repulsive, consisting of blasphemous, obscene thoughts, doubts, or fears that invade the patient's consciousness. There are five major categories of obsessions and in descending order of frequency these include: (1) dirt, germs, and contamination; (2) aggressive behavior; (3) orderliness of inanimate objects; (4) sexual behavior; and (5) religious matters.

A *compulsion* is a recurring impulse to perform some act that cannot be resisted. It is, in a sense, an obsession in action. The two primary forms of compulsive behavior are excessive cleaning or washing and the checking of inanimate objects. Compulsive behavior tends to relieve anxiety that would be overwhelming for the individual if restrained from performing the activity.

The two behaviors may be combined in an obsessive-compulsive reaction. For example, the person who compulsively washes his hands might also experience obsessive thoughts relating to dirt and germs. Here again the repeated thought or act defends the person against experiencing severe anxiety. The important element with these disorders is that the person does not want to repeat the act or thought, but feels compelled to do so.

■ **POST-TRAUMATIC STRESS DISORDER.** The essential feature of this disorder is the development of characteristic symptoms following a psychologically traumatic event that is generally outside the range of usual human experience. The characteristic symptoms involve reexperiencing the traumatic event; a numbing of responsiveness or reduced involvement with the external world; recurrent, distressing dreams of the event; and autonomic, depressed, or anxious symptoms.

■ **GENERALIZED ANXIETY DISORDER.** The essential feature is generalized, persistent anxiety of at least 6 months' duration about two or more life circumstances without the specific symptoms that characterize panic disorders, obsessive-compulsive disorders, or anorexia nervosa. The diagnosis is not made if the disturbance is caused by another physical or mental disorder. Mild depressive symptoms are common.

■ **ANXIETY DISORDER NOS.** This is a residual category for disorders involving prominent anxiety or phobic avoidance that are not classified as a specific anxiety disorder or as an adjustment disorder with anxious mood.

❧ Planning and implementation

■ Goal setting

The overall goal of the nurse working with an anxious patient is not to free him totally from anxiety but rather to help him develop the capacity to tolerate mild anxiety and to use it consciously and constructively. In this way his self will become stronger and more integrated and, as he uses these experiences as learning experiences, he will move on in his development. The patient will be able to meet anxiety constructively if he has sound, firm, and flexible values and if he is convinced that the values to be gained in moving ahead are greater than those to be gained by escape. If one views anxiety as a war between the threat and the values a person identifies with his existence, then maladaptive behavior means that the struggle is won by the threat, whereas the constructive approach to anxiety means that the struggle is won by the person's values. Thus a general nursing goal is to help the patient evolve sound values. This does not mean that the patient assumes the nurse's values. Rather, the nurse works with the patient to sort out his own values, which transcend the present situation and extend toward the good of the community.

Anxiety can also be an important factor in the patient's decision to seek treatment. No one wants anxiety, but if it is present, then the lessening of it is desirable. If the patient's coping mechanism or symptom is not successful in minimizing his anxiety, his motivation for treatment will be increased. Conversely, anxiety about the therapeutic process can also contribute to its being delayed, impeded, or deterred.

The patient should be an active participant in the phases of planning and implementation. If the patient is actively involved in identifying relevant stressors and planning possible solutions, the success of the implementation phase will be maximized. Patients in extreme anxiety will not, initially, be able to participate in the problem-solving process. However, as soon as their anxiety is reduced, the nurse should incorporate them in her care to establish mutuality of approach and reinforce the fact that they are responsible for their own growth and personal development.

In formulating a plan of care for the patient the nurse first attends to the creation of nursing goals. Goals such as "decrease anxiety" and "minimize anxiety" lack specific behaviors and evaluation criteria, which minimizes their usefulness in guiding nursing care and evaluating its effectiveness. The long-term goals for the patient should relate to the nursing diagnosis. They should reflect the significant reduction or elimination of the problematic behavior identified in the nursing diagnosis as well as the learning of new, more constructive coping mechanisms. The short-term goals should break this down into discrete, more readily attainable steps. Short-term goals are important to provide smaller but significant progress toward the long-term goal accomplishment. Both these factors allow the nurse and patient to see progress throughout the relationship even if the ultimate goal still appears to be distant.

When the nursing diagnosis describes the patient's anxiety at the severe or panic levels, the highest priority short-term goals should address the lowering of the anxiety level. Only after this has been achieved can additional progress be made. The reduced level of anxiety should be evident in a reduction of behaviors associated with the severe or panic levels. The reduction of these behaviors, then, forms part of the content for the short-term goals. Following are examples of short-term goals for a particular patient.

After 10 days Mr. Jones will

1. Attend and remain seated during all ward meetings
2. Participate at least three times during each meeting
3. Discuss one topic for a minimum of 10 minutes when meeting with his nurse
4. Attend all occupational therapy sessions
5. Sleep a minimum of 6 hours a night

When these goals are met, the nurse can assume and validate that the patient's level of anxiety has been reduced and the nurse may then develop new short-term goals that may be directed toward insight or relaxation therapy. Throughout the nursing process, it will be necessary for the nurse to continually reevaluate the level of the patient's anxiety. Kristic's study[17] of the anxiety level of hospitalized psychiatric patients throughout their total hospitalization found three specific crisis periods of increased anxiety. These were at the time of admission, after the fifth day of the hospitalization, and on discharge. She notes that not only is

there need for intensive intervention at these times, but that nurses would have the greatest opportunity for implementing them. Studies such as these may provide a basis for prediction of periods of particular stress for patients that have direct implications for the planning and implementing of therapeutic nursing care.

◾ Intervening in severe and panic levels of anxiety

◾ **ESTABLISHING A TRUSTING RELATIONSHIP.** The patient experiencing severe or panic levels of anxiety may be hospitalized. To reduce this patient's level of anxiety, most of the nursing actions will be supportive and protective. Initially, the nurse wishes to establish an open, trusting relationship. To accomplish this, she should actively listen to the patient and encourage him to discuss his feelings of anxiety, hostility, guilt, and frustration. She should answer his questions directly and offer unconditional acceptance of him. Both her verbal and nonverbal communications should convey awareness of the patient's feelings and acceptance of them. The patient might express himself in rapid, disjointed speech, hostile outbursts, or crying episodes. She should remain available to the patient and respect his use of personal space. In this regard research indicates that a 180-cm (6-foot) distance in a small room may create the optimum condition for openness and discussion of fears.[19] The more this distance is increased or decreased, the more anxious the patient may become.

◾ **SELF-AWARENESS.** The nurse's own feelings are of particular importance when working with a highly anxious patient. The nurse may find herself being unsympathetic to the patient, impatient with him, and frustrated by him. These are common feelings of reciprocal anxiety that the nurse should be aware of and accepting of when they are elicited. If the nurse is alert to the development of anxiety in herself, she can learn from it and use it therapeutically within the nurse-patient relationship. It may, for example, be indicative of some important emotional issue that the patient is unable to identify and verbalize. Or it may reflect a conflict within the nurse that is interfering with her ability to be therapeutic. She should therefore be alert to the signs of anxiety in herself, accept them, and attempt to explore their cause. What is threatening her? Is this patient a source of reflected esteem for her? Has she failed to live up to what she imagines is the patient's ideal? Is she comparing herself to a peer or another health professional? Is the patient's area of conflict one that she has not resolved for herself? Is her anxiety related to something that will or may happen in the future? Is her patient's conflict really one of her own that she is projecting onto him?

If the nurse does not explore the reasons for her own anxiety and instead denies it, it can have detrimental effects on the nurse-patient relationship. Because of her own anxiety she may be unable to differentiate between levels of anxiety in others. She may also transfer her own fears and frustrations to the patient, thus compounding his problem. Finally, her anxiety will arouse defenses in other patients and staff that will severely interfere with her therapeutic usefulness. She should strive to accept her patient's anxiety without reciprocal anxiety by continually clarifying her own feelings and role (see Clinical example 12-1).

■ **PROTECTING THE PATIENT.** Another major area of intervention is providing for and reassuring the patient of his safety. One way of decreasing his anxiety is by allowing the patient to determine what stress he can handle at the time. The nurse should not force or probe the severely anxious patient into situations he is not able to handle. She should not attack his coping mechanism or attempt to strip him of it. Rather, she should attempt to protect his defenses. The coping mechanism or symptom is attempting to deal with an unconscious conflict. The patient does not understand why the symptom has developed nor what he is gaining from it. What he does believe is that the symptom relieves some of the intolerable anxiety and tension. If he is unable to release this anxiety, his tension will mount to the panic level and he could lose control. It is also important to remember that the severely anxious patient has not worked through his area of conflict and therefore has no alternatives or substitutes for his present coping mechanisms.

This principle also applies to severe levels of anxiety, such as obsessive-compulsive reactions and phobias. The nurse should not initially interfere with the repetitive act or force the patient to confront the phobic object. She should not ridicule the nature of his defense or attempt to argue with him about it or reason him out of it. He needs this coping mechanism to keep his anxiety within tolerable limits. With time, however, the nurse can place some limits on the patient's behavior and attempt to help him find satisfaction with other aspects of life. It is also important not to reinforce the phobia, ritual, or physical complaint by focusing attention on it and devoting a great deal of time to talking about it.

■ **MODIFYING THE ENVIRONMENT.** If the patient is hospitalized, the nurse can consult with other members of the health team to identify anxiety-producing situations for the patient and attempt to reduce them. She can set limits by assuming a quiet, calm manner, decreasing environmental stimulation, and limiting the patient's interaction with other patients to minimize

---

CLINICAL EXAMPLE 12-1

Ms. R was a 35-year-old married woman and mother of three children, ages 4, 6, and 9. She was a full-time housewife and mother. Her husband was a salesman and spent about two nights each week out of town. She came to the clinic complaining of severe headaches that "come upon me very suddenly and are so terrible that I have to go to bed. The only thing that helps is for me to lie down in a dark and absolutely quiet room." She said that these headaches were becoming a real problem for everyone in the family, and her husband told her that she "just had to get over them and get things back to normal."

Mr. W, a psychiatric nurse, offered to see Ms. R in therapy once a week. After 4 weeks, he was asked to present his evaluation, treatment plans, and progress report to the clinic staff at their regular weekly team conference. Mr. W began his presentation by stating, "This case is really a tough nut to crack. I'll start with the progress report and say that there is none, because I can't seem to get past all of the complaining this patient does!" He then went on to discuss his evaluation and treatment plan in depth. It became obvious to the other members of the staff that Mr. W saw his patient as a woman who was not living up to her roles and responsibilities. He defended Ms. R's husband even though the husband had refused to come to the sessions with his wife. When the psychiatrist asked about the possibility of a medication evaluation for Ms. R, the nurse replied, "Everyone gets headaches. I don't think we should reward or reinforce this woman's complaints."

In reviewing this case, the staff noted that Mr. W appeared to have problems relating empathically to his patient because of her particular set of problems and some of his own values and perceptions. Mr. W agreed with this and said he had thought of asking someone else to work with Ms. R. Mr. W's supervisor observed that the nurse had problems with this type of patient in the past, and a more constructive approach would be to increase his supervision on this case, focusing on the dynamics between the patient and nurse that were blocking learning and growth for both of them. Mr. W and his supervisor then set a time when they could begin to meet with this purpose in mind.

---

the contagious aspects of anxiety. Supportive physical measures may also be helpful in decreasing a patient's anxiety, such as warm baths, massages, or whirlpool baths.

■ **ENCOURAGING ACTIVITY.** The nurse should also encourage the patient's interest in activity outside himself. The rationale for doing this is to limit the time he has available for his destructive coping mechanisms and to increase his participation in and enjoyment of other aspects of life. Within the hospital setting he may become engaged in simple games, concrete tasks, or occupational or art therapy. It would be most beneficial if the nurse shared some of these activities with him to provide him with support and reinforce socially productive behavior. She might also schedule vigorous physical activities for him, such as walking, a sport, or an active hobby. This kind of physical exercise is helpful in the dissolution of anxiety because it provides an emotional release or discharge and directs the patient's attention outward. In a recent study, participation in a jogging program resulted in the reduction of anxiety for chronically distressed community clients; these gains were maintained 15 months after the completion of the study.[20]

Similar interventions can be implemented with the severely anxious patient who is not hospitalized. The nurse and patient can plan a daily schedule or a list of activities that he can carry out in the community. Family members may be involved in the planning, since they can be very supportive in setting limits and stimulating outside activity.

Some nursing interventions can be detrimental and serve to increase the already high anxiety of severely anxious patients. These include pressuring the patient to change prematurely, being judgmental and verbally disapproving of the patient's behaviors, asking the patient a direct question that places him on the defensive, focusing in a critical way on the anxious feelings of the patient with other patients present, lacking awareness of one's own behaviors and feelings, and withdrawing from the patient.

■ **INTERVENING WITH MEDICATION.** Another possible area for nursing intervention is the administration of tranquilizing drugs to the highly anxious patient. Because anxiety is a pervasive problem, large portions of the population take tranquilizers. Americans are now spending over $500 million each year for drugs to relieve anxiety. Among the minor tranquilizers, the benzodiazepines are the drug treatment of choice in the management of anxiety. They are the most widely prescribed drugs in the world, and they have almost replaced the barbiturates in the treatment of anxiety due to their effectiveness and wide margin of safety. Use of these drugs, however, in combination with alcohol may result in a serious or even fatal sedative reaction. Antipsychotic drugs, or major tranquilizers, are frequently prescribed for those patients who are experiencing a panic level of anxiety that is of psychotic proportions.

Although some patients may need to take antianxiety drugs for extended periods of time, these drugs are not without their drawbacks and should always be used together with nonpharmacological treatments. Potential dangers include withdrawal syndrome side effects and addiction. It should be emphasized that psychopharmacology is an adjunct to, and not a substitute for, an ongoing therapeutic relationship. In fact, the effect of a therapeutic relationship may be enhanced if the chemical control of painful symptoms allows the patient to direct his attention more freely to the conflicts underlying his anxiety. More detailed information on antianxiety and antipsychotic medications is presented in Chapter 23. Table 12-6 summarizes the principles, rationale, and nursing interventions in severe and panic levels of anxiety.

■ **Intervening in a moderate level of anxiety**

All the nursing interventions previously mentioned are supportive interventions and are directed toward the general short-term goal of reducing the anxiety of a severely anxious or panicky patient. When the patient's anxiety is reduced to a moderate level, the nurse can develop additional goals to aid the patient in his problem-solving efforts to cope with the stress. Long-term goals that are directed toward helping the patient understand the cause of his anxiety and learn new ways of controlling it are insight oriented or reeducative in nature.

A most important aspect of promoting the patient's adaptive responses to anxiety is that of patient education. The nurse can identify relevant health teaching needs of each patient and then formulate an individualized teaching plan to meet those needs. Such a teaching plan should be designed to increase the patient's knowledge of his own predisposing and precipitating stressors, coping resources, and adaptive and maladaptive responses. Alternative coping strategies can be identified and explored. Health teaching by the nurse should also address the beneficial aspects of mild levels of anxiety in motivating learning and producing growth and creativity.

The specific interventions used by the nurse when intervening in a moderate level of anxiety were originally described by Peplau[26] and Burd[8] and reflect the problem-solving process. Short-term goals may be written for each step of this process, including recognition of anxiety, insight into the anxiety, and coping with the threat. These interventions can be implemented in any setting—psychiatric, community, or general hospital.

TABLE 12-6

SUMMARY OF NURSING INTERVENTIONS IN SEVERE AND PANIC LEVELS OF ANXIETY
Goal—Support and protect the patient and reduce his anxiety to a moderate-mild level

Principle	Rationale	Nursing interventions
Establish an open trusting relationship	Reduce the threat that the nurse poses to the highly anxious patient	Listen to the patient Encourage the patient's discussion of feelings Answer questions directly Offer unconditional acceptance Be available to the patient Respect his use of personal space
Awareness and control of nurse's own feelings	Anxiety is communicated interpersonally; reciprocal anxiety in the nurse can interfere with her ability to be therapeutic	Openness to one's own feelings Acceptance of both positive and negative feelings, including the development of anxiety Explore the cause of one's feelings Use this understanding of one's feelings in a therapeutic way
Reassure the patient of his safety and protect his defenses and coping mechanisms but do not focus on or reinforce the presenting maladaptive behaviors	Severe and panic levels of anxiety can be reduced by initially allowing the patient to determine what stress he can handle If the patient is unable to release his anxiety, his tension may mount to the panic level and he may lose control; at this time, he has no alternatives for his present coping mechanisms	Initially accept and support, rather than attack, the patient's defenses Acknowledge the reality of the pain associated with the patient's present coping mechanisms but do not focus on the phobia, ritual, or physical complaint itself Give feedback to the patient about his behavior, stressors, appraisal of stressors, and coping resources Reinforce the idea that one's physical health is related to one's emotional health and that this is an area which will need exploration in the future In time, begin to place limits on the patient's maladaptive behavior in a supportive way
Identify and attempt to reduce anxiety-provoking situations for the patient	The patient's behavior may be modified by altering his environment and his interaction with it	Assume a calm manner with the patient Decrease environmental stimulation Limit the patient's interaction with other patients to minimize the contagious aspects of anxiety Identify and modify anxiety-provoking situations for the patient Administer supportive physical measures, such as warm baths and massages
Encourage the patient's interest in activity outside himself	By encouraging outside activities, the nurse acts to limit the time the patient has available for his destructive coping mechanisms, while increasing his participation in and enjoyment of other aspects of life	Initially share an activity with him to provide support and reinforce socially productive behavior Provide for physical exercise of some type Plan a schedule or list of activities that can be carried out daily Involve family members and other support systems as much as possible
Promote the patient's physical health and well-being	The effect of a therapeutic relationship may be enhanced if the chemical control of symptoms allows the patient to direct his attention to underlying conflicts	Administer medications that help reduce the patient's discomfort Observe for medication side effects and initiate relevant health teaching

■ **RECOGNITION OF ANXIETY.** After analyzing the patient's behaviors and determining his level of anxiety, the nurse helps the patient to recognize he is anxious. She helps him explore his underlying feelings with such questions as "Are you feeling anxious now?" or "Are you uncomfortable?" It is also helpful for the nurse to identify the patient's behavior and link it to the feeling of anxiety (e.g., "I noticed you smoked three cigarettes since we started talking about your sister. Are you feeling anxious?"). In this way the nurse acknowledges the patient's feeling, attempts to label it for the patient, encourages the patient to describe it further, and relates it to a specific behavioral pattern. She is also validating her inferences and assumptions with the patient.

The patient's goal, however, is often to avoid or negate his anxiety. He therefore might use any of the following resistive approaches described by Meares[22]:

1. **Screen symptoms.** In this case the patient focuses his attention on minor physical ailments. The purpose of these apparently unrelated complaints is to avoid acknowledging his anxiety and conflict areas.

2. **Superior status position.** The patient attempts to control the interview by questioning the nurse's abilities or asserting the superiority of his own knowledge or experiences. It is important that the nurse not respond emotionally to this approach. She should not accept the patient's challenge and compete with him, since a conflict of this kind would serve only to further avoid the issue of anxiety.

3. **Emotional seduction.** By means of this technique the patient attempts to manipulate the nurse and to elicit feelings of pity or sympathy.

4. **Superficiality.** The patient relates on an obvious level and resists any attempts by the nurse to explore underlying feelings or analyze issues.

5. **Circumlocution.** In this case the patient gives the pretense of answering questions asked of him, but he succeeds instead in talking around the topic and actually avoiding it.

6. **Amnesia.** This is a type of purposeful "forgetting" of a certain incident or event to avoid confronting and exploring it with the nurse.

7. **Denial.** The patient may use this approach only when discussing significant issues with the nurse or may generalize his denial to all others including himself. His purpose is often to avoid humiliation.

8. **Intellectualization.** The patient who utilizes this technique usually has some knowledge of

CLINICAL EXAMPLE 12-2

Mr. T was a 28-year-old male who was transferred from the neurological unit to the psychiatric unit where Ms. P was assigned to be his primary nurse. Ms. P was 24 years old and had been working on the unit for 3 years. In completing her nursing assessment of Mr. T, the nurse noted that he was experiencing a paralysis of his legs, which began gradually approximately 4 weeks previously. All neurological tests were negative, and he was transferred to the psychiatric unit for evaluation and treatment. He was an only child, unmarried, and had been living at home with his parents. He had completed college and was employed in the postal service. He had been dating one girl for 2 years and had recently proposed to her. She had told him that she was not ready to get married yet but she did want to continue seeing him. Mr. T had a small group of close friends, males and females, and they visited him often in the hospital, as did his family.

Ms. P had established a good relationship with her patient and spent much time with him. She found his friends to be kind and jovial and noted that one of Mr. T's strengths was his sense of humor and "ready smile." She observed, however, that his girl friend never visited with him alone. Mr. T, meanwhile, had many cards, gifts, and visitors and appeared to be most appreciative of everything done for him.

A physical therapist came to work with Mr. T on a regular basis, and this was a very difficult time of the day for him. While watching them work together one day, Ms. P remarked how impersonal and brusque the physical therapist was in relating to her patient. In discussing this observation in nursing rounds the next day, Ms. P began to realize that some of her actions were being influenced by her feelings of sympathy and pity for the patient and blame she had been unconsciously projecting onto his girl friend. She wondered if his joviality, agreeable nature, and professed signs of gratitude were not indications of his manipulation of her and emotional seduction of her feelings toward him. The more she thought about this possibility, the more likely it seemed. At the end of the nursing rounds that morning, she requested that she be able to present his case in the staff treatment meeting the next day. Other staff were also feeling frustrated in their care for him and agreed that the conference would be most valuable.

psychology or medicine. He is able to verbalize appropriate insights and analysis yet lacks personal involvement in the problem he describes. He is not actually participating in the problem-solving process.

9. **Hostility.** The patient believes that offense is the best defense. He therefore relates to others in an aggressive defiant manner. The greatest danger in this situation is that the nurse will take his behavior personally and respond, in turn, with anger. This serves to reinforce the patient in avoiding the exploring of his anxiety.

10. **Withdrawal.** The patient may resist the nurse by replying in vague, diffuse, indefinite, and remote ways.

All these resistive approaches may create feelings of frustration, irritation, or reciprocal anxiety in the nurse. It will be important for her to recognize her own feelings and identify the behavior pattern of the patient that might be causing them (see Clinical example 12-2).

In attempting to deal with these patient defenses and intervene successfully, the importance of a trusting relationship becomes evident. If the nurse establishes herself as a warm and responsive listener, gives the patient adequate time to respond, and is supportive of his self-expressions, she will become less threatening to him. In helping him recognize his anxiety, the nurse should use open questions that move from nonthreatening topics to central issues of conflict. It may be helpful to vary the amount of anxiety to enhance the patient's motivation. In time, supportive confrontation may be used in reflecting back to the patient his repeated use of a particular resistive pattern. If, however, the patient's level of anxiety begins to rapidly rise, the nurse might choose to refocus the patient to a previous discussion topic.

■ **INSIGHT INTO THE ANXIETY.** Once the patient is able to recognize his anxiety, the subsequent nursing interventions strive to expand the present context of the patient. The patient may be asked to describe the situations and interactions that immediately precede the increase in anxiety. Together the nurse and patient make inferences about the precipitating causes or biopsychosocial stressors.

The nurse then helps the patient see which of his values are being threatened. It is possible to link the threat with underlying causes and to analyze how the conflict developed. To do this, the patient's present experiences are related to his past ones. The depth of this analysis depends on the nurse's educational and professional experiences. It is also important to explore how the patient reduced anxiety in the past. How did he handle anxiety, and what kinds of actions produced relief?

■ **COPING WITH THE THREAT.** If previous coping responses have been adaptive and constructive, the patient should be encouraged to utilize them. If not, the nurse can point out their maladaptive or destructive effects. She can share her perception with the patient that his present way of life is apparently unsatisfactory and distressing to him and he does not attempt to change things for the better. The patient needs to assume responsibility for his own actions and realize that he has placed limitations on himself; other people are not doing it to him. In this phase of intervention the nurse assumes an active role as she interprets, analyzes, confronts, and correlates cause and effect relationships. She should proceed clearly so that the patient can follow while maintaining his anxiety within appropriate limits. If his anxiety becomes too severe, she may change topics temporarily.

There are various ways the nurse can help the patient in his problem-solving efforts. One way of helping the patient cope is to reevaluate the nature of the threat or stressor. Is it as bad as the patient perceives it? Is his cognitive appraisal realistic? Together they might discuss his fears and feelings of inadequacy and analyze his projective identification. Does he fear others are as critical, perfectionistic, and rejecting of him as he is of others? Is his conflict based in reality, or is it the result of unvalidated, isolated, and perhaps distorted thinking? By sharing his fears with family members, peers, and staff, the patient frequntly sees his own misperceptions, and with their support he can validate his ideas, values, and goals.

Another approach is to help the patient modify his behavior and learn new ways of coping with stress. He may decide to restructure his goals or evolve different values based on feedback from those around him. Or he might consider alternatives to mastering the situation. The nurse may act as a role model in this regard or engage the patient in role playing to decrease his anxiety about new responses to problematical situations. One nursing function therefore is to educate the patient in aspects of mild anxiety that can be constructive and growth producing. Physical activity should be encouraged as a way to discharge anxiety. Interpersonal resources such as family members or close friends should be incorporated into the nursing plan of care to provide the patient with support.

Frequently the cause for anxiety will arise from an interpersonal conflict. In this case, analyzing the situation with the patient by himself is significantly less help-

TABLE 12-7

MENTAL HEALTH EDUCATION PLAN—THE RELAXATION RESPONSE

Content	Instructional activities	Evaluation
Describe the characteristics and benefits of relaxation	Discuss physiological changes associated with relaxation and contrast these with the behaviors of anxiety	Patient identifies own responses to anxiety Patient describes elements of a relaxed state
Teach deep muscle relaxation through a sequence of tension-relaxation exercises	Engage the patient in the progressive procedure of tensing and relaxing voluntary muscles until his body as a whole is relaxed	Patient is able to tense and relax all muscle groups Patient identifies those muscles that become particularly tense for him
Discuss the relaxation procedure of meditation and its components	Describe the elements of meditation and assist the patient in using this technique	Patient selects a word or scene with pleasant connotations and engages in relaxed meditation
Assist in overcoming anxiety-provoking situations through systematic desensitization	With patient, construct a hierarchy of anxiety-provoking situations or scenes Through imagination or reality work through these scenes using relaxation techniques	Patient identifies and ranks anxiety-provoking situations Patient exposes himself to them while remaining in a relaxed state
Allow the rehearsing and practical use of relaxation in a safe environment	Role play stressful situations with the nurse or other patients	Patient becomes more comfortable with new behavior in a safe and supportive setting
Encourage patient to use relaxation techniques in life	Assign homework of using the relaxation response in everyday experiences Support success of patient	Patient utilizes relaxation response in life situations Patient able to regulate anxiety response through use of relaxation techniques

ful than including the involved persons and opening communication between them. In this way cause and effect relationships are more open to examination, and coping patterns can be examined in light of their effect on others as well as the patient himself.

Working through this problem-solving or reeducative process with the patient will take time. He has to accept it on an intellectual and an emotional level, and breaking previous behavioral patterns can be difficult. Throughout the implementation phase the nurse needs to be patient and consistent in her approach and continually reappraise her own anxiety.

■ **PROMOTE THE RELAXATION RESPONSE.** In addition to the problem-solving function of coping addressed previously, one can also cope with stress by regulating the emotional distress associated with it. Long-term goals that are directed toward helping the patient regulate emotional distress are supportive or palliative. Although distress can be regulated in maladaptive ways, such as taking drugs, denying the facts, or withdrawing, only the adaptive responses will be described in this chapter. These include the relaxation techniques of systematic desensitization, meditation, and the use of biofeedback. All human beings have a natural and protective mechanism against "overstress," which Benson calls the "relaxation response."[5,6] This response brings about a decreased heart rate, lower metabolism, and decreased respiratory rate. Relaxation, therefore, is the ultimate stress management technique because the relaxation response is the physiological opposite of the fight or flight, or anxiety, response.

Relaxation techniques are useful nursing interventions when the patient's level of stress interferes with his ability to function and be productive. They have long been used in helping women deal with childbirth because they form the basis for childbirth education.

TABLE 12-8

MANIFESTATIONS OF RELAXATION

Physiological	Cognitive	Behavioral
Decreased pulse Decreased blood pressure Decreased respirations Decreased oxygen consumption Decreased metabolic rate Pupil constriction Peripheral vasodilation Increased peripheral temperature	Altered state of consciousness, usually alpha level Heightened concentration on single mental image Receptivity to positive suggestion	Lack of attention to and concern for environmental stimuli No verbal interaction No voluntary change of position Passive movement easy

From DiMotto, J.: Am. J. Nurs. **1984**:754, June 1984.

However, new ways are presently being discovered of using relaxation techniques with all kinds of people in various stress situations. These include helping patients handle pain; overcome test anxiety; sleep better; overcome side effects related to chemotherapy, surgery, or myocardial infarctions; handle various medical, nursing, and dental procedures; monitor the emotional triggers associated with chronic illnesses, such as asthma, muscle tension, ulcers, hypertension, tension headaches, or colitis; and deal with anger more constructively.

Relaxation can be taught in many ways, individually, in small groups, or even in larger group settings.[7] A mental health education plan to teach the relaxation response is presented in Table 12-7. It is within the scope of nursing practice and, as a group of interventions, requires no special equipment, does not need a physician's supervision, and can be implemented in a variety of settings. A major benefit of relaxation interventions for the patient is that after a number of training sessions, the patient can practice the techniques on his own. This puts the control in the patient's hands and increases his self-reliance.

In 1929, relaxation training was originated by a physiologist named Edmunt Jacobson[16] who developed a method of combating tension and anxiety by instructing patients to tense and relax various muscle groups in the body systematically. The philosophy of the method is that it is physically impossible to be "nervous" in a part of the body if in that part the person is completely relaxed. The aim of the training was not for people to be devoid of stress, but rather to feel comfortable with themselves and alert to their internal and external environment. Relaxation did not become popular in psy-

chiatric circles until the late 1950s when Wolpe[34] developed the procedure called "systematic desensitization" and produced research evidence demonstrating its effectiveness in treating phobic patients.

The various relaxation procedures are very similar. They all involve rhythmic breathing, reduced muscle tension, and an altered state of consciousness.[10] Clinical experience suggests there are individual differences in people's experiences of relaxation and not everyone will demonstrate all characteristics of a relaxed psychophysiologic state. The physiological, cognitive, and behavioral manifestations of relaxation are presented in Table 12-8.

All these relaxation techniques require a thorough assessment of oneself and one's patient. It is essential that the nurse learn how to relax herself because it is impossible for a tense person to teach another tense person to relax. The nurse should also remember that relaxation is a learned skill that develops over time. Trying "too hard" is a deterrent and can actually create tension, whereas an open willingness to relax is most effective. A complete assessment of the patient must also be done with particular focus given to where the patient experiences anxiety in his body. Relevant muscle groups should be identified and given emphasis in the relaxation interventions.

Systematic desensitization. The goal of systematic desensitization is to help the patient to change his response to the threatening stimulus. To be successful, the person must have sufficient skills for coping with whatever he fears. For example, a person may be afraid of driving, but he can, in fact, drive and is limited only by his fear. This is different from the person who fears heterosexual contacts, but actually lacks the social skills in this regard. This technique involves the pairing of deep muscle relaxation with imagined scenes depicting situations that cause the patient to feel anxious. The assumption is that if the person is taught relaxation rather than anxiety while imagining such scenes, the real-life situation that the scene depicted will cause much less anxiety.

One of the important parts of systematic desensitization is deep muscle relaxation. As a therapeutic tool it is very effective and can be utilized by itself to decrease tension and anxiety. It can also be combined with other types of interventions such as supportive or insight therapy. The basic premise is that muscle tension is related to anxiety, and if tense muscles can be made to relax, the person will experience a reduction in anxiety. The method used for relaxing the muscles involves the tensing and relaxing of voluntary muscles in an orderly sequence until the body, as a whole, is helped.

Rimm and Masters[28] describe the procedure. The patient should be seated in a comfortable chair in an open and unrestricted manner. The environment may contain soft music or pleasant visual cues. Before beginning the exercises, a brief explanation should be given that relates anxiety to muscle tension and describes the relaxation procedure about to be begun. The patient should take a deep breath and exhale slowly. A sequence of tension-relaxation exercises is then initiated. The patient is instructed to tense each muscle group for about 10 seconds while the nurse describes how tense and uncomfortable this body part feels. He then is asked to relax this muscle group as the nurse comments, "Notice how all the hardness and tension is draining from your hands. Now notice how they feel warm, soft, and calm. Compare this feeling to when they were tense and see how much better they feel now." The patient should be reminded to tense only the muscle group named and not other muscles.

The patient then proceeds to the next muscle group in the following sequence.

1. **Hands.** First the fists are tensed and relaxed. Then the fingers are extended and relaxed.
2. **Biceps and triceps.** These are tensed and relaxed.
3. **Shoulders.** They are pulled back and relaxed and then pushed forward and relaxed.
4. **Neck.** The head is turned slowly as far to the right as possible and relaxed, turned to the left and relaxed, and then brought forward until the chin touches the chest and relaxed.

5. **Mouth.** The mouth is opened as wide as possible and relaxed. The lips form a pout and then relax. The tongue is extended out as far as possible and relaxed and is then retracted into the throat and relaxed. It is pressed hard into the roof of the mouth and relaxed and then is pressed hard into the floor of the mouth and relaxed.
6. **Eyes.** They are opened as wide as possible and relaxed and then closed as hard as possible and relaxed.
7. **Breathing.** The patient inhales as deeply as possible and relaxes. He then exhales as much as possible and relaxes.
8. **Back.** The trunk of the body is pushed forward so the entire back is arched, and then it is relaxed.
9. **Midsection.** The buttock muscles are tensed and relaxed.
10. **Thighs.** The legs are extended and raised about 6 inches off the floor and then relaxed. The backs of the feet are pressed into the floor and relaxed.
11. **Stomach.** It is pulled in as much as possible and relaxed and is then extended and relaxed.
12. **Calves and feet.** With legs supported, the feet are bent with the toes pointing toward the head and then relaxed. Feet are then bent in the opposite direction and relaxed.
13. **Toes.** The toes are pressed into the bottom of the shoes and relaxed. They are then bent to touch the top inside of the shoes and relaxed.

The final exercise asks the patient to become *completely* relaxed, beginning with his toes and following the sensation up through his body to his eyes and forehead. When the patient learns the procedure, he can eliminate some of the exercises and employ them only on the muscles that usually become tense. This is individual for each person and may include the shoulders, forehead, back, or neck. He may also eliminate the tensing exercises and perform only the relaxation ones.

The procedure may be followed or replaced by another approach to evoke the relaxation response—meditation. The basic components for meditation include the following[5]:

1. A quiet environment
2. A passive attitude
3. A comfortable position
4. A word or scene to focus on

The first three components are necessary elements for any relaxation procedure. The fourth component in meditation refers to the process in which the patient is asked to select a cue word or scene with pleasant connotations. He is then instructed to close his eyes, relax each of the major muscle groups, and then begin repeating the word silently to himself each time he exhales.

Another method of tension reduction is the use of biofeedback. During a biofeedback training session small electrodes connected to the biofeedback equipment are attached to the patient's forehead. The patient is then instructed to concentrate on relaxing, which will reduce the pitch of the biofeedback tone created by his tension. The higher the pitch, the more muscle tension. Once he has developed the ability to relax, the patient is then encouraged to apply the technique in stressful situations.

If systematic desensitization is employed, the patient must be able to attain muscle relaxation. Additional steps are then undertaken. A hierarchy, or graded series, of situations or scenes is identified. They must be realistic, concrete situations created by the patient. They are then ranked from 1 to 10, with a rating of 1 evoking little or no anxiety and a rating of 10 evoking intense or severe anxiety. These feared situations may then be worked with either through imagination (in vitro) or in reality (in vivo). In vivo exposure is widely considered to be the treatment of choice for simple and social phobias, as well as obsessive-compulsive disorders.

For example, with in vitro exposure the patient is asked to imagine the scenes, beginning with the first anxiety-provoking one, and use his ability to relax. If he experiences no anxiety, he continues on to the next scene. If he experiences anxiety, he stops and restores himself to the state of relaxation. This procedure is implemented repeatedly until the hierarchy is completed. This method of intervention appears to be successful because it indirectly encourages patients to expose themselves to objects or situations that are actually feared, and it is most effective in the treatment of phobias.

Additional steps may also be taken. The patient may role play the stressful situation with the nurse or other patients. While role playing, he is asked to identify the location and level of his anxiety and practice relaxing it away. The patient can practice relaxing while at home, as well as when in proximity to feared situations. These exercises teach the practical use of relaxation and allow the patient to rehearse them with some safety. Ideally, he will learn to recognize when and how his body responds to stress and will initiate relaxation exercises accordingly. The final step is to regulate one's response

when actually coping with the stressor and to maintain these new relaxation skills. This will require nursing care feedback and follow-up and perhaps the development of personalized stress management programs for the patient.

As with any other nursing intervention, problems can arise in the teaching, learning, and practicing of these relaxation techniques. If a little is good, it should not be assumed that a lot is even better. It has been observed that when the response was elicited for two limited daily periods of 20 to 30 minutes, no adverse side effects resulted. However, when elicited more frequently, some patients might experience a "withdrawal from life" that can complicate or compound previous psychiatric problems.[6] Furthermore, relaxation techniques should not be used to insulate oneself from the outside world. Mild levels of anxiety are growth producing and the fight or flight response is often appropriate and essential for survival. Other common problems specific to relaxation training are summarized in Table 12-9. Table 12-10 summarizes the nursing interventions that help the moderately anxious patient in his problem-solving efforts to cope with stress.

 Evaluation

Evaluation is an ongoing process engaged in by the nurse and patient that is part of each phase of the nursing process. Even before she begins to formulate the nursing diagnosis, the nurse should ask herself: "Did I critically observe my patient's physiological and psychomotor behaviors? Did I listen to his subjective description of his experience? Did I fail to see the relationships between his expressed hostility or guilt and his underlying anxiety? Did I assess his intellectual and social functioning?" In concluding her collection of data, the nurse should analyze the data she has collected. Was she able to identify the precipitating stressor for the patient? What was his perception of the threat? How was this influenced by his physical health, past experiences, and present feelings and needs? Did she correctly identify the patient's level of anxiety and try to validate it with him? Was she able to identify the patient's coping mechanisms and determine if they were constructive or destructive in nature? The diagnosis itself should be stated clearly and precisely. It should include the patient's problematical behavior pattern and his level of anxiety.

Nursing goals should be mutually determined and should describe what the nurse wishes to accomplish within a designated time span. Her plan of action explains how and why. When using the criteria of ade-

TABLE 12-9

COMMON PROBLEMS AND SOLUTIONS ASSOCIATED WITH RELAXATION TRAINING

Problem	Solution	Problem	Solution
Muscle cramps	Ask the patient to generate less tension in these areas for shorter periods of time and to tense and relax the muscles more slowly; if cramps do occur, let the patient manipulate the cramped muscle, wait a few minutes, and then continue	**Inability to relax certain muscle groups**	Work with the patient to evaluate the technique and develop an alternate tensing strategy
Movement, such as stretching, yawning, or shifting position	Sometimes this is to help the patient assume a more relaxed position and should be encouraged; if it is disruptive, review the specific relaxation technique being used and evaluate its effectiveness	**Strange or unfamiliar feelings, such as floating, lack of body perception, etc.**	This is a common occurrence if relaxation techniques are new to the patient; convey this to him, ask him to open his eyes and look around and become oriented; encourage the patient to respond to relaxation as an enjoyable, rather than fearful, experience
Laughter or talking	Initially this may indicate embarrassment or nervousness over a new situation; since doing the facial exercises may create "funny-looking" expressions, it may be helpful for the nurse to do them with the patient	**Sense of "losing control"**	Sometimes these exercises focus directly on issues of control that may be problematic in themselves for the patient; if so, spend more time discussing his subjective experience, introduce the exercises more gradually, and spend more time ensuring that the positive expectancies established earlier are fulfilled
Noise	Initially a quiet room is best, which minimizes the disruptions associated with phones ringing, clocks ticking, and doors slamming; gradually, the patient should be helped to relax with some background noise, since the everyday world is filled with sounds	**Sense of "internal arousal" or inside tension despite external relaxation**	Explain to the patient that these exercises effect voluntary muscle control, whereas internal tension results from involuntary muscles also; however, voluntary and involuntary control are interrelated and, with practice, the patient should feel decreased internal tension
Intrusive thoughts	If intrusive thoughts result in anxiety or discomfort for the patient, the nurse can either increase dialogue or help the patient select a new group of thoughts or images; if the intrusive thoughts involve sexual arousal, the nurse can note that this is not unusual and continue to focus on other images	**Failure to follow instructions**	Identify and analyze the underlying cause, has the patient forgotten or misunderstood the directions, or is he trying to control the nurse and therapy situation

TABLE 12-9—cont'd

COMMON PROBLEMS AND SOLUTIONS ASSOCIATED WITH RELAXATION TRAINING

Problem	Solution	Problem	Solution
Sleep	This is *not* a desired outcome; the nurse should be careful not to use the word sleep, but rather "relaxed but very awake"; the patient can also be asked to focus on the sound of her voice	Problems with practicing	Assist the patient in arranging his work and home schedules to allow for two 20-minute sessions per day; if a problem continues, the patient's lack of cooperation and resistance should be discussed
Coughing and sneezing	This is usually only a problem with heavy smokers; in this case, the nurse should not encourage very deep breaths because they might cause the smoker to cough	Words and phrases to avoid	Assess the patient before and during the exercises for phrases that appear to be annoying or tension producing for him; these should be avoided in the first few sessions

Adapted with permission from Bernstein, D., and Borkovec, T.: Progressive relaxation training, Champaign, Ill., 1973, Research Press.

TABLE 12-10

SUMMARY OF NURSING INTERVENTIONS IN A MODERATE LEVEL OF ANXIETY
Goal—Help the patient in his problem-solving efforts to cope with stress

Principle	Rationale	Nursing interventions
Establish and maintain a trusting relationship	Reduce the threat the nurse poses to the patient	Be a warm and responsive listener Give the patient adequate time to respond Be supportive of the patient's self-expressions.
Awareness and control of the nurse's own feelings	Resistance by the patient may produce negative feelings in the nurse that can block future progress	Recognize own feelings Identify the behavior pattern or resistive approach of the patient that might be causing them Explore the patient's behavior and the nurse's response to them with the patient to learn and grow from them
Help the patient recognize his anxiety	To adopt new coping responses the patient first needs to be aware of his feelings and to overcome his conscious or unconscious denial and resistance	Help the patient to identify and describe his underlying feelings Link the patient's behavior with his feeling Validate all inferences and assumptions with the patient Use open questions to move from non-threatening topics to issues of conflict Vary the amount of anxiety to enhance the patient's motivation In time, supportive confrontation may be used judiciously

Continued.

TABLE 12-10—cont'd

SUMMARY OF NURSING INTERVENTIONS IN A MODERATE LEVEL OF ANXIETY
Goal—Help the patient in his problem-solving efforts to cope with stress

Principle	Rationale	Nursing interventions
Expand the patient's insight into the development of his anxiety	Once the patient recognizes his feelings of anxiety, he needs to be helped to understand its development, including precipitating stressors, appraisal of the stressor, and resources available to him	Help the patient describe the situations and interactions that immediately precede his anxiety Review with the patient his appraisal of the stressor, which of his values are being threatened, and the way in which the conflict developed Relate his present experiences with relevant ones from the past
Help the patient learn new adaptive coping responses	New adaptive coping responses can be learned through analyzing coping mechanisms used in the past, reappraising the stressor, utilizing available resources, and accepting responsibility for change	Explore how the patient reduced anxiety in the past and what kinds of actions produced relief Point out the maladaptive and destructive effects of present coping responses Encourage the patient to use adaptive coping responses that have been effective in the past Focus responsibility for change on the patient Assume an active role with the patient correlating cause and effect relationships while maintaining his anxiety within appropriate limits Assist the patient in reappraising the value, nature, and meaning of the stressor when appropriate Help the patient identify ways he can restructure goals, modify behavior, utilize resources, and test out new coping responses Utilize role playing if appropriate Educate the patient in the growth-producing aspects of mild anxiety Encourage physical activity to discharge energy Include significant others as resources and social supports in helping the patient learn new coping responses Allow the patient time to implement new adaptive coping responses
Promote the relaxation response	One can also cope with stress by regulating the emotional distress that accompanies it through the use of stress management techniques	Utilize relaxation techniques to reduce the patient's level of stress Teach the patient relaxation exercises to increase his control and self-reliance

quacy, effectiveness, appropriateness, efficiency, and flexibility in judging the nursing goals and actions, the following questions can be raised:

- Were the planning and implementation a mutual process as much as possible?
- Were my goals and actions adequate in number and sufficiently specific to minimize my patient's level of anxiety?
- Did I work through all the stages of the problem-solving process with my patient?
- Were his maladaptive responses reduced?
- Did he learn new adaptive coping responses?
- Was the care plan reasonable in terms of our mutual constraints of time, energy, and expense?
- Were my many inferences, such as anxiety level, stressors, and coping patterns, appropriately validated with the patient and other staff members?
- Was I accepting of the patient and did I critically monitor my own anxiety level throughout the relationship?
- Was I able to modify my interventions on the basis of the patient's changing needs and feelings?
- Did I include the patient in the evaluation process?

Answering these questions will allow the nurse to review the total care she provided. Additional patient needs may become evident at this time. The nurse will also identify personal strengths and limitations in working with the anxious patient. Plans may then be made for overcoming the areas of limitation and further improving the quality of the nursing care provided. Throughout this process the nurse supports the belief that the "clarification of anxiety makes possible expanded awareness and an expansion of the self, which means the achievement of emotional health."[21:150]

■ SUGGESTED CROSS-REFERENCES ■

The nursing model of health-illness phenomena with a detailed discussion of precipitating stressors, appraisal of the stressors, and coping resources is discussed in Chapter 3. Interventions related to preventive mental health nursing are discussed in Chapter 9. Crisis intervention is discussed in Chapter 10. Physical illness as a response to stress is discussed in Chapter 13. Nursing interventions in psychotic panic states are discussed in Chapters 14 and 17. Antianxiety drugs are discussed in Chapter 23.

DIRECTIONS FOR FUTURE RESEARCH

The following are some of the nursing research problems raised in Chapter 12 that merit further study by psychiatric nurses:

1. Empirical validation of the four levels of anxiety and their effects on the individual as described by Peplau
2. Exploration of the relationships between anger and anxiety and self-esteem and anxiety
3. Early life experiences that predispose the individual to high levels of anxiety later in life
4. Knowledge by psychiatric nurses and nurses in other specialties of the physiological, behavioral, cognitive, and affective behaviors that are associated with anxiety
5. Personality characteristics associated with use of the various types of coping mechanisms
6. The ability of psychiatric nurses and nurses in other specialties to diagnose maladaptive anxiety responses to physical and psychological illnesses
7. The validity of the NANDA nursing diagnoses for problems of anxiety
8. The relationship between medical and nursing diagnoses associated with anxiety
9. The ability of psychiatric nurses to distinguish among anxiety, depression, and fear
10. Analysis of the role anxiety plays in the patient's decision whether or not to seek treatment
11. Levels of anxiety of patients during the course of the nurse-patient relationship
12. Therapeutic use of personal space by staff working with patients experiencing various levels of anxiety
13. The effectiveness of various types of supportive physical measures in decreasing a patient's anxiety
14. Knowledge by psychiatric nurses of the indications, actions, and possible side effects of the minor tranquilizers
15. Effective nursing actions for dealing with the resistance of patients to recognizing anxiety and conflict areas
16. Evaluation of the short- and long-term effectiveness of relaxation techniques with different patient groups

■ SUMMARY ■

1. Anxiety was defined as diffuse apprehension that is vague in nature and is associated with feelings of uncertainty and helplessness. It is an emotion without an object that is subjective in nature and communicated interpersonally. The capacity to be anxious is necessary for survival. Four levels of anxiety were identified and described: mild, moderate, severe, and panic. Mild anxiety increases one's perceptual field, motivates learning, and can produce growth and creativity in the individual.

2. Predisposing factors may be related to the threat of deprivation, the emotional conflict between the id and superego, the fear of interpersonal disapproval and rejection, low self-esteem, frustration, a learned response to avoid pain, conflict situations involving avoidance, family background, and biological factors. There are two major types of precipitating factors: threats to one's physical integrity and threats to one's self-system.

3. Data collection by the nurse should include both behavioral responses and coping mechanisms. Physiological responses associated with anxiety are primarily mediated through the autonomic nervous system. They are predominantly sympathetic in nature and serve to activate body processes in a "fight or flight" reaction. Behavioral responses reflect increased activity and restlessness. Withdrawal and decreased personal involvement are common social manifestations of high levels of anxiety. Affective responses convey apprehension and vague fears and may also include feelings of anger, boredom, depression, worthlessness, and helplessness. As anxiety increases, cognitive functioning is characterized by a decreased perceptual field, poor concentration, and errors in judgment.

4. The individual uses various coping mechanisms to deny or allay his anxiety. Mild levels of anxiety are often handled without conscious thought, and their effects can be minimized with little effort. Task-oriented reactions and ego-oriented reactions are coping mechanisms used with moderate and severe levels of anxiety.

   a. Task-oriented reactions are conscious attempts to realistically meet the demands of the stress situation. They are action-oriented responses and include *attack, withdrawal,* and *compromise.*

   b. Ego-oriented reactions, or *defense mechanisms,* serve as one's first line of psychic defense, since they protect the person from feelings of inadequacy and anxiety. Thirteen specific defense mechanisms were defined and described.

5. The position of anxiety within the larger perspective of the model of health-illness phenomena was described. Constructive coping mechanisms lead to adaptive responses, whereas destructive coping mechanisms lead to maladaptive responses and can be expressed as either neurotic or psychotic health problems. Formulating a nursing diagnosis requires that the nurse determine the quality (appropriateness) of the patient's response, the quantity (level) of his anxiety, and the nature of the coping mechanism mobilized.

6. Nursing and medical diagnoses were related. The overall goal of the nursing intervention is to help the patient develop the capacity to tolerate mild anxiety and use it consciously and constructively.

7. The highest priority nursing goals should address lowering the patient's severe or panic levels of anxiety, and related nursing interventions should be supportive and protective. The development of a therapeutic relationship is necessary in which the nurse critically monitors her own anxiety level. The patient's needs are met through the protection of his defenses and providing for the discharge of anxiety through physical activity. Supportive medications may also be administered.

8. When the patient's anxiety is reduced to the mild or moderate level, insight-oriented or reeducative nursing interventions may be implemented. This involves the patient in a problem-solving process that includes the following steps: recognition of anxiety, insight into the anxiety, and coping with the threat.

Nursing interventions that help the patient cope with stress by regulating the emotional distress associated with it were also described. These included the relaxation techniques of systematic desensitization, meditation, and the use of biofeedback.

9. In evaluating the nursing care given, the nurse reviews and analyzes each phase of the nursing process. By examining her effectiveness in working with an anxious patient, the nurse enlarges her own self-awareness and increases her therapeutic potential.

■ REFERENCES ■

1. Akiskal, H.: Anxiety: definition, relationship to depression, and proposal for an integrative model. In Tuma, A., and Maser, J., editors: Anxiety and the anxiety disorders, Hillsdale, N.J., 1985, Lawrence Erlbaum Associates Publishers.
2. American Psychiatric Association: Draft of the DSM-III-R in Development (subject to change), as proposed by the Work Group to Revise DSM-III. October 1985, The Association.
3. Arieti, S.: Anxiety and beyond in schizophrenia and psychotic depression, Nurs. Digest **2:**70, March 1974.
4. Beck, A., and Emery, G.: Anxiety disorders and phobias, New York, 1985, Basic Books.
5. Benson, H.: The relaxation response, New York, 1975, William Morrow & Co., Inc.
6. Benson, H., et al.: The relaxation response, Psychiatry **37:**37, Feb. 1974.
7. Bernstein, D., and Borkovec, T.: Progressive relaxation training, Champaign, Ill., 1973, Research Press.
8. Burd, S.: Effects of nursing intervention in anxiety of patients. In Burd, S.F., and Marshall, M.A., editors: Some clinical approaches to psychiatric nursing, New York, 1963, Macmillan, Inc.
9. Caplan, G.: Mastery of stress: psychosocial aspects, Am. J. Psychiatry **138**(4):413, 1981.

10. DiMotto, J.: Relaxation, Am. J. Nurs., **1984**:754, June 1984.
11. Dollard, J., and Miller, N.: Personality and psychotherapy, New York, 1950, McGraw-Hill Book Co.
12. Dzegede, S., Pike, S., and Hackworth, J.: The relationship between health-related stressful life events and anxiety: an analysis of a Florida metropolitan community, Community Ment. Health J. **17**(4):294, Winter 1981.
13. Elliott, S.: Denial as an effective mechanism to allay anxiety following a stressful event, J. Psychiatr. Nurs. **18**(10):11, 1980.
14. Freud, S.: Problem of anxiety, New York, 1936, W.W. Norton & Co., Inc.
15. Freud, S.: A general introduction to psychoanalysis, New York, 1969, Pocket Books.
16. Jacobson, E.: Progressive relaxation, ed. 3, Chicago, 1974, Univesity of Chicago Press.
17. Kristic, J.: Anxiety levels of hospitalized psychiatric patients throughout total hospitalization, J. Psychiatr. Nurs. **17**(7):33, 1979.
18. Lagina, S.: A computer program to diagnose anxiety level, Nurs. Res. **20**:491, 1971.
19. Lassen, C.: The effect of proximity in the psychiatric interview, J. Abnorm. Psychol. **82**:226, June 1973.
20. Long, B.: Stress-management interventions: a 15-month follow-up of aerobic conditioning and stress innoculation training, Cognitive Therapy Research **9**(4):471, 1985.
21. May, R.: The meaning of anxiety, New York, 1950, Ronald Press Co.
22. Meares, A.: The management of the anxious patient, Philadelphia, 1963, W.B. Saunders Co.
23. Mendels, J., Weinstein, N., and Cochrane, C.: The relationship between depression and anxiety, Arch. Gen. Psychiatry **27**:649, 1972.
24. Menninger, K., Maymann, M., and Rugyser, P.: The vital balance, New York, 1963, The Viking Press.
25. Oden, G.: Individual panic: elements and patterns. In Burd, S., and Marshall, M., editors: Some clinical approaches to psychiatric nursing, New York, 1963, Macmillan, Inc.
26. Peplau, H.: Interpersonal techniques: the crux of psychiatric nursing, Am. J. Nurs. **62**:53, June 1962.
27. Peplau, H.: A working definition of anxiety. In Burd, S., and Marshall, M., editors: Some clinical approaches to psychiatric nursing, New York, 1963, Macmillan, Inc.
28. Rimm, D., and Masters, J.: Behavior therapy, New York, 1974, Academic Press, Inc.
29. Shand, J., and Grau, B.: Perceived self and ideal self ratings in relation to high and low levels of anxiety in college women, J. Psychol. **87**:55, Jan. 1977.
30. Sullivan, H.S.: The interpersonal theory of psychiatry, New York, 1953, W.W. Norton & Co., Inc.
31. Tillich, P.: The courage to be, New Haven, Conn., 1952, Yale University Press.
32. Weissman, M.: The epidemiology of anxiety disorders: rates, risks and familial patterns. In Tuma, A., and Maser, J., editors: Anxiety and the anxiety disorders, Hillsdale, N.J., 1985, Lawrence Erlbaum Associates Publishers.
33. Will, O.: Psychotherapy in reference to the schizophrenic reaction. In Stein, M., editor: Contemporary psychotherapies, New York, 1961, The Free Press of Glencoe.
34. Wolpe, J.: The practice of behavior therapy, New York, 1973, Pergamon Press, Inc.

■ ANNOTATED SUGGESTED READINGS ■

Beck, A., and Emery, G.: Anxiety disorders and phobias: a cognitive perspective, New York, 1985, Basic Books.

This recent text is a good presentation of various aspects of anxiety disorders. The focus of treatment is on cognitive therapy and it is clearly written and clinically useful.

*Bell, J.: Stressful life events and coping methods in mental illness and wellness behaviors, Nurs. Res. **26**:136, Mar.-Apr. 1977.

This descriptive comparative study examines not only the relationship between stressful life events and mental illness and wellness behaviors but also the coping methods used by individuals exhibiting each behavior. Data collection included the use of the Holmes and Rahe Social Readjustment Rating Scale. The author summarizes her study with implications for nursing and health care.

*Breeden, S., and Kondo, C.: Using biofeedback to reduce tension, Am. J. Nurs. **75**:2010, 1975.

This brief article supports the use of biofeedback training to reduce stress and relieve stress-related illness. It describes how biofeedback works and briefly reviews three clinical experiences in biofeedback training sessions.

*Burd, S.: Effects of nursing intervention in anxiety of patients. In Burd, S.F., and Marshall, M.A., editors: Some clinical approaches to psychiatric nursing, New York, 1963, Macmillan, Inc.

Following the approach outlined by Peplau, the author uses the problem-solving and learning process to develop a framework for intervening with anxious patients. The article reports the results of a small study conducted to examine the framework; principles as well as techniques are described.

*Davis, J.: Treatment of a medical phobia including desensitization administered by a significant other, J. Psychosoc. Nurs. Ment. Health Serv. **20**(8):6, Aug. 1982.

This is an account of a young woman's fear of physicians and medical treatments and how it was helped through teaching her boyfriend systematic desensitization techniques.

Fischer, W.: Theories of anxiety, New York, 1970, Harper & Row, Publishers, Inc.

Freudian, neo-Freudian, learning theory, physiological, and existential formulations of anxiety are clearly synthesized and impartially described. An attempt is also made to integrate the theories based on common experiential phenomena. This is a good source book for a more detailed comparison of the various theories of anxiety.

---

*Asterisk indicates nursing reference.

*Garrison, J., and Scott, P.: A group self-care approach to stress management, J. Psychiatr. Nurs. **17**(6):9, 1979.

A procedure is described for teaching patients the use of relaxation as a coping skill. Each of the three components of this group training is clearly defined in the article, including progressive relaxation and clinical meditation.

*Hawkrigg, J.J.: Agoraphobia. I and II, Nurs. Times **71**:1280, 1337, 1975.

Agoraphobia is defined and pertinent clinical features are described. The article reports the results of a research project on treating agoraphobia and compares the treatment modalities of relaxation, systematic desensitization, behavioral counseling, reinforced graded practice, and stress inoculation.

*Hays, D.: Teaching a concept of anxiety, Nurs. Res. **10**:108, Spring 1961.

This article summarizes a small study that involved teaching patients about anxiety. It relates levels of anxiety, perceptual and behavioral changes, and learning tasks of the anxious person.

Jenike, M., et al., editors: Obsessive compulsive disorders: theory and management, Littleton, Mass., 1986, PSG Publishing Co.

This text presents current state of the art in the treatment of obsessive-compulsive disorders. Researchers and clinicians contribute to describing various therapies; neurobiology, management issues, and related illnesses.

*Jones, P., and Jakob, D.: Nursing diagnosis: differentiating fear and anxiety, Nurs. Papers **3**:20, Winter 1981.

This paper describes a research project to collect data related to the differential diagnosis of fear and anxiety by nurses. It summarizes the literature and explores the implications for nursing care of patients experiencing either human coping response. Additional studies of this nature are needed to further define and validate accepted nursing diagnoses.

*Kristic, J.: Anxiety levels of hospitalized psychiatric patients throughout total hospitalization, J. Psychiatr. Nurs. **17**(7):33, 1979.

Nurses interested in conducting research in psychiatric nursing will benefit from reading the report of this clinical study for the research process it describes, the findings it reveals, and the implications for nursing care it discusses.

May, R.: The meaning of anxiety, New York, 1950, Ronald Press Co.

This book brings together various theories of anxiety, synthesizes common elements of these theories, and suggests some constructive methods for dealing with anxiety. It incorporates philosophy, culture, biology, and psychology in its discussion and supports its analysis of anxiety with pertinent clinical studies. It is an excellent text and a "classic" in the field.

*Oden, G.: Individual panic: elements and patterns. In Burd, S.F., and Marshall, M.A., editors: Some clinical approaches to psychiatric nursing, New York, 1963, Macmillan, Inc.

The author explores the questions "What is panic?" and "What happens during a panic episode?" She reviews the literature on both individual and group panic and presents the results of her research study related to the identification of the elements and patterns of individual panic. Seven case studies are described.

*Olson, L.: Intervention in a pathological cycle of anxiety, J. Psychiatr. Nurs. **12**:21, Mar. 1974.

This is a case presentation of a 13-year-old girl hospitalized with myasthenia gravis and experiencing high levels of anxiety. The plan of care developed with the aid of a nursing consultant is described, and it includes problems, goals, and nursing approaches.

*Roncoli, M.: Bantering: a therapeutic strategy with obsessional patients, Perspect. Psychiatr. Care **12**:171, Oct.-Dec. 1974.

The author explores the strategy of the therapist as a psychological humorist who assists the obsessional patient to gain insight through the use of bantering. Bantering is defined as ridiculing lightly and good naturedly. The purpose is to release the patient's aggression and anger and the therapist's feelings of exasperation.

Salzman, L., and Thaler, F.: Obsessive-compulsive disorders: a review of the literature, Am. J. Psychiatr. **138**(3):286, 1981.

The authors reviewed the studies on obsessive-compulsive disorders published from 1953 to 1978. They report on various theories of the etiology of the disorders and treatment modalities used and conclude that, although the disorders are prevalent, there are little new data concerning their treatment, and serious questions about the effectiveness of the various treatment approaches remain.

*Sheer, B.: The effects of relaxation training on psychiatric inpatients, Issues Mental Health Nurs. **2**(4):1, 1980.

The purpose of the author's research was to determine if psychiatric inpatients who receive relaxation training as a part of their nursing care show a decrease between pretest and posttest scores on an anxiety scale. Although the results of the data did not support this hypothesis, this article is worth reading for the research process it describes.

*Sutterly, D., and Donnelly, G., editors: Coping with stress: a nursing perspective, Germantown, Md., 1981, Aspen Systems Corp.

This text is a collection of articles about stress and nursing organized around the following areas: models of stress, stress and life events, stress of illness, self-regulation of stress, and stress and the caregiver.

Tillich, P.: The courage to be, New Haven, Conn., 1952, Yale University Press.

This book is concerned with anxiety, its conquest, and the meaning of courage. Tillich believes anxiety comes from the loss of the meaning of life, whereas the "courage to be" involves participation as well as individualization. This distinguished book is a classic in the field.

*Trygstad, L.: Simple new way to help anxious patients, R.N. **43**(12):28, 1980.

This brief article is useful for the relaxation techniques and model scripts described by the author.

Tuma, A., and Maser, J.: Anxiety and the anxiety disorders, Hillsdale, N.J. 1985, Lawrence Erlbaum Associates Publishers.

This is a collection of perspectives on the anxiety disorders. It is a complete analysis from psychodynamic, biological, evaluation, and treatment points of view. It is highly recommended reading for the interested nurse.

Turner, S.: Behavioral theories and treatment of anxiety, New York, 1984, Plenum Press.

A nurse who is interested in refining a behavioral approach to patients with anxiety would find this text to be most valuable. It is organized around medical diagnoses and contains useful clinical examples.

White, R., and Gilliland, R.: Elements of psychopathology, New York, 1975, Grune & Stratton, Inc.

All the basic information needed to understand the mechanisms of defense is brought together in a readable form from a psychoanalytical frame of reference. Each defense mechanism is organized into general comments, definition, clinical examples, clinical syndromes that illustrate the mechanism, and examples of the use of the mechanisms in normal behavior. This book is of value to the student and is also an excellent review for the clinician.

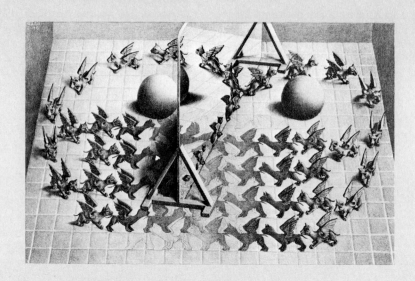

Every affection of the mind that is attended with either pain or pleasure, hope or fear, is the cause of an agitation whose influence extends to the heart.

William Harvey, 1628

CHAPTER 13

PSYCHOPHYSIOLOGICAL ILLNESS

LEARNING OBJECTIVES

After studying this chapter, the student should be able to:

- describe the stress response.

- discuss the relationship among intrapsychic conflict, anxiety, stress, and psychophysiological illness.

- discuss the predisposing factors that have been proposed for psychophysiological illnesses.

- analyze precipitating stressors that contribute to the development of psychophysiological illness.

- identify the physiological, psychological, and interpersonal behaviors that are associated with the development of psychophysiological illnesses.

- identify and describe coping mechanisms commonly used by persons with psychophysiological illnesses.

- analyze psychophysiological illness relative to the nursing model of health-illness phenomena.

- formulate individualized nursing diagnoses for patients with psychophysiological illnesses.

- assess the relationship between nursing diagnoses and the medical diagnoses of somatoform disorder and psychological factors affecting physical condition.

- develop long-term and short-term individualized nursing goals with patients who are experiencing psychophysiological illness.

- apply therapeutic nurse-patient relationship principles with an appropriate rationale in planning the care of a patient with a psychophysiological illness.

- describe nursing interventions appropriate to the needs of the patient who is experiencing a psychophysiological illness.

- develop a mental health education plan to assist a patient to develop more effective methods of coping with stress.

- assess the importance of the evaluation of the nursing process when working with patients who have a psychophysiological illness.

- identify directions for future nursing research.

- select appropriate readings for further study.

Continuum of psychophysiological responses

Throughout human history, philosophers and scientists have debated the nature and extent of the relationship between the mind *(psyche)* and body *(soma)*. In ancient times, physical illness was thought to be the result of possession by evil spirits, possibly related to misbehavior on the part of the victim. Shamans, witch doctors, and medicine men used potions and incantations to eliminate the evil. The continued use of these approaches, in some parts of the world to the present time, bears testimony to their success in many cases. The cures effected by primitive methods have not been explained scientifically. However, it is possible that absolute belief in the power of the healer has a curative effect on the physical disorder, through some as yet undefined mind-body interaction.

The Greek philosophers searched for the meaning of life, or *logos*. While Plato pursued meaning through mathematics, Aristotle focused his search on language.

According to Lynch,[13] these divergent belief systems had a profound effect on the development of medical theory. During the Renaissance, Descartes and Pascal continued the pathways initiated by Plato and Aristotle. Pascal believed in the importance of the emotional dimension of the human experience, while Descartes focused on the mathematical, or the rational. As a result of his reasoning about the nature of being human, Descartes concluded that people differ from animals in their ability to think, which is related to the existence of the soul. However, physiological functioning among people and animals was thought to be essentially the same and based on mechanical principles. The result of this widely accepted approach was to divorce the thinking and feeling aspects of human functioning from the body. This attitude is still reflected in modern medical thinking when physical disorders are addressed with little or no thought given to the interaction of mind and body.

Kaplan[10] cites the contribution of Freud in linking

physical and mental processes. Freud's theory of psychosexual development describes developmental tasks related to specific areas of physical functioning. For instance, the meeting of oral needs for nurturance is related to the development of the capacity to trust. Freud also studied extensively disorders that he labeled "conversions." These were physical illnesses that had no demonstrable organic pathological changes. Freud documented that psychoanalysis was an effective treatment for these patients. He concluded that the physical disruption symbolized an intrapsychic conflict related to failure to successfully resolve the conflicts associated with an early developmental stage. For example, a young woman suffering from paralysis of her legs beginning the day after her engagement had not resolved issues related to the oedipal stage of development. Therefore, she became paralyzed so she literally could not "walk down the aisle" and assume the sexual role of an adult woman.

Recently, there has been a renewed interest in exploring the Aristotelian approach to human nature. The growing popularity of holistic health practices attests to the recognition that mental processes influence physical well-being and vice versa. Research is attempting to identify the links between thoughts, feelings, and somatic functioning. In particular, there is great interest in the role of the endocrine and immune systems in the development of psychophysiological disorders. There is even a belief by some that all illness has a psychophysiological component—that physically manifested disorders include a psychological component and mental disorders include a physical one.

Much of the current thinking relative to psychophysiological behavior is related to an increased understanding of the role of stress in human life. In 1929, Walter Cannon[5] published his landmark work, *Bodily Changes in Pain, Hunger, Fear and Rage*. Based on research on animal physiology, he described the "fight-or-flight" response. The physiological behaviors associated with this reaction to stress are described in Chapter 12 (see Table 12-1). In response to Cannon's research, other investigators began to study physical responses to a variety of stressors, including psychological ones. For instance, in 1951, Wolf and colleagues[17] reported their research on the connection between stress and hypertension. They found that emotional arousal did lead to elevations in blood pressure.

Stress theory was significantly advanced when Hans Selye[15] published *The Stress of Life* in 1956. Selye described the stress response in detail, creating a greater understanding of the impact of stressful experiences on somatic functioning. He identified a three-stage process of response to stress which has overwhelmed the adaptive capacity of a localized area. This generalized response is called the general adaptation syndrome (GAS). These levels of response are:

1. *The alarm reaction.* This is the immediate response to a stressor which has not been eliminated locally. Adrenocortical response mechanisms are mobilized, resulting in the behaviors associated with the fight-or-flight response.
2. *Stage of resistance.* There is some resistance to the stressor. The body adapts at a lower than optimal level of functioning, requiring greater than usual expenditure of energy for survival.
3. *Stage of exhaustion.* The adaptive mechanisms become worn out and fail. The negative effect of the stressor spreads to the entire organism. If the stressor is not removed or counteracted, death will ultimately result.[15]

Selye's formulation has been invaluable to investigators in psychophysiology as they attempt to identify more specific mental-physical interactions and interventions in stress responses.

Any experience that is perceived by the individual to be stressful may result in a psychophysiological disorder. The stress does not need to be recognized consciously and in fact, most frequently is not. If the person does recognize that he is under stress, he is often unable to connect the cognitive understanding of feeling stress with the physical symptoms of the psychophysiological disorder. Fig. 13-1 illustrates the range of possible psychophysiological responses to stress, based on Selye's theory.

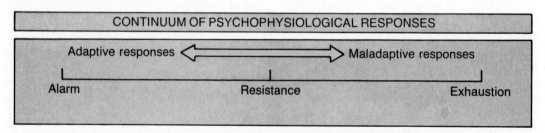

Fig. 13-1. Continuum of psychophysiological responses.

Assessment

Predisposing factors

A number of biopsychosocial factors are believed to influence the individual's psychophysiological response to stress. Because most of the specific relationships between physical and mental processes are still not well described, it is particularly important for the nurse to consider all possibilities when assessing factors that might predispose the patient to a particular disorder.

BIOLOGICAL FACTORS. One line of reasoning that has been applied to the predisposition to psychophysiological illness is that biological factors may be involved. Knapp[12] has described several theories of biological influences. Endocrine activity has been noted to exert an effect on the person's personality. However, although efforts have been made to link specific hormones and emotions, there has been little success. Genetic factors have also been considered. It has been speculated that a biological tendency for particular psychophysiological responses could be inherited. Unanswered questions related to this theory include concerns about the specificity of the biological tendency. Alexander[1] believed that target organs were related to specific stressors. He theorized that conflict was experienced as stress, and this resulted in the transmission of nerve impulses to the associated organ. This theory has not been supported by research, but does represent an early effort to establish a mind-body connection.

Recently, more sophisticated research has taken place regarding the biological factors that underlie psychophysiological illness. One focus has been on the new field of psychoneuroimmunology.[3] It has been demonstrated that the immune response can be modified by use of behavior modification techniques. Researchers are now investigating the possibility of modifying the immune response in the treatment of autoimmune illnesses, such as rheumatoid arthritis, systemic lupus erythematosus, myasthenia gravis, and pernicious anemia. Other related research is exploring the relationship among the immune system, stress, and cancer. It has been suspected that high stress, especially if prolonged, can decrease the ability of the immune system to destroy neoplastic growths. Unfortunately, this is an extremely difficult area in which to conduct research, since there has not been enough time to conduct prospective studies of this hypothesis. Retrospective studies are compromised by the subject's stress response to the diagnosis of cancer, which makes it impossible to measure pre-existing stress levels accurately.

PSYCHOLOGICAL FACTORS. Clinical observation has led to the theory that there is a relationship between personality type and specific psychophysiological disorders. Probably the best known of these descriptions is the "Type A" personality as identified by Friedman and Rosenman.[7] The type A person is more likely than others to develop stress related cardiac symptomatology. This person is described as being tense, ambitious, impatient, achievement oriented, irritable, and aggressive. He tends to be successful in work, but is frequently less successful interpersonally. Although most type A's tend to be men, as women's roles change, more of them are also beginning to fit this personality type. Initially, a type B was also identified as the polar opposite of the type A. More recently, it has become apparent that it is misleading to try to polarize all people into one of two personality types. Type B identification has less potential for practical application and is seldom used.

Lynch[13] has described the personality characteristics frequently observed in people who have migraine headaches. They tend to be "meticulous, perfectionistic, conscientious, intelligent, neat, inflexible, rigid, resentful, guilt-ridden, and compulsive." He also described the personality of the hypertensive person as being conflicted over the expression of hostile and aggressive feelings. In addition, the person struggles with dependency needs which conflict with his need to achieve. Interpersonally, he fears exposure of these conflicts, so represses them, leading to hypertension. As one reviews the adjectives used to describe the heart disease–prone person, the migraine sufferer, and the hypertensive person, the role of stress in the psychophysiological reaction again becomes clear. None of these people can be described as relaxed, calm, or secure.

Not only do people with psychophysiological disorders have difficulty dealing with feelings, they also resist acknowledging the role that emotions play in their illnesses. This led Sifneos[16] to coin the term, *alexithymia*. It means "no words for feelings." These individuals can describe feelings and discuss them intellectually, but they do not experience them and therefore do not convey the affective experience. Interpersonally, they are perceived as being cold and aloof. It is not possible to empathize with them, because the emotional component is missing.

Some people exhibit symptoms of physical illness with no evidence of organic impairment. These disorders, which are termed "somatoform" by psychiatrists, are assumed to represent a response to an underlying psychological conflict. Psychoanalysts believe that the physical symptoms of a conversion reaction symbolically represent unacceptable impulses that have been repressed. For instance, a woman who becomes angry with her child experiences paralysis of her arm. This prevents her from acting on her rage which she unconsciously believes to be murderous. The symptom protects her from experiencing the overwhelming anxiety she would feel if she were consciously aware of her rage. Another psychoanalytic approach to psychophysiologic problems focuses on the patient's dependency needs. In this case, the person is unaware of his wish to be dependent and to recreate the mother-infant relationship. Physical illness is an acceptable expression of that need.

■ **SOCIAL FACTORS.** There is current research on psychophysiological disorders focused on the influence of the social system. Lynch[13] has been investigating the effect of interaction on various psychophysiological disorders, particularly hypertension and migraine headaches. He has discovered that most of his patients are out of touch with their bodies. They are unaware of the response of body functions to social interaction and are resistant to admitting that they have interpersonal problems. When hypertensive persons are attached to a monitor during an interaction, they are able to see blood pressure changes related to interpersonal relationships. Their blood pressure rises when talking and rises still more if discussing stressful experiences. Observations such as this assist individuals to recognize the need for life-style changes to control their physical problems. Similarly, migraine patients are amazed to see the fluctuations in skin temperature that take place as their peripheral blood vessels constrict in response to interpersonal interactions.

Precipitating stressors

Any experience that is perceived by the individual to be stressful may lead to a psychophysiological response. Some of these are relatively mild and transient, related to the stimulation of the fight-or-flight reaction. Examples include diarrhea before an important examination or a dry mouth when speaking before a large group of people. Sometimes the response is more serious and indicates a higher level of anxiety. For instance, a person might feel panicky and experience tachycardia when boarding an airplane. Because the psychophysiological disorder is an attempt to deal with anxiety, it is recommended that information on stressors related to anxiety (Chapter 12) be reviewed.

One type of stressor that has been demonstrated to cause physical illness and even death is the loss of a significant interpersonal relationship. It has been observed that there is an increased mortality rate in recently widowed people. Similar observations have been made relative to people who have been admitted to institutions such as nursing homes, thereby experiencing separation from significant others. Children who have been separated from their mothers, especially if placed in an impersonal environment, also suffer a decline in physical

health. Illnesses and deaths related to loss of a loved person seem to represent the exhaustion phase of the general adaptation syndrome.

Sometimes a psychophysiological problem is a response to an accumulation of relatively small stressors. A patient may find it hard to identify one specific stressor that preceded his problem, but careful assessment may reveal a pattern of overwork and overcommitment or a series of seemingly minor events that all required extra effort. The use of a tool such as the Holmes and Rahe Social Readjustment Rating Scale described on p. 74 may be helpful in assessing the impact of accumulated stressors. Most of the psychophysiological disorders are characterized by remissions and exacerbations. This may be related to fluctuations in the person's stress level. When the cumulative stress gets too high, the body "calls time out" by developing physical symptoms.

Behaviors

■ **PSYCHOLOGICAL FACTORS AFFECTING PHYSICAL CONDITION.** The primary behaviors observed with psychophysiological illnesses are the somatic symptoms. These are the disruptions that are experienced by the patient and lead him to seek health care. Psychological factors affecting the physical condition may involve any body part. The most common reactions involve the following:

Skin (allergic eczema, hives, and acne)
Respiratory system (asthma, sinusitis, and bronchial spasms)
Cardiovascular system (hypertension and migraine headaches)
Musculoskeletal system (backaches and muscle cramps)
Gastrointestinal system (colitis, gastritis, constipation, hyperacidity, duodenal ulcer, obesity, and anorexia)
Genitourinary system (menstrual disturbances, impotence, and vaginismus)

Some would add cancer to this list. The list changes periodically, because no specific psychological-biological connection has been scientifically established for any of them. All the above disorders are associated with demonstrable organic disease, and it is suspected that most result from difficulties in coping with psychological stress.

The person is usually reluctant to believe that the problem is related to psychological factors. In part, this is because it is much more socially acceptable to be physically ill than it is to be mentally ill. The problem is compounded because the patient really does have physical symptoms. Denial of the psychological component of the illness may lead to "doctor shopping" as the patient searches for someone who will find an organic cause for the illness. Clinical example 13-1 illustrates this problem.

Mr. R is typical of many people with stress-related psychophysiological disorders. He is reluctant to admit

---

CLINICAL EXAMPLE 13-1

Mr. R was a successful 42-year-old executive who had risen quickly to the top of his company. He worked long hours and had difficulty delegating any of his responsibilities. He set high standards for his employees and was believed to be insensitive to human concerns. He viewed himself as "tough, but fair." However, he had little sympathy for a worker who requested extra time off for personal business.

Mr. R was married, but saw little of his family. He expected his wife and children to do their part to maintain his standing in the community by associating with "the right people." He seldom interacted with his children except to reprimand them if they disturbed his concentration while he was working. His wife reported that their sexual relationship was unsatisfying to her because he used it for physical release for himself, but was not concerned about meeting her needs. She suspected that he was involved in an extramarital affair, but did not want to endanger the marriage by confronting him.

Mr. R was expecting to be named to the board of directors of a prestigious philanthropic foundation. He anticipated that this would add to his social prominence in the community. Shortly before the announcement was to be made, his 14-year-old son was arrested in a drug raid in a lower middle class part of town. Mr. R did not get the appointment. He was furious with his son, but dealt with his anger by withdrawing still more. One day at work, he experienced an episode of dizziness, followed by a severe headache. He attributed it to tension, took some aspirin, and continued to work. However, after several similar episodes, he decided to consult his family doctor. The physician arrived at a diagnosis of essential hypertension. He tried to discuss work, family, and social behavior with Mr. R, but was frustrated by superficial responses. Although concerned about Mr. R's condition and stress level, the doctor gave in to Mr. R's demand for medication to lower his blood pressure. He also advised Mr. R to exercise and to find a relaxing activity, but did not really expect him to comply with those suggestions.

---

to a lack of control over his mind and body. He expects a magical cure that will allow him to pursue his usual life-style without interruption. It is likely that he will discontinue his medication as soon as he feels better. Distance from the stressor that caused the recent episode of symptoms will probably allow him to function for a while without overt symptoms of his hypertension. Sooner or later, however, a new stressor or the accumulation of smaller stressors will lead to another dizzy spell, headaches, or possibly myocardial infarction or cerebrovascular accident.

In his studies of hypertension, Lynch[13] has found that people with psychophysiological problems are unable to share feelings with others. The person who is not aware of or comfortable with his own feelings has trouble communicating, because sharing of personal pain would result. Speech is used to hide rather than reveal. When that mechanism fails, the cardiovascular system goes out of control. Lynch describes this as the "loneliest loneliness."

Pines[14] has reported work done by Kobasa and Maddi to define "hardiness," a behavioral characteristic that seems to assist people to resist stress. Hardiness consists of three components. The first is the perception of change as a challenge, rather than a threat. Second, there is a sense of commitment to people or a cause. Finally, hardy people have a sense of control over their lives. One study compared hardiness and frequency of illness in lawyers and businesspeople. Lawyers had the lower rate of illness episodes. It was suspected that this was related to the professional socialization of the lawyer to expect stress and to function in a stressful environment. On the other hand, businesspeople are influenced by mass media information that defines stress as harmful and to be avoided. This research seems to indicate that attitude toward stress is also influential in determining the individual's response. Of course, one can also speculate that a person who selects a law career is already someone who enjoys working under stress.

■ **SOMATOFORM DISORDERS.** Some people experience physical symptoms without the presence of any organic impairment. These are termed *somatoform disorders*. They include somatization disorder, in which the person presents multiple physical complaints; conversion disorder, involving a loss or alteration of physical functioning; idiopathic pain disorder, in which pain is the only symptom; and hypochondriasis, the fear of or belief that one has an illness. Clinical example 13-2 is a case history of a person with a medical diagnosis of somatization disorder.

Ms. O demonstrates the dependent behavior that is often characteristic of people who somaticize their intrapsychic conflicts. Her many symptoms allowed her to be taken care of and to avoid the demands of adult responsibility. Her needs to be cared for were congruent with her mother's needs to nurture. Therefore, she received little encouragement to give up her symptoms. A periodic hospital stay served to reinforce the serious-

ness of her problem. Secondary gain related to the gratification of dependency needs is a powerful deterrent to change in many patients.

Another type of somatoform disorder is the conversion disorder, in which symptoms of some physical illness appear without an underlying organic pathological condition. This leads to the reduction of anxiety, and the organic symptom usually symbolizes the conflict. For example, a patient who has an impulse to harm his domineering mother may develop paralysis of his arms and hands. The primary gain the patient receives from his symptom is that he is unable to carry out his impulses. This person also may experience secondary gain in the form of attention, manipulation of others, freedom from responsibilities, and economic compensation. Conversion symptoms might include the following:

1. Sensory symptoms, such as areas of anesthesia, blindness, or deafness
2. Motor symptoms, such as paralysis, tremors, or mutism
3. Visceral symptoms, such as urinary retention, headaches, or difficulty breathing

It is frequently difficult to diagnose this reaction. Other patient behaviors may be helpful in this regard. Often patients have a bland attitude toward the conversion symptom and the disability produced by it. They tend to display little anxiety or concern and the classic term for describing this lack of concern is *la belle indifference*. There is also a tendency for the patient to seek attention in a pervasive way not limited to the actual symptom.

Hypochondriasis is another type of somatoform disorder. It is characterized by an exaggerated concern with one's physical health that is not based on a real organic pathological condition. The person fears presumed diseases of various organs and is not helped by reassurance. These people tend to seek out information about diseases and use that information to reinforce their contention that they are probably ill or about to become so. This reaction differs from the conversion reaction in that there is no actual loss or distortion of function. The patients appear worried and anxious about their symptoms. This concern may be based on physical sensations overlooked by normal persons or on symptoms associated with minor physical illness that the patient exaggerates out of proportion. This is frequently a chronic pattern for the individual, and it is often accompanied by a history of visits to numerous physicians.

Of course, hypochondriacal behavior is not related to a conscious decision. If a person decides to feign

---

CLINICAL EXAMPLE 13-2

Ms. O is a 28-year-old single woman who is admitted to the medical unit of a general hospital for a complete medical workup. When asked about her main problem during the nursing assessment, she replies, "I've never been very well. Even when I was a child I was sick a lot." While the admitting nurse was assessing biological functioning, Ms. O revealed multiple complaints. These included palpitations, dizzy spells, menstrual irregularity, painful menses, blurred vision, dysphagia, backache, pain in her knees and feet, and a variety of gastrointestinal symptoms including stomach pain, nausea, vomiting, diarrhea, flatulence, and intolerance to seafood, vegetables of the cabbage family, carbonated beverages, and eggs. None of the symptoms were constant, with the exception of the food intolerances. However, they occurred unpredictably, making her fearful of going out of her home.

The psychosocial assessment revealed that Ms. O lived with her parents. She was the youngest of three children. Her siblings were living away from the parental home. She had graduated from high school, but had poor grades because of her frequent absences. She had tried to work as a clerk in a retail store, but was asked to leave because of absenteeism. She did not seem particularly bothered about the loss of her job. She had never tried to find other work, although she had been unemployed for 8 years. When asked how she spent her time, she said that she did some gardening and some housework when she felt well enough. However, she spent most of her time watching television.

Ms. O's parents visited her most of every day. Her mother inquired about whether she would be able to spend the night in her daughter's room and was most displeased when told that this would not be possible. The O family had numerous complaints about the quality of the nursing care, mostly related to failures to anticipate the patient's needs. Extensive diagnostic studies failed to reveal any organic basis for her physical complaints. When informed that the problem was most likely psychological and advised to obtain psychotherapy, the O's protested angrily and refused a referral to a psychiatric clinic. Ms. O was discharged and returned to her parents' home.

illness, the behavior is referred to as *malingering*. This is usually done to avoid responsibilities and obligations that the person perceives as burdensome. Many otherwise healthy people malinger at one time or another. For instance, a person who was involved in an automobile accident may feign neck pain in order to receive insurance compensation. Frequently, the person exaggerates his symptoms, is evasive, and contradicts himself.

The behaviors associated with psychophysiological disorders are many and varied. The process of assessment must be carefully conducted so that actual organic problems are defined and treated. This type of illness should never be dismissed as "only psychosomatic" or "all in his head." Serious psychophysiological disorders can be fatal if not treated adequately.

■ Coping mechanisms

The psychophysiological disorders may be viewed as attempts to cope with the anxiety associated with overwhelming stress. Unconsciously, the person binds the anxiety to the physical illness. As described above, the secondary gain then adds to the psychological relief experienced.

Several of the defense mechanisms described in Chapter 12 may be observed to be operating in psychophysiological disorders. Repression of feelings, conflicts, and unacceptable impulses often leads to expression through physical symptoms. The maintenance of repression over long periods of time requires a great deal of psychic energy. As the system approaches a state of exhaustion, the physical symptomatology occurs. Denial is apparent when the patient is confronted with the psychological component of his illness. It indicates that the person is unable to handle the anxiety that would be released if he acknowledged the psychic conflicts that are being repressed. The need for this defense should be respected.

Some individuals respond to psychophysiological illness with compensation. They attempt to prove that they are actually healthy by being more active and exerting themselves physically even if told to rest. This coping style is typical of the type A person, who needs desperately to prove that he is in control of his body, not that he is controlled by it. The opposite of this reaction is the person who uses regression as a coping mechanism. This individual becomes dependent and embraces the sick role as a way of avoiding responsibility and dealing with conflictual issues.

It can be seen that the commonality among these attempts to cope is the need not to confront the basic conflict that is leading to stress and anxiety. This need is so strong that premature challenging of the coping mechanism with attempts to convince the person of his psychological conflicts may result in the substitution of a less adaptive coping mechanism for a more adaptive one. In extreme cases, if the person is stripped of all his efforts to cope and not provided with a substitute, death can result. This may be related to worsening of the organic disorder when one is present or by suicide.

 ## Nursing diagnosis

The nursing diagnosis must reflect the complexity of the biopsychosocial interaction that is the hallmark of psychophysiological disorders. The individual's effort to cope with stress-related anxiety may result in numerous somatic and emotional disorders. Care must be taken to consider all the possible disruptions when formulating a complete nursing diagnosis.

The model of health-illness behavior (Fig. 13-2) may serve as a helpful guide to the diagnostic process. A comprehensive interview will reveal many of the predisposing factors and precipitating stressors that are pertinent to the individual. The nurse must be careful to use good communication skills during the interview, to enable the patient to share his experience as completely as possible. Areas of resistance and gaps in information should be noted as possibly indicative of a conflict. These may be explored more completely as trust is established in the nurse-patient relationship. Questions related to life-style and usual activities may be helpful in identifying precipitating stressors as well as coping behaviors. It is particularly important to have the patient describe his perception of what is happening to him. This will provide valuable information about his awareness of the relationship between his mind and body. Nonverbal behaviors also provide clues about the patient's concerns. Apparent lack of concern may reveal the use of denial that is typical of a person with a conversion disorder.

As the diagnosis is formulated, the nurse needs to consider the individual's coping in the context of the stress response. Is he in a stage of alarm with many coping resources at hand? Or, is he in the stage of resistance, utilizing coping mechanisms but depleting his energy resources? Has he reached the stage of exhaustion, needing intensive intervention to maintain life? The determination of the level of stress and coping in operation will have an influence on the interventions that are initiated for patient care. The box on page 385 presents primary NANDA diagnoses and complete nursing diagnoses for patients with psychophysiological disorders. Medical and nursing diagnoses for these patients are described in Table 13-1.

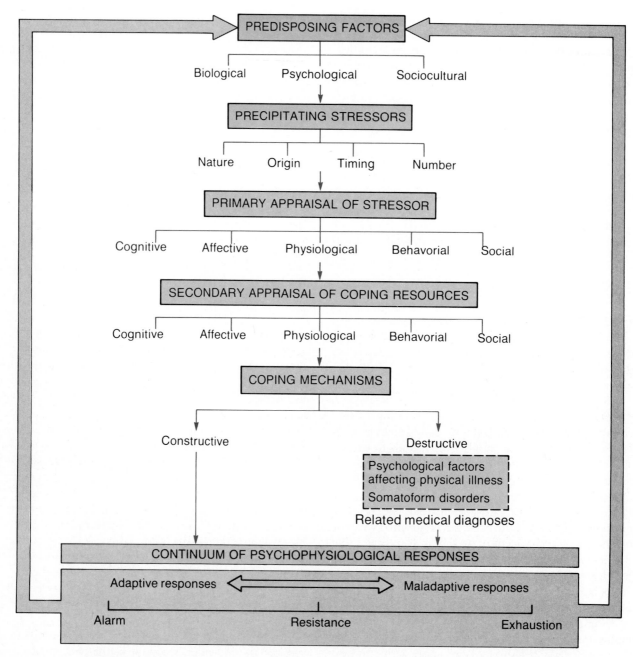

Fig. 13-2. Nursing model of health-illness phenomena with psychophysiological responses.

■ Related medical diagnoses

Medical disorders related to psychophysiological illnesses are classified under the general headings of somatoform disorders and other disorders associated with physical condition. Specific diagnostic criteria for disorders classified as psychological factors affecting physical condition in the Draft of the DSM-III-R in Development[2] are found in the International Classification of Diseases, edition 9 (ICD-9). These disorders and related nursing care are described in great detail in medical and surgical nursing textbooks and will not be repeated here.

TABLE 13-1

MEDICAL AND NURSING DIAGNOSES RELATED TO PSYCHOPHYSIOLOGICAL ILLNESS

Medical Diagnostic Class

Somatoform disorders
Other disorders associated with physical condition

Psychiatric Nursing Diagnostic Class

Psychophysiological illness

Related Medical Diagnoses (DSM-III-R)*

Somatization disorder
Conversion disorder
Idiopathic pain disorder
Hypochondriasis
Psychological factors affecting physical condition

Related Nursing Diagnoses (NANDA)

Altered comfort: chronic pain
Anxiety
Bowel elimination, alteration in: diarrhea
Bowel elimination, alteration in: constipation
Comfort, alteration in: pain
†Coping, ineffective individual
Family process, alteration in
Fear
Gas exchange, impaired
Mobility, impaired physical
Nutrition, alteration in: less than body requirements
Powerlessness
Self-care deficits
Self-concept, disturbance in
Skin integrity, impairment of: actual
Sleep pattern disturbance
Social isolation

*From American Psychiatric Association: Draft of the DSM-III-R in Development (subject to change), as proposed by the Work Group to Revise DSM-III. American Psychiatric Association, October 1985.
†Indicates primary nursing diagnosis for psychophysiological illness

---

■ **SOMATIZATION DISORDER.**[2] The essential features of somatization disorder include a history of multiple somatic complaints, beginning before age 30 and potentially involving several organ systems. There must be no associated demonstrable organic pathology. In addition, the symptoms do not occur only during a panic attack and do cause an alteration in life-style or require medical attention or medication.

■ **CONVERSION DISORDER.**[2] The essential features of conversion disorder include lost or altered physical functioning suggestive of a physical disorder, but which ensues soon after an identifiable stressor has occurred. The disorder is not intentionally produced and cannot be explained by organic pathology. It is not limited to pain or alterations in sexual functioning.

■ **IDIOPATHIC PAIN DISORDER.**[2] The essential features of idiopathic pain disorder include pain that has persisted for more than 6 months without demonstrable organic pathology or in excess of that usually associated with the pathological condition.

Nursing Diagnoses Related to Psychophysiological Illness

Primary NANDA nursing diagnosis

Coping, ineffective individual

Examples of complete nursing diagnoses

Ineffective individual coping related to inability to express hostile and aggressive feelings evidenced by labile hypertension
Ineffective individual coping related to fear of assuming adult responsibilities evidenced by multiple somatic complaints
Ineffective individual coping related to repressed sexual impulses evidenced by urinary retention with no organic cause

■ **HYPOCHONDRIASIS.**[2] The essential features of hypochondriasis include preoccupation with fear of illness or the belief that the individual has an illness based on interpretation of physical signs or sensations. There is no evidence of a related illness on physical examination, but the concern persists. The disturbance must have lasted at least 6 months and must be unrelated to any major mental illness.

■ **PSYCHOLOGICAL FACTORS AFFECTING PHYSICAL CONDITION.**[2] The essential features include a temporal relationship between psychologically meaningful stimuli and the development of organic pathology (recorded on Axis III). The condition must not meet the criteria for any of the somatoform disorders.

❦ Planning and implementation

■ Goal setting

The primary goal for the patient with a psychophysiological disorder is to consciously experience feelings and to be able to share them with others. This is a very long-term goal, and for some may never be reached. However, an increased level of self-awareness is also beneficial and should be achievable to some extent by all patients. Reduction of the need for repression related to an improved ability to deal with conflict will decrease stress and allow the patient to function with fewer episodes of somatic illness.

The establishment of mutual goals with these patients is a problem. The patient's primary goal is to alleviate the physical manifestations of his illness. He expects that this will be done by medical or surgical treatment. Exploration of psychological conflicts is likely to be regarded as unnecessary. This resistance is related to the need to maintain defenses against the extreme anxiety that has led to the illness. The nurse needs to identify the treatment goals about which she and the patient can agree. The nurse also wants the patient to obtain relief from physical symptoms. Many patients will receive medical or surgical treatment and related nursing care. At the same time, the nurse should concentrate on building a trusting relationship, so she can assist the patient to begin to feel safe in exploring interpersonal conflicts and feelings.

Significant others must also be considered in developing the plan of care. It is important to explore their understanding of the patient's problem. They can be valuable allies in encouraging the patient to change his life-style if this is necessary. At the same time, the nurse must recognize that a change in one family member requires a change in all the others. The family may be active participants in the patient's pathological behavioral style. In this case, goals should be included to address the family relationship with the patient.

Care plans for these patients may turn out to be rather lengthy. This is because the nurse must attend to the whole complex of the patient's biopsychosocial needs. Most patients, although having needs in all spheres, have their most urgent needs in a more limited area of functioning. Patients with psychophysiological disorders are likely to have urgent needs in all three functional areas. Physical disorders are usually disabling and may be life threatening. Psychosocial problems will stand in the way of significant recovery from the physical illness and therefore must also be given immediate attention.

Long-term goals for the patient should focus on either decreasing the frequency of or eliminating the physical disorder. Short-term goals provide the milestones along the way to long-term goal achievement. They assure a logical approach to goal achievement and provide periodic reinforcement that the therapeutic interventions are being successful. This keeps the patient involved in the therapeutic program and decreases the possibility of noncompliance.

Long- and short-term goals for a patient with migraine headaches might be

Long-term goal:
   The patient will no longer experience migraine headaches.
Short-term goals:
   In 1 week, the patient will:
   1. Describe the activity that immediately preceded a migraine attack, identifying possible stressors
   2. Agree to learn relaxation exercises
   In 3 weeks, the patient will:
   1. Practice relaxation exercises daily and whenever involved in a stressful situation
   2. While relaxed, label the feelings experienced prior to a migraine attack
   3. Identify at least one alternative way to deal with stressful situations
   In 5 weeks, the patient will:
   1. Report at least one stressful situation that did not result in a migraine attack
   2. Identify and practice additional positive responses to stress
   In 1 year the patient will report absence of migraine attacks for at least 6 months.

A similar approach may be used with patients with other psychophysiological problems that involve organic pathology. The specific approaches and time intervals must be individualized depending on the patient's physical condition, receptiveness to treatment approaches, and the severity and tenacity of the underlying psychological conflicts. Many of these patients will require intensive insight-oriented psychotherapy which may be provided only by nurses with graduate education in psychiatric nursing.

When the patient has no organic pathology, the nurse must remember that the symptoms are still very real to the person. Psychogenic pain is no less painful than organic pain. Goals for the care of these patients must also be directed toward enabling them to give up the physical symptom by developing healthier coping mechanisms. This, too, frequently requires insight-oriented psychotherapy.

Long- and short-term goals for a patient with psychogenic pain might be

Long-term goal:
    The patient will only experience pain related to organic disorders.
Short-term goals:
    In 1 week the patient will:
    1. Identify one nonmedication approach to pain relief
    2. Talk with the primary nurse for at least 30 minutes daily
    In 2 weeks the patient will:
    1. Practice a nonmedication approach to pain relief between doses of medication
    2. Talk with the primary nurse for at least 30 minutes daily, with at least 15 minutes of that time focused on issues other than pain
    In 1 month the patient will:
    1. Delay use of pain medication at least 15 minutes by using a nonmedication approach to pain relief
    2. Carry on a conversation for at least 30 minutes without mentioning pain
    3. Discuss with the primary nurse the impact of the pain on his life

The above progression of goals would continue until the patient had achieved recognition of the role pain played in his life and could maintain control of pain with minimum medication. Goals for patients with other somatoform disorders would have the same dual focus of learning to control physical functioning while simultaneously beginning to examine the effects of the illness on the person's life-style.

■ Intervening in psychophysiological illnesses

Patients with psychophysiological illnesses are most frequently encountered in general hospital and outpatient settings. They usually seek health care because of symptoms related to physiological functioning. It is only after a thorough medical examination that the role of psychosocial stressors in the disorder may be evaluated.

In some cases, there will be a pathophysiological disruption that requires physical nursing intervention. If the physical condition is life-threatening, intervention in this area is given highest priority. For instance, a person with a bleeding ulcer needs intensive intervention to maintain his life. However, once the physical crisis is past, the nurse needs to intervene to assist the patient to avoid similar problems in the future. For physical illnesses that have psychosocial etiologies, this requires implementation of psychiatric nursing approaches using the medium of the interpersonal relationship.

Provision of skilled and compassionate nursing care directed toward the patient's physical needs is the first step in establishing the trusting relationship. A person who is in pain, bleeding, or covered with a rash is in no position to discuss emotions or interpersonal relationships. The cardinal principle to follow with patients who have psychophysical disorders is to assess the patient's stress level and, whenever possible, act to reduce it. Stress and anxiety are at the root of the patient's problem. Therefore, the nurse must attend to immediate needs before addressing less obvious ones.

■ **INTERPERSONAL APPROACHES.** The psychophysiological symptom, whether with or without organic pathology, serves to defend the person from overwhelming anxiety. It provides some patients with a way to receive help and nurturance without admitting the need for it. Others are protected from expressing frightening aggressive or sexual impulses. Recognizing the defensive nature of the symptom, the nurse should never try to convince the patient that his problem is entirely psychological. Likewise, the attitude that the patient only needs to get his life under control to get better is not therapeutic. The patient has not made a conscious choice to be hypertensive or to develop a conversion disorder. The dilemma of these disorders is that the patient consciously would like nothing more than to be cured, but unconsciously is unable to give up the symptom. Conscious recognition of the psychological role of the symptom defeats its purpose and is therefore vigorously resisted. An example of this resistance is illustrated in Clinical example 13-3.

It is not unusual for a person with a conversion disorder to substitute another symptom if the original one is taken away. This happens because the basic conflict still remains and the ego still needs to be defended from experiencing repressed anxiety. The patient really needs assistance in dealing with the conflict. When this is resolved, the symptom will disappear because there is no longer a need for it.

Great skill is needed to intervene psychotherapeu-

CLINICAL EXAMPLE 13-3

Ms. W was a 20-year-old woman who was admitted to the general hospital with a history of sudden onset of blindness. There was no evidence of any pathophysiological process affecting her eyes. Assessment revealed that she had witnessed her father's suicide by gunshot at the age of 5, although she claimed to have no memory of this. Her boyfriend had recently been expressing suicidal thoughts to her.

It seemed clear that the blindness was a conversion reaction. In order to confirm the diagnosis, the physician decided to interview Ms. W while she was sedated with amobarbital sodium. The interview was videotaped. During the interview, Ms. W was able to see. She read the day's menu and told the time by looking at a clock across the room. She also described the incident with her father. However, when the sedation wore off, Ms. W was again blind.

The decision was made to show her the videotape, so she would recognize the psychogenic nature of her blindness. As she watched the tape, she did indeed regain the ability to see. However, when it reached the part in which she described her father's suicide, she became deaf.

tically with these patients. Graduate education in psychiatric mental health nursing is required to be qualified to provide insight-oriented psychotherapy. The nurse who is not prepared at this level can be of assistance by being supportive and available to talk with the patient in addition to providing the necessary physical nursing care. She should be familiar with the therapeutic process so she can encourage the patient and understand behavioral changes that may occur. See Table 13-2 for nursing interventions used in psychophysiological illnesses. Kaplan[11] has described the process of insight-oriented therapy for patients with psychophysiological disorders. The patient's underlying anger must be recognized and confronted supportively. As the patient becomes aware of anger, he may have difficulty expressing it appropriately. The nurse should accept the patient's attempts to express anger as healthy and provide feedback. Sometimes patients who are in this phase of their therapy are labeled as hostile or demanding and avoided by nursing staff. This only reinforces their conviction that angry feelings are unacceptable.

The next step in therapy is to identify and explore the patient's defenses. The therapist proceeds very carefully in this area, helping the patient to discover and test new, more adaptive coping mechanisms as the dysfunctional ones are relinquished. The nurse can again be helpful by supporting the patient in attempting new behaviors. Spending time with the patient and appreciating his positive qualities will help build his self-esteem and give him confidence. The nurse should be alert to indications of increased anxiety and report these immediately to the psychotherapist. An exacerbation of the physical disorder may occur if the therapy progresses too rapidly. The therapist may decide to recommend changes in the patient's environment to assist him to function more comfortably. If the patient needs to consider a job change or another change in life-style, the nurse can offer time to talk about alternatives.

The patient may also need help in explaining changes in himself or his life-style to his significant others. The family is a system, and a change in one component of the system requires adjustment of all the other parts. For instance, if a man who was very involved in his job and out several nights a week agreed to limit himself to 8-hour work days, this would affect the rest of the family. Although his wife may have protested for years that he spent too much time away from home, in reality she built her life around his schedule. She, too, may have spent several evenings a week in other activities. If he were to be at home every evening, she would have to reevaluate her activities and decide whether she should go out or be with him. These are not easy decisions for family members to make. It is important that any underlying feelings of resentment be revealed and discussed to prevent indirect expression, which would create a new stressor for the patient. Family therapy may be necessary if family members have been supporting the patient's pathology. For instance, families sometimes become adjusted to having a dependent member and unwittingly sabotage efforts to foster independence.

Nurses need to be aware that countertransference is frequently an issue with these patients. They may be impatient and demanding. In general, it is easier to care for them when they are seriously physically ill. However, it is easy to become impatient with a demanding patient who is not acutely ill when there are sicker patients also needing nursing care. Reacting to this behavior by avoidance or anger only adds to the patient's anxiety and makes the situation worse. Clinical supervision with an experienced psychiatric nurse is highly recommended for nurses who work with these difficult patients. Frequent nursing care conferences including the nursing staff who usually care for the patient are also helpful. If possible, a limited number of staff members should be assigned to the care of these patients. This fosters the development of a trusting relationship.

TABLE 13-2

SUMMARY OF NURSING INTERVENTIONS IN PSYCHOPHYSIOLOGICAL ILLNESSES

Goal—Assist the patient to consciously experience feelings and to be able to share them with others

Principle	Rationale	Nursing interventions
Maintain biological integrity	Highest priority is given to nursing interventions that preserve life and safety	Based on the patient's physical pathology, provide for adequate nutrition, hygiene, elimination, and safety needs
Establish a trusting relationship	Psychosocial nursing intervention is based on the therapeutic nurse-patient relationship	Meet the patient's stated needs; establish mutual goals; empathize with the patient; utilize therapeutic communication skills
Support the psychotherapeutic process	Conflict aroused in psychotherapy leads to increased anxiety and possible exacerbation of psychophysiological symptoms	Schedule time to interact with the patient; encourage to continue to work in therapy; observe changes in symptoms; report increases to therapist; give patient positive feedback for new, healthier behaviors
Assist the patient to develop new ways to cope with stressful situations	Inability to deal with intrapsychic conflict leads to anxiety and stress, resulting in physiological dysfunction	Assist to identify stressful situations; explore alternative coping behaviors; teach various approaches to stress management; support patient in testing new behaviors
Assist significant others to support the patient's behavioral changes	Change in one part of a system affects all the other parts; systems tend to resist change	Explain the plan of care to significant others; involve them in the patient's care whenever possible; teach stress management techniques

■ **EDUCATIONAL APPROACHES.** Health education is an important aspect of the nursing care of the patient with a psychophysiological disorder. The patient who has organic pathology will almost certainly need instruction about medications, treatments, and life-style changes. He and his family will need information about follow-up care and crisis management. In addition to this, patients should be offered education about ways to cope with stress. It may be possible to increase acceptance of this idea by linking it to the general concern about stress management that the holistic health movement has engendered in American society. Group classes on stress management may be productive, enabling patients to share experiences and make suggestions to each other about coping behaviors. Former patients who have made successful life adjustments can also be effective teachers of coping strategies. Table 13-3 presents a mental health education plan for stress management.

It is adapted from the work of Hoover and Parnell.[9] This approach would be most effective with a small group of patients, but could be used with an individual if the nurse participated actively in suggesting and demonstrating coping strategies.

■ **ALTERNATIVE APPROACHES.** The approach to relaxation described by Benson[4] and presented in Chapter 12 is also helpful for patients with psychophysiological disorders. The relaxation response helps decrease tension. Physiologically, it is the opposite of the fight-or-flight response. Therefore, it decreases the sympathetic nervous system activity that leads to many of the physiological problems that these patients experience. It is also helpful to patients who dislike the idea of medication, and want to be able to counteract stress when it occurs. Relaxation requires no special equipment and is not difficult to learn. The nurse will find that this is a useful intervention with many patients with

---

TABLE 13-3

MENTAL HEALTH EDUCATION PLAN—TEACHING COPING STRATEGIES

Content	Instructional activities	Evaluation
Definition of stress	List feelings that indicate stress Discuss behaviors that are associated with elevated stress	The student will identify behaviors that are associated with stressful situations
Recognition of stressful situations	Ask learners to describe situations that they have experienced as stressful Role play the situation (with videotape if possible) Discuss stress-related behaviors observed and feelings experienced	The student will correctly identify a stressful experience
Description of common life stressors	Ask each learner to describe one situation in his life that produces stress Conduct discussion about common elements of stressful experiences	The student will identify stressful aspects of his life
Identification of coping mechanisms	Review the role-played stressful situations Discuss alternative ways to cope with the stressors Role play at least one coping mechanism Provide feedback about the effectiveness of the selected coping mechanism	The student will identify and practice alternative coping mechanisms The student will select an appropriate coping mechanism when experiencing stress

Adapted from Hoover, R.M., and Parnell, P.K.: J. Psychosoc. Nurs. **22**:17, June 1984.

---

a variety of nursing care problems. Hartl[8] also suggests that nurses may find it helpful to practice relaxation when they themselves are under stress.

Meditation and hypnosis are closely related to relaxation therapy. Both involve the induction of deep states of relaxation by altering the state of consciousness. In meditation, the person concentrates on a word or phrase and clears his mind to convey a sense of peace to himself. Hypnosis may be induced by oneself or another. Posthypnotic suggestions are often effective in strengthening healthy coping mechanisms. Hypnosis should not be attempted by anyone who has not had extensive training and supervision in its use. Zahourek[18] describes the use of hypnosis with patients who are experiencing pain. She found that it was most helpful in cases of acute pain. People with psychogenic pain were too fearful of giving up their pain, but it was sometimes possible to modify it. The best candidates for hypnosis were emotionally healthy, intelligent, and motivated persons.

Biofeedback may also be used successfully in conjunction with the relaxation response as described in Chapter 12. This approach is used by Lynch[13] in work with hypertensive and migraine headache patients. The blood pressure and pulse of hypertensive patients is monitored during an interpersonal interaction. Fluctuations in these values are pointed out. As the patient is able to tolerate the information, the connection is made between the content of the conversation and the change in vital signs. This helps him recognize the role played by stress in his problem. He is then taught to express the feelings he has been repressing and to accept social support. Improvement is demonstrated by positive changes in the monitored physical signs. A similar approach is used with migraine headache patients, except that peripheral skin temperature is monitored.

Other approaches to stress management have been described by Charlesworth and Nathan.[6] For instance, physical activity is very relaxing for some people. Ideally, it is an activity that the person enjoys and can share with others. Patients needs medical permission before being encouraged to participate in strenuous physical activity. Diet may also be helpful in building the person's coping ability. People who are under stress should be advised to avoid overuse of dietary stimulants, such as caffeine. They may need education about the elements of a healthful diet. If the patient has been relying on alcohol or other drugs to cope with stress, he should be encouraged to find less destructive coping mechanisms. Specific information on alcohol and drug abuse will be found in Chapter 20.

Evaluation

The evaluation of the nursing care of the patient with psychophysiological illness is based on the identified patient care goals. If goal achievement is not attained, the nurse needs to ask the following questions:

Was the assessment complete enough to correctly identify the problem?

Did the patient agree with the goal?

Was enough time allowed for goal achievement?

Was I skilled enough to carry out the desired intervention?

Were there environmental constraints that affected goal accomplishment?

Did additional stressors change the patient's ability to cope?

Was the goal achievable for this patient?

What alternative approaches should be tried?

It is very important that neither the patient nor the nurse interpret the lack of goal achievement as a failure. The nurse should try to experience it as a challenge and convey that attitude to the patient. It is not at all helpful to add failure to achieve a goal to the patient's collection of stressors. The care of these patients is exceedingly complex. The nurse may expect to modify the treatment plan several times before finding a successful approach. The most important thing is to keep trying and to encourage the patient to persist in his efforts to find health.

■ SUGGESTED CROSS REFERENCES ■

The nursing model of health-illness behavior is discussed in Chapter 3. The therapeutic nurse-patient relationship is discussed in Chapter 4. Anxiety and coping responses are discussed in detail in Chapter 12. Problems with the expression of anger are discussed in Chapter 18. Liaison nursing is discussed in Chapter 26.

■ SUMMARY ■

1. A historical perspective was provided on the progression of understanding of the relationship between the

---

DIRECTIONS FOR FUTURE RESEARCH

The following are some of the nursing research problems raised in Chapter 13 that merit further study by psychiatric nurses:

1. The effect of feeling states on biological parameters
2. The relationship between the stress state of the nurse and her response to patient demands
3. Nursing interventions that assist Type A patients to modify their behavior
4. Validation of nursing diagnoses that are related to level of coping ability
5. Behaviors that patients interpret as indicative of increased stress
6. The relationship between personality characteristics and acceptance of various stress management approaches
7. Impact of having family members participate in a stress management program with the patient
8. Relationship between various dietary patterns and coping ability
9. Characteristics of activities that are perceived as being relaxing
10. Responses of nurses to patients with psychophysiological illnesses in medical as opposed to psychiatric settings
11. Analysis of the effect of offering relaxation training to all patients on a general hospital unit

---

mind and the body. A dualistic approach was identified as being the major influence on modern medical thinking. More recently, a holistic influence has begun to be accepted.

2. The stress response was described as identified by Selye. It consists of three phases: alarm, resistance, and exhaustion.

3. Predisposing factors were discussed relative to biological, psychological and sociocultural influences. Biological factors included the target organ theory and the possibility of genetic influences. Psychological factors include the possible influence of developmental experiences, unresolved dependency needs, and the inability to recognize, identify, or express feelings. Personality traits thought to be related to selected psychophysiological disorders were described. Sociocultural factors include lack of social support systems and the loss of significant others.

4. Precipitating stressors were related to the experiencing of a crisis or to the gradual accumulation of a number of small

stressors. Loss of defense mechanisms can also lead to the development of physical disorders.

5. Behaviors were discussed in terms of the meaning of the primary symptom to the patient. Somatoform disorders which do not involve organic impairment were compared to psychological factors affecting physical condition, which do. Feelings associated with psychophysiological disorders include anger, dependency, and sexual impulses which are unacceptable to the person. Depression and anxiety are also present.

6. Coping mechanisms associated with psychophysiological illnesses were identified as repression, regression, denial, and compensation. The function of the illness itself as a coping mechanism was also discussed.

7. Nursing and medical diagnoses related to psychophysiological illnesses were presented.

8. Long- and short-term goals were suggested for patients with psychophysiological illnesses.

9. Nursing interventions were discussed. These included interpersonal approaches of a supportive nature, educational approaches, and alternative approaches of relaxation, meditation, hypnosis, biofeedback, activity, and nutrition. A mental health education plan was presented.

10. Evaluation of the nursing care is based on the identified goals. Several questions were proposed that will assist the nurse to assess lack of goal accomplishment.

■ REFERENCES ■

1. Alexander, F.: Psychosomatic medicine: its principles and application, New York, 1950, W.W. Norton.
2. American Psychiatric Association: Draft of the DSM-III-R in Development (subject to change), as proposed by the Work Group to Revise DSM-III. Washington, D.C., 1985, The Association.
3. Anderson, A.: How the mind heals, Psychol. Today, **16**:50, Dec. 1982.
4. Benson, H.: Behavioral medicine: a perspective from within the field of medicine, Nat. Forum **60**:3, Winter, 1980.
5. Cannon, W.B.: Bodily changes in pain, hunger, fear and rage, New York, 1929, Appleton-Century-Crofts.
6. Charlesworth, E.A., and Nathan, R.G.: Stress management: a comprehensive guide to wellness, New York, 1982, Atheneum.
7. Friedman, M. and Rosenman, R.H.: Type A behavior and your heart, Greenwich, Conn., 1974, Fawcett.
8. Hartl, D.E.: Stress management and the nurse, Adv. Nurs. Sci. **1**:91, July 1979.
9. Hoover, R.M., and Parnell, P.K.: An inpatient education group on stress and coping, J. Psychosoc. Nurs. **22**:17, June 1984.
10. Kaplan, H.I.: Psychological factors affecting physical conditions (psychosomatic disorders). In Kaplan, H.I., Freedman, A.M., and Sadock, B.J., editors: Comprehensive textbook of psychiatry, ed. 3, Baltimore, 1980, The Williams & Wilkins Co.
11. Kaplan, H.I.: Treatment of psychosomatic disorders. In Kaplan, H.I., Freedman, A.M., and Sadock, B.J., editors: Comprehensive textbook of psychiatry, ed. 3, Baltimore, 1980, The Williams & Wilkins Co.
12. Knapp, P.H.: Current theoretical concepts in psychosomatic medicine. In Kaplan, H.I., Freedman, A.M., and Sadock, B.J., editors: Comprehensive textbook of psychiatry, ed. 3, Baltimore, 1980, The Williams & Wilkins Co.
13. Lynch, J.J.: The language of the heart, New York, 1985, Basic Books, Inc.
14. Pines, M.: Psychological hardiness: the role of challenge in health, Psychol. Today **14**:34, Dec. 1980.
15. Selye, H.: The stress of life, New York, 1956, McGraw-Hill Book Co.
16. Sifneos, P.: The prevalence of "alexithymic" characteristics in psychosomatic patients, Psychother. Psychosom. **22**:255, 1973.
17. Wolf, S., et al.: Life stress and essential hypertension, Baltimore, 1955, The Williams & Wilkins Co.
18. Zahourek, R.P.: Hypnosis in nursing practice—emphasis on the "problem patient" who has pain, Part II, J. Psychosoc. Nurs. **20**:21, Apr. 1982.

■ ANNOTATED SUGGESTED READINGS ■

Charlesworth, E.A., and Nathan, R.G.: Stress management: a comprehensive guide to wellness, New York, 1984, Atheneum.

This book is a useful reference for the nurse who is looking for information on a variety of approaches to stress management. It would be particularly helpful to recommend it to patients who were interested in learning more about stress.

Cousins, N.: Anatomy of an illness, New York, 1979, W.W. Norton Company.

The author demonstrates through an account of a personal experience that patients should assume a partnership role in the health care relationship. Through the use of a stress management approach, he actively participated in his own recovery from a progressive and potentially fatal illness. The author has many provocative observations about the health care system.

*Hartl, D.E.: Stress management and the nurse, Adv. Nurs. Sci. **1**:91, July 1979.

Nurses are not immune from stress. In fact, nursing is a relatively stressful profession. The author of this article suggests stress management approaches that nurses might find helpful in their personal and professional lives.

*Lessman, M.: A painful chronicle, Am. J. Nurs. **85**:551, May 1985.

A nursing student reflects on his experience as an adolescent being treated for Crohn's disease. He reminds the reader of the need to reach out to frightened adolescents and to allow them the time to understand the alien experience of hospitalization and surgery.

---

*Asterisk indicates nursing reference.

Lynch, J.J.: The language of the heart, New York, 1985, Basic Books, Inc.

The author shares his observations of patients who suffer from psychophysiological disorders and his approaches to their treatment. He believes that these patients need help in developing an awareness of their feelings and in reaching out to other people. He works in partnership with a clinical nurse specialist who carries out much of the intervention.

Selye, H.: The stress of life, New York, 1956, McGraw-Hill Book Company.

This classic work set forth the description of the stress response. It is a pioneering work with which every nurse should be familiar.

Sontag, S.: Illness as metaphor, New York, 1977, Vintage Books.

This small, but thought-provoking book uses the examples of tuberculosis and cancer to demonstrate the many meanings that are attributed to illness. The author suggests that metaphorical thinking relative to illness may stand in the way of successful coping.

*Sparacino, J., et al.: Psychological correlates of blood pressure: a closer examination of hostility, anxiety and engagement, Nurs. Research **31**:143, May/June 1982.

This article describes nursing research related to blood pressure in response to hostility and anxiety. A possible relationship was described. Further research in this area was recommended.

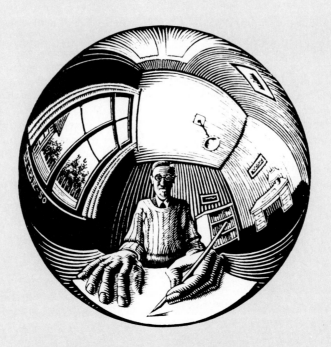

To venture causes anxiety, but not to venture, is to lose one's self. And to venture in the highest sense is precisely to be conscious of one's self.

Sören Kierkegaard

C H A P T E R   1 4

ALTERATIONS IN SELF-CONCEPT

LEARNING OBJECTIVES

After studying this chapter, the student should be able to:

- define the following terms: self-concept, body image, self-ideal, self-esteem, role, and identity.

- discuss factors and experiences throughout the life cycle that influence each of the above concepts.

- describe the characteristics of a healthy personality structure.

- analyze the predisposing factors and precipitating stressors affecting self-concept.

- identify and describe behaviors and coping mechanisms that are associated with alterations in self-concept.

- formulate individualized nursing diagnoses for patients with alterations in self-concept.

- assess the relationship between nursing diagnoses and medical diagnoses associated with alterations in self-concept.

- develop long-term and short-term individualized nursing goals for patients who are experiencing alterations in self-concept.

- apply therapeutic nurse-patient relationship principles with appropriate rationale in planning the care of the patient who is experiencing an alteration in self-concept.

- describe the progressive levels of nursing interventions appropriate to the needs of the patient who is experiencing an alteration in self-concept.

- develop a mental health education plan to promote a patient's adaptive self-concept responses.

- assess the importance of the evaluation of the nursing process when working with patients with alterations in self-concept.

- identify directions for future nursing research.

- select appropriate readings for further study.

Of all man's attributes, the self appears to be the most complex and most intangible. One can neither see nor touch a self-concept, yet it has been a topic of concern to behavioral scientists since the late 1800s. The concept of self is not clearly defined, has various meanings, and is used in many different ways. But the self is the most real thing in one's experience and it is the frame of reference through which a person perceives, conceives, and evaluates the world around him. Self-concept can be defined as all the notions, beliefs, and convictions that constitute an individual's knowledge of himself and influence his relationships with others. It includes the perceptions of one's characteristics and abilities, one's interaction with other people and the environment, one's values associated with experiences and objects, and one's goals and ideals.

Helping professionals of all backgrounds have increasingly come to view the self-concept as a critical and central element for the understanding of people and their behavior, and it is now the subject of an enormous body of theory and research. This inquiry has given rise to a theoretical school know as "self theory," which is based on the principle that man's behavior is always meaningful and that a person reacts to the world in terms of the way he perceives it. No two people have identical self-concepts. The self-concept emerges or is learned as a result of each person's unique experiences within himself, with other people, and with the realities of the world. Because it is the frame of reference through which the person interacts with the world, it is a powerful influence on human behavior. Self theorists believe it is impossible to understand a person fully or to accurately predict his behavior without understanding his internal frame of reference. This involves sharing his own private perceptual world and his views of himself. Thus understanding a patient's self-concept is a necessary component of all nursing care.

Continuum of self-concept responses

■ Developmental influences

Although theories of self-concept development vary considerably, there is general agreement that the self-concept does not exist at birth. The self develops gradually as the infant recognizes and distinguishes others and vaguely begins to differentiate himself as a separate individual. The boundaries of the self are defined as a result of exploratory activity and experience with his own body as the infant interacts with this environment. At first, the process of self-differentiation is slow, but with the development of language, the process becomes accelerated. Language helps to clarify the concept of the self, and the child's own name is a major linguistic aid. The use of a proper name helps the child identify himself and perceive himself as someone special, unique, and independent. In general, the ability to use language enables the child to make clear distinctions between himself and the rest of the world and to symbolize and understand his experiences. Once the infant has begun to differentiate himself from other people and the environment, the continued process of self-concept development is greatly benefited by the following:

- Interpersonal and cultural experiences that generate positive feelings and a sense of value and worth
- Perceived competence in areas that are valued by the individual and society
- Self-actualization, or the implementation and realization of one's true potential

■ **SIGNIFICANT OTHERS.** The self-concept is learned in part through accumulated social contacts and experiences with other people. Sullivan[45] called this development "learning about self from the mirror of other people." What a person believes about himself is a function of his interpretation of how others see him, which he infers from their behavior toward him. His concept of self therefore rests in part on what he thinks others think of him. "Significant others" in the life of a child particularly affect the development of self-concept, and, for a young child, the most significant others in his life are his parents. How they help him grow and react to his experiences has a tremendous influence on him. According to Combs and Snygg:

No experience in the development of the child's concepts of self is quite so important or far-reaching as his earliest experiences in his family. It is the family which introduces a child to life, which provides him with his earliest and most permanent self definitions. Here it is that he first discovers those basic concepts of self which will guide his behavior for the rest of his life.[13:134–135]

They believe that the family provides the individual with his earliest experiences of (1) feelings of adequacy or inadequacy, (2) feelings of acceptance or rejection, (3) opportunities for identification, and (4) expectancies concerning acceptable goals, values, and behaviors. Studies indicate that parental influence is strongest during early childhood and continues to have a significant impact through adolescence and young adulthood.[18]

However, with age, the power and influence of friends and other adults increase, and they now become significant others to the individual. Parents and immediate family therefore are crucial to the initial development of the self-concept, and the continuing development and change in self-perceptions are influenced by countless experiences with many other people.

Culture and socialization practices also affect self-concept and personality development. An understanding of the dominant cultural patterns of the individual's environment gives important clues to the sources of personality formation. General culture patterns as well as cultural subdivisions, such as social class membership, have formative influences on the individual's view of self. According to Combs and Snygg:

The culture in which we move is so completely a part of our experience as to overshadow almost all else in determining the nature of the self. Even our definitions and values are not left entirely to our own experience but are colored, interpreted and valued one way or another by the culture into which we are born, as they are interpreted to us by the acts of the people who surround us.[13:86]

■ **SELF-PERCEPTIONS.** A person's view of himself is not exclusively a collection of the views, expectations, and desires of others. Each person can observe his own behavior the same way that others do and form opinions about himself. One's perception of reality is selective, however, according to whether the experience is consistent with one's current concept of self. The way a person behaves is a result of how he perceives the situation, and it is not the event itself that elicits a specific response but rather the individual's subjective experience of the event. An individual's needs, values, and beliefs strongly influence his perceptions. One more readily perceives that which is meaningful and consistent with present needs and personal values. Similarly, people behave in a manner that is consistent with what they believe to be true. In this case, a fact is not what is but what one believes to be true. Once perceptions are acquired and incorporated into one's self-system, they can be difficult to change. There are ways, nonetheless, to change or modify one's perceptions, and these can include modification of cognitive processes, exposure to drugs, sensory deprivation, and biochemical changes within the body.

As the self-concept develops, it brings with it a unique perspective in viewing one's relationship with the world. What a person perceives and how he interprets what he perceives are conditioned by his concepts of self. A person with a weak or negative self-concept and who is unsure of himself is likely to have a narrowed or distorted perceptual field. Because he feels easily

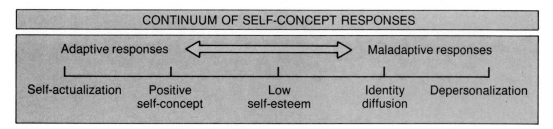

Fig. 14-1. Continuum of self-concept responses.

threatened, his anxiety level will rise quickly and he will become preoccupied with defending himself. In contrast, a person with a strong or positive self-concept can explore his world openly and honestly because he has a background of actual experiences of acceptance and success. Positive self-concepts are the result of actual positive experiences that lead to perceived competence.

In conclusion, it can be stated that self-concept is a critical and central variable in human behavior. Individuals with positive self-concepts function more effectively, which is evident in interpersonal competence, intellectual efficiency, and environmental mastery. In contrast, negative self-concept is correlated with personal and social maladjustment. Like the other nursing problems described in this text, it is possible to view one's self-concept responses along the health-illness continuum of coping responses described in Chapter 3. Fig. 14-1 describes the range of self-concept responses from the most adaptive state of self-actualization to the most maladaptive response of depersonalization.

Precisely because one's self-concept pervades every aspect of life, therapeutic interventions related to self-concept are a core element in psychiatric nursing practice. This requires an understanding of the various components of the self, including the concepts of body image, self-ideal, self-esteem, role, and identity, which will now be briefly discussed. The chapter will then focus on the nursing therapeutic process model for maladaptive responses related to self-concept.

■ **Body image**

The concept of one's body is central to the concept of self. The body can be thought of as a capsule in which one is permanently enclosed and through which one interacts with the world. One lives with his body 24 hours a day from birth until death. It is the most material and visible part of the self, and, although it alone never accounts for one's entire sense of self, it remains a life-long anchor for self-awareness. An individual's attitude toward his body may mirror important aspects of his identity. A person's feelings that his body is big or small,

attractive or unattractive, or weak or strong also reveal something about his self-concept.

Body image can be defined as the sum of the conscious and unconscious attitudes the individual has toward his body. It includes present and past perceptions as well as feelings about size, function, appearances, and potential. Body image is a dynamic entity because it is continually being modified by new perceptions and experiences. It serves as a target or screen on which the person projects significant personal feelings, anxieties, and values.

■ **DEVELOPMENTAL INFLUENCES.** One is not born with a body image. The infant receives input from his body but reacts to it in a global, undifferentiated way. As he gradually explores parts of his body, receives sensory stimulation from others, and begins to manipulate the environment, he becomes aware of the separateness of his own body from others. In the development of body awareness, the external body, that is, the body that can be seen and felt to the touch, is easier to learn about and is discovered earlier than the inner body. This recognition grows out of pleasurable and painful experiences. Actually, pain becomes the more dominant learning experience because pain sensory endings are distributed over the total surface of the body while sensations of pleasure are concentrated in a few erotic zones. For the preschooler the exploration of genitals and the discovery of anatomical differences between the sexes becomes especially important. The body occupies a middle position between the external world and the self as the agent of one's perceiving, thinking, and acting. The body can be viewed more externally and objectively than one's inner tensions, thoughts, and feelings. With increasing age there is a further differentiation of the self as a body and the self as a mind that can solve problems, make decisions, and experience feelings.

During the age of adolescence the physical self is of more concern than during any other period of life except, perhaps, old age. Basic physical changes force the body into the adolescent's awareness. He has lost the security of a familiar body. New sensations, features, and body proportions have emerged. Height, weight, and physical strength increase, and the growth of secondary sex characteristics may be troublesome or embarrassing. The development of breasts, menarche, growth of pubic and facial hair, and voice changes must be integrated into the individual's evolving body image. Physical changes at adolescence also symbolize the end of childhood; maturity is just over the horizon. Adult proportions begin to emerge, although it is impossible to be certain of the nature, extent, or duration of changes still to come. Soon the outline of mature features will be complete. So the adolescent is anxious—will his mature physical self become reasonably close to his ideal? One's body image during adolescence is a crucial element in shaping his self-concept and in facilitating or retarding his attainment of status and adequate social relations.

Early adulthood sees some stability of body change. For the healthy adult, the body experience is a moment-to-moment, highly flexible aspect of his daily life pattern. As he has grown older, his view of the importance of his body experience has changed. It can be truly said that the child "lives in his body," as compared to the adult who lives in his mind. To the child, eating, crawling, walking, and defecating can be all consuming, as can coughing and being febrile, congested, or constipated. They can occupy his sense of reality totally. The intensity of the child's involvement with his body, however, must be diminished in the course of his developing into an adult with a broadening sense of what is real. The diminution must be selective, since the emerging adult needs to retain a flexible potential fullness of awareness of direct body sensation and a blending in of body awareness into all aspects of his life. Many parts of his body experience must achieve the autonomy of automatic responses, such as walking and breathing. Other aspects of the body experience must emerge as flexibly adjusted pleasures, such as eating, orgasm, and exercise.

Middle age brings new challenges as different body parts age at different rates. The individual realizes his body is not functioning as well as it previously had. The later years of life accelerate the decline in physical abilities and can severely influence one's life-style and self-concept. As one's body image develops, extensions of the body become important, and anything that extends the effectiveness or control of one's body function can be called one's own. Clothes become identified closely with the body, and in the same way toys, tools, and possessions serve as extensions of the body and help to widen one's sense of self. Still later, position and wealth serve similar functions.

When the individual values his body and acts to preserve and protect it, the body image becomes the basis of sympathy through which the bodies and possessions of others are also valued. Body image, appearance, and positive self-concept are related. Studies have indicated that the more a person accepts and likes his body, the more secure and free from anxiety he feels.[27,43] It has also been shown that people who accept their bodies are more likely to manifest high self-esteem than people who dislike their bodies.[22] Thus the concept of body image is a central one to understanding self theory, and the relationship between the two will have implications for developing and implementing nursing care.

■ Self-ideal

The self-ideal is the individual's perception of how he should behave based on certain personal standards. The standard may be either a carefully constructed image of the kind of person one would like to be or merely a number of aspirations, goals, or values that one would like to achieve. The self-ideal creates self-expectations that are based in part on society's norms and to which the person tries to conform. The formation of the self-ideal begins in childhood and is influenced by significant others who place certain demands or expectations on the child. With time, the child internalizes these expectations, and they form the basis of his own self-ideal. New self-ideals that may persist throughout life are taken on during adolescence, and they are formed from identification with parents, teachers, clergy, and age contemporaries. In old age additional adjustments must be made that reflect diminishing physical strength and changing roles and responsibilities.

There are a number of factors that influence one's self-ideal. The first is that a person tends to set goals within a range determined by his abilities. One does not ordinarily set a goal that is accomplished without any effort nor one that would be entirely beyond one's abilities. Self-ideals are also influenced by cultural factors as the person compares his self-standards with those of his peers so that his behavior will be consistent with his culture. Other influencing factors would include one's ambitions and the desire to excel and succeed, the need to be realistic, the desire to avoid failure, and the presence of feelings of anxiety and inferiority. Based on these factors, one's self-ideal may be clear and realistic and thus facilitate personal growth and relations with others, or it may be vague, unrealistic, and demanding. The adequately functioning individual, however, demonstrates congruence between his perception of self and his self-ideal. That is, he sees himself as being very much like the person he would like to be.

In summary, self-ideals are important in maintaining mental health and balance. They serve as internal regulators and help a person maintain an even course in the face of conflicting or confusing circumstances. For mental health the self-ideal must not be too high and too demanding nor too vague and shadowy, and yet it must be high enough to give continuous support to self-respect.

■ Self-esteem

Self-esteem is the individual's personal judgment of his own worth obtained by analyzing how well his behavior conforms to his self-ideal. The frequency with which his goals are achieved will directly result in the development of feelings of superiority (high self-esteem) or inferiority (low self-esteem) (Fig. 14-2). If a person is repeatedly successful, he tends to feel superior, but if he fails to live up to his expectations, he feels inferior. High self-esteem is a feeling rooted in unconditional acceptance of self, despite mistakes, defeats, and failures, as an innately worthy and important being. It involves accepting complete responsibility for one's own life.

Self-esteem is derived from two primary sources: the self and others. It is first of all a function of being loved and of gaining the respect of others. Self-esteem is lowered when love is lost and when one fails to receive approval from others. Conversely, it is raised when love is regained and when one is applauded and praised. The origins of self-esteem can be traced to childhood and are based on acceptance, praise, and respect. Coopersmith[14] described the four best ways to promote a child's self-esteem as follows:

1. Providing him with success
2. Instilling ideals
3. Encouraging his aspirations
4. Helping him build defenses against attacks of his self-perceptions

This should provide him with a feeling of significance—success in being accepted and approved of by others, a feeling of competence—ability to cope effectively with life, and a feeling of power—control over one's own destiny.

Self-esteem increases with age, although it is most threatened during adolescence. At this time, concepts of self are being modified and many self-decisions need to be made. The adolescent has to make an occupational choice and decide if he is good enough to succeed in a given career. He has to decide whether he is able to participate or is accepted in various social activities. Heterosexually, is he attractive enough to interest and attract a desirable member of the opposite sex? Will he succeed in marriage? Does he have the courage to carry out his convictions? Is he capable of performing the roles assigned to him?

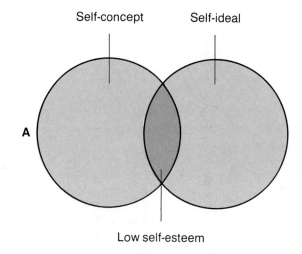

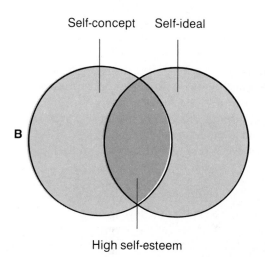

Fig. 14-2. A, Individual with a low level of self-esteem caused by a large discrepancy between self-concept and self-ideal. **B,** Person with greater conformity of self-concept and self-ideal and therefore a person with a high level of self-esteem. (From Sundeen, S.J., Stuart, G., et al.: Nurse-client interaction: implementing the nursing process, ed. 3, St. Louis, 1985, The C.V. Mosby Co.)

With adulthood the self-concept stabilizes, and maturity provides a clearer picture of self. The adult tends to be more self-accepting and less idealistic than the adolescent. He has learned to cope with many of his self-deficiencies and maximize his self-strengths. Of course, not all adults attain maturity, and some continue to function as adolescents for many of their adult years. In later life, self-esteem problems again arise due to the new challenges posed by menopause, retirement, loss of spouse, and physical disability.

Recent research shows clear relationships between self-reported physical health and self-esteem.[3] The report of a health problem, regardless of its type or severity, was associated with significantly lower self-esteem than was the report of no health problem. Severity of reported health problems was also related to lower levels of self-esteem. Finally, perception of ill health was negatively related to self-esteem.

High self-esteem has similarly been correlated with low anxiety, effective group functioning, and acceptance of others. According to Maslow, it is a prerequisite to self-actualization; once self-esteem is achieved, the individual is free to concentrate on achieving his potential.[35] Low self-esteem has been correlated with poor interpersonal relations, and a sense of low self-worth is particularly prominent in schizophrenia and depressive disorders.

■ Role performance

Roles are sets of socially expected behavior patterns associated with an individual's function in various social groups. Identity emerges from self-concept and is evident in the form of role behavior.[25] Roles can provide a means for social participation and a way to test out identities for consensual validation by significant others. The individual assumes various roles that he attempts to integrate into one functional pattern. Because these roles overlap and intertwine, an understanding of the person requires the nurse to see him in the context of the several roles he occupies. On the basis of his perception of role adequacy in the most "ego-involved" roles, the individual develops a level of self-esteem. High self-esteem results from roles that meet our needs and are congruent with our self-ideal. Many factors, including the following, influence an individual's adjustment to the role he occupies:

1. The clarity of the behaviors appropriate to the role and his knowledge of specific role expectations
2. The consistency of the response of significant others to his role
3. The compatibility and complementarity of his various roles
4. The congruency of cultural and his own expectations for role behavior
5. The segregation of situations that would create incompatible role behaviors

There are two basic types of roles. The first is an ascribed role over which the individual has no choice. Examples of ascribed roles include age and sex. The second is an assumed role that the individual selects or achieves by choice. These roles include occupation and marital or family roles.

Sex roles are important roles that affect one's per-

formance in other roles. They are particularly significant for the performance of family roles, but they permeate most other roles as well and are frequently the cause of role conflict or disturbance. Another difficult role problem faced by the individual growing up in contemporary society is that of emancipation from one's parents and the establishment of an independent life. This primarily occurs during adolescence and early adulthood when there is marked ambiguity in role definitions. The social roles of child and adolescent make it difficult to prepare oneself for adulthood. The child is not expected to be responsible; the adult is. The child is expected to be submissive; the adult dominant. The child is expected to be asexual; the adult is expected to be sexually mature and maintain intimate sexual relationships. Yet there are few transitional procedures or "rites of passage" to help the adolescent shift his role behavior. A final crisis is faced during old age when role behavior must again be changed by aging parents who rely on their children and yet strive to balance their lives by maintaining a sense of independence and a high level of self-esteem. It is obvious that role behavior is intimately related to self-concept and identity, and role disturbances frequently involve conflicts between independent and dependent functioning.

■ Personal identity

The word identity is derived from the Latin root *idem,* meaning the same. It is the organizing principle of the personality system that accounts for both the unity and continuity of the personality. Identity is the awareness of the process of "being oneself," which is derived from self-observation and judgment. It is the synthesis of all self-representations into an organized whole, and it is not associated with any one accomplishment, object, attribute, or role assumed by the individual. It is different from self-concept in that it refers to a feeling of distinctness from others. It implies consciousness of oneself as an individual with a definite place in the general scheme of things. The person with a sense of identity feels integrated, not diffuse. When a person acts in accordance with his self-concept, his sense of identity is reinforced; when he acts in ways contrary to his self-concept, he experiences anxiety and apprehension. Behavior that conforms with the self-concept may thus be viewed as behavior that preserves one's sense of identity.

The person with a strong sense of identity sees himself as a unique individual. Indeed, the very word individual, as a synonym for person, implies a universal need to perceive oneself as separate from others. This depends in part on a sense of self-perceived consistency, not only at a particular moment, but also over time. One needs to perceive the person he is today as, if not the same person he was yesterday, at least similar to and having links with the person he was yesterday. This does not imply, however, that one attains a stable, fixed identity. Rather, as Bugenthal says, "to be human is . . . to be incomplete, needing; for life to be ever open, uncertain. Only as I allow full awareness of my needs and wants can I approach real wholeness."[11:276]

Identity combines many conscious and unconscious elements. It connotes autonomy as a person, based on understanding of, and confidence in, self. In this sense autonomy arises from feelings of self-respect, competency, and mastery over one's destiny. Autonomy implies self-government and self-acceptance with a tendency toward self-assertion and self-expansion. Identity also includes a person's body image, his own perceptions of his role performance, and the definitions of self contained in these roles.

■ **DEVELOPMENTAL INFLUENCES.** The concept of ego identity was developed by Erikson[17] and built within his formulation of the eight stages of development in the human life cycle. For each stage, Erikson describes a "psychosocial crisis" that must be resolved for further growth and personality development. It is in adolescence that the crisis of "identity versus identity diffusion" occurs. The process of identity formation, however, does not begin in adolescence. Rather, the groundwork is laid in infancy and evolves through the steps of introjection and identification. Introjection, or incorporation, depends on a mutually satisfying relationship between the infant and the mothering one. The safety of this relationship allows the child to reach out for his first "love objects." Through the process of identification the child further broadens and expands his sense of self as he identifies with parents, peers, teachers, and folk heroes. But identity is more than the process of successive identifications. It is, rather, the capacity to synthesize successive identifications into a coherent, consistent, and unique whole.

Identity formation begins where the usefulness of identification ends and is the major task of the adolescent period. At no other phase of the life cycle are the promise of finding oneself and the threat of losing oneself so closely aligned. The adolescent's task is one of self-definition as he strives to integrate significant identifications and previous roles into a unique and reasonably consistent sense of self. Just as the process of identity formation did not begin in adolescence, neither does it end there. It is an evolving configuration, and the circumstances in later periods of life greatly influence one's sense of identity.

An important aspect in achieving identity is the issue of one's sexuality. Sexual identity is the image one has of oneself as a male or a female and convictions about what membership in that group implies. "What does it feel like to be a girl?" "Do I like being a boy?" The answers to these questions are built up gradually from infancy as the result of learned conceptions about males and females. Society's ideals of masculinity and femininity provide important standards for judging oneself as good, bad, inferior, superior, desirable, or undesirable. These ideals are passed down from generation to generation and become an important part of the culture that transmits expectations to males and females. If males in a society are defined as superior, this idea becomes part of the self-image of both males and females. If passivity and obedience are feminine ideals in a society, most little girls will be taught and expected to be unassertive and obedient.

It is recognized that men and women differ from each other anatomically, hormonally, and genetically. Anatomical differences involving strength, ratio of muscle to fat, and reproductive organs are obvious. Hormone and chromosome differences between the sexes are less obvious. The question of the relationship of these differences to personality, sexual behavior, and conceptions of masculinity and femininity is controversial and still open for question. How much weight do chromosomal and hormonal factors have versus environment and learning? One psychologist, John Money,[38] who has done extensive research into sexual behavior, has concluded that sexual identity and sex-typed behavior are established primarily by learning experiences in the first 3 years of life. This area merits further research, which will hopefully yield greater freedom and experimentation in the expression of sexuality in society. This is an important element of the personality because the security of one's sexual identity is a cardinal factor in the achievement of a stable ego identity.

In addition, much of one's identity is expressed in relationships with others. How a person relates to other people is a central personality characteristic. This presents a paradox in that everyone is a part of humanity and yet each person is also separate from all others, and the achievement of identity is both the precursor to and partial prerequisite for the establishment of an intimate interpersonal relationship. Research has shown that only after a stable sense of identity has been established can one engage in genuinely intimate, mature, and successful relationships.[40]

Meier identified the following six attributes of ego identity, which can serve to summarize this discussion:

1. The individual recognizes himself as an intact body organism, separate from other organisms.

2. The individual acknowledges his sexuality.
3. The individual regards the various aspects of himself, such as roles, values, and actions, as compatible.
4. The individual's regard for himself is congruent with the way in which he is regarded by society.
5. The individual is aware of the relationships between past, present, and future.
6. The individual has goals of value that can be realized.[36:65]

Meier notes that not all these attributes are of equal importance nor are they always present to the same degree. Rather, the individual's quest for identity is an evolving one, whereby new elements of identity are in the process of being added or changed as one attempts to answer the question "Who am I?"

■ **The healthy personality**

It is possible to describe the healthy personality according to developmental theory and the dynamics of the self. This description may help to give perspective to the many aspects of the self previously discussed. An individual with a healthy personality would experience the following:

1. **A positive and accurate body image.** Body image is the sum of the conscious and unconscious attitudes the individual has toward his body. It includes present and past perceptions, as well as his feelings about size, function, appearance, and potential. A healthy body awareness would be based on self-observation and appropriate concern for one's physical well-being.
2. **A realistic self-ideal.** Self-ideal is the individual's perception of how he should behave or the standard by which he appraises his behavior. An individual with a realistic self-ideal would have attainable life goals that are valuable and worth striving for.
3. **A positive self-concept.** Self-concept consists of all the aspects of the individual of which he is aware. It includes all of his self-perceptions, which direct and influence his behavior. A positive self-concept implies that the individual expects to be successful in life. It includes the acceptance of the negative aspects of the self as part of the individual's personality. Such a person believes he can master his environment. He does not fear rejection but feels secure and accepted. He faces life openly and realistically and affirms his own existence.
4. **A high self-esteem.** Self-esteem is the individual's personal judgment of his own worth, obtained by analyzing how well he matches up to his own standards and how well his performance compares with others. It is evolved through the comparison of the individual's self-ideal and self-concept. A person with high self-esteem views himself as someone worthy of respect and dignity. He believes in his own self-worth, and he approaches life with aggressiveness and zest. The individual with a healthy personality is one who sees himself to be very much like the person he would like to be.
5. **Satisfying role performance.** The individual with a healthy personality has the ability to relate to others intimately and receives gratification from enacting various social and personal roles. Through open and honest communication he can trust others and enters into mutual and interdependent relationships. His capacity for sharing enables him to enter into a relationship with another person and experience love, freedom, interdependence, and high role adequacy.
6. **A clear sense of identity.** Identity is the integration of inner and outer demands in the individual's discovery of who he is and what he can become. It is the realization of personal consistency. The individual with a clear sense of identity experiences a unity of personality and perceives himself to be a unique individual. His "sense of self" gives his life direction and purpose.

An individual with these qualities is able to perceive himself and his world accurately. His insight into himself creates a feeling of harmony and inner peace.

 # Assessment

■ **Predisposing factors**

■ **AFFECTING SELF-ESTEEM.** Problems with self-concept can be contributed to by predisposing factors that originate in early childhood experiences. Because the infant initially views himself as an extension of his parent, he is very responsive to both his parents' own self-hate and any perceived feelings of hatred toward himself. Parental rejection is an important factor in that it causes the child to be uncertain of himself and other human relationships. As a result of his failure to be loved, the child fails to love himself and is unable to reach out with love to others.

As he grows older, the child may experience lack of recognition and appreciation by parents and significant others as an intrinsically valuable and important individual. He may learn to feel inadequate because he is not encouraged and motivated to be independent, to think for himself, and to take responsibility for his own needs and actions. Overpossessiveness, overpermissiveness, or overcontrol, exercised by one or both parents, can nurture a feeling of unimportance and lack of esteem in the child. Harsh and demanding parents can set unreasonable standards, often raising them before the child has developed the ability to meet them. Parents may also subject their children to unreasonable harsh criticism and inconsistent punishment. These actions can cause early frustration, defeatism, and a destructive sense of inadequacy and inferiority. Another factor in creating such feelings may be the rivalry or unsuccessful emulation of an extremely bright sibling or of a prominent parent, which can often generate a sense of hopelessness and inferiority. In addition, repeated defeats and failures can also destroy one's sense of self-worth. In such an instance the failure, in itself, does not produce a sense of helplessness but the internalization of the failure as proof of personal incompetency does.

Unrealistic self-ideals. With age, additional factors emerge that can both cause and perpetuate feelings of low self-esteem. The individual who lacks a sense of meaning and purpose in life also fails to accept responsibility for his own well-being. He becomes dependent on others and self-indulgent and fails to develop his inherent capabilities and innate potential. He denies himself the freedom to full expression, including the right to make mistakes and fail, and becomes impatient, harsh, and demanding with himself. He sets standards that cannot be met. Examinations are constructed that cannot be passed. Self-consciousness and observation then turn to self-contempt and an underlying sense of self-defeat. This results in a further loss of self-trust.

These self-ideals or goals are often silent assumptions and the person may not be immediately aware of them. They reflect high expectations for oneself and are unrealistic in relation to one's proved capacities. When the individual judges his performance by these unreasonable and inflexible standards, he cannot live up to his ideals and, as a result, experiences feelings of guilt and low self-esteem. Horney[24] has described these inner dictates as the "tyranny of the shoulds" and has identified some of the common ones:

1. I should be the utmost of generosity, considerateness, dignity, courage, unselfishness.
2. I should be the perfect lover, friend, parent, teacher, student, spouse. Everyone should love me.
3. I should be able to endure any hardship with equanimity.
4. I should be able to find a quick solution to every problem.
5. I should never feel hurt; I should always be happy and serene.
6. I should know, understand, and foresee everything. I should be competent in all ways.
7. I should always be spontaneous; I should always control my feelings.
8. I should assert myself; I should never hurt anybody else.
9. I should never be tired or get sick.
10. I should always be at peak efficiency. I should not make mistakes.

The person who overemphasizes these rules or ideals often makes the following series of deductions: "Everyone should love me . . . If he doesn't love me, I have failed . . . I have lost the only thing that really matters . . . I am unlovable . . . There is no point in going on . . . I am worthless." This inner punishment results in feelings of depression and despair because the demands on self are those no human being could fulfill, and they reflect a disloyalty to what one can feel or do as he is at present. Obviously, slavishly striving for these ideals frequently interferes with other activities, such as living a reasonably healthy, tranquil life and having satisfying relationships with other people. These predisposing factors lay the groundwork for potential feelings of low self-esteem.

■ AFFECTING ROLE PERFORMANCE

Sex roles. A particularly relevant source of potential role strain in contemporary American society is derived from the values, beliefs, and behaviors related to sex roles. The differences between male and female body structures have given rise to a number of theories or propositions. Freud gave a great deal of weight to biological factors in the determination of both male and female sexuality. Erikson supported his belief that anatomy predestined the individual to certain types of behavior. These psychoanalytical views have come under attack in recent years for their theories of femininity and masculinity, and for the effects these theories are believed to have had on sexuality and role behavior. They largely ignore the influence of culture and learning on one's self-perceptions.

Despite this, research demonstrates the continued existence of clearly defined sex-role stereotypes for men and women. Broverman's work[10] indicates that women are perceived as relatively less competent, less independent, less objective, and less logical than men. Men are perceived as lacking interpersonal sensitivity, warmth, and expressiveness in comparison to women. Moreover, stereotyped masculine traits are more often perceived to be desirable than stereotyped feminine characteristics.

To the extent that these results reflect societal standards of sex-role behavior, both women and men are put in role conflict by the difference in the standards. If a woman adopts the behaviors specified as desirable for a man, she risks censure for her failure to be appropriately feminine; if she adopts the behaviors designated as feminine, she is deficient in the valued behaviors associated with masculinity. So, too, if a man adopts the behaviors specified as desirable for a woman, his masculinity and sexuality may be questioned and his contributions may be devalued or ignored; if he adopts the behaviors associated with masculinity, he risks alienating attributes of his personality associated with warmth, tenderness, and responsiveness. Thus when a woman steps out of her home, where her sex role has traditionally been defined and confined, and enters the world of work, she may expect to experience heightened role strain. Similarly, the man who arrives home from work in the evening may feel uncertain or conflicted about how he should relate to his school-age son, infant daughter, or working wife.

Most important, both men and women incorporate both the positive and negative traits of the appropriate stereotype into their self-concepts. Since more feminine traits are negatively valued than are masculine traits, women tend to have more negative self-concepts than do men. Women also have higher rates of mental illness than men and are more likely to become depressed. Grove and Tudor[21] suggest a number of possible reasons for this:

1. Many women are restricted to a single, major social role as housewife, whereas most men have two roles—household and work—and therefore two sources of gratification.
2. Some women find their role expectations regarding raising children and keeping house to be limiting and frustrating and wish to work but are unable to, whereas other women are forced to work for financial reasons at jobs that are not gratifying and would rather remain at home caring for their house and children. In either situation, one's role preferences are not being met.
3. The housewife role is unstructured and invisible and often perceived to be of low status, particularly with the current value and status placed on "career women."
4. Even when a married woman works, she is often in a less satisfying position than a man because of discrimination and limited opportunity.
5. Expectations confronting women are unclear and diffuse and may result in an unclear female identity.

Role conflict and role ambiguity therefore arise from the biological factors and social expectations set for men and women. Role overload can also occur for the woman who has numerous, often conflicting, roles imposed on her. The existence of a women's movement in many countries of the world can be viewed as an attempt by women to examine their own identities and determine appropriate role behavior. According to a Labor Department survey, "The old-fashioned 'typical American family' with a breadwinner husband, a homemaker wife, and two children, now makes up only 7 percent of the nation's families."[7] Thus the interaction of marriage, parenting, and employment emerges as a likely source of role strain for women.

Work roles. Work does not imply, however, a singular social role. It is possible to distinguish between women who perceive their employment as careers and those who view their work as a job. Women are still in the minority of most high-status occupations. Only 9.2% of physicians, 4.7% of lawyers, 1.6% of engineers, and 28.7% of college and university teachers were women according to the 1970 census. Most of the women in these fields, moreover, are clustered near the bottom in terms of professional status and financial reward. Holahan and Gilbert[23] conducted a study that compared role conflict experienced by career and noncareer (job) women in relationship to the roles of worker, spouse, parent, and self as a self-actualizing person. Greater role conflict was reported by the job versus career group, particularly involving the parent versus self and spouse versus self roles. The career group reported receiving significantly more life satisfaction from both work and self roles than the job group.

This and other studies suggest that work which is viewed as desirable, valuable, and adequately compensated for by the woman can bring greater life satisfaction. Hunt has listed the needs of women that may be met by work as those for "money, identity, achievement, status, personal pride, inner joy, and for many a woman, whether she realizes it or not, a means of achieving a lasting peace rather than a cease-fire within marriage."[41] Furthermore, a large scale study conducted by the Department of Health, Education, and Welfare found housewives had higher symptom rates then employed women, and professionally employed women had lower symptom rates than those in other occupational categories.

The problem appears to be the lack of support received by women who are performing multiple roles. This lack of support is reflected in amount of payment received, willingness by other family members to share family tasks, and encouragement for the woman pursuing her own life goals. At present, in American society, women are being socialized to seek an ideal that includes marriage, children, higher education, and satisfying work outside the home, and they are increasingly being expected to perform in both the "feminine" and "masculine" spheres.

This potentially has both positive and negative aspects. First, it can be argued that it merely replaces the traditional woman's role with another equally confining one. By valuing the new role, the traditional role of wife and mother assumed by women becomes devalued. Second, although women are expected to assume more "masculine" qualities, a corresponding trend for men to assume more "feminine" role behaviors is not obvious. Third, the woman who wishes to seek such an expanded role is faced with the task of reconciling the often conflicting goals of work, marriage, homemaking, and parenting. Yet there is little organized support by society to aid the woman, and thus her task can be formidable or overwhelming.

Despite social and economic changes, there is often little sharing of tasks when men and women are both gainfully employed. Rather, most industrial societies have witnessed a gradual change in the obligations of women, who now perform a double, or "dual," role—outside employment and continued responsibility for home and children. The expectation exists that the woman will make the adjustments needed both at home and in her career, including housekeeping and managing; arranging meals, lessons, and appointments; entertaining; caring for the sick; and communicating with the family. There is also the traditional expectation that the wife will be the primary caretaker of the child and will subsume other activities to this end. Johnson and Johnson[26] report that the wives and mothers of dual-career families with young children experience difficulties with the growing of role demands in both home and job situations. The greatest strain was in the maternal role, where guilt and anxiety predominated.

Although it may appear that attitudes toward sex roles are changing, the division of household labor within the family is not. In Berk's study[5] wives reported that they did 86% of the kitchen cleaning, 92% of the laundry tasks, 88% of the meal preparation, 89% of the straightening tasks, 74% of the outside errands, and 76% of "other" household tasks. Even in the stereotypically husbandly duties of taking out the garbage and paying the bills were generally done by wives (60% and 62%, respectively). Furthermore, married women employed outside the home were not found to do a significantly smaller proportion of household work. Neither did the presence of preschool children affect the division of labor. They conclude that women with small children at home just work harder.

Given these factors, it is understandable that Weissman[46] found that the search for work by the young educated housewife is associated with a moderate degree of stress and mild depressive symptoms. On the one hand they wanted to find self-expression through work outside the home, and, on the other hand, they held traditional values about marriage and children; thus career adaptations had to be made to fit personal and family needs. One attempted solution to this role strain is for the woman to try to become "superwoman" and do everything well. Not only is this virtually impossible, but the attempt is exhausting and self-defeating.

Bailyn[4] compares this situation to that of a man. He too is faced with different values in his work and family, and some degree of conflict along the same lines also exists for him. His situation is eased, however, by the existence in his environment of a hierarchy of values that precludes the necessity of conscious decision. Unless family needs reach crisis proportions, the demands of his work come first. Very little is written about paternal role strain, accommodation, or the career and homemaking changes made by men in a dual career family. Comparatively, the role set of women appears far more complex, and, in light of these findings, the increased susceptibility of women to the stress of role strain seems hardly surprising at all.

One might conclude, therefore, that sex and work roles will continue to be a source of role strain until care of one's children, home, and career are viewed as equally valuable and important by both sexes and until gender is regarded as irrelevant to the abilities, personalities, and activities of the individuals involved. Such a change in attitude should begin with nurses and other mental health clinicians who, by accepting the stereotyped views of society, indirectly serve to increase role strain. Broverman's research[9] shows that clinicians have different concepts of health for men and women and that these differences parallel the sex-role stereotypes prevalent in our society. The cause of mental health may be better served if both men and women were encouraged by psychiatric clinicians toward maximum realization of individual potential, rather than to an adjustment to existing restrictive sex roles.

■ **AFFECTING PERSONAL IDENTITY.** Constant parental intervention interferes with adolescent choices. In our culture this is related to the fact that there is no cutoff point and no fixed limit to parental intervention. Parental distrust leads a child to wonder whether his own choices are correct and to feel guilty if he goes against parental ideas. Parental distrust implies belittlement of the child because it devalues the child's opinions, and belittlement leads inevitably to indecisiveness, feelings of nothingness, exasperated impulsiveness, and acting out in an attempt to achieve some identity. When the parent does not trust the child, the child ultimately loses respect for the parent. It has been found that parents and children do not disagree on significant issues, such as war, peace, race, or religion. Instead, personal and narrow concerns—fads, dating, a party, the car, curfews, doing homework—create the conflict between parents and youth. Here parental intervention interferes with option choices and identity.

Peers also add to the problems of identity. The adolescent wants to belong, to feel needed and wanted. The peer group, with its rigid standards of behavior, gives him this feeling. It provides a bridge between childhood and adulthood. The adolescent loses himself in the fads and the language of the group. However, because all the members of the peer group are searching to define their identity and are beset by the pressures and frustrations of a complex society, the peer group is often a cruel testing ground that hurts as much as it helps. Taught to be competitive, the young person competes with his friends, "putting them down" to bring himself up. Membership in the peer group is bought at a high price; the adolescent must surrender much of his identity to get in. Often there is open destruction of self-esteem and ferocious insistence on conformity. In sexual relationships, adolescents introduce further uncertainty into their lives, which can interfere with the development of a stable self-concept.

■ **Precipitating stressors**

Specific problems are initiated or precipitated by almost any difficult or stressful situation for which the person does not have the capacity to adjust. During his lifetime, the individual is faced with numerous role transitions or changes in role relationships, expectations, or abilities. These role transitions may require the person to incorporate new knowledge and alter his behavior. Meleis[37] has identified three categories of role transitions: (1) developmental, (2) situational, and (3) health-illness. Developmental transitions are normative changes associated with growth. Situational transitions involve the addition or subtraction of significant others, which may occur through birth or death. An example of this transition is the change from nonparental to parental status. Health-illness transitions result from moving from a well state to an illness state. Each of these role transitions can precipitate a threat to the individual's self-concept.

■ **ROLE STRAIN.** People who experience stress associated with expected roles or positions are said to experience role strain.[20] Role strain is experienced as frustration, since the person may feel torn in opposite directions or feel inadequate or unsuited to performing

certain roles. Over time, role strain places a considerable burden on the person, and the individual will tend to act to alleviate role strain and heighten the gratification of high role adequacy. Role strain, as a general term, incorporates the concepts of role conflict, role ambiguity, and role overload.[6]

Role conflict is said to occur when a person is subjected to two or more contradictory expectations that the person cannot simultaneously meet in behavior. Conflict can arise because two internal needs, drives, or motives are incompatible, or because an internal need, drive, or motive opposes an external demand. For example, role conflict can occur because there are cultural expectations that certain attributes go with certain roles. In this case the role conflict is caused by the incongruency between the individual's and society's expectations for specific role behavior. This is evident in a society's sex-role stereotyping and may be experienced by the woman who enters a traditionally male occupation or vice versa. Another source of conflict is different perceptions of appropriate role-related behavior among individuals. An example of this is evident in family roles. Each adult brings to a marriage a set of perceived family roles that have been greatly influenced by their own upbringing. Often the individuals' perceptions may be contradictory and pose problems within the marriage.

Role ambiguity appears when shared specifications set for an expected role are incomplete or insufficient to tell the involved individual what is desired or how to do it. This lack of knowledge of specific role expectations and confusion regarding appropriate role behavior can be very stressful for the individual. This is particularly evident among adolescents, since society's demands have become stronger, more diversified, and more immediate and often produce feelings of confusion, frustration, alienation, and violence. Adolescents are pressured to play different roles by their parents, the mass media, and their peers. They are expected to "earn their own keep," yet are unable to find jobs in times of high unemployment and economic inflation. They are confused by the discrepancy they see between the reality of the practiced morality of society and the morality they learned as a child and accepted as reality. Some young people turn to violence as a way of asserting themselves, whereas others become apathetic and alienated in response to their perceived role ambiguity.

A final type of role strain is **role overload**, which occurs when a person is faced with a role set that is too complex. The person lacks the adequate or appropriate resources that may be physical, intellectual, emotional, or economic for performing the necessary role requirements. Each of the roles undertaken by the individual may be making legitimate discreet demands, but together the expectations are overwhelming and perhaps impossible to carry out. An example of this is the numerous roles of the contemporary woman—wife, cook, mother, employee, chauffeur, maid, lover, etc.

■ **DEVELOPMENTAL TRANSITIONS.** Various developmental stages can precipitate threats to one's identity. Adolescence is perhaps the most critical, since it is a time of upheaval, change, anxiety, and insecurity. Adolescents are modifying their concepts of self, and they are more analytical about not only themselves but also the world in general. Adolescents are faced with many important decisions. They have to make an occupational choice and decide if they are good enough to succeed in a given career. They must determine if they have the ability to participate in various social activities. Are they attractive enough heterosexually to interest and succeed with a member of the opposite sex? Will they succeed in marriage? Do they have the courage to carry out their convictions as an individual apart from the crowd while remaining a member of the crowd? Are they a leader, follower, or coward? Are they satisfied with their roles and can they implement them comfortably?

An adult's problems of identity are simpler than those of an adolescent. Maturity stabilizes self-concept and provides a firmer picture of self. A serious threat to identity in adulthood is cultural discontinuity. This occurs when a person moves from one type of cultural setting to another and experiences the emotional upheaval that accompanies the change to a new cultural milieu. When faced with differing cultural standards, many people have difficulty maintaining their self-system. In addition, problems within the social structure, such as political upheavals, economic depression, and high unemployment, can pose threats to the identity of individuals.

Cultural stressors confront a person in challenging personal values: conforming versus individuality, cowardice versus bravery, winning versus losing, career versus marriage, equality versus superiority, cooperation versus competition, dependence versus independence, intelligence versus feeling. Although these values are not necessarily opposite nor mutually exclusive, they raise fundamental questions that the individual must resolve and integrate into his personality structure. One's sexual identity can also be influenced by cultural pressures, which can control both the way in which one expresses sexuality and the way in which it is a part of one's self-system. Definitions of acceptable approaches to both sexes, the values placed on virility, the necessity for procreation as proof of virility, the definitions of suitable sex partners, and the values concerning marital fidelity may all be culturally determined.

In late maturity and in old age, identity problems again arise. New problems and roles result from the process of aging and from the view of the elderly held by the more youthful members of society. Menopause, retirement, and increasing physical disability are problems for which the aging person, as he enters his declining years, must work out adaptive coping behavior.

■ **HEALTH-ILLNESS TRANSITIONS.** There are some specific stressors that can cause disturbances in body image and related changes in self-concept. One threat is the loss of a major body part, such as an eye, breast, or leg. Disturbances also may occur following a surgical procedure in which the relationship of body parts is disturbed. The results of the surgical intervention may be either visible, as with a colostomy or gastrotomy, or invisible, as with a hysterectomy or gallbladder removal. Changes in body size, shape, and appearance can threaten one's self-perceptions. These changes can be the result of a rapid weight gain or loss, a skin infection, or even plastic surgery. Threats to body image can occur because of a pathological process that causes changes in the structure or function of one's body, such as arthritis, multiple sclerosis, Parkinson's disease, cancer, pneumonia, and heart disease. The failure of a body part to function, as experienced by the paraplegic or the patient recovering from a stroke, is particularly difficult to integrate into one's self-perceptions. The physical changes associated with normal growth and development may pose problems for the individual, as might some potentially threatening medical or nursing procedures, such as enemas, catheterizations, suctioning, radiation therapy, dilation and curettage, and organ transplantation.

All of these stressors can pose a threat to one's body image with resultant changes in levels of self-esteem and role perception. In fact, any threat to body integrity is interpreted as a threat to self and increases one's anxiety level. How the individual perceives the seriousness of the threat determines the type of coping mechanism called into play. Factors that influence the degree of threat to one's body image have been identified by Norris[39]:

1. The meaning of the stressor for the individual. Does it threaten his ideal of youth and wholeness and act to decrease his self-esteem?
2. The degree to which his pattern of adaptation is interrupted. Does it jeopardize his security and self-control?
3. The coping capacities and resources available to him. What response is elicited from significant others, and what help is offered him?
4. The nature of the threat, extent of change, and

rate at which it occurs. Is the change one of many small adjustments over time or a great and sudden readjustment?

Finally, there may also be physiological stressors that disturb one's sense of reality, interfere with an accurate perception of the world, and threaten the maintenance of one's ego boundaries and identity. Such stressors include oxygen deprivation, hyperventilation, biochemical imbalances, severe fatigue, and sensory and emotional isolation. Alcohol, drugs, and other toxic substances may also produce self-concept distortions. Usually these stressors produce only temporary changes within the individual.

Whether the problem in self-concept is precipitated by psychological, sociological, or physiological stressors, the critical element is the patient's perception of the threat. As the nurse assesses pertinent behaviors and formulates a nursing diagnosis, she must continue to validate her observations and inferences to establish a mutual and therapeutic relationship with the patient.

■ Behaviors

Assessing the various components of a patient's self-concept will present a challenge to the nurse. Because self-concept is the cornerstone of the personality, it is intimately related to states of anxiety and depression, problems in interpersonal relationships, and acting out and self-destructive behavior. All behavior is motivated by a desire to enhance, maintain, or defend the self; so the nurse will have a wealth of information to evaluate. There is a need, however, for the nurse to delve beyond the objective and observable behaviors to the subjective and internal world of the patient. Only when the nurse explores this realm will the patient's actions be given meaning.

The nurse can begin the assessment by observing the patient's appearance. The person's posture, cleanliness, makeup, and clothing all provide data. She might discuss his appearance with him to determine his values and ideals related to his body image. Observing or inquiring about his eating, sleeping, and hygiene patterns gives clues to his biological gratifications and tendencies toward self-preservation. These initial observations should lead the nurse to ask, "What does my patient think about himself as a person?" She might ask him to describe himself or how he feels about himself. What strengths does he think he has? What does he see as his areas of weakness? What is his self-ideal? Does he conform to it? Does fulfillment of his self-ideal bring him satisfaction? Does he value his strengths? Does he view his weaknesses as important personality deficits or are they relatively unimportant to his self-concept? What

are his priorities? Is he a participant in life or an observer? Does he feel unified and self-directed or diffuse and other directed?

The nurse can then compare the patient's responses to his behavior, looking for inconsistencies or contradictions. How does he relate to other people? How does he respond to compliments and criticisms? She can also examine her affective response to the patient. Is it one of hopelessness, despair, anger, or anxiety? The nurse's own response to the patient is often a good indication of the quality and depth of the patient's pain.

■ **ASSOCIATED WITH LOW SELF-ESTEEM.** Low self-esteem is a major problem for many people, and it can be expressed in moderate and severe levels of anxiety. It involves negative self-evaluations and is associated with feelings of being weak, helpless, hopeless, frightened, vulnerable, fragile, incomplete, worthless, and inadequate. Low self-esteem is a major component of depression, which acts as a kind of punishment and anesthesia for the individual. Low self-esteem indicates self-rejection and self-hate, which may be a conscious or unconscious process and may be expressed in direct or indirect ways.

Direct expressions of self-hate or low self-esteem may include any of the following behaviors:

1. **Self-derision and criticism.** The patient has a negative cognitive set and believes he is doomed to failure. Although the expressed purpose of the criticism may be self-improvement, there is no constructive value to it and the underlying goal is to demoralize oneself. This occurs when the individual places himself in a situation he cannot handle and then subjects himself to ridicule. He might describe himself as "stupid," "no good," or a "born loser." He views the normal stressors of life as impossible barriers and becomes preoccupied with self-pity.

2. **Self-diminution.** The minimizing of one's ability, which is accomplished by avoiding, neglecting, or refusing to recognize one's real assets and strengths.

3. **Guilt and worrying.** A destructive activity by which the individual terrorizes and punishes himself. It may be expressed through nightmares, phobias, obsessions, or the reliving of painful memories and indiscretions. It indicates self-rejection.

4. **Physical manifestations.** These might include hypertension, psychosomatic illnesses, and the abuse of various substances, such as alcohol, drugs, tobacco, or food.

5. **Postponing decisions.** A high level of ambivalence or procrastination produces an increased sense of insecurity.

6. **Denying oneself pleasure.** The self-rejecting person feels the need to punish himself and expresses this through denying himself the things he finds desirable or pleasurable. This might be a career opportunity, a material object, or a desired interpersonal relationship.

7. **Disturbed interpersonal relationships.** The person may be cruel, demeaning, or exploitive with other people. This may be an overt process, or he might develop a passive-dependent pattern of relating, which indirectly exploits others. Another behavior included in this category is withdrawal or social isolation, which arises from his feelings of worthlessness.

8. **Withdrawal from reality.** When the anxiety resulting from self-rejection reaches the severe or panic levels, the individual may dissociate and experience hallucinations, delusions, and feelings of suspicion, jealousy, or paranoia. Such withdrawal from reality may be a temporary coping mechanism or a long-term behavior pattern, indicating a profound problem of identity confusion.

9. **Self-destructiveness.** Self-hatred can be expressed through accident proneness or attempting dangerous feats. Extremely low levels of self-esteem can lead to the ultimate act of rejection, which is suicide.

10. **Other destructiveness.** People who have overwhelming consciences may choose to act out against society. This activity serves to paralyze their own self-hate and displaces or projects it on victims in their environment.

There are also indirect forms of self-hate that complement and supplement the direct forms. They may be chronic patterns for the individual and difficult to change in therapy:

1. **Illusions and unrealistic goals.** Self-deception is the core element; the individual refuses to accept a limited here and now. Illusions increase the possibility of disappointment and further self-hate. The illusions or goals frequently involve money, love, power, prestige, marriage, sex, children, family, success, and parenthood. Examples of illusions are "If I were married, I would be happy" and "Money brings fulfillment." This indirect form of low self-esteem may make the person sensitive to criticism or overresponsive to flattery. It may also be evident in the defensive mechanisms of blaming others for one's failures and becoming hypercritical with others to create the illusion of superiority.

The individual may also attempt to compensate by expressing an exaggerated opinion of his ability. He may continually boast, brag of his prowess and exploits, or claim possession of extraordinary talents. An extreme compensatory behavior for low esteem is grandiose thinking and related delusions.

Yet another example of unrealistic goals is evident in the perfectionist whose standards are high beyond reach or reason. Such individuals strain compulsively and unremittingly toward impossible goals and measure their own worth entirely in terms of productivity and accomplishment. The result of such striving, however, is often vulnerability to emotional turmoil and impaired productivity. This tendency may further serve as a predisposing factor toward the development or recurrence of depressive illnesses.[12]

2. **Boredom.** This involves the rejection of one's possibilities and capabilities. The individual may neglect or reject aspects of himself that have great potential for future growth.

3. **Polarizing view of life.** In this case the individual has a simplistic view of life in which everything is worst or best, wrong or right. He tends to have a closed belief system that acts as a defense against a threatening world. Ultimately this view of life will lead to confusion, disappointment, and alienation from others.

The behaviors associated with low self-esteem are described in Clinical example 14-1 and are summarized in the box on page 411.

In this clinical example, Mrs. G's favorable perception of self was closely related to her ability to work. Her retirement created role changes for her, and she found it difficult to adapt to them. This example points out the close relationship that exists between feelings of low self-esteem and role strain. The situation was further compounded by her husband's retirement. Mrs. G's feelings of low self-esteem were evident in her self-criticism, refusal to recognize her own strengths, worrying, physical complaints, reduced social contacts, and unrealistic expectations of her family. Her diagnosis of major depressive episode was based on the severity of her feelings of self-depreciation, somatic problems, saddened emotional tone, history of losses, and absence of a manic episode.

Low self-esteem is also a major dynamic element occurring with problems of disturbed body image. Clin-

CLINICAL EXAMPLE 14-1

Mrs. G was a 66-year-old woman who was admitted to the psychiatric hospital with the diagnosis of major depressive episode. She told the admitting nurse that "things have been building up for some time now" and she had been seeing a private psychiatrist for the past 6 months who suggested she enter the hospital. Mrs. G slowly recounted an extensive medical history with numerous gastrointestinal problems. These did not, however, significantly interfere with her functioning. She had been employed in a community college as a librarian until 18 months previously when she was forced to retire. Mrs. G said she had been married for 39 years and had two grown children who were married and lived out of state. Her husband worked as an accountant but had retired a month previously. She said that since her retirement she had felt "useless and lost and closed in by their apartment." She seldom left the apartment, however, and had lost contact with many of her friends. She said she worried a great deal about their financial situation, especially now that her husband was also retired. He has repeatedly reassured her that they have sufficient funds, but she cannot stop worrying about it. She said her children called her weekly, but she thought they did this only out of duty and were not "really interested" in her or her husband. She thought that if they did love her and were concerned about her, they would never have moved out of state.

Mrs. G said that she liked her job very much and thought she was good at it. A younger woman took her place at the library, and Mrs. G was very bitter when talking about her. She said that, little by little, this woman took over duties Mrs. G was responsible for and one day even cleaned out Mrs. G's desk and took it as her own. Since her retirement, she said "things have been going downhill steadily." She said she is not a good housewife and she dislikes cooking. These tasks had become even more difficult since her husband retired because he is "always underfoot and criticizing what I do." In the past couple of weeks, she had had great difficulty sleeping, a decreased appetite, fatigue, and little interest in her personal appearance. She said that it seemed to her that all she had to do was to "wait around to die."

CLINICAL EXAMPLE 14-2

Mrs. M was a 29-year-old married woman who was admitted to the general hospital for a total hysterectomy. Her history was presented in a nursing care conference because she was making many demands on the nursing staff and the head nurse noticed that many of the staff were avoiding caring for her. Mrs. M had been married for 2 years and did not have any children. It was observed that Mr. M seldom visited his wife, although the staff noticed that she spoke to him over the phone almost daily. Mrs. M complained that she was unable to sleep at night and often rang for the nurses with apparently minor requests. She appeared to have established a relationship with one of the evening nurses who was able to describe some of Mrs. M's concerns.

Mrs. M appeared to have a severe level of anxiety about her hysterectomy. She feared the effect of the operation on her sexual desires, sexual attractiveness, ability to have intercourse, and ability to respond to her husband. Without her reproductive organs she said she felt "inadequate and no longer like a woman." She said that she and her husband always planned on having children and she wondered if her husband might leave her in the future. She also feared that she would look older and that having the hysterectomy would cause her to lose her beauty and youth.

When the nursing staff became aware of Mrs. M's many fears and concerns, they were better able to understand her behavior and plan appropriate nursing care. They discussed with her the physiological implications of a hysterectomy and encouraged her to openly verbalize her feelings. Mr. M was not aware of his wife's concerns, and the nursing staff supported open discussions between them. As the staff were able to identify Mrs. M's specific concerns, they realized that some of their previous avoidance behavior was due to their own fears and discomfort. The female nurses had identified with her as a patient, and the hysterectomy, in some ways, threatened their own concepts of self, body integrity, and sexual identity.

Behaviors Associated with Low Self-Esteem

Criticism of self and/or others	Physical complaints
Decreased productivity	Polarizing view of life
Destructiveness toward others	Rejection of personal capabilities
Disruptions in relatedness	Self-derision
Exaggerated sense of self-importance	Self-destructiveness
Feelings of inadequacy	Self-diminution
Guilt	Social withdrawal
Irritability or excessive anger	Substance abuse
Negative feelings about one's body	Withdrawal from reality
Perceived role strain	Worrying
Pessimistic view of life	

---

ical example 14-2 illustrates the effect of the loss of a body part on a person's self-concept.

■ **ASSOCIATED WITH IDENTITY DIFFUSION.** The term "identity diffusion" was first used by Erikson to denote the failure, in certain individuals, to integrate various childhood identifications into a harmonious adult psychosocial identity.[16] Individuals with identity diffusion manifest incompatible personality attributes. For example, they can exhibit both marked tenderness and extreme indifference toward others. Other contradictory character traits that coexist include: naivete and suspiciousness, greed and self-denial, and arrogance and timidity.[1]

An important group of behaviors that relate to identity diffusion include disruptions in interpersonal relationships or problems of intimacy. The presenting behavior may be one of withdrawal or distancing. If a person is experiencing an undefined identity, he may wish to ignore or destroy those people who threaten him. The problem is one of gaining intimacy, but it is reflected in the behaviors of isolation, denial, and withdrawal from others. Such patients lack the condition for normal empathy.

A contrasting behavior that may be evident is one of personality fusing. Erikson has pointed out that true intimacy involves a sense of mutuality, which implies a firm self-delineation of the partners and not a diffused merger of two people. If a person is struggling to cope with a weak or undefined identity, however, he may try to establish his sense of self by fusing or belonging to someone else. This may occur in formal relationships, intense friendships, or brief affairs, since each can be seen as a desperate attempt to outline one's own identity. This non-autonomous fusion, however, leads to a further loss of identity. Some of these behaviors will be evident in Clinical example 14-3.

CLINICAL EXAMPLE 14-3

Mrs. P was seen by a psychiatric nurse in the psychiatric outpatient department of a general hospital. She was a well-dressed 24-year-old woman who had numerous somatic complaints, including decreased appetite, frequent headaches, fatigue, and difficulty falling asleep. She reported she had no energy or interest in doing anything or being with people. She said she dreaded each new day and felt abandoned and all alone.

She was married at the age of 17 to the only boy she ever dated in high school. He was 19 at the time and she "looked up to him tremendously." He established a successful career in the insurance business and she stayed at home to care for the house. She described herself as "centering my whole world around him." Three months previously he had told her that he wanted a separation and suggested she begin making a new life for herself. He said he intended to move out of the house at the end of the present month, but Mrs. P said that she hoped he would not do that when he saw how much she loved and needed him.

Mrs. P also described feelings of being unloved and unlovable. She said she "felt empty inside" and "didn't really know who she was." She complained about her appearance and expressed much fear about living alone, finding a job, and getting along with people, especially men.

Many of the behaviors displayed by Mrs. P reflect the problem of *identity diffusion*. She married at an early age before defining her own sense of self as an autonomous individual. Her only experience in a close relationship was with her husband, and she attempted to establish her own identity by living through his. Within the security of the marriage she managed to avoid any self-analysis, but the reality of the impending separation brought forth her fears and self-doubts. She displayed a low level of self-esteem and an unresolved conflict between dependence and independence.

Personality fusion and problems with identity have serious implications also for the larger family system. Dysfunctional families are frequently characterized by a fusion of ego mass that may be evident in severe symptomatology by one or more family members. This may be expressed in some form of family violence or abuse described in Chapter 32 or in the scapegoating of one family member who may become the "diagnosed" or "symptomatic" psychiatric patient as described in Chapter 29.

Identity diffusion can also be expressed as pathological narcissism in which the individual has an exaggerated sense of self-importance manifested as extreme self-absorption. The person has an unrealistic idealized self that is based in illusion rather than reality. He believes he has solved his search for identity, but his idealized notion of self reflects a kind of alienation of his own being. In narcissism, according to Kernberg, "The normal tension between actual and ideal self . . . is eliminated by the building up of an inflated self-concept in which the actual self and ideal self . . . are confused."[29:238] Thus unlike the person with low self-esteem who keenly perceives the discrepancy between his actual self and self-ideal, the narcissist rejects the reality of who he really is by subscribing to an idealized self. His resulting state of identity confusion may be characterized by fantasies of unlimited success, an insatiable need for attention and admiration, exploitative interpersonal relationships, feelings of entitlement, and the lack of empathy for others.

An additional behavior is the lack of temporal continuity in oneself. The past, present, and future are not integrated into a smooth continuum of remembered, felt, and expected existence for these patients. Time is fragmented, and all real experience is confined to the present. This may be manifested as an inability to make goals and to project into the future. Fragmentation is also evident in these patients' lack of authenticity and susceptibility to external influence. These experiences result in a sense of inner aloneness and feelings of emptiness. These should be distinguished from the feeling of loneliness which is alive with fantasies and emotions.

In contrast, emptiness in this sense is a more deeply frightening and dehumanizing experience.

Individuals with identity diffusion display weak gender identity or more apparent gender confusion. They also lack an historical-cultural basis of identity and thus display a peculiar lack of ethnicity. It is evident in their sense of history, cultural norms, group affiliations, object choices, life-style, and child-rearing practices. A related behavior is that of the absence of an inner moral code or of any genuine inner value. These behaviors characteristic of identity diffusion are summarized in the accompanying box.

■ **ASSOCIATED WITH DEPERSONALIZATION.** A more maladaptive response to problems in identity involving withdrawal from reality occurs when the individual experiences panic levels of anxiety. This panic state produces a blocking off of awareness, a collapse in reality testing, and feelings of depersonalization. Depersonalization is a feeling of unreality in which one is unable to distinguish between inner and outer stimuli. It is, in essence, a true alienation from oneself. The individual has great difficulty distinguishing self from others, and one's body has an unreal or strange quality about it. It is the subjective experience of the partial or total disruption of one's ego and the disintegration and disorganization of one's self-concept. Because of this, it is the most frightening of human experiences. It develops as an outcome of uncertainties in human relationships. The individual has a not-loved feeling and, as a result of his failure to be loved, he fails to love himself. Depersonalization serves as a defense, but it is destructive in nature because it masks and immobilizes anxiety without in any way diminishing its intensity. It can occur in a variety of clinical illnesses, including depression, schizophrenia, manic states, and organic brain syndromes, and it represents the advanced state of ego breakdown associated with psychotic states.

There are many behaviors associated with depersonalization. The primary one is that the patient experiences feelings of estrangement as though he were hiding something from himself. He experiences a lack of inner continuity and sameness and feels as if life is happening *to* him rather than his living by his own initiative. The patient may say that the world appears queer, dreamlike, or frightening. He may experience a loss of identity and express confusion regarding his own sexuality. He may describe related feelings of insecurity, inferiority, frustration, fear, hate, shame, and a loss of self-respect and be unable to derive a sense of accomplishment from any activity.

In depersonalization there may be a loss of impulse control and an absence of feeling and emotion that is manifested in impersonality, stiffness, formality, and

---

Behaviors Associated with Identity Diffusion

Absence of moral code
Contradictory personality traits
Exploitative interpersonal relationships
Feelings of emptiness
Fluctuating feelings about self
Gender confusion
High degree of anxiety

Inability to empathize with others
Lack of authenticity
Pathological narcissism
Problems of intimacy
Temporal fragmentation and discontinuity
Unrealistic idealized self

---

rigidness in social situations. The individual may become lifeless and lack spontaneity and animation. He may plod through each day in a state of numbness and may respond to situations ordinarily eliciting emotion without characteristic love, hate, anxiety, or guilt. A heightened sense of isolation may mark his interpersonal relationships. The individual may become increasingly passive, as shown by withdrawing from social contacts, failing to assert himself, losing interest in his surroundings, and allowing others to make decisions for him.

Another sign of depersonalization is a disturbance in the individual's perception of time and space. He may become disoriented with regard to time and be unable to correctly recognize events as pertaining to yesterday or tomorrow or to plan his activities with reference to a time schedule. There may be a disturbance of memory characterized by aphasia, amnesia, or memory distortion. His thinking and judgment may be impaired and reflect great confusion and distortion or focus on trivial details. Problems in information processing can be evident in visual hallucinations, and disturbed interpersonal relationships may be reflected in delusions, auditory hallucinations, and incongruent or idiosyncratic communication.

A final common behavior associated with depersonalization is a confused or disturbed body image. The person may have a feeling of unreality about parts of his body. He may describe the feeling that his limbs are detached, the size of his body parts is changed, or he is unable to tell where his body leaves off and the rest of the world begins. Some patients describe the feeling that they had stepped outside their bodies and were observing themselves as detached and foreign objects. The many behaviors associated with depersonalization are summarized in Table 14-1. Clinical example 14-4 may further help to clarify the problem of depersonalization.

It is obvious from this example and the previous

CLINICAL EXAMPLE 14-4

Mr. S was a 40-year-old man who had no previous history of psychiatric hospitalization. Two months before his present admission, he was severely burned while on the job as an employee of a steelmaking plant. He received second- and third-degree burns over his face, hands, chest, and back, and was treated in the burn center of a large university hospital. Three days before he was to be discharged from the burn unit, he experienced a psychotic episode. He reported hearing voices telling him to kill himself, and he was unable to recall any events surrounding the accident that produced his burns. He said he "felt his arms were withering away and his eyes were falling into his skull." He was unable to change the dressing on his burns even though he had been able to do this previously. When looking at his arms or chest, his face remained impassive and he showed no emotion. He began to talk continuously about returning to work but was unable to identify how long he had been out on sick leave or the amount of time recommended by his doctor for recovery.

With the onset of these symptoms he was transferred from the burn unit to the psychiatric unit of the hospital. He remained socially isolated on the unit and refused to participate in ward meetings and group activities. At times he would wander into other patients' rooms and take pieces of their clothing. He would later be seen wearing this clothing on the unit and the staff would intervene to return it to its owner.

TABLE 14-1

BEHAVIORS ASSOCIATED WITH DEPERSONALIZATION

Affective	Perceptual	Cognitive	Behavioral
Experiences loss of identity	Auditory and visual halluci-	Confusion	Blunting of affect
Feelings of alienation from self	nations	Disoriented to time	Emotional passivity and
Feelings of insecurity, inferiority,	Confusion regarding one's	Distorted thinking	nonresponsiveness
fear, shame	sexuality	Disturbance of memory	Incongruent or idiosyncratic
Feelings of unreality	Difficulty distinguishing self	Impaired judgment	communication
Heightened sense of isolation	from others		Lack of spontaneity and an-
Lack of sense of inner continuity	Disturbed body image		imation
Unable to derive pleasure or a	Experiences the world as		Loss of impulse control
sense of accomplishment	dreamlike		Loss of initiative and deci-
			sion-making ability
			Social withdrawal

discussion that the various feelings and perceptions associated with depersonalization represent extreme defenses against threats to self that do not serve to alleviate the anxiety and, in fact, may add to it by the frightening nature of the experience. The patient views his own behavior as foreign, and he sees himself as a strong, unknown, and unpredictable being whom he does not recognize. As both a participant and a spectator, he observes himself with great fear, since he is unable to control his own impulses. He cannot completely escape the pain of self-awareness. He therefore disowns his behavior, feelings, thoughts, and body and becomes alienated from his true self and personal identity.

■ Coping mechanisms

Erikson identified the normative crisis of **identity confusion** as a normal phase of increased conflict occurring during adolescence that is characterized by a high growth potential.[16,17] The transitory stage of acute identity confusion poses the possible failure to achieve integration and continuity of one's self-images. Adolescents may appear excessively self-conscious because of their extreme self-doubt. They may also display a diffused time perspective, which consists of a sense of great urgency and yet also of a loss of consideration for time as a dimension of living. They may feel very young and very old simultaneously and ambivalently hope and fear that change will come with time. These contradictory feelings may be displayed in a general slowing of activities, which reflects an underlying sense of despair. A diffused sense of industry is also often present, which is evident in inability to concentrate on the work they

are supposed to be doing. This may be accompanied by a distaste for competition. Although they may be intelligent and previously successful in office work, schoolwork, and sports, adolescents may lose the capacity for work, exercise, and sociability.

■ **SHORT-TERM DEFENSES.** The identity crisis of adolescence is a transitory one and may be resolved in a number of ways. It is possible to view these resolutions as either short-term or long-term ego-oriented coping mechanisms to ward off the anxiety and uncertainty of identity confusion. Logan[33] has described the following four broad categories of short-term defenses:

- Activities that provide temporary escape from the identity crisis
- Activities that provide temporary substitute identities
- Activities that serve temporarily to strengthen or heighten a diffuse sense of self
- Activities that represent short-term attempts to make an identity out of the fact of meaningless and identity diffusion itself—that try to assert that the meaning of life is meaningless itself

The first category of temporary escape includes any of a number of activities that seem to provide intense immediate experiences, experiences which so overwhelm the senses that when one is involved in them, the issue of identity literally does not exist because one's entire being is taken up with "right now" sensations. Examples of this might include drug experiences, loud rock concerts, fast car and motorcycle riding, some forms of hard physical labor, exercise, or sports, and even obsessive television watching.

The category of temporary substitute identity is derived from being a "joiner"; the identity of a club, group, team, movement, or gang may function as one's basis for self-definition. The individual temporarily adopts the group definition as his own identity, in a kind of totalistic devotion to the larger entity. The adolescent's need to join and "belong" makes him particularly vulnerable to being manipulated by various religious groups and political sects. Being a devoted "follower" and imitator of an idolized figure, such as a guru, rock star, sect leader, or life-style rebel, can also provide a temporary substitute identity for those who may not actually "join" a group. Temporary substitute identities can also be obtained by playing a certain role within a group, such as clown, bully, or chauffeur, or by purchasing objects that are marketed with ready-made identities. Thus a certain type of cologne, make of car, or article of dress imply built-in personalities that the person can adopt as his own.

The third category of defenses involves the idea of "putting oneself up against something" to feel more intensely alive. This is evident in risk taking for its own sake, which creates a feeling of heroic bravado and notoriety. Engaging in competitive activities, such as sports, academic achievement, and popularity contests can also fit into this category. The idea here is that competition and comparison with an outsider more sharply define one's own sense of self. Another example of this is the use of bigotry and prejudice. By adopting a bigoted stance toward some outgroup or scapegoat one can temporarily strengthen one's own sense of esteem or ego integrity. Superpatriots, youth gangs, and cliques are all examples of this temporary defense.

The final category helps to explain the fads adolescents indulge in with such fervor and that seem so meaningless to others. It is suggested that the sheer force of commitment to the fads is an attempt to transform them into something meaningful. It is obvious, however, that all of these categories of short-term coping mechanisms do overlap and can be used to compound the overall effect. Logan emphasizes this point in analyzing the problem of drug abuse and the powerful hold it has on some adolescents:

One may take drugs for the intense, immediate experience and the escape from worldly concerns into heightened sensations that they provide. The very acts of procuring, smuggling, selling, and taking drugs provide challenging risks of harm, arrest, and illness that may make one feel more daringly and rebelliously alive. The taking of drugs may also be the initiation ceremony for "joining," and the badge of membership for belonging to the group and life-style from which one derives a temporary identity. A sense of identity may also be derived from the role of freak, head, or pusher that one plays within the drug culture. The drug culture may also be a vehicle for bigotry and prejudice—the contemptuous "put-down" of the "straight" world for its narrow-minded rejection of drugs helping to boost the self-esteem of drug users. One might speculate that a kind of identity might be derived from the kind of "stuff" one habitually purchases and uses. Finally, one even might argue that drugs may be taken because of the faddish meaninglessness of the act—as a kind of final affirmation and flinging in the face of society that, yes, life is meaningless, so meaningless, in fact, that the drug-taker makes a career of meaninglessness.[33:506-507]

■ **LONG-TERM DEFENSES.** Any of these short-term defenses may develop into a long-term one that will be evident in maladaptive behavior. Other resolutions or long-term defenses are also possible for the adolescent. A positive resolution or adaptive response is one that produces an integrated ego identity and unified self, as has previously been described. Another type of long-term resolution has been identified as that of **identity foreclosure**.[34] This occurs when a young person adopts "ready made" the kind of identity desired by his elders without really coming to terms with his own desires, aspirations, or potential. This is a less desirable long-term resolution as is that of adopting a deviant, or negative identity.

A **negative identity** is one that is at odds with the values and expectations of society. This choice of delinquent roles may be caused by pressing demands made on the adolescent by parents or significant others to adopt a particular self-definition. The individual may think his autonomy is in jeopardy or he may not value social norms. He then attempts to define the self in a nonprescribed or antisocial manner. The choice of a negative identity represents an attempt to retain some mastery in a situation in which a positive identity does not seem possible or desirable. It is like saying, "I would rather be somebody bad than nobody at all." Clinical example 14-5 describes the negative identity assumed by an adolescent with a medical diagnosis of conduct disorder—undersocialized, aggressive.

Ken displays many of the behaviors characteristic of a negative identity. His actions seem to challenge the accepted activities of youth. The nurse working with Ken explored with him his underlying feelings and self-perceptions. Great anger with his father began to surface and Ken was able to verbalize about it. Because he was the only son, he felt like he was competing with his father and had to live up to his father's ideals. Ken feared failing in trying to adopt a positive identity, and he resented the identity his father was trying to impose on him. He thought he had no part in defining it and it did not represent his real self.

This example demonstrates that although identity

CLINICAL EXAMPLE 14-5

Ken was a 17-year-old boy who was referred to the local community mental health center by his high school nurse. She made the referral after attending a team conference at school concerning Ken's repeated behavioral problems. He had a history of aggressive and destructive behavior in school, poor peer relationships, and low academic performance. The school had suspended him on three occasions previously, and the result of the team conference was to expel him for the remainder of the school year.

Mr. P, a psychiatric nurse at the mental health center, established a contract to work with Ken and his family. He noted that Ken was an obese young man (112.5 kg [250 pounds]) who took little interest in his appearance. His dress was sloppy, his complexion unclean, and his hair oily. He sat slumped in the chair in a disinterested and slightly defiant posture.

As Ken talked about himself, he complained of many pressures he experienced in his part-time job at a local hardware store. He thought the work was too difficult and tiring and that he was qualified for better and more prestigious work. When asked for specifics, he could not identify another job in particular. He also expressed a great deal of harassment from his family. His mother and father had been married for 31 years, and he was the only child of the marriage. His mother worked part time at a bakery, and his father was recently retired from his job as a supervisor at a local utility company where he was highly regarded.

Ken said that his father "always had things for me to do." He described how his father signed him up for various team sports—baseball, basketball, football—without acknowledging how much Ken hated sports and how uncoordinated he was. His father also stressed good grades and "the necessity of college" for success in life. Ken described his mother as passive and polite and said he had little respect for her. He said his aggressive outbursts occurred both at home and at school—whenever he was frustrated. People reacted by staying out of his way. He said he never hurt anyone with his temper. He mostly destroyed property and objects.

Ken avoided the subject of peers but, when asked about friends, said that there were a couple of boys in the neighborhood he "hung out with." They were older than he was. Most had dropped out of high school and were employed in odd jobs. He denied drug use but said they drank heavily, especially on the weekends. He said he had no girl friends and "wasn't interested in complicating my life with some broad."

confusion is a normative crisis of adolescence, the adoption of a negative identity can establish a maladaptive coping response which continues throughout life. So, too, problems of identity diffusion may emerge at any point during one's adult years.

■ **EGO DEFENSE MECHANISMS.** In later life, patients with alterations in self-concept may use a variety of defense mechanisms to protect themselves from confronting their own inadequacies. However maladaptive, the defenses represent attempted solutions to inner problems and perceived deficiencies. Typical defense mechanisms include fantasy, dissociation, isolation, projection, displacement, splitting, turning anger against the self, and acting out.

 Nursing diagnosis

■ Identifying nursing problems

The nature of an individual's self-concept is a critical aspect of his overall personality adjustment. Problems with self-concept are associated with feelings of anxiety, hostility, and guilt. These often create a circular and self-propagating process for the individual that ultimately results in maladaptive coping responses (Fig. 14-3).

Most individuals who express dissatisfaction with life, display deviant behavior, or have difficulty functioning in social or work situations have problems related to self-concept. The nature of the patient's problem, the degree of disruption, and his level of anxiety will be determined by the patient and nurse together on the basis of the behavioral or objective data the nurse has collected, as well as the subjective responses and description of the patient. In completing an assessment the nurse attempts to identify relevant stressors and link these to the problem the patient is experiencing related to self-concept.

The formulation of a nursing diagnosis should specify the nature of the nursing problem, the relevant stressors, and the patient's maladaptive coping response. The primary NANDA nursing diagnosis related to alterations in self-concept is that of self-concept, disturbance in: body-image, self-esteem, role performance, and personal identity.[30] Examples of complete nursing diagnoses related to self-concept are presented in the box shown on page 418. However, alterations in self-concept affect all aspects of an individual's life. One would expect, therefore, that many additional nursing problems would be identified by the nurse. Nursing diagnoses related to the range of possible maladaptive responses of the patient are identified in Table 14-2.

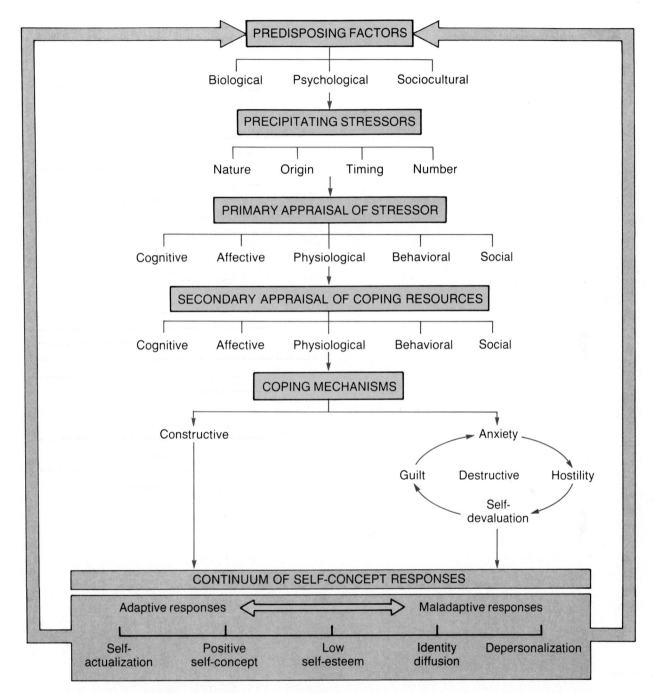

Fig. 14-3. Nursing model of health-illness phenomena related to self-concept responses.

■ Related medical diagnoses

In practice, maladaptive responses indicating alterations in self-concept can be seen in a wide variety of people experiencing threats to their physical integrity or self-system. It is a nursing diagnosis that is by no means limited to the psychiatric setting, and it does not have a discrete category of medical diagnoses associated with it. Because it pertains to one's basic personality structure and feelings about oneself, it is a nursing diagnosis that can emerge with a number of neurotic and psychotic disorders. In fact, it potentially could be related to all of the diagnostic categories identified in the Draft of the DSM-III-R in Development,[2] since the psychodynamics of all of these disorders ultimately reflect on one's view of self. A number of specific medical diagnoses do deserve particular attention, however,

Nursing Diagnoses Related to Self-Concept

Primary NANDA nursing diagnosis

Self-concept, disturbance in: body image; self-esteem; role performance; personal identity

Examples of complete nursing diagnoses

Disturbance in self-concept: body image related to fear of becoming obese evident by refusal to maintain body weight at normal limits

Disturbance in self-concept: body image related to leukemia chemotherapy evidenced by negative feelings about one's body

Disturbance in self-concept: body image related to cerebral vascular accident evidenced by lack of acceptance of body limitations

Disturbance in self-concept: self-esteem related to death of spouse evidenced by withdrawal from others and feelings of hopelessness

Disturbance in self-concept: self-esteem related to overly high self-ideals evidenced by depressed mood and withdrawal from activities

Disturbance in self-concept: role performance related to incompatibility of newly assumed work and family roles evidenced by self-criticism and feelings of inadequacy

Disturbance in self-concept: role performance related to incongruency of cultural and self role expectations about aging evidenced by feelings of frustration and criticism of others

Disturbance in self-concept: personal identity related to unrealistic parental expectations evidenced by running away from home

Disturbance in self-concept: personal identity related to drug toxicity evidenced by confusion and loss of impulse control

---

since their dominant features include alterations in self-concept. They are listed in Table 14-2 and will now be briefly described.[2]

■ **PSYCHOGENIC AMNESIA.** The essential feature includes a temporary disturbance in the ability to recall important personal information that is too extensive to be explained by ordinary forgetfulness. It typically has a sudden onset and is the most common dissociative disorder.

■ **PSYCHOGENIC FUGUE.** The essential feature is sudden, unexpected travel away from home or one's customary place of work, with an inability to recall one's past. A partial or complete new identity is assumed, and the patient is unaware that he has forgotten anything.

■ **MULTIPLE PERSONALITY.** The essential feature is the existence within the individual of two or more distinct personalities or personality states. Each personality has a full or nearly full range of mental functions, each with its own pattern of perceiving, relating to, and thinking about the environment and one's self. Each of these personality states at some time takes full control of the individual's behavior and the transition from one to the other is sudden. Amnesic barriers are found between one personality and another.

■ **DEPERSONALIZATION DISORDER.** The essential feature is an alteration of the perception or experience of the self, with loss of the sense of one's own reality and associated changes in body image. All of a person's mental operations and behavior may feel alien to him. There is a loss of the capacity to express emotions, and feelings of unreality and strangeness invade the patient's perceptions of the objects and people in the world around him.

■ **TRANCE/POSSESSION DISORDER** (under consideration). Either one may be the predominant disturbance. A trance is an altered state of consciousness with markedly diminished responsivity to environmental stimuli. A possession is the belief that one has been taken over by some spirit or person.

■ **DISSOCIATIVE DISORDER NOS.** This is a residual category to be used for disorders in which the predominant feature is a dissociative symptom that does not meet the criteria for a specific dissociative disorder.

■ **NARCISSISTIC PERSONALITY DISORDER.** The essential feature is excessive self-involvement, hypersensitivity to the evaluation of others, and lack of empathy. There is a grandiose sense of self-importance, demands for constant attention, and the taking advantage of others to achieve one's own ends.

■ **BORDERLINE PERSONALITY DISORDER.** The essential feature is an instability of mood, interpersonal relationships, and self-image. There is a marked and persistent lack of a consistent sense of identity, recurrent suicidal threats and self-destructive acts, and problems with the expression of anger and impulse control. Interpersonal relationships are exploitive and characterized by manipulation and splitting, with intense shifts between the extremes of overidealization and devaluation. This disorder has received greater attention recently because of the challenge it presents to the psychiatric clinician.

TABLE 14-2

MEDICAL AND NURSING DIAGNOSES RELATED TO SELF-CONCEPT

Medical Diagnostic Class

Dissociative disorders
Personality disorders

Psychiatric Nursing Diagnostic Class

Alterations in self-concept

**Related Medical Diagnoses
(DSM-III-R)***

Psychogenic amnesia
Psychogenic fugue
Multiple personality
Depersonalization disorder
Trance/possession disorder
Dissociative disorder
Narcissistic personality disorder
Borderline personality disorder

**Related Nursing Diagnoses
(NANDA)**

Altered sexuality patterns
Anxiety
Communication, impaired: verbal
Coping, ineffective: individual
Grieving, dysfunctional
Hopelessness
Impaired adjustment
Impaired social interaction
Powerlessness
Self-care deficit
†Self-concept, disturbance in: body image, self-esteem, role performance, personal identity
Sensory-perceptual alteration
Social isolation
Spiritual distress
Thought processes, alteration in
Violence, potential for

*From American Psychiatric Association: Draft of the DSM-III-R in Development (subject to change), as proposed by the Work Group to Revise DSM-III. American Psychiatric Association, October 1985.
†Indicates primary nursing diagnosis for alterations in self-concept

 Planning and implementation

■ Goal setting

Research indicates that patients with negative self-concepts believe their illnesses have a greater negative effect on their lives, have less hope and optimism about the future, and are more anxious about their illnesses.[43] These findings support the need for effective nursing intervention related to problems with self-concept.

The general goal of the nursing intervention is to facilitate the person's self-actualization by helping him grow, develop, and realize his potential while compensating for his impairments. The nurse's focus is to help the individual understand himself more fully and accurately so he can direct his own life in a more satisfying way. In a sense, nursing intervention concerns all that is involved in promoting the patient's self-realization. This means helping him strive toward a clearer and deeper experience of his feelings, wishes, and beliefs; toward a greater ability to tap his resources and to use them for constructive ends; and toward a clearer perception of his direction in life with the assumption of responsibility for himself and his decisions. It involves replacing repression with consciousness and unreality with reality. Sustaining, protecting, and enhancing the self results in increased self-esteem and self-acceptance, which is the essence of personality integration. A positive therapeutic outcome results in greater self-direction, tolerance, flexibility, and risk taking. A reorganization of the self will result in a change in behavior, and changes in behavior are outcomes of changes in the concept of the self.

Self-awareness is a crucial aspect in bringing about changes in self-concept, but people usually spend little time in introspection. Certain conditions or events, however, do stimulate self-awareness. This may occur when stimuli from the body are intensified, as in states of pain, fatigue, or anger, or when stimuli from the environment are decreased, as in sensory deprivation or states of isolation. Self-awareness may be triggered when something unexpected or extraordinary takes place, when the person has succeeded well or failed miserably, or when the person is confronted with himself by looking in a mirror, listening to his voice on a tape recorder, or reading an old letter. Special occasions, such as birthdays, anniversaries, New Year's Eve, or a death may stimulate introspection, and it may also be initiated when others direct their attention to the person through conversation or touch.

Once the person begins to look at and analyze himself, changes in the self become possible. Frequently they are the result of feelings of failure, unhappiness, anxiety, inadequacy, doubt or perplexity, or perceived discrepancies between one's concept of self and the demands of the environment or the expectations of others. Usually changes in the self occur only as a result of experiences and they take place gradually. Occasionally, however, a change may take place suddenly when a person has a traumatic experience that forces him to face the fact that he is inadequate or out of step with his peers and that something drastic must be done to remedy the situation.

The nurse should take all these factors into consideration when planning nursing care. Since the goal is to increase the patient's self-realization and acceptance, he must be an active participant in the formulation and implementation of specific plans. The nurse therefore must move with the patient and assess his readiness for growth within the therapeutic relationship. Together they formulate long-term goals that should reflect a positive resolution of the problem and the stressor identified in the nursing diagnosis. Short-term goals should be as clear and explicit as possible. They should identify realistic steps that the patient can accomplish. In this way the patient's self-confidence will increase, and this will directly affect his feelings of self-esteem. These goals should emphasize his strengths instead of his pathological condition, and, if they are mutually identified, they will serve to motivate him and help him assume increased responsibility for his own behavior. Following are examples of goals related to role conflict:

Long-term
Mrs. P will resolve role conflict by achieving greater congruency between work and family roles.
Short-term
After 1 week:

1. Mrs. P will describe her responsibilities in both her work and home roles.

2. She will identify aspects of these roles that provide her with satisfaction.
3. She will identify areas of role incompatibility.

After 2 weeks:
1. She will describe three alternative ways of increasing the complementarity of the roles.
2. She will discuss the advantages and disadvantages of each alternative.

After 3 weeks:
1. Mrs. P will take the necessary measures to implement one of the above alternatives.

Following are examples of goals related to disturbed body-image:

Long-term
Mr. B. will accept his modified body image after treatment with chemotherapy for leukemia.
Short-term
After the first phase of chemotherapy:

1. Mr. B will identify the medications he is receiving.
2. He will describe the effect they have on his illness and related body systems.
3. He will express his feelings (e.g., anger, sadness) about his illness and therapy.
4. He will identify three positive aspects of his modified body image.

■ Intervening in alterations in self-concept

The mutually identified goals can be accomplished by a problem-solving approach that focuses primarily on the present, removes much of the responsibility from the nurse, and actively engages the patient in working on his difficulties. This approach increases the patient's self-confidence and self-esteem. It requires that the patient first develop **insight** into his problems and life situation and then take **action** to effect lasting behavioral change. The nurse must thus incorporate both the responsive dimensions (insight oriented) and the action dimensions (action oriented) of the therapeutic relationship as described in Chapter 4 in implementing her nursing care.

The focus of this approach is on the patient's cognitive appraisal of his life, which may contain faulty perceptions, beliefs, and convictions. The patient's awareness of his feelings and emotions is also important, since they may be subject to misconceptions that arise from the acceptance of his cognitive analysis. Often the patient's display of affect is a clue to significant problem areas. Only after examining his cognitive appraisal of the situation and related feelings can he gain insight into the problem and bring about behavioral change. Adaptive behavior is based both on insight and on actually carrying out an appropriate solution to the presenting problem.

It is possible therefore to describe principles of nursing care that are applicable to the various problems with self-concept. These principles will be incorporated within a problem-solving approach and will be presented as progressive levels in the sequence in which they occur. It should also be noted that these principles focus primarily on the level of the individual. They may, however, be implemented in conjunction with group- or family-level interventions, and it is expected that the nurse would include the patient's family, significant others, and community supports whenever possible. Such a mobilization of the patient's possible coping resources can have both preventive and curative effects.

■ **LEVEL 1—EXPANDED SELF-AWARENESS.** A consistent picture of the self is necessary for security, and most people, to avoid anxiety, resist change. The ego resists change because any change becomes a threat to its stability and integration. Furthermore, the closer a deviant perception of the self is to the core of the self-concept, the more difficult it is to change. In general, change in the self is easier when there is an absence of threat. Threat forces a person to defend himself, and under threat, perceptions are narrowed and it becomes difficult for the person to form new perceptions of himself.

To expand the patient's self-awareness and reduce the element of threat, the nurse should adopt an accepting attitude toward the patient. Acceptance by the nurse allows the patient the security and freedom to examine all aspects of himself as a total human being with both positive and negative qualities. The basis of a therapeutic relationship will be established by listening to the patient with understanding, responding nonjudgmentally to him, expressing genuine interest in him, and conveying a sense of caring and sincerity. Creating a climate of acceptance allows previously denied experiences to be brought into consciousness and explored. This broadens the patient's concept of self and helps him to accept all aspects of his personality. It also indicates to him that he is a valued individual who is responsible for himself and able to help himself. This is important because the nurse must work through whatever ego strength the patient possesses. To the extent that a person has certain elements of ego strength—the capacity for self-control, some adeptness at reality testing, and a degree of ego integration—there is a foundation on which to build.

Most patients seen in clinics, the general hospital, and the community setting will possess a fair amount of ego strength. Hospitalized individuals, however, might have limited ego resources with which to work.

Psychotic patients who are experiencing feelings of depersonalization and identity confusion are often difficult challenges for the nurse. They tend to isolate themselves and withdraw from reality so that there is little ego strength available for problem solving. For this type of patient, expanding self-awareness means first confirming the patient's identity. The nurse should attempt to provide supportive measures to decrease the panic level of anxiety experienced by this fragile and vulnerable patient. Her nursing actions will be more active while they exert less pressure on the patient. Additional interventions related to anxiety and psychotic states are described in Chapters 12 and 17.

The nurse can spend time with the patient in an undemanding way and approach him in a nonaggressive manner. Initially she may accept his need to remain nonverbal and attempt to clarify and understand his verbal communication even though it may be distorted or lacking in apparent logic. She should prevent him from isolating himself from others and establish a simple routine for him. If the patient displays bizarre behavior, such as inappropriate laughing or mannerisms, she can provide control for him and set limits on his behavior. It is important to orient him frequently to reality and reinforce appropriate behavior.

The patient should be helped to increase the activities that provide positive experiences for him. This may involve the use of occupational therapy, recreational therapy, or activity groups. It has been shown that success at tasks and increased involvement with objects can increase self-esteem.[32] Movement therapy or body ego technique provides a special goal-directed way to facilitate the development of identity, body image, and ego structure and bring about changes in experiences that are necessary for ego growth. It is predominantly a nonverbal therapy because the emphasis is on movement and not on what the person says.[42]

The patient experiencing depersonalization often exhibits poor hygiene and an unkempt personal appearance. The nurse who is aware of her own value system regarding cleanliness and grooming can assist the patient who is unable to care for himself. She can use patience and repetition to establish health routines and kindly but firmly encourage the patient to care for himself. By her verbal and nonverbal messages she can encourage the patient to take pride in his appearance and reinforce any progress made in this area. Another possible nursing intervention in the area of body image is to use photographic self-image confrontation. This involves taking photographs of the patient and discussing them with him. Spire[44] found that this intervention produced positive behavioral changes with schizophrenic patients and provided a means for establishing a nurse-patient relationship and mutually exploring some aspects of the self.

Mutuality is often difficult to establish with a patient experiencing depersonalization. Initially the nurse will determine appropriate activities and incorporate the patient into them without asking for a response. Gradually, however, the nurse can expect greater participation and involve the patient in decision making that affects his care. Table 14-3 summarizes the nursing interventions appropriate to level 1.

Sometimes the attitude or behavior of the nurse can actually block or prevent the patient from expanding his self-awareness. This can be done in the form of criticism, belittlement, condemnation, condescension, indifference, or insincerity. If the nurse has an impersonal attitude or ignores the patient, it can decrease his self-esteem. Excessive demands on the patient or direct challenges to his self-concept at this time can result in his further withdrawal. The nurse should not allow him to remain alone or inactive, attempt to shame him into improving his habits, or assume total care for him. If the nurse avoids these attitudes and behaviors and strives for acceptance, she removes herself as a source of threat and encourages the patient to lower his defenses. He is then prepared to undertake the next step in the problem-solving approach.

■ **LEVEL 2—SELF-EXPLORATION.** At this level of intervention the nurse encourages the patient to ex-

---

TABLE 14-3

SUMMARY OF NURSING INTERVENTIONS IN ALTERATIONS IN SELF-CONCEPT AT LEVEL 1
Goal—Expand the patient's self-awareness

Principle	Rationale	Nursing interventions
Establish an open, trusting relationship	Reduces the threat that the nurse poses to the patient and helps him to broaden and accept all aspects of his personality	Offer unconditional acceptance Listen to the patient Encourage discussion of his thoughts and feelings Respond nonjudgmentally Convey to the individual that he is a valued person who is responsible for himself and able to help himself
Work with whatever ego strength the patient possesses	Some degree of ego strength, such as the capacity for reality testing, self-control, or a degree of ego integration, is needed as a foundation for later nursing care	Identify the ego strength possessed by the patient Guidelines for the patient with limited ego resources are as follows: 1. Begin by confirming his identity 2. Provide support measures to reduce his panic level of anxiety 3. Approach him in an undemanding way 4. Accept and attempt to clarify any verbal or nonverbal communication 5. Prevent him from isolating himself 6. Establish a simple routine for him 7. Set limits on inappropriate behavior 8. Orient him to reality 9. Reinforce appropriate behavior 10. Gradually increase activities and tasks that provide positive experiences for him 11. Assist him in personal hygiene and grooming 12. Encourage the patient to care for himself
Maximize the patient's participation in the therapeutic relationship	Mutuality is necessary for the patient to assume ultimate responsibility for his own behavior and maladaptive coping responses	Gradually increase the patient's participation in decisions that affect his care Convey to the patient that he is a responsible individual

amine his feelings, behavior, beliefs, and thoughts, particularly in relationship to the current stressful situation. The patient's feelings may be expressed verbally, nonverbally, symbolically, or directly. Acceptance continues to be important in this level because when the nurse accepts the patient's feelings and thoughts, she is helping him to accept them also. The nurse should facilitate the expression of strong emotions, such as anger, sadness, and guilt. In a sense, the patient's emotions or affect serve as clues to the exploration of inner thoughts and the examination of current behavior.

As the patient is helped to focus his attention on the meaning that experiences have for him, he is clarifying his perceptions and concept of himself and his relationship to the people and events around him. The nurse can elicit his perception of self-strengths and weaknesses and have him describe his self-ideal. He can be made aware of his self-criticisms. Frequently recognition in itself is a powerful therapeutic tool that motivates the patient to change. Jourard[28] has noted that many patients will experience a reduction in anxiety following the experience of full self-disclosure to an interested nurse. He believes patients withhold self-disclosure because of anxiety and the belief that no one is really interested in them.

It is important for the nurse to accept and deal with her own feelings before involving herself in the self-exploration of others. Her self-awareness will limit the potential negative effects of countertransference in the relationship. It will also allow her the freedom to manifest authentic behavior, which she, in turn, can elicit and reinforce in the patient. Often patients will experience great difficulty in discussing or describing their feelings. This might be because society tends to discourage self-revelation or because the patient is honestly out of touch with his own inner self. In this case the nurse can use herself therapeutically by sharing her own feelings with the patient, verbalizing how she might feel in the situation, or mirroring her perception of the patient's feelings. In this way, the nurse can help the patient explore his maladaptive thinking patterns including:

- Catastrophizing—the tendency to think the worst about what will happen in the future
- Minimizing and maximizing—the tendency to minimize the positive and magnify the negative
- Black-and-white thinking—the tendency to see things as belonging to one of two extremes without any middle ground
- Overgeneralization—the tendency to believe that since something happened once it will always happen

- Self-reference—the tendency to believe that everyone is concerned with their thoughts and actions and is particularly aware of their mistakes
- Filtering—the process of supporting one's beliefs by selectively pulling certain details out of context and neglecting other more positive facts[15]

The nurse can facilitate the patient's thinking by using reflection to paraphrase and sharpen the meanings in the patient's discussion. Validation and empathic responses are essential to guide the patient to the next level of nursing intervention. In all these ways the nurse provides encouragement, since most patients have strong tendencies to avoid thinking and talking about disturbing aspects of their problems. In addition, the nurse's reflections or clarifications of meaning help the patient to perceive more precisely what he has been discussing. Verbalized thoughts that have been responded to by the nurse often become more concrete and tangible. Reflected responses can also provide subtle guides for the patient because they often emphasize particular verbal content whose significance may have escaped the patient's attention.

In implementing these actions the nurse must be careful not to reinforce the patient's self-pity by responding with sympathy. Patients frequently disclaim any personal responsibility for their "plight," and they fail to see how their own behavior precipitates the very things about which they complain. Examples of this are patients who seek treatment because of things that happened *to* them, such as their wife left them, their husband beats them, or their boss fired them, and patients who seek help because of things that have *not* happened, such as not being happy or not having friends. These patients fail to see that they have a choice in life and that personal growth and satisfaction involve both risk and responsibility.

The nurse can clarify with the patient that he is not helpless or powerless in the face of difficulties. He is powerless when he sees himself as such and gives up control and responsibility for his behavior. Each person is responsible for his own behavior, including the things he decides to do and those which he decides not to do. One must also accept the responsibility for the logical consequences of those behaviors which one selects. Only if a patient fully understands the implications of his actions and the scope of his choices can he proceed to set goals, explore alternatives, and effect change.

In stressing the importance of behavior, the nurse helps the patient see that he chooses to behave in certain ways. If the patient projects his problems onto the environment, she can discuss with him the difficulty in changing situations and other people and instead explore the posibilities of changing his own self. This means helping the patient realize that when he says "I can't" he really means "I don't want to." The nurse should not give the impression that she has the power to change a patient's life. That power lies with him alone. She can, however, help him to maximize his strengths, utilize available resources, and see that there is more to life than being involved with misery and pain.

Self-exploration need not take place solely within the one-to-one relationship. Family sessions and group meetings can be helpful to clarify how the individual appears to others. These meetings can supplement the individual sessions with the patient, or similar nursing interventions can be applied within a regular family therapy or group therapy situation. Regardless, the nurse will be collecting information on the patient's thinking about himself, his use of logical or illogical reasoning, and his reported or observed emotional reactions. Interventions at this level should see the patient progress from denying or attributing contradictory feelings to the external situation, to realizing his own conflict in the particular situation, to recognizing a major conflict within himself (Table 14-4).

■ **LEVEL 3—SELF-EVALUATION.** This level involves hard work for the patient as he critically examines his own behavior, accepts the consequences for it, and judges it on the basis of whether it is his best possible choice. At this point, the problem should be clearly defined, and the patient should be helped to understand that his beliefs influence both his feelings and his behavior. It is only by actively and systematically challenging his faulty beliefs and perceptions that he can hope to alter his feelings and change his behavior. Previously identified misperceptions and distortions should be evaluated. Irrational beliefs, such as the following, should be brought to light and analyzed:

- Everyone must love me.
- I must be competent and adequate in all ways.
- I am unable to control my own happiness and destiny.
- I should condemn myself for making mistakes.
- I am better off if I avoid responsibilities rather than trying to face them.
- I am controlled by my past and can never break free of it.
- If I worry about potential problems, my anxiety will prevent their occurrence.
- My life is a disaster if it doesn't work out exactly as I had planned.

The patient's hopelessness should be countered by exploring areas of realistic hope. It is important to point out the mature part of the patient's personality and contrast it to the childhood part that causes problems. The behaviors that interfere with effective functioning have to be put in perspective so that the patient can clearly see that his maladaptive behavior is only a small part of his total personality.

Sometimes the patient is unable to identify any strengths and few may be readily obvious to the nurse. This requires additional thinking on her part. All people, no matter how disturbed their behavior, have some areas of personal strength. The nurse should examine the following areas:

1. Hobbies
2. Skills
3. School
4. Work
5. Character traits
6. Interpersonal skills
7. Personal qualities, such as loyalty and honesty
8. Appearance

As she is able to see positive aspects of the individual, she should share them with him to expand his own awareness.

The concepts of success and failure need to be placed in proper perspective. Failures occur every moment of every day, and they are a natural consequence of human activity. As long as people strive to achieve, they will frequently not reach their goals. The only way to avoid failure is to do absolutely nothing. Failure may be caused by one's own mistakes; it may be a result of lack of motivation; or it may be due to circumstances beyond one's control. But failure is the unavoidable outcome of human effort. The problem arises when individuals are labeled or label themselves as failures merely because they fail. This is illogical and potentially destructive. As an inherent aspect of life, failure should be viewed as a neutral concept rather than a negative one. If misperceptions such as this and unrealistic goals can be changed in the direction of greater accuracy where reality is concerned, maladaptive behavior and feelings of self-depreciation are likely to be reduced.

Unrealistic self-ideals, dependency patterns, and denial are all potential areas that can be analyzed. The patient can be helped to realize that all behavior and coping responses have both positive and negative consequences. Contrasts can be drawn between behavior that is destructive, inhibitory, or sabotaging, and that which is productive, enhancing, and growth producing. It is important for the patient to see that he acts in self-

TABLE 14-4

SUMMARY OF NURSING INTERVENTIONS IN ALTERATIONS IN SELF-CONCEPT AT LEVEL 2
Goal—Encourage the patient's self-exploration

Principle	Rationale	Nursing interventions
Assist the patient to accept his own feelings and thoughts	When the nurse shows interest in and accepts the patient's feelings and thoughts, she is helping him to do so also	Attend to and encourage the patient's expression of his emotions, beliefs, behavior, and thoughts—verbally, nonverbally, symbolically, or directly Utilize therapeutic communication skills and empathic responses Note his use of logical and illogical thinking and his reported and observed emotional responses
Help the patient to clarify his concept of self and his relationship to others through self-disclosure	Self-disclosure and understanding one's self-perceptions are prerequisites to bringing about future change; this may, in itself, produce a reduction in anxiety	Elicit his perception of self-strengths and weaknesses Assist him to describe his self-ideal Identify his self-criticisms Help him to describe how he believes he relates to other people and events
Be aware and have control of your own feelings	Self-awareness allows the nurse to model authentic behavior and limits the potential negative effects of countertransference in the relationship	Openness to one's own feelings Acceptance of both positive and negative feelings Therapeutic use of self by: 1. Sharing one's own feelings with the patient 2. Verbalizing how another might have felt 3. Mirroring one's perception of the patient's feelings
Respond empathically, not sympathetically, emphasizing that the power to change lies with the patient	Sympathy can reinforce the patient's self-pity; rather, the nurse should communicate that the patient's life situation is subject to his own control	Use empathic responses and monitor oneself for feelings of sympathy or pity Reaffirm to the patient that he is not helpless or powerless in the face of his problems Convey verbally and behaviorally that the patient is responsible for his own behavior, including his choice of maladaptive or adaptive coping responses Discuss with him the scope of his choices, his areas of ego strength, and coping resources that are available to him Utilize the support systems of family and groups to facilitate the patient's self-exploration Assist the patient in recognizing the nature of his conflict and the maladaptive ways in which he tries to cope with it

defeating ways because there is some "pay-off" or personal gain in it for him. The drawbacks or disadvantages to the patient's maladaptive coping responses will probably be well known to him. The payoffs, or secondary gains, may be more obscure and well repressed. Following are some commonly experienced payoffs[31]:

- Procrastination
- Avoiding risks
- Retreating from the present
- Not having to accept responsibility for one's actions
- Avoiding working or having to change

More specific payoffs should be identified by the nurse and patient together, relative to his particular problem. For example, possible secondary gains that can be derived from being obese include having people feel sorry for you, having an excuse for not dating or being married, being the focus of dieting attention, or being easily recognized and noticed when with other people. Possible secondary gains for an adult remaining dependent on his parents might include not having to make one's own decisions, having someone else to blame if things go wrong, being protected from having to take risks and venture out in the world on one's own, having an excuse for not establishing lasting intimate relationships with one's peers, or not having to establish one's own identity, but rather adopting the values and goals of others. Such payoffs can be identified for each nursing diagnosis formulated by the nurse.

The nurse becomes more active in this level of intervention. She begins confronting, interpreting, persuading, and challenging the patient. Her goal is to increase the patient's objectivity in dealing with the stressors he perceives. For example, the nurse can work to show the borderline patient that the negative and positive characteristics of people can be integrated. Thus, the same person can nurture and gratify as well as anger and frustrate, since both negative and positive qualities can coexist in the same person.

A number of techniques may be utilized by the nurse at this time. In interpretation and confrontation, the nurse offers information that the patient may not have or does not recognize as relevant. Supportive confrontation may be particularly effective in calling to the patient's attention inconsistencies in words and actions that he has not seen. The climate of acceptance established by the nurse in level 1 and the empathic communication developed in level 2 provide a basis for confrontation in level 3. This groundwork is necessary to prevent premature confrontation, which can be destructive.

The use of reflection allows the nurse to restate the meaning or emphasize the significance of the patient's revelations. It functions to inform the patient that the nurse understands what is being said, and it encourages him to continue his self-evaluation. Reflections and confrontations are often phrased in the form of questions, and the use of questions can also encourage the patient to search for additional information. In this regard the questions should be specific and not vague or overwhelming, which occurs when one repeatedly asks "Why?" Suggestion can be used to introduce alternative ways of thinking or behaving.

The nurse may use various aspects of role theory during this level of intervention. She may assist the patient in role clarification, which is the gaining of knowledge, information, and cues needed to perform a role. It involves the identification of appropriate behaviors, clarification of expectations, and specification of goals relative to the role, taking into consideration the influence of significant others and the context of the situation. Role clarification therefore reduces the potential for, or existence of, role strain. The nurse can also encourage the patient to participate in any activity in which he can observe his own behavior. The use of role playing may be particularly effective in providing the patient with feedback and increasing his insight. Through it, he may be able to gain objectivity toward the irrationality and self-destructiveness of his self-criticisms.

The nurse-patient relationship provides a rich source of information for the patient. Within this relationship he is enacting and experiencing many of his problem areas and the nurse can use this as a "study in miniature." The nurse can assist the patient in observing how he reacts in the one-to-one situation. She can share her reactions with him to give him feedback on how he affects others and openly disclose some of her own feelings about the patient's behavior. The analysis and use of transference and countertransference reactions comprises the nurse's "therapeutic use of self." When a block arises within the relationship or the nurse experiences increased anxiety, she should use this opportunity to explore its meaning with the patient. She should confront the problem and openly discuss it with him. This can also be done in family therapy or group therapy sessions.

Psychodrama, a special form of group therapy, provides the patient with an additional opportunity to gain self-insight. In psychodrama the therapist organizes the events so that the patient has an audience to whom he plays a role structured for him by the therapist. In this therapy modality the audience acts as a standard against which the patient can obtain evidence for the social adequacy of his own reactions and behavior.

During this level of intervention the patient and nurse critically evaluate his behavior (Table 14-5). Misperceptions, unrealistic goals, and distortions of reality are explored. This provides the patient with sufficient knowledge to progress to the next level of the problem-solving process.

■ **LEVEL 4—REALISTIC PLANNING.** The nurse and patient are now ready to formulate possible solutions or alternatives. This begins by investigating what solutions were attempted in the past and evaluating their effectiveness. When inconsistent perceptions are held by the individual, he is faced with a number of choices. He can change his perceptions and beliefs to bring them closer to the reality that cannot be changed. Or he may seek to change his environment to bring it in line with what he believes. When his behavior is not consistent with his self-concept, he can change his behavior to conform to his self-concept, change the beliefs underlying his self-concept so that they include his behavior, or change his self-ideal while leaving his self-concept intact.

At this time, all possible solutions should be openly discussed with the patient. The nurse must be careful not to use her influence to persuade the patient to do anything that represents her own values rather than the patient's. She should help him conceptualize his goals. If they are within his reach, she can support his efforts to reach them. If the patient has conflicting goals, she

---

TABLE 14-5

SUMMARY OF NURSING INTERVENTIONS IN ALTERATIONS IN SELF-CONCEPT AT LEVEL 3
Goal—Assist the patient's self-evaluation

Principle	Rationale	Nursing interventions
Help the patient to clearly define the problem	Only after the problem is accurately defined can alternative choices be proposed	Identify relevant stressors with the patient and his appraisal of them Clarify to the patient that his beliefs influence both his feelings and behaviors Mutually identify faulty beliefs, misperceptions, distortions, illusions, and unrealistic goals Mutually identify areas of strength Place the concepts of success and failure in proper perspective Explore with the patient his use of coping resources
Explore the patient's adaptive and maladaptive coping responses to his problem	It is then necessary to examine the coping choices the patient has made and evaluate both the positive and negative consequences of them	Describe to the patient how all coping responses are freely chosen and have both positive and negative consequences Contrast adaptive and maladaptive responses Mutually identify the disadvantages of the patient's maladaptive coping responses Mutually identify the advantages or "payoffs" of the patient's maladaptive coping responses Discuss how these payoffs have perpetuated the maladaptive response Utilize a variety of therapeutic skills, such as the following: 1. Facilitative communication 2. Supportive confrontation 3. Role clarification 4. The transference and countertransference reactions occurring in the one-to-one relationship 5. Psychodrama

helps him identify which ones are more realistic or obtainable by discussing the emotional and practical consequences of each goal.

The nurse can work with the patient in various ways. He may be encouraged to give up superhuman standards by which he judges his behavior. These standards may set him up for failure and create a pathological cyclical pattern that will need to be broken. Together they may work at destroying illusions that are not part of his authentic self. Perhaps the patient will need to lower his self-ideal and limit his personal goals to make them consistent with what is humanly possible. He should be encouraged to renew involvement with life and enter new experiences for their growth potential.

The techniques of role rehearsal, role modeling, and role playing may be employed. In role rehearsal the person imagines how a particular situation might take place and how his role might evolve. He mentally enacts his role and tries to anticipate the responses of significant others. Role rehearsal is important in anticipating and planning the course of future action. Role modeling occurs when the individual observes someone else playing a certain role so that he is able to understand and emulate the behaviors in that role. The person he observes may be the nurse, a family member, a group member, or peer. The nurse can be important in assisting the patient in his role learning. She can model behavior that may be posing problems for the patient, such as the appropriate expression of feelings, specific socialization skills, or realistic self-expectations. Proceeding one step further, the nurse and patient may role play certain situations to conceptualize alternative solutions.

Visualization can also be used to enhance self-

TABLE 14-6

SUMMARY OF NURSING INTERVENTIONS IN ALTERATIONS IN SELF-CONCEPT
AT LEVEL 4
Goal—Assist the patient in formulating a realistic plan of action

Principle	Rationale	Nursing interventions
Help the patient identify alternative solutions	Only when all possible alternatives have been evaluated can change be affected	Help the patient understand that he can only change himself, not others If the patient holds inconsistent perceptions, help him to see that he can change the following: 1. His beliefs or ideals to bring them closer to reality 2. His environment to make it consistent with his beliefs If his self-concept is not consistent with his behavior, he can change the following: 1. His behavior to conform to his self-concept 2. The beliefs underlying his self-concept to include his behavior 3. His self-ideal Mutually review how coping resources may be better utilized by the patient
Help the patient conceptualize his own realistic goals	Goal setting that includes a clear definition of the expected change is necessary	Encourage the patient to formulate his own (not the nurse's) goals Mutually discuss the emotional, practical, and reality-based consequences of each goal Help the patient clearly define the concrete change to be made Encourage the patient to enter new experiences for their growth potential Utilize role rehearsal, role modeling, role playing, and visualization when appropriate

esteem through goal setting.[15] Through the conscious programming of desired change with positive images, expectations are molded. Strong, positive expectations can then become self-fulfilling. To use visualization, the nurse should

1. Ask the patient to select a positive, specific goal statement, such as: "I will call a friend and suggest we go out together."
2. Help the patient to relax using an appropriate relaxation technique (see Chapter 12).
3. Have the patient repeat the goal phrase several times slowly.
4. Instruct the patient to close his eyes and visualize the goal written on a piece of paper.
5. While relaxed, have the patient imagine accomplishing the goal.

The patient should then describe how he feels when the desired goal is accomplished, and how other people are responding to him. In this way, the patient can be helped to gain positive control over his life.

Nursing actions appropriate to this level of intervention are summarized in Table 14-6. Ultimately, the patient should decide on a plan of action that includes a clear definition of the concrete change to be achieved. Converting a "talking decision" into an "action decision" is the final, but obviously most important, step.

■ **LEVEL 5—COMMITMENT TO ACTION.** The nurse assists the patient to become committed to his decision and then achieve his own goals. The patient's development of self-awareness, self-understanding, and insight is not the ultimate desired outcome of the nursing therapeutic process. Insight alone does not make problems disappear or transform one's world in magical ways. Although a patient may have obtained a high level of insight, he may nevertheless continue to function at a minimal level. Such a patient may be able to intellectually discuss with great ease the nature of his problem and the influences contributing to it. But the problem itself continues to be unresolved. Some patients actually use their insights to resist moving forward and avoid the hard work involved in making behavioral changes. The value of having the patient gain insight and increase his self-understanding is so that he can gain perspective on why he behaves the way he does and what must be done to break the maladaptive coping pattern.

Providing opportunity for the patient to experience success becomes essential at this time. To help him commit himself to his goal, the nurse can relate to the patient how she sees him, correcting his own poor self-image. In this mirroring technique she can openly and honestly describe to the patient the normal healthy parts of his personality and how by using these parts he can achieve his goal. She should reinforce his strengths or skills and provide him with opportunities to use them whenever possible.

Sometimes the lack of vocational or social skills may be a causative factor for low self-esteem. If so, nursing intervention can be directed toward gaining vocational assistance for the patient. Group involvement may be instrumental in raising self-esteem.[19] The experience of being accepted by others, the sense of belonging and being important to others, and the opportunity to develop interpersonal competence can all enhance self-esteem.

In a similar way, the family of origin is the source of most people's self-esteem. The key relationships for improving basic self-differentiation are those with parents and siblings, even in adulthood. These relationships involve the unresolved emotional fusion that influences many interactions an individual has with others. Adult contact with parents and siblings can correct misconceptions underlying low self-esteem, and allow for the development of more positive beliefs. Learning to interact with family members with appropriate closeness, but without counterproductive kinds of fusion and emotionality, can enable a more mature interactional pattern to develop. Family relationships would therefore be an appropriate focus for patient education by the nurse. A mental health education plan using Bowen's theory of family systems is presented in Table 14-7.[8] Chapter 29 presents a more detailed discussion of family systems theory and family therapy.

At this point the individual needs a great deal of support and positive reinforcement in affecting and maintaining change. For many patients this will mean breaking chronic behavior patterns and exposing themselves to real risk. A person must actively maintain the processes learned to avoid slipping back to the old behavior. Doing this is difficult and requires that the patient build on the progress he has made in the other levels. Successful change is a continuing process of modifying not only one's behavior but one's environment to help ensure that the change to new ways of behaving is permanent. Otherwise there will be a relapse.

The nurse serves as a transition between the pain of the past and the positive gratification the future holds. It is important that both the nurse and patient allow sufficient time for change. A significant amount of time may be required for patterns that developed over months or years to be broken and new ones established. The nurse's role now becomes less an active and directive one, but rather one of confirming the value, potential, and accomplishments of the patient (Table 14-8).

TABLE 14-7

MENTAL HEALTH EDUCATION PLAN—FAMILY RELATIONSHIPS[8]

Content	Instructional activities	Evaluation
Define the concept of self-differentiation within one's own family of origin	Discuss the differences between high and low levels of self-differentiation Ask the patient to identify level of functioning among own family members	Patient identifies his functioning level in his family of origin
Describe the characteristics of emotional fusion, emotional cutoff, and triangulation	Analyze types and patterns of family relationships Use paper and pencil to diagram family patterns	Patient describes interactional patterns within his own family Patient identifies his own roles and behavior
Discuss the role of symptom formation and symptom bearer in a family	Sensitize the patient to family dynamics and manifestations of stress Encourage communication with family of origin	Patient recognizes family contribution to the stress of individual members Patient contacts family members
Describe a family genogram and show how it is constructed	Use a blackboard to map out a family genogram Assign family genogram as homework	Patient obtains factual information about own family Patient constructs family genogram
Analyze need for objectivity and responsibility for changing one's own behavior and not that of others	Role play interactions with various family members Encourage testing out new ways of interacting with family members	Patient demonstrates a higher level of differentiation in family of origin

---

 Evaluation

Problems with self-concept are prominent in many psychological disorders. Changes in self-concept are accompanied by greater self-realization and self-acceptance and lead to behavioral changes and improved personality adjustment. To evaluate the success or failure of the nursing care given in this area, each phase of the nursing process should be reviewed and analyzed by the nurse and patient.

The nurse's assessment should include both the objective and observable behaviors as well as the subjective perceptions of the patient. Did she explore his areas of strengths and weaknesses and elicit his self-ideal? Was information obtained on his body image, feelings of self-esteem, role satisfaction, and sense of identity? Did she compare his responses to his behavior, and were any inconsistencies or contradictions identified? Was she

aware of her own affective response to the patient, and how did this affect her ability to be therapeutic?

Before formulating a nursing diagnosis, the nurse should have discussed with the patient his appraisal of stressful life events and the nature of the threat they posed to him. Did they determine his level of anxiety and was he able to express related feelings, such as hostility, sadness, or guilt? Were the therapeutic goals realistic, explicit, adequate, and efficient? Were the patient's coping resources well assessed and utilized?

The nurse should have adopted a problem-solving approach that placed responsibility for growth on the patient. The most fundamental nursing action should have been to create a climate of acceptance that confirmed the patient's identity and conveyed a sense of value or worth. In expanding the patient's self-awareness, how effective was the nurse in promoting the patient's full and pertinent self-disclosure? Was he able to

---

TABLE 14-8

SUMMARY OF NURSING INTERVENTIONS IN ALTERATIONS IN SELF-CONCEPT AT LEVEL 5

Goal—Assist the patient to become committed to his decision and achieve his own goals

Principle	Rationale	Nursing interventions
Help the patient take the necessary action to change maladaptive coping responses and maintain adaptive ones	The ultimate objective in promoting the patient's insight is to have him replace the maladaptive coping responses with more adaptive ones	Provide opportunity for the patient to experience success Reinforce the strengths, skills, and healthy aspects of the patient's personality Assist the patient in gaining the assistance he might need (vocational, financial, and social services) Utilize groups to enhance the patient's self-esteem Promote the patient's self-differentiation in his family of origin Allow the patient sufficient time to change Provide the appropriate amount of support and positive reinforcement for the patient to help him maintain his progress

---

listen more fully to himself and others? What behaviors or attitudes did the nurse display that prevented the patient from expanding his self-awareness? Was the nurse able to manifest authentic behavior in the relationship and share thoughts and reactions with the patient? What interventions were used and which ones proved to be beneficial—validation, reflection, confrontation, suggestion, role clarification, or role playing? Did the nurse progress on the basis of the patient's readiness and motivation?

What was the outcome of the patient's cognitive analysis and exploration of feelings? Was he able to transfer his new perceptions into possible solutions or alternative behavior? How did the nurse help him implement his plans? What success did he experience? Did they both allow sufficient time for changes to occur? The degree of overall success achieved through nursing care can be determined by eliciting the patient's perception of his own growth and comparing his behavior to the characteristics of the healthy personality as described in this chapter. Not everyone will achieve all these characteristics, but success has been achieved if the patient's potential has been maximized.

■ SUGGESTED CROSS-REFERENCES ■

Definitions of mental health are discussed in Chapters 2 and 3. Therapeutic relationship skills are discussed in Chapter 4. Interventions with family and group support systems and other coping resources are discussed in Chapters 9 and 11. Interventions related to anxiety are discussed in Chapter 12. The relationship of role strain and low self-esteem to depression is discussed in Chapter 15. Self-destructive behaviors, including anorexia, obesity, and suicide are discussed in Chapter 16. Nursing intervention in psychotic panic states is discussed in Chapter 17. Family therapy is discussed in Chapter 29. The family dysfunctions of violence and abuse are discussed in Chapter 32.

■ SUMMARY ■

1. Self-concept is defined as all the notions, beliefs, and convictions that constitute an individual's knowledge of himself and influence his relationships with others. One's self-concept does not exist at birth but is learned as a result of a person's unique experiences within himself, with significant others, and with the realities of the world.

2. Body image is the sum of the conscious and unconscious attitudes the individual has toward his body. It includes present and past perceptions, as well as feelings about size, function, appearance, and potential. It is continually modified by new perceptions and experiences.

3. Self-ideal is the individual's perception of how he should behave based on certain personal standards, aspirations, goals, or values. Mental health is associated with a clear, realistic self-ideal and congruence between one's perception of self and his self-ideal.

4. Self-esteem is the individual's personal judgment of his own worth obtained by analyzing how well his behavior conforms to his self-ideal. High self-esteem is a feeling rooted in unconditional acceptance of self, despite mistakes, defeats, and failures, as an innately worthy and important being.

5. Roles are sets of socially expected behavior patterns associated with an individual's function in various social groups. Ascribed roles are assigned roles over which the person has no choice. Assumed roles are those selected or chosen by the person.

6. Identity is the organizing principle of the personality that accounts for the unity, continuity, consistency, and uniqueness of the individual. In connotes autonomy and includes perceptions of one's sexuality. Identity formation begins in infancy and proceeds throughout life but is the major task of the adolescent period.

7. Individuals with positive self-concepts function more effectively, which is evident in interpersonal competence, intellectual efficiency, and environmental mastery. Because negative self-concept is correlated with personal and social maladjustment, self-concept change is a core element in psychiatric nursing practice.

8. Predisposing factors and precipitating stressors related to alterations in self-concept were identified and briefly described.

9. Data collection by the nurse should include objective and observable behaviors as well as the subjective and internal world of the patient. Behaviors relative to problems with self-concept were identified and described in clinical examples.

10. The formulation of a nursing diagnosis should specify the nature of the nursing problem, the related stressor, and the patient's maladaptive coping response. Nursing diagnoses associated with alterations in self-concept were presented and related to selected medical diagnoses.

11. The goal of nursing intervention is to facilitate the person's self-actualization by helping him grow, develop, and realize his potential while compensating for his impairments. Changes in the self occur only as a result of experiences and they take place gradually. If the goals are clear, realistic, and mutually identified, they will serve to motivate the patient and help him assume increased responsibility for his own behavior.

12. Nursing intervention helps the patient examine his cognitive appraisal of the situation and his related feelings to help him gain insight, and then take action to bring about behavioral change. This problem-solving approach includes the following levels of intervention: (a) expanded self-awareness, (b) self-exploration, (c) self-evaluation, (d) realistic planning, and (e) commitment to action. It can be used with individuals, families, or groups.

13. A climate of acceptance was noted to be of particular importance in broadening the patient's concept of himself, helping him to accept all aspects of his personality, and conveying to him that he is a valued individual who is responsible for himself and able to help himself. Confirming the patient's identity is particularly important with problems of identity confusion and depersonalization.

14. The nurse and patient together evaluate the success of the nursing care in each step of the nursing process. The degree of overall success can be determined by eliciting the patient's perception of his own growth and comparing his behavior to the characteristics of the healthy personality as described in this chapter.

■ **REFERENCES** ■

1. Akhtar, S.: The syndrome of identity diffusion. Am. J. Psychiatry **141**(11):1381, Nov. 1984.
2. American Psychiatric Association: Draft of the DSM-III-R in Development (subject to change), as proposed by the Work Group to Revise DSM-III. American Psychiatric Association, October 1985.
3. Antonucci, T., and Jackson, J.: Physical health and self-esteem, Family and Community Health **6**(2):1, Aug. 1983.
4. Bailyn, L.: Notes on the role of choice in the psychology of professional women. In Lifton, R., editor: The woman in America, Boston, 1967, Beacon Press.
5. Berk, S., Berk, R., and Berheide, C.: The non-division of household labor. In Fisher, A., editor: Women's worlds, NIMH Supported Research on Women, Rockville, Md., 1978, National Institute of Mental Health.
6. Biddle, B.: Role theory: expectations, identities, and behaviors, New York, 1979, Academic Press, Inc.
7. Boston Globe, March 8, 1977.
8. Bowen, M.: Family therapy in clinical practice, New York, 1978, Jason Aronson.
9. Broverman, I., et al.: Sex-role stereotypes and clinical judgments of mental health, J. Consult. Clin. Psychol. **24**:1, Jan. 1970.
10. Broverman, I., et al.: Sex-role stereotypes: a current appraisal, J. Soc. Issues **28**:59, Feb. 1972.
11. Bugenthal, J.: The search for existential identity, San Francisco, 1976, Jossey-Bass, Inc., Publishers.
12. Burns, D.: The perfectionist's script for self-defeat, Psychol. Today **14**(11):34, 1980.
13. Combs, A., and Snygg, D.: Individual behavior: a perceptual approach, New York, 1959, Harper & Row, Publishers, Inc.
14. Coopersmith, S.: The antecedents of self-esteem, San Francisco, 1967, W.H. Freeman & Co., Publishers.
15. Crouch, M., and Straub, V.: Enhancement of self-esteem in adults, Fam. Community Health **6**(2):65, Aug. 1983.
16. Erikson, E.: The problem of ego-identity, J. Am. Psychoanal. Assoc. **4**:56, Jan. 1956.
17. Erikson, E.: Childhood and society, New York, 1963, W.W. Norton & Co., Inc.
18. Fitts, W.: The self concept and self actualization, Nashville, Tenn., 1971, Dede Wallace Center Monograph No. 3.
19. Goldberg, C., and Stanitis, M.A.: The enhancement of self-esteem through communication in group therapy, J. Psychiatr. Nurs. **15**(12):5, 1977.
20. Goode, W.: A theory of role strain, Am. Sociol. Rev. **25**:438, 1960.
21. Grove, W., and Tudor, J.: Adult sex roles and mental illness, Am. J. Sociol. **78**:812, 1973.
22. Hamachek, D.: Encounters with the self, New York, 1971, Holt, Rinehart & Winston, Inc.
23. Holahan, C., and Gilbert, L.: Interrole conflict for working women: careers versus jobs, J. Appl. Psychol. **64**:86, 1979.
24. Horney, K.: Neurosis and human growth, New York, 1950, W.W. Norton & Co., Inc.
25. Horrocks, J., and Jackson, D.: Self and role: a theory of self-process and role behavior, Boston, 1972, Houghton Mifflin Co.
26. Johnson, C., and Johnson, F.: Attitudes toward parenting in dual-career families, Am. J. Psychiatry **134**:391, 1977.
27. Jourard, S.: Personal adjustment: an approach through the study of the healthy personality, New York, 1963, Macmillan, Inc.
28. Jourard, S.: The transparent self, New York, 1971, Litton Educational Publishing, Inc.
29. Kernberg, O.: Borderline conditions and pathological narcissism, New York, 1975, Jason Aronson, Inc.
30. Kim, M., McFarland, G., and McLane, A.: Pocket guide to nursing diagnoses, St. Louis, 1984, The C.V. Mosby Co.
31. Kottler, J.: Promoting self-understanding in counseling: a compromise between the insight and action-oriented approaches, J. Psychiatr. Nurs. **17**(12):18, 1979.
32. Lancaster, J.: Activity groups as therapy, Am. J. Nurs. **76**:947, 1976.
33. Logan, R.: Identity diffusion and psychosocial defense mechanisms, Adolescence **13**(51):503, 1978.
34. Marcia, J.: Development and validation of ego-identity status, J. Pers. Soc. Psychol. **3**:551, 1966.
35. Maslow, A.: Motivation and personality, New York, 1954, Harper & Row, Publishers, Inc.
36. Meier, E.: An inquiry into the concepts of ego identity and identity diffusion, Soc. Casework **13**:63, Feb. 1964.
37. Meleis, A.: Role insufficiency and role supplementation: a conceptual framework, Nurs. Res. **24**:264, 1975.
38. Money, J., and Ehrhardt, A.: Man & woman, boy & girl, Baltimore, 1972, Johns Hopkins University Press.
39. Norris, C.: The professional nurse and body image. In Carlson, C., editor: Behavioral concepts and nursing intervention, Philadelphia, 1970, J.B. Lippincott Co.
40. Orlofsky, J., Marcia, J., and Lesser, I.: Intimacy vs. isolation: crisis of young adulthood, J. Pers. Soc. Psychol. **27**:211, 1973.
41. Rostow, E.: Conflict and accommodation. In Lifton, R., editor: The woman in America, Boston, 1967, Beacon Press.
42. Salkin, J.: Body ego technique, Springfield, Ill., 1973, Charles C Thomas, Publisher.
43. Schwab, J., Clemmons, R., and Morder, L.: The self-concept: psychosomatic applications, Psychosomatics **7**:1, Jan.-Feb. 1966.
44. Spire, R.: Photographic self-image confrontation, Am. J. Nurs. **73**:1207, 1973.

45. Sullivan, H.S.: The interpersonal theory of psychiatry, New York, 1963, W.W. Norton & Co., Inc.
46. Weissman, M. et al.: The educated housewife: mild depression and the search for work, Am. J. Orthopsychiatry **43**:565, 1973.

■ ANNOTATED SUGGESTED READINGS ■

Berne, E.: Games people play, New York, 1964, Grove Press, Inc.

This well-known book is divided into three sections. In Part I the theory behind transactional analysis is presented. Part II contains descriptions of various interpersonal games, and Part III explores the possibility of being game free. Berne's theory of TA has implications for problems with self-concept and is recommended reading for all nurses.

*Bonham, P., and Cheney, A.: Concept of self: a framework for nursing assessment. In Chinn, P., editor: Advances in nursing theory development, Rockville, Md., 1983, Aspen.

This chapter briefly reviews the literature and proposes a model to define a nursing focus for self-concept. Utilizing a systems approach, the authors apply the model to nursing and address future implications.

Burns, D.: The perfectionist's script for self-defeat, Psychol. Today **14**(11):34, 1980.

This article describes the price perfectionists pay in the compulsive striving toward impossible goals. A treatment approach, which uses cognitive therapy or thought reform, is also discussed.

Dellas, M., and Gaier, E.: The self and adolescent identity in women: options and implications, Adolescence **10**:399, 1975.

In light of the changing sex role standards and the reassessment of the status of women in society, the authors explore three possible female identity patterns—traditional role and stereotype, achievement and role success, and bimodal. Problems related to each are also discussed.

Ellis, A.: Humanistic psychotherapy: the rational-emotive approach, New York, 1974, McGraw-Hill Book Co.

This text introduces the idea of rational-emotive therapy (RET). It is a cognitive therapeutic approach in which Ellis works with patients to change their irrational belief systems.

Erikson, E.: Identity: youth and crisis, New York, 1968, W.W. Norton & Co., Inc.

Erikson's extensive formulations on the adolescent crisis of identity are presented in this text. His stages of the life cycle are briefly reviewed, and the pathology of identity confusion is explored through theory and case history. This is an important work on a previously unexplored developmental stage.

Family and Community Health **6**(2), Aug. 1983.

The entire volume of this journal is devoted to self-esteem. This is highly recommended reading for all the various articles:

Physical health and self-esteem
Self-esteem through the life span
The evaluation of self-esteem
Enhancement of self-esteem in children and adolescents
Enhancement of self-esteem in adults
Future needs for self-esteem research and services

Glasser, W.: Reality therapy, New York, 1965, Harper & Row, Publishers, Inc.

This text introduces the reader to a therapeutic approach called reality therapy. It is based on three elements: reality, responsibility, and right and wrong. The author presents the basic formulations of his theory and applies them in specific clinical examples.

*Gruendemann, B.: The impact of surgery on body-image, Nurs. Clin. North Am. **10**:635, 1975.

This article summarizes the impact of surgery on the patient's view of himself and his body. It presents aids to a nursing assessment, guides to formulating nursing goals, and methods for nursing intervention.

*Hauser, M.: Cognitive commands change, J. Psychiatr. Nurs. **19**(2):19, 1981.

A nurse therapist reviews three specific techniques for working with parent-child interpersonal and behavioral problems: (1) Ellis' restructuring beliefs, (2) Meichenbaum's coping via internal speech, and (3) Gordon's problem solving. All of these are cognitive techniques that are aligned with social learning theory.

*Journal of Psychosocial Nursing and Mental Health Services, **23**(4), Apr. 1985.

The entire edition of this journal is devoted to the borderline patient. Multiple perspectives and techniques are presented with implications for nursing.

Kanfer, F., and Goldstein, A., editors: Helping people change, New York, 1975, Pergamon Press, Inc.

A number of authors contributed excellent articles that deal with such topics as cognitive change, self-management, modeling, and role play.

*Kerr, N.: Pathological narcissism, Perspect. Psychiatr. Care **18**(1):29, 1980.

The author reviews the many facets of narcissism including its development, psychodynamics, and interpersonal aspects. It includes a good bibliography for further reading on the problem.

*Kjervik, D.: Dual personality: assessment and reintegration, J. Psychosoc. Nurs. **17**(7):28, 1979.

This is one of the few articles in the nursing literature that discusses the phenomenon of multiple personalities. Theoretical considerations are presented; then practical application of the theory is made to a case of dual personality.

Meier, E.: An inquiry into the concepts of ego integrity and identity diffusion, Soc. Casework **13**:63, Feb. 1964.

This article is recommended for its description of the attributes and behaviors associated with ego identity. Those associated with identity diffusion as a result of the stress of cultural changes are also presented.

*Meleis, A.: Role insufficiency and role supplementation: a conceptual framework, Nurs. Res. **24**:264, 1975.

This article offers a theoretical basis for the diagnosis of nursing problems related to role insufficiency. The basis for nursing intervention is role supplementation, and appropriate strategies are described. The role of the nurse is discussed, and a predictive and prescriptive paradigm is presented.

---

*Asterisk indicates nursing reference.

Money, J., and Ehrhardt, A.: Man & woman, boy & girl, Baltimore, 1972, Johns Hopkins University Press.

One of the authors, John Money, is a significant researcher in the field of sex behavior. This text describes how sex roles are learned, how boys become masculine and girls feminine, and what the results of the failure to learn the role are. Also included is a discussion of some of the findings in hormonal research.

*Moscato, B.: Sex-role stereotyping. In Kneisl, C.R., and Wilson, H.S., editors: Current perspectives in psychiatric nursing, vol. 2, St. Louis, 1978, The C.V. Mosby Co.

Various aspects of sex-role stereotyping are presented—historical considerations, stereotypical patterns, implications for the mental health care delivery system, and behaviors evidenced by nurses. This is a highly recommended reading.

*Platt-Koch, L.: Borderline personality disorder: a therapeutic approach, Am. J. Nurs. **1983**:1666, Dec. 1983.

The author describes her work with a borderline patient. Underlying dynamics and therapeutic strategies are clearly integrated in this article.

Raimy, V.: Misunderstandings of the self, San Francisco, 1975, Jossey-Bass, Inc., Publishers.

The premise of this book is that misunderstandings of the self may be major hindrances to personal and social adjustment. The author presents an approach to psychotherapy that is an application of self-concept theory and describes faulty beliefs or misconceptions as responsible for psychological disturbances. The text is easy to read and integrates sophisticated features of various psychotherapies that involve cognitive change. It is also provocative for the advanced reader.

Rogers, C.: On becoming a person, Boston, 1961, Houghton Mifflin Co.

Personal growth is the focus of this text, and Rogers discusses it from the point of view of the individual as well as the therapist in a helping relationship. The text is a compilation of important papers that are addressed to a variety of mental health disciplines. It is highly recommended reading.

Rubin, T.: Compassion and self-hate, New York, 1975, David McKay Co., Inc.

Two opposing forces are explored in this text—compassion and self-hate. The author believes that a therapeutic relationship that reduces self-hate and enhances compassion contributes to human growth and the enhancement of inner peace. The text is written in a conversational manner but is provocative and stimulating in content.

Salkin, J.: Body ego technique, Springfield, Ill., 1973, Charles C Thomas, Publisher.

Body ego technique represents an educational and therapeutic approach to the normal development of body image and self-identity. The author gives an in-depth account of procedures, materials, and technique and describes how to use the elements of movement, rhythm, space, and force to facilitate the development of ego strength. The text is explicit and is a useful reference for interventions related to dance and body movement.

Searles, H.: Anxiety concerning change, as seen in the psychotherapy of schizophrenic patients—with particular reference to the sense of personal identity, Int. J. Psychoanal. **42**:74, Feb. 1961.

The author proposes that change for the schizophrenic patient threatens his sense of identity, which is tenuous and precarious. Developmental factors are explored, and implications for therapy are presented. It is advanced reading for the nurse therapist.

Stein, M., Vidich, A., and White, D., editors: Identity and anxiety, New York, 1960, The Free Press of Glencoe.

This book explores contemporary threats to authentic identity. Part I defines and examines identity and anxiety. Part II traces the threats to stable identity imposed by political and social upheavals. Part III explores the challenge of evolving a personal style within a mass society. This is substantial reading for the advanced student or practitioner.

Yorburg, B.: Sexual identity, New York, 1974, John Wiley & Sons, Inc.

The author draws on biology, anthropology, history, psychology, and sociology to explore the conceptions of ideal masculine and feminine behavior and emotions. Her belief is that in any particular society these learned, sex-typed role definitions and expectations result in differing basic self-images or sexual identities for men and women. The particular ramifications of the contemporary sexual identity of women are analyzed.

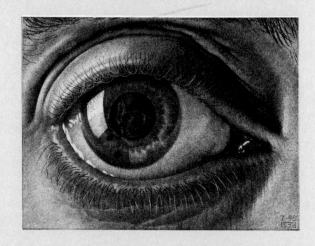

Lying awake, calculating the future,
Trying to unweave, unwind, unravel
And piece together the past and the future,
Between midnight and dawn, when the
past is all deception,
The future futureless . . .

T.S. Eliot

CHAPTER 15

DISTURBANCES OF MOOD

LEARNING OBJECTIVES

After studying this chapter, the student should be able to:

- define mood, its four adaptive functions, and the continuum of emotional responses.

- identify the characteristics that lead to the recognition of severe disturbances of mood.

- describe the concepts of grief, the delayed grief reaction, depression, and mania.

- discuss the predisposing factors that have been proposed for the origin of disturbances of mood.

- analyze precipitating stressors that contribute to the development of disturbances of mood.

- state the value of a unified multicausal model of disturbances of mood.

- identify and describe behaviors and coping mechanisms that are associated with uncomplicated grief reactions, delayed grief reactions, depression, and mania.

- formulate individualized nursing diagnoses for patients with disturbances of mood.

- assess the relationship between nursing diagnoses and medical diagnoses associated with disturbances of mood.

- develop long-term and short-term individualized nursing goals for patients who are experiencing disturbances of mood.

- apply therapeutic nurse-patient relationship principles with appropriate rationale in planning the care of a patient who is experiencing a disturbance of mood.

- describe nursing interventions appropriate to the needs of the patient who is experiencing an uncomplicated grief reaction, depression, or mania.

- develop a mental health education plan to promote a patient's adaptive emotional responses.

- assess the importance of the evaluation of the nursing process when working with patients with disturbances of mood.

- identify directions for future nursing research.

- select appropriate readings for further study.

Variations or fluctuations in mood are a dominant feature of human existence. They indicate that a person is perceiving his world about him and responding to it on some level. Extremes in mood have also been linked with extremes in the human experience, such as creativity, madness, despair, ecstasy, romanticism, personal charisma, and interpersonal destructiveness. These extremes in mood appear to have captured the interest, fascination, and curiosity of scientists, philosophers, and novelists alike, who romanticize, study, and exaggerate the possible alliance between mood, deep emotional experience, and talent.

In this text, **mood** refers to a prolonged emotional state that influences one's whole personality and life functioning. It pertains to one's prevailing and pervading emotion and is synonymous with the terms of affect, feeling state, and emotion. As with other aspects of the personality, emotions or moods serve an adaptive role for the individual.

The four adaptive functions of emotions have been identified as social communication, physiological arousal, subjective awareness, and psychodynamic defense.[36] The components of affective communication, such as crying, posture, facial expression, and touch, promote early mother-child attachment and the later formation of other interpersonal bonds. Depressive mood states also initiate physiological arousal involving the central nervous system, biogenic amines, and neuroendocrine systems. Theories regarding the protective function of the resulting conservation-withdrawal response with decreased activity have been postulated. The subjective components of human emotions are believed to play important functions in goal setting and in the monitoring of current behavior, particularly in judging personal reality against internalized values and goals. Finally, the fourth adaptive function of emotions is in aiding one's psychodynamic defense on both the conscious and unconscious levels.

Continuum of emotional responses

The variety of emotions one can experience, such as fear, joy, anxiety, love, anger, sadness, and surprise, are all normal accompaniments of the human condition. The problem arises in trying to evaluate when a person's mood or emotional state is maladaptive, abnormal, or unhealthy. Grief, for example, is a healthy adaptive separative process that attempts to overcome the stress of a loss. Grief work, or mourning, therefore, is not a pathological process. It is an adaptive response to a real stressor. The absence of grieving in the face of a loss is suggestive of maladaptation.

If one views the expression of emotions on a continuum of health and illness, some relevant parameters become apparent (Fig. 15-1). At the adaptive, or healthy, end is emotional responsiveness. This involves being affected by, and being an active participant in, one's internal and external worlds. It implies being open to one's feelings and aware of them. If used in such a way, feelings provide us with valuable learning experiences. They are barometers that give a person feedback about himself and his relationships with others, and they help a person function more effectively in his world. Also adaptive in the face of stress is an uncomplicated grief reaction. Such a reaction implies that the person is facing the reality of his loss and is immersed in the work of grieving.

A maladaptive response would be the suppression of emotions. This may be evident as a denial of one's feelings, a detachment from them, or an internalization of all aspects of one's affective world. Although a transient suppression of feelings may, at times, be necessary to cope, such as in an initial response to a death or tragedy, prolonged suppression of emotions, such as in delayed grief reaction, will ultimately interfere with effective functioning.

The most maladaptive emotional responses or severe mood disturbances can be recognized by their intensity, pervasiveness, persistence, and interference with usual social and physiological functioning. These characteristics apply to the severe emotional states of depression and mania, which complete the maladaptive end of the continuum of emotional responses.

Nursing intervention in disturbances of mood requires an understanding of a range of emotional states. To assist in this process, the phenomena of grief, the delayed grief reaction, depression, and mania will now be briefly described.

■ Grief

Grief is the subjective state that follows loss. It is one of the most powerful emotional states experienced by an individual and it affects all aspects of one's life. It forces the person to stop his normal activities and to focus on his present feelings and needs. Most commonly, it is the response to loss of a loved person through death or separation, but it also occurs following the loss of something tangible or intangible that is highly regarded. It may be a valued object, a cherished possession, an ideal, a job, or status. As a response to the loss of a loved one, grief is a universal reaction experienced by everyone at some time in life. As one's interdependence on others grows, there is an increased chance that one must face loss, separation, and death, which elicits intense feelings of grief. The capacity to form warm satisfying relationships with others also makes one vulnerable to sadness, despair, and grief when those relationships are terminated.

As a natural reaction to a life experience, grief is universal. It involves stress, pain, and suffering and an impairment of the capacity to function that can last for days, weeks, or months. The understanding of grief and its manifestations has become of great practical importance. As Noyes commented:

With research linking bereavement to increased morbidity and mortality, grief has emerged as a model of psychosocial stress to be understood in terms of its impact on physical and emotional health.[48:137]

The ability to experience grief is gradually formed in the course of normal development and is closely related to the acquisition of the capacity for developing

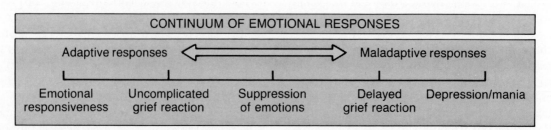

Fig. 15-1. Continuum of emotional responses.

meaningful object relationships. The process of growth and development is a series of goal attainments marked by emotional withdrawals from previous positions and reinvestment in new prospects that are thought to offer increased security. Progress is stimulated by physiological growth, which provides new abilities, strengths, and skills, as well as by encouragement and reinforcement from parents and significant others. Goals become more complex, and conflicts in life's choices create inner stress, turmoil, pressure, and unrest. Energies previously turned inward are projected to external objects. If the gratification obtained from the external object is relatively complete and fulfilling, the external object is valued as necessary to the self and is loved. If there is a change in the object, gratification ceases and readjustment is necessary. The person may withdraw within himself, feel isolated, and become preoccupied with his own person and feelings. This is a part of the grieving process. It is resolved only when the lost object is internalized, bonds of attachment are loosened, and new object relationships are established.

Grief responses may be either uncomplicated and adaptive or morbid and pathological. Uncomplicated grief runs a consistent course that is modified by the abruptness of the loss, one's preparation for the event, and the significance of the lost object. It is a self-limited process of realization; it makes real the fact of the loss.

■ Delayed grief reaction

A maladaptive, or pathological, response to loss implies that something has prevented it from running its normal course. Two types of pathological grief reactions have been identified by Lindemann—the delayed reaction and the distorted reaction.[42] Depression is one type of a distorted grief reaction.

Persistent absence of any emotion may signal an undue delay in the work of mourning, or a delayed grief reaction. The delay may occur in the beginning of the mourning process or become evident in a retarding of the process once it has begun or both. The delay and rejection of grief may occasionally involve many years. The underlying emotions associated with the loss may be triggered by a deliberate recall of circumstances surrounding the loss or by a spontaneous occurrence in the patient's life. A classic example of this is the anniversary reaction in which the person experiences incomplete or abnormal mourning at the time of the loss only to have the grieving response recur at anniversaries of the original loss.

■ Depression

The individual who does not engage in the process of mourning can experience a pathological grief reaction known as depression, or melancholia. It is an abnormal extension or overelaboration of sadness and grief. Depression is the oldest and most frequently described psychiatric illness. It has been recognized and described since as early as 1500 BC, and it appears to be part of the human condition that is familiar to all and yet mysterious to many. The term "depression" is used in a variety of ways. It can refer to a sign, symptom, syndrome, emotional state, reaction, disease, or clinical entity. In this chapter it will be viewed as a clinical entity that is severe, abnormal, maladaptive, and incapacitating in nature.

The Wall Street Journal called depression the disease of the 1970s, and some mental health workers consider it to cause more total suffering and anguish in the world than any other single medical or psychiatric illness. Depression may range from mild and moderate states to severe states with psychotic features. Psychotic depression is relatively uncommon, however, accounting for less than 10% of all depressions. It is estimated that 15% to 30% of adults experience clinical depressive episodes, most often of moderate severity, at some point in their lives, with the onset of depressive illness peaking in the 40s and 50s. However, only 25% of persons with depressive symptoms seek mental health professional attention. Furthermore, 50% to 80% of all suicides are attributed to depression, and perhaps as much as 75% of all psychiatric hospitalizations.[63]

There is also an almost universal trend, independent of country, of the greater prevalence of depression among women than among men in a fairly consistent female-to-male ratio of 2:1. Other risk factors for depression are having a family history of depression or alcoholism; having childhood experiences in a disruptive, hostile, and generally negative home environment; having had recent negative life events, particularly exits; lacking an intimate, confiding relationship; and having had a baby in the past six months.[54,71]

Research has also revealed the high incidence of depression among patients hospitalized for medical illnesses, as well as the fact that these depressions are largely unrecognized and hence untreated by health care personnel. Depression is found in all severities of medical illness, although its intensity and frequency were higher in patients who were more severely ill. Certain types of diseases are frequently associated with depression, especially gastrointestinal (35%), neurological (21%), and respiratory (20%).[63] This research suggests that depression is undoubtedly a common accompaniment of any major medical illness.

At first glance, the grieving person and the depressed person may seem indistinguishable. Both are in despair. Both are unable to be interested in the world around them. Neither can believe the pain and sadness will ever cease. Both may feel life is finished or wish it were, and for both, time is meaningless.

However, there are differences between the states of mourning and depression. Drake and Price[22] believe the difference is the quality of the individual's attachment to the loved object. The degree and nature of the attachment determines the nature of the loss phenomenon and the extent of the depressive reaction to the loss. The disruption of a "normal" attachment results in a sense of loss and grief that is resolved in simple mourning and bereavement. In contrast, disruption of an "inordinate" attachment results in a grieving process that leads into a cycle of depression, since the person is unable to cope with life and function effectively.

Freud made the following distinction between mourning and melancholia:

The distinguishing mental features of melancholia are profoundly painful rejection, abrogation of interest in the outside world, loss of capacity to love, inhibition of all activity, and a lowering of self-regarding to a degree that finds utterances in self reproaches and culminates in a delusional expectation of punishment. . . . with one exception, the same traits are met with in grief. The fall in self-esteem is absent in grief.[25:246]

Many theorists disagree with Freud's position and believe the lowering of self-esteem and ambivalence toward the loved object are present in both reactions. A difference is acknowledged, however, in the level of regression experienced in both reactions as the depressed individual regresses more deeply and fully in response to the loss.

A final difference is apparent in the acknowledgment of the loss. The mourner attends to all things that are connected in any way with the person he mourns.

Although his pain is heightened, it is not meaningless; rather, it is an acknowledgment of the loss, and positive feelings toward the lost object predominate. The depressed individual wishes to deny the loss and separation. Even though his affective responses express sorrow, he continues to deny his need to mourn or even that a need to mourn exists.

■ Mania

In addition to the severely depressed disturbance of mood, one may also experience manic episodes. These episodes, like those of depression, can vary in intensity and accompanying level of anxiety from moderate manic states to severe and panic states with psychotic features. Basically, mania is characterized by a mood that is elevated, expansive, or irritable. The term, **hypomania,** is used to describe a clinical syndrome that is similar to, but not as severe as, that described by the term mania or manic episode.

In the Draft of the DSM-III-R in Development[4] both manic episodes and depressive episodes are contained under the category of mood (affective) disorders. Mania, however, is not given a separate category of classification as is depression. Rather, the major affective disorders are separated into two subgroups—bipolar and depressive disorders—based on whether or not manic and depressive episodes are involved longitudinally (Table 15-1).[4] In this classification, major depression may involve either a single episode or a recurrent depressive illness, but without manic episodes. When there has been one or more manic episodes, with or without a major depressive episode, the category of bipolar disorder is used. Bipolar disorders are subdivided according to the symptoms of the current episode as manic, depressed, or mixed.

TABLE 15-1

CLASSIFICATION OF MOOD (AFFECTIVE) DISORDERS IN DSM-III-R* RELATIVE TO DEPRESSIVE AND MANIC EPISODES

	Depressive disorders		Bipolar disorders		
	Single	Recurrent	Manic	Depressed	Mixed
Depressive episode	Yes	Yes	—	Yes-present	Yes-present
Manic episode	No	No	Yes-present	Yes-past	Yes-present

*American Psychiatric Association: Draft of the DSM-III-R in Development (subject to change), as proposed by the Work Group to Revise DSM-III. American Psychiatric Association, October 1985.

Thus if one experiences a depressive episode with no manic episodes, it would be classified as a depressive disorder. If one experiences a depressive episode with a history of manic episodes in the past or at present, it would be classified as a bipolar disorder.

Although bipolar affective disorders are far less common than depressive disorders, it has been estimated that 0.6% to 0.88% of the adult population has the disorder. Risk factors for bipolar disorder are being female and having a family history of bipolar disorder. The data suggest that people under the age of 50 are at higher risk of a first attack, whereas someone who already has the disorder faces an increased risk of a recurrent manic or depressive episode as he or she grows older.[54]

 ## Assessment

The existence of severe disturbances of mood, such as in depressive and manic episodes, has been accounted for by numerous theories or models of causation. These models identify a variety of predisposing and precipitating factors that may affect the individual's coping response and adjustment. Some of the theories are in conflict with each other, some are not supported by research, and certainly all of them are not applicable to each person. Rather, they present the range of causative factors that may be operative in severe disturbances of mood.

■ Predisposing factors

■ **GENETIC FACTORS.** The first theory addresses genetic aspects of depression. There is wide agreement that both heredity and environmental factors play an important role in depressive illness.[74] Genetic factors related to severe mood disturbances have been investigated in Scandinavia, Germany, Great Britain, and the United States. Four basic techniques of genetic investigation are used: (1) familial aggregation studies, comparing illness rates within and between generations of a particular family; (2) twin studies comparing illness rates in monozygotic and dizygotic twins; (3) general population surveys, comparing illness rates of relatives of depressed patients with those of the general population; and (4) linkage studies, using known genetic markers, such as blood type or color blindness.[36]

Studies using only familial aggregations do not necessarily demonstrate the role of genetics, since the resulting disturbances may be the result of nutritional, infectious, or psychological factors. However, studies using genetic markers, such as blood type or color blindness, suggest that bipolar affective disorder is transmitted by an X-linked dominant gene. There is controversy about the mode of genetic transmission in affective disorders, however, since the findings from other studies contradict this hypothesis and suggest a multifactorial mode of transmission. Most recent research studies suggest that there are different forms of genetic transmission for different forms of mood disorders.

Other evidence from investigations supporting genetic transmission includes an increased frequency of the illness in relatives of the patient compared with the population, a greater concordance rate for the disease in monozygotic twins than in dizygotic twins, an increased frequency of psychiatric abnormalities in relatives of the affective disorder patient than in the general population, and onset of the illness at a characteristic age without any evidence of a precipitating event. One might conclude by saying that good evidence exists for the role of genetic factors in affective disturbances. Additional studies continue to be made in this important area of psychiatric research.

■ **AGGRESSION-TURNED-INWARD THEORY.** The anger-turned-inward theory of Freud[25] views depression as the inward turning of the aggressive instinct, which for some reason is not directed at the appropriate object, with accompanying feelings of guilt. The process is initiated by the loss of an ambivalently loved object. The person feels both angry and loving toward the object at the same time, but he is unable to express his angry feelings because he may be suppressing them, think they are inappropriate or irrational, or may have developed a pattern throughout life of containing feelings, especially ones he views in a negative way. He then directs his angry feelings inward and turns them toward himself. Freud believed that if one went so far as to commit suicide, the self-destructive act was a strike against the hated and loved object as well as against the self.

This theory does not lend itself to empirical verification. Even though it is one of the most widely quoted theories of depression, there is little systematic evidence to substantiate it. Some researchers have identified patients suffering from depression who outwardly express their anger and hostility. Furthermore, the redirection of hostility at outside objects has not been consistently correlated with clinical improvement. In some instances it may actually have negative effects on the patient's view of self and problem resolution. It should therefore be viewed as one possible theory of causation that is not applicable to all people experiencing disturbances of mood.

■ **OBJECT LOSS THEORY.** The object loss theory of depression has been advanced by Bowlby,[13,14] Robertson and Robertson,[58] and Spitz,[66] and it refers to the traumatic separation of the person from significant objects of attachment. Two interrelated issues are important to this theory: loss during childhood as a predisposing factor for the occurrence of adult depressions and separation in adult life as a precipitating stress for depression.

The first issue proposes that a child has ordinarily formed a tie to a mother figure by 6 months of age, and once that tie is ruptured, the child experiences separation anxiety, grief, and the process of mourning. Furthermore, this mourning process of the early years of life frequently affects future personality development and predisposes the child to psychiatric illness. As Bowlby states:

Unfavorable personality development is often to be attributed to one or more of the less satisfactory responses to loss having been provoked during the years of infancy and childhood in such degree, over such length of time, or with such frequency, that a disposition is established to respond to all subsequent losses in a similar way.[14:22]

Evidence for this model was reported by Spitz[66] in 1942 when he described a deprivational reaction in infants separated from their mothers in the second half of the first year of life. The reaction was characterized by apprehension, crying, withdrawal, psychomotor slowing, dejection, stupor, insomnia, anorexia, and gross retardation in growth and development. This syndrome is called anaclitic depression, and it has been questioned whether it is caused by the separation or the adverse effects of institutionalization in an orphanage. A similar separation reaction was described by Robertson and Robertson[58] and Bowlby[13] in older children. They identified three stages of response:

1. A "protest" stage in which the child appeared restless and tearful and searched for his mother
2. A "despair" stage of apathetic withdrawal
3. A "detachment" stage seen in some children who rejected their mothers on reunion

From a research point of view, the connection between early object loss and adult depression can be considered to be unproved. Robertson and Robertson[58] cast doubt on the universality of the behavioral responses described and suggest that appropriate mothering during the separation period can prevent their occurrence. Although studies indicate that, as a group, depressive patients seem to experience more parental loss from death, separation, and other causes than do normal and other diagnostic groups, that factor alone does not seem sufficiently universal to account for all forms of depression. There is even speculation about the beneficial or immunizing effects of having successfully coped with a loss early in development.

■ **PERSONALITY ORGANIZATION THEORY.** Another psychodynamic view of depression focuses on the major psychosocial variable of low self-esteem. The patient's problem of self-concept is an underlying issue, regardless of whether this is expressed as dejection and depression, or overcompensated with an air of supreme competence as displayed in manic and hypomanic episodes. Threats to self-esteem arise for the individual from poor role performance, perceived low-level everyday functioning, and the absence of a clear self-identity.[68]

Three forms of personality organization that could lead to depression have been identified by Arieti.[5] One form of depression, that based on the "dominant other," occurs because the patient has relied on an esteemed other for self-esteem. Satisfaction is experienced only through an intermediary. Clinging, passivity, manipulativeness, and avoidance of anger characterize the person with this type of depression. There is a noticeable lack of personal goals and a predominant focus on problems.

Another form results when a person realizes he may never be able to accomplish a desired, but unrealistic, goal. This is the "dominant goal" type of depression. This person is usually seclusive, arrogant, and often obsessive. He has set unrealistic goals for himself and evaluates them with an all-or-nothing standard. He spends an inordinate amount of time engaged in wishful thinking and introverted searches for meaning.

The third type of depression is manifested as a constant mode of feeling. These patients "inhibit any form of gratification because of strongly held taboos." They experience emptiness, "hypochondriasis, pettiness in interpersonal relationships, and a harsh critical attitude toward themselves and others."[5]

This view of depression looks at the patients' belief systems in relation to their experiences. Even in the absence of an apparent precipitating stressor, their depression appears to be preceded by a severe blow to their self-esteem. It emphasizes the crucial position of one's self-concept in determining adaptation or maladaptation and the importance of the patient's appraisal of his life situation.

■ **COGNITIVE MODEL.** The cognitive model of Beck[7,8,10] proposes that people experience symptoms of depression because their thinking is disturbed. He proposes that depression is a cognitive problem that is dominated by the patient's negative evaluation of himself, his world, and his future. This theory is in contrast to other theories that propose that the depressive affect is primary and the negative cognitive set is secondary. Beck suggests that in the course of his development certain experiences sensitize the individual and make him vulnerable to depression. He also acquires a tendency to make extreme, absolute judgments; loss is viewed as irrevocable and indifference as total rejection.

The depression-prone person, according to this theory, is likely to explain an adverse event as a personal shortcoming. For example, the deserted husband believes "She left me because I'm unlovable," instead of considering the other possible alternatives, such as personality incompatibility, the wife's own problems, or her change in feelings toward him. As he focuses on his personal deficiencies, they expand to the point where they completely dominate his self-concept. He can think of himself only in a negative way and is unable to acknowledge his other abilities, achievements, and attributes. This negative set is reinforced when he interprets ambiguous or neutral experiences as additional proof of his deficiencies. Comparisons with other people further lower his self-esteem, and thus every encounter with others becomes a negative experience. His self-criticisms increase as he views himself as deserving of blame.

Depressed patients become dominated by pessimism; they expect future adversities and experience them as though they were happening in the present or had already occurred. Their predictions tend to be overgeneralized and extreme. Since they view the future as an extension of the present, they expect their failure to continue permanently. Thus pessimism dominates their activities, wishes, and future expectations.

Beck proposes that the constellation of negative thoughts which characterize depression remains relatively dormant until a person becomes depressed. Depressed individuals are capable of logical self-evaluation when not in a depressed mood or when only mildly depressed. When depression does occur, after some precipitating life stressors, the long-dormant negative cognitive set makes its appearance. As depression develops and increases, the negative idiosyncratic thinking increasingly replaces objective thinking.

Although the onset of the depression may appear to be sudden, Beck suggests it develops over weeks as each experience is interpreted as further evidence of failure. As a result of this "tunnel vision," the individual becomes hypersensitive to experiences of loss and defeat and oblivious to experiences of success and pleasure. He has difficulty acknowledging anger, since he thinks he is responsible for, and deserving of, insults from others and problems in living. Along with low self-esteem, he experiences feelings of apathy and indifference. He is drawn to a state of inactivity and withdraws from life. He lacks all spontaneous desire and only wishes to remain passive. Because he expects failure, he lacks the ordinary mobilization of energy to make an effort to achieve.

Suicidal wishes can be viewed as an extreme expression of the desire to escape. The patient sees his life as filled with suffering with no chance of improvement. Given this negative set, suicide seems to be a rational solution. It promises to end his misery and relieve his family of a burden, and he begins to believe that everyone would be better off if he were dead. The more he considers the alternative of suicide, the more desirable it may seem, and as his life becomes more hopeless and painful, the stronger his desires become to end his life.

Naturalistic, clinical, and experimental studies have provided substantial support for this model of depression.[9] The nurse, using this theoretical model in her practice, will find it useful in understanding the personal world of the depressed person and organizing her observations regarding the depressed person's idiosyncratic logic and thinking.

■ **LEARNED HELPLESSNESS MODEL.** The learned helplessness model evolved from Seligman's research with dogs, from which he postulated a theory of human depression. He defines helplessness as a "belief that no one will do anything to aid you and hopelessness a belief that neither you nor anyone else can do anything."[64] His theory proposes that it is not trauma per se that produces depression, but the belief that one has no control over the important outcomes in one's life and therefore the person refrains from making adaptive responses. Learned helplessness is both a behavioral state and a personality trait of a person who believes that he has lost control over the reinforcers in his environment. These negative expectations lead to hopelessness, passivity, and an inability to assert oneself.

Seligman suggests that people resistant to depression have experienced mastery in life. Their childhood experiences proved that their actions were effective in producing gratification and removing annoyances. In contrast, those susceptible to depression have had lives devoid of mastery. Their experiences proved that they were helpless to influence their sources of suffering and gratification or they controlled too many reinforcers that did not allow for the development and use of their coping responses against failure.

Abramson, Seligman, and Teasdale[1] proposed an attributional reformulation of the learned helplessness hypothesis. According to the attributional reformulation, the kinds of causal attributions people make for lack of control influence whether or not their helplessness will entail low self-esteem and whether or not their symptoms of helplessness will generalize across situations and time. According to the reformulation, three attributional dimensions are crucial for explaining human helplessness and depression: internal-external, stable-unstable, and global-specific.

In brief, the reformulated model postulates that attributing lack of control to internal factors leads to lowered self-esteem, whereas attributing lack of control to external factors does not. Attributing lack of control to stable factors should lead to an expectation of uncontrollability in future situations and, consequently, helplessness deficits extended across time. Similarly, attributing lack of control to global factors should lead to an expectation of uncontrollability in other situations and, consequently, helplessness deficits extended across situations. Alternatively, attributing lack of control to unstable specific factors should lead to short-lived situation-specific helplessness deficits.

Abramson, Seligman, and Teasdale summarized the implications of the attributional reformulation for the helplessness model of depression:

1. Depression consists of four classes of deficits: motivational, cognitive, self-esteem, and affective.
2. When highly desired outcomes are believed improbable or highly aversive outcomes are believed probable, and the individual expects that no response in his repertoire will change their likelihood (helplessness), depression results.
3. The generality of depressive deficits will depend on the globality of the attribution for helplessness, the chronicity of the depression deficits will depend on the stability of the attribution for helplessness, and whether self-esteem is lowered will depend on the internality of the attribution for helplessness.
4. The intensity of the deficits depends on the strength, or certainty, of the expectation of uncontrollability and, in the case of the affective and self-esteem deficits, on the importance of the outcome.[1:68]

In concluding a discussion of this model, three points are worth noting. The first is that the attributional reformulation of helplessness and depression bears a significant similarity to Beck's cognitive model of depression previously described. The second point is that this model is proposed as a sufficient, but not necessary, condition for depression, which means that other physiological and psychological factors can produce the symptoms of depression in the absence of an expectation of uncontrollability. Finally, it must be emphasized that the reformulation model is still in the process of being empirically validated.

■ **BEHAVIORAL MODEL.** The behavioral model studied by Lewinsohn[41] is derived from a social learning theory framework in which the cause of depression is assumed to reside in the person-behavior-environment interaction. Social learning theory assumes that psychological functioning can best be understood in terms of continuous reciprocal interactions among personal factors, such as cognitive processes, behavioral factors, and environmental factors, all operating as interdependent determinants of one another. The relative influences exerted by these interdependent factors differ in various settings and for different behaviors.

This theory views people as being capable of exercising considerable control over their own behavior. They do not merely react to external influences. They select, organize, and transform incoming stimuli. Thus people are not viewed as powerless objects controlled by their environments, but neither are they absolutely free to do whatever they choose. Rather, people and their environment are reciprocal determinants of one another.

The concept of reinforcement is crucial to this view of depression. Reinforcement is defined in terms of the quality of one's interactions with one's environment. Person-environment interactions with positive outcomes constitute positive reinforcement. Such interactions strengthen the person's behavior. The experience of little or no rewarding interaction with the environment causes the person to feel sad or blue. Thus the key assumption in this model is that a low rate of positive reinforcement is the historical antecedent of depressive behaviors.

Two particular variables are important in this regard. One is that the individual may fail to provide the appropriate responses to initiate positive reinforcement. The other is that the environment may fail to provide the reinforcement and thus worsen the patient's condition. These variables are often apparent, since depressed patients have been shown to be deficient in the social skills needed to interact effectively with others. In turn, other people find the behavior of the depressed person to be distancing, negative, or offensive and avoid him as much as possible.

Depression is likely to occur if certain positively reinforcing events are absent; particularly those which fall into the following categories[40]:

Positive sexual experiences
Rewarding social interaction
Enjoyable outdoor activities
Solitude
Competence experiences

These may be described as "being sexually attractive," "being with friends," "being relaxed," "doing my job well," and "doing things my own way." It also occurs in the presence of certain punishing events, particularly those which fall into three categories:

Marital discord
Work hassles
Receiving negative reactions from others

This model of depression emphasizes an active, rather than passive, approach to the person and relies heavily on an interactional view of personality. Within this model, social interpersonal behavior, cognitive factors, and self-regulatory mechanisms play important roles, and treatment is aimed at assisting the person to increase the quantity and quality of positively reinforcing interactions with the environment and decrease aversive interactions.

■ **BIOLOGICAL MODEL.** Another major area of research on depression involves a biological model, which explores chemical changes in the body that take place during depressed states. Whether these chemical changes cause depression or are a result of the depression is not yet clearly understood. However, significant abnormalities can be demonstrated in the functioning of many body systems during a depressive illness.[54] These include electrolyte disturbances, especially of sodium and potassium; neurophysiological alterations based on findings from electrophysiological studies using electroencephalography and evoked potential methods; dysfunction and faulty regulation of autonomic nervous system activity; adrenocortical, thyroid, and gonadal changes; and neurochemical alterations in the neurotransmitters, especially in the biogenic amines, which serve as central nervous system and peripheral neurotransmitters.[6] The biogenic amines include three catecholamines—dopamine, norepinephrine, and epinephrine—as well as serotonin and acetylcholine.

Catecholamines. The catecholamine hypothesis states that depression is associated with a deficiency of catecholamines, particularly of norepinephrine, in the central nervous system, and that mania is associated with an excess of catecholamine. This hypothesis is derived in part from the observations that certain drugs, such as the MAO inhibitors and tricyclic antidepressants, which potentiate or increase brain catecholamines, stimulate behavior and relieve depression. In contrast, lithium carbonate, a drug that is effective in the treatment of mania, acts by decreasing the release of norepinephrine and increasing its reuptake. One of the metabolites of norepinephrine, MHPG, has been found to be decreased in the cerebrospinal fluid and urine of depressed patients, thus further supporting this hypothesis. The biogenic amine model is particularly important since it provides links between clinical observations and pharmacological agents that have emerged as effective treatments in mood disorders.

Endocrine dysfunction. The possibility of hormonal causes of depression has been considered for many years. Some of the symptoms of depression that suggest endocrine changes are: decreased appetite, weight loss, insomnia, diminished sex drive, gastrointestinal disorders, and variations of mood. New assay techniques have recently detected alterations of hormone activity concurrent with depression. Mood changes have also been observed with a variety of endocrine disorders including Cushing's disease, hyperthyroidism, and estrogen therapy. Further support for this theory is evident in the high incidence of depression in the postpartum period, when hormonal levels change.

Cortisol. Many depressed patients exhibit hypersecretion of cortisol, and this has been used in the dexamethasone suppression test (DST) (dexamethasone is an exogenous steroid that suppresses the blood level of cortisol). The DST is based on the observation that in patients with biological depression, late afternoon cortisol levels are not depressed after a single dose of dexamethasone. However, many physical illnesses and some medications can interfere with the test results, and thus these results should be viewed only as a research tool at this time.

Biological rhythms. Mood disorders are also typified by periodic variations in physiological and psychological functions. Circadian rhythm shows a periodicity of about 24 hours. All-night sleep studies of depressed patients show some basic abnormalities in their sleep patterns. There is decreased total sleep time, an increased percentage of dream time, difficulty in falling asleep, an increased number of spontaneous awakenings, and a shortened period between sleep onset and the first dreaming period (REM latency period). This last finding is a valuable biological diagnostic index for depression.

Research on the biological model has been extensive and of high quality. It has lent support to a biological basis for mood disorders and suggested biological markers of clinical usefulness in diagnosis and treatment. These tests, such as the urinary MHPG, DST, and REM latency measure are described in greater detail in Chapter 23 of this text under the discussion of antidepressant drugs.

The discovery of neuropharmacological abnormalities is not surprising, nor does it preclude psychological causes as well. Furthermore, a biochemical model based on one amine is undoubtedly an oversimplification. According to Akiskal and McKinney, "biochemical statements that propose a causal relationship between a chemical event in the brain and a set of observable behaviors or subjective experiences present serious philosophical problems,"[3] since neurobiology has dismissed the possibility of such a direct one-to-one relationship.

Although the research in this model of depression is conflicting at times, there is sufficient evidence to suggest that a variety of precipitating stressors can induce changes in biogenic amines, and the neuropharmacological mechanisms that have been investigated might form final common pathways for both psychological and biological causes. Some depressions might be due primarily to neuropharmacological dysfunctions, resulting in reduced norepinephrine; others might be due to events whose psychological effect would presumably have parallel neurophysiological phenomena resulting in reduced release of norepinephrine. In other cases both effects might apply, the life event tipping the balance more easily into depression because activity of the norepinephrine-producing system was already reduced.

■ Precipitating factors

Disturbances of mood are a specific response to stress. Although this statement is undoubtably true, its simplicity tends to mask the full implications of it. For example, there are two major types of stress that a person may experience. The first is the stress of major life events that are evident to others. The second type of stress may not be obvious at all to others, but it is the minor stress or irritations of daily life. These are the small disappointments, frustrations, criticisms, and arguments that, when accumulated over time, and in the absence of compensating positive events produce a major and chronic negative impact. McLean notes:

Nondepressed persons also report high rates for these kinds of stressors, but the critical difference is that, on the average, nondepressed persons experience compensating numbers of positive events and outcomes within the same time period that effectively offset the negative impact of the routine stressors. It is the ratio between negative and positive events and outcomes that is decisive for mood determination.[45:186]

It is appropriate, therefore, to examine in more detail some of the sources of life stressors that may produce disturbances of mood. Five such sources include loss of attachment, major life events, roles, coping resources, and physiological changes.

■ LOSS OF ATTACHMENT.

Loss in adult life can be a precipitating stressor for depression. The loss may be real or imagined and may include the loss of love, a person, physical functioning, status, or self-esteem. Many losses take on importance because of their symbolical meaning, which makes the reactions to them appear to be out of proportion to reality. In this sense, even an apparently pleasurable event, such as moving to a new home, may involve the loss of old friends, warm memories, and neighborhood associations. Loss of hope is another significant loss that is often overlooked. Because of the actual and symbolical elements involved in the concept of loss, the patient's perception takes on primary importance.

The individual is constantly experiencing losses and thus continually struggling with the tasks of integrating them. The intensity of a person's grief reaction only becomes meaningful when one understands his earlier losses and separations. A person who is reacting to a recent loss is behaving as he did in previous separations. The intensity of the present reaction therefore becomes more understandable when one realizes that the reaction is not only to the present loss but to earlier losses as well. Loss by definition is negative, a deprivation. But the ability to sustain, integrate, and recover from loss is a sign of personal maturity and growth.

Uncomplicated grief reactions can be considered to be the process of normal mourning or simple bereavement. Mourning includes a complex sequence of psychological processes and their behavioral manifestations. It is accompanied by the subjective experiences of anxiety, anger, pain, despair, and hope. The sequence is not a smooth unvarying course, however. It is filled with turmoil, regressions, and potential problems. Certain factors have been identified that influence the outcome of the mourning process[50]:

Childhood experiences (especially the loss of significant others)

Losses experienced later in life

Previous history of psychiatric illness (especially depression)

Life crises prior to the loss

Nature of the relationship with the lost person or object, including kinship, strength of attachment, security of attachment, dependency-independency bonds, and intensity of ambivalence

Process of dying (when applicable), including age of deceased, timeliness, previous warnings, preparation for bereavement, expression of feelings, and preventability of the loss

Social support systems

Secondary stresses

Emergent life opportunities

These should be assessed by the nurse for each person experiencing a loss. Two of the factors—the nature of the relationship with the lost person or object, and the mourner's perception of the preventability of the loss—have been identified as prime predictors of the intensity and duration of the bereavement.[17] Concurrent crises, the circumstances of the loss, and a pathological relationship with the lost person or object are all factors that contribute to a failure to successfully resolve grief.[43]

Inhibiting factors. Loss of a loved one has been identified as a major precipitating stressor for grief reactions. Most individuals resolve this loss through simple bereavement and do not experience pathological grief reactions or depression. A number of external and internal factors, however, can inhibit the process of mourning. An external factor may be the immersion of the mourner in practical, necessary tasks that accompany the loss but which are not directly connected to the emotional fact of the loss. These tasks may include funeral arrangements, completing the unfinished business of the deceased, or being forced to search for immediate employment and sources of support. All these tasks foster denial of the loss, which also may be encouraged by cultural norms that minimize or negate the finality of the loss. The American norm of "courage in the face of adversity" can prevent the mourner from any open display of grief.

Mourning may also be inhibited when the bereaved does not receive support from his social network or support systems. Nonsupportiveness that suppresses grieving can be evident when significant others inhibit the mourner's expression of sadness, anger, and guilt, block his review of the lost relationship, and attempt to orient him too quickly to the future. Finally, the widespread use of tranquilizers and antidepressant medications may serve to suppress normal grief and encourage the development of pathological grief reactions.

Internal factors that inhibit mourning are often fostered by social learning that encourages the control and hiding of feelings. Crying, for example, may be seen as a sign of weakness and something to be avoided, especially in men. Two emotions are particularly repressed and suppressed in our society—grief and anger—and this may create many emotional problems for the individual. Another inhibiting factor is the belief that the quantity and quality of emotion is so unique that it cannot be effectively communicated through verbal or nonverbal channels. Both these factors lead to suppression of the mourning process and rely heavily on the intellectual concepts of behavior.

In concluding this discussion of loss as a precipitating stressor, it is necessary to place it in proper perspective based on research in this area. Some studies have failed to demonstrate a relationship between loss and depression.[18] Other studies support the relationship but suggest that depression may be the cause of alienation and object loss and not vice versa.[31] Thus the following conclusions may be proposed:

1. Loss and separation events are prominent among the possible precipitating stressors of depression.
2. Loss and separation are not universal in all depressions.
3. Not all people who experience loss and separation will develop depressions.
4. Loss and separation are not specific to depression but may serve as precipitating events for a wide variety of psychiatric and medical illnesses.
5. Loss and separation may result from depression.

■ **MAJOR LIFE EVENTS.** Holmes and Rahe[29] did the pioneering work in this area with the development of the Social Readjustment Rating Scale described in Chapter 3. Subsequently, others have used this approach for measurement of stress concentrations experienced by people who have become depressed shortly thereafter.

Research conducted by Paykel and co-workers[52] on life events and depression reveals that, on the average, depressed patients reported the occurrence of nearly three times as many important life events during the 6 months before the onset of their clinical depressive episode as did normal subjects. The events included loss of self-esteem, interpersonal discord, socially undesirable occurrences, and major disruptions of life patterns. The authors found that those events perceived as undesirable were most often the precipitants of depression. He further categorized the events into "exit" events, which involved separation and interpersonal losses, and "entrance" events, which involved the introduction of a new person into the social sphere of the subject. Analysis of the data showed that exit events more frequently than entrance events were followed by worsening of psychiatric symptoms, physical health changes, impairment of social role performance, and depressive illnesses in particular. The concept of exit events in his study overlaps with the psychiatric concept of loss.

Most psychiatric clinicians are convinced that a relationship does exist between stressful life events and depression. Some believe that life events play the primary or major role in depression; others are more conservative, limiting the role of life events to that of contributing to the onset and timing of the acute episode. Any definitive conclusions, however, should be made with caution. The fact is that all people experience stressful life events, but not all people become depressed. This suggests that specific events can contribute only partially to the onset or the development of depression. Wender[72] noted that, when the incidence of a single event to account for the disease is low, as with affective disorders, the power of a single event to account for the disease is relatively limited. Thus, in an analysis of loss in relation to depression, exits from the social field occurred in 25% of depressives and 5% of controls. Exits preceded depression in only a small, although substantial, number of depressive cases. Furthermore, less than 20% of the population experiencing exits became clinically depressed. This evidence suggests that other factors

TABLE 15-2

SUMMARY OF ILFELD'S FINDINGS ON SOCIAL ROLE STRESSORS AND DEPRESSION

	Employed married fathers	Employed married mothers	Unemployed married mothers	Employed single men	Employed single women
Stressors (in degree of magnitude)	Marriage Job Financial Parental Neighborhood	Marriage Parental Financial Neighborhood Job Homemaking	} equal } equal	< Marriage Homemaking < Parental < Financial Neighborhood	Singlehood Financial Neighborhood Job	Financial Singlehood

Data from Ilfeld, F.: Am. J. Psychiatry **134**:161, Feb. 1977.

must also be significant in the development of disturbances of mood.

A recent study supporting such a conclusion was conducted by Nezu and Ronan, who proposed a conceptual model in which the negative life events experienced by an individual influence depression directly as well as indirectly through their impact on the frequency of current problems and one's level of problem-solving ability.[47] Their model was supported as a strong predictor of depressive symptoms, and has implications for nurses engaged in treatment and prevention activities.

■ **ROLES.** The relationship between role strain and depression has gained popularity with the emergence of the women's movement in American society. Women have higher rates of depression, and various theories have been proposed linking depression with various aspects of women's lives. For example, Beck[11] examined learned helplessness and prejudice as possible explanations for depression in women. Very few research studies, however, have explored the relationship between role strain and depression.

The most notable work in this area has been done by Ilfeld who developed nine scales to measure current social stressors defined as "those circumstances or conditions of daily social roles which are generally considered to be problematic or undesirable."[32] These scales measure ongoing stressful experiences instead of single "events" that occurred in the past. They include stressors from the social role areas of neighborhood, job, financial affairs, homemaking, parenting, marriage, singlehood, unemployment, and retirement. The survey population was divided into five subgroups to compare the relative potency of different social stressors and the differential

effects of any one stressor across each population. He found that current social stressors are significantly related to depressive symptoms for each of the five groups.

Table 15-2 presents a summary of the five subgroups and a ranking of the stressors for each group in order of magnitude of stress from the greatest to the least.[33] These findings indicate that current marital/singlehood stressors have the highest correlation for all groups except single employed women. Parenting, job, and financial stressors were intermediate in association. The parenting scale, however, was constructed only for parents who had a child 6 years or older. Therefore they did not assess the role strain associated with parenting children under 6 years of age. Also, homemaking was not assessed for men, only women.

Marriage. It is possible to analyze each social role stressor in more detail. It becomes obvious in doing so that much of the literature focuses on women. This is a reflection of the predominance of depression among women as compared to men and the increasing interest in women's changing roles in contemporary society. Role strain associated with marriage emerges as a major stressor related to depression for both men and women. Jacob and co-workers[34] studied role expectation and role performance in distressed and nondistressed couples and found that nondistressed couples reported (1) greater satisfaction, pleasure, and fidelity in sexual relationships with spouses, (2) more shared activities and positive emotional interchanges, and (3) greater wife influence in various areas of family decision making. Gove[27] studied the rates of mental illness among married men and women. He found higher rates of mental illness for married women, whereas single, divorced, and widowed women have lower rates than men. From this, he concludes that being married has a protective effect for males but a detrimental effect for females.

Parenting. Another explanation for differences in rates of mental illness, particularly depression, between men and women may be the role strain inherent in parenting. LeMasters[38] and Dyer[23] found an "extreme crisis reaction" to the birth of the first child in many young mothers, particularly those with extensive professional training or work experience. Cohen[20] found more pregnancy-related emotional problems in multiparas than in primiparas, commenting that it looked as though these mothers had realized that pregnancy and parenting were sources of conflict and dissatisfaction.

An interesting finding in this regard reported by Ilfeld[33] is the relatively low position of parenting as a social role stressor for employed married men and unemployed married women as compared to its primary ranking along with marriage as a social role stressor for employed married women (Table 15-2). This finding is interesting, especially since it includes only those individuals with children over 6 years of age. It suggests an interaction and possible role strain between parenting and employment for women.

Work. Additional research also shows that married career women have, or need, supportive husbands.[55,56] The nature of this support, however, is not clearly described in the literature. Much of the literature on two-career families directly documents the additive nature of the mother's role, that is, the assumption of a career role in addition to her domestic role.[30] Ilfeld[33] did not even include homemaking as a social role for men. Division of household labor did emerge as an important aspect of Rosenfield's study.[61] She examined the relationship between depressive symptoms and traditional and nontraditional sex-role relationships in the family in terms of division of labor. In nontraditional relationships, males were found to have higher levels of depressive symptoms than females. She suggests that this gives further support to a sex-role basis for sex differences in depressive symptoms.

In a nursing research study, Woods explored employment, family roles, and mental health in young married women.[75] She found that the number of women's roles was not associated with poorer mental health, nor was there a clear relationship between employment or parenting and mental health. She did find, however, that women who had traditional sex role norms, little task-sharing support from a spouse, and little support from a confidant had poorer mental health than their counterparts. In addition, for women who were both spouse and parent, support from a confidant was most important. Task-sharing support was the most important for

women who were employed but not parents, and nontraditional sex role norms had the most important protective effects on mental health for women who had multiple roles as spouse, employee, and mother.

Clearly, the relationship between role strain and depression merits further exploration. Research in this area, however, must take into account the complexity of factors involved in causal or interactive relationships. Stuart has identified these as follows[67]:

1. *Predisposing factors.* Important variables include sex, marital status, income, age, education, type of occupation, social position, level of social integration, past experiences (particularly history of disturbances of mood), and a sense of mastery over one's own fate or locus of control.

2. *Role strain as a precipitating stress.* Measurements should provide for identification of roles; type of role strain experienced (role conflict, ambiguity, discontinuity, or overload); magnitude, intensity, and unpredictability of strain; degree of control over roles; duration of role strain (short term vs. habitual pattern or personality characteristic); and interaction among roles.

3. *Affective significance of role strain.* The meaning or significance of the role strain experienced should be placed within the context of the need-value system of the individual.

4. *Coping-defensive patterns available.* Focus should be placed on the individual's social support systems that might act as buffers, including family members and a community of significant others who express shared values. The marital relationship merits particular emphasis through examining the supportiveness of the spouse, ways in which this support is expressed, power relationships within the marriage, and levels of marital satisfaction and intimacy.

5. *Illness outcome.* In addition to depressive symptoms, one might assess the length and intensity of disability, areas of impaired functioning, and long-term consequences of the depression (i.e., role strain that induces depression might serve to legitimize future role failure).

6. *Adaptive outcome.* Research in this area would assess specific coping strategies used by individuals to handle role strain, including division and delegation of responsibilities, changing expectations, clarifying goals, and use of social resources. Research of this nature would have direct implications for planning and implementing preventive and therapeutic interventions in the future.

■ **COPING RESOURCES.** Life stress may also take the form of inadequate coping resources. Personal resources available to individuals include their socioeconomic status (income, occupation, social position, and education), families (nuclear and extended), interpersonal networks, and the secondary organizations provided by the broader social environment. The far-ranging effects of poverty, discrimination, inadequate housing, and social isolation cannot be ignored or taken lightly. The results of three studies are relevant in this regard.

In the first study Myers, Lindenthal, and Pepper[46] report that the level of social integration is associated with the relationship between life events and psychiatric symptoms and changes in that relationship over 2 years. In particular, those who report few life events but significant symptoms are less well integrated than those who report few symptoms but many events. Three particular deficiencies in social networks or support systems serve to increase the individual's vulnerability to stress—social isolation, social marginality, and status inconsistency.

The second study, which takes into consideration these issues, was reported by Brown and Harris.[15] Using data collected from a community survey in London, they examined the relationship between psychosocial stress and subsequent affective disorders among women. They found that working-class married women with young children at home had the highest rates of depression. They were five times more likely to become depressed than middle-class women given equal levels of stress. Four factors were found to be significant in this regard: loss of a mother in childhood, three or more children under age 14 living at home, absence of an intimate and confiding relationship with a husband or boyfriend, and lack of full- or part-time employment outside the home. The first three factors were more frequent among working-class women. Confidants other than a spouse or boyfriend did not have a protective effect. Rather, an important factor in preventing depression in the presence of stress was the amount of emotional support the husband or boyfriend gave the woman and the general levels of satisfaction and intimacy inherent in the relationship. Employment outside the home was seen to provide a protective effect by alleviating boredom, increasing self-esteem, improving financial affairs, and increasing social contacts. This is the type of research needed to answer etiological questions regarding life stress and illness.

A final and most important study was conducted by Warheit[70] on the relationship between life-event losses, coping resources, and depressive symptoms. The major findings of the research can be summarized as follows:

1. Persons having high life-event loss scores had higher depression scores than those with low to moderate loss scores.
2. The presence of a spouse was significantly correlated with lower depression scores for all groups. The presence of relatives nearby was not significant. The availability of friends was significantly correlated with lower depression scores for the high-loss group.
3. Low socioeconomic status (SES) was significantly correlated with higher depression scores. It was also found that 64.8% of those in the low SES group were in the high-loss group, compared with 31.1% of those in the high SES group. The data suggest that low SES places persons in double jeopardy; they have fewer resources with which to cope and experience more losses.
4. A series of regression equations showed that losses, absence of resources, and preexisting depressive symptoms were powerful predictors of depression scores. Of these variables, the most powerful predictor was preexisting depressive symptoms, followed by absence of resources (including personal, familial, social, cultural, and socioeconomic status). Life-event loss scores had the lowest predictive value.

The author concludes that these data illustrate the complex nature of the interrelationships between life events, coping resources, and depressive symptoms:

The findings suggest that while life-event losses and the absence of personal and social resources are related to high depression scale scores, other factors are statistically (and probably theoretically) more important sources of explanation of depressive symptomatology. The findings also suggest that for some persons, at least, depressive symptomatology is a trait condition that may predispose them to life events which in turn exacerbate their preevent levels of psychiatric distress. The data also indicate that life-event losses are mitigated somewhat by the availability of personal, familial, interpersonal, and other resources; this finding has implications for early therapeutic intervention designed to assist those experiencing significant life-event losses.[70:507]

■ **PHYSIOLOGICAL CHANGES.** Disturbances in mood may also occur as a response to physiological changes produced by drugs or a wide variety of physical illnesses. These are summarized in Table 15-3. Drug-induced depressions have been noted to occur following treatment with various antihypertensive drugs, partic-

---

TABLE 15-3

PHYSICAL ILLNESSES AND DRUGS ASSOCIATED WITH DEPRESSIVE AND MANIC STATES

	Depression	Mania
Infectious	Influenza	Influenza
	Viral hepatitis	St. Louis encephalitis
	Infectious mononucleosis	Q fever
	General paresis (tertiary syphilis)	General paresis (tertiary syphilis)
	Tuberculosis	
Endocrine	Myxedema	Hyperthyroidism?
	Cushing's disease	
	Addison's disease	
Neoplastic	Occult abdominal malignancies (e.g., carcinoma of head of pancreas)	
Collagen	Systemic lupus erythematosus	Systemic lupus erythematosus
		Rheumatic chorea
Neurological	Multiple sclerosis	Multiple sclerosis
	Cerebral tumors	Diencephalic and third ventricular tumors
	Sleep apnea	
	Dementia	
	Parkinson's disease	
	Nondominant temporal lobe lesions	
Nutritional	Pellagra	
	Pernicious anemia	
Drugs	Steroidal contraceptives	Steroids
	Reserpine	Levodopa
	Alpha-methyl-dopa	Amphetamines
	Physostigmine	Methylphenidate
	Alcohol	Cocaine
	Sedative-hypnotics	Monoamine oxidase inhibitors
	Amphetamine withdrawal	Tricyclics
		Thyroid hormones

From Whybrow P., Akiskal, H., and McKinney, W.: Mood disorders: toward a new psychobiology, New York, 1984, Plenum Press.

---

ularly reserpine, and the abuse of addictive substances, such as amphetamines, barbiturates, and alcohol.[73] Depression may also occur secondary to a wide variety of medical illnesses, for example, viral infections, nutritional deficiencies, endocrine disorders, anemias, and central nervous system disorders, such as multiple sclerosis, tumors, and cerebral vascular disease. Most chronic debilitating illnesses—whether physical or psychiatric—that cause pain and limit one's functioning and social interaction are also frequently accompanied by depression.

The depressions of the elderly are particularly complex because the differential diagnosis often involves organic brain damage and clinical depression. The diagnostic differentiation is complicated by the fact that persons with early signs of senile brain changes, vascular disease, or other neurological diseases associated with age may be more at risk for depression than is the general population. In the United States there has been a tendency to overdiagnose arteriosclerosis and senility in persons over 65, without recognizing that depression may manifest itself by a slowing of psychomotor activity, a reduction of intellectual functioning, a decrease in concentrating ability, and a loss of interest in sex, hobbies, and activities, changes that may be taken as signs of brain damage.[36]

Mania has also been found to occur secondary to drugs, particularly steroids, amphetamines, and tricyclic antidepressants. It can also be triggered by infections, neoplasms, and metabolic disturbances. The evidence that mania can result from a variety of pharmacological, structural, and metabolic disturbances suggests that ma-

---

TABLE 15-4

SUMMARY OF MODELS OF CAUSATION OF SEVERE MOOD DISTURBANCES

Model	Mechanism
Genetic	Transmission through heredity and family history
Aggression turned inward	Turning of angry feelings inward against oneself
Object loss	Separation from loved one and disruption of attachment bond
Personality organization	Negative self-concept and low self-esteem influence one's belief system and appraisal of stressors
Cognitive	Hopelessness experienced because of negative cognitive set
Learned helplessness	Belief that one's responses are ineffectual, and reinforcers in the environment cannot be controlled
Behavioral	Loss of positive reinforcement in life
Biological	Impaired monoaminergic neurotransmission
Life stressors	Response to life stress from five possible sources: loss of attachment, major life events, roles, coping resources, and physiological changes
Integrative	Interaction of chemical, experiential, and behavioral variables acting on the diencephalon

---

nia, like depression, is a clinical syndrome with multiple causes. The diversity of causes probably involves more than one pathophysiological pathway and challenges any unitary model of causation, whether the proposed factor of causation be biochemical, psychological, genetic, or structural.

■ Integrative model

There is continuing debate throughout psychiatry over the nature of depression—that is, whether depression is a single illness with different signs and symptoms or whether there are several different diseases. This discussion of the various models or theories of causation of severe mood disturbances also suggests the controversies in psychiatric research and practice. Each of these theories contributes to an understanding of mood disturbances. It it obvious that many of them overlap and interrelate. It is also clear from recent research that there are multiple causes for mood disturbances involving an interactive effect among predisposing and precipitating factors that are biological and psychosocial in origin. Thus a unitary theory is not possible, but perhaps a unified theory is. Table 15-4 summarizes these major theories on causation.

Akiskal and McKinney and Whybrow[2,3,73] have presented a unified model of mood disorders that attempts to integrate the various conceptual models which now exist. They view depression as the feedback interaction of three sets of variables at the chemical, experiential, and behavioral levels, with the diencephalon serving as the field of action. They propose that impairment in one of the variables affects the other two. Thus any one of the three variables can contribute to a depression and produce changes in the other two areas. For example, a chemical imbalance can result in distorted perceptions, or a major life change can cause a chemical imbalance. In their model, depressive illness is the culmination of various processes that converge in those areas of the diencephalon that modulate arousal, mood, motivation, and psychomotor functions. As depicted in Fig. 15-2, the specific form the illness will take depends on the interaction of the following factors:

1. Genetic vulnerability—important particularly in recurrent and manic-depressive illnesses
2. Developmental events—early object loss that may sensitize the individual to future stress, create negative cognitive sets, and originate experiences resulting in learned helplessness
3. Physiological stressors—stimuli such as viral infections and childbirth that induce biochemical changes
4. Psychosocial stressors—stressful life events that overwhelm the coping mechanisms of the individual

This integrative multicausal model presents a useful frame of reference for the nurse because it is holistic in nature and encourages the assessment of behavior in developing appropriate nursing interventions. It also presents a variety of causative factors and stresses the interrelationship of them in explaining present behavior. Obviously predisposing factors are important, and the way in which they interact with the precipitating event is crucial in determining whether a severe mood disturbance will result. Such an integrated model is most valuable for the nurse to utilize when completing a patient assessment and implementing nursing care.

■ Behaviors

■ ASSOCIATED WITH UNCOMPLICATED GRIEF REACTIONS.

The successful resolution of uncomplicated grief reactions follows, to some degree, a sequence of phases or steps by which the nurse can determine if healing is occurring. Knowledge of behaviors associated with the normal process of mourning allows the nurse to provide supportive interventions, as well as identify maladaptive responses, if they should occur. Various theorists have identified stages of grief and mourning, including Bowlby,[14] Kübler-Ross,[37] and Engel,[24] and there are many similarities among these stages.

A cross-cultural study of grief and mourning in 78 cultures indicated that the mourning process and the accompanying state of grief represent a universal human response.[60] The specific form of emotional expression varies from culture to culture, but an emotionless reaction to the loss of a loved person is rare. Bowlby's phases present a comprehensive review of the process of mourning and they can be applied to losses of any type. These phases of mourning are (1) the urge to recover the lost object, (2) disorganization, and (3) reorganization. Each phase and its emotional component of mourning are briefly described.

Phase 1 is characterized by disequilibrium. Initially the survivor experiences feelings of shock and disbelief. This reaction is followed by a numbed sensation in which the survivor does not acknowledge the reality of the death and hopes to recover his loss. Two of the major affective components of this phase are weeping and anger. Tears are evoked by loss, and crying fulfills an important function in the work of mourning. Crying involves both an acknowledgment of the loss and a regression to a more childlike state. Tears among the survivors are generally accepted, and they elicit certain kinds of support and help from the group, although this varies greatly from culture to culture.

Anger is the other major component of this stage. It may erupt toward nurses or other health care personnel whom the survivor associates with the death. The mourner may also turn this anger on himself, particularly if he feels the death was his responsibility in any way. Guilt is a related emotion as the survivor berates himself for failing to do right by the lost one. The greater the survivor's ambivalence toward the deceased, the greater will be his sense of guilt.

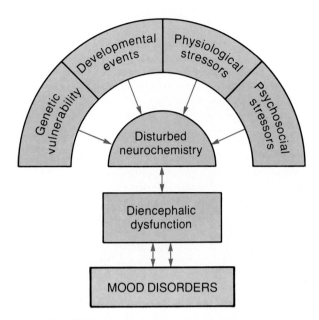

Fig. 15-2. Unified model of mood disorders.

Phase 2 is characterized by disorganization. When the survivor realizes the loss is permanent, despair sets in and his behavior becomes increasingly disorganized and restless. He experiences a loss of self-esteem, and profound feelings of loneliness, fear, and helplessness overwhelm him. This phase is a painful and alarming one for the individual, and he might use the mechanism of denial to protect himself. Symptoms of somatic stress might appear. Lindemann[42] identified the most common ones: (1) the tendency to sighing respirations, (2) the complaint of lack of strength and exhaustion, and (3) the occurrence of digestive difficulties, such as loss of appetite and feeling of emptiness in the stomach. There may be the reactivation of old conflicts such as dependence vs. independence and trust vs. mistrust.

The sensorium is generally altered, and there is a slight feeling of unreality, emotional distance from others, and a preoccupation with the image of the deceased. There may be a recurrent experience of tearful longing for the deceased associated with thoughts, memories, or mental images of him. They may be triggered by any reminder of the lost one and may be especially intense and painful at night. Many survivors have illusions of seeing or feeling the presence of the dead person. In extreme cases this experience takes the form of frank but transient hallucinations. There may be much random activity but an inability to organize and complete specific tasks. Life is devoid of enthusiasm and daily activities proceed in an automatic manner. Social interaction is greatly reduced, and feelings of helplessness may complicate the process of mourning

---

CLINICAL EXAMPLE 15-1

Mrs. G was a 38-year-old married woman who had no history of previous depression. She came to the local community mental health center complaining of "severe throbbing headaches, difficulty falling asleep, fitful and disturbing dreams when asleep, and poor appetite." She said she felt "disgusted" with herself and "useless" to her family. At present she was living alone with her husband.

Her family history revealed that she had three children—two boys and a girl. Her eldest son, age 20, was attending college out of state, and her daughter, 19 years of age, was living with a girl friend in an apartment in the same city. Her youngest son was killed in an automobile accident 2 years ago when he was 15 years old. She described him as her "baby" and expressed much guilt for contributing to her son's death. She scolded herself for allowing him to drive to the shore for the weekend with friends, and said she now worries a great deal about her other two children. She said she was trying to protect them from the dangers of the world, but they resented her advice and concern. On questioning by the nurse, Mrs. G reported that these feelings of sadness and guilt had emerged in the last month and seemed to be triggered by the graduation of her son's high school class.

---

in two ways: there is a sense of powerlessness over restoring the lost person and a helplessness in the face of continuing life without the companionship of the deceased.

Phase 3 is one of reorganization. The survivor no longer lives in the past and begins to break his attachment to the lost person. He establishes new goals and interpersonal relationships. He may incorporate the values, behaviors, and goals of the deceased in an appropriate and satisfying way. He tests out new behavior and expands his own sense of identity.

The successful work of mourning takes 6 months to a year, with the intensity of the initial reaction subsiding after a couple of weeks. Like any other process, it can take one of several courses. Those which enable the individual ultimately to relate to new objects and to find satisfaction in them are commonly judged to be adaptive, or healthy. Those which fail in this outcome are believed to be maladaptive, or pathological.

In recent years attention has been focused on the development of somatic illness and increased mortality as a consequence of the death of or separation from a loved object. The loss of a loved person has been identified as a precipitating factor in the onset or the identification of such diverse diseases as asthma, pulmonary tuberculosis, peptic ulcer, ulcerative colitis, diabetes, coronary occlusion, myocardial infarction, cardiac failure, thyrotoxicosis, pernicious anemia, leukemia, and multiple sclerosis.[49]

Psychiatric illness can also be a sequel to loss. Parkes and Brown,[51] in an investigation of the relationship between bereavement and mental illness, found that 2.9% of 3245 admissions to psychiatric hospitals took place within 6 months of the death of a close relative. The frequency of admission after the death of a spouse was six times greater than would be expected by chance alone. Although the bereaved patients proved to have a variety of psychiatric illnesses, the most common diagnosis was depression. Although the evidence relating object loss to somatic symptom formation does not prove a cause-and-effect relationship, it strongly suggests that grief related to object loss may contribute to a number of diverse somatic reactions.

■ **ASSOCIATED WITH DELAYED GRIEF REACTIONS.** The designation of grief as pathological indicates that something has prevented it from running its normal course. The defenses that were used successfully in the uncomplicated grief reaction become exaggerated or maladaptive in the pathological reaction. The result may be a delayed grief reaction or a distorted reaction, such as in depression or mania. Delayed grief reactions may be indicated by excessive hostility and grief, prolonged feelings of emptiness and numbness, an inability to weep or express emotions, low self-esteem, use of the present tense instead of the past when speaking of the loss, persistent dreams about the loss, retention of the clothing of the deceased, an inability to visit the grave of the deceased, and the projection of living memories into an object that is held in place of the lost one. Clinical example 15-1 illustrates some of the behaviors associated with a delayed grief reaction.

In this example Mrs. G was experiencing a delayed grief reaction that was precipitated by the emotionally invested event of her deceased son's would-be graduation. She had failed to progress through the process of mourning at the time of her son's death and was beginning to engage in the "grief work" at the present time. The behaviors she displayed were consistent with the state of depression she was experiencing.

Because feelings of sadness, disappointment, and frustration are normal accompaniments of human life, the boundary between normal and abnormal mood is often difficult to define. Basically, behaviors associated with severe mood disturbances or affective disorders reflect an increase in the intensity or the duration of

TABLE 15-5

BEHAVIORS ASSOCIATED WITH DEPRESSION

Affective	Physiological	Cognitive	Behavioral
Anger	Abdominal pain	Ambivalence	Aggressiveness
Anxiety	Anorexia	Confusion	Agitation
Apathy	Backache	Inability to concentrate	Alcoholism
Bitterness	Chest pain	Indecisiveness	Altered activity level
Dejection	Constipation	Loss of interest and motiva-	Drug addiction
Denial of feelings	Dizziness	tion	Intolerance
Despondency	Fatigue	Self-blame	Irritability
Guilt	Headache	Self-depreciation	Lack of spontaneity
Helplessness	Impotence	Self-destructive thoughts	Overdependency
Hopelessness	Indigestion	Pessimism	Poor personal hygiene
Loneliness	Insomnia	Uncertainty	Psychomotor retardation
Low self-esteem	Lassitude		Social isolation
Sadness	Menstrual changes		Tearfulness
Sense of personal worthlessness	Nausea		Underachievement
	Overeating		Withdrawal
	Sexual nonresponsiveness		
	Sleep disturbances		
	Vomiting		
	Weight change		

otherwise normal emotions. They may range from behaviors associated with moderate anxiety (and indicative of neurotic health problems) to those associated with panic levels of anxiety (and indicative of psychotic health problems). In severe forms, disturbances of mood can be recognized as being maladaptive because of their intensity, pervasiveness, persistence, and interference with effective daily functioning. This may be reflected in impaired body functioning; the inability to perform expected social roles, such as at work, in the family, or at school; suicidal thoughts; and interference with reality testing, such as delusions, hallucinations, or confusion.

■ **ASSOCIATED WITH DEPRESSION.** The behaviors associated with depression are varied. Sadness and slowness may predominate, or there may be states of agitation. The key element to a behavioral assessment is change—the individual changes his usual behavioral patterns and responses. Research indicates that the individual working through the normal mourning process responds to his loss with a set of psychological symptoms that are often indistinguishable from depression but are accepted by him and by his environment as normal. In contrast, patients with depression experience their condition as a "change" unlike their usual self, which often leads them to seek help.[19]

A number of behaviors are associated with states of depression. These may be divided into affective, physiological, cognitive, and behavioral manifestations (Table 15-5). Obviously, some of these behaviors are contradictory and incompatible. The lists are intended to describe the spectrum of possible behaviors, acknowledging that not all individuals experience all of them.

The most common and central behavior is that of the depressive mood. This is not necessarily described by the patient as "depression" but as feeling sad, blue, down in the dumps, unhappy, or unable to enjoy life. Crying commonly occurs. On the other hand, some depressed persons do not cry, and describe themselves as "beyond tears." The mood disturbance of the depressed patient resembles that of normal unhappiness multiplied in intensity and pervasiveness. Another mood that often accompanies depression is anxiety—a sense of fear and intense worry. Both depression and anxiety may show diurnal variation, that is, a pattern of change whereby certain times of the day, such as morning or evening, are consistently worse or better.

In the literature there is a lack of agreement on which behaviors typically reflect depression and which are most significant for assessment, treatment, and prognosis. Neither are the identified behaviors exclusive to depression; they may also appear in other kinds of health

TABLE 15-6

SYMPTOMS OF DEPRESSION AND THEIR PREVALENCE

Symptom	Sources using symptom[39] (%)	Measurement instruments monitoring symptom[39] (%)	Severely depressed patients showing symptom[8] (%)
Self-devaluation	54	100	81
Dejected mood	92	87	88
Suicidal thoughts	100	81	74
Pessimism, feelings of hopelessness	77	81	87
Loss of appetite	77	75	72
Sleep disturbance	77	75	87
Loss of libido	84	44	61
Fatigability	46	81	78
Loss of interest, enjoyment	46	62	92
Guilt feelings	70	62	60
Social withdrawal	38	69	64
Crying spells	38	44	83
Indecisiveness	30	50	76
Constipation	30	44	52
Psychomotor retardation	30	81	87
Loss of motivation	46	62	86
Diurnal mood variation	40	20	37
Feelings of inadequacy, helplessness	30	20	90

problems. Levitt and Lubin[39] reviewed the literature and listed the symptoms of depression cited in at least 2 of 13 selected sources published between 1961 and 1969. They also reviewed the symptoms of depression appearing in at least 2 of 16 depression measurement instruments. Of the 24 self-rating measures of depression, the following five are most commonly used: the Minnesota Multiphasic Personality Inventory (MMPI) depression scale, the Beck Depression Inventory, the Hamilton Rating Scale for Depression, the Zung Self-Rating Depression Scale, and the Depression Adjective Checklist. Beck[7] provided further data by reviewing the proportions of depressed patients manifesting various symptoms. Table 15-6 selectively summarizes the findings of Levitt and Lubin and Beck. Using patient reporting as the criterion reference (Beck's data on severely depressed patients), the cardinal symptoms of a depressive syndrome, as defined by their presence in at least 75% of cases, include feelings of inadequacy and helplessness, loss of motivation, psychomotor retardation, indecisiveness, crying spells, loss of interest and enjoyment, fatigability, sleep disturbance, pessimism, dejected mood, and self-devaluation.

Finally, the potential for suicide should always be assessed in severe mood disturbances. Suicide and other self-destructive behaviors are discussed in detail in Chapter 16. The intensity of the feelings of anger, guilt, and worthlessness may precipitate suicidal thoughts, feelings, or gestures, as illustrated in Clinical example 15-2.

This example dramatically emphasizes three important points. First, the experience of a medical illness frequently involves a loss of some type for the individual—loss of function, body part, or appearance. Therefore all patients should be assessed for the presence of depression. Second, all people experiencing states of depression and despair have the potential for suicide. Third, nurses can intervene in a variety of ways to support the grieving and mourning process whether it is of an uncomplicated or pathological nature. Nursing actions can be preventive, curative, or rehabilitative, based on the nursing assessment and diagnosis.

■ **ASSOCIATED WITH MANIA.** The essential feature of mania is a distinct period of intense psychophysiological activation. Some of the behaviors associated with it are given in Table 15-7. In this state the predominant mood is either elevated or irritable accompanied by one or more of the following symptoms: hyperactivity, the undertaking of too many activities, lack of judgment of the consequences of actions, pres-

TABLE 15-7

BEHAVIORS ASSOCIATED WITH MANIA

Affective	Physiological	Cognitive	Behavioral
Elation or euphoria	Dehydration	Ambitious	Aggressive
Expansive	Inadequate nutrition	Denial of realistic danger	Excessive spending of money
Humorous	Needs little sleep	Distractibility	Grandiose acts
Inflated self-esteem	Weight loss	Flight of ideas	Hyperactivity
Intolerant of criticism		Grandiosity	Increased motor activity
Lack of shame or guilt		Illusions	Irresponsible
		Lack of judgment	Irritable or argumentative
		Loose associations	Poor personal grooming
			Provocative
			Sexually overactive
			Socially active
			Verbose

sure of speech, flight of ideas, distractibility, inflated self-esteem, and hypersexuality.

If the mood is elevated or euphoric, it is often infectious in nature. Patients report feeling happy, unconcerned, carefree, and devoid of problems. Although such experiences would seem enviable, these affects are exhibited without any concern for reality or the feelings of others. Mood is often expansive, and some patients have extraordinary delusional notions about their power and importance. They characteristically involve themselves in various seemingly senseless and risky enterprises.

Alternately, the mood may be irritable, especially when the patient's plans are thwarted. In such a case they can be contentious and readily provoked by seemingly harmless remarks. Self-esteem is inflated during a manic episode, and, as the activity level increases, the feelings about the self become increasingly disturbed. Delusional grandiose symptoms are in evidence, and the patient is willing to undertake any project possible.

In contrast to depressed patients, manic patients are extremely self-confident, with an ego that knows no bounds; they are "on top of the world." Accompanying this magical omnipotence and supreme self-esteem is an equally inordinate lack of guilt and shame. Often there is a denial of realistic danger. The patient's boundless energy, cunning, planning, scheming, and inability to forecast resulting consequences frequently lead to irresponsible enterprises and excessive spending, as well as to misdemeanors of a sexual, aggressive, or possessive nature. In contrast to the depressed state, patients in the manic state have heightened libidinal drives, with

CLINICAL EXAMPLE 15-2

Mr. W was a 60-year-old man who lived alone. His son and daughter were married and lived in the same state. His wife died 2 years ago, and since that time his children had often asked him to move in with either of them. He had consistently refused to do this, believing that both he and his children needed privacy in their lives. Six months ago he was diagnosed as having advanced prostatic cancer with metastasis. After the diagnosis was made and because of increasing disability, he left his job and began to receive disability compensation. He visited his children and their families on the average of twice a month and kept his regularly scheduled visits with the medical clinic. The nurses and physicians at the clinic noted he was "despondent and withdrawn" but viewed this as a normal reaction to his diagnosis and family history. No interventions were implemented based on his emotional needs. A week after attending the clinic for a routine, follow-up visit, he went to the cemetery where his wife was buried and at her gravestone shot himself in the head. A grounds keeper of the cemetery heard the shot, discovered what had happened, and called an ambulance. Mr. W was taken to the emergency room of the nearest hospital and, with prompt medical care, survived the suicide attempt.

abounding energy and a heightened sexual appetite. Characteristic physical changes can be related to the basic affect: inadequate nutrition, partly because manic patients have no time to eat, and serious loss of weight in conjunction with their insomnia and overactivity. In severe cases, there may be dehydration, which requires prompt attention.

In addition to mood disturbance, speech is often disturbed. As the mania gets more intense, formal and logical speech is displaced, and speech becomes loud, rapid, and difficult to interpret. As the activated state increases, speech becomes full of plays on words and irrelevancies that can increase to loosened associations and flight of ideas. Some of these behaviors are evident in Clinical example 15-3.

Associated behaviors found in mania include lability of mood with rapid shifts to brief depression. Such behavior accounts for those patients who have loosened associations and alternately laugh and cry. In addition, hallucinations of any type, ideas of reference, and frank delusions may be present with predominant feelings of guilt and thoughts of suicide. Manic episodes have a high tendency toward recurrence, only about 25% of manic patients have only one episode, and almost all individuals with manic episodes also have depressive episodes. However, there is a variation in the duration

---

CLINICAL EXAMPLE 15-3

Mr. B was a 30-year-old single man who was admitted to the psychiatric unit of the local community hospital. He had been hospitalized 2 years ago for problems related to alcoholism. He was accompanied to the hospital by a friend who lived with him. His friend said that for the past 2 months Mr. B had been "running on ten cylinders instead of four." He slept and ate little and talked constantly, sometimes so fast that no one could understand what he was trying to say. He had redecorated his bedroom in the apartment twice and had gone into debt buying a new "mod" wardrobe. His friend brought him in because his behavior was becoming more erratic and his physical condition was failing.

The nurse who admitted Mr. B asked about his social relationships. He revealed that his girl friend of 7 years had left him 6 months ago for another man. He said that initially he thought she would "see the light," but she had refused to see him since them. Mr. B said this "upset" him a little at the time, but he was sure it was "for the best and there were plenty other women out there just waiting for him."

---

and severity of the manic episode and in the intervals between relapses and recurrences.

All of these clinical examples illustrate the interrelatedness of disturbances of mood with the problem of self-esteem and disrupted interpersonal relationships. Because of the intensity of the reaction, multiple aspects of the individual's life are affected. This may also include his physical health, as reflected in the lists of physiological behaviors. Another effect on physical functioning is the possible onset of psychosomatic illness. Hypertensive crises, irritable bowel syndromes, coronary occlusions, rheumatoid arthritis, migraine headaches, and various dermatological conditions can occur in conjunction with severe mood disturbances.

■ Coping mechanisms

Uncomplicated grief reactions can be considered to be the process of normal mourning or simple bereavement. Mourning includes all the psychological processes set in motion within the individual by the loss. The psychological symptom of increased preoccupation with all the detailed memories of the lost object is the work of mourning. Freud[25] described it as the painful and necessary work of readjustment to the loss. As mourning is extended over time, there is a "working through" of an affect that, if released in its full strength, would overwhelm the ego.

The mourning process begins with the introjection of the lost object. When a person grieves, his feelings are directed to the mental image he possesses of the loved one. Thus the mechanism of introjection serves as a buffering mechanism. Through reality testing, the individual realizes that the love object no longer exists, and he withdraws his emotional investment from it. This is accompanied by an internal struggle because the individual does not willingly abandon a source of personal gratification. The ultimate, productive outcome is that reality wins out, but this is accomplished slowly over time. When the mourning work is completed, the ego becomes more free and uninhibited to invest in new objects.

Although the specific reactions to grief may vary, it has to be worked out. If not, the person will continue to experience emotional conflict. Hodge has explained it as follows:

The problem must be brought into the open and confronted, no matter how unpleasant it may be for the patient. *The grief work must be done.* There is no healthy escape from this. We might even add that the grief work *will* be done. Sooner or later, correctly or incorrectly, completely or incompletely, in a clear or a distorted manner, *it will be done.* People have a natural protective tendency to avoid the unpleasantness of the grief work, but it is necessary and the more actively it is done, the shorter will be the period of grief. If the grief work is not actively pursued, the process may be fixated or aborted or delayed, with the patient feeling that he may have escaped it. However, almost certainly a distorted form of the grief work will appear at some time in the future.[28:230]

A delayed grief reaction, therefore, reflects the exaggerated use of the defense mechanisms of denial and suppression in an attempt to avoid the intense distress associated with grief. The distorted grief reaction of depression is, in a sense, abortive grieving. The specific defenses that are used to block the mourning process are repression, suppression, denial, and dissociation. There may even be the unconscious wish to be rewarded for suffering by the restoration of the lost object. Because this is impossible, the depressed person's hopelessness takes on an added dimension. The denial of the loss in depression results in profound feelings of guilt, anger, and despair that focus on one's own unworthiness. Thus, the cycle of depression is reinforced and perpetuated in a self-defeating way.

Manic and hypomanic episodes occur more rarely than depressive states. Some believe that mania is a mirror image of depression and that, even though the behaviors are dissimilar, the dynamics and coping mechanisms are related. According to this view, manic behavior is a defense against depression, as the individual attempts to deny his feelings of worthlessness and helplessness. His elation and hyperactivity are an appeal for love and a protection from depression.

 # Nursing diagnosis

■ Identifying nursing problems

The diagnosis of disturbances of mood depends on an understanding of many interrelated concepts, including anxiety, self-concept, and hostility. One task of the nurse in formulating a diagnosis is to decide if the patient is experiencing primarily a state of anxiety (Chapter 12) or depression. It is often difficult to distinguish between them because they may coexist in one patient and present similar behaviors. Crary and Crary[21] suggest some comparative observations that may be helpful to the nurse. They note that the depressed patient is often slowed down in speech and movements, whereas the anxious patient often responds normally or more actively. The depressed patient is reluctant to discuss his problems or symptoms, while the anxious patient is more likely to discuss his symptoms and related topics. The depressed patient has decreased his outside interests, whereas the anxious patient usually retains interest in some things. The depressed patient has diffi-

culty enjoying things, but the anxious patient can enjoy some activities. The depressed patient usually feels worse in the morning or after sleep, whereas the anxious patient usually feels worse in the evening and better after sleep or rest; and the depressed patient usually has a decreased appetite and enjoyment of food, while the anxious patient usually eats intermittently and generally enjoys at least some foods.

An appropriate nursing diagnosis should include the patient's maladaptive coping response and related stressor. Fig. 15-3 presents the nursing model of health-illness phenomena with the continuum of emotional responses. The maladaptive responses are a result of feelings of anxiety, hostility, self-devaluation, and guilt. This model suggests that nursing care will be centered around increasing self-esteem and encouraging the appropriate expression of emotions.

Nursing Diagnoses Related to Mood Disturbances

Primary NANDA nursing diagnoses

Coping, ineffective individual
Grieving, anticipatory
Grieving, dysfunctional
Hopelessness
Powerlessness
Spiritual distress
Violence, potential for self-directed

Examples of complete nursing diagnoses

Ineffective individual coping related to discovery of spouse's extramarital affair evidenced by euphoric state, hyperactivity, and lack of judgment
Anticipatory grieving related to son's impending departure from home evidenced by sadness and loss of interest in daily events
Dysfunctional grieving related to death of sister evidenced by self-devaluation, sleep disturbance, and dejected mood
Hopelessness related to loss of job evidenced by feelings of despair and development of ulcerative colitis
Powerlessness related to new role as parent evidenced by apathy, uncertainty and overdependency
Spiritual distress related to loss of child in utero evidenced by self-blame, somatic complaints and pessimism about the future
Potential for self-directed violence related to rejection by boyfriend evidenced by self-destructive acts

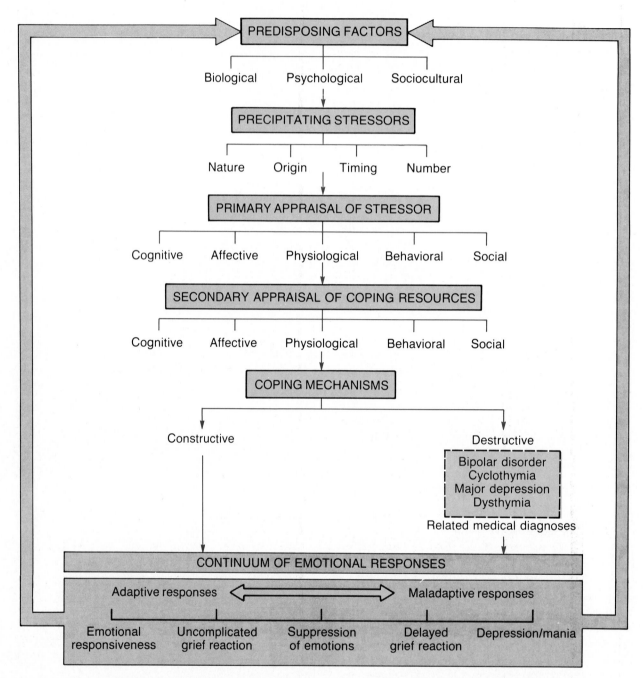

Fig. 15-3. Nursing model of health-illness phenomena related to emotional responses.

There are many NANDA nursing diagnoses that would be appropriate for an individual experiencing a disturbance of mood. Primary NANDA nursing diagnoses and examples of complete nursing diagnoses related to mood disorders are presented in the box on page 459. A complete nursing assessment would incorporate the many related human responses in one's diagnostic formulations. Table 15-8 presents the nurs-

ing diagnoses related to the range of possible maladaptive responses of the patient with a mood disorder.

■ **Related medical diagnoses**

The model also identifies some medical diagnoses that are appropriate to disturbances of mood or affective disorders. The psychiatric classification of affective disorders has reflected, to a large extent, the controversies

TABLE 15-8

MEDICAL AND NURSING DIAGNOSES RELATED TO MOOD DISTURBANCES

Medical Diagnostic Class	**Psychiatric Nursing Diagnostic Class**
Mood (affective) disorders	Disturbances in mood
Related Medical Diagnoses (DSM-III-R)*	**Related Nursing Diagnoses (NANDA)**
Bipolar disorder	Anxiety
Cyclothymia	Communication, impaired: verbal
Bipolar disorder NOS	†Coping, ineffective individual
Major depression	†Grieving, anticipatory
Dysthymia	†Grieving, dysfunctional
Depressive disorder NOS	†Hopelessness
	Injury, potential for
	Nutrition, alteration in
	†Powerlessness
	Self-care deficit
	Self-concept, disturbance in
	Sexual dysfunction
	Sleep pattern disturbance
	Social isolation
	†Spiritual distress
	Thought processes, alteration in
	†Violence, potential for self-directed

*From American Psychiatric Association: Draft of the DSM-III-R in Development (subject to change), as proposed by the Work Group to Revise DSM-III. American Psychiatric Association, October 1985.
†Indicates primary nursing diagnoses for disturbances in mood

surrounding the nature, cause, and treatment of these disorders. Although these traditional labels are no longer used in the Draft of the DSM-III-R in Development,[4] nurses should be familiar with them because they may continue to have some research and clinical value.

One traditional distinction has been to separate patients into **psychotic vs. neurotic affective states.** Unfortunately these terms have acquired multiple meanings and have lost their precision in defining clinical or research practice. Another traditional distinction has been between **endogenous vs. reactive, or exogenous, types of depression.** Endogenous depressions were believed to have resulted from early personality development and intrinsic biological processes, whereas exogenous, or reactive, types were believed to have occurred in response to external environmental stress, such as recent loss or disappointment. Research, however, has failed to verify the existence of these traditional distinctions. Thus the psychotic-neurotic distinction and the endogenous-reactive dichotomy are better regarded as continuums along which patients may be placed. Most patients are intermediate on the continuum and few are at the ex-

tremes. Neither classification is used in the Draft of the DSM-III-R in Development.[4]

Another classification system developed by Robins and Guze[59] avoids the controversial endogenous-reactive and psychotic-neurotic dichotomies. They propose a distinction between **primary and secondary affective disorders** based on two criteria, chronology and the presence of associated illnesses. "Primary" affective disorders are the disorders in patients who have been well or whose only previous episodes of psychiatric disease were mania or depression. "Secondary" affective disorders include feelings of sadness, inadequacy, and hopelessness that occur with another preexisting psychiatric disorder, such as anxiety reactions. It also includes symptoms secondary to medical illnesses.

A final distinction is the **bipolar-unipolar affective states.** It proposes the separation of depressed patients with a history of manic episodes (the bipolar group) from those patients who have had only recurrent episodes of depression (the unipolar group). Among the newer approaches; the bipolar-unipolar distinction has achieved considerable acceptance. There are two major categories of mood or affective disorders identified in the Draft of theDSM-III-R in Development:[4] bipolar disorders and depressive (unipolar) disorders (Table 15-8). The specific disorders identified under each will now be briefly described.

■ **BIPOLAR DISORDER.** The essential feature of bipolar disorder is a current or past experience of a manic episode lasting at least 1 week when one's mood was abnormally and persistently elevated, expansive, or irritable. The episode of mood disturbance is sufficiently severe to cause marked impairment in social or occupational functioning. Bipolar disorders may be classified as manic (limited to only manic episodes), depressed (a history of manic episodes with a current depressive episode), or mixed (a mixed presentation of both manic and depressive episodes).

■ **CYCLOTHYMIA.** The essential feature of cyclothymia is a history of 2 years of hypomania in which there have been numerous periods with abnormally elevated, expansive, or irritable moods that did not meet the criteria for a manic episode, and numerous periods of depressed mood that did not meet the criteria of a major depressive episode.

■ **BIPOLAR DISORDER NOS.** This is a residual category for hypomanic episodes that are not part of bipolar disorder mixed, manic or depressed, or cyclothymia.

■ **MAJOR DEPRESSION.** The essential feature of major depression is the presence of at least five symptoms during the same 2-week period with one being either depressed mood or loss of interest or pleasure. Other symptoms might include weight loss, insomnia, psychomotor agitation or retardation, fatigue, feelings of worthlessness, diminished ability to think, and recurrent thoughts of death. Major depressions may be classified as single episode or recurrent.

■ **DYSTHYMIA.** The essential feature of dysthymia is a history of at least 2 years of experiencing, more often than not, a depressed mood and at least one of the symptoms mentioned above without meeting the criteria for a major depressive episode.

■ **DEPRESSIVE DISORDER NOS.** This is a residual category for disorders with depressive features that do not meet the criteria for any other affective disorder or adjustment disorder with depressed mood.

🌿 Planning and implementation

■ Goal setting

The general goal of the nurse working with a patient who is experiencing an uncomplicated grief reaction is to support the patient in the subjective experience of his grief work or to help the person mourn. This means helping the person know what has been lost, that his pain is worthy of his own respect, and that real hope lies in acknowledging rather than denying his loss. He needs to extricate himself from his bondage to the lost object and find new patterns of rewarding interaction. In this way he copes with the loss, integrates it into his past, and grows from the experience. The content of the mutual long-term goals will therefore refer to the patient's completing the process of grieving, mourning, or bereavement. This may take 6 months to a year or possibly longer, since the duration of the grieving process varies considerably among different cultural groups. Short-term goals are necessary to identify specific realistic steps the patient can take as he works through the mourning process. They should reflect progression through Bowlby's[14] phases: (1) the urge to recover the lost object, (2) disorganization, and (3) reorganization. Possible short-term goals may include the following:

> The patient will:
> 1. Express feelings of sorrow caused by the loss of her husband within 10 days
> 2. Describe her ambivalence (love and anger) toward her husband by the end of 1 month
> 3. Review her relationship with her husband, including shared pleasures, regrets, etc.

When the patient is experiencing a maladaptive disturbance of mood, the long-term goals may be directed toward reinitiating a delayed grief reaction or exploring areas of conflict underlying a depressive or manic state. When nursing intervention is planned, psychotherapeutic, sociotherapeutic, and somatotherapeutic factors should be considered collectively and conjointly. The long-term goals of nursing care for the patient with a severe mood disturbance have the following aims:

1. To allow for the recognition and continuous expression of feelings, including denial, hopelessness, anger, guilt, blame, helplessness, regret, hope, and relief within a supportive therapeutic atmosphere
2. To allow for the gradual analysis of the stressors the individual is experiencing while strengthening his self-esteem
3. To increase the patient's sense of identity, control, awareness of choices, and responsibility for behavior
4. To encourage the establishment of healthy interpersonal ties with others
5. To promote the understanding of the nature of one's maladaptive emotional responses and acquire more adaptive coping responses to life stressors

Specific short-term goals should be generated from the behaviors displayed by the patient, present areas of difficulty, and relevant stressors. Goal setting should involve a holistic view of the patient and his world. It is probable that goals will need to be developed regarding the patient's self-concept, physical status, behavioral performance, expression of emotions, and interpersonal relationships. All these areas can directly relate to the disturbance of mood displayed by the patient. The participation of the patient in setting these goals can be a significant first step in regaining mastery over his own life.

■ Intervening in uncomplicated grief reactions

The overall goal of the nurse is to assist the patient who has experienced a loss to work through the process of grieving or mourning and to prevent maladaptive emotional responses. The grieving process is resolved when the lost object is internalized, bonds of attachment are loosened, and new object relationships are established. Grief reactions most commonly occur as a response to separation. They may also occur, however, following the loss of something tangible or intangible that is highly regarded. Thus loss of a body part or function, job, opportunity, relationship, family possessions through an accident, or status and regard among one's peers can all precipitate grief reactions.

Nurses frequently care for patients who have experienced losses related to the body and its parts and functions. Such losses inlude body parts (amputation and mastectomy), internal organs, sensory loss (vision and hearing), sexual function (impotence and menopause), and aging (mental functioning and physical strength). More than 40,000 limb amputations are performed annually in the United States. Breast amputation is a major approach to the treatment of mammary cancer, a disease that accounts for 25% of all malignancies in women. Such partial loss of the body is an increasingly common experience, and it often results, at least temporarily, in a disturbance in body image (Chapter 14). The nature of the patient's reaction to a loss of body part may be comparable to the loss of a significant person. Consequently, a process of mourning is initiated and grief is the normal emotional response.

In a larger sense, loss and separation are the recurrent themes of human life, and all change can be regarded as loss—the loss of the past in the movement to something new. This new area can be anticipated or feared, valued or dreaded. It can also be a normal developmental change, such as entering school or getting married. Even if society regards the event as a positive one, the significance of it for the individual may be quite different. Thus both the nature of the change or loss, as well as the significance of it, needs to be appropriately assessed by the nurse. The principles underlying therapeutic nursing interventions in uncomplicated grief reactions are the same, however, regardless of the exact nature of the loss.

■ **SELF-AWARENESS.** Before the nurse becomes actively involved with the bereaved, she must have an understanding of her own feelings and reactions to loss. Time should be spent recalling previous losses in her own life, examining related feelings, and resolving areas of conflict. If she is uncomfortable or ambivalent about death or has delayed the grief work involved in a personal loss, she will be unable to be therapeutic with the bereaved she hopes to help. Hope is an essential quality for the nurse to possess. Her hope and commitment in the future can be transmitted to the bereaved. Hope also involves sharing and a sense of partnership. These are demonstrated in the nurse-patient relationship as the nurse shares the grief work of the bereaved. Finally, nurses working with patients in the process of mourning need support systems of their own. Nursing peers, supervisors, and other professionals can provide formal or informal opportunities for ventilation and rejuvenation. This is essential because assisting the bereaved in the process of mourning can be psychologically draining and interpersonally painful at times.

■ **OFFER ANTICIPATORY GUIDANCE.** Interventions in this area can be initiated through anticipatory guidance even before the loss occurs. This involves talking about the impending loss with the individual and his family, if appropriate. Past losses may be reviewed and analyzed to clarify the meaning of the present loss. Since losses are present in all aspects of life and in all settings, any nurse may implement these interventions. For example, the industrial nurse may discuss the impending retirement of an employee; an office nurse may discuss the implications of a scheduled hysterectomy for a young woman; or a public health nurse may focus on a mother's feelings about her youngest child starting school. Many opportunities for interventions in this area are overlooked by nurses and yet their preventive potential is immeasurable.

■ **SUPPORT THE PATIENT AND FAMILY.** Engel[24] identifies a number of preventive actions the nurse can implement in working with a dying patient and his family. He suggests that news of death or impending death should be communicated to a family group, rather than an individual alone, in a private setting. The nurse should be prepared for the possibility of staying with and comforting the bereaved at least until a friend or clergyman arrives. The survivor's need to see the dying or dead patient should be met whenever possible because this is helpful in facing the reality of death.

When the nurse is confronted with an angry hostile reaction from the survivor, two considerations should be kept in mind. First, the person could be justified, but, if not, he may be trying to deal with his own anger and guilt toward the dying person. In this case the reaction is not directed toward the nurse as a person, but it serves as an important coping mechanism in the initial stage of mourning. Another defense that may be displayed by the survivor after hearing the news is disbelief and distraught behavior. The nurse should find a place for the survivors to cry and express their feelings, since this is an important need of the bereaved. The nurse should also be considerate of the cultural, religious, and social customs of the mourners, regardless of how different they may be from her own. Finally, Engel stresses the importance of the need for the patient to grieve for himself. This point is emphasized by Kübler-Ross[37] in her work with dying patients.

■ **IDENTIFY THOSE AT HIGH RISK.** The principal task of the nurse is to support the process of normal mourning, and her effectiveness will be increased if she is able to identify those individuals who are likely to experience difficulty in this task. The factors used in the nursing assessment will be helpful in this regard. Childhood experiences and later losses provide information about early separations that predispose the individual to renewed conflicts and unresolved feelings which may surface in the present loss or disruption. Previous history of psychiatric illness alerts the nurse to recurrent depressive episodes or decreased coping abilities. Information about life crises prior to the loss reveals the amount of stress previously experienced and the quantity of adaptive resources available at present. The nature of the relationship with the lost person or object is a critical factor. A close interpersonal relationship, a strong attachment, a high degree of dependency, and great ambivalence are all factors that will make the mourning process more complex and painful. As Bugen states, "Individuals who believe that they now have no life of their own or who cling to symbolic vestiges of the deceased will perceive their world only through grief-colored glasses."[17:205]

When the separation occurs through death, the process of dying is also crucial. A sudden death poses greater problems for the bereaved, as do a denial of emotions in the early mourning phase, the death of a child or young adult, and a belief that the death was preventable. Bugen asserts that the belief that the death was preventable is the "single most influential factor contributing to the prolongation of the human grief response."[17:202] The bereaved's support systems, secondary stresses, and future opportunities are relevant factors in planning interventions and promoting future growth.

■ **ASSIST IN GRIEF WORK.** The core nursing interventions are directed toward helping the patient go through the "grief work" by helping him experience the feelings and emotions connected with the loss and eventually find new patterns of rewarding interaction. He needs to accept the reality of the loss and realize that grieving is appropriate and sharing it makes it less painful. In establishing a contract, the nurse can explain that she would like to help the bereaved talk over any feelings and difficulties he might have related to the loss. Many people find it is easier to talk to an impartial "outsider" about painful memories, ambivalent feelings, and problems that threaten self-esteem. With the nurse the bereaved does not have to fear alienation from the family. In addition, it is important for the nurse, in establishing the contract, to convey her belief in the person's recovery and future coping ability.

Initially the person may be in a dazed or numbed condition. If so, he will need help in making even simple decisions. He will also need time to organize his ideas and take in what has happened. After the initial reaction has subsided, it will be possible to explore the loss, related memories, and affect of the bereaved. A useful beginning point is a discussion of the circumstances and nature of the loss. This often mobilizes the expression of significant and related feelings and reveals those which are absent or inappropriately expressed, such as sadness or anger. Many bereaved people are surprised and frightened by the intensity of their emotions. They may ask, "Is this normal?" or "Am I going mad?" Distractability, difficulty remembering, and a sense of unreality may cause worry and concern. Reassurance that they are not going mad and that such feelings are normal is helpful, particularly if the nurse does not seem frightened or alarmed by them. Nurses can show by their willingness to reveal their own feelings that they are not ashamed of them or rendered useless by them.

Guilt, anger, and sadness are all important emotions to be explored. Crying is an effective emotional release that can communicate strong feelings and drain off immobilizing energy or tension. At times, the values of the nurse or society may negate crying as an emotional outlet because it is viewed as a sign of weakness or causes discomfort in others. Nurses need to guard against these prejudices and encourage crying as an acceptable emotional release. In these instances silence and companionship are often the most therapeutic responses. The appropriateness of sadness and the common occurrence of anger and guilt need to be communicated to allow the free expression of these emotions. Asking how the person feels about a certain event, suggesting the way the person may have felt ("that must have made you feel angry"), or describing how another person would feel in the situation ("that would make me feel isolated and forgotten") may help the bereaved person explore his emotions. In the beginning the bereaved may test out the nurse for the clichés of reassurance used by others. The person may be exploring whether the nurse can confront the loss. If the nurse does not respond in a stereotyped and superficial way, the bereaved may begin to express "bad" memories as well as "good."

Initially, defenses need to be supported, but with time they should be analyzed and released. Denial needs to be changed to developing awareness. Reaction formation may lead to idealization of the lost one and may have to be dealt with by releasing the negative emotions involved. In projective identification the anger and guilt are acknowledged in another but not as part of oneself, and the concern is with the other. With this defense the nurse needs to promote more direct expression of feeling. The goal is to place the loss in perspective and loosen the bonds of attachment.

A number of resistances may appear. Early resistance shows as attempts to concentrate on the practical or financial problems rather than the emotional. The bereaved may ask help in getting a job or collecting the insurance. The nurse can offer appropriate assistance or referral in these areas while also encouraging the expression of grief and promoting the mourning. The nurse must not join with the bereaved in avoiding the grief. Another resistance occurs when the person shuts out the nurse through such statements as "No one really knows what I'm going through" or "You're so young, how can you possibly understand what it's like?" Other resistances occur when the person focuses on the nurse's losses as a way of escaping his own or when he claims that his grief is resolved, although the nurse realizes it is a premature resolution.

■ **SUPPORT SOCIAL SYSTEMS.** It may be necessary for the nurse to work directly or indirectly to promote an appropriate social network support, that is, support that will promote the expression of grief. The nurse may modify the bereaved's support system or may mobilize various significant others, such as the clergy. The nurse may hold a conjoint interview with the family to open up channels of communication and break the conspiracy of silence that frequently blocks grief.

The use of daytime sedatives and tranquilizers should be avoided. They may help the person maintain a calm appearance and avoid crying, but they artificially extend the period of denial and suppress the normal process of mourning. With the suppression of these emotions the balance of normal ambivalence may be tipped to its extreme, producing depression instead of mourning with its greater degree of maladaptation.

They can also encourage the development of patterns of drug dependence, sedation, and inhibition of grief in response to stress.

As the grief process is resolved, the person will be seen investing himself in new situations and relationships. The loss is placed in perspective, the attachment bonds are released, and energy is directed back out into the world. New patterns of rewarding interaction should be encouraged and reinforced.

It is important that in terminating the nurse-patient relationship, sufficient time is allowed for dealing with the loss termination imposes. The person may wish to continue the relationship as a substitute for the previous loss. Awareness of these issues will allow the nurse to confront them and encourage the independence of the bereaved.

Other therapeutic nursing interventions look to society in general. The nurse can work to encourage others in her community to accept the open expression of grief and the display of emotions. If these are accepted and supported, one type of stress can be avoided. In addition to changing attitudes, the nurse can facilitate the growth of organizations for the bereaved. The effectiveness of widow-to-widow groups, colostomy associations, and single-parent groups has been well established. Support groups play a significant role in preventing maladaptive emotional responses and are an appropriate area for nursing intervention. These interventions related to uncomplicated grief reactions are summarized in Table 15-9.

■ Intervening in depression and mania

Maladaptive emotional responses may emerge at unpredicted moments, can vary in intensity from mild to severe, and can be transitory, recurrent, or more stable trait conditions. Episodes of depression and mania can occur in any setting and can arise in conjunction with existing medical problems. So too, the treatment of mood disturbances can take place in various settings—at home, at an outpatient department, or in a hospital. The choice of where the patient can be best treated depends on the severity of the illness, available support systems, and resources of the treatment center. In timing one's intervention the nurse should remember that help given when maladaptive patterns of thought and behavior are developing is likely to be more acceptable and effective than help given a long time after these maladaptive patterns have been established. Thus early diagnosis and treatment are associated with more positive outcomes.

The nursing interventions that will be described relative to severe mood disturbances are based on a unified, multicausal, and interactive model of affective

TABLE 15-9

SUMMARY OF NURSING INTERVENTIONS IN UNCOMPLICATED GRIEF REACTIONS
Goal—Assist the patient who has experienced a loss to work through the process of grieving or mourning and prevent maladaptive emotional responses

Principle	Rationale	Nursing actions
Awareness and control of nurse's own feelings	Self-awareness is a prerequisite for the "therapeutic use of self" in working with those experiencing loss	Understand one's own feelings and reactions to loss Recall previous losses and resolve areas of conflict Communicate hope in the future and commitment to the work of grieving in the nurse-patient relationship Utilize one's own personal and professional support systems for ventilation and rejuvenation
Grieving can be facilitated by anticipating losses and their consequences	Anticipatory guidance by the nurse can be an effective intervention in primary prevention	Discuss impending losses and their significance with the patient and family Review past losses
Support the patient and family at the time of the loss	Therapeutic interventions at the time of the loss can prevent future maladaptive responses	Be prepared to stay with and comfort the bereaved until others arrive Use the family group or significant others as a coping resource to provide initial support for those experiencing the loss Provide the bereaved a place to express their feelings Unconditionally accept the emotional responses of those grieving Incorporate the cultural, religious, and social customs of those grieving in one's nursing care
Identify those persons at high risk for maladaptive responses	Nursing interventions will be more effective if adapted to a person's unique needs	Individuals at high risk for maladaptive responses should be identified by assessing factors that significantly influence the outcome of the mourning process
Help the patient go through the "grief work"	This will help him accept the reality of the loss and realize that grieving is an appropriate and healthy response	Convey belief in the person's recovery and future coping ability Initially assist the patient in immediate decision making if necessary Explore the circumstances and nature of the loss Facilitate the patient's expression of feelings, including guilt, anger, and sadness Offer acceptance and assurance of the appropriateness and commonality of the patient's positive and negative emotions Initially support the patient's ego defense mechanisms; with time, encourage his analysis and release of them by placing the loss in perspective and loosening bonds of attachment Work through any resistances that may occur in the nurse-patient relationship New patterns of rewarding interactions should be encouraged and reinforced Deal with the loss imposed by the termination of the nurse-patient relationship
Promote social network support as a coping resource	The positive role social support plays in dealing with loss has been well established in both research and clinical practice	Mobilize a social support system for the patient that is appropriate to his needs (i.e., family, clergy, and community agency) Facilitate the formation and growth of organizations that act as support groups to others

disorders. Such a model dismisses the notion of either one cause or one cure modality for the range of maladaptive emotional responses. Rather, it proposes that affective problems have many determinations and many dimensions that affect all aspects of a person's life. Thus a single approach to nursing care would be inadequate. Nursing interventions must instead reflect the complex nature of the model and address all maladaptive aspects of a person's life. Intervening in as many areas as possible should have the maximum effect in modifying maladaptive responses and alleviating severe mood disturbances. The ultimate aim of these nursing interventions is to teach the patient adaptive coping responses and increase the satisfaction and pleasure he receives from his world.

These nursing actions can be implemented in any setting. They are described on the basis of patients' needs in the following areas:

1. Environmental
2. Nurse-patient relationship
3. Affective
4. Cognitive
5. Behavioral
6. Social
7. Physiological

The specific interventions that will now be described are derived from an integration of the model of the causation of severe mood disturbances presented earlier in this chapter.

■ **ENVIRONMENTAL INTERVENTIONS.** Environmental interventions are useful when the patient's environment is highly dangerous, impoverished, aversive, or lacking in personal resources. In caring for the patient with a severe mood disorder, high priority should be given to the potential for suicide. Hospitalization is definitely indicated when there is a suicidal risk. In the presence of a history of rapidly progressing symptoms and the absence or rupture of the usual support systems in the environment, hospitalization is strongly indicated. Nursing care in this case means protection and assuring the patient he will not be allowed to harm himself. Specific interventions related to the suicidal patient are described in Chapter 16.

The depressed patient must always be assessed for possible suicide. The patient is at particular risk for suicide when he appears to be coming out of his depression because he may then have the energy and opportunity to kill himself. Acute manic states are also life threatening. These patients show poor judgment, excessive risk taking, and an inability to evaluate realistic danger and the consequences of their actions. In an acute manic episode immediate environmental measures must be instituted to prevent a fatal outcome.

Another kind of environmental intervention involves changing the physical or social setting by assisting the patient to move to a new environment. Sometimes a change in the patient's general pattern of living is indicated, such as a leave of absence from work, a change of jobs, a new peer group, or leaving one's family setting. Environmental changes such as these serve to decrease the immediate stress and mobilize additional support systems.

■ **NURSE-PATIENT RELATIONSHIP.** Both depressed and manic patients present unique challenges to the nurse who wishes to engage them in a therapeutic alliance. Depressed patients resist involvement through the defenses of withdrawal and nonresponsiveness. Because of their negative view of life they tend to remain isolated, verbalize little, feel they are unworthy of help, and form dependent attachments to others.

In working with depressed patients, the nurse's approach should be a quiet, warm, and accepting one. She should demonstrate the qualities of honesty, empathy, and compassion. Admittedly, it is not always easy to give warm, personal care to a person who is unresponsive and detached. The nurse may feel angry or resentful of his helplessness or fear rejection by him. The nurse needs patience and a belief in the potential of each person to grow and change. If this is calmly communicated to the patient, both verbally and nonverbally, in time he may begin to respond to the nurse's perceptions.

The nurse should avoid assuming an overaggressive or lighthearted approach with the depressed individual. Comments such as "You have so much to live for," "Cheer up—things are sure to get better," or "You shouldn't feel so depressed" convey little understanding of and respect for the patient's feelings. They will create more distance between the nurse and patient and block the formation of a potential relationship. Neither should the nurse sympathize with the patient. Subjective overidentification by the nurse can cause her to experience similar feelings of hopelessness and helplessness and seriously limit her ability to be therapeutic.

Rapport is best established with the depressed patient through shared time, even if the patient talks little, and supportive companionship. The very presence of the nurse indicates that she believes the patient is a valuable person. The nurse should adjust to the depressed patient's pace by speaking more slowly and allowing him sufficient time to respond. She should address him by name, talk to him, and listen to him. By studying the life and interests of the patient, the nurse might select topics that can serve as points of entry and lay the foundation for more meaningful discussions.

In contrast, elated patients may be very talkative and need simple explanations and concise truthful answers to questions. Although the manic patient might appear to be very willing to talk, he resists involvement through the defenses of manipulation, testing limits, and superficiality. His hyperactivity, short attention span, flight of ideas, poor judgment, lack of insight, and rapid mood swings all present special problems to the nursing staff.

Manic patients can be very disruptive to a unit and resist engagement in the work of therapy. They may dominate group meetings or therapy sessions by their excessive talking and manipulate the nursing and medical staff or patient group. By identifying a vulnerable area of another person or a group's area of conflict, manic patients are able to exploit and manipulate others. This provokes defensive and angry responses in others. Nurses are particularly susceptible to these feelings, since they often have the most contact with patients and the responsibility for coordinating and maintaining the psychiatric unit. When anger is generated, there is a breakdown of coordinated therapeutic care. Thus the maneuvers of manic patients serve as diversionary tactics. By alienating themselves they can avoid exploring their own problems.

It is important for nurses to understand how manic patients are able to manipulate others and their reasons for doing so. The treatment plan for these patients should be thorough, well coordinated, and consistently implemented. Constructive limit setting on manic patients' behavior is an essential part of the therapeutic plan. The entire treatment team must be consistent in their expectations of these patients and progressive limits set as situations arise. Other patients may also be encouraged to carry out the limits decided on. Pressure applied by peers can sometimes be more effective than pressure applied by the staff. Frequent staff meetings are recommended to reduce faulty communication, share in understanding the manic patient's behavior, and assure steady progress toward therapeutic goals.

One goal of nursing care is to ultimately increase the patient's self-control, and this should be kept in mind when setting limits with manic patients. They need to see that they have the ability to monitor their own behavior and that the staff is there to help them in this area. Also, it should be pointed out that there are many positive aspects to their behavior. The ability to be outgoing, expressive, and energetic are coping strengths that can be maximized in the therapeutic process.

■ **AFFECTIVE INTERVENTIONS.** Affective interventions are necessary because patients with mood disturbances have difficulty identifying and expressing feelings. Feelings that are particularly problematic are hopelessness, sadness, anger, guilt, and anxiety. A range of interventions are available to the nurse in meeting the patient's need in this area.

Intervening in the area of emotions requires self-understanding in the nurse. Whether or not the nurse's interventions will be therapeutic depends greatly on her values regarding the various emotions, her own emotional responsiveness, and her ability to offer genuine respect and nonjudgmental acceptance. The nurse must be able to experience feelings and express them herself if she expects to help her patient in this important aspect of his life.

Initially, the nurse must hope for depressed patients. They have a genuine need for repeated reassurance. The nurse can reinforce the fact that depression is a self-limiting disorder and things will be better in the future. The nurse can express this calmly and simply. Her intent is not to cheer the patient but to reassure him that, although recovery is a slow process involving weeks or months to complete, he will feel progressively better and will not remain at his current level of depression. Related to this, the nurse may acknowledge the patient's inability to take comfort from this reassurance. For him, only the depression is real; past or future happiness is an illusion. However, by affirming her belief, she may make his existence more tolerable.

This initial reassurance is a way of acknowledging the patient's pain and despair, while also conveying to him the nurse's sense of hope in his recovery. It is not the premature reassurance of "Don't worry—everything's going to be just fine." It is an openness to his feelings and acknowledgment of them. This is a very important first step. It also tells him that his present state is not permanent but is changeable. For the depressed patient who lacks a perspective of time, it directs his thoughts beyond the present time and into the future with genuine hopes for tomorrow.

Nursing actions in this area should convey that expressing feelings is normal and necessary. Blocking or repressing emotions is partly responsible for his present plan. She can help him to realize that his overwhelming feelings of dejection and worthlessness are defenses that serve to prevent him from dealing with his problems. Encouraging a patient to express his unpleasant or painful emotions through verbalizing them can reduce their intensity and make the person feel more alive and masterful. Thus the nursing actions should be directed toward first helping the patient experience his feelings and then express them. These actions are prerequisite to implementing interventions in the cognitive, behavioral, or social areas.

When the nurse accepts without criticism the anger,

despair, or anxiety expressed by the patient, he sees that expressing feelings is not destructive or a sign of weakness. Sometimes, however, the expression of anger by the patient changes his cognitive set from self-blaming to other blaming. It may allow him to see himself as more effective because it connotes power, superiority, and mastery. How this anger is expressed is important because aggressive behavior can be destructive and serve to further isolate him interpersonally. Many patients experiencing both depressive and manic emotional states have problems with the expression of anger and need to learn effective assertive behavior. This important area of nursing intervention is explored in more depth in Chapter 18.

Relaxation techniques may also be useful in helping both manic and depressed patients deal with their anxiety and tension and obtain more pleasure from life. Reducing anxiety to tolerable levels broadens the individual's perceptual field and allows the nurse to introduce interventions in the cognitive and behavioral areas. Nursing actions to reduce anxiety are described in Chapter 12.

To successfully implement any of these nursing actions related to the patient's affective needs, the nurse must utilize a variety of facilitative communication skills and responsive and action dimensions in the therapeutic nurse-patient relationship. These are described in Chapter 4. Particularly important among these are empathy skills, reflection of feeling, open-ended feeling-oriented questions, validation, self-disclosure, and confrontation. Feelings are the essence of empathy and, as such, make empathy an essential therapeutic quality. The various other communication skills must also be used to focus on feelings rather than facts. The patient with a severe mood disturbance will challenge the nurse's therapeutic skills and stringently test the level of her caring and commitment.

■ **COGNITIVE INTERVENTIONS.** When intervening in the cognitive area, the nurse has three major aims, which require that the nurse begin with the patient's conceptualization or definition of his problem:

1. To increase the patient's sense of control over his goals and behavior
2. To increase the patient's self-esteem
3. To assist the patient in modifying his negative expectations

Depressed patients usually see themselves as victims of their moods and environment. They do not view their behavior and their interpretation of events as possible causes of depression. They assume a passive stance and wait for someone or something to come along that will lift their mood. One task of the nurse, therefore, is to move the patient beyond his limiting preoccupation with his mood to a recognition of other aspects of his world that are related to it. To do this, the nurse will progress gradually with the patient. The first step is to help him explore his feelings. This is followed by eliciting his view of the problem. In so doing the nurse accepts the patient's perceptions but need not accept his conclusions. Together they need to define the problem so as to give the patient a sense of control, a feeling of hope, and a realization that change may indeed be possible.

Nursing actions may then be focused on modifying the patient's thinking. Depressed patients are noticeably dominated by negative thoughts. The effect of this is that often, despite a successful performance, the patient will view it negatively because of his pessimistic world view. Cognitive changes may be brought about in a number of ways.[7–10,76]

Frequently, negative thinking is an automatic process of which the patient is not even aware. The nurse can therefore assist him in identifying his negative thoughts and decreasing them through thought interruption or substitution. Concurrently, the patient can be encouraged to increase his positive thinking by reviewing his personal assets, strengths, accomplishments, and opportunities. Next the patient can be assisted in examining the accuracy of his perceptions, logic, and conclusions. In so doing, misperceptions, distortions, and irrational beliefs become evident. The patient should be helped to move from unrealistic to realistic goals and attempt to decrease the importance of unattainable goals. All of these actions serve to enhance the patient's self-understanding and increase his level of self-esteem. More detailed interventions in this area are explored in Chapter 14, which addresses alterations in self-concept—a problem inherent in disturbances of mood.

Also, because the depressed patient tends to be overwhelmed by his despair, it is important to limit the amount of negative personal evaluation he engages in. One way this can be accomplished is by involving the patient in productive tasks or activities; another way is to increase his level of socialization. These benefit the patient in two complementary ways: they limit the time he can spend on brooding and self-criticism, and they provide positive reinforcement in themselves.

A final consideration in this area is that the nurse needs to realize the meaning, nature, and value the patient places on his behavior and mood change. Most research has been focused on the psychopathologic nature of affective disorders. One study that explored the positive aspects of them found that patients with bipolar illnesses receive pronounced short- and long-term positive effects from their manic-depressive illness.[35] The patients reported short- and long-term increases in productivity, creativity, sensitivity, social outgoingness, and sexual intensity. It is important for the nurse to understand these attributions because they suggest that disturbances of mood can produce powerful reinforcers of a maladaptive response and thus make change more difficult. It would appear that for some patients, the positive consequences of an illness may outweigh their perception of negative outcomes.

■ **BEHAVIORAL INTERVENTIONS.** Successful behavior is a powerful antidepressant. This idea, however, seldom occurs to depressed patients who use their despondent mood as a rationalization for inactivity. They believe, instead, that once their mood lifts, they will be able to be productive once again. Such an idea is consistent with a negative cognitive set and a sense of helplessness over one's life. But inactivity prevents the patient from obtaining satisfaction and receiving social recognition. So, in actuality, it serves to reinforce one's depressive state.

Nursing interventions in this area therefore focus on activating the patient in a realistic, goal-directed way to move the patient in the direction of adaptive coping responses. The assignment of therapeutic tasks can be viewed as directed activities, strategies, or homework assignments mutually determined by the nurse and patient based on their long-term treatment goals. They are action-oriented and behavior focused and allow the patient to explore alternative coping responses. Some of the benefits derived from assigning therapeutic tasks as identified by Goldberg include the following:

1. The client continues to be involved with the therapist even when not in therapy, thus strengthening the therapeutic relationship.
2. The responsibility for change is the client's.
3. The implication is that the client can change, which instills hope.
4. If successfully completed, therapeutic tasks tend to enhance the client's self-esteem.
5. They help restructure a system.
6. They teach problem-solving skills by providing the client an opportunity for experiential learning.
7. They test the flexibility of a person or system and reveal areas of resistance to change.
8. They encourage the generalization of therapeutic gains beyond the therapy session.[26:157]

Many depressed patients benefit from nursing actions that encourage them to redirect their self-preoccupation to interests in the outside world. The timing of these interventions is crucial. The patient should not be forced into activities initially. Neither will he benefit from coming into contact with too many people too soon. Rather, the nurse should encourage activities

gradually and suggest escalating involvement on the basis of the mobilization of his energy.

For severely depressed hospitalized patients a structured daily program of activities can be beneficial. Because these patients lack motivation and direction, they are reticent to initiate actions. In this case the nurse should provide a tangible structure for activities, taking into consideration the patient's tolerance to stress and probability of succeeding. The particular task should not be too difficult nor too time consuming. Success tends to increase the patient's expectations and the possibility of future success. Failure tends to increase his feelings of worthlessness and hopelessness.

The elated patient usually needs little encouragement to become involved with others. Because of his short attention span and restless energy, however, he cannot deal with complicated projects. He needs tasks that are simple and that can be completed quickly. In his environment he needs room to move about and furnishings that do not overstimulate him.

The patient's ability to accomplish tasks and be productive will depend on a number of factors. First, expectations and goals for him should be small enough to ensure successful performance, relevant to his needs, and focused on positive activities. Following is a positive activities list* that contains categories of rewarding or potentially rewarding activities.[57]

1. Planning something you will enjoy
2. Going on an outing (e.g., a walk, a shopping trip downtown, a picnic)
3. Going out for entertainment
4. Going on a trip
5. Going to meetings, lectures, classes
6. Attending a social gathering
7. Playing a sport or game
8. Spending time on a hobby or project
9. Entertaining yourself at home (e.g., reading, listening to music, watching TV)
10. Doing something just for yourself (e.g., buying something, cooking something, dressing comfortably)
11. Spending time just relaxing (e.g., thinking, sitting, napping, daydreaming)
12. Caring for yourself, making yourself attractive
13. Persisting at a difficult task
14. Completing a routine task or unpleasant task
15. Doing a job well
16. Cooperating with someone else on a common task
17. Doing something special for someone else, being generous, going out of your way

---

*From Rehm, L.: A self-control therapy program for treatment of depression. In Clarkin, J., and Glazer, H., editors: Depression: behavioral and directive intervention strategies, New York, 1981, Garland Publishing, Inc.

18. Seeking out people (e.g., calling, stopping by, making a date or appointment, going to a meeting)
19. Initiating conversation (e.g., at a store, party, or class)
20. Discussing an interesting or amusing topic
21. Expressing yourself openly, clearly, or frankly (e.g., opinion, criticism, anger)
22. Playing with children or animals
23. Complimenting or praising someone
24. Physically showing affection or love
25. Receiving praise, compliments, attention

Next, attention should be focused on the task at hand, not what has yet to be done or was done incorrectly in the past. Finally, positive reinforcement should be based on actual performance. If such an approach is used consistently over time, the nurse can expect the patient to demonstrate increasing amounts of productive behavior.

When considering possible activities for the patient, occupational and recreational ones are usually easily identified by the nurse. These can be most valuable and are well represented in the positive activities list. Another source of accomplishment is in the area of movement and physical exercise. Brown[16] has made the following observations about the relationship between mood and movement:

- Physical fitness is often associated with a feeling of well-being and reduced depression and anxiety.
- Fitness appears to be associated with physical and psychological benefits regardless of the subject's age.
- The biological benefits of exercise may be associated in part with changes produced among brain amines, salt metabolism, muscle neuronal activity, and striatal functions.
- A comprehensive history of the depressed patient's motor activity is useful in prescribing an exercise regimen of maximum benefit.

Jogging, walking, swimming, bicycling, and aerobics are popular forms of exercise that may be incorporated in a regular program of physical activity for the patient. They are beneficial because they improve the patient's physical condition and provide a release of emotions and tensions.[62,65]

■ **SOCIAL INTERVENTIONS.** Evidence from diverse sources indicates that social factors play a major role in the causation, maintenance, and resolution of affective disorders, particularly depression. Socialization serves to moderate the experience of depression by providing an experience that is incompatible with depressive withdrawal and by providing a source of increased self-esteem through the social reinforcers of approval, acceptance, recognition, and support.

A major problem in the social area is that patients with maladaptive emotional responses have fewer interpersonal skills and are less accomplished in social interaction. In addition, they may be avoided by others because of their self-absorption, pessimism, or elation. One nursing action to counteract this problem is to help the patient improve his interpersonal style and increase his social skills. A mental health education plan for enhancing social skills is presented in Table 15-10. It involves a sequential learning process that includes the following:

1. Assessing the patient's social skills, supports, and interests
2. Reviewing existing and potential social resources available to the patient
3. Instructing and modeling of effective social skills
4. Role playing and rehearsal of troublesome social situations and interactions
5. Feedback and positive reinforcement of effective interpersonal skills
6. Encouraging the initiation of socialization in an expanded social arena

This final accomplishment often proves to be difficult for depressed patients who report they are unable to meet new people and engage in an active social life. Thus increasing a patient's social activities is another area of nursing intervention. Involvement with others often is a result of shared activities. The nurse can work with the patient to identify recreational, career, cultural, religious, and personal interests and how to best pursue these interests through community groups, organizations, and clubs. Women's groups, single parents groups, jogging clubs, church groups, and neighborhood associations are all possible opportunities for expanding one's social network. Although this may appear to be a relatively simple nursing intervention, it is often one that taxes the nurse's knowledge of resources and creativity.

Family involvement. In addition to a one-to-one relationship, patients with maladaptive emotional responses can also benefit from family and group therapy. In the context of family therapy the behaviors of depression can be interpreted as signs of dependency, which is contributed to and supported by other family members. The patient's sense of powerlessness in human relationships is examined in light of family patterns, and all family members are expected to take responsibility for their share of the continuing pattern.

The notion that friends and partners often reinforce

TABLE 15-10

MENTAL HEALTH EDUCATION PLAN—ENHANCING SOCIAL SKILLS

Content	Instructional activities	Evaluation
Describe behaviors interfering with social interaction	Instruct the patient on corrective behaviors	Patient identifies problematic and more facilitative behaviors
Discuss components of social performance relevant to the patient's situation	Model effective interpersonal skills for the patient	Patient describes specific skills he could acquire
Analyze the way in which the patient could incorporate these specific skills	Use role-play and guided practice to allow patient to test out these new behaviors	Patient shows beginning skill in assumed social behaviors
Encourage patient to test out new skills in other situations	Give homework assignments for the patient to do in his natural environment	Patient discusses his ability to complete the assigned tasks
Discuss generalization of new skills to other aspects of the patient's life and functioning	Give feedback, encouragement, and praise for newly acquired social skills and their generalization	Patient able to integrate the new social behaviors in his social interactions with others

and support the patient's depression has been well documented. When a person gets depressed, he usually receives a lot of attention and secondary gain from others who respond by being helpful, nurturing, or annoyed. But when the patient acts in a nondepressed way, there is little attention paid to him. Therefore one goal of family therapy is to have the family reinforce adaptive nondepressed behavior and ignore his maladaptive depressive responses.

There is also a need for family interventions with manic patients. In one study that followed the families of patients with bipolar manic-depressive illness, the authors noted the following:

The recurring psychopathology of manic-depressive patients has significant effects on the psychosocial adaptation of their spouse and children. Not only is the genetic predisposition handed down over generations, but the environment may have long-term detrimental effects on the children's personality.[44:1537]

The "wavering capacity for interpersonal relatedness" on the part of the patient with a mood disturbance and other family members is a clear indication for nursing interventions at the family level of care.

Group treatment. Group therapy can also provide multiple benefits. Knowledge that others have ambivalence and the sharing of guilt concerning this, as well as the realistic sympathy and support of the group members, enable the depressed patient to lessen his guilt, give up his maladaptive behavior patterns, and develop more satisfying relationships with others in the group. Van Servellen and Dull developed a format for group treatment of women with major depressive illness. The overall aim is to increase self-worth and self-esteem through identification with the group and awareness of personal strengths. The depressed women in Van Servellen and Dull's group[69] identified several general goals:

1. Learning more about their individual behavior and relationships with others based on feedback from members and group process
2. Increasing social support through group relatedness
3. Gaining a heightened sense of identity, self-understanding, and control over their own lives
4. Realizing that other people have problems similar to their own, which helps to reduce their sense of loneliness and isolation, thereby also decreasing feelings of hopelessness, helplessness, and powerlessness
5. Learning new ways to cope with stress from others in the group
6. More realistically modifying their perceptions and expectations of self and others
7. Allowing for the expression of feelings of hopelessness and frustration within the supportive context of the group

An essential part of any therapeutic intervention is the evaluation of its effectiveness. The authors also present a format for evaluation that can be used to measure change in the specific patients in group treatment. Research in comparing and evaluating various therapeutic modalities used by nurses continues to be a high priority in the future.

■ **PHYSIOLOGICAL INTERVENTIONS.** Interventions in this area include both physical care and somatic therapies. They begin with a thorough physical examination and health history to determine present health status, past and present health problems, and the presence of current treatments or medications that may be affecting the patient's mood state.

In depression, physical well-being may be forgotten or the patient may not be capable of caring for himself. The more severe the depression, the more important is the physical care. For example, the anorexic patient may need to have his diet monitored. Staying with the patient when he is eating, arranging for preferred foods, and encouraging frequent small meals may be helpful. Recording his intake and output and weighing him daily will help in evaluating this need.

Sleep disturbances are common. It is best to plan activities according to each patient's energy levels; some feel best in the morning and others in the evening. A scheduled rest period may be helpful, but patients should not be encouraged to take frequent naps or remain in bed all day. Patients with depression experience less stage III and stage IV sleep, and since these stages are dependent on the period of wakefulness, napping may actually exacerbate sleep disturbances. For many patients, eating regularly, staying active during waking hours, and cutting back on caffeine—especially late in the day—may promote more normal sleep patterns.[53]

The patient's appearance may be neglected and all his movements slowed. If it is necessary to assist the hospitalized patient with bathing or dressing, it should be done matter of factly with the explanation that he is being helped because he is unable to do it for himself at the present time. Cleanliness and interest in appearance can be noticed and praised. It is important for the nurse to allow the patient to help himself whenever possible. Often the nurse might rush the patient or do a task herself to save time, but these do not facilitate the patient's recovery and should be avoided.

The manic patient primarily needs protection from himself. He may be too busy to eat or take care of himself. Eating problems can be handled in the same way as with the depressed patient. Sleep is scarce; so rest periods should be provided along with supportive interventions, such as baths, soft music, and whirlpools. The manic patient may also need help in selecting appropriate clothes and carrying out hygiene activities. Setting limits and firm decisive actions are effective ap-

proaches to the physical care of the patient with a severe mood disturbance.

Somatic and drug therapies. Over the past 25 years, there has been much progress in the somatic and pharamacological treatment of affective disorders. Recent developments include biological markers of clinical value in the diganosis and treatment of disturbances in mood. One test for somatically treatable depression is the dexamethasone suppression test (DST) mentioned previously in this chapter and described in detail in Chapter 23. It is an easy, relatively inexpensive test that poses minimal risk to the patient. It is most useful in identifying patients who do not display all the typical behaviors of depression but who are likely to respond to somatic treatments, such as antidepressant therapy or ECT. It may also be useful in monitoring recovery from depression and of value in the decision about when to stop maintenance antidepressant therapy.

Antidepressant medications are frequently administered to elevate the mood of the depressed patient. At this time no single drug has been found to be effective for all kinds of depressions. Of the two types of antidepressants—tricyclics and monoamine oxidase (MAO) inhibitors—the former are used more commonly. Tricyclic drugs appear to be the most effective class of antidepressants. They pose a smaller risk of side effects than the MAO inhibitors and appear to be useful against relapses of depression. Lithium carbonate is considered by many to be the drug of choice in the treatment of mania. Some believe that it not only produces a remission of symptoms but also actually prevents a recurrence of the manic state. The overall success rate of drugs for the treatment of depression is 60% to 80%.

Despite their success, antidepressant drugs are far from ideal. Their therapeutic effects begin only after 2 to 6 weeks, and they have numerous side effects, which deter some patients from maintenance. This increases the need for patient education by nurses. Youssef reports that a directive patient-education group conducted by nurses resulted in a significant difference in medication compliance among psychiatric outpatients with affective disorders.[77] Additional programs and research by nurses in this area is needed to monitor and evaluate patient progress.

Another major problem with antidepressant medications is their toxicity. They are lethal at high doses which makes these drugs particularly dangerous for people most in need of them—suicidal patients. In addition, antidepressant medications do not help everyone, and it is difficult to predict who will respond to which drug. Fortunately, those who do not benefit from one type of antidepressant frequently do well on another type.

Electroconvulsive therapy (ECT) is also used with

depressed patients, particularly those with recurrent depressions and those who are resistant to drug therapy. ECT is regarded by many as a specific therapy for those severe depressions characterized by somatic delusions and delusional guilt, accompanied by a lack of interest in the world, suicidal ideation, and weight loss. A more detailed discussion of antidepressant medication and electroconvulsive therapy is presented in Chapters 22 and 23.

Sleep deprivation therapy may also be effective in the treatment of depression. Research indicates that depriving some depressed patients of a night's sleep will bring about an improvement in their clinical condition.[12] The means by which sleep deprivation works is not known, and the duration of the improvement varies greatly. Further developments in somatic therapies will have direct implications for nursing care.

All of the previously described nursing interventions in depression and mania are summarized in Table 15-11. It appropriately reflects the holistic nature of the nursing care given to patients with disturbances of mood.

 Evaluation

The effectiveness of nursing care is determined by changes in the patient's maladaptive emotional responses and the effect they have on his present functioning. Problems related to self-concept and interpersonal relationships merge and overlap. Since all individuals experience life stress and related losses, one of the fundamental questions the nurse can ask related to evaluation is "Did I assess my patient for problems in this area?"

Of particular significance with this problem are the many special aspects of transference and countertransference that may occur. The patient's heightened attachment and dependency behaviors and his lowered defensiveness can lead to intense transference reactions that should be worked through. Themes of loss and fear of loss, control of emotions and lack of control, and ambivalence predominate. Termination of the nurse-patient relationship may be difficult, since the patient experiences it as another loss that requires mourning and integration.

Countertransference issues can be related to the nurse's own bereavements, her attitudes about anger, guilt, sadness, and despair, her ability to confront these emotions openly and objectively, and, most important, her own conflicts about death and loss. Difficulties related to any of these issues can be evident in avoidance behavior, preoccupation with fantasies, blocking of feelings, or shortening of sessions. The nurse can expect to review and perhaps rework her feelings about personal bereavement. Her nursing care will be more appropriate and effective if she is aware of these issues and sensitive to her own feelings and conflicts regarding loss. Supervision and peer support groups can be of great help to her in this area.

DIRECTIONS FOR FUTURE RESEARCH

The following are some of the nursing research problems raised in Chapter 15 that merit further study by psychiatric nurses:

1. Nursing interventions that facilitate a healthy experience of grief
2. Development and validation of an assessment instrument that will identify individuals who are at risk for complicated grief reactions
3. Comparison of the nature of the grief process when it is mediated by the administration of psychopharmacological agents and when it is not, including behavioral outcomes
4. The relationship between various life events, the production of biogenic amines, and the occurrence of disturbances of mood
5. Family studies of patients with affective disorders with psychosocial, biologic, and genetic markers
6. Outcomes associated with nursing interventions related to patients' sleep patterns
7. The relationship between social role, role strain, and the occurrence of depression
8. Identification of nursing interventions that are effective in the primary prevention of disorders of mood
9. Development and refinement of a nursing diagnostical nomenclature relative to disturbances of mood
10. Exploration of the outcomes of various approaches to nursing intervention with individuals who are experiencing a mood disturbance
11. Description of the common characteristics of self-help groups for individuals who have experienced a loss
12. Identification of children at risk for developing affective disorders
13. The effect of patient education by nurses on medication compliance
14. Structured social interventions used by nurses working with depressed and manic patients

TABLE 15-11

SUMMARY OF NURSING INTERVENTIONS IN DEPRESSION AND MANIA

Goal—Teach the patient adaptive emotional responses and increase the satisfaction and pleasure he receives from his world

Principle	Rationale	Nursing action
Modify the patient's environment if it is dangerous, impoverished, aversive, or lacking in personal resources	All patients with severe mood disturbances are at high risk for suicide; environmental changes can protect the patient, decrease the immediate stress, and mobilize additional resources	Continually evaluate the patient's potential for suicide Hospitalize the patient when there is a suicidal risk Assist the patient to move to a new environment when appropriate (i.e., new job, peer group, family setting)
Establish and maintain a therapeutic nurse-patient relationship	Both depressed and manic patients resist becoming involved in a therapeutic alliance; acceptance, persistence, and limit setting are necessary	Utilize a warm, accepting, empathic approach Be aware of and in control of one's own feelings and reactions (i.e., anger, frustration, sympathy) With the depressed patient: 1. Establish rapport through shared time and supportive companionship 2. Allow the patient time to respond 3. Personalize his care as a way of indicating his value as a human being With the manic patient: 1. Give simple truthful responses 2. Be alert to possible manipulation 3. Set constructive limits on negative behavior 4. Use a consistent approach by all health team members 5. Maintain open communication and sharing of perceptions among team members 6. Reinforce the patient's self-control and positive aspects of his behavior
Assist in the patient's recognition and expression of emotions	Patients with severe mood disturbances have difficulty identifying and expressing feelings	Demonstrate emotional responsiveness and acceptance Utilize facilitative communication skills and the responsive and action dimensions described in Chapter 4 Respond empathically with a focus on feelings rather than facts Acknowledge the patient's pain and convey a sense of hope in his recovery Help the patient experience his feelings and then express them Assist the patient in the appropriate expression of anger Reduce the patient's anxiety to mild-moderate levels
Aid the patient in modifying his negative cognitive set	This will help to increase his sense of control over his goals and behaviors, enhance his self-esteem, and modify his negative expectations	Review with the patient his conceptualization of the problem but do not necessarily accept his conclusions Identify the patient's negative thoughts and help him to decrease them through thought interruption or substitution Help him increase his positive thinking Examine the accuracy of his perceptions, logic, and conclusions

Continued.

TABLE 15-11—cont'd

SUMMARY OF NURSING INTERVENTIONS IN DEPRESSION AND MANIA
Goal—Teach the patient adaptive emotional responses and increase the satisfaction and pleasure he receives from his world

Principle	Rationale	Nursing action
Aid the patient in modifying his negative cognitive set—cont'd		Identify misperceptions, distortions, and irrational beliefs Help him move from unrealistic to realistic goals Decrease the importance of unattainable goals Limit the amount of negative personal evaluations he engages in Realize the meaning, nature, and value the patient places on his behavior and mood change
Activate the patient in a realistic goal-directed way	Successful behavioral performance counteracts feelings of helplessness and hopelessness	Assign appropriate action-oriented therapeutic tasks Encourage activities gradually, escalating them as the patient's energy is mobilized Provide a tangible structured program when appropriate Set goals that are realistic, relevant to the patient's needs and interests, and focused on positive activities Focus on present activities, not past or future activities Positively reinforce successful performance Attain mutuality whenever possible Incorporate physical exercise in the patient's plan of care
Enhance the patient's establishment of interpersonal relationships	Socialization is an experience that is incompatible with withdrawal and increases self-esteem through the social reinforcers of approval, acceptance, recognition, and support	Assess the patient's social skills, supports, and interests Review existing and potential social resources Instruct and model effective social skills Use role playing and rehearsal of social interactions Give feedback and positive reinforcement of effective interpersonal skills Encourage increasing socialization in an expanded social arena Intervene with families to have them reinforce adaptive emotional responses of the patient Support or engage in family and group therapy when appropriate
Promote the patient's physical health and well-being	Physiological changes occur in disturbances of mood; physical care and somatic therapies are required to overcome problems in this area	Complete a nursing assessment of the patient's physiological health status Assist the patient to meet his self-care needs, particularly in the areas of nutrition, sleep, and personal hygiene Encourage the patient's independence whenever possible Administer prescribed medications and treatments

■ SUGGESTED CROSS-REFERENCES ■

The model of health-illness phenomena, including precipitating life stressors is described in Chapter 3. Therapeutic relationship skills and self-awareness of the nurse are discussed in Chapter 4. Strengthening coping resources through health education, environmental change, and supporting social systems is presented in Chapter 9. Interventions related to self-concept and cognitive therapy are discussed in Chapter 14. Interventions with the suicidal patient are discussed in Chapter 16. Disruptions in interpersonal relationships are discussed in Chapter 17. Problems with anger and limit setting are discussed in Chapter 18. Somatic therapy is discussed in Chapter 22. Psychopharmacology is discussed in Chapter 23. Group therapy is discussed in Chapter 28. Family therapy is discussed in Chapter 29.

■ SUMMARY ■

1. Mood refers to a prolonged emotional state that influences one's whole personality and life functioning. It pertains to one's prevailing and pervading emotion and is synonymous with the terms affect, feeling state, and emotion. Four adaptive functions of mood and a continuum of emotional responses were described. Severe mood disturbances can be recognized by their intensity, pervasiveness, persistence, and interference with usual social and physiological functioning.

   a. Grief is an individual's subjective response to the loss of a person, object, or concept that is highly valued. Uncomplicated grief is a healthy, adaptive, reparative response that is closely related to the acquisition of the capacity for developing meaningful object relationships. An uncomplicated grief reaction is the process of normal mourning. Mourning is resolved only when the lost object is internalized, bonds of attachment are loosened, and new object relationships are established. The work of mourning may take 6 months to a year. If grief is not worked through, delayed grief reactions and depression can occur.

   b. Depression was distinguished from grief by the attachment to the loved object, degree of regression, acknowledgment of the loss, and intensity of emotions over time.

   c. Mania is characterized by a mood that is elevated, expansive, or irritable. Hypomania is similar to mania but less severe. The prevalence of depression and mania was described, as well as their classification in the Draft of the DMS-III-R in Development.[4]

2. Stressors affecting the grief reaction and factors that place a person at high risk for maladaptive responses were identified. Ten models of causation of severe mood disturbances were discussed. These included the genetic, object loss, aggression turned inward, personality organization, cognitive, learned helplessness, behavioral, biochemical, life stressors, and integrated models. An integrated multicausal model is the most valuable for the nurse to use when implementing nursing care.

3. The phases associated with the process of mourning as described by Bowlby were presented. These are the urge to recover the lost object, disorganization, and reorganization. They can be applied to losses of any kind. Behaviors associated with delayed reactions, depression, and mania, were identified. The key element of a behavioral assessment is change in the person's usual patterns and responses.

4. Maladaptive emotional responses were related to feelings of anxiety, hostility, self-devaluation, and guilt. The psychiatric classification of affective disorders was discussed. Selected nursing diagnoses were related to appropriate medical diagnoses from the Draft of the DSM-III-R in Development.[4]

5. The general goal of the nurse when working with a patient who has experienced loss is to support the patient in the subjective experience of grief work. He needs to extricate himself from his bondage to the lost object and find new patterns of rewarding interaction. When the patient is experiencing a maladaptive disturbance of mood, the long-term goals may be directed toward reinitiating a delayed grief reaction or exploring areas of conflict underlying a depressive or manic state. Psychotherapeutic, sociotherapeutic, and somatotherapeutic factors should be considered collectively and conjointly. More specific short-term goals should be identified with the patient based on his behavior, present area of difficulty, and relevant stressors.

6. Interventions in uncomplicated grief reactions were described as anticipatory guidance, supporting the process of normal mourning, and social system intervention. Interventions in depression and mania were presented in the environment, nurse-patient relationship, affective, cognitive, behavioral, social, and physiological areas. Intervening in as many areas as possible should have the maximum effect in modifying maladaptive responses and alleviating severe mood disturbances.

7. When evaluating the nursing care, the nurse should pay particular importance to problems with transference and countertransference. Supervision and peer support groups can be helpful to the nurse in working with patients experiencing grief reactions.

■ REFERENCES ■

1. Abramson, L., Seligman, M., and Teasdale, J.: Learned helplessness in humans: critique and reformulation, J. Abnormal Psychol. **87**:49, 1978.
2. Akiskal, H., and McKinney, W.: Depressive disorders: toward a unified hypothesis, Science **182**:20, Oct. 5, 1973.
3. Akiskal, H., and McKinney, W.: Overview of recent research in depression, Arch. Gen. Psychiatry **32**:285, 1975.
4. American Psychiatric Association: Draft of the DSM-III-R in Development (subject to change), as proposed by the Work Group to Revise DSM-III. American Psychiatric Association, October 1985.
5. Arieti, S., and Bemporad, J.: The psychological organization of depression, Am. J. Psychiatry **137**:1360, 1980.

6. Baldessarini, R.: Biogenic amine: hypotheses in affective disorders, In Flach, F., and Draghi, S., editors: The nature and treatment of depression, New York, 1975, John Wiley & Sons, Inc.

7. Beck, A.: The diagnosis and management of depression. Philadelphia, 1973, University of Pennsylvania Press.

8. Beck, A.: Cognitive therapy and emotional disorders, New York, 1976, International Universities Press.

9. Beck, A., and Rush, A.: Cognitive approaches to depression and suicide. In Servan, G., editor: Cognitive defects in development of mental illness, New York, 1977, Brunner/Mazel, Inc.

10. Beck, A. et al.: Cognitive therapy of depression, New York, 1979, The Guilford Press.

11. Beck, C.: The occurrence of depression in women and the effect of the women's movement, J. Psychiatr. Nurs. 17(11):14, 1979.

12. Bhanji, S.: Treatment of depression by sleep deprivation, Nurs. Times 73:540, 1977.

13. Bowlby, J.: Grief and mourning in infancy and early childhood, Psychoanal. Study Child 15:9, 1960.

14. Bowlby, J.: Processes of mourning, Int. J. Psychoanal. 42:22, 1961.

15. Brown, G., and Harris, T.: Social origins of depression, London, 1978, Tavistock Publications, Ltd.

16. Brown, R., Ramirez, D., and Taub, J.: The prescription of exercise for depression, Physician Sports Med. 6(12):34, 1978.

17. Bugen, L.: Human grief: a model for prediction and intervention, Am. J. Orthopsychiatry 47:196, Apr. 1972.

18. Cadoret, R. et al.: Depressive disease: life events and onset of illness, Arch. Gen. Psychiatry 26:133, 1972.

19. Clayton, P. et al.: Mourning and depression: their similarities and differences, Can. Psychiatr. Assoc. 19:309, 1974.

20. Cohen, M.: Personal identity and sexual identity, Psychiatry 29:1, 1966.

21. Crary, W., and Crary, G.: Depression, Am. J. Nurs. 73:472, 1973.

22. Drake, R., and Price, J.: Depression: adaptation to disruption and loss, Perspect. Psychiatr. Care 13:163, Oct.-Dec. 1975.

23. Dyer, E.: Parenthood as crisis: a restudy, Marriage Family Living 25:196, 1963.

24. Engel, G.: Grief and grieving, Am. J. Nurs. 64:93, Sept. 1964.

25. Freud, S.: Mourning and melancholia. Standard edition of the complete psychological works of Sigmund Freud, vol. 14, London, 1957, Hogarth Press.

26. Goldberg, C.: Therapeutic tasks: strategies for changes, Perspect. Psychiatr. Care 18(4):156, 1980.

27. Gove, W.: The relationship between sex roles, marital status, and mental illness, Soc. Forces 51:34, Sept. 1972.

28. Hodge, J.: They that mourn, J. Relig. Health 11:229, 1972.

29. Holmes, T., and Rahe, R.: The social readjustment rating scale, J. Psychosom. Res. 2:213, 1967.

30. Holmstrom, L.: The two-career family, Cambridge, Mass., 1972, Schenkman Publishing Co., Inc.

31. Hudgens, R., Morrison, J., and Barchha, R.: Life events and onset of primary affective disorders, Arch. Gen. Psychiatry 16:134, 1967.

32. Ilfeld, F.: Characteristics of current social stressors, Psychol. Rep. 39:1231, 1976.

33. Ilfield, F.: Current social stressors and symptoms of depression, Am. J. Psychiatry 134:161, Feb. 1977.

34. Jacob, T. et al.: Role expectation and role performance in distressed and normal couples, J. Abnorm. Psychol. 87:286, 1978.

35. Jamison, K. et al.: Clouds and silver linings: positive experiences associated with primary affective disorders, Am. J. Psychiatry 137(2):198, Feb. 1980.

36. Klerman, G.: Overview of affective disorders. In Freedman, A., Kaplan, H., and Sadock, B., editors: Comprehensive textbook of psychiatry, vol. 2, Baltimore, 1980, The Williams & Wilkins Co.

37. Kübler-Ross, E.: On death and dying, New York, 1969, The Macmillan Publishing Co., Inc.

38. LeMasters, E.: Parenthood as crisis, Marriage Family Living 19:352, 1957.

39. Levitt, E., and Lubin, B.: Depression: concepts, controversies, and some new facts, New York, 1975, Springer Publishing Co., Inc.

40. Lewinsohn, P., and Amenson, C.: Some relations between pleasant and unpleasant mood related activities and depression, J. Abnorm. Psychol. 87:644, 1978.

41. Lewinsohn, P., Youngren, M., and Grosscup, S.: Reinforcement and depression. In Depue, R., editor: The psychobiology of the depressive disorders, New York, 1979, Academic Press, Inc.

42. Lindemann, E.: Symptomatology and management of acute grief, Am. J. Psychiatry 101:141, Sept. 1944.

43. Maddison, D., and Walker, W.: Factors affecting the outcome of conjugal bereavement, Br. J. Psychiatry 113:1057, 1967.

44. Mayo, J., O'Connell, R., and O'Brien, J.: Families of manic-depressive patients: effect of treatment, Am. J. Psychiatry 136:1535, 1979.

45. McLean, P.: Remediation of skills and performance deficits in depression. In Clarkin, J., and Glazer, H., editors: Depression: behavioral and directive intervention strategies, New York, 1981, Garland Publishing, Inc.

46. Myers, J., Lindenthal, J., and Pepper, M.: Life events, social integration, and psychiatric symptomatology, J. Health and Soc. Behav. 16:421, 1975.

47. Nezu, A., and Ronan, G.: Life stress, current problems, problem solving, and depressive symptoms: an integrative model, J. Consult. Clin. Psychol. 53(5):693, 1985.

48. Noyes, R.: Book review of grief and mourning in cross-cultural perspective, Am. J. Psychiatry 135:137, 1978.

49. Parens, H., McConville, B., and Kaplan, S.: Prediction of frequency of illness from the response to separation, Psychosom. Med. 28:162, 1966.

50. Parkes, C.: Bereavement: studies of grief in adult life, New York, 1972, International Universities Press.

51. Parkes, C., and Brown, R.: Health after bereavement: a controlled study of young Boston widows and widowers, Psychosom. Med. **34:**449, 1972.

52. Paykel, E. et al.: Life events and depression, Arch. Gen. Psychiatry **21:**753, 1969.

53. Plumlee, A.: Biological rhythms and affective illness, J. Psychosoc. Nurs. Ment. Health Serv. **24**(3):12, Mar. 1986.

54. Post, R., and Ballenger, J.: Neurobiology of mood disorders, Baltimore, Md., 1984, The Williams & Wilkins Co.

55. Rapoport, R., and Rapoport, R.: Dual career families, London, 1971, Penguin Books, Ltd.

56. Rapoport, R., and Rapoport, R.: Early and later experiences as determinants of adult behavior: married women's family and career patterns, Br. J. Sociol. **22:**16, Mar. 1971.

57. Rehm, L.: A self-control therapy program for treatment of depression. In Clarkin, J., and Glazer, H., editors: Depression: behavioral and directive intervention strategies, New York, 1981, Garland Publishing, Inc.

58. Robertson, J., and Robertson, J.: Young children in brief separation: a fresh look, Psychoanal. Study Child **26:**264, 1971.

59. Robins, E., and Guze, S.: Establishment of diagnostic validity in psychiatric illness, Am. J. Psychiatry **126:**983, 1970.

60. Rosenblatt, P., Walsh, R., and Jackson, D.: Grief and mourning in cross-cultured perspective, New Haven, Conn., 1976, HRAF Press.

61. Rosenfield, S.: Sex differences in depression: do women always have higher rates? J. Health Soc. Behav. **21:**33, Mar. 1980.

62. Sachs, M.: Running therapy for the depressed client, Topics Clin. Nurs. **3**(2):77, 1981.

63. Secunda, S., editor: The depressive disorders, special report 1973, U.S. Department of Health, Education, and Welfare, National Institute of Mental Health.

64. Seligman, M.: Helplessness: on depression, development and death, San Francisco, 1975, W.H. Freeman and Co., Publishers.

65. Smith, A., and Brandt, S.: Physical activity: a tool in promoting mental health, J. Psychiatr. Nurs. **17**(11):24, 1979.

66. Spitz, R.: Anaclitic depression, Psychoanal. Study Child **2:**313, 1942.

67. Stuart, G.W.: Role strain and depression: a causal inquiry, J. Psychosoc. Nurs. **19**(12):20, 1981.

68. Van Servellen, G.: Women treating women for depression, J. Psychosoc. Nurs. **19**(8):22, 1981.

69. Van Servellen, G., and Dull, L.: Group psychotherapy for depressed women: a model, J. Psychosoc. Nurs. **19**(8):25, 1981.

70. Warheit, G.: Life events, coping stress, and depressive symptomatology, Am. J. Psychiatry **136**(4B):502, 1979.

71. Weissman, M., and Klerman, G.: Sex differences and the epidemiology of depression, Arch. Gen. Psychiatry **34:**98, Jan. 1977.

72. Wender, P.: On necessary and sufficient conditions in psychiatric exploration, Arch. Gen. Psychiatry **16:**41, 1967.

73. Whybrow, P., Akiskal, H., and McKinney, W.: Mood disorders: toward a new psychobiology, New York, 1984, Plenum Press.

74. Winokur, G.: Heredity in the affective disorders. In Anthony, E., and Benedek, T., editors: Depression and human existence, Boston, 1975, Little, Brown & Co.

75. Woods, N.: Employment, family roles, and mental health in young married women, Nurs. Res. **34**(1):4, 1985.

76. Wright, J., and Beck, A.: Cognitive therapy of depression: theory and practice, Hosp. Community Psychiatry **34**(12):1119, Dec. 1983.

77. Youssef, F.: Compliance with therapeutic regimens: a follow-up study for patients with affective disorders, J. Adv. Nurs. **8:**513, 1983.

■ ANNOTATED SUGGESTED READINGS ■

Akiskal, H., and McKinney, W.: Overview of recent research in depression, Arch. Gen. Psychiatry **32:**285, 1975.

This article translates data from psychodynamic, sociobehavioral, and neurobiological research into a clinically meaningful framework. Ten models of depression are described and an integrated model is presented that incorporates and synthesizes findings from different schools. This is advanced reading with an extensive bibliography for the interested nurse.

*Authier, J., Authier, K., and Lutey, B.: Clinical management of the tearfully depressed patient: communication skills for the nurse practitioner, J. Psychiatr. Nurs. **17**(2):34, 1979.

The first section of this article deals with the management of the patient who has a legitimate reason to be depressed, followed by a discussion of the more complex management of "illegitimate" tears in a categorization of personality types.

*Baker, B., and Lynn, M.: Psychiatric nursing consultation: the use of an inservice model to assist nurses in the grief process, J. Psychiatr. Nurs. **17**(5):15, 1979.

The authors relate an account of their consultation with medical-surgical nurses in relation to their feelings of caring for the dying via the development, implementation, and evaluation of an inservice model.

Beck, A., Rush, A., Shaw, B., and Emery, G.: Cognitive therapy of depression, New York, 1979, The Guilford Press.

This primary reference describes cognitive therapy and combines both theory and clinical practice. It is necessary reading for nurses who wish to utilize this approach.

Belmaker, R., and von Praag, H.: Mania: an evolving concept.

This text surveys the rapidly developing area of primary affective disorders. Good reference source.

Bowden, C.: Current treatment of depression, Hosp. Community Psychiatry **36**(11):1192, Nov. 1985.

---

*Asterisk indicates nursing reference.

This important article reviews current medical treatments for depression emphasizing biological therapies, including drug selection, newer antidepressants, usefulness of plasma levels, and ECT. This should be read by all nurses working with depressed patients.

Bowlby, J.: Processes of mourning, Int. J. Psychoanal. **42:**317, 1961.

Bowlby describes the object loss model of depression and his stages of mourning in this important article. This is a "classic" in the field and highly recommended as a primary reference.

Clarkin, J., and Glazer, H.: Depression: behavioral and directive intervention strategies, New York, 1981, Garland Publishing, Inc.

This highly recommended text is quite comprehensive in behavioral intervention in depression. Its four parts include assessment of depression, major behavioral models, clinical treatment strategies (including suicide and somatic treatments), and special groups (such as children and the elderly).

*Dealing with death, Am. J. Nurs. **76:**1486, 1976.

This is a series of three articles discussing adaptation to death. Two are particularly good—"The Grieving Patient and Family" and "The Grieving Nurse." The last article contends that nurses who work with the dying also go through a grieving process and explains this process within the stages of dying described by Kübler-Ross.

*Field, W.: Physical causes of depression, J. Psychosoc. Nurs. Ment. Health Serv. **23**(10):7, 1985.

This article summarizes the major physical causes of depression including brain diseases, drugs, electrolyte disorders, postsurgical phenomena and other physiological relationships.

*Freihofer, P., and Felton, G.: Nursing behaviors in bereavement: an exploratory study, Nurs. Res. **25:**332, Sept.-Oct. 1976.

Terminally ill patients and their families were studied to determine nursing behaviors that offer greatest support, comfort, and ease of suffering to loved ones. The behaviors were categorized and have implications for nursing care.

Gaylin, W.: Feelings: our vital signs, New York, 1979, Harper & Row, Publishers, Inc.

This text attempts to analyze and describe feelings. The author contends that feelings are important and serve a purpose; they provide for our survival both as individuals and as a species.

*Goldberg, C.: Therapeutic tasks: strategies for change, Perspect. Psychiatr. Care **18**(4):156, 1980.

The value of therapeutic action-focused tasks is well described in this article through the effective use of clinical examples. Practical, pertinent, and clearly written by the nurse author.

*Gordon, V., and Ledray, L.: Depression in women: the challenge of treatment and prevention, J. Psychosoc. Nurs. Ment. Health Serv. **23**(1):26, Jan. 1985.

Theories of etiology of depression as applied to women are described in this article with implications for treatment and depression. It is a thorough review of the field.

*Harris, E.: The dexamethasone suppression test, Am. J. Nurs. **82:**784, 1982.

This brief article describes the indications and procedures related to this recently developed test for somatically treatable depression.

*Hauser, M., and Feinberg, D.: An operational approach to the delayed grief and mourning process, J. Psychiatr. Nurs., **14:**29, July, 1976.

The authors describe Bowlby's phases of mourning and identify psychological components related to each phase. They identify appropriate nursing interventions based on their model. It is a well-written article with direct clinical application.

*Jacobson, A.: Melancholy in the 20th century: causes and prevention, J. Psychiatr. Nurs. **18**(7):11, 1980.

The nurse author examines the detrimental aspects of depression for both individuals and society. Her unique contribution, however, is her focus on primary prevention activities that may be implemented by nurses. Well researched, well conceived, and well written.

Kiev, A.: Somatic manifestations of depressive disorders, Princeton, N.J., 1974, Excerpta Medica Foundation.

This brief text reviews the various physical behaviors associated with depression. Individual chapters discuss the gastrointestinal tract, sleep, sexual dysfunction, and pain.

Lindemann, E.: Symptomatology and management of acute grief, Am. J. Psychiatry **101:**141, Sept. 1944.

In this "classic" article Lindemann describes the course and management of normal and abnormal grief reactions on the basis of his observations of 101 patients. It is an important work in the study of grieving.

*Mandel, H.: Nurses' feelings about working with dying, Am. J. Nurs. **81:**1194, 1981.

The value of this brief article is in the elaboration of feelings and attitudes expressed by nurses who are working with the chronically and terminally ill. These feelings can serve as a good starting point for increasing one's self-awareness and in stimulating the need for support systems for nurses working with the dying.

*Manderino, M.: Mobilizing depressed clients: cognitive nursing approaches, J. Psychosoc. Nurs. Ment. Health Serv. **24**(5):23, 1986.

Cognitive-behavioral interventions are described in detail by the authors. This article will be particularly helpful to practitioners who would like to see specific examples of the application of the cognitive therapy approach to depression.

Post, R., and Ballenger, J.: Neurobiology of mood disorders, Baltimore, Md., 1984, The Williams & Wilkins Co.

This text is an encyclopedia of present knowledge of the neurobiology of affective disorders with implications for diagnosis, treatment, etiology, and prevention. It is advanced reading for the nurse specialist.

*Rankin, N.: Name that feeling! An innovative teaching tool, J. Psychosoc. Nurs. Ment. Health Serv. **19**(12):37, 1981.

This article describes a simple but innovative teaching strategy for promoting awareness of different kinds of feelings to beginning nursing students.

*Rogers, C., and Ulsafer-Van Lanan, J.: Nursing interventions in depression, Orlando, Fl., 1985, Grune & Stratton.

This nursing text describes the treatment of people with affective disorders in a variety of age groups and treatment settings. It is one of the few books devoted entirely to depressed patients and it is recommended for its incorporation of recent research and biological aspects of affective disorders.

Scarf, M.: Unfinished business: pressure points in the lives of women, New York, 1980, Doubleday and Co., Inc.

Using 10 case studies, the journalist author describes the causes and consequences of female depression. Readable and provocative.

*Schneider, J.: Hopelessness and helplessness, J. Psychiatr. Nurs. **18**(3):12, 1980.

The concepts of hopelessness and helplessness are thoroughly described in this article along with the effect of the concepts on patients in a general hospital setting. Valuable suggestions for nursing intervention are proposed and demonstrated in case examples.

Schoenberg, B. et al., editors: Bereavement: its psychosocial aspects, New York, 1975, Columbia University Press.

This is an excellent collection of essays that uses a multidisciplinary approach. Bereavement is examined in light of sociological research, clinical studies, and theoretical designs. Support systems, the role of health professionals, and therapeutic interventions are also described. It is useful reference for nurses.

Stotland, E.: The psychology of hope, San Francisco, 1969, Jossey-Bass, Inc., Publishers.

This text presents a theory of motivation and hope. It explores the relationship of hope to action, anxiety, and psychosis and outlines a form of therapy using the element of hope.

*Van Servellen, G., and Dull, L.: Group psychotherapy for depressed women: a model, J. Psychosoc. Nurs. Ment. Health Serv. **19**(8):25, 1981.

The authors present a useful format for group treatment of depressed women along with a research design to evaluate the effectiveness of therapy.

Whybrow, P., Akiskal, H., and McKinney, W.: Mood disorders: toward a new psychobiology, New York, 1984, Plenum Press.

This text reviews historical and clinical perspectives on mood disorders and the present knowledge of etiologic factors. It then presents a model of psychobiological integration that views affective illness as a final common path to adaptive failure. Highly recommended reading.

Wright, J., and Beck, A.: Cognitive therapy of depression: theory and practice, Hosp. Community Psychiatry **34**(12):1119, Dec. 1983.

This excellent article summarizes the salient features of the theory and practice of cognitive therapy, including supportive research. It is highly recommended to nurses interested in this topic.

*Wright, L.: Life threatening illness, J. Psychosoc. Nurs. Ment. Health Serv. **23**(9):6, 1985.

This article describes a nursing approach to working with patients and family members confronted with a life-threatening illness. Care is described according to three phases of dying identified by the author.

*Youssef, F.: Compliance with therapeutic regimens: a follow-up study for patients with affective disorders, J. Adv. Nurs. **8**:513, 1983.

This is one of the few research articles to report on a patient education intervention by nurses and its effect on patient compliance. More studies like this should be conducted by nurses.

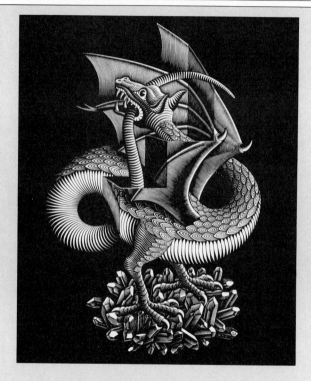

Out, out brief candle!
Life's but a walking shadow, a poor player
That struts and frets his hour upon the stage
And then is heard no more. It is a tale
Told by an idiot, full of sound and fury,
Signifying nothing.

William Shakespeare, Macbeth, Act V

C H A P T E R   1 6

SELF-DESTRUCTIVE BEHAVIOR

LEARNING OBJECTIVES

After studying this chapter, the student should be able to:

- describe the continuum of coping responses related to self-enhancing/self-destructive behavior.

- compare and contrast indirect and direct self-destructive behavior.

- discuss the predisposing factors that place a person at risk for self-destructive behavior.

- identify individuals who represent a high suicide risk.

- analyze precipitating stressors that contribute to the development of self-destructive behavior.

- identify the behaviors of an individual that are indicative of direct or indirect self-destructive activity.

- differentiate suicide threats and attempts as related to the concepts of ambivalence and hostility.

- analyze coping mechanisms related to indirect and attempted direct self-destructive behavior.

- formulate individualized nursing diagnoses for patients with direct and indirect self-destructive behavior.

- assess the relationship between nursing diagnoses and medical diagnoses associated with self-destructive behavior.

- develop long- and short-term nursing goals that take into account the need to protect the patient from self-destructive impulses and promote self-enhancing behavior.

- apply therapeutic nurse-patient relationship principles with appropriate rationale in planning the care of the patient with self-destructive behavior.

- describe nursing interventions appropriate to the needs of the patient who is experiencing self-destructive behaviors.

- develop a mental health education plan to assist patients and family members to understand self-destructive behavior.

- assess the importance of the evaluation of the nursing process when working with patients who have self-destructive behaviors.

- identify directions for future nursing research.

- select appropriate readings for further study.

Continuum of self-enhancing to self-destructive responses

Many daily activities involve an element of risk. For instance, riding in an automobile exposes a person to the risk of physical injury if the car is involved in an accident. Even if no accident occurs, there is increased stress from exposure to hazardous situations that creates anxiety and requires the use of coping mechanisms. As another example, choice of diet may indicate a willingness to take risks. A family that lives on a farm and uses organic methods to raise most of their food is exposed to a much lower level of potentially harmful chemicals then the family that usually eats commercially prepared foods.

Since life is characterized by a pervasive element of risk, each individual must choose the amount of potential danger to which he is willing to expose himself.

Sometimes these choices are conscious and rational. For instance, the elderly person who decides to stay in the house on an icy day has chosen not to risk falling and possibly fracturing a bone. Other risk-taking behavior is unconsciously determined. The soldier who volunteers for a suicide mission is probably unaware of his motivation, although if asked, he would be likely to cite patriotism or concern for his comrades. Most people go through life accepting some risks as part of their daily routine, while carefully avoiding others. The person who constantly takes chances while driving may refuse to fly in an airplane because he feels unsafe.

Even though life is risky, there is a norm in most societies that defines the degree of danger to which the person may expose himself. This norm varies according to the age, sex, socioeconomic status, and occupation of the individual. For instance, there is great reluctance in contemporary American society to allow women to

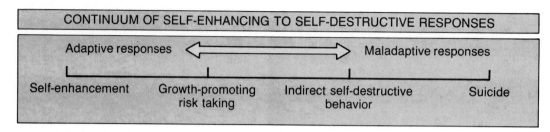

Fig. 16-1. Continuum of self-enhancing to self-destructive behaviors.

participate in "contact" sports with men. Although this attitude is undoubtedly determined by many factors, the reason that is usually given is that women are not strong enough to compete with men and would get hurt. In general, the very young, the old, and women are viewed as needing to be protected from harm.

There is great ambivalence toward those who engage in potentially self-destructive behavior. Some risk takers are greatly admired, particularly athletes, members of the military services, those with dangerous occupations, and those who place themselves in danger to help others. At the same time, feelings of admiration may be accompanied by fear and perplexity about the danger-seeking behavior. The varying attitudes toward cigarette smoking provide another example of cultural ambivalence. On one hand, smoking is viewed as mature behavior, denoting sophistication and social acceptability; on the other, it is seen as socially alienating, immature, and inconsiderate of the needs of others.

■ Types of self-destructive behavior

Although there has been an awareness of the range of self-destructive behavior from subtle to overt, until recently, there has been little systematic attention given to the covert and generally long-term end of the continuum. Farberow[11] has differentiated indirect from direct self-destructive behavior. Direct self-destructive behavior (DSDB) includes any form of suicidal activity, such as suicide threats, attempts, gestures, and completed suicide. The intent of this behavior is death and the individual is aware of this as the desired outcome. Indirect self-destructive behavior (ISDB) is any activity that is detrimental to the physical well-being of the person and potentially has the outcome of death. However, the person is unaware of this potential and will generally deny it if confronted. Examples of ISDB that will be used in this chapter include eating disorders, such as obesity, anorexia nervosa, and bulimia, and noncompliance with medical treatment. Abuse of alcohol and drugs is also self-destructive in nature. This behavioral disruption is discussed in detail in Chapter 20. Other ISDBs identified by Farberow[11] include cigarette smok-

ing, automobile accidents, self-mutilation, gambling, criminal activity and socially deviant behavior, stress-seeking behavior, and participation in high-risk sports.

Theories of self-destructive behavior are intertwined with those of self-concept and alterations in mood. Understanding of the behaviors to be discussed in this chapter will be enhanced by careful study of Chapters 14 and 15. To contemplate or initiate destruction of the self, one must have low regard for the self. Low self-esteem leads to depression, which is always present to some extent in self-destructive behavior. The range of behaviors related to the self that includes self-destructive behavior is illustrated in Fig. 16-1.

It should be noted that the levels of behavior in the continuum overlap. This indicates that growth-promoting risk-taking behavior may be self-enhancing. For instance, the young girl who learns and excels at gymnastics is building her self-esteem and projecting a positive self-concept. However, if she attempts to do stunts for which she is not prepared and does not take safety precautions, her behavior becomes indirectly self-destructive. Similarly, there are times when ISDB may merge into DSDB. For instance, a diabetic who has never complied completely with his prescribed diet and medication regimen may become very discouraged and intentionally take an overdose of insulin. The nurse must be aware of this tendency and be alert to subtle shifts in the mood and behavior of self-destructive patients.

Assessment

■ Predisposing factors

■ **AFFECTING INDIRECT SELF-DESTRUCTIVE BEHAVIOR.** ISDB may be differentiated from DSDB, or suicidal behavior, by its duration and by the individual's awareness of the purpose of the behavior. ISDB is usually long term and repetitive, whereas suicidal behavior, if not interrupted, leads rapidly to death. This distinction differentiates between the individual who is involved in numerous traffic accidents as the result of drinking and driving (ISDB) and the person who is killed while sober by driving his car into a wall at a high rate of speed (DSDB). Although the latter situation is usually classified as accidental, it may be assumed that many one-car accidental deaths are really suicidal in nature.

The other cardinal feature of ISDB is the person's use of the mechanism of denial, frequently accompanied by rationalization. If the dangerous nature of the behavior is recognized intellectually, it is not taken seriously. For instance, a hypertensive person may avoid salting food and adding salt while cooking, but eat potato chips, cured meats, and processed foods with a high sodium content. The patient may respond to confrontation about this behavior by saying, "I know I shouldn't eat those foods, but I feel good. A little bit once in a while can't hurt me." Another example is the anorexic person who is a student of nutrition but refuses to acknowledge her own starvation. This recognition of potential harmfulness without any change in behavior, or actual denial of any danger is typical of the indirectly self-destructive person. It should also be recognized that denial can help the individual to function. Everyone engages in risky activities on a daily basis. Denial controls the anxiety that would interfere with activities of daily living if there was complete awareness of the dangers of everyday life. The failure of this mechanism may lead to maladaptive neurotic behaviors, such as phobias. The nurse must assess whether the individual is using denial in a healthy adaptive manner, or if it is interfering with adaptation and healthier coping mechanisms must be explored.

Noncompliance. Nurses are frequently involved in caring for patients who are resistant to recommended self-care activities. It has been estimated that at least 50% of patients do not comply with health care providers' recommendations.[19] Since our society is characterized by an increasing elderly population, there is also an increase in the incidence of chronic diseases, such as cardiovascular disease, cancer, cerebrovascular accident, renal disease, and diabetes mellitus. The medical and nursing care of all these conditions requires self-care activities on the part of the patient. Diet, activity, and medications must be controlled. Good health practices are necessary to prevent complications or the development of additional illnesses. To support the patient in performing self-care, the nurse must understand the underlying emotional issues and assist the patient to deal with them.

Eating disorders. Sociocultural factors are believed to play an important role in the development of eating disorders. Family eating patterns are transmitted to children beginning even before birth. The nutritional status of the mother has a direct effect on the health of the infant. Sociocultural factors influence dietary patterns.

Ethnic background may affect a mother's decision to breast feed or bottle feed. It has been demonstrated that bottle fed babies have a higher tendency to be overweight. Ethnicity also has an influence on food preferences. People of Italian descent become accustomed to high carbohydrate diets, whereas people with Oriental backgrounds tend to consume more seafood and vegetables. Economic status also affects diet. In affluent societies, obesity tends to be more prevalent among the poor. Anorexia nervosa, on the other hand, occurs more frequently in the upper middle and upper classes.

Powers[24] has applied Minuchin's description of psychosomatogenic families to the understanding of the eating disorders. The characteristics of this type of family include a special configuration and functioning, child involvement in parental conflicts, and the presence of a physiological vulnerability in the child. There are four characteristics of the family configuration. The first is enmeshment. This means that individuality is lost within the identity of the family group. Autonomy is not encouraged. Role confusion results from lack of clear boundaries among family members. Emotionally, there is overinvolvement and intrusion on the thoughts and feelings of other members. The second characteristic is overprotectiveness and the third is rigidity. Finally, there is conflict avoidance, which results in a lack of resolution of conflicts. Conflict may be denied, or there may be continuous fighting without addressing the real problem. Family conflicts are focused on the problematic member, thus avoiding confrontation with the real issue. The true conflict may really lie between the parents, but is acted out by the physiologically vulnerable child.

Anorexia nervosa is a condition that occurs primarily among young women. Only 5% to 10% of all cases of anorexia nervosa have been identified in young men.[2] It has been described by Bruch as "the relentless pursuit of excessive thinness."[5] The incidence of anorexia nervosa in the United States has been increasing for the last 20 years. Prior to 1960, it was rarely seen. Recent estimates of prevalence are 1.3 to 2.4 per 100,000 total population. However, there have been reports of a prevalence of one in 250 in white females who are in the high-risk age group of 12 to 18 years old.[24] Most anorectic people are members of upper or upper middle class families. It is extremely rare in situations where food is scarce and is also rarely seen in blacks.[24]

Researchers have developed profiles of those who are predisposed to developing anorexia nervosa. Doyen[9] describes them as "overly sensitive, introverted, secretive, perfectionistic, selfish, and extremely stubborn." The anorectic males studied by Andersen and Mickalide[2] were found to be perfectionistic and self-critical. Their families are of a higher socioeconomic status, and there was a positive history for affective or eating disorders. These men were frequently involved in an occupation or sport that valued thinness. Both men and women often become anorectic when they continue with a weight reduction diet after they have achieved a normal weight.

Another eating disorder that is similar in some respects to anorexia nervosa is **bulimia.** The bulimic patient experiences episodes of binge eating, frequently followed by vomiting. Binge eating is compulsive intake of food that is stopped only when the person vomits, experiences pain, runs out of food, or is interrupted. This disorder is also almost exclusively one of white, socioeconomically secure, young women. The age of onset is usually between 17 and 25 years, somewhat

older than that of anorexia nervosa. It is differentiated from anorexia nervosa by the fact that severe weight loss is not generally seen and the individual is well aware that her behavior is abnormal.[24] Bulimic patients are usually able to maintain a more normal weight by alternating binging and vomiting or by eating very little between binges.

The third eating disorder that is indirectly self-destructive is **obesity.** There is no generally accepted definition of obesity. A guideline is that obesity is considered to be present when the person weighs more than 20% over his ideal weight; overweight is defined as 10% above the ideal weight. The problems with this criterion are that height and weight charts have not been developed scientifically, and individual characteristics, such as proportion of muscle mass to total body weight are not considered. When it is performed correctly, mea-

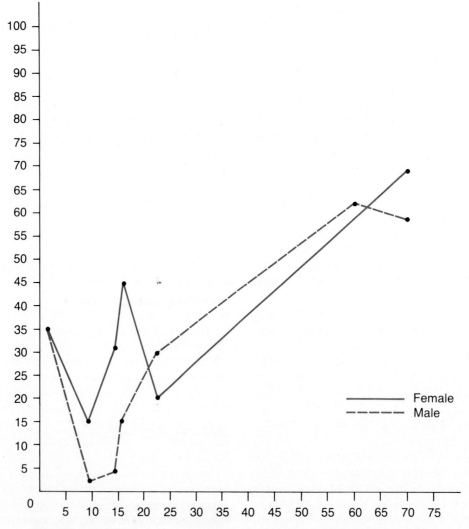

Fig. 16-2. Prevalence of overweight in males and females from infancy to age 69.

surement of skinfold thickness over the midtriceps area is a more accurate way to determine the presence of obesity.[24] It has been estimated that one third of the population of the United States is overweight. Obesity is sometimes described as a disorder that is characteristic of an affluent society. In reality, there is a higher prevalence of overweight and obesity among the poor in affluent societies. Low-calorie foods, such as meat, seafood, fruits, and vegetables, are expensive. Poor people tend to eat diets that are high in carbohydrates, leading to weight gain. Obesity is also related to low activity levels. Figure 16-2 illustrates the prevalence of overweight and obesity by age and sex in the United States.[8] No definite correlation has been found between obesity and educational level. However, there is a lower prevalence among people who achieve a higher socioeconomic status than that of their parents. The inverse is also true. In terms of the major religious groups, prevalence is highest among Jews, followed by Roman Catholics, and lowest among Protestants.

Familial tendencies toward obesity and overweight have been identified. However, it is premature to assume that this is due to heredity. It may be more related to sociocultural dietary patterns. It is difficult to identify a familial tendency for anorexia nervosa because the disorder has been so rare in the past that there are few longitudinal data on the children of anorectic women.

Research has revealed that overweight and obese people tend to have more fat cells than thin people. Fat cells develop during the last trimester of intrauterine life, the first 6 to 8 months after birth, and again during the adolescent growth spurt.[24] Children who gain weight at these critical times are at greater risk for obesity as adults. These data have implications for health education and primary prevention, particularly for nurses working in community health settings or schools. It has also been determined that there is a relationship between weight and activity level. Overweight people have been observed to be less active, even when engaged in sports, than people of normal weight.[24] Obesity is clearly a major public health problem that is a significant risk factor for the development of other serious health problems, including heart disease, hypertension, some forms of cancer, and diabetes mellitus.

■ **AFFECTING DIRECT SELF-DESTRUCTIVE BEHAVIOR.** The ultimate level of self-destructiveness is suicidal behavior. The stigma attached to suicide makes it difficult to determine the magnitude of the problem. The reported suicide rate in the United States in 1975 was 12.6 per 100,000 population. The rate for males of all ages was 18 per 100,000 and for females was 6.6.[28] The recent increase of suicide by adolescents in the United States has been a source of great concern to mental health care providers. For females aged 15 to 25, the suicide rate per 100,000 increased from 2 in 1955 to 4.3 in 1980. For males in the same age group the increase was from 6.3 per 100,000 in 1955 to 20.2 in 1980. Since 1980, the adolescent suicide rate has remained stable.[16]

Many deaths that appear to be accidental may in reality be suicidal. Inferences about the motivation for accidental death can sometimes be made based on a "psychological autopsy." This is a retrospective review of the individual's behavior for the time preceding his death and is accomplished by tracing the person's activities and interviewing those with whom the dead person had contact just prior to death.

Suicidology has become an important subspecialty in psychiatry. Specialists in this field have done much work in an effort to identify groups of people who are at risk for suicide. It has been possible to develop profiles of high-risk groups. In general, males commit suicide more frequently than females (a ratio of about 3:1), and women attempt suicide more frequently than men (also about 3:1).[27] Suicide rates also vary with age. For example, the rate for white men increases steadily with age. Although white males over 50 years old constitute only 10% of the United States population, they represent 28% of the total deaths by suicide.[16] In contrast, the rate for white women peaks at age 45 to 54 and then declines. In general, married people have the lowest rates, those never married are next, and divorced or widowed people have the highest rate, with the exception of older, never-married white men.[21] Table 16-1 summarizes the risk factors associated with suicidal behavior.

■ **Precipitating stressors**

Self-destructive behavior may result from almost any stress that is experienced by the individual as overwhelming. Therefore stressors are to some extent individualized, as is the person's ability to tolerate stress. All self-destructive behaviors may be viewed as attempts to escape from life situations that have become uncomfortable or intolerable. Anxiety is therefore central to the cause of self-destructive behavior.

The anxiety that is associated with a deliberate attempt at self-destruction is overwhelming. It is difficult to imagine if it has not been experienced. Most people cringe from contemplating their own deaths, much less initiating the destruction of the self. In fact, Shneidman[27] believes that self-death is experienced differently from the death of another, since self-death literally cannot be experienced. Therefore, in a sense, the person who destroys himself actually destroys everything else *but* himself.

TABLE 16-1

RISK FACTORS FOR SUICIDAL BEHAVIOR*

Factor	High risk	Low risk
Age	Over 45 years or adolescent	25 to 45 years or under 12 years
Sex	Male	Female
Marital status	Divorced, separated, or widowed	Married
Socialization	Isolated	Socially active
Occupation	Professional workers (medicine, dentistry, or law) or student	Blue collar workers
Employment	Unemployed	Employed
Physical illness	Chronically or terminally ill	No serious medical problems
Mental illness	Depression, delusions, or hallucinations	Personality disorder
Drug and alcohol use	Intoxicated and/or addicted	Neither intoxicated nor addicted
Previous attempts	At least one	None
Plan	Definite plan specified	Vague plan
Method	Violent means: shooting, hanging, or jumping	Nonviolent means: drugs, poison, or carbon monoxide
Availability of means	Readily available	Not yet obtained

*Risk factors are relative and intended as a guide to assessment. **Low** risk never means **no** risk.

In contrast, people who are engaged in gradually self-destructive behavior tend to deny their eventual deaths, usually believing that they can assume control at any time. This fantasy of being able to control, although it alleviates anxiety, also helps to perpetuate the behavior. Such activities as overeating may also decrease anxiety and thus are difficult to change. The anxiety that leads to self-destructive behavior may evolve from a variety of sources: physiological, psychological, and sociocultural.

■ AFFECTING INDIRECT SELF-DESTRUCTIVE BEHAVIOR

Physiological stressors. There is no definitive research indicating a direct relationship between a biological factor and most forms of ISDB. Some forms of obesity do seem to be biologically determined. Endocrine disorders, such as hypothyroidism, hypercortisolism (Cushing's syndrome), the Stein-Leventhal syndrome, and hypogonadism[8] result in obesity. The latter three disorders are quite rare, and known physiological stressors account for very few instances of obesity. Endocrinological disorders have been explored in conjunction with anorexia nervosa. However, most studies have been done after the condition is well advanced and may be the result, rather than the cause, of starvation. There is some suggestion that dopamine may play a role in the development of this disorder. Dopamine is known to be an appetite depressant, so elevated dopamine levels could contribute to anorexia nervosa.[24] However, the fact that most anorectic persons experience extreme hunger would tend to negate this theory.

Psychological stressors. Psychologically, one of the antecedents of self-destructive behavior is **depression.** Filstead[13] has identified that despair is usually present when ISDB occurs. He describes despair as "a psychosocial state that people experience when they are trying to resolve what has become a serious personal problem . . . and realize that there does not appear to be any way to resolve it."[13] The ISDB may be serving as a defense against underlying despair. For instance, a person who is obese may overeat to overcome anxiety related to an inadequate self-concept. However, the behavior is self-defeating and does not resolve the problem. As self-dissatisfaction increases, despair may break through into awareness. If this happens, the person is at high risk for suicidal behavior.

Low self-esteem and depression contribute to the development of anorexia nervosa. This problem occurs at a point in psychosexual development that is characterized by emotional upheaval. Adolescents must establish a personal identity and become independent of parental control. Bruch[5] believes that anorectic behavior may follow a new experience that is viewed as threatening or may even be precipitated by a casual remark that is perceived as being critical of the patient's weight. She observes that, "they act as if no one had ever told them that developing curves and roundness is part of normal puberty."[5] Young women who are anorectic reject their growing feminine body configuration and strive for a childlike smallness. This lack of acceptance of the self leads to low self-esteem and depression that contributes to the continuation of the problem. It is interesting that obese young people may reflect the opposite pole of the same problem. They avoid the threat of growing sexuality by becoming unattractive and maintain a regressive childlike role by relating to the world through food. Parents may perpetuate the problems of children who have eating disorders by reinforcing dependency through their involvement in trying to persuade the child to eat or not to eat.

Adult obese persons are also frequently dependent people who feel insecure. Food may represent the security they felt during infancy. Comparisons have been made to alcoholism and the alcoholic's use of alcohol to protect him from the stresses of life. Alienation of others from the obese person often results in loneliness, adding to insecurity and depression, which leads to continued overeating.

Another issue that is prominent in relationship to ISDB is one of **control.** Whatever the risky behavior that is being performed, it is under the control of the actor. In addition, there are frequently power struggles between the person who is performing the behavior and significant others who recognize the perilous nature of the behavior and try to change it. For instance, the parents of anorectic patients become very worried as their daughter becomes more and more emaciated. As they try to persuade or force her to eat, she becomes more and more determined to circumvent their efforts. If forced to eat, the anorectic person will induce vomiting, take laxatives or diuretics, or exercise frantically, thus continuing to maintain control. The control issue is clearly reflected in this statement by Annie Ciseaux, the pseudonym of a nurse who is also anorectic: "The moment I surrendered myself to my parents' wishes that I eat—in other words when I refused to be responsible any more for what I was to become: a fat powerless person—I felt my self-esteem evaporate."[7]

Obese people again reflect the opposite side of the same behavioral pattern. As others try to persuade them to lose weight, they control the situation by sneaking food. This behavior leads to remorse, which causes anxiety, resulting in further eating. The motivation for dieting must come from within the dieter if weight loss is to occur.

Control is also a theme that is relevant to noncompliant behavior. The person who has a chronic illness often feels betrayed by his body, which, in the past, has been under his control. Compliance with a therapeutic regimen may be perceived as an admission that a problem exists and that the person cannot manage the problem without help. Refusal to perform required self-care activities returns a sense of control. As long as overt symptoms do not occur or can be ignored, the person maintains an illusion of health. As in the situations described, significant others may become concerned about the implications of noncompliant behavior. However, if they try to intervene, the sense of loss of control is increased and the person may become even more resistant. Powerful emotions, including anger, fear, and depression, underlie the overt behavior of self-control. If the person is not assisted to cope with these feelings, the ISDB will continue, or it may progress to more directly suicidal behavior.

Sociocultural stressors. Disorders of eating are influenced by the cultural definition of ideal body image. In the contemporary United States, thinness is valued, particularly for women. Pubertal girls who begin to develop rounded body contours may interpret this as fatness and attempt to counteract the effects of normal growth and development by dieting. This behavior sometimes leads to anorexia nervosa. The idealization of slimness can also assist the anorectic girl to justify her behavior by entering modeling, the theater, or the dance.

The adolescent must assimilate new behaviors and roles as a part of the developmental process. Demands from parents and peers can create increased anxiety and lead to eating disorders. Doyen has noted that anorexia nervosa may be precipitated by exposure to new social situations that require skills that the young person has not had an opportunity to master. Relative to young anorectic males, Andersen and Mickalide found that onset was sometimes preceded by "social disappointment, major life change, or a temporary illness that led to weight loss."[2]

Sociocultural factors also influence the occurrence of noncompliance with treatment. Leventhal[20] points out that most people develop their concept of the experience of illness through childhood episodes of acute infectious diseases. Treatment is instituted to cure the illness and when the symptoms disappear the treatment is discontinued. This conceptualization is not applicable to chronic illness, but is still the expectation of many patients. Many chronic diseases are characterized by episodic exacerbations of overt symptoms during a long-term covert disease process. If the acute illness model is applied, the patient assumes that the periods of time when no symptoms are experienced are times of wellness. Therefore, treatment is unnecessary. Leventhal[20] and others have also found that patients have difficulty identifying symptoms of chronic health problems, such as hypertension, except when they are severe. These findings have serious implications for the health care of the chronically ill.

Chronic illness also does not fit the pattern of sick role behavior that is acceptable in our society. The sick person is expected to acknowledge his illness, comply with treatment, and then recover. When recovery does not take place, the lack of conformity with cultural norms regarding sickness can lead to guilt and contribute to reluctance to comply with health care needs. Patient education programs must provide adequate information about the nature of the health problem, but must also recognize and attend to the patient's emotional responses to the illness experience.

■ **AFFECTING DIRECT SELF-DESTRUCTIVE BEHAVIOR.** When the sense of self-worth is extremely low, self-destructive behavior reaches its peak. It is at this point that suicidal behavior is likely to take place. Suicide implies a loss of the ability to value the self at all. This, in turn, may be related to unresolved grief, a perceived failure in life, or anger at the self.

Intrapsychic stressors. Unexpressed anger at others may lead a person to vent these feelings on himself. The individual may feel that his anger is not justified and then become guilty or may not be able to direct appropriate feelings outward. Since feelings must be attended to, the direction may be changed, with the self bearing the brunt of the attack. Some people with this problem may exhibit masochistic behavior. Masochism relates to the need to inflict pain on the self. Others may derogate the self or may underachieve. Still others may be so angry that they try to kill themselves.

Freudian theorists have viewed self-destructive behavior as the direction of hostile feelings toward an internalized love object. Ambivalence was an important component of the theory. More recently additional emphasis has been placed on the importance of the feelings of helplessness, hopelessness, and dependency in self-destructive behavior.

These feelings will be recognized as characteristics of depression. Individuals who are severely depressed are always suicidal risks. The extreme outcome of the self-directed anger that is believed to be present in depression is suicide. This is also the ultimate way of expressing hostility toward significant others. However, it is believed that there is always a kernel of hope that help will arrive, and someone will rescue the suicidal person by demonstrating that they really do care.

Bahra[3] has identified four psychological mechanisms that lead to suicide: ego destruction, ego withdrawal, displaced hostility, and response to hallucinations or delusions. Ego destruction refers to loss of self-esteem resulting in self-condemnation and guilt.

This becomes a vicious circle that strikes at the integrity of the ego. Ego withdrawal occurs as the result of a buildup of stress. Withdrawal is difficult to maintain. Frequently the stress is a major loss, leading to a feeling of isolation. Displaced hostility is manifest in two different patterns: the first is a need to punish a significant other and the second is a hostile response to a real or imagined threat.

Biological stressors. Another precursor to self-destructive behavior may be extreme confusion or personality disorganization.[3] This may be related to organic mental disorder, psychosis, or ingestion of hallucinogenic drugs. Many times, self-destructive behavior that is caused by one of these problems occurs inadvertently. The young person who is under the influence of PCP (phencyclidine) may feel invincible and walk in front of a truck or jump out a window. The psychotic person may harm himself because he is hearing voices that tell him to do so. The person may be quite unaware of the ultimate implications of his behavior.

Socioeconomic stressors. Patients with chronic, painful, or life-threatening illnesses may engage in self-destructive behavior. Frequently these people consciously choose to kill themselves. Quality of life becomes an issue that does, at times, supersede quantity of life. There may be an ethical dilemma for the nurse who becomes aware of the patient's choice to engage in one of these behaviors. There are no easy answers to the question of how to resolve this conflict. Each nurse must do so according to his or her own belief system.

Self-destructive behavior may also be related to a multiplicity of social and cultural factors. Durkheim,[10] in his pioneer study of suicidal behavior, identified three subcategories of suicide, based on the individual's motivation:

1. *Egoistic suicide* results from the individual's being poorly integrated into society.
2. *Altruistic suicide* results from obedience to customs and habit.
3. *Anomic suicide* results when society is unable to regulate the individual.

It is clear that in Durkheim's opinion the structure of society has a great influence on the individual and may either help or sustain him or lead him to destroy himself.

Choron[6] points out the importance of loneliness as a stressor related to suicide. This may refer either to the existential loneliness experienced by the psychotic individual or the loneliness that results from the loss of a loved one or self-esteem. He adds that interpersonal conflicts may also be stressors. Therefore the mere existence of relatedness is not sufficient to prevent suicides. The quality of the relationship must also be considered.

Interpersonal stressors. A related concept is the interpersonal frustration theory of suicide developed by Krauss.[19] This theorist agrees that interpersonal relationships are influential on suicidal behavior. He identified several propositions based on this belief:

1. Some people are more vulnerable to interpersonal frustration. These people tend to direct aggression inward and have a history of problems with interpersonal relationships.
2. The more meaningful the frustration is to the person, the more intense the feelings and the more serious the consequences.
3. Some cultures seem to produce greater occurrence of interpersonal frustration and thus have higher suicide rates.
4. Cultures that support positive interpersonal relationships tend to have lower suicide rates.

At this time it seems likely that self-destructive behavior is determined by a variety of factors, probably differing from one person to the next. For this reason it is extremely important to completely assess the patient's medical, psychological, and social history. Identification of probable causative factors leads to individualized planning for nursing care.

■ Behaviors

■ **ASSOCIATED WITH INDIRECT SELF-DE-STRUCTIVE BEHAVIOR.** The common characteristics of all varieties of ISDB are that it is progressively or potentially detrimental to the individual, the individual is intellectually aware that his behavior is risky, and he denies that he will suffer significant negative consequences from his behavior. This complex of behaviors will be examined for the examples of eating disorders, including overweight/obesity and anorexia nervosa/bulimia, and noncompliance with prescribed health care practices.

Eating disorders. Overweight and **obesity** generally result from an imbalance between calories consumed and energy expended. The exception to this rule occurs when a disruption in endocrine functioning causes disordered metabolism. It has been theorized that people who have a larger number of fat cells have a greater tendency to obesity than those with fewer fat cells. Longitudinal research is in progress to validate this theory.[24] However, it has been established that fat babies have a greater tendency to be fat children, and fat children tend to become fat adolescents and adults. Hence good nutrition and encouragement of activity in infancy and childhood leads to a tendency for normal weight in adulthood.

Some obese people experience a body image dis-

tortion. This is more frequently a problem for people who have had early onset of overweight problems. The body image disturbance takes the form of an inaccurate perception of body appearance combined with a feeling of dislike for the self. An interesting feature of this behavior is that it tends to persist even after weight has been lost. Many formerly obese people continue to view themselves as fat, even though they are cognitively aware that their weight is normal.

Contributing to the negative self-concept of overweight people is the commonly encountered belief that overweight is evidence of a moral defect related to the sin of gluttony. It may be viewed as a controllable problem, by the patient as well as others, resulting in guilt that compounds the problem. Guilt and self-dislike may lead to sporadic self-denial interspersed with episodes of binge eating. Some people become night eaters.[24] These people are able to control their eating all day, but then consume huge numbers of calories during the evening or night. A similar pattern is that of stringent dieting alternating with overeating, leading to a fluctuating weight pattern. People who fall into this category are susceptible to fad diets that promise quick weight loss with minimum deprivation. They are also vulnerable to using drugs to aid weight loss. Fad diets and diet pills do not assist the person to change basic eating patterns. Thus future weight gain is inevitable because the person returns to old habits as soon as a few pounds have been lost.

Food has multiple meanings for people. To assist an obese individual, it is necessary to discover the meaning of food for that person. For some, food represents love, particularly the unconditional love of infancy. Giving up food is then experienced as a severe deprivation. For these people, eating may also serve as consolation and is indulged in when stress is increased. Food also represents a cultural identity. People with strong ethnic ties find it hard to follow a diet that does not consider their cultural dietary patterns. There are also status implications associated with food and eating. The upper class places a great value on thinness, but also values indulgence, including appreciation of gourmet foods. Behaviors relative to eating patterns and weight reflect the individual's perception of food and eating.

Perception is also an important aspect of the behavior of young women with **anorexia nervosa.** These people perceive that they are fat and literally starve themselves to achieve their goal of being thin. However, because of the distortion in body image that they experience, the goal is unattainable. Even when emaciated to the point that their appearance is skeletal, they will maintain that they are fat and persist in their attempt to lose weight.

Bruch[5] describes the typical anorectic process as beginning with a diet. Initially, the dieter experiences a sense of deprivation and difficulty in maintaining the restrictions. However, she then enters a stage of pride in her accomplishment and this perpetuates the behavior. At the same time, biological effects of starvation cause distortions in perception of body sensations. There is a heightening of sensory experience and a feeling that has been compared to intoxication. As the condition progresses, the patient begins to feel special and different because of her superhuman effort and extraordinary accomplishment. This results in her alienation and isolation from others who fail to understand her behavior and its meaning to her. She then becomes increasingly absorbed in her own world and her behavior assumes even greater importance to her.[5]

Anorexia nervosa is really a misnomer. Anorexia means lack of appetite. People with anorexia nervosa do experience hunger, and it is the victory over hunger that provides their reward. Anorectic persons are often fascinated with food and cooking, becoming students of nutrition. They may compulsively loiter in places where food is sold or served and watch other people eat. Their life becomes centered around food and the avoidance of eating. Anorectic persons go to extremes to avoid weight gain. They will induce vomiting, take diuretics and laxatives, and exercise strenuously. If they are forced to eat, these associated behaviors are exacerbated. Ciseaux[7] described her discovery of vomiting to compensate for eating and her compulsion to vomit as soon as she had eaten.

In addition to the disturbance in body image, Bruch[5] describes decreased internal awareness and a sense of ineffectiveness as characteristics of anorexia nervosa. Decreased internal awareness refers to both emotional awareness and recognition of body sensations. Bruch believes that this results from the parents' failure to respond to the patient's needs during infancy. Since feeding was not directly related to hunger when she was an infant, the adolescent is also less aware of the relationship. The sense of ineffectiveness leads to the great need of anorectic persons to control at least one aspect of their lives. Hence, they focus all their attention on mastery of their weight and eating.[5]

As the disorder continues, signs of starvation become more evident. Amenorrhea occurs early in the course of the illness. It is now believed that the menarche is triggered by body size. Frisch[14] has identified that the mean body weight at menarche is 48 kg, and the weight range for 50% of girls is 43 to 51 kg. This research is being validated by the study of recovering anorectic patients. It was believed that amenorrhea was a symptom of anorexia nervosa. It is now believed that it is

secondary to weight loss. Early symptoms of anorexia nervosa are difficult to identify because the problem is usually not recognized until a significant weight loss has already occurred. Therefore initial assessment reveals symptoms of starvation as well as those of the anorexia itself.

Feighner[12] is another theorist who has described behaviors characteristic of anorexia nervosa. The six criteria identified include onset prior to age 25; weight loss of at least 25% of preillness weight; a distorted attitude toward food, eating, or weight, despite attempts to change this behavior; no known medical illness that would cause weight loss; no known psychiatric illness, such as depression, that would result in anorexia; and at least two of the behaviors of amenorrhea, lanugo, bradycardia, episodes of overactivity, episodes of bulimia, and vomiting (including self-induced). The behaviors identified by Feighner[12] are compared to those recommended for diagnosis of anorexia nervosa by the Draft of DSM-III-R in Development[1] in Table 16-2. The Feighner criteria are widely used in settings where anorexia nervosa research is taking place. Clinical example 16-1 illustrates behaviors that are characteristic of anorexia nervosa.

The prognosis for anorexia nervosa is unclear at the present time. Powers reports a mortality of 10% to 20%.[24] Bruch believes that psychotherapists must identify the patient's concerns and avoid dealing exclusively with eating patterns if there is to be any long-term change.[5] Longitudinal studies are clearly needed to determine whether the body image distortions and disordered eating patterns are overcome when weight is gained.

People with **bulimia** differ from anorectic persons in several respects. They tend to be older at onset. They are usually aware that they have a behavioral problem and may be embarrassed about it. They experience physical and psychological discomfort related to their bulimic behavior. These people tend to be more outgoing socially than anorectic persons, and frequently are able to become involved in heterosexual relationships.[17]

The typical bulimic pattern is to follow a normal dietary pattern for a period of time, followed by an episode of binging and purging. For this reason, they frequently are able to maintain a relatively normal weight and do not experience the physical symptoms of starvation that are characteristic of the anorexic. However, the binging and purging behavior leads to other physical disorders. Herzog and Copeland[17] describe these as menstrual irregularities; gastric dilatation, sometimes with rupture of the stomach; and aspiration leading to pneumonia. Vomiting can also cause enlarged parotid glands, dental caries, esophagitis, and tears or rupture of the esophagus. Hypokalemia can result from vomiting and abuse of laxatives or diuretics. Poisoning from overdose of ipecac, an emetic agent, may lead to potentially fatal myocardial dysfunctions. Therefore, although bulimics may not appear to be as physically ill as anorexics, they are really at great risk for serious physical illness.

Noncompliance. People who are noncompliant with recommended health care activities are generally aware that they have chosen not to care for themselves. They usually have a reason for noncompliance, such as being asymptomatic, not being able to afford the treatment they need, not understanding the activity they are to perform, or not having time. These are rationalizations and help to alleviate the underlying anxiety that is really causing the noncompliance. Patients may also minimize the seriousness of their problems. Many

chronic illnesses are characterized by long periods of stability, during which the person may not be aware of discomfort. This reinforces the noncompliant behavior.

Patients with chronic illnesses frequently hunt for health care providers who will prescribe other, less disruptive, treatment plans than the ones they are trying to avoid. They are susceptible to questionable practices such as miracle cures and faith healing in their search

---

TABLE 16-2

COMPARISON OF FEIGHNER AND DSM-III-R* CRITERIA FOR THE DIAGNOSIS OF ANOREXIA NERVOSA

Feighner[12]	DSM-III-R*
Onset before 25 years old	Unrelenting fear of obesity
Loss of at least 25% of preillness weight	Disturbed body image
Distorted attitude toward food, eating, or weight	Refusal to maintain weight within norms for age and height
No known medical illness causing weight loss	In females, at least three missed menstrual periods
No known psychiatric illness causing anorexia	
At least two of the following:	
1. Amenorrhea	
2. Lanugo	
3. Bradycardia	
4. Episodic overactivity	
5. Episodic bulimia	
6. Vomiting (may be self-induced)	

*From American Psychiatric Association: Draft of the DSM-III-R in Development (subject to change), as proposed by the Work Group to Revise DSM-III. American Psychiatric Association, October 1985.

CLINICAL EXAMPLE 16-1

Ms. L was a 17-year-old, white unmarried woman who was admitted to a general hospital medical unit with a diagnosis of malnutrition. On admission, she was 5 feet, 5 inches (162.5 cm) tall and weighed 92 pounds (40.4 kg). She told Ms. B, her primary nurse, that she was on a special diet. She ate no breakfast, a carrot for lunch, and an apple for dinner. She also said that she would be jogging in the halls twice a day. It was very important that she maintain her exercise routine of running 10 miles daily. Physical assessment revealed the presence of lanugo, especially on the arms and buttocks, amenorrhea of 8 months' duration, and dry skin and mucous membranes. At lunchtime, Ms. L offered her tray to another patient, and then watched her while she ate. Soon after this, she began to jog up and down the hall.

Ms. B tried to communicate to Ms. L her concern that she was starving and could die. Ms. L said, "You sound just like my parents. You want me to be fat just like they do. You're jealous that I can control my body." When her parents visited, they were observed to be a well-dressed, upper middle class couple. They gave Ms. L a box of candy. She became furious, throwing the candy on the floor and demanding that they tell the nurses to give her the carrots and apples that she had requested. The parents told Ms. B that they were frustrated and frightened. They recognized that their daughter's irrational behavior could be fatal. They said that she began to diet after her physical education teacher told her she was getting too large to compete in gymnastics. She had always been athletic and had won several prizes for her gymnastic ability. The L's were unconcerned at first, but then realized that she had nearly stopped eating. Coercion did not persuade her to eat. After many family arguments, they forced her to see the family physician who recommended hospitalization.

A diagnosis of anorexia nervosa was made, and Ms. L was transferred to the psychiatric unit for treatment.

CLINICAL EXAMPLE 16-2

Ms. C was a 61-year-old, white married woman who had been in good health most of her life. She had three grown children who had left home and established their own families. She had been a homemaker since her marriage at age 19. She and her husband were both looking forward to his retirement in 6 months. They planned to buy a recreational vehicle and travel around the United States.

Ms. C visited the gynecologist regularly. She was very concerned about having annual Pap smears. Since she was receiving no other regular health care, the nurse practitioner who worked with this physician did a complete physical examination each time Ms. C was seen. On her most recent visit, laboratory studies revealed an elevated blood glucose level. She was then referred to an internist for a more thorough examination. The new physician hospitalized her for a short time. Her diagnosis was diabetes mellitus, adult onset. Ms. C was told that her condition was not serious and could be controlled by diet. She was 20 pounds (9 kg) overweight and was advised that she needed to lose the excess weight. Before discharge, she was instructed about her diet, how to test her urine, and about possible complications of diabetes. A public health nursing referral was made.

Ms. C was frightened about her condition but did not mention this because no one else seemed very concerned. When she first arrived home, she was conscientious about following her diet and testing her urine. She felt very well and was proud when she lost 5 pounds. When the public health nurse visited, she congratulated Ms. C on how well she was doing. As time went on, Ms. C began to wonder if she was really so sick. She had never felt ill. On her husband's birthday, she fixed a special dinner and baked a cake. She decided she deserved a reward for "being good" and did not follow her diet. She anxiously tested her urine at bedtime and it was negative. Then her son and his family visited the C's for a week. She fixed all their favorite foods and ate with them. She still felt fine and decided she did not need to test her urine. When it was time for her next checkup, she postponed calling the physician. She was very busy preparing for retirement travel.

The public health nurse contacted the physician's office to find out about the results of Ms. C's visit. When she discovered that Ms. C had not been seen, she made a home visit. Ms. C talked with her, but was not very receptive to her expressed concern. Ms. C said she would try to diet, but emphasized that she really felt well and was not sure if the diet was realistic in view of her travel plans. She agreed that she would see her physician immediately if she developed any signs of illness and that she would make an appointment for a physical examination at her convenience. The public health nurse's plan was to visit Ms. C again in a month. However, she noted that it was unlikely that Ms. C would observe her treatment plan until she experienced overt behavioral disruption related to her illness.

---

for the return of complete health. Patients who are receiving chemotherapy or radiation for cancer become frustrated with the side effects of the treatment. They are easily victimized by those who promote "cures" that involve no discomfort, but have no scientifically proven effectiveness. The popular literature is constantly reporting miraculous new treatments for chronic diseases. Most of these are invalid and lead to more suffering for those who become hopeful and are then disappointed.

The most prominent behavior associated with noncompliance is refusal to acknowledge the seriousness of the health problem. This denial interferes with acceptance of treatment. However, at the same time, it protects the ego from the anxiety that recognition of impaired health will create. The greater the threat imposed by the illness, the greater will be the tenacity of resistance to treatment. Many chronic illnesses are associated with advancing age. Anxiety is increased because admission of illness also implies recognition that one is growing older. In a society that values youth, this behavior is not surprising. If one considers the resistance of middle-aged people to admitting that they need bifocals, refusal to acknowledge hypertension or diabetes mellitus should be anticipated. Societal attitudes reinforce the behavior of the noncompliant individual.

An unfortunate aspect of noncompliance is that guilt about not following health care recommendations may also interfere with obtaining regular care. The hypertensive person who has not been taking his medication will be reluctant to have his blood pressure checked because an elevated reading will undermine his defensive system. If the medical system treats these people like children and chastises them for their behavior, they feel even guiltier and are more reluctant to seek routine health care.

Noncompliant people are also struggling for control. Serious illness is often perceived as an attack on the person and a betrayal by his body. The patient needs to reassert his control and prove that he is still the master of his fate. The diabetic who cheats on his diet is gambling that he still has control over his body and can resist his problem by will. Most chronically ill people need to test the limits of their control and the validity of the prescribed self-care regimen. Clinical example 16-2 illustrates the problem of noncompliance with a prescribed health care regimen.

■ **ASSOCIATED WITH DIRECT SELF-DESTRUCTIVE BEHAVIOR (SUICIDE)**

Types of suicidal behavior. Suicidal behavior is usually broken down into the categories of suicide threats, suicide attempts, and successful suicide. In addition, certain suicide attempts may be referred to as **suicide gestures.** The gesture is described as a suicide attempt that is primarily directed toward the goal of receiving attention rather than actual destruction of the self. Use of this term is questionable because it has acquired a pejorative connotation. The implication is often that it is *only* an attention-seeking behavior and should not be taken seriously. All suicidal behavior is serious, whatever the intent, and deserves the serious consideration of the nurse. Therefore suicide gestures will be included in the general category of suicide attempts.

The **suicide threat** may be veiled but usually occurs before overt suicidal activity takes place. Verbally, the suicidal person may make a statement such as "Will you remember me when I'm gone?" or "Take care of my family for me." If taken in the context of recent stressors and the person's life situation, statements such as these may be ominous. Nonverbal communication is frequently the vehicle for the suicide threat. The person may give away prized possessions, make a will or funeral arrangements, or systematically withdraw from all friendships and social activities. Sometimes a person may make a direct verbal suicidal threat, but this is less common. The threat is an indication of the ambivalence that is usually present in the suicidal behavior. It represents the hope that someone will recognize the danger and rescue the person from his self-destructive impulses. It may also represent an effort to discover whether anyone cares enough to prevent the individual from harming himself.

Jourard[18] has presented an interesting analysis of suicidal behavior related to the wish for rescue. He believes that suicide is sometimes the result of an "invitation to die" extended by significant others. The invitation may be communicated by failure to respond to a suicide threat or, at times, even more directly. For instance, a woman was admitted to the hospital following the ingestion of iodine. She was severely depressed and highly suicidal. After a course of electroconvulsive therapy she recovered and went home. The social history revealed that her husband's occupation was tombstone carver. He reportedly had prepared a tombstone for the patient with only the date of death missing and kept it in a back room of their house. A few months after discharge the patient successfully committed suicide.

Suicide attempts include any actions taken by the individual toward himself that will lead to death if not interrupted. In the assessment of suicidal behavior much emphasis is placed on the lethality of the suicidal method that is threatened or used. Although all suicide threats and attempts are to be taken seriously, more vigorous and vigilant attention is indicated when the person is planning or tries a highly lethal means such as gunshot, hanging, or jumping. Less lethal means include carbon monoxide and drug overdose, which allow time for discovery once the suicidal action has been initiated. Assessment of the suicidal person also includes the factors of whether the person has made a specific plan and whether the means to carry out the plan are available. The most suicidal person would be one who plans a violent death (e.g., gunshot to the head), has a specific plan (e.g, as soon as his wife goes shopping), and has the means readily available (e.g., a loaded gun in a desk drawer). This person is exhibiting little ambivalence about his plan. On the other hand, the person who thinks he might take a bottle of aspirin if the situation at work does not improve soon is communicating an element of hope and is really asking for help in coping with his work situation.

Assessment instrument. Several assessment instruments, or lethality scales, have been developed by staff members at suicide prevention centers. One good example is the Assessment of Suicidal Potentiality form developed by the Los Angeles Suicide Prevention Center (see box on pages 496-497). It takes into consideration risk factors, stressors, the lethality of the method, coping mechanisms, and support systems to arrive at an overall rating of suicide potential.

Clinical example 16-3 illustrates the behavior of a suicidal person. It may be used in conjunction with the Assessment of Suicidal Potentiality if the student wishes to practice assessment skills as related to the suicidal patient.

Assessment of Suicidal Potentiality

Name _____ Age _____ Sex _____ Date _____

Rater _____ Evaluation _____

1 2   3 4 5 6 7 8 (9)
Low Medium High

Suicide potential

Age and sex _____   Resources _____   Total _____
Symptoms _____   Prior suicidal behavior _____
Stress _____   Medical status _____   Number of categories related _____
Acute vs. chronic _____   Communication aspects _____
Suicidal plan _____   Reaction of significant other _____   Average _____

Rating for category   **Rating for category**

1. Age and sex (1-9)   ( )   **3. Stress (1-9)**   ( )

   Male   Loss of loved person by   ( )
     50 plus (7-9)   ( )   death, divorce,
     35-49 (4-6)   ( )   separation (5-9)
     15-34 (1-3)   ( )   Loss of job, money,   ( )
   Female   prestige, status (4-8)
     50 plus (5-7)   ( )   Sickness, serious illness,   ( )
     35-49 (3-5)   ( )   surgery, accident, loss of
     15-34 (1-3)   ( )   limb (3-7)
                                              Threat of prosecution,   ( )
2. Symptoms (1-9)   ( )   criminal involvement,
                                                  exposure (4-6)
   Severe depression: sleep   ( )   Change(s) in life,   ( )
     disorder, anorexia,   environment, setting (4-
     weight loss, withdrawal,   6)
     despondent, loss of   Success, promotion,   ( )
     interest, apathy (7-9)   increased responsibilities
   Feelings of hopelessness,   ( )   (2-5)
     helplessness, exhaustion   No significant stress (1-3)   ( )
     (7-9)   Other (describe):   ( )
   Delusions, hallucination,   ( )
     loss of contact,   **4. Acute versus chronic**   ( )
     disorientation (6-8)   **(1-9)**
   Compulsive gambler (6-8)   ( )
   Disorganization, confusion,   ( )   Sharp, noticeable, and   ( )
     chaos (5-7)   sudden onset of specific
   Alcoholism, drug   ( )   symptoms (1-9)
     addiction, homosexuality   Recurrent outbreak of   ( )
     (4-7)   similar symptoms (4-9)
   Agitation, tension, anxiety   ( )   Recent increase in long-   ( )
     (4-6)   standing traits (4-7)
   Guilt, shame,   ( )   No specific recent change   ( )
     embarrassment (4-6)   (1-4)
   Feelings of rage, anger,   ( )   Other (describe):   ( )
     hostility, revenge (4-6)
   Poor impulse control, poor   ( )   **5. Suicidal plan (1-9)**   ( )
     judgment (4-6)   Lethality of proposed   ( )
   Frustrated dependency   ( )   method—gun, jump,
     (4-6)   hanging, drowning,
   Other (describe):   ( )   knife, poison, pills,
                                                  aspirin (1-9)

From Los Angeles Suicide Prevention Center: Assessment
of suicidal potentiality, Los Angeles, The Center.

Assessment of Suicidal Potentiality—cont'd

Rating for category

Availability of means in
    proposed method (1-9)   ( )

Specific detail and clarity in
    organization of plan (1-9)   ( )

Specificity in time planned
    (1-9)   ( )

Bizarre plans (4-6)   ( )

Rating of previous suicide
    attempt(s) (1-9)   ( )

No plans (1-3)   ( )

Other (describe):   ( )

6. Resources (1-9)   ( )

No sources of support
    (family, friends, agencies,
    employment) (7-9)   ( )

Family and friends available,
    unwilling to help (4-7)   ( )

Financial problem (4-7)   ( )

Available professional help,
    agency, or therapist (2-4)   ( )

Family and/or friends
    willing to help (1-3)   ( )

Stable life history (1-3)   ( )

Physician or clergy
    available (1-3)   ( )

Employed (1-3)   ( )

Finances no problem (1-3)   ( )

Other (describe):   ( )

7. Prior suicidal behavior (1-7)   ( )

One or more prior
    attempts of high
    lethality (6-7)   ( )

One or more prior attempts
    of low lethality (4-5)   ( )

History of repeated threats
    and depression (3-5)   ( )

No prior suicidal or
    depressed history (1-3)   ( )

Other (describe):   ( )

8. Medical status (1-7)   ( )

Chronic debilitating illness
    (5-7)   ( )

Pattern of failure in
    previous therapy (4-6)   ( )

Many repeated
    unsuccessful experiences
    with doctors (4-6)   ( )

Rating for category

Psychosomatic illness (e.g,
    asthma, ulcer, etc.) (2-4)   ( )

Chronic minor illness
    complaints,
    hypochondria (1-3)   ( )

No medical problems (1-2)   ( )

Other (describe):   ( )

9. Communication aspects (1-7)   ( )

Communication broken
    with rejection of efforts
    to reestablish by both
    patient and others (5-7)   ( )

Communications have
    internalized goal (e.g.,
    declaration of guilt,
    feelings of worthlessness,
    blame, shame) (4-7)   ( )

Communications have
    interpersonalized goal
    (e.g., to cause guilt in
    others, to force
    behavior, etc.) (2-4)   ( )

Communications directed
    toward world and
    people in general (3-5)   ( )

Communications directed
    toward one or more
    specific persons (1-3)   ( )

Other (describe):   ( )

10. Reaction of significant other (1-7)   ( )

Defensive, paranoid, rejected,
    punishing attitude (5-7)   ( )

Denial of own or patient's
    need for help (5-7)   ( )

No feelings of concern
    about the patient; does
    not understand the
    patient (4-6)   ( )

Indecisiveness, feelings of
    helplessness (3-5)   ( )

Alternation between feelings
    of anger and rejection
    and feelings of responsi-
    bility and desire to help (2-4)   ( )

Sympathy and concern plus
    admission of need for
    help (1-3)   ( )

Other (describe):   ( )

CLINICAL EXAMPLE 16-3

Mr. Y was a 52-year-old black man who was employed in the foundry of a large steel mill. He had worked for the company for 20 years. He lived in a rented room in a blue collar neighborhood near the mill. Most of his neighbors were Appalachian white and southern black families who had moved to the community to work at the mill. There was an undercurrent of racial tension in the neighborhood, but Mr. Y was not involved in conflicts with his neighbors. He had separated from his wife before moving to the community and had no close friends or family. The separation resulted from his violent behavior related to drinking binges.

Mr. Y was seen by the occupational health nurse, Ms. G, when he came to the employee health clinic following a 6-week absence from work. He had been hospitalized for broken ribs and a concussion after he had been beaten and robbed by a gang of adolescents in an alley behind his home. Ms. G was familiar with this employee because he had been a participant in the company's Employee Assistance Program for alcoholics. When she saw him in the clinic, she immediately noted that he appeared depressed. His face was expressionless, his posture slumped, and he had lost weight. He appeared disheveled, which was a change from his usual neat appearance. He said he did not feel ready to return to work, but had received a letter from the personnel office requesting that his condition be evaluated by the company's physician. His speech was slow and halting and so soft that he could barely be heard. He told Ms. G that he had a request to make of her. He knew from past conversations that she was an animal lover. He wanted her to take his pet dog because he did not feel able to care for it adequately and the neighbors who kept it while he was in the hospital had neglected it.

Ms. G was very concerned about Mr. Y and asked him how he was spending his time. He said he kept the television on and he thought a lot. When asked, he said he felt "too shaky" to go outside unless he absolutely had to. He thought the boys who attacked him were still in the neighborhood. Ms. G asked if he had thought about harming himself. Mr. Y looked startled, then admitted that he saw no other solution to his problem. "It makes sense. I don't have anybody. If you take Rover, I can go." With further questioning, he admitted that he had a loaded revolver at home and planned to use it after he left the clinic. Ms. G realized that Mr. Y needed help immediately. She asked the clinic secretary to sit with him while she discussed his situation with the physician.

Completed suicide may take place after warning signs have been missed or ignored. Some people do not reveal any easily recognizable warning signs. Research that has been done on completed suicide has of necessity been retrospective. However, it can be informative to interview survivors. This procedure is referred to as the psychological autopsy. The information obtained from these inquiries can be used to better understand suicidal behavior and to enhance the effectiveness of primary prevention activities.

Significant others of suicidal people, including survivors, have many feelings about this behavior. There is a significant element of hostility inherent in suicidal behavior. Frequently the message to significant others, stated or implied, is "You should have cared more." At times, when the person survives the attempt, this message may be transmitted in a manipulative way. An example is the adolescent girl who discovers that her boyfriend is dating someone else and takes an overdose of over-the-counter sleeping pills. If she sets the scene so she will almost inevitably be discovered and makes sure that her boyfriend hears of her behavior, she is behaving in a hostile manipulative way. A remorseful response by the boyfriend would be reinforcing and increase the likelihood that the behavior will be repeated in the future. It is important to treat these attempts seriously and help the patient develop healthier communication patterns. Persons who do not really intend to die may do so if they are not discovered in time.

When suicide is successful, the survivors are left with many feelings that they cannot communicate to the involved object, the dead person. This may lead to an unresolved grief reaction and depression. Some suicide prevention centers have become involved in what Shneidman[27] refers to as postvention to assist people to deal with this dilemma. Survivors are assisted either individually or in groups to express their feelings and work through their grief.

■ Coping mechanisms

The most prominent coping mechanism relative to ISDB is **denial**. Even though the individual may verbalize that his behavior is potentially harmful, direct injury to the self is denied. For instance, the overweight person will remark, "I shouldn't do this—but I will" as he cuts a large slice of cake. Most obese people can recite all the risks associated with obesity, but there is no sense of immediate personal threat.

Other people who engage in risk-seeking behavior enjoy the feeling of challenging fate and gambling that they will overcome danger. Daredevils, soldiers, and people who participate in dangerous sports deny the importance of the risk involved. The sense of mastery they feel when they win the gamble reinforces future repetition of the behavior.

Rationalization is another coping mechanism that is often present with ISDB. The noncompliant patient may give numerous reasons for his inability to comply with his health care plan. These explanations are really ways of decreasing the anxiety and fear that are related to recognition of a serious illness.

Many patients also use **intellectual defenses.** Anorectic and overweight people may become students of nutrition, thus gaining a sense of mastery over their behaviors. Noncompliant patients may seek out information about their illness and then use conflicts among the experts to justify their reluctance to accept treatment.

Regression is another characteristic of these patients. Eating disorders frequently have a relationship to the feeding patterns that the person experienced during infancy. Overeating may be pleasurable because having a good appetite was rewarded during childhood. Anorectic patients often begin dieting when confronted with the need to behave in a more adult manner. It is as if maintaining a childlike appearance will allow the continuation of childlike behavior. The occurrence of amenorrhea reinforces this perception. ISDB also invites parental interaction from significant others who try to persuade the person to behave in a self-enhancing way.

It must be remembered that these coping mechanisms may be standing between the person and self-destruction. They are defending him from strong emotional responses to life events that are a serious threat to the ego. If challenged too strongly without provision of other means of coping, underlying depression will become overt and may lead to suicidal behavior.

Suicidal behavior indicates the imminent failure of the coping mechanisms. A suicidal threat may be a last-ditch effort to get enough help to be able to cope. Completed suicide represents the failure of the coping and adaptive mechanisms.

 Nursing diagnosis

When considering the nursing diagnosis of self-destructive behavior, the nurse must incorporate information about the seriousness and immediacy of the patient's harmful activity. The nurse must take into consideration the information obtained in the assessment in order to accurately identify the patient's need for nursing intervention. It is necessary to review the stressors that are being experienced by the person and his

> ### Nursing Diagnoses Related to Self-Destructive Behavior
>
> #### Primary NANDA nursing diagnoses
> Noncompliance
> Nutrition, alteration in: less than body requirements
> Nutrition, alteration in: more than body requirements
> Violence, potential for: self-directed
>
> #### Examples of complete nursing diagnoses
> Noncompliance with taking antihypertensive medication related to asymptomatic behavior evidenced by unchanged elevation in blood pressure
> Noncompliance with 1800 calorie per day diabetic diet related to denial of illness evidenced by gain of 10 pounds since last clinic visit
> Alteration in nutrition: less than body requirements related to conflict over sexual maturation evidenced by loss of 30% of preillness weight
> Alteration in nutrition: less than body requirements related to prolonged dieting evidenced by refusal to eat any food other than green salads
> Alteration in nutrition: more than body requirements related to maternal rejection evidenced by hoarding and binging on food
> Alteration in nutrition: more than body requirements related to embarrassment about secondary sex characteristics evidenced by weight 25% above the norm for age and height
> Potential for self-directed violence related to loss of spouse evidenced by purchase of a gun
> Potential for self-directed violence related to phencyclidine (PCP) abuse evidenced by extreme psychotic disorganization

coping mechanisms. Formal assessment tools may help in organizing data so that the nursing diagnosis may be formulated.

Validation of the nursing diagnosis with the patient may additionally ensure the accuracy of the diagnostic statement. However, denial is a prominent defense with most of the self-destructive disorders, and the patient may not be able to concur with a statement that confronts this behavior. The primary concern is to communicate through the diagnosis the level of need for protection. In the case of self-destructive behavior, caution is recommended in determining the level of risk. It is better to respond to the patient more intensively than necessary than it is to allow serious injury to occur.

TABLE 16-3

MEDICAL AND NURSING DIAGNOSES RELATED TO SELF-DESTRUCTIVE BEHAVIOR

Medical Diagnostic Class

Eating disorders
Mood (affective) disorders

Psychiatric Nursing Diagnostic Class

Self-destructive behavior

Related Medical Diagnoses (DSM-III-R*)

Anorexia nervosa
Bulimic disorder
Bipolar disorder
Major depression
Dysthymia
Noncompliance with medical treatment

Related Nursing Diagnoses (NANDA)

Anxiety
Coping, ineffective: individual
Family process, alteration in
Fluid volume deficit, potential
†Noncompliance
†Nutrition, alteration in: less than body requirements
†Nutrition, alteration in: more than body requirements
Self-concept, disturbance in
†Violence, potential for: self-directed

*American Psychiatric Association: Draft of the DSM-III-R in Development (subject to change), as proposed by the Work Group to Revise DSM-III. American Psychiatric Association, October 1985.
†Indicates primary nursing diagnoses for self-destructive behavior

A complete nursing diagnosis is individualized and related to the total constellation of the patient's behaviors and nursing needs. Primary NANDA nursing diagnoses and examples of complete nursing diagnoses related to self-destructive behavior are presented in the box on page 499. Because of the nature of the disorders associated with self-destructive behavior, several other NANDA diagnoses will frequently be applied in the nursing care of these patients. These closely related nursing diagnoses related to self-destructive behavior are listed in Table 16-3. In addition, many of these patients will receive a psychiatric assessment and be given a DSM-III diagnosis. The psychiatric diagnoses that are most closely related to self-destructive behavior are also represented in Table 16-3.

Nursing diagnoses for these patients will generally also refer to other behavioral problems that have been discussed in other sections of this book, including anxiety, communication, unresolved grief, self-concept disorders, and anger. Self-destructive behavior generally evolves from other behavioral problems. Figure 16-3 relates self-destructive behavior to the nursing model of health-illness phenomena.

■ Related medical diagnoses

Several medical diagnostic classifications include actual or potential self-destructive behavior among the defining criteria. Suicidal behavior is not separately identified as a diagnostic category. Therefore, medical diagnoses in which this type of behavior is listed as possible are included in this section. Additional description of the affective disorders will be found in Chapter 15. The disorders to be included in this section are described in the Draft of the DSM-III-R in Development[1] and are listed in Table 16-3.

■ **ANOREXIA NERVOSA.** The essential features are fear of obesity, unrelated to actual body weight; disturbed body image; refusal to maintain weight within norms for age and height; in females, at least three missed menstrual periods.[1]

■ **BULIMIC DISORDER.** The essential features include recurrent binge-eating; self-induced vomiting, laxative abuse or excessive exercise to counteract binging; and a perceived inability to control binging.

Weight may fluctuate related to binges and fasts. Bulimics may feel that conflicts about eating dominate their lives.

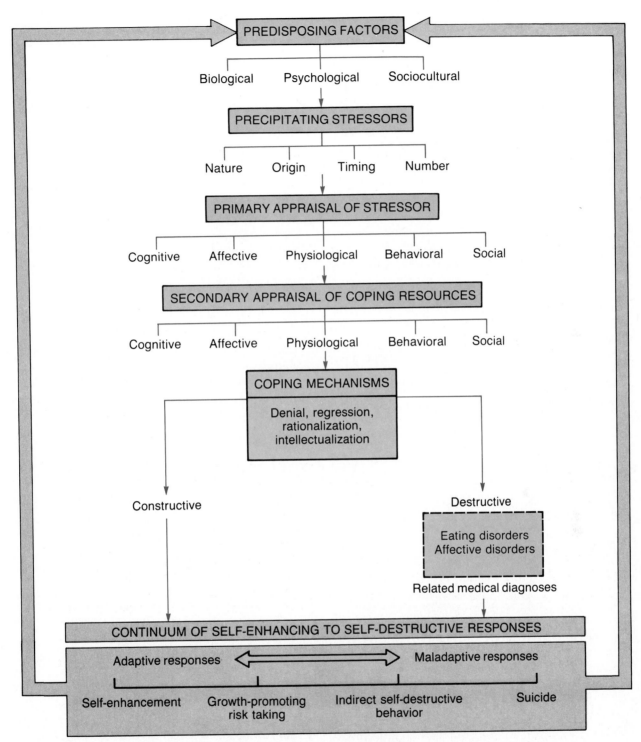

Fig. 16-3. Nursing model of health-illness phenomena related to self-destructive behavior.

■ **BIPOLAR DISORDER.** The essential feature of bipolar disorder is a current or past experience of a manic episode lasting at least 1 week when one's mood was abnormally and persistently elevated, expansive, or irritable. The episode of mood disturbance is sufficiently severe to cause marked impairment in social or occupational functioning. Bipolar disorders may be classified as manic (limited to only manic episodes), depressed (a history of manic episodes with a current depressive episode), or mixed (a mixed presentation of both manic and depressive episodes).[1]

Although the outstanding characteristic of bipolar disorder in the manic phase is expansiveness, there is a threat of suicidal behavior related to the extreme lability of mood, resulting in depression and thoughts of suicide. The patient's lack of control may lead to impulsive suicide attempts.

■ **MAJOR DEPRESSION.** The essential feature of major depression is the presence of at least five symptoms during the same 2-week period with one being either depressed mood or loss of interest or pleasure. Other symptoms might include weight loss, insomnia, psychomotor agitation or retardation, fatigue, feelings of worthlessness, diminished ability to think, and recurrent thoughts of death. Major depressions may be classified as single episode or recurrent.

■ **DYSTHYMIA.** The essential feature of dysthymia is a history of at least 2 years of experiencing, more often than not, a depressed mood and at least one of the symptoms mentioned above without meeting the criteria for a major depressive episode.[1] There may be recurrent thoughts of suicide or death.

■ **NONCOMPLIANCE WITH MEDICAL TREATMENT.** This category can be used when a focus of attention or treatment is noncompliance with medical treatment that is apparently not due to a mental disorder. Examples include behavior that results from denial of illness, religious beliefs or personal values.[1]

❧ Planning and implementation

■ Goal setting

Careful attention must be given to the assignment of priorities in setting goals with the self-destructive patient. Highest priority should be given to goals that are relevant to the preservation of life. In terms of this constellation of behaviors, further consideration must be given to first identifying goals related to immediately life-threatening behavior. For example, the actively suicidal person must first be prevented from acting on his impulses. At a later time attention can be given to the development of insight into the suicidal behavior and

substitution of healthy coping mechanisms. The anorectic person must be prevented from starving to death as the highest priority goal.

ISDBs also serve as coping mechanisms. Therefore there is great resistance to changing these behaviors. Goals must incorporate the development of new ways of coping that will replace the old self-destructive ones.

In dealing with self-destructive behavior, it may appear that the nurse and the patient are pursuing incompatible goals. Suicidal patients may resist attempts to protect them and may actively try to evade their observers. However, most of these patients have some ambivalence. The nurse, in setting positive, life-preserving goals, is appealing to the healthy part of the person's self that wants to survive and be better able to cope with life. The very act of seeking help is an expression of this healthy aspect of the personality. The positive attitude of the nurse in setting constructive goals conveys a sense of hope to a patient who may be feeling hopeless.

Following are examples of goals related to DSDB:

Long-term
By 2 weeks before discharge from the hospital, the patient will refrain from attempts to inflict physical harm on himself.

Short-term
1. In 3 days the patient will voluntarily remain within the view of a staff member.
2. In 1 week the patient will inform a staff member when he feels like hurting himself.
3. In 2 weeks the patient will state two reasons why he does not want to hurt himself.
4. In 3 weeks the patient will list three good things about himself.

Following are examples of goals related to ISDB:

Long-term
The patient will take prescribed medications and perform self-care activities independently as recommended by the health care team.

Short-term
1. In 2 weeks, the patient will verbalize feelings related to his medical diagnosis.
2. In 4 weeks, the patient will describe the relationship between the medical diagnosis and the recommended self-care activities.
3. In 4 weeks, the patient will describe the consequences of failure to carry out self-care activities.
4. In 6 weeks, the patient will verbally accept responsibility for his health care behavior and will participate in self-care activities on his own initiative.
5. In 6 weeks, the patient will have stable biopsychosocial functioning based on compliance with an individualized self-care treatment plan.

If the patient is made aware of a treatment plan of this type, he can actively engage in evaluating his progress and modifying the plan. This again reinforces the message of confidence that the patient will be able to change his behavior and find more satisfaction in life.

■ Intervening in self-destructive behavior

There are common elements in nursing intervention with all patients who exhibit self-destructive behavior. The first important matter for the nurse to consider is her own response to people who are trying to destroy themselves. It can be difficult for a person who is happy and involved in life to imagine the depth of despair that leads to suicidal impulses or the lack of caring for the self that results in behavior which is physically, psychologically, and socially damaging, even if it is not immediately lethal. On the other hand, a nurse who is depressed and dissatisfied with her own life may be threatened by interacting with patients who are more upset because she may fear similar consequences for herself. The latter nurse may also overidentify with the patient. This limits one's ability to help the patient because of the tendency to assume that the patient's situation and one's own are exactly alike, whereas in reality this is probably not so. A therapeutic approach is empathic and nonjudgmental, with limitation of subjective responses through awareness of one's own attitudes.

Hamel-Bissell[15] has studied the reactions of nurses to long-term work with suicidal individuals. She has identified four stages of reaction.

1. *Stage of naïveté*—In the first exposure to suicidal behavior, the nurse experiences feelings of "shock, lack of understanding, avoidance, and denial."[15]
2. *Stage of recognition*—In the first work experience with a suicidal patient, the nurse undergoes a recapitulation of the stage I feelings, only they are stronger. The forced confrontation of these feelings leads to the next feeling cycle of "fear, anxiety, hopelessness, and confusion."[15]
3. *Stage of responsibility*—The nurse experiences conflict over the need to protect the patient combined with realization of her limitations to control the behavior of another person. The feelings associated with this stage are "responsibility, guilt, and anger."[15]
4. *Stage of individual choice*—The nurse achieves a realistic understanding of the patient's responsibility for his own life. There is an acceptance of the possibility of loss of a suicidal patient.

The recognition of the patient's ultimate responsibility for determining his own fate does not imply a fatalistic or unconcerned attitude on the part of the nurse. All possible efforts are made to protect the patient and to motivate him to choose life. Blythe and Pearlmutter[4] suggest that the nurse align herself with the patient's wish to live and then assist the patient to be responsible for his own behavior. However, nurses must understand that some patients will choose death despite their best efforts to intervene. For the nurse's own emotional health, she must recognize when this has happened. Hamel-Bissell found that nurses took from 2 to 10 years to reach the stage of individual choice.

■ **PROTECTION.** The highest priority nursing activity with the self-destructive patient is to protect him from inflicting further harm on himself and, if suicidal, from killing himself. The message of protection is conveyed to the patient verbally and nonverbally. Verbally, the patient is informed of the nurse's intention not to allow harm to come to the patient.

To the anorectic patient, she might say, "We will not allow you to starve yourself to death. You may choose whether to eat voluntarily or to be fed by us, but you will be prevented from starving to death." To the suicidal patient she might say, "I understand that you are feeling impulses to harm yourself. I will be here with you to help you control those impulses and I will do whatever is necessary to protect you. I'd like to talk with you about how you are feeling whenever you feel able to share that with me." The nonverbal communications should reinforce and be congruent with the verbal. Obviously, dangerous objects such as belts, sharp implements, glass, and matches should be taken from the suicidal patient. It is recognized that it is impossible to render an environment perfectly safe. Even walls and floors can inflict injury if the patient throws himself against them. However, the removal of dangerous objects gives a message of concern. One-to-one observation of the extremely suicidal individual also communicates caring. This observation should be carried out with sensitivity, the nurse neither hovering over the patient nor remaining aloof from him. The patient's nonverbal cues can guide the one-to-one interaction. It is important to remain alert until the mental health team and the patient agree that the self-destructive crisis is over. Suicidal patients may appear to be feeling much better immediately prior to making an attempt. This is attributed to the feeling of relief that is experienced when the decision has been made and the plans have been finalized. Nurses have been fooled by this behavior pattern, relaxing their vigilance, only to have the patient kill himself when he is allowed to be alone for a moment.

If anorectic patients are being forced to eat, they must be observed carefully following a meal to prevent induced vomiting. Vigilance during meals is necessary because anorectic patients are usually very accomplished at hiding food in napkins, giving it to other patients, burying it in plants, and other means of disposing of it without eating it. They also require limits on activity and close observation of bowel and bladder functioning to be sure that they are not secretly taking laxatives or diuretics.

■ **INCREASING SELF-ESTEEM.** Self-destructive people have low self-esteem. The nurse may intervene in this area by treating the patient as someone who is deserving of attention and concern. Positive attributes of the patient should be recognized with genuine praise. An attempt to manufacture reasons to praise the patient is usually recognized as artificial and has the effect of lowering the patient's self-esteem. The message is that the patient is so bad that one has to search for positive characteristics.

Overweight people frequently have low self-esteem. They perceive their inability to achieve a normal weight as a character flaw and feel shame about their size. The nurse can help them identify their positive attributes. Recognition for success in weight loss is also helpful and provides motivation for continued dieting and exercise.

Andersen and Mickalide[2] suggest a similar approach to the male anorectic patient. They recommend that the primary therapeutic interventions be educational and supportive with encouragement of the patient to give up his attitude of guilt and blame.

As the nurse gets to know the patient, she should be alert to strengths that can be built on to provide the patient with positive experiences, as illustrated in Clinical example 16-4.

■ **REINFORCING HEALTHY COPING.** Closely related to the building of self-esteem is the reinforcement of healthy coping mechanisms. Ms. P's bread making was a way for her to express her anger more productively than by pacing. If past healthy coping mechanisms can be identified, these may be reinforced. In addition, growth may take place through the learning and practice of new adaptive behaviors.

Behavior modification programs may be initiated to teach new coping patterns. Eating disorders are often approached in this way. Many of the popular weight loss groups are built around behavior modification principles. Public weighing in results in group approval for weight loss and disapproval for failure to lose. Other diet plans recommend techniques, such as saving a dollar for each pound lost and buying a (nonfood) treat when

---

CLINICAL EXAMPLE 16-4

Ms. P was an extremely suicidal woman who was very depressed. She spoke little and spent much of her time pacing in an agitated manner. Her husband was distressed about her condition and was willing to share with the nurse a description of Ms. P when she was well. He revealed that Ms. P loved to bake and had never bought anything from a bakery. The nurse arranged to get the ingredients for Ms. P to show her how to bake bread. Ms. P did so reluctantly but put a great deal of energy into beating and kneading the dough. As she did so, she explained her activity to the nurse. She received sincere praise for the completed bread from the nurse and from other patients with whom it was shared. The nurse incorporated the baking activity as a regular part of her intervention with Ms. P.

---

the goal is reached, or buying an article of clothing in a smaller size that will fit when excess weight is lost. Posting an unflattering photograph on the refrigerator door deters the obese person from eating. Changes in eating habits are also recommended. These include eating slowly and chewing food well, eating only in a designated place, putting the fork down between bites, and refraining from other activities while eating.

Principles of behavior modification are also recommended by some anorexia nervosa treatment programs. Privileges may be granted for pounds gained. For instance, a patient may be confined to her room until she gains 2 pounds, restricted from visitors until 5 pounds have been gained, and so on. Some programs use feeding by nasogastric intubation as a type of aversive stimulus. Tube feeding is initiated if the patient fails to consume the required number of calories in a specified period of time or if weight declines by a predetermined amount. Other programs avoid tube feeding except in emergency situations. These health care providers feel that the insertion of a feeding tube reinforces the patient's low self-esteem and may be interpreted as punishment for misbehavior rather than an effort to be helpful. Activity limitations and constant observation by staff are also unpleasant conditions that the patient can change only by altering her behavior. Some treatment teams also advocate refusing to inform the patient of either her present or her goal weight. This avoids endless arguments about desirable weight and decreases to some extent the anxiety the patient feels about increasing weight. Behavior modification programs are structured to allow the patient to assume more responsibility for her behavior as she demonstrates her ability to behave responsibly. Group interaction and peer support are encouraged.

Potts[23] has suggested a behavior modification program to assist bulimic patients to gain control over their binging and purging behavior. Intake is recorded, and a regular eating pattern is maintained. Alternative activities are explored to keep the patient busy and distracted from eating. Other interventions are directed toward altering the attitude about the self and food. The patient is assisted to learn alternative coping mechanisms. The eating of small amounts of "forbidden foods" is encouraged to demonstrate that the patient can avoid binging. Self-help groups are advised to obtain peer support.

■ **EXPLORATION OF FEELINGS.** For noncompliant patients, healthy coping implies the assumption of responsibility for self-care. Interventions must be directed toward the development of understanding of the meaning of the illness experience to the patient.

It may be helpful to assist the patient to explore the predisposing and precipitating factors influencing his behavior. Once the acute crisis is over, understanding the underlying feelings and realizing how they developed and got out of control may help the person to change his behavior in the future. The nurse without advanced preparation in psychiatric nursing should not probe for feelings that the patient is reluctant to discuss and should avoid making interpretations of behavior. These approaches can be very stressful and have the potential to precipitate a new crisis, which the inexperienced nurse may be unable to handle.

If the self-destructive behavior represents a response to other behavioral disruptions, appropriate nursing interventions should be directed toward these problems. The angry patient must be helped to deal constructively with his anger. The patient who has physiological needs must be helped to meet those needs. For example, the anorectic patient who is in a state of starvation is unable to think rationally and interpret sensations correctly until she has been stabilized metabolically. Attempts to help her develop insight during the period of starvation are certain to fail. When she is physiologically stable, psychotherapy may be initiated.

■ **LIMIT SETTING AND CONTROL.** Issues of control are usually present when self-destructive behavior occurs. A person may be so determined to demonstrate control of his life that he participates in harmful behavior because it is discouraged by others. Bruch[5] has observed that this is a characteristic of anorectic patients. Schlemmer and Barnett[26] describe the manipulative behavior that they have experienced in their work with

anorexia nervosa patients. They note that manipulation seems to occur in response to limits. For instance, self-induced vomiting, which is a common behavior of anorectic patients, occurred in only one patient. The treatment program had no limits specified relative to vomiting. Patients who were being treated with behavior modification were more manipulative than those who were not. The behavior modification treatment plan was very structured and initially involved strict limits. The authors advise that nurses respond to manipulation with consistent enforcement of limits. They observed that as patients grew to trust the reliable response of the staff, manipulation decreased. They also made it clear to the patients that they retained control of their weight gain or loss. It was recommended that nursing staff meet together regularly to express their feelings and provide group support. The constant limit testing of a self-destructive patient can be frustrating to nursing staff.[26] All forms of self-destructive behavior are controlling in nature. In effect, the patient challenges others to try to stop him from harming himself, although in reality everyone knows that the patient retains the right to choose growth-promoting or harmful behavior.

■ **MOBILIZATION OF SOCIAL SUPPORT.** Frequently, self-destructive behavior reflects a lack of both internal and external resources. Mobilization of social support systems is an important aspect of nursing intervention. Significant others probably have many feelings about the self-destructive behavior of the patient. They need an opportunity to express their feelings and to make realistic plans for the future. Family members need to be made aware of control issues and helped to encourage self-control of the behavior by the patient. Both the patient and the family may need assistance in seeing that caring can be expressed by fostering self-care, as well as by providing care. Families of suicidal patients may be frightened of future suicidal activity. They need to be aware of behavioral clues to suicide and of community resources that can assist with crises. In reality, suicidal behavior frequently recurs. False reassurance should be avoided. A better approach is to foster improved communication patterns and an ability to cope in the family. The nurse may help people sort out their feelings and frequently may want to refer significant others for social work intervention or initiate a referral for family therapy.

Community resources may also be important for the long-term care of the self-destructive person. Self-help groups such as Weight Watchers, Diet Workshop, TOPS, and Recovery, Inc. may provide the recovering patient with needed peer support. Family therapy may assist in the reintegration of a family group that has

TABLE 16-4

MENTAL HEALTH EDUCATION PLAN—COUNSELING OBESE PATIENTS

Content	Instructional activities	Evaluation
Identify the basic four food groups	Show slides of foods included in basic four Provide handout listing foods in each group	Patient names the correct group when presented with a food
Compare and contrast a menu from a typical day with the basic four food groups	Record all foods eaten on a typical day Discuss the number of foods eaten from each of the basic four	Patient identifies the correct group for each food listed and states which foods were missing or overrepresented
Identify the nutrients present in foods	Define and discuss proteins, fats, carbohydrates, vitamins, and minerals Analyze food labels based on nutrient content	Patient defines each type of nutrient Patient describes a packaged food's nutritional value based on package labeling
Describe low-calorie, nutritionally balanced meal plans	Plan one day's menus, including attention to the patient's food preferences	Patient selects foods that are acceptable to him and are low-calorie and nutritionally balanced
Design a low-calorie diet pattern, based on weight loss goals and medical condition	Refer to patient dietitian	Patient attends counseling session with dietitian
Teach the importance of regular exercise	Discuss the influence of exercise on weight loss Demonstrate exercises, based on patient's physical condition	Patient returns demonstration of exercises Patient reports exercising for 20 minutes at least every other day
Assist patient identify sources of peer support in the community	Describe self-help groups that assist with weight loss Provide written descriptions of community self-help groups, including instructions for joining the group	Patient joins a self-help group and attends at least once a week

been disrupted by the patient's recent experiences. Public health nurses, clergy, and other community-based helping people can provide the patient and family with day-to-day support. The nurse may be active in explaining resources to the patient and in initiating referrals to other agencies.

■ **MENTAL HEALTH EDUCATION.** Patient education is another important aspect of nursing intervention. The nutritional knowledge of patients with eating disorders should be assessed. Dieters, in particular, may be helped by learning about the nutritional values of various foods. Meal planning based on a food exchange system or on calorie counting gives the patient a feeling of control. Others respond better to following a diet pattern that has been designed by someone else. In either case, referral to a nutritionist for diet teaching is advisable. Questions about fad diets should be answered honestly. Analysis of the nutritional value of the diet by the nurse or nutritionist and the patient may help the

patient assess diet plans more accurately in the future. Health teaching for overweight patients should also emphasize the importance of exercise as a way of improving general health and maximizing weight loss. Community resources for exercise, such as adult education classes, YWCA and YMCA exercise programs, and aerobic dance programs can be identified and information provided to the patient. Table 16-4 presents a health education plan for an obese patient. Patients who are noncompliant with prescribed health care regimens may not understand the nature of their problem. Knowledge should be assessed and appropriate teaching initiated. Many patients are willing to participate in self-care if it makes sense to them. Teaching ways to monitor health status may also be helpful. For instance, if a hypertensive patient can check his own blood pressure, he can learn to associate his health care activities with his physiological response. Powers and Wooldridge[25] studied factors influencing knowledge, attitudes, and compliance

TABLE 16-5

SUMMARY OF NURSING INTERVENTIONS IN SELF-DESTRUCTIVE BEHAVIOR

Goal: Prevention of infliction of physical harm to self

Principle	Rationale	Nursing action
The patient must be protected from harming himself	Highest priority is given to life-saving patient care activities The patient's behavior must be supervised until self-control is adequate for safety	Close observation Removal of harmful objects Provision of a safe environment Provision for basic physiological needs
Increase self-esteem	Self-destructive behavior reflects underlying depression related to low self-esteem and anger directed inward	Identify patient strengths Encourage patient to participate in activities that he likes and does well Encourage good hygiene and grooming Foster healthy interpersonal relationships
Reinforcement of healthy coping mechanisms	Maladaptive coping mechanisms must be replaced with healthy ones to manage stress and anxiety	Assist the patient to recognize unhealthy coping mechanisms Identify alternative means of coping Reward healthy coping behaviors

Goal: Acceptance of help from family and community support systems

Principle	Rationale	Nursing action
Mobilization of social support systems	Social isolation leads to low self-esteem and depression, perpetuating self-destructive behavior	Assist significant others to communicate constructively with the patient Promote healthy family relationships Identify relevant community resources Initiate referrals to community resources
Patients and significant others should receive education about identified health care needs	Understanding of and participation in health care planning enhances compliance	Involve patient and significant others in care planning Explain characteristics of identified health care need, nursing care needs, medical diagnosis, and recommended treatment and medications Elicit response to nursing care plan Modify plan based on patient feedback

of hypertensive patients. They found that educational programs presented by nurses were effective in increasing patients' understanding of their illnesses and medications. There was also a significant decrease in the blood pressure of patients who participated in the study. Patients who are on medication regimens, such as psychotropic medication for the previously suicidal patient, should know the prescribed dosage, frequency, and side effects of the medication. Information about how to handle any future crises should be provided to the patient. If there has been an explanation of the possible reason for the patient's behavior, this may be reinforced

with him at termination to help him integrate his experience into his self-concept. Helping a patient to work through his self-destructive behavior can be an extremely rewarding aspect of psychiatric nursing. Table 16-5 summarizes nursing interventions for patients with self-destructive behavior.

 Evaluation

Powers and Wooldridge[25] have identified one of the difficulties in evaluating nursing intervention with noncompliant patients. The most intensive level of intervention is often the most effective in creating behavioral change. It is also the most expensive. In an era of cost containment, it is very difficult to support the advantages of improved quality of care relative to the added cost of providing that care. Longitudinal studies must be conducted to demonstrate the effectiveness of nursing intervention in preventing deterioration of the patient's condition and rehospitalization.

Problems have also been identified related to anorexia nervosa research. Following an extensive review of the literature, Doyen[9] identified the following factors that make it difficult to compare research studies:

1. Lack of consistent diagnostic criteria.
2. Use of subjects with different levels of severity of illness.
3. Different post-treatment follow-up intervals.
4. Mixing a variety of treatment approaches within the same study.
5. Lack of consistent criteria for recovery.
6. Varied methods of collecting follow-up data. None were found with the validity or reliability of the methodology established.

Problems such as these must be resolved if clinical research is to be useful for evaluating patient care programs.

Hendin[16] has identified the following changes in approaches to research on suicide in the last 20 years:

1. Exploration of the differentiation of suicidal subgroups in diagnostic categories
2. Consideration of the role of genetic factors
3. Reconsideration of the inverse relationship between overt aggression and suicide
4. Abandonment of the search for universal models of suicide
5. More attention given to cultural influences

Nurses need to contribute to research on the various forms of self-destructive behavior. As more nurses with graduate preparation in clinical nursing become active researchers, they will assist all nurses to be evaluators of patient care by developing and validating criteria.

Evaluation of the nursing care of the self-destructive patient requires careful monitoring of the patient's behavioral status on a daily basis. Involvement of the patient in evaluation of his progress can provide reinforcement and an incentive to work toward a goal. Modifications of the plan of care are frequently necessary as the patient reveals more of himself and his needs to the nurse. As soon as possible, the patient should become a participant in the planning, evaluation, and modification process.

Unfortunately, self-destructive behavior has a ten-

dency to recur. Nurses sometimes become discouraged and angry with patients who return again and again with the same behavior. When this occurs, the nurse may be caught in the trap of feeling responsible for the patient's behavior. Once the nurse has given the best nursing care she knows how to give, she has done as much as she can for the patient. It is impossible to change a patient's total life situation for him. The nurse can only help to identify alternative behaviors and provide encouragement for change. If the patient returns, the nursing process must be reinitiated with an attitude of hope that this time the patient will learn and grow more and be better able to live a satisfying life.

DIRECTIONS FOR FUTURE RESEARCH

The following are some of the nursing research problems raised in Chapter 16 that merit further study by psychiatric nurses:

1. Longitudinal study of the eating patterns of children of women who have a diagnosis of anorexia nervosa
2. Comparison of alterations in body image, self-concept, and eating patterns to weight gain by recovering anorexia nervosa patients
3. The relationship between nurses' experiences with and attitudes toward death and their ability to intervene therapeutically with self-destructive patients
4. The ability of nurses to identify the characteristics of indirectly self-destructive behaviors
5. Health education approaches that enhance or inhibit the likelihood of compliance with a prescribed health care plan
6. The effectiveness of family therapy in decreasing the occurrence of future episodes of self-destructive behavior
7. Patient responses to one-to-one observation for the prevention of suicidal behavior
8. Nursing staff attitudes toward persistently self-destructive patients
9. The relationship of various staffing patterns to the occurrence of episodes of self-destructive behavior in the hospital setting
10. Identification of behavioral responses to the physiological condition of starvation
11. Comparison of the relative effectiveness of nursing interventions with self-destructive patients when the health care process is controlled by the nurse, patient, or is collaborative in nature
12. Identification of primary prevention nursing activities that decrease the incidence of self-destructive behavior in a community

■ SUGGESTED CROSS-REFERENCES ■

The model of health-illness phenomena is discussed in Chapter 3. Therapeutic relationship skills are discussed in Chapter 4. The phases of the nursing process are discussed in Chapter 5. Mobilization of social support systems and health education are discussed in Chapters 9, 10, and 11. Interventions related to low self-esteem are discussed in Chapter 14. Depression is discussed in Chapter 15. Substance abuse is discussed in Chapter 20. Behavior modification approaches are discussed in Chapter 27.

■ SUMMARY ■

1. Self-destructive behavior varies in degree from slow and insidious (overeating) to immediate and dangerous (suicide attempts).

2. Stereotypes of self-destructive people are usually misleading. The majority of people engage in some form of self-destructive behavior.

3. Descriptive information was presented about indirect self-destructive behavior. The examples of this behavior that were used throughout the chapter were obesity, anorexia nervosa, bulimia, and noncompliance with a prescribed health care plan.

4. Data were presented about identification of groups at high risk for suicide.

5. The continuum of coping responses from self-enhancing behavior to suicide was presented. Anxiety and the attempt to escape from it are central to the occurrence of self-destructive behavior.

6. Other behavioral disruptions, including psychosis, may lead to self-destructive behavior.

7. Depression related to low self-esteem and unexpressed anger is intimately related to self-destructive behavior.

8. Issues of control are prominent relative to self-destructive behavior.

9. Social factors, such as loneliness, interpersonal frustration, family communication patterns, cultural changes, and patterns of a subculture may lead to self-destructive behavior.

10. Behaviors characteristic of indirect self-destructive behavior, including anorexia nervosa, obesity, and noncompliance were discussed, including the core behavior of denial of potential personal harm.

11. Characteristics of suicidal threats, attempts, and completed suicide were discussed, including warning signs, assessment of suicidal risk, and the necessity to understand ambivalence as it relates to suicidal behavior. The function of hostility in suicidal behavior was discussed.

12. Coping mechanisms related to indirect self-destructive behavior include denial, rationalization, intellectualization, and regression. Suicide represents the failure of all coping attempts.

13. Nursing diagnoses and related medical diagnoses relative to self-destructive behavior were presented.

14. Initially, it may be necessary to set goals for self-destructive patients, but they should be encouraged to participate as soon as possible. Highest priority is given goals that preserve the person's life. An example of long- and short-term goals was presented.

15. Nursing interventions should focus on protecting the patient, increasing self-esteem, reinforcing healthy coping mechanisms, understanding the underlying problem, mobilization of environmental resources, and patient education.

16. The nurse must explore her own feelings relative to the self-destructive behavior of patients.

17. Evaluation is based on the patient's increasing ability to behave in a self-enhancing manner. An attitude of hopefulness is necessary even when patients revert to their self-destructive behaviors and require readmission.

■ REFERENCES ■

1. American Psychiatric Association: Draft of the DSM-III-R in Development (subject to change), as proposed by the Work Group to Revise DSM-III. American Psychiatric Association, October 1985.
2. Andersen, A.E., and Mickalide, A.D.: Anorexia nervosa in the male: an underdiagnosed disorder, Psychosomatics **24**:1066, Dec. 1983.
3. Bahra, R.J.: The potential for suicide, Am. J. Nurs. **75**:1782, 1975.
4. Blythe, M.M., and Pearlmutter, D.R.: The suicide watch: a re-examination of maximum observation, Perspect. Psychiatr. Care **21**:90, July-Sept. 1983.
5. Bruch, H.: The golden cage: the enigma of anorexia nervosa, Cambridge, Mass., 1978, Harvard University Press.
6. Choron, J.: Suicide, New York, 1972, Charles Scribner's Sons.
7. Ciseaux, A.: Anorexia nervosa: a view from the mirror, Am. J. Nurs. **80**:1468, 1980.
8. Douglass: Endocrinology and other uncommon causes of obesity. In Powers, P.S.: Obesity: the regulation of weight, Baltimore, 1980, The Williams & Wilkins Co.
9. Doyen, L.: Primary anorexia nervosa: a review and critique of selected papers, J. Psychosoc. Nurs. Ment. Health Serv. **20**:12, June 1982.
10. Durkheim, E.: Suicide, New York, 1951, The Free Press. (Translated by J.A. Spaulding and G. Simpson.)
11. Farberow, N.L., editor: The many faces of suicide: indirect self-destructive behavior, New York, 1980, McGraw-Hill Book Co.
12. Feighner, J.P. et al.: Diagnostic criteria for use in psychiatric research, Arch. Gen. Psychiatry **26**:57, 1972.
13. Filstead, W.J.: Despair and its relationship to indirect self-destructive behavior. In Farberow, N.L., editor: The many faces of suicide: indirect self-destructive behavior, New York, 1980, McGraw-Hill Book Co.
14. Frisch, R.E.: Critical weight at menarche, initiation of adolescent growth spurt, and control of puberty. In Grumbach, M.M., Grave, G.D., and Mayer, F.E., editors: Control of the onset of puberty, New York, 1974, John Wiley & Sons, Inc.
15. Hamel-Bissell, B.P.: Suicidal casework: assessing nurses' reactions, J. Psychosoc. Nurs. Ment. Health Serv. **23**:20, Oct. 1985.
16. Hendin, H.: Suicide: a review of new directions in research, Hosp. Community Psychiatry **37**:148, Feb. 1986.
17. Herzog, D.B., and Copeland, P.M.: Eating disorders, N. Engl. J. Med. **313**:295, Aug. 1985.

18. Jourard, S.: Suicide: an invitation to die, Am. J. Nurs. **70**:269, 1980.
19. Krauss, H.H.: Suicide: a psychosocial phenomenon. In Wolman, B.B., editor: Between survival and suicide, New York, 1976, Gardner Press, Inc.
20. Leventhal, H.: Wrongheaded ideas about illness, Psychol. Today **16**:48, 1982.
21. Linden, L.L., and Breed, W.: The demographic epidemiology of suicide. In Shneidman, E.S., editor: Suicidology: contemporary developments, New York, 1976, Grune & Stratton, Inc.
22. Los Angeles Suicide Prevention Center: Assessment of suicidal potentiality, Los Angeles, The Center.
23. Potts, N.L.: The secret pattern of binge/purge, Am. J. Nurs. **84**:32, Jan. 1984.
24. Powers, P.S.: Obesity: the regulation of weight, Baltimore, 1980, The Williams & Wilkins Co.
25. Powers, M.J., and Wooldridge, P.J.: Factors influencing knowledge, attitudes and compliance of hypertensive patients, Res. Nurs. Health **5**:171, 1982.
26. Schlemmer, J.K., and Barnett, P.A.: Management of manipulative behavior in anorexia nervosa patients, J. Psychiatr. Nurs. **15**:35, Nov. 1977.
27. Shneidman, E.S., editor: Suicidology: contemporary developments, New York, 1976, Grune & Stratton, Inc.
28. Wekstein, L.: Handbook of suicidology: principles, problems and practice, New York, 1979, Brunner/Mazel, Inc.

■ ANNOTATED SUGGESTED READINGS ■

*Abercrombie, R.K., and Thielemann, P.: Suicide: two views, Am. J. Nurs. **84**:597, May 1984.

This presentation of a dilemma in practice compares the beliefs of two people regarding suicide as a response to chronic debilitating illness. The viewpoints are "a compassionate solution" and "a chilling encounter." The issues that are raised would provide material for a stimulating debate.

Alvarez, A.: The savage god, New York, 1971, Bantam Books.

This well-written book presents suicide against a historical and literary background. The author was acquainted with Sylvia Plath, a writer who committed suicide. He writes about his experiences with her and his observations of her behavior.

Andersen, A.E., and Mickalide, A.D.: Anorexia nervosa in the male: an underdiagnosed disorder, Psychosomatics **24**:1066, Dec. 1983.

The authors compare and contrast anorexia nervosa in males and females. Although there are many similarities between the groups, it is important for the nurse to be aware of the differences and integrate them into the patient's nursing care.

*Ciseaux, A.: Anorexia nervosa: a view from the mirror, Am. J. Nurs. **80**:1468, 1980.

This author, using a pseudonym, describes her personal experience with anorexia nervosa. She provides insight into the anorectic person's view of her behavior and her interpretations of the responses of others to her. The article is illustrated with a fascinating self-portrait accompanied by the author's explanation of the meaning of the picture.

Cohen, F., and Lazarus, R.S.: Coping with the stress of illness. In Stone, G., editor: Health psychology: a handbook, San Francisco, 1979, Jossey-Bass, Inc., Publishers.

The authors present an analysis of coping and adaptation behaviors related to the experience of serious physical illness. They discuss the complexity of coping processes and review current research. They conclude by making recommendations for future study. Many of the issues that they delineate have implications for patient compliance with health care regimens. This work is appropriate for graduate level study.

*Doyen, L.: Primary anorexia nervosa: a review and critique of selected papers, J. Psychosoc. Nurs. **20**:12, June 1982.

This excellent article reviews research on anorexia nervosa. The author analyzes study designs and results related to diagnosis, etiology, and approaches to treatment. She makes recommendations regarding the design of future studies.

Durkheim, E.: Suicide, New York, 1951, The Free Press. (Translated by J.A. Spaulding and G. Simpson.)

This is a classic that identified demographic factors which apply to suicidal behavior. Durkheim also described types of suicidal behavior that are still discussed in contemporary literature. This study is also of note because it was one of the first attempts to apply research techniques to a sociological study.

*Evans, D.L.: Explaining suicide among the young: an analytical review of the literature, J. Psychosoc. Nurs. Ment. Health Serv. **20**:9, Aug. 1982.

The author provides a critical overview of the literature on child and adolescent suicide. He concludes that there is little consistency among studies, resulting in difficulty conceptualizing the problem. He particularly notes the lack of nursing research on this topic.

Farberow, N.L., editor: The many faces of suicide: indirect self-destructive behavior, New York, 1980, McGraw-Hill Book Co.

This book is highly recommended as a resource on a variety of indirectly self-destructive behaviors. The contributors are knowledgeable about their topics and discuss them in relationship to the characteristics of this behavioral pattern. Included are the problems of noncompliance with therapeutic plans, drug abuse, alcohol abuse, hyperobesity, cigarette smoking, self-mutilation, automobile accidents, gambling, criminal and deviant activity, stress-seeking behaviors, and high-risk sports.

Frances, A., and Clarkin, J.F.: Considering family versus other therapies after a teenager's suicide attempt, Hosp. Community Psychiatry **36**:1041, Oct. 1985.

This case study illustrates the possible relationship between the suicide attempt of a child and family stress. The author illustrates the utilization of both family and individual therapy to intervene in this situation.

Hendin, H.: Suicide: a review of new directions in research, Hosp. Community Psychiatry **37**:148, Feb. 1986.

Recent research in suicide has challenged some of the assumptions regarding etiology, demographics, and psychodynamics of suicidal behavior. The author presents a thorough review

---

*Asterisk indicates nursing reference.

of current research in comparison with past assumptions and suggests directions to be pursued in the future.

Herzog, D.B., and Copeland, P.M.: Eating disorders, N. Engl. J. Med. **313**:295, Aug. 1985.

This is an extremely thorough review of current research related to eating disorders. It is particularly strong in the area of analyzing the physical disruptions related to anorexia nervosa and bulimia.

*Jourard, S.: Suicide: an invitation to die, Am. J. Nurs. **70**:269, 1970.

This provocative article connects family process to suicidal behavior. It leads the reader to consider the broader social system, which usually affects the behavior of the identified patient.

*Kiecolt-Glaser, J., and Dixon, K.: Postadolescent onset male anorexia, J. Psychosoc. Nurs. Ment. Health Serv. **22**:11, Jan. 1984.

These authors use literature review and case material to support their contention that males who become anorectic following adolescence are different in personality characteristics from females and younger males. This observation is an important one for treatment planning. Further study would be beneficial.

*Mahan, L.K.: A sensible approach to the obese patient, Nurs. Clin. North Am. **14**:229, June 1979.

This is a thorough review of contemporary views of obesity. A convenient table describes various treatments for obesity. There is a good description of the behavior modification approach to treatment. The author also discusses the importance of activity and the components of a healthy reducing diet.

Menninger, K.: Man against himself, New York, 1938, Harcourt, Brace & World, Inc.

This classic work investigated self-destructive behavior long before it was fashionable to do so. Menninger took a psychoanalytical approach to suicidal behavior and identified several levels of attempts at self-destruction.

*Moore, J.A., and Coulman, M.V.: Anorexia nervosa: the patient, her family and key family therapy interventions, J. Psychosoc. Nurs. Ment. Health Serv. **19**:9, May 1981.

In this article, anorexia nervosa is discussed in the context of family dynamics. The presentation is based on the theoretical framework of structural family therapy. Concepts are illustrated with clinical vignettes. This is a clear presentation of the involvement of the family in the anorectic patient's illness.

Morgan, H.G.: Death wishes? The understanding and management of deliberate self-harm, New York, 1979, John Wiley & Sons, Inc.

This book provides an excellent comparison of the characteristics of suicide and nonfatal deliberate self-harm. Reports of recent research are included. Studies cited address such issues as epidemiological factors, treatment, and implications for prevention. The author clarifies the need for further study of this phenomenon. This book is particularly recommended for readers who have an interest in research.

*Neville, D., and Barnes, S.: The suicidal phone call, J. Psychosoc. Nurs. Ment. Health Serv. **23**:14, Aug. 1985.

The authors discuss issues related to interacting with a suicidal person on the telephone. They recommend information that should be collected, as well as helpful and unhelpful responses.

Of particular value is the attention given to the need for peer support of the telephone counselor.

Niswander, G.D., Casey, T.M., and Humphrey, J.A.: A panorama of suicide, Springfield, Ill., 1973, Charles C Thomas, Publisher.

A fascinating collection of psychological autopsies is presented here. Reading them adds depth to one's understanding of the many facets of suicidal behavior.

*Potts, N.L.: The secret pattern of binge/purge, Am. J. Nurs. **84**:32, Jan. 1982.

The author presents an overview of issues related to bulimia including assessment, possible etiology, and treatment approaches. The article includes useful information differentiating bulimia from anorexia nervosa.

Powers, P.S.: Obesity: The regulation of weight, Baltimore, 1980, The Williams & Wilkins Co.

The author has included a wealth of information on obesity and other eating disorders in this volume. A particular strength is the inclusion of reports of relevant research with critical evaluation of the results. Extensive bibliographies are also an asset.

Pretzel, P.W.: Understanding and counseling the suicidal person, New York, 1972, Abingdon Press.

This author takes a philosophical approach to the problem of suicide in this deeply humanistic view of the subject. Although intended for clergy, there are approaches to counseling that are equally applicable to nursing.

*Price, J.H., and Pritts, C.: Overweight and obesity in the elderly, J. Gerontol. Nurs. **6**:341, 1980.

This article focuses on factors related to obesity in the elderly. However, the principles that are included are applicable to the understanding and treatment of overweight individuals in all age groups. This is a readable article that covers the topic quite thoroughly.

*Sanger, E., and Cassino, T.: Avoiding the power struggle, Am. J. Nurs. **84**:31, Jan. 1984.

This is a description of a treatment program that has been successful in helping anorectic patients. This program is structured to use a behavior modification approach with defined outcomes. Behaviors associated with anorexia are not addressed directly by nursing staff.

*Santora, D., and Starkey, P.: Research studies in American Indian suicides, J. Psychosoc. Nurs. Ment. Health Serv. **20**:25, Aug. 1982.

This article demonstrates the value of exploring sociocultural influences on behavior. Studies of suicide in several American Indian tribes are reviewed, enabling the reader to identify similarities and differences.

Schwartz, D.A.: The suicidal character, Psychiatr. Q. **51**:64, Winter, 1979.

The author describes the development of a characterological suicidal trait that may result from the secondary gain related to long-term suicidal behavior. In this case, the nurturing behavior that is usually provided to the suicidal person perpetuates the dysfunctional behavior. The patient and the care provider become enmeshed in a life and death power struggle. The danger is that the patient will need to demonstrate his control by carrying out his suicidal threat.

Shneidman, E.S., editor: Suicidology: contemporary developments, New York, 1976, Grune & Stratton, Inc.

This anthology is edited by one of the United States' most respected suicidologists. The information included is well selected and may be particularly useful to the experienced practitioner who may want to gain more depth in knowledge of suicidal behavior.

*Stanitis, M.A., and Ryan, J.: Noncompliance: an unacceptable diagnosis? Am. J. Nurs. **82**:941, June 1982.

The authors challenge the acceptability of the nursing diagnosis of noncompliance. They point out that this is a value-laden term which may result in the development of negative attitudes toward the patient. They also question whether compliance with a medical regimen is always a positive behavior. This article could be assigned as a stimulus for group discussion.

Wekstein, L.: Handbook of suicidology: principles, problems and practice, New York, 1979, Brunner/Mazel, Inc.

This well-written book provides an extensive examination of suicidal behavior. The author is knowledgeable about the use of psychotherapy with suicidal patients. He includes some suggested experiential learning activities and illustrates theory with case histories. He also includes current research in suicidology. This is a useful reference for both the student and the practitioner of psychiatric nursing.

*White, J.H.: Bulimia: utilizing individual and family therapy, J. Psychosoc. Nurs. Ment. Health Serv. **22**:22, Apr. 1984.

This case study demonstrates the application of individual and family therapy to the treatment of bulimia by a nurse psychotherapist. The author describes the use of the interpersonal individual and structural/functional family therapy models. The theory is well integrated with the clinical material.

Wolman, B.B., editor: Between survival and suicide, New York, 1976, Gardner Press, Inc.

This anthology includes chapters by several of the more controversial psychiatric theorists. The volume is stimulating and thought provoking, because many of the writers take unique approaches to their subject matter.

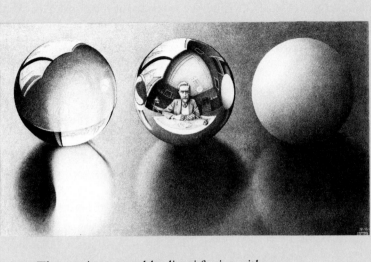

The emptiness caused by dissatisfaction with mere achievement and the helplessness that results when the channels of relation break down have brought forth a loneliness of soul such as never existed before.

Karl Jaspers, Existenzphilosophie*

CHAPTER 17

DISRUPTIONS IN RELATEDNESS

*Translated by Kaufmann, F. In Kaufmann, W., editor: Existentialism from Dostoevsky to Sartre, New York, 1956, Meridian Books.

LEARNING OBJECTIVES

After studying this chapter, the student should be able to:

- describe the characteristics of a healthy interpersonal relationship.

- discuss the development of relatedness throughout the life cycle.

- identify five possible disruptions that can occur in the process of relatedness.

- compare and contrast the states of aloneness and existential loneliness.

- describe predisposing factors that may lead to problems with interpersonal relationships.

- analyze the developmental, sociocultural, biochemical, and psychodynamic stressors that contribute to the development of disruptions in relatedness.

- identify and describe behaviors that are associated with disruptions in relatedness, including impaired communication, withdrawal, suspicion, dependency, and manipulation.

- discuss the manifestation of impaired relationship behaviors in patients with medical diagnoses of paranoid schizophrenia, catatonic schizophrenia, dependent personality disorder, borderline personality disorder, and antisocial personality disorder.

- formulate individualized nursing diagnoses for patients with disrupted relationship patterns.

- assess the relationship between the nursing and medical diagnoses of individual patients.

- identify the individual's attempts to cope with the anxiety created by the inability to establish healthy interpersonal relationships.

- develop long-term and short-term individualized nursing goals with patients who are experiencing disruptions in relatedness.

- apply therapeutic nurse-patient relationship principles with an appropriate rationale to the care of the patient who is unable to establish healthy relationships.

- analyze nursing interventions appropriate to the needs of the patient who is suspicious, dependent, withdrawn, manipulative, or who is unable to communicate effectively.

- develop a mental health education plan to assist patients to understand and participate in the treatment of their relationship problems.

- assess the importance of the evaluation of the nursing process when working with patients who experience disrupted interpersonal relationships.

- identify directions for future nursing research.

- select appropriate readings for further study.

Continuum of social responses

■ Positive interpersonal relationships

Human beings are socially oriented and to achieve satisfaction with life, they must be able to establish positive interpersonal relationships. A healthy interpersonal relationship is one in which the individuals involved experience intimacy with each other while maintaining separate identities. According to Sullivan,[42] intimacy is characterized by sensitivity to the needs of the other person and mutual validation of personal worth. There may or may not be a sexual component to the intimate relationship. Other characteristics of healthy relatedness as delineated by Rogers[35] include open communication of feelings, acceptance of the other as a valued separate person, and deep empathic understanding. To achieve this depth of involvement with another person, there must be willingness to take the risk of self-revelation. This can be a frightening experience, particularly if either individual has been more reserved about expressing feelings. Fear of exposure of the self frequently inhibits people from developing intimate relationships.

Issues of control are also involved when people relate to each other. There are times when it is necessary to subordinate individual needs to the needs of the other individual or to the demands of the relationship itself. At other times it may be more important to the individual to be self-assertive and to set aside the needs of others. The mature person must be able to sort out priorities of needs and to share with others the rationale for his behavior. Within the context of any relationship there is a continuum of dependent to independent behavior on the part of each participant. Ideally, there should be some balance between these behaviors within the relationship. This balance can be described as interdependence. The interdependent person identifies areas where there is a need to rely on others and experience the caring aspects of dependency. There are also times when it is appropriate and gratifying to self-esteem to function independently. In addition to behaving in this flexible way, the interdependent person can allow another to be dependent on him or independent of him, according to the other person's need. In this case each individual assumes responsibility for control of his own behavior but also receives support and assistance from significant others when it is needed.

Every person has the potential to be involved in relationships at many levels, from the intimacy just described to superficial transient contacts. Intimate and interdependent relationships provide a secure base from which the person derives self-confidence in coping with the various demands of day-to-day life. A lack of intimacy with family members and friends leaves only a series of superficial encounters, depriving the person of many of life's most meaningful experiences. The support of significant others frees energy for involvement with social groups, work groups, and the community. The mature adult is able to maintain involvement at all these levels and feel satisfied with the quality of his relationships with others.

■ Life cycle development of relatedness

■ **INFANCY.** Learning to relate to others in a mature way is a growth process that takes place throughout the developmental cycle. The infant is by necessity dependent on others for meeting all its biological and psychosocial needs. A consistent reliable relationship with a mothering person resulting in the establishment of trust is essential at this stage of the growth process. People who fail to accomplish the task of establishing basic trust are handicapped in relating to others as they continue to grow and develop.

■ **CHILDHOOD.** As a child grows older and develops motor skills, independence becomes a possibility and he strives to establish himself as an individual, separate from the mothering person who has been meeting all his needs. This leads to conflict as more powerful adults set limits on behavior, often frustrating the child's efforts toward independence. Loving, consistent limit setting, however, communicates caring and provides the beginning of the development of a capacity for interdependence. As the child grows older, the parents' guidelines for behavior are internalized, and a value sys-

tem begins to emerge. At this point the child enters school and begins to learn interdependent concepts of cooperation, competition, and compromise. Peer relationships become important, as does the approval of adults from outside the family group, such as teachers, scout leaders, and parents of friends.

■ **PREADOLESCENCE AND ADOLESCENCE.** By preadolescence, the individual becomes involved in an intimate relationship with a friend of the same sex, a "best friend." This relationship is characterized by sharing and offers another opportunity for clarification of values and recognition of individual differences. This is usually also a very dependent relationship and intrusions by others are actively resisted. However, as adolescence develops, the dependence on a close friend of the same sex usually yields to a heterosexual relationship, also very dependent in nature. Simultaneous with these dependent relationships with peers, the individual vigorously asserts independence from parents. This striving for independence, often marked by rebellious behavior, is supported by peers who are engaged in the same struggle. Parents can facilitate growth by consistent limit setting and a caring tolerance of the adolescent's rebellious outbursts. As the individual learns to balance parental demands and peer group pressures, another step toward mature interdependence is taken.

■ **YOUNG ADULTHOOD.** The adolescent period ends when the person is able to be self-sufficient, maintaining an interdependent relationship with parents and peers. Decisions are now made independently, with the advice and opinions of others taken into account. The individual may marry and begin a new family unit. Occupational plans are made and implemented. The mature person will demonstrate self-awareness by balancing dependent and independent behavior and by allowing others to be dependent or independent as appropriate. Sensitivity to and acceptance of the feelings and needs of oneself and of others is critical to this level of mature functioning. Interpersonal relationships are characterized by mutuality.

■ **MIDDLE ADULTHOOD.** Parenting and adult friendships will test the person's ability to foster independence in others. This involves a need to give up some dependence on the other person so he may grow. Children gradually separate from parents as they grow and friends may move away or drift apart. The mature person must then be self-reliant and find other supports to augment those which have diminished or been lost. Pleasure can be found in the development of an interdependent relationship with children as they grow. The freedom that results from decreased dependent demands by children can be used for new activities which promote self-growth.

■ **LATE ADULTHOOD.** As adulthood continues, change continues to occur. There are losses, such as the physical changes of aging, the death of parents, loss of occupation through retirement, and later the deaths of friends and of one's spouse. The need for relatedness must still be satisfied. The mature person grieves over these losses and recognizes that others can help resolve the grief. However, there are also new possibilities even in the face of loss. Old friends and relatives cannot be replaced, but new relationships can develop. Grandchildren may become important to the grandparent, who may delight in spending time with them that was never available for children. The aging person may also find a sense of relatedness to the culture as a whole. Life assumes deeper meaning in relation to the individual's perception of his accomplishments and contributions to the welfare of the whole. The mature older person can accept whatever increase in dependence is necessary but also retain as much independence as possible. Even loss of physical health need not necessarily force the person to give up all independence. Self-esteem is enhanced by the ability to maintain mature relatedness throughout life.

■ **Disruptions in relatedness**

Disruptions can occur in the development of mature interdependent interpersonal relationships. Some individuals find it difficult to establish or maintain close relationships. They may **withdraw** from other people, sometimes to the point where they are unable to maintain themselves in the community. A similar situation can occur when a person is isolated by others. In other cases individuals may experience excessive **dependency** on other people, draining the resources of those to whom they relate and potentially inviting rejection by friends and relatives. A third disruption in relatedness is **manipulation** of other people. In this case closeness is not established and other people are treated as objects to be maneuvered to meet the needs of the manipulator. Individuals who are experiencing problems in the area of relatedness are likely to have difficulty in experiencing basic trust in others. Therefore there is generally some degree of **suspicion** present along with any of the behaviors described. Another behavior that frequently accompanies disruptions in relatedness is **impaired communication.** Verbal and nonverbal communication patterns may be distorted or incongruent, thus keeping others at a safe distance and preventing the development of intimacy.

In addition, loneliness is likely to be a component of the lives of these people. The loneliness of lack of intimacy with others is pervasive and painful. This is difficult to imagine if it has not been experienced. The pain of loneliness can be shared empathically to some extent and often arouses anxiety in the person with whom it is shared. Biographical accounts of experiences of a psychiatric patient, such as *I Never Promised You a Rose Garden* by Joanne Greenberg or *The Bell Jar* by Sylvia Plath, also communicate some of the character of this existential pain. Frieda Fromm-Reichman conceptualized extreme loneliness as she worked with many withdrawn patients. She hypothesized that it should be differentiated from anxiety and that perhaps it is an even more frightening experience than anxiety. She describes loneliness as a state in which past relationships are for the most part forgotten and there is little hope of any future relationship.[14] It is a difficult concept to study because the person who is lonely is unable to communicate about it, the person who has been lonely does not usually want to remember what it was like, and the person who is studying it becomes anxious when he tries to understand it. Loneliness of this kind must be differentiated from aloneness and solitude. The latter conditions may be sought out by individuals from time to time and may be conducive to contemplation, creativity, and the growth of self-awareness.

■ **Continuum of social responses**

Behaviors that are related to interpersonal relationships may be represented on a continuum that ranges from healthy interdependent interactions to those which involve no real contact with other people. This continuum of coping responses is illustrated in Fig. 17-1.

Progression from the adaptive to the maladaptive end of the continuum reflects an increase in the seriousness of the relationship disorder. The medical diagnoses used in this chapter to demonstrate these behaviors include schizophrenic disorders and selected personality disorders. These illnesses also present the patient with a range of problems of varying intensity. The goal of nursing intervention is to assist the patient to shift his interpersonal behavior toward the adaptive end of the continuum.

 Assessment

■ **Predisposing factors**

A variety of factors—within the individual, between the individual and significant others, and environmental—may lead to disrupted interpersonal relationships. Although a great deal of research is directed toward the disorders to be considered in this chapter, no conclusions have been reached about the specific conditions that lead to interpersonal problems. In all likelihood, a combination of factors result in the individual's experiencing difficulties in his interpersonal relationships.

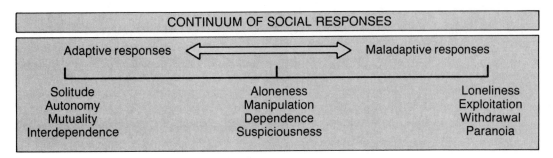

Fig. 17-1. Continuum of social responses.

The nurse needs to recognize this and be sure to explore all relevant areas during the nursing assessment.

■ **DEVELOPMENTAL FACTORS.** Since the capacity for relatedness is the result of a developmental process, anything that inhibits the accomplishment of relevant developmental tasks will also decrease the individual's ability to develop healthy interpersonal relationships. The family is the unit within which the first experiences with closeness to others take place. Lack of maternal stimulation or attention deprives the infant of a sense of security and there is failure to establish basic trust. This can lead to a suspicious attitude toward others that may continue throughout life. The quality of mothering attention is also important. A child may be adequately fed and receive impeccable physical care but without any communication of maternal caring. A child who is treated like an object may well become an adult who treats others like objects. Rather than responding to personal expressions of caring, the person may rely on material possessions to feel secure. Early experiences of maternal deprivation also frequently lead to severe depression in the child, as demonstrated in the studies of Spitz.[41] Without corrective experiences, and provided he survives, the child will probably develop into a withdrawn and chronically depressed adult. Early experiences such as these can lead to the most serious of psychiatric disorders and frequently to chronic institutionalization.

Between the ages of 3 and 18 months, the infant is in the symbiotic stage of development.[29] During this time, it is very important for the mothering person to perform ego functions for the child, including orienting him to reality. This forms the basis for future interpersonal relationships in terms of being able to empathize and understand the position of others.

Another group of potential problems arises as the child begins to strive for independence. Masterson[29] calls this the separation-individuation stage, occurring between 18 months and 3 years of age. The develop-ment of autonomy is the goal of this phase. Inhibition of the toddler's efforts to develop autonomy can result in excessive dependency that may continue into adulthood, resulting in a fearful, clinging person. Inconsistent limits or lack of limits can interfere with the person's ability to perceive the needs and rights of others, thus blocking the ability to achieve intimacy in relationships. The mothering person and child must learn to tolerate separation from each other for periods of time, and the child must develop confidence that the nurturer will return after an absence. At the same time, the mothering person must adjust to the child's increased independence that comes with walking and increased mobility. The child must also learn to perceive significant others as whole objects, with both good and bad characteristics. Interference with the process at this stage may result in the severe interpersonal limitations that are characteristic of the person with the medical diagnosis of borderline personality disorder. By the end of this phase of development, the child differentiates himself from others. The ego functions that have developed include reality testing, impulse control, frustration tolerance, and the beginning of object constancy.[29]

The value system that is held by the parents is communicated to the preschool and school-aged child. In addition, the exposure to other ideas that comes about as school begins and the child's world expands to include parts of the community broadens his developing value system. Congruency between parental and community values facilitates this process for the child. Lack of clarity about values may result in confusion in adulthood, with vulnerability to compliance with the ideas of others rather than a healthy personal decision-making ability. It is also possible that value confusion may lead to antisocial behavior by a person who has a flexible value system that encompasses a variety of possible behaviors based on the individual's self-interest.

■ **FAMILY COMMUNICATION FACTORS.** Family communication patterns may also be factors leading to disruptions in relationships. Patients with a medical diagnosis of schizophrenia are frequently members of families with identifiably disturbed communication patterns. In a survey of current family research relative to schizophrenia, Wynne, Toohey, and Doane[53] identify the following three types of family communication patterns that are being investigated by schizophrenia researchers: communication deviance studies, initiated by Wynne and his associates[52,53]; the expressed emotion studies of Brown, Vaughn, and Leff[44,53]; and the family relationship test investigated by Scott and colleagues.[53] The communication deviance studies use projective tests, such as the Rorschach and the Thematic Apperception Test (TAT), to study the communication patterns of identified schizophrenic patients and their immediate family members. These studies have demonstrated that deviant patterns of communication exist in families in which a child becomes schizophrenic. The expressed emotion studies[44] analyze interviews with family members of schizophrenic patients in terms of the frequency of critical comments about the patient, as well as assigning a global rating for the amount of hostility, warmth, or overinvolvement expressed by the relative. These characteristics were related to the future course of the illness. It was found that a high amount of expressed emotion by relatives is associated with a higher frequency of relapses. The Family Relationship Test[53] measures family members' perceptions of interpersonal relationships by use of an adjective checklist. It was found that patients who view their parents as "well" have a better prognosis than those who perceive their parents as "ill."

The role of the family in producing impaired interpersonal relationships has been studied extensively by Bateson and his associates.[3,4] These theorists state that basic intrafamilial relationship problems frequently become manifest in the symptomatic behavior of one family member. This deviant behavior develops when the family is subjected to intolerable levels of stress. Satir[36] notes that a family member who acts "crazy" may serve the function of keeping the family system intact. This is further supported by the frequent observation that, as the "family symptom bearer" gets better, other family problems get worse.[36] Satir further states that the family system operates within a set of rules that concern communication and "it is the rigidity or restrictions of these rules and the consequent distortions which ultimately create the need for symptoms."[36] For example, if there is a family rule that hostility is never expressed directly between family members, and the parents are involved in a conflict which they may not confront, tension will build up within the family system. One of the children may respond to this tension by "acting crazy" and performing destructive acts in the home. Family tension is then kept in control by identifying the symptom bearer as the cause of the problem and justifying his behavior as the result of his "illness," whereas in reality he is expressing the conflict between the parents.

Another family communication pattern that has been linked to the development of psychotic behavior is the double-bind theory developed by Bateson and associates.[4] The components of the double bind are described as follows:

1. The presence of two or more persons, one of whom is the "victim"
2. Repeated experience with the process so that it becomes the expected pattern of communication
3. A "primary negative injunction" that promises punishment either for performance of a given action or for failure to perform a given action; punishment being described as "withdrawal of love. . . . expression of hate or anger—or most devastating—the kind of abandonment that results from the parent's expression of extreme helplessness"[4]
4. A "secondary injunction" that conflicts with the primary injunction at a more abstract level, with similar threats of punishment; usually transmitted nonverbally and may negate any or all parts of the message in the primary injunction
5. A "tertiary negative injunction" that forbids the victim to escape[4]

In the following example of communication that follows the double-bind pattern, a hospitalized schizophrenic man in his early twenties is being visited by his parents. As they arrive, the mother says, "Aren't you glad to see us, dear?" As the son says, "Yes, I am" and moves forward to embrace his mother, she turns away to her husband and remarks about the dreariness of the hospital. The son then withdraws and waits passively for his parents to continue the interaction. In this case the primary injunction was to be glad to have a parental visit. However, when the son tried to demonstrate his gladness, the mother's nonverbal communication of turning away communicated her displeasure at his action and a secondary injunction not to initiate closeness. This nonverbal message was enhanced by her remark about the dreariness of the setting, which at another level could be interpreted as a rebuke to her son whose illness brought her there. Also coexisting in this scene is the double message "You should be glad to see me, but I'm not glad to see you." It should also be noted that a lack of response to the first statement, "Aren't you glad to see us, dear?" would not be a solution to the problem because this directly challenges the primary injunction and will also be dealt with by punishment. Therefore the young man, who has no way of being rewarded for his behavior, protects himself by withdrawing from the situation.

Although the mother in this scene seems like a villain, complementing the son's role of victim, any family member can be cast in any role and multiple victimizers may exist. Unfortunately the mother is sometimes stereotyped as the one who always creates double binds for psychotic children. The other misconception that can occur easily is that this behavior is intentional and maliciously directed toward the defenseless child. Parents are not usually aware of double-binding behavior and when confronted about it tend to respond defensively. The problem lies within the family system and the total communication process which occurs within that system. For instance, the father in the example, who stood by while his wife set up the double bind, is equally responsible for doing nothing to clarify the confused communication.

Social relationships outside of the family may also be disrupted and have a lasting effect on behavior. Families of persons who develop a borderline personality disorder often discourage relationships with others. Failure to develop intimacy with peers, first of the same sex and later of the opposite sex, leads to social isolation in adulthood. Such an individual may appear cool and aloof and is likely to become involved in superficial relationships. There is likely to be a romanticized idea of heterosexual relationships and disappointment when this does not materialize. This person may also become depressed as an adult because of a vague sense of what an intimate relationship could be like compared to the reality of what the person is experiencing. Involvements with others may be transient and characterized by approach-avoidance behavior as the person tries to pursue closeness. The individual who has difficulty establishing intimacy may also be extremely dependent, clinging to any relationship that may potentially bring fulfillment but frightened to take the risk of self-disclosure, which would lead to a truly mature involvement.

■ **SOCIOCULTURAL FACTORS.** Sociocultural factors can also influence the person's ability to establish and maintain relatedness. In contemporary culture there are many forces that tend to make the individual feel isolated and lonely. Cultural mores discourage reaching out to casual acquaintances. Friendships are often transient because of the mobility involved in many occupations. Packard[32] studied transient populations and found higher rates of mental hospital admissions, more aggressive behavior, and more marital discord in this group. Even family relationships acquire an ephemeral quality as children move from place to place, frequently seeing parents only occasionally. Friends are often closer than siblings, at times creating a vague discomfort and a cultural nostalgia for the "good old days" of the close-knit extended family.

Certain groups within the culture are particularly vulnerable to isolation. The elderly are frequently ignored in our production-oriented culture. Older people are takers of material goods and the young must be the givers. We have little tolerance as a society for those who are not actively involved in the economic system. Paradoxically, even if older people have the ability to be active, they are pushed out of the system to make room for the young.

Involuntary social isolation also happens to the handicapped and chronically ill of any age. People with terminal illnesses or disfiguring disorders are frequently avoided by others. This is also true for people with long-term psychiatric problems. Although there has been an effort to decrease chronic institutionalization, there is great resistance to integration of the disabled into the community. This externally imposed isolation may result in withdrawal, depression, dependency, suspicion, impaired communication, manipulative behavior, or any combination of these as the individual tries to cope with loneliness.

Other sociocultural factors are related to the cultural norms present in contemporary society. For instance, there is an idealized expectation that people will be involved in "meaningful" relationships, which is constantly reinforced through the media. Heterosexual relationships in particular are romanticized, which is perhaps reflected in the increasing numbers of adolescent out-of-wedlock pregnancies and early marriages leading to divorce. This cultural attitude leads to the experience of loneliness as described by Gordon: "the sense of deprivation that comes when certain *expected* human relationships are absent."[15:26] For the purpose of this discussion, the term "aloneness" will be used to differentiate this degree of loneliness from the existential kind of loneliness described earlier. The dynamics of aloneness as experienced by many Americans include the following[15]:

1. Feelings of hopelessness
2. Escape into unsatisfying relationships
3. Fear of experiencing lonely feelings
4. Denial of loneliness
5. Feelings of worthlessness and failure

A spiral of repetitive behavior often results, with feelings of helplessness, hopelessness, and worthlessness accumulating until the person in desperation often resorts to self-destructive behavior.

Some groups in society prey on the alone and the lonely. In recent years there has been a flood of various planned group experiences that are advertised as therapeutic. Most of them promise a degree of intimate human experience. Encounter groups, when under the direction of a skilled therapist, often can be helpful to the isolated person. However, there is danger that the group leader may be untrained and unsophisticated in dealing with emotional problems. Another cultural development that attracts those who are lonely, particularly the young, is the various religious cults, which offer the attraction of a close-knit community and a sense of commonality of belief and effort. This sense of belonging is so important that cult members may sever all ties with family and friends and behave in compliance with the demands of the group, even if this is in conflict with a previous value system.

Although closeness is an ideal that is viewed as positive in this culture, a different message is given at the same time. This message is that it is acceptable to be selectively intimate, but most people should not be trusted and it is important to be careful in interpersonal contacts. This attitude can create confusion and a sense of insecurity. In a relatively short period of time, people have gone from leaving houses unlocked all the time to installing several locks on each door, burglar alarms, and guard dogs. Rising crime rates cause fear and more reluctance on the part of many people to risk closeness or contact with strangers. Some urban residents, particularly the elderly, become virtual prisoners in their homes and experience loneliness and all the associated behaviors.

■ **BIOLOGICAL FACTORS.** Biological factors are genetic tendencies that may predispose the person to experience interpersonal problems. This has been investigated relative to the identification of populations at risk for schizophrenia. In general, it has been found that monozygotic twins, even when adopted at birth by different parents and raised separately, show greater concordance for the occurrence of schizophrenia than do dizygotic twins.[8] Other studies have demonstrated that first-degree relatives (parents, siblings, and children) of schizophrenic patients also are at greater risk than the general population, but less so than monozygotic twins. Because these results are found even when environmental influences are controlled, as in the twin-separation studies, there is strong evidence for a genetic aspect to at least some forms of schizophrenia.[8]

Recently, neuroscientists have begun to use brain imaging techniques, such as computerized axial tomography (CT scan) and positron emission tomography (PET scan) to study structural characteristics of the brains of schizophrenic persons. Weinberger and Kleinman[45] report that of over thirty CT studies, the majority have found structural abnormalities. The most common defects include enlarged lateral and third ventricles and dilated cortical fissures and sulci. The process of alteration in brain structure seems to be neither progressive nor reversible. It is not known how the changes relate to symptoms of schizophrenia. However, it appears that structural changes are related to fewer positive (abnormal or excessive behaviors) and more negative (decreased or absent behaviors) symptoms. In addition these changes are linked with more neurological impairment, poor premorbid social adjustment, and less response to neuroleptic medication. These observations have led to hope that enlarged ventricles may be a marker for one subtype of schizophrenia.

■ **Precipitating stressors**

Disruptions in relatedness evolve as the result of various experiences that influence the growth of the individual. In most instances, a series of life events predisposes a person to difficulty with interpersonal relationships. Many people cope with their interpersonal problems and describe themselves as reasonably satisfied with this aspect of life. However, additional stress can cause a marginally satisfying interpersonal life to become grossly disrupted. Response to various stressors is highly individualized. However, the factors to be discussed are likely to cause some degree of interpersonal disruption for most people. It is also essential to remember that an increase in the level of stress is experienced by the individual as anxiety, which is at the root of the behavioral disruptions.

The person who reaches maturity with a capacity for healthy interpersonal relationships is still vulnerable to psychological stressors that may interfere with his success. Either a series of losses or a single significant loss may lead to difficulty in establishing future intimate relationships. The pain of a loss can be so great that the individual will withdraw from future involvements rather than risk a repetition of pain. This response is of course enhanced if the person had difficulty during any of the developmental tasks pertinent to relatedness. Losses of significant others may cause difficulty with future relationships, but so may other kinds of losses. The loss of a job decreases a person's self-esteem and can also result in future withdrawal and problems with relatedness unless the person has a well-established interpersonal support system.

■ **SOCIOCULTURAL STRESSORS.** Stressors leading to interpersonal relationship difficulties may be sociocultural. For instance, there are indications that the family unit is becoming less stable. The divorce rate has been rising. Mobility has broken up the extended family, depriving people of all ages of an important support system. This has resulted in less contact between the generations, with young people losing the wise advice of grandparents and older people missing the stimulation of youth. Tradition, which provides a powerful link with the past and a sense of identity, is also less observed when the family is fragmented. The current resurgence of interest in ethnicity and "roots" may reflect the striving of isolated people to associate themselves with a specific identity. The many stresses on the family system have made it more difficult for family members to accomplish the developmental tasks relevant to intimacy.

Nurses frequently encounter patients with behaviors related to disrupted interpersonal relationships in the general hospital setting. Even a reasonably well-adjusted person may have difficulty maintaining a satisfactory level of intimacy while hospitalized. The hospital environment tends to be impersonal, which enhances the patient's sense of isolation. Patients who must be isolated because of concern about infection or, in the psychiatric setting, to control behavior are susceptible to the effects of sensory deprivation and need creative nursing care to lessen this problem. On the other hand, patients in critical care areas may experience sensory overload, which may also lead to a feeling of loneliness and separation from others.

■ **BIOCHEMICAL STRESSORS.** There is a strong probability that there are biochemical stressors associated with difficulty in establishing and maintaining effective interpersonal relationships. For instance, people with a medical diagnosis of one or another form of schizophrenia are generally withdrawn, dependent, exhibit unusual communication patterns, and may be suspicious of other people. A great deal of research is presently being directed toward discovering a biochemical disorder associated with at least some of the schizophrenic disorders. This research tends to be confusing because various studies frequently contradict each other. It should also be noted that even if a particular biochemical disruption is discovered, it will not explain the origin of schizophrenia, but will be evidence of some other, more basic, problem which may still be unidentified. For example, knowing that a person who exhibits the behaviors associated with diabetes mellitus has hypoglycemia does not define the real cause of the problem, which is a deficit in insulin production by the pancreas related to heredity, diet, or some other basic stressor.

At the present time, there seems to be a rapidly growing amount of evidence that at least some cases of schizophrenia are related to an excess of dopamine in key areas of the brain, probably the mesocortical and mesolimbic nerve tracts. The excessive dopamine may result from increased production, increased release, or turnover of dopamine, or an increased number or activity of receptors.[6] Identification of the cause of dopamine excess would assist greatly in discovering the cause of schizophrenia. The dopamine hypothesis[30,46] has been supported by (1) noting that the administration of dopaminergic agents (amphetamines, L-dopa, or apomorphine) leads to initiation or exacerbation of psychotic behavior and (2) ascertaining that neuroleptic drugs (phenothiazine) act at the synapse by binding dopamine receptor sites. This theory is viewed as the most promising one and is being studied intensively by biochemical researchers.

Another biochemical theory that continues to be investigated is the platelet monoamine oxidase (MAO) theory,[3] which hypothesizes that schizophrenics have lower levels of MAO in the bloodstream than do others. This theory is related to the amine theory, in that MAO is an enzyme that deactivates brain cell amines, including dopamine. Low levels of MAO, then, would lead to high levels of dopamine. However, there have been many methodological problems associated with the platelet MAO research.

Another theory is the indolamine hypothesis. This theory suggests that a defect in the metabolism of the indolamine serotonin results in the production of the hallucinogenic substances bufotenine and dimethyltryptamine (DMT). Evidence that supports this hypothesis includes the presence of bufotenine in the urine of schizophrenic patients. Researchers have also induced an excited state in normal persons or recurrence of psychosis in schizophrenics by producing an excess of substrate through administration of the amino acids tryptophan and methionine. Methyl groups combine with the substrate to produce bufotenine and DMT.[21]

The transmethylation hypothesis links schizophrenia to an abnormality in the transmethylation of catecholamines, resulting in the production of dimethoxyphenylethylamine (DMPEA), which is similar to mescaline. Findings in terms of this theory are equivocal at this point, but the possibility is still under consideration.[21,30]

Biochemical research is important not only because it may reveal clues to the cause or, more likely, causes of schizophrenia but also because understanding of biochemical processes may provide important guidelines to treatment. In addition, the identification of measurable biochemical imbalances, such as low platelet MAO, could lead to simple tests to identify at-risk populations, ultimately leading to methods of preventing the onset of some types of schizophrenia.

■ **BIOLOGICAL-SOCIOENVIRONMENTAL MODELS.** Modern day researchers emphasize that socioenvironmental and biochemical studies constantly reinforce the assumption that interaction between the individual and his environment is necessary for the manifestation of schizophrenic behavior. For instance, while some monozygotic twins are concordant for schizophrenia, others are not. This implies that environmental factors in some way modify or interact with the individual's inherited biological makeup. Liberman and colleagues[26] cite the *stress-diathesis* model of schizophrenia, which relates the occurrence of symptoms to the relationship between the stress experienced by the individual and an internal stress tolerance threshold.

Similarly, McGlashan[28] describes the *vulnerability-stress* model. Vulnerability is viewed as a developmental process that is relatively stable. It may be genetic to some extent. The role of perinatal factors is also being considered. Stressors can cause symptoms in a vulnerable person. Coping mechanisms act to decrease vulnerability. The following general areas of vulnerability have been described:

1. Difficulty processing complex information, focusing attention, discriminating relevant versus irrelevant stimuli, and thinking abstractly
2. Psychophysiological disruptions including decreased sensory inhibition and impaired autonomic response, especially to aversive stimuli
3. Decreased social competence reflected by difficulty processing interpersonal messages, poor eye contact, lack of assertiveness, and limited conversational skills
4. Deficits in coping skills such as inability to correctly assess threats, underestimating coping abilities, or overuse of denial[28]

Figure 17-2 demonstrates the relationship between stress, vulnerability, personal strengths, and environmental supports and the occurrence of schizophrenia.

■ **PSYCHOLOGICAL STRESSORS.** Many psychological theories have been advocated as causes of disturbances in the ability to establish and maintain satisfying relationships. Psychologically, it is known that high anxiety levels result in an impaired ability to relate to others. As has been described in the chapter on anxiety, the level of anxiety experienced determines the degree of difficulty that may occur. Prolonged and/or extremely intense anxiety, together with a limited ability to cope, is believed to be the cause of relationship difficulties of psychotic proportions. This theory will be further explored from the psychoanalytical and interpersonal points of view.

Psychoanalytical theory states that schizophrenic behavior results when the ego can no longer withstand the pressures emanating from the id and from external reality. The ego of the psychotic person has limited ability to cope with stress because of serious deficiencies in the symbiotic mother-child relationship that inhibited psychological development. The initial response to high levels of stress and anxiety is to employ ego defense mechanisms pathologically in an effort to control unacceptable impulses and thoughts. An example of this is the development of paranoid delusions, a pathological manifestation of the mechanism of projection. So much libido (psychic energy) is invested in the maintenance of repression that there is little left to invest in the performance of activities of daily living. Therefore the person withdraws from usual activities and has difficulty maintaining basic physiological needs such as nutrition and hygiene. If stress continues and the anxiety level is unabated, ego functioning may deteriorate further. The person then has difficulty maintaining repression and may be flooded with frightening and primitive thoughts and impulses. There is also difficulty differentiating self from environment as ego identity disintegrates. Communication at this point is confused, garbled, and highly symbolic, reflecting primary process thought, which is usually kept unconscious. There is little capacity for relatedness with others.

Will states the interpersonal view of schizophrenia as, "the expression of complicated patterns of behavior adopted by the organism in an effort to deal with a gross inadequacy in relating to other humans."[49] Will further states that the behavior is a response to stress, demonstrates a disordered personality structure, involves communication, and provides some degree of security and comfort.

The mother-infant relationship sets the stage for later behavioral problems. The mother's extreme anxiety is communicated empathically to her child. Confusing and conflicting messages are received from significant others before the child has developed enough skill in communication to clarify meanings. There is lack of a feeling of continuity in the relationship with significant others, leading to incorporation of behavior that seems to be unacceptable into the "not-me" component of the self-system. This results in a distorted view of reality. Anxious family members teach the child a distorted perception of the culture. Fear of people also develops, which inhibits learning and restricts the use of consensual validation. Adolescence brings many anxiety-provoking experiences related to the need to develop a

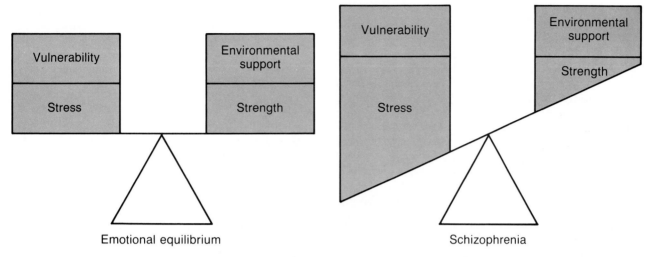

Fig. 17-2. Vulnerability-stress model of schizophrenia.

firm sense of identity. Normal developmental experiences lead to extreme anxiety and loneliness. The person is then trapped in a conflict between a longing for intimacy and a fear of the loss of the limited human contact he has.[49]

Masterson[29] has described the process of development of the borderline personality disorder as rooted in the mother-child relationship. The mother, who frequently is borderline herself, resists signs of independence and autonomy in the child. If the child tries to individuate, the mother withdraws from him emotionally. This creates a conflict for the child who, on the one hand, wants to grow in autonomy, but on the other, fears losing his mother's love. In most cases, the child suppresses his individuality and clings to his mother. In later life, the borderline person relates to others in a hostile, dependent, or manipulative way. The dilemma of dependence versus independence continues to be reflected in his interpersonal relationships.

Stressors that may lead to impairments in interpersonal relationships have been discussed. The interplay among these factors leads to the behavior that the nurse observes while relating to an individual, family, or group. It is essential to consider each of these areas when performing a thorough nursing assessment.

■ **Behaviors**

The behaviors that are observed in response to disruptions in relatedness are representative of the individual's attempt to cope with the anxiety arising from the feeling of loneliness and the related feelings of fear, anger, shame, guilt, and insecurity. Frequently occurring behaviors include impaired communication, withdrawal, suspicion, dependency, and manipulation.

■ **ASSOCIATED WITH SCHIZOPHRENIA**

Schizophrenia, paranoid type. Disruptions in communication accompanied by withdrawal and suspicion are evident in the thought process and interaction patterns of patients who have the medical diagnosis of schizophrenia, paranoid type.[1] Clinical example 17-1 illustrates this disruption.

From the description of Mr. D's hospitalization experience, it is apparent how disrupted communication can interfere with the ability to function. Mr. D was placed in an impossible communication situation by his parents when forced to choose between them. The timing of this family upheaval could well have been related to Mr. D's recent improvement and his move toward more independent behavior by entering the vocational rehabilitation program. If the family equilibrium depended on Mr. D's being the symptom bearer, the pressure from his parents was that he should continue in his role. Their perception of the reason for Mr. D's becoming upset further supports this hypothesis. They attributed his problem to the vocational rehabilitation plan, which was moving him away from the family, and not their argument, which essentially pulled him back.

Mr. D, in his distress, most likely experienced ambivalent feelings toward his parents. He was very dependent on them so feared angering them and risking rejection. At the same time, he became very angry because of the demands they made on him but was blocked in expressing his anger by his need for them. He was able to resolve this problem only by withdrawing and, at an unconscious level, by relying on repression, regression, and projection to handle the unacceptable impulses aroused by the conflict situation.

Mr. D is a 24-year-old single man who was admitted for the third time to the psychiatric unit of an acute general hospital. His diagnosis was chronic schizophrenia, paranoid type. His other admissions had been at ages 19 and 22 and had each lasted a month. His outpatient treatment since the last admission had consisted of individual supportive therapy provided by the clinical nurse specialist, chemotherapy, and family therapy provided by the social worker. He had also been referred to the vocational rehabilitation counselor and was about to start a job training program.

Mr. D was brought to the hospital by his parents. They expressed great disappointment in his readmission because they had hoped that he was "finally going to lick this thing." They thought that the recurrence of his psychotic behavior was probably related to his impending involvement in the job training program. They could identify no other recent stressors that might have upset him.

Mr. D's nurse therapist, Ms. T, evaluated his condition soon after his admission to the hospital. He appeared frightened and was curled up in a chair when she approached him. He did not look at her when she greeted him and seemed preoccupied with his own thoughts. Ms. T was not sure that he was aware she was there. She sat down a few feet away from him and again stated his name. He looked at her blankly for a brief moment, said, "hello," and then went back to staring into space. When asked what brought him to the hospital, he replied, "My father's car." Ms. T observed that Mr. D seemed rather upset and asked if something was bothering him. He told her nothing could bother him because God had told him that he was invincible. He knew many people were jealous of his powers and were trying to destroy him, but he had special protection. He then showed her a rabbit's foot that was sent to him by God to protect him from "evil forces." As Ms. T reached out to touch the rabbit's foot, Mr. D pulled it away and shouted angrily, "Don't touch that! It's mine! They want you to take it away to destroy my powers, but I won't let you!" Ms. T assured Mr. D that she would not take away his rabbit's foot, since it had great importance to him. He gradually relaxed. She asked if he could say more about the contact he thought he had had with God. He replied that God had spoken to him and told him about the evil forces. He knew these forces existed because they put bad thoughts in his head. He also heard people talking about him and commenting on his behavior. There were several voices, and he thought he recognized the voices of his father

and Dr. M, who saw him once a month to evaluate his medications. He denied any visual hallucinations. His speech was disjointed and at times difficult to follow because of loose associations. For instance, he said, "Mother brought me here . . . birth . . . rebirth . . . deliverance . . . didn't like that movie." As Ms. T attempted to explore his feelings about his parents' returning him to the hospital, he turned away and angrily told her to leave him alone because she was "one of them, those g ____ d ____ f ____ liars." Ms. T responded that she would continue to work with him to help him regain control of his life while he was in the hospital. However, she added that she could see he was tired and upset so she would leave and see him again later.

For his first 3 days in the hospital, Mr. D continued to be hostile, refusing to eat or drink and not sleeping except when under the influence of medication, which he took reluctantly when presented with the clear alternative of state hospital commitment. The content of his speech revolved around the messages he received from God and the evil forces who were trying to destroy him. He would tolerate only brief interactions with his therapist and other staff members. He did not interact at all with other patients, whom he believed to be staff members and "undercover agents" who were supposed to report on his behavior. He totally refused to see his parents, consistently referring to his mother as "That b ____."

With the assistance of consistent interpersonal support and medication, Mr. D gradually began to gain control over his thoughts. There was a steady decline in the amount of delusional speech, and although the auditory hallucinations continued, he was able to ignore them or block them out by talking with someone. He revealed to Ms. T that he became upset after his parents had a violent argument and threatened to divorce each other. They pulled him into their conflict by demanding to know with whom he would choose to live and he was unable to respond to that demand except by becoming psychotic. He was disappointed that he had missed the beginning of his job training program and was hopeful that he would still be able to start vocational rehabilitation soon. Ms. T gently helped Mr. D to look at his feelings toward his parents and also informed the family therapist of the events preceding his admission. His discharge plan was for referral to a day treatment program for a short stay until the vocational rehabilitation referral was again available. Individual therapy, pharmacotherapy, and family therapy were all to continue.

■ **HALLUCINATIONS.** Hallucinations, such as Mr. D's experiences of hearing God and of hearing people talk about him, frequently occur in schizophrenic patients. A hallucination is a sensory perception that takes place without external stimuli. The biochemical theorists suspect that hallucinatory experiences result from a metabolic response to stress that results in the release of hallucinogenic neurochemicals, such as bufotenine and DMT. Psychoanalytical theorists view hallucinations as an attempt by the ego to defend against alien impulses that have been repressed but are threatening to enter awareness. The mechanism of projection allows the ego to deal with the impulses as threats from the outside, thus alleviating some of the anxiety. Stated in the framework of interpersonal psychiatry, the hallucination is the autonomous expression of a specific zone of interaction, usually auditory, which symbolically represents the dissociated processes of the person's personality.[31] These dissociated experiences are included in the "not-me" component of the personality, which includes those experiences arousing such great anxiety that they were not integrated into awareness within the self-system. When the self-system is flooded with anxiety, as it is during an acute schizophrenic episode, the usual security operations are not adequate. The dissociated thoughts that come into awareness are then dealt with by means of projecting them as the verbalizations of others.[31]

■ **DELUSIONS.** Both psychodynamic theories relate hallucinatory experiences to efforts to alleviate panic levels of anxiety and both identify projection as the mechanism that is used to accomplish this goal. Delusions may be explained in a similar way. A delusion is a fixed false belief. Some delusions are suspicious in nature, or **paranoid,** such as Mr. D's belief that evil forces wanted to destroy him. In this instance, unacceptable (ego-alien) aggressive impulses are projected outside the individual and perceived as being directed toward him. Paranoid delusions may also include a sexual component if the ego defense is directed toward sexual impulses. For instance, a woman who believes that the man next door wants to break into her house and rape her may be projecting her own unconscious sexual feelings for him. Paranoid delusions with homosexual content also occur with schizophrenic patients. This indicates a defense against an onslaught of homosexual impulses that are very frightening to the patient. If the patient is confronted with unavoidable close contact with a member of the same sex, homosexual panic can occur. When this happens, the patient enters a panic state with lack of impulse control and frequently very aggressive behavior.

Other delusions are **grandiose** in nature. Mr. D's belief that God had singled him out and given him special powers was a grandiose delusion. Grandiosity occurs in schizophrenic patients but is particularly marked in patients with a diagnosis of manic episode; bipolar disorder, mixed; or bipolar disorder, manic. Delusions of grandeur may endow the person with a special power or talent or may identify him with a famous or powerful person, such as God, a political leader, or a sports hero. This is an example of the pathological use of the mechanism of identification. It usually reflects a low self-esteem and a poorly formed ego identity. In this case increased anxiety brings about a sense of powerlessness. Identification with a powerful entity such as God allows the ego to acquire some of the power that is lacking within the personality structure. It is also a means of dealing with extreme fear. People with grandiose delusions may feel invincible and involve themselves in dangerous situations. It is important to keep in mind that the identification process takes place at an unconscious level and that the patient really believes he is God or the president of the United States.

Somatic delusions focus on the body and usually include the conviction that the person is the victim of a frightening disease. The person may believe that he is becoming incapacitated or that parts of his body are dead or rotting away. A variation of the somatic delusion is the belief that all or part of the body is distorted or misshapen. An attractive young male patient with this type of delusion refused to turn on the light when he used the bathroom because he feared what he might see in the mirror. Bizarre somatic delusions are associated with schizophrenia. Delusions of fatal or debilitating illness are frequently associated with depression, as are **delusions of poverty.** The person is convinced that he is penniless and is responsible for the downfall of his family. This is a reflection of a pervasive sense of guilt and low self-esteem. These patients may make remarks such as "Everything I touch turns to ashes."

The nature of delusional thinking is such that it defies conventional logic. Its function is a protective one in helping the person cope with anxiety that would otherwise be overwhelming.

Schizophrenia, catatonic type. Clinical example 17-2, in contrast with that of Mr. D, deals with Ms. W, who is psychotically withdrawn and has a medical diagnosis of schizophrenia, catatonic type.[1]

Ms. W was a rigid, inhibited young woman who had built her personal security around her relationship to her parents, assuming the role of a perfect daughter. Any threat to that relationship threatened the foundation of her security as well, giving rise to extreme anx-

---

CLINICAL EXAMPLE 17-2

Ms. W is a 26-year-old single childless woman who lives with her parents. She was brought by ambulance to the emergency room of a large university hospital and referred to the psychiatric service for evaluation. The evaluator, a psychiatric nurse, observed Ms. W immobile, lying propped up in a hospital bed. She was totally mute and kept her eyes fixed straight ahead. She did not move voluntarily, and when moved by the examiner, offered some resistance. However, when she had been moved, she would maintain the new position. For instance, the nurse raised Ms. W's right arm 6 inches above the bed. When she let go of the arm, the patient did not move it for 5 minutes, at which time the nurse moved it back to a resting position on the bed.

Ms. W had been accompanied to the hospital by her parents, who gave the following history. Mr. and Mrs. W had been married for 20 years before their daughter was born and they had despaired of ever having a child. They had lavished her with anything she wanted and had also set high standards for her behavior. She had always been a well-behaved child, rarely requiring punishment by her parents. In fact, she was very sensitive to criticism and would burst into tears at a harsh word. She had had few friends, sharing the family feeling that most other people did not have their high standards for behavior. She was particularly uncomfortable around young men, although she spoke of wanting to marry someday. She had attended an exclusive women's college, majoring in biology. At the time of her hospitalization, she was working as a research assistant in a cancer research laboratory. She was responsible for the care of laboratory rats being used for a study of suspected carcinogenic agents. She was a steady worker and apparently had performed adequately on the job, since she had recently received a merit raise.

About a month prior to admission Ms. W had mentioned that a new laboratory assistant had been hired. This was a young man who began asking her to have lunch with him. She had told her parents that she mistrusted his motives, and she started to find reasons not to eat lunch. The quality of her work began to deteriorate. She attempted to avoid this man at work, but he persisted in his attentions and the day before admission asked her out to dinner and a movie the following weekend. She refused. That evening she seemed preoccupied and spent the evening reading. Her parents noticed that she rarely turned a page. The next morning she did not get up when called for work. When her parents entered her room, they found her much as she was on admission, immobile and mute. They tried all day to arouse her but finally called their family physician, who advised them to take her to the emergency room.

iety. This dependency on her parents interfered with Ms. W's ability to develop an adult level of relatedness. She was unable to establish intimacy with anyone outside her own family circle. Intellectually, she was aware of this problem and had rationalized that she owed a great deal to her aging parents and should repay them by continuing to share her life with them. She therefore placed plans for marriage and a family far into the future. The intrapsychic conflict between her wish for closeness and her wish not to displease her parents by leaving them created a large amount of anger, which was not compatible with her self-concept of the dutiful and obedient daughter. She defended against the anxiety this aroused by using repression and reaction formation. However, when an attractive young man began to exhibit interest in her, her usual defenses crumbled and she was overwhelmed by anxiety and primitive anger. She then resorted to extreme withdrawal as a way of controlling her frightening feelings. At an unconscious level she feared that any voluntary movement whatsoever would lead to uncontrolled eruption of all her feelings, which she viewed as exceedingly destructive. Her behavior therefore was self-protective.

Ms. W's behavior is characteristic of a conflict that Burnham, Gladstone, and Gibson have termed the **need-fear dilemma**.[7] She is strongly drawn toward wanting intimacy and dependency on others (the need), but is ambivalent because she also fears being engulfed and losing her own identity. This is an example of the approach-avoidance type of conflict described in Chapter 12. This dilemma is one of the most common characteristics of most types of schizophrenia.

Many theorists have attempted to identify patterns of behavior that would be diagnostic of schizophrenia. However, these efforts have been confounded by the identification of a variety of types of schizophrenia. In the Draft of the DSM-III-R in Development,[1] the American Psychiatric Association has divided schizophrenia into the following types: paranoid, catatonic, disorganized, undifferentiated, and residual. Further description of the characteristics of each of these categories, as well as of schizophrenia in general, is included in the nursing diagnosis section of this chapter.

The behaviors that have been described as criteria for the medical diagnosis of schizophrenia have evolved over the course of many years and will continue to evolve as more is learned about this syndrome. Because of this evolutionary process, nurses will hear discussions of other classifications of behavior. Some with historical or current significance include Bleuler's primary (the four A's) and secondary symptoms of schizophrenia, Schneider's first- and second-rank symptoms, and the diagnostic criteria developed by the International Pilot Study of Schizophrenia.

■ **BLEULER'S FOUR A's.** The first effort to identify a group of behaviors typical of schizophrenia was that of Eugen Bleuler, who also renamed the disorder which was once known as "dementia praecox." Bleuler identified primary and secondary symptoms of schizophrenia. Primary symptoms, frequently called the four As, include an *a*ffective disturbance, disordered *a*ssociation of thought, *a*utism, and *a*mbivalence.[25]

Affect. One disturbance in affect is a "blunting" or shallowness of affective expression, demonstrated by minimal change in facial expression and a monotonous tone of voice. Hostility may be expressed if the patient feels threatened. This may be directly or symbolically expressed and may seem out of proportion to the situation. Some patients use cursing or obscene language as a means of expressing hostile feelings. Another affective disturbance is the expression of affect inappropriate to the subject being discussed. For instance, a patient describing her impulse to murder her children begins to giggle.

Associations. Associations between thoughts are often disrupted in schizophrenic patients. Sometimes **blocking of thoughts** occurs. In this case the patient begins to speak but then stops and loses track of the meaning of the statement. **Looseness of association** is revealed when the patient makes a statement that sounds jumbled, such as in the following example:

NURSE: **How can we improve your nursing care, Mr. J?**
MR. J: **Improve? Can't improve. Can't prove a thing. Got me in this jail, but can't prove anything.**

Mr. J seems to drift away from the topic, but reveals that he views the hospital as a jail and suspects he is there because he has been accused of something. It is up to the nurse at this point to explore further the meaning of his statement. This loosely connected speech is frequently highly symbolical. Although the patient's own speech may be highly symbolical, he tends to interpret the speech of others very literally. An example follows:

NURSE: **How are you feeling, Mr. J?**
MR. J: **(Touches various parts of his body) I guess I feel OK.**

This is often referred to as **concrete** thought and speech. Speech may also be lacking in goal direction, as in **tangential speech** when the person begins to respond to a question but follows with a series of related topics, never really getting to the point of the original statement. **Circumstantial speech** is an instance in which the person does get to the point but only after adding many unnecessary details to the response. **Perseveration** is a pattern of speech in which the person repeats the same word or phrase over and over again. The word or phrase chosen may have symbolical significance to the patient. There are other speech patterns in which it is more difficult to grasp the patient's meaning. Sometimes patients respond by rhyming, which is called **clang association.** A patient might say, "Play ball, call, fall, tall, etc." Another disrupted attempt at communication is **echolalia,** in which the patient repeats whatever he hears. The following is an example of echolalia:

NURSE: **How are you today, Mr. J?**
MR. J: **How are you today, Mr. J?**

A related behavior is **echopraxia,** in which the patient mimics the body position of another person. In **word salad** the patient expresses a random jumble of words, apparently aimless and meaningless.

Autism. Autism refers to a preoccupation with the self and with inner experience. The person may withdraw from any voluntary contact with others and seem to go inside a shell. Speech is highly personalized and may include **neologisms,** which are made-up words understood only by the patient. Some patients create and populate whole imaginary worlds. An example of this is Yr, created by Debbie in *I Never Promised You a Rose Garden.* As Debbie became more involved in the real world, she found that she had to give up Yr and its people. Nonverbal behaviors associated with autism include rocking, head banging, stroking or fondling the self, and sometimes curling up in a fetal position.

Ambivalence. Ambivalence results in difficulty with decision making. Schizophrenics may debate endlessly about the alternatives in a situation that requires making a choice. They may also have strong simultaneous positive and negative feelings about a situation, which can be confusing and frightening. This may be reflected particularly in their response to significant others, who may be loved and hated with equal intensity at the same time.

Functions of symptoms. All these behaviors are reflective of the degree of disruption of ego function being experienced by the patient. Problems of affect demonstrate compromised ability of the ego to inhibit impulses unless the control is absolute, resulting in no expression of feeling. Problems in association indicate the intrusion of primary process thinking from the id, which results in much use of symbolism and in difficulty in maintaining a logical thought sequence. Autism reveals a disturbance of ego boundaries with decreased ability to distinguish between reality and fantasy and need to identify the self in concrete ways, by touching and feeling. It also represents an effort to decrease stim-

TABLE 17-1

BEHAVIORS CHARACTERISTIC OF SCHIZOPHRENIA ACCORDING TO BLEULER, SCHNEIDER, AND THE IPSS

Bleuler[25]	Schneider[24]	IPSS[2]
Primary behaviors Affective disturbance Ambivalence Autism Disordered thought association **Secondary behaviors** Delusions Hallucinations Negativism Stupor	**First-rank behaviors** Auditory hallucinations commenting on behavior Belief that actions are controlled or influenced from outside Belief that one's thoughts are controlled Belief that one's thoughts can spread to others Delusions Hearing thoughts spoken aloud **Second-rank behaviors** Depression Emotional blunting Euphoria Other hallucinations Perplexity	Bizarre delusions Hearing thoughts spoken aloud Incoherent speech Nihilistic delusions No depressed facies No early waking No elation Poor insight Poor rapport Restricted affect Unreliable information given Widespread delusions

uli by withdrawing into the self. Ambivalence represents an inability to use secondary process thought for logical decision-making purposes. It also indicates confusion and fear about strong conflicting feelings, which may give rise to frightening impulses.

In a relationship context this complex of behaviors may serve a protective function. The schizophrenic person has difficulty controlling impulsive behavior. This is easier when others are not around. He also has trouble differentiating himself from others and may not be sure where he ends and the other person begins. He is usually not able to trust others and becomes frightened that he will be harmed in some way when others are around. Communication patterns that are hard to understand and sometimes threatening in content tend to drive people away. The inherent problem in this for the ambivalent schizophrenic is that he feels less threatened with people at a distance but abandoned if they get too far away.

Bleuler also listed secondary symptoms of schizophrenia that he considered to be less specific to the condition and less essential for making the diagnosis. They include such behaviors as delusions, hallucinations, stupor, and negativism.[25]

■ **SCHNEIDER'S FIRST AND SECOND RANK SYMPTOMS.** Another description of behaviors typical of schizophrenia has been developed by Kurt Schneider. He has divided them into first- and second-rank symp-

toms. Schneiderian first-rank symptoms include hearing one's thoughts spoken aloud, auditory hallucinations commenting on one's behavior, somatic hallucinations, the belief that one's thoughts are controlled, the belief that one's thoughts can be spread to others, delusions, and outside control or influence of one's actions.[24]

Second-rank symptoms include other hallucinations, depression, euphoria, perplexity, and emotional blunting.[24] Schneider has emphasized that none of the behaviors he has identified are absolutely indicative of schizophrenia but that the presence of a number of them in the absence of any other identifiable pathological condition makes the diagnosis of schizophrenia probable. The clinical and family history must also be considered. It seems unlikely that specific behavioral criteria for schizophrenia will be developed until more is understood about the stressors that cause this disruption in behavior.

■ **INTERNATIONAL PILOT STUDY OF SCHIZOPHRENIA.** The International Pilot Study of Schizophrenia (IPSS) was initiated by the World Health Organization[50,51] as an effort to obtain new knowledge about the epidemiology of schizophrenia. The countries involved included Denmark, India, Colombia, Nigeria, England, the Soviet Union, Taiwan, the United States, and Czechoslovakia. A major problem in the crosscultural interpretation of epidemiological studies has been doubt as to whether diagnosticians in various settings have used the same diagnostic criteria. For instance, schizophrenia is diagnosed far more frequently in the United States than it is in Great Britain. Therefore one of the major objectives of the IPSS was to develop and standardize diagnostic criteria that could be used in all nine countries participating in the study and have as high a degree of reliability and validity as possible. Bartko[2] reports a twelve-point diagnostic system that was derived from the work of the IPSS. The twelve signs and symptoms include restricted affect, poor insight, hearing one's thoughts spoken aloud, absence of early waking, poor rapport, lack of depressed facies, lack of elation, widespread delusions, incoherent speech, unreliable information given, bizarre delusions, and nihilistic delusions. Carpenter[9] points out that use of a diagnostic system such as that presented by Bartko does not preclude the necessity for the clinician to learn to know the patient as a person. Knowledge of strengths, as well as symptoms, is essential for the clinician to be of assistance to the person who seeks therapy. Table 17-1 summarizes the criteria cited by Bartko in comparison with those of Bleuler and Schneider.

The IPSS[50,51] represents a major step forward in the epidemiological study of mental illnesses. The study included a 2-year follow-up of the patients who were included in the initial study population. A high percentage of patients were interviewed a second time, providing valuable information about the course of the illness in the nine cultures. One most interesting conclusion was that subjects who live in developing nations seemed to fare better than those from the more highly developed societies. This study has laid the foundation for future important epidemiological studies.

Some investigators are looking for other ways to differentiate and possibly identify subtypes of schizophrenia. Pfohl and Andreasen[33] have noted a trend toward differentiation on the basis of positive and negative symptoms. Positive symptoms are characterized by abnormal or excessive mental functioning, such as hallucinations, delusions, or agitation. Negative symptoms reflect a deficit or absence of function, such as lack of energy, poverty of speech, lack of affect, and decreased socialization. Pfohl and Andreasen describe positive symptom schizophrenics as having "a relatively acute onset, a course marked by exacerbations and remissions, good premorbid functioning and reasonably intact social functioning."[33] They also have a normal brain structure, normal cognition, and respond well to neuroleptics. This type of schizophrenia may be related to an increased dopamine level. In contrast, negative symptom schizophrenics have "an insidious onset, a history of poor premorbid functioning, and a chronic or deteriorating course."[33] There is evidence of cognitive im-

pairment, more frequently enlarged ventricles, and less response to neuroleptics. It is suspected that this constellation of behaviors could be related to a decrease in dopamine. Clearly, research linking brain structure, neurochemical functioning, and behavior will play an important role in identifying and classifying the various types and manifestations of schizophrenia.

■ **ASSOCIATED WITH SUSPICION.** Schizophrenia is a severe mental disorder. Many people experience disruptions in interpersonal relationships that are less severe. Sometimes these disruptions are characterized by suspiciousness. A suspicious person is exhibiting a problem with the ability to trust. This may derive from the earliest life experiences as related to the basic sense of trust described by Erikson or may be the result of disruptive experiences later in life, as will be demonstrated in Clinical example 17-3.

Mr. J is a person who has become suspicious primarily in response to sociocultural and environmental stressors. His own personal experience of being mugged and the reinforcement he receives from the television news lead him to believe that he lives in a basically hostile environment. Most of his suspiciousness is probably also based on reality. The nurse, of course, will validate as much of the information he gave as possible so that her assessment will be accurate. Mr. J's feelings of vulnerability are probably also related to the frailty associated with aging, which was reinforced by his recent experience of illness and hospitalization. His suspiciousness is functional for him in that it protects him from the dangers in his environment and reduces the anxiety arising from his feeling of vulnerability. It is not functional insofar as it is extending to his children, who probably could be more supportive if they knew he was in need and could possibly persuade him that they wanted him to live with one of them because they cared for him and his safety. His possession of a gun is also potentially harmful to him, since a young intruder could probably overpower Mr. J and would be more likely to harm him if he were armed.

Many people in this society, young and elderly, are isolated from others and know little of their neighbors. Isolation from others can lead to fear and misunderstanding, resulting in an attitude of suspicion. It is obvious how this can develop into a vicious circle, thus leading to a major social problem.

Suspiciousness may be considered in terms of a continuum from completely trusting to completely distrusting. Of course, most people fall somewhere between the extremes. Behavior at either extreme can be problematical. Complete naiveté can result in others taking advantage of the individual. Such people are usually described as gullible and are ineffectual in influencing

CLINICAL EXAMPLE 17-3

Mr. J is an 80-year-old man who lives by himself in the ghetto of a large city. He was referred to a community health nurse following a 2-week hospitalization. He was admitted to the hospital after being arrested for "intoxication" when he was found unconscious on the street. Fortunately, he was taken to a hospital where they discovered that he was comatose because of diabetic acidosis. An attempt was made to refer Mr. J to a nursing home, but he vehemently insisted on returning to his own home. The purpose of the community health nursing referral was to evaluate his ability to cope at home and to assess his ability to manage his American Dietetic Association diet and oral hypoglycemic medication.

Ms. B, the community health nurse, made her first visit the day following Mr. J's discharge from the hospital. When she knocked at his door, there was a long pause and then a feeble voice asked who was there. When she identified herself, the door opened a crack and Mr. J peeked out at her. He said he recognized her blue uniform and would let her in his apartment. There was another pause punctuated with the sound of several locks being undone. At last Ms. B was face-to-face with a withered old man. His apartment was sparsely furnished but neat. The one comfortable chair faced a battered black and white television set. The shades at the window were drawn, leaving most of the room in shadows. A brief inspection of the kitchen revealed sparsely stocked cupboards. There was no evidence of insects or rats. A scrawny cat rubbed against the nurse's leg. Mr. J introduced him as "Tiger."

Ms. B sat down to talk with Mr. J and learn more about his perception of his condition. He knew about his diabetes and seemed to understand his diet but doubted that he could comply with it. He said that he usually ate sweet rolls and coffee for breakfast, soup for lunch, and cereal with milk for dinner. He shopped at a small corner grocery store and bought only what he could carry home. Meats were expensive and he had little money left for food after he paid his rent and utility bills. He was also hesitant to go out very often because he had been knocked down and robbed earlier in the year.

Mr. J said he had lived in the neighborhood many years and stayed there because of his memories of happier times. However, he thought the area had gone downhill. Most of his friends had died or moved away. His children lived in the suburbs, and were "too busy" to see him often, although they had asked at times for him to live with them. He doubted their motives, saying that he thought they probably wanted control of his Social Security checks, his only income.

Ms. B asked if he knew about the senior citizens center two blocks away where they served a hot meal daily and had many activities. He said he had heard about it but had no desire to socialize with the people who went there, since the others in the neighborhood were "not his kind." He also suspected that they would not serve foods that he liked. He again expressed his feelings about the lack of safety in the neighborhood and said that was the reason for his many locks. He watched the news on television every day and there were always stories about thefts and muggings of elderly people. He then confided that he also kept a gun near his bed so if "they" came in at night he would be able to defend himself.

Ms. B spent a little more time on diabetic teaching, trying to help Mr. J find ways to manage his diet within his real social and economic limitations. She planned eventually to introduce the idea of "Meals on Wheels" but realized that she needed to gain his trust first. As she left, she promised to return in 2 days to see how he was doing. Mr. J's response was, "That's up to you. I don't know why you should bother. Nothing will change much."

others. Extreme suspiciousness, on the other hand, results in behavior that is usually described as paranoid and is of psychotic proportions. The paranoid person uses the mechanism of projection to attribute his own unacceptable impulses to other real or imaginary people and feels that he is being persecuted.

■ **ASSOCIATED WITH DEPENDENCY.** Behaviors of withdrawal and suspiciousness alleviate anxiety by decreasing interpersonal contacts. Sometimes people who have disrupted intimate relationships deal with their anxiety by behaving in an excessively dependent way. This type of behavior is demonstrated by Clinical example 17-4 of a patient with a medical diagnosis of dependent personality disorder and panic disorder.[1]

Ms. R later discussed Ms. J with the nursing staff. She explained that the patient was a very dependent woman who had for many years lived vicariously through her family, especially her daughter. When her daughter married, Ms. J felt abandoned but could not express her feelings directly. Her dependent style of

CLINICAL EXAMPLE 17-4

Ms. R, the psychiatric liaison nurse, was called to see Ms. J, a patient on the medical service of a general hospital. Ms. J had been admitted to the hospital complaining of attacks of dizziness, tremulousness, dyspnea, and diaphoresis. She stated the fear that she was "losing her mind." The nurses on the medical unit had called Ms. R because, although the medical workup was almost completed and the results were entirely negative, the patient continued to complain of the same symptoms. The nurses were frustrated because Ms. J was constantly asking to have her bed adjusted, her water refreshed, her bedroom slippers found, and similar requests. In addition, she would have attacks of panic with hyperventilation during which she needed close nursing observation and help rebreathing into a paper bag to prevent loss of consciousness. Through careful nursing observation, the nurses were able to identify that the panic attacks occurred most frequently during visits from family members and often when her demands of the hospital staff were not complied with readily. The nurses were also aware that their frustration with Ms. J's constant demands and lack of response to their nursing intervention was interfering with their ability to give her good nursing care.

When Ms. R interviewed Ms. J, she observed that the patient lay curled on the bed and spoke in a soft, barely audible tone. She teared frequently during the conversation. She spoke readily of her past when questioned but quickly refocused the discussion to her present complaints. Ms. J revealed that she was 45 years old, married, and the mother of a daughter, age 23. She said that she felt very close to her daughter who had married and moved away from home 3 months ago. The attacks began

soon after she left. Her daughter now lived about a mile from Ms. J and was described as devoted to her mother. Mr. J was employed as a pharmacist and was required to work some evenings. Ms. J said she had not minded this until her daughter had left home. She then began to find the evenings that her husband worked to be difficult because she felt lonely and did not want to bother her daughter with visits or phone calls. She said that her family was her whole life. Ms. R asked Ms. J about other interests that she might have. She said that her main diversion was watching television, although she also read a few magazines and did a little sewing. She enjoyed cooking for others but not herself, and usually did not eat when her husband was working. She was on speaking terms with her neighbors but not really friendly with them. Because of her husband's objections, she had never worked outside of the home.

As she spoke with the nurse, Ms. J began to appear more and more anxious. She became tremulous and started to breathe rapidly. Ms. R helped her to rebreathe and comforted her by talking soothingly and patting her on the shoulder. After Ms. J seemed calmer, Ms. R asked if she thought her behavior was related to the topics that they had been discussing. Ms. J said that she could see no connection and stated that her symptoms were real to her, not just in her head, which was what people kept telling her. Ms. R assured her that she could see that she was indeed uncomfortable but that very nervous people sometimes showed their nervousness in physical ways. Soon after this Ms. R had to leave. As she left the room, Ms. J asked her if she would be back.

relating blocked her from assertively reaching out for other activities to gratify her need for relatedness. Her frustration and loneliness caused anxiety. Her coping response took the form of a physiological conversion. This behavior was reinforced when she received a great deal of attention focused on her illness. Thus her hospitalization was providing her with not only the primary psychological gain of knowing that her symptoms were being explored and treated but also the secondary gain of the renewed attention and consideration from her family. Her symptoms were not conscious behaviors on her part but were her response to her anxiety. Therefore she could not understand why people kept suggesting

that there was really no physical basis for her illness. Any increase in her anxiety level, then, caused an increase in her symptoms and in her dependent behavior. Ms. J needed help with this problem because, although people were initially sympathetic to her need for dependency gratification, they would soon become frustrated with her, as is demonstrated by the response of the nursing staff.

■ **ASSOCIATED WITH MANIPULATION.** The disruptions in relatedness discussed so far have involved either too much distance from other people or the need for too much closeness to others. Another disruption in relatedness focuses on individuals who are superfi-

CLINICAL EXAMPLE 17-5

Mr. Y is a 20-year-old single man who was committed to an inpatient psychiatric unit by a judge for a psychiatric evaluation. He had been charged with sale of illicit drugs, statutory rape of his 15-year-old pregnant girl friend, and contributing to the delinquency of a minor. He had been arrested on the grounds of a junior high school where he was selling PCP and barbiturates to a group of young teenagers.

In jail, Mr. Y had been observed to be "crazy" by the guards. He paced his cell, chanted, and threw his food on the floor. On the basis of this behavior, the judge was requested to order a psychiatric evaluation and did so. On arrival at the psychiatric unit, Mr. Y continued to behave in the same manner. However, his behavior did not seem typical of psychosis. There was no evidence of hallucinations or disorders of thought or affect. When unaware that he was observed, Mr. Y seemed relaxed and was noted at one time to be conversing with another patient. By the day after admission he seemed to be free of his symptomatic behavior. At this point the staff began to describe him as a "nice guy." He complimented female staff members and behaved toward them in a pleasantly seductive manner. He was deferential to the physicians and readily agreed to abide by all the rules. He was helpful with other patients. In group meetings he admitted that he had behaved badly in the past and described how he had been led astray by his friends. He said he became involved in drugs because he wanted to be "one of the gang" and he "needed the bread" so he "had to" start selling drugs. By the end of his first week in the hospital he had elicited the sympathy of all the other patients and of the staff. However, an interview with his parents revealed that he had had a stormy adolescence, including arrests for vandalism and expulsion from school at age 14 for drug use and fighting. They said he had become involved with friends who were a bad influence. His family was glad he was getting help, because they had always known he was "sick."

Nine days after admission, following visiting hours, it was noted that Mr. Y and two other patients looked lethargic. Their speech was slurred, and their gaits were ataxic. The nursing staff immediately collected urine and blood specimens for toxicological analysis. The unit was searched for hidden drugs, but none were found. The results of the toxicology screening tests, however, were positive for barbiturates. Suspicion was immediately focused on Mr. Y, since the other patients involved were young adolescents with no history of drug abuse. When confronted, he seemed amazed that he could be suspected and pointed out his past behavior as a model patient. He acknowledged that he had behaved strangely and said he had wondered if someone had "slipped" him some drugs. He was convincing but was warned that if he was seen to be involved in any way with drugs, he would be sent directly back to jail.

As part of the evaluation, the social worker had been working with Mr. Y's pregnant girl friend. As the girl began to trust the social worker, she confided that she was not sure that Mr. Y had fathered her child, since she had had to turn to prostitution to help support them. Mr. Y, who had been unemployed for a year, had been angry when told of her pregnancy because it meant a reduction in his income, and he had pressured her to have an abortion. She had refused because she hoped it was his baby and that he would decide to marry her once he saw the child. However, when she told him that her decision to have the baby was final, he assaulted her and then told her he did not want to see her again.

Mr. Y began to pressure the physicians for their decision on his ability to be held responsible for his actions. He seemed to be actively engaged in therapy and promised to continue with outpatient treatment if recommended for probation. He also convinced his family of his good intentions and they agreed to allow him to move into their house. On the basis of these indications of positive behavioral change, Mr. Y did receive a recommendation for probation, which was carried out by the judge.

Three months after discharge from the hospital Mr. Y and a friend were arrested for operating a PCP-manufacturing lab in the friend's garage.

cially involved with others. These are people who use manipulative behaviors, treating others as objects. The patient who demonstrates this in Clinical example 17-5 has a history of multiple drug abuse and a medical diagnosis of antisocial personality.[1]

The manipulative person presents a particularly difficult nursing problem. There is frequently little motivation for change because, as is demonstrated in the case of Mr. Y, manipulative behavior has inherent rewards to the individual with antisocial personality dis-

CLINICAL EXAMPLE 17-6

Ms. S is a 23-year-old woman who was admitted to an acute psychiatric unit in a general hospital following three episodes of superficially lacerating her wrists within the week prior to admission. Each time, she had telephoned her therapist, a psychiatric clinical nurse specialist, immediately following the self-mutilating behavior. Because her therapist was about to leave for a month's vacation, she decided to arrange to have Ms. S hospitalized.

Upon admission, Ms. S appeared mildly depressed and gave the impression of a guilty child who had been chastised by a parent. She denied any current self-destructive ideation. During the physical examination, it was noted that there were numerous scars on her body. When asked about these, she claimed to have been abused as a child. The records of the referring therapist described the scars as the result of many instances of self-mutilation, beginning at the age of 16. In fact, this had been the main reason for her seeking therapy. There was also a history of sexual promiscuity. She had been arrested 2 years earlier for possession of cocaine. She described herself as a failure, stating that she had "the best parents in the world, but they did not get the daughter they deserve." She said she was a drifter, who had never been able to settle on a career, a lifestyle, or any consistent friends. She didn't know who or what she was. When asked how she felt, she responded, "Most of the time, I don't feel anything, just empty." There were no signs of psychosis.

Ms. S was placed on constant observation, in order to prevent further cutting. All sharp objects were removed from her room. Initially, she was very cooperative with the rules of the milieu and superficially friendly to the other patients. Because of her uneventful adjustment, the constant observation was discontinued after 3 days. She was also presented with a schedule of activities and informed that she was responsible for following it. The next day, an Exacto knife was missing from the activities therapy room. When a search was initiated, Ms. S was found in the bathroom, bleeding from several small cuts on her ankles. This sequence was repeated several times. Each time the constant observation was discontinued, the patient would find a sharp object and cut herself. She was also observed to be very labile emotionally. In particular, she had unpredictable outbursts of anger, which were similar to temper tantrums. However, these outbursts passed as quickly as they came, never lasting more than several minutes. In addition, she began to categorize the staff as "good guys and bad guys." When she was around staff members she liked, she was generally pleasant, complimenting them on their kind and understanding attitudes toward her. With the staff she disliked, she was sullen and uncooperative, comparing them unfavorably to the other staff members. Eventually, the staff began to bicker about her care, some believing she was spoiled and others that she was neglected. When her parents visited, they participated in the staff splitting by complaining about the staff that Ms. S disliked and bringing small gifts to those she liked.

Ms. S remained in the hospital for the whole month of her therapist's absence. When she returned, the patient initially refused to see her and the frequency of angry outbursts increased dramatically. However, following regular and frequent visits from her therapist, she began to request discharge. Behavioral criteria for discharge were set, including at least a week of no self-mutilation and no temper tantrums. She met the criteria and was discharged back to outpatient treatment.

---

order. It helps him accomplish a desired goal. The manipulator is goal oriented or self oriented, not other oriented. However, this person is skilled at giving the impression of involvement with others and may be charming to gain the confidence of the other. Mr. Y was able to gain the confidence of the staff and knew that he needed to do so to have the support he needed in court. Another prominent characteristic of the antisocial personality is an absence of awareness of the lack of relatedness to others and the assumption that all interpersonal relationships are opportunistic in nature.

This person cannot imagine an intimate, sharing relationship because he assumes that if he does not maintain control, the other person will take advantage of or control him. Shostrom[39] sees this issue of controlling or being controlled as central to manipulative behavior. He adds that these same issues are primary in actualizing behavior, but the actualizer expresses manipulative behavior creatively, whereas the manipulator is self-defeating.

Individuals with the medical diagnosis of borderline personality disorder[1] are also frequently perceived as manipulative. This type of disruption in interpersonal relatedness is illustrated by Clinical example 17-6.

The manipulation of the borderline patient results from an arrest in psychosocial development leading to an inability to participate in mature interpersonal relationships. Ms. S demonstrates this problem when she describes herself as a drifter and when she divides the staff into good and bad. Gunderson[17] describes the behaviors characteristic of the borderline personality as follows:

1. Interpersonal relationships are intense and unstable at the same time. Interpersonal behavior is characterized by devaluation, manipulation, dependency, and masochism.
2. Manipulative suicide attempts are designed to ensure rescue by significant others.
3. Intolerance of aloneness related to failure to develop a sense of object constancy and fear of abandonment result from an unstable sense of self.
4. Negative affects, including anger, sustained dysphoria, and depression, reflecting a basic sense of "badness."
5. Occasional ego-dystonic psychotic experiences, characterized by paranoia, regression, and dissociation.
6. Impulsivity with episodic substance abuse and promiscuity.
7. A history of low achievement.[17]

Masterson[29] also notes the failure of the borderline person to achieve object constancy during the separation-individuation stage of psychosocial development. Because of this the person relates to others as parts, rather than wholes. When the other person fails to meet the borderline's needs, the relationship is likely to end. In addition, the borderline person cannot evoke the image of a significant other who is absent and is not able to mourn the loss of another person. For individuals who fail to complete separation from the mother and the development of autonomy there is often a recapitulation of this developmental crisis at adolescence. Behaviors characteristic of this phase include clinging; depression accompanied by rage and defended by acting out or neurotic behavior; and detachment and withdrawal.

Many of these behaviors can be seen in the description of Ms. S's hospitalization. Because of their tendency to be manipulative and their inability to become involved in reciprocal interpersonal relationships, these patients are frustrating for nursing staff. It must be remembered that their behavior is not consciously planned, but is an attempt to defend against a pervasive fear of existential loneliness.

The major behaviors representative of disruptions in relatedness have been presented. Individual patients frequently experience combinations of these behaviors and the nurse must be able to identify the complex spectrum of behavior that any person may exhibit when confronted with high levels of stress and anxiety. In some cases a usual mode of behavior, such as manipulation, may be exaggerated or combined with a change in behavior. For instance, a manipulative person may withdraw when confronted by his manipulations and may be rejected by those he has been trying to manipulate. In other instances the behavior that appears in response to stress may be different from the individual's usual style of relatedness. A person who is usually gregarious may withdraw when under great stress. It is helpful to include in the nursing assessment a description of the patient's usual interpersonal relationships to provide a baseline of normal behavior for that individual. This helps to avoid measuring the patient's progress against the nurse's rather than the patient's norm.

■ **Coping mechanisms**

The behaviors associated with disruptions in relatedness are in themselves attempts to cope with the anxiety that is associated with threatened or actual existential loneliness. Unfortunately, as demonstrated by the case studies presented in this chapter, these attempts to cope may lead to a marginal adjustment and may, at times, serve to drive people even farther away. Thus the person is always caught in the approach-avoidance conflict of the need-fear dilemma, seeking some degree of human contact on the one hand and pushing people away on the other.

The dependent person copes by clutching others and refusing to let go, inviting rejection when others feel smothered by clinging behavior. This person has no faith at all in his ability to rely on himself. Dependent behavior is often reciprocal with the dominant behavior of a partner. Reaction formation may be a coping mechanism that is used to avoid confrontation of the anger that results from feeling unable to become involved in self-actualizing activities. The withdrawn person craves interpersonal contact but fears rejection even more. Retreat into a shell is protective but is also a deprivation and therefore not rewarding. Extremely withdrawn people are using the mechanism of regression. Suspicious people keep others at arm's length by refusing to believe that they are to be trusted. This is frequently a defense against confronting the lack of a more basic trust in the self. Such a confrontation would result in intolerable anxiety and ego disintegration. Projection is the coping mechanism underlying suspicious behavior.

Manipulative people view other people as inanimate objects. Their defenses protect them from potential psychological pain related to the loss of a significant other. Reid[34] has described the defenses used by the individual with antisocial personality disorder as projection and splitting. Projection allows the person to deny responsibility for negative consequences of his antisocial behavior. For instance, a patient may excuse his use of drugs by saying, "Everybody I know uses heroin. Why shouldn't I?" Splitting is characteristic of individuals with borderline personality disorder as well. Gunderson[17] defines this as the inability to synthesize the good and bad aspects of oneself and of objects. In this case, an object is anything outside of the self, animate or inanimate, to which the person has an attachment. An object could be a parent, a friend, or a teddy bear. Gunderson describes Kernberg's formulation of the manifestations of splitting. These are:

1. Alternately expressing opposite sides of a conflict while appearing unconcerned about the contradiction
2. Inconsistent lack of impulse control with periodic expression of primitive impulses that do not cause anxiety at the time
3. Dividing external objects into those that are "all good" and those that are "all bad"
4. Vacillation between "all good" and "all bad" perceptions of others[17]

Masterson adds several other defense mechanisms which are characteristic of individuals with borderline personality disorder. These include "acting out, reaction formation, obsessive-compulsive mechanisms, projection, isolation, detachment and withdrawal of affect." Yet another set of coping mechanisms related to the borderline personality have been identified by Danziger.[11] In addition to splitting, she includes the following:

1. Denial of responsibility for acting out behavior and of painful or threatening feelings
2. Devaluation of another which makes the borderline person appear good by contrast
3. Projective identification in which the individual criticizes his own shortcomings in another
4. Idealization of positive traits of others, which when combined with identification results in good feelings[11]

Although there are several approaches to defining the defensive structure of the borderline patient, all of the defenses reflect the person's severe difficulty separating

himself from others and participating in authentic relationships.

People with schizophrenia rely on coping mechanisms that tend to be primitive and sometimes only marginally effective in controlling their interpersonal anxiety. Searles[38] has delineated several aspects of schizophrenic communication that are used as coping mechanisms.

The first mechanism described by Searles is displacement. This results in the direction of the communication toward an object that is not the real stimulus for the response. There may also be a temporal discrepancy between the conscious and unconscious objects. For example, a patient who is angry at the nurse may talk about a past quarrel with a close friend. Searles[38] relates this to the person's poor differentiation of "perceptual-conceptual" experience, which leads him to perceive similar objects as identical.

Projection is a mechanism discussed earlier as it relates to the development of paranoid delusions and auditory hallucinations. Aside from projective verbalizations, schizophrenic patients frequently also project meaning to the nonverbal communication of others, which reflects the meaning attached to the person's own nonverbal behavior. Projection can reveal a great deal about a person's world view and about which aspects of existence are difficult for him to handle.

Another coping mechanism used by schizophrenic patients is introjection. Searles believes that this mechanism is at the root of the patient's feeling he is controlled or influenced by others. The behavior and even sometimes the unconscious impulses of the other person are experienced by the patient as his own and reflected in his behavior. For instance, the patient may act out an unconscious wish of a significant other person that is transmitted nonverbally.

Condensation entails the concentration of several thoughts and feelings into a relatively simple verbal or nonverbal message. This may be expressed as a repetitive statement or gesture, which may assume a variety of meanings, as if the person has very limited resources of communication. Searles believes that this is related to a lack of differentiation of concrete figurative meanings. For example, a statement that seems to be clear and straightforward may also be highly complex and symbolical.[38] The patient may be unaware of the hidden meanings, and the nurse may need supervisory help to interpret the communication.

Patients may unconsciously protect themselves from experiencing overwhelming emotion by means of isolation. Much of this may be related to ambivalent feelings and helps the individual cope with the anxiety aroused by these conflicting feelings.[38]

As can be seen from this discussion, many coping mechanisms may be reflected in impaired communication patterns. Behavior that is symptomatic of a high level of anxiety may also be reflective of the person's attempt to cope with the anxiety. The nurse must understand this complex interrelationship between anxiety, coping, and observable behavior to plan appropriate nursing interventions.

 Nursing diagnosis

When diagnosing a disruption in an individual's relatedness, the nurse should take into account the degree of disruption experienced by the patient, the behaviors that demonstrate the presence of the disruption, and the predisposing factors and the precipitating stressors that are leading to the disruption. Generally, there are multiple patient problems that must be considered when one is planning nursing care; so the diagnosis should be thorough and should reflect depth in understanding the patient's life situation. The nurse may formulate a nursing diagnosis by using the model of health-illness phenomena (Fig. 17-3) as a guide. When usual coping mechanisms fail, the patient will exhibit behaviors related to a personality disorder or to a psychosis. The category of behavior is not directly related to its severity. A person with a first episode of a psychosis who receives adequate psychopharmacological and interpersonal intervention may be less disabled than someone who has a severe personality disorder. However, accurate observation of behavior and data analysis will ensure that appropriate nursing intervention may be initiated promptly.

A complete nursing diagnosis includes the statement of the nursing problem, the identified stressor related to that problem and the observed behavioral response. It is preferable to validate the essential features of the diagnosis with the patient, if he is able to participate in a discussion of his condition. If the patient is too suspicious or withdrawn to participate actively, significant others may be involved, unless it is determined that it is in the patient's best interest to minimize their involvement in decisions about his life. An example of the latter situation is that of the borderline patient who has not accomplished the developmental task of separation-individuation. Even if the patient refuses to participate in treatment planning, it is not a good idea to confuse him about the boundary between him and his parents by asking them to participate in his stead. Primary NANDA nursing diagnoses and examples of complete nursing diagnoses related to disruptions in relatedness are presented in the box above. Persons with

---

Nursing Diagnoses Related to Disruptions in Relatedness

Primary NANDA nursing diagnoses
Coping, ineffective: individual
Social isolation
Thought processes, alteration in

Examples of complete nursing diagnoses
Ineffective individual coping related to lack of trust in others evidenced by refusal to take medicine
Ineffective individual coping related to lack of confidence in decision-making ability evidenced by referring all questions to husband
Social isolation related to inadequate interpersonal skills evidenced by inappropriate sexual advances
Social isolation related to inability to accept shortcomings in others evidenced by excessive criticism of friends
Alteration in thought processes related to projection of aggressive impulses evidenced by delusion that the communists are looking for him
Alteration in thought processes related to physiologic changes evidenced by neologisms and dissociated speech

---

serious mental disorders frequently have other health problems. Although only those nursing diagnoses that are frequently related to interpersonal problems are presented here, the nurse is responsible for identifying and documenting all relevant nursing diagnoses for each patient. Table 17-2 identifies nursing and medical diagnoses related to disorders leading to disruptions in relatedness.

■ Related medical diagnoses

The major categories of medical diagnosis that relate to disruptions in relatedness are schizophrenia and several of the personality disorders. There are general criteria for the diagnosis of schizophrenia (see the box on page 539). Subtypes of schizophrenia are further defined in terms of the essential features that differentiate one from the other.

■ **SCHIZOPHRENIA, PARANOID TYPE.** The essential features include preoccupation with systematized delusions or auditory hallucinations. There is no evidence of incoherence, loose associations, affective disturbances, catatonia or gross disorganization.[1]

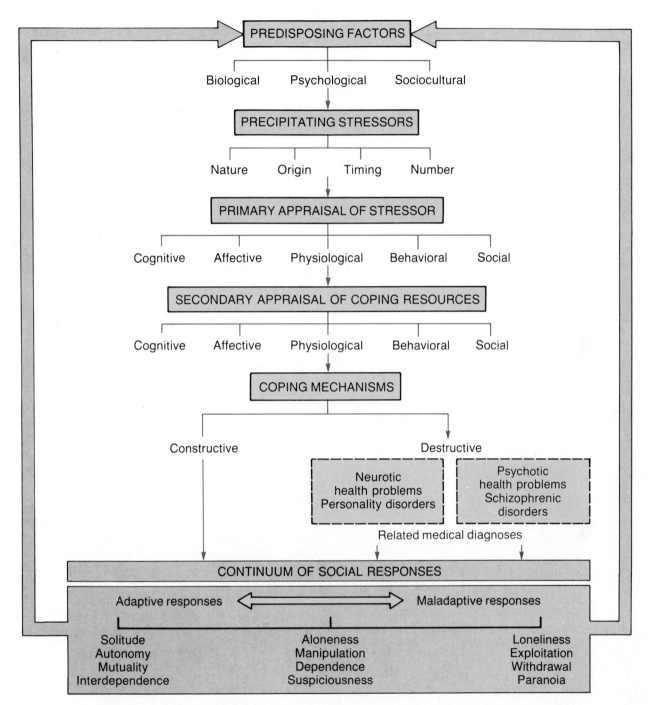

Fig. 17-3. Nursing model of health-illness phenomena related to interpersonal relationships.

TABLE 17-2

MEDICAL AND NURSING DIAGNOSES RELATED TO DISRUPTIONS IN RELATEDNESS

Medical Diagnostic Class
Schizophrenic disorders
Personality disorders

Related Medical Diagnoses (DSM-III-R)*

Schizophrenia
   Paranoid type
   Catatonic type
   Disorganized type
   Undifferentiated type
   Residual type
Personality disorders
   Paranoid
   Schizoid
   Schizotypal
   Antisocial
   Borderline
   Dependent

Psychiatric Nursing Diagnostic Class
Disruptions in relatedness

Related Nursing Diagnoses (NANDA)

Anxiety
Communication, impaired: verbal
Coping, ineffective: family
[†]Coping, ineffective: individual
Family process, alteration in
Impaired adjustment ·
Impaired social interaction
Self-care deficit
Self-concept, disturbance in ·
Sensory-perceptual alteration
[†]Social isolation
[†]Thought processes, alteration in

*American Psychiatric Association: Draft of the DSM-III-R in Development (subject to change), as proposed by the Work Group to Revise DSM-III. American Psychiatric Association, October 1985.
[†]Indicates primary nursing diagnosis for disruption in relatedness.

■ **SCHIZOPHRENIA, CATATONIC TYPE**

The clinical picture is dominated by any of the following:
1. Catatonic stupor or mutism
2. Catatonic negativism (resistance to all instructions or attempts to be moved)
3. Catatonic rigidity
4. Catatonic excitement
5. Catatonic posturing (voluntary assumption of inappropriate or bizarre posture)[1]

■ **SCHIZOPHRENIA, DISORGANIZED TYPE.** The essential features include incoherence and flat or inappropriate affect.[1]

■ **SCHIZOPHRENIA, UNDIFFERENTIATED TYPE.** The essential features include delusions, hallucinations, incoherence or grossly disorganized behavior.[1]

■ **SCHIZOPHRENIA, RESIDUAL TYPE.** The essential features include the presence of residual symptoms as described in the accompanying box without evidence of delusions, hallucinations, incoherence or gross disorganization.[1]

■ **GENERAL CHARACTERISTICS OF PERSONALITY DISORDERS.** Personality disorders are defined by Hirschfeld as "mental disorders in which personality traits are inflexible and maladaptive and cause either significant impairment in social or occupational functioning, or cause subjective distress." Personality is composed of temperament, which comprises the inherited aspects, and character, which is learned. In general, the distinguishing characteristics of the personality disorders are that they are chronic and long standing; a basic dysfunction which is not imposed on a basically sound structure; hard to change; and ego-syntonic.

Siever and Klar[40] have sorted the personality disorders into clusters, based on the predominant characterological feature. These clusters are

1. Odd: schizoid, schizotypal, and paranoid
2. Dramatic: borderline, antisocial, histrionic, and narcissistic
3. Anxious: avoidant, dependent, compulsive, and passive-aggressive.

The schizoid, schizotypal, paranoid, borderline, antisocial, and dependent types will be described by the Draft of the DSM-III-R in Development[1] diagnostic criteria.

■ **SCHIZOID PERSONALITY DISORDER.** The essential features include social detachment and restricted expression of emotions. Specific symptoms may include

General Criteria for the Diagnosis of Schizophrenia

A. Either 1, 2, or 3 for at least 2 weeks:
  1. Two of the following:
    a. delusions
    b. prominent hallucinations (throughout the day for several days or several times a week for several weeks and each hallucinatory experience is not limited to a few brief moments)
    c. incoherence or marked loosening of associations
    d. catatonic behavior
    e. flat or grossly inappropriate affect
  2. Bizarre delusions (i.e., involving a mechanism that the individual's subculture does not acknowledge as existing, such as thought broadcasting or mind control)
  3. Prominent auditory hallucinations (as defined in 1b. above) of a voice with content having no apparent relation to depression or elation, or a voice keeping up a running commentary on the individual's behavior or thoughts, or two or more voices conversing with each other
B. During the course of the illness, functioning in such areas as work, social relations, and self-care is significantly below the highest level achieved prior to the illness (or with onset in childhood or adolescence, failure to achieve expected level of social development).
C. Major depressive or manic syndrome, if present during the active phase of the illness (symptoms in A), was brief relative to the duration of the illness.
D. Continuous signs of the illness for at least 6 months. The 6-month period must include an active phase of at least 2 weeks during which there were psychotic symptoms characteristic of Schizophrenia, with or without a prodromal or residual phase, as defined below.
  Prodromal phase: A clear deterioration in functioning before the active phase of the illness, not due to a disturbance in mood or to a Psychoactive Substance Use Disorder, and involving at least two of the symptoms noted below
  Residual phase: Following the active phase of the illness, persistence of at least two of the symptoms noted below, not due to a disturbance in mood or to a Psychoactive Substance Use Disorder

Prodromal and residual symptoms

1. Marked social isolation or withdrawal
2. Marked impairment in role functioning as wage-earner, student, or homemaker
3. Markedly peculiar behavior (e.g., collecting garbage, talking to self in public, or hoarding food)
4. Marked impairment in personal hygiene and grooming
5. Blunted, flat, or inappropriate affect
6. Digressive, vague, overelaborate, or circumstantial speech, or poverty of speech or poverty of content of speech
7. Odd or bizarre ideation, or magical thinking (e.g., superstitiousness, clairvoyance, telepathy, sixth sense, others can feel my feelings), overvalued ideas, ideas of reference
8. Unusual perceptual experiences (e.g., recurrent illusions, sensing the presence of a force or person not actually present)
9. Apathy or lack of initiative
  Examples: Six months of prodromal symptoms with 2 weeks of symptoms from A; no prodromal symptoms with 6 months of symptoms from A; no prodromal symptoms with 2 weeks of symptoms from A and 6 months of residual symptoms.
E. Not due to any Organic Mental Disorder
F. If a history of Autistic Disorder, the additional diagnosis of Schizophrenia is made only if prominent delusions or hallucinations are also present.

From American Psychiatric Association: Draft of the DSM-III-R in Development (subject to change), as proposed by the Work Group to Revise DSM-III. American Psychiatric Association, October 1985. Used with permission.

lack of close relationships, aloofness, indifference, little interest in sexual experiences, denial of experiencing anger, and lack of interest in others' responses or feelings.[1]

■ **SCHIZOTYPAL PERSONALITY DISORDER.** The essential features include relationship deficits combined with peculiar ideation, affect, and behavior.[1]

■ **PARANOID PERSONALITY DISORDER.** The essential features include an unwarranted tendency to interpret the actions of people and events as threatening. Typical behaviors may include suspicion of the actions or motivations of others, holding grudges, and sensitivity to perceived slights.[1]

■ **BORDERLINE PERSONALITY DISORDER.** The essential features include instability of mood, interpersonal relationships and self-image. Characteristic behaviors may include unstable relationships, exploitation of others, impulsive behavior, labile affect, problems expressing anger appropriately, self-destructive behavior, and identity disturbances.[1]

■ **ANTISOCIAL PERSONALITY DISORDER.** The essential features include current age at least 18 and evidence of conduct disorder before that age. Conduct disorders are characterized by truancy, school behavior problems, arrests, running away, lying, substance abuse, and general disregard for rules. After age18, characteristic behaviors include a poor work record, disregard for social norms, aggressiveness, financial irresponsibility, impulsiveness, lying, recklessness, and inability to maintain close relationships or to meet responsibilities for significant others.[1]

■ **DEPENDENT PERSONALITY DISORDER.** The essential features include dependent and submissive behavior.

❧ Planning and implementation

■ Goal setting

■ **MUTUALITY.** It can be difficult to set mutual goals with a patient in the area of relatedness. This is in part because mutuality must be based on a strong nurse-patient relationship, and it is, of course, difficult to develop a strong relationship with a patient who has problems establishing intimacy. In addition, the setting of a goal implies a commitment to change. Many patients who have disruptions in human relationships are reluctant to commit themselves to change. Since most of these behavioral disruptions are also serving as coping mechanisms, there is additional resistance to change.

For these reasons, even though it is desirable to have the patient's full participation in goal setting, it may be necessary for the nurse to set initial goals. This must be done with consideration to all the data collected

in the nursing assessment and should be based on the nursing diagnosis. Environmental constraints also need to be considered, especially since to overcome a problem with relatedness, the person must be involved with others. At first, the other person may be the nurse, but eventually the behaviors learned in the nurse-patient relationships should be transferred to other interpersonal relationships.

■ **LONG- AND SHORT-TERM GOALS.** Long-term goals should be directed toward alleviation of the patient's particular problem with relatedness. For instance, a goal for a withdrawn patient might be to inquire about the activities of other family members. For a suspicious patient, it might be to initiate a new relationship with a co-worker. A goal for a dependent person could be to join a new social activity group in an area of interest, such as a sport or a craft and attend regularly. A long-term goal for a manipulative patient might be to spontaneously ask about the welfare of another person. For a person who exhibits impaired communication, a goal might be to use logical and coherent speech when relating to others. Each of these long-term goals must be approached by a series of short-term goals. For instance, the long-term goal for the dependent person to join an activity group might be broken down as follows:

1. After 1 week of contact with the nurse the patient will attend an activity group accompanied by the nurse and observe the group meeting.
2. After observing two group sessions with the nurse the patient will participate in one simple individual activity within the group setting.
3. After two individual activity sessions the patient will attend the group session with the nurse and participate in an activity with one other group member.
4. After two sessions of participating in an activity with one other member the patient will attend with the nurse and join in an activity involving the whole group.
5. After two sessions of whole-group activity the patient will attend the group accompanied by another member and join in whole-group activity.
6. After two sessions accompanied by another member the patient will attend the group alone and participate fully in activities.
7. The patient will join a new social activity group in an area of interest and attend regularly (original long-term goal).

This kind of stepwise progression gradually exposes the patient to more complex interactions and decreases the involvement of the nurse. The timing may require modification depending on the patient's response, but a time sequence should be included to stimulate progress.

■ **REALISTIC EXPECTATIONS.** Goals that are developed with patients who have impaired relationships may take a long time to accomplish. These patients frequently use bizarre communication patterns to avoid intimate relationships, so are usually reluctant to take the risk of communicating more directly. However, it is still possible to develop goals directed toward modification in disrupted communication patterns. Grosicki and Harmonson[16] demonstrate this in their nursing action guide for dealing with hallucinating patients. The long-term goals they developed focus on involvement in satisfying interpersonal relationships and on learning more effective methods of coping with anxiety. The short-term goals focus on relating first to an individual and later to groups and on verbalizing the occurrence and content of the hallucination. Goals with these patients may also focus on the modification of specific communication patterns. For example, the patient will use nonverbal communication that is congruent with the verbal content of his speech. Another example of a goal for a patient with impaired communication is "The patient will verbally identify angry feelings when they occur during a one-to-one interaction." These goals need to be developed with the active participation of the patient and must be congruent with his ability to tolerate anxiety, since learning to relate more directly and openly is an anxiety-provoking experience. Increasing the anxiety level before the patient has increased coping ability and environmental supports may only reinforce his use of dysfunctional coping behaviors.

■ **Intervening in withdrawal**

The interpersonal relationship between the nurse and the patient is central to the practice of psychiatric nursing. In the case of a patient who has a disruption in the area of relatedness, it is even more complicated than it is with other patients to establish and maintain a therapeutic relationship. The disrupted behavior will also be experienced in the context of the therapeutic nursing relationship. The nurse therefore has the additional challenge of establishing a relationship with a patient who already has problems relating to others. It takes a great deal of sensitivity and self-awareness to do this successfully. Kahn[20] has described the therapeutic approach to the schizophrenic patient as characterized by "non-intrusive availability, compassionate limit setting, establishment of realistic expectations, and self-care."

One of the most frustrating, but also one of the most potentially rewarding, experiences for the psychiatric nurse is that of intervening therapeutically with a withdrawn patient, particularly one who is psychotic. Withdrawn patients do not often respond quickly to nursing intervention. They usually need consistent, repeated approaches by the nurse to convince them of sincere concern.

■ **MEETING BIOLOGICAL NEEDS.** The extremely withdrawn patient may be mute and immobile, challenging the nurse's ingenuity in giving nursing care that attends to all the biological, psychological, and social needs. In her classic article on the nursing care of the withdrawn patient, Will[48] cites three general focuses for nursing intervention. These include the fulfillment of the patient's needs, the facilitation of communication, and the facilitation of social participation. Frequently the highest priority must first be given to the fulfillment of biological needs. Food and fluid intake must be carefully monitored to maintain adequate nutrition and hydration. If the patient is relatively immobile, intravenous or gavage feeding may be necessary. This should be explained to the patient in terms of the need to maintain his health, as opposed to it being seen as a punitive measure. It is equally important to record urinary output and frequency of defecation. Urinary retention with bladder distention and fecal impaction are complications that can be avoided by good nursing care. If the patient refuses to move voluntarily, positioning and skin care are other nursing concerns. Even if the patient will respond to direction from the nurse, reminders to attend to personal hygiene will probably be required. Although withdrawn people may appear indifferent to others, it must be remembered that this apparent lack of concern is probably a defense. Even people who seem completely oblivious to their surroundings are likely to be aware of everything that happens. Frequently a patient who has recovered from a state of catatonic stupor is able to describe in detail conversations and events that occurred during the stupor. Empathy can help the nurse to understand how the patient may feel about being fed, bathed, and dressed. These activities are best carried out in a matter-of-fact way and with the attitude conveyed that the nurse is sensitive to the patient's needs and feelings. Patients who do not perform self-care should still be given the opportunity to do so by being instructed to perform simple tasks. The patient who is being bathed can be given a soaped washcloth and asked to wash himself. In this way the nurse may assess the patient's progress. As the patient can perform one task, another should be introduced, with the nurse developing a hierarchy of successively more complex tasks for the patient to master with the ultimate goal of achieving maximum possible responsibility for meeting his own biological needs.

■ **VERBAL COMMUNICATION.** Communicating with the withdrawn patient demands great patience on the part of the nurse. It can be uncomfortable to sit in silence with a mute person if one is accustomed to the more usual action-oriented role of the nurse. There may be a temptation to chatter aimlessly, to make trite remarks, or to fidget. As always, the nurse needs to analyze her own response to the situation and be sure that her nursing interventions are goal directed. For instance, if the nurse has assessed the patient's baseline interests and knows that he is a football fan, telling him about a big game can be a way of stimulating his interest in his environment. However, if she tells the patient the details of her date the night before, she is more likely trying to make herself less anxious by filling up the silence. Constant chatter also conveys to the patient the message that there is no expectation for him to verbalize. It is much more therapeutic to make open-ended statements followed by pauses so the patient may respond if he feels inclined to do so. Direct questions may be experienced as intimidating or intrusive by the patient and should be used judiciously. Questions giving a choice should be used only if there is a choice to be made. Asking a patient if he wants his medication when he should definitely take it is not a clear message and should be avoided. Statements should be clear and concise but not infantilizing. Information from the nursing assessment can guide the nurse in selecting language appropriate to the sociocultural background of the patient.

■ **NONVERBAL COMMUNICATION.** Awareness of nonverbal communication is particularly important in interacting with a withdrawn patient. Even a totally silent patient may communicate a great deal through body language and gestures. Feelings may be communicated nonverbally, sometimes more accurately than by verbalization. For instance, a tense person who holds his body rigidly and glares at the nurse may be angry but may not feel able to tell her this. Depressed people often communicate the depth of their despair by a body position that looks tired, droopy, and bent as if to ward off unexpected assaults. Anxiety is communicated nonverbally and may contribute to the nurse's discomfort when interacting with a withdrawn patient.

The withdrawn person may also indicate increased accessibility to others nonverbally. The establishment of eye contact by a person who has usually avoided it may signal the beginning of a relationship. Reaching out or the acceptance of a touch may have the same meaning. Relaxation of a usually tense body posture can be the first sign of increased comfort with the nurse. Other nonverbal signs of decreasing withdrawal include attention to personal appearance and initiation of interpersonal contacts in other activity.

The nurse's own nonverbal activity is also an integral part of the relationship. Many times, gestures and grimaces may be automatic, but they convey a message to the other person. Since the withdrawn patient is usually still very sensitive to events in the environment, the nurse needs to develop an awareness of habitual body language. Feedback from colleagues and supervisors can be helpful in this respect and should be encouraged by the nurse. If videotape is available, it can provide immediate input about nonverbal and verbal communication and can be a helpful tool in supervision. If videotaping is done with a patient, it should, of course, be carefully planned and done only with the patient's informed consent. Role play with other professionals can often be equally useful and eliminate the concern about adversely influencing the therapeutic relationship.

Nonverbal means of communicating can be therapeutic in the nursing care of the withdrawn patient. Looking directly at a patient when greeting him may convey concern. A gentle touch can establish contact with a withdrawn depressed person. Leaning toward a patient but maintaining a comfortable distance screens out other people and transmits the message that the nurse is focusing attention on the patient only. Caring for physiological needs is a powerful means of expressing caring. An attitude of concerned, but not intrusive, interest allows the patient to control the pace of the development of closeness. The process of relating to a withdrawn patient requires much sensitivity of the nurse.

■ **INVOLVING OTHERS WITH THE PATIENT.** The initial intervention with a person who is socially isolated or withdrawn is generally most effective as a one-to-one relationship between the nurse and the patient. However, the ultimate goal is to facilitate the patient's ability to establish healthy interpersonal relationships with a variety of other people to experience a fulfilling life. As the nurse and patient begin to relate more comfortably, others should gradually be included in the patient's social sphere. The nurse can help the patient try to relate to others. Another person can be invited to join a card game or to share in a discussion. In the hospital setting the nurse is often in a good position to introduce the patient to others with whom he might have something in common, since she has knowledge of others in the environment. In the community the nurse can utilize knowledge of community resources and refer the patient to a social group that is likely to be compatible with his needs and interests. As the process of expanding the patient's sphere of relationships is taking place, the nurse must be careful not to give the impression that the goal is to reject the patient. Time for individual interaction should still be scheduled on a regular basis so the therapeutic relationship can continue to grow.

Brown, Cornwell, and Weist[5] describe the ways that the elderly in institutions are depersonalized, leading to their alienation from the social system. These staff behaviors include impersonal communication, such as not using the correct name; material depersonalization, such as not allowing personal objects to be kept; routinization of life activities; and deprivation of protection, exemplified by leaving the windows open in cold weather. In contrast, Carter and Galliano[10] describe a personalizing intervention with a group of elderly nursing home residents who were isolating themselves as a protection from the pain of potential losses.

■ **FAMILY INTERVENTION.** For many patients the family is the focus of much of the interpersonal difficulty. Frequently family therapy is indicated and should be undertaken only by a therapist who is especially trained for this modality. However, the nurse who is working with the patient can assist the family to understand the patient's needs. If the patient does not want to visit with the family, the nurse may help them to maintain the relationship by demonstrating her concern for the family members and by suggesting things they can do for the patient, such as bringing favorite foods or taking care of errands. Sometimes a family needs help in seeing small signs of progress. Often family members have questions about the patient's care. The nurse can be helpful by educating the family about the treatment process. Of course, the patient should be included in this teaching and should be informed about contacts between the nurse and the family.

Nursing intervention with the withdrawn patient should be directed toward the accomplishment of reasonable goals. A shy person should not be expected to become a gregarious one. Knowledge of the person's usual personality is helpful in setting expectations. However, the patient is the best source of information about goal accomplishment. The individual's comfort or discomfort with his life-style and interpersonal relationships should always be the primary criterion for therapeutic progress.

■ **TERMINATING THE RELATIONSHIP.** Terminating a relationship with a withdrawn patient may be difficult for the nurse. The patient is likely to resist termination from a person to whom he has become close after a time of loneliness and isolation. He may be frightened that he will not be able to maintain the ability to form healthier relationships. New problems are often brought up at termination and usually indicate an attempt to prolong an important relationship. The nurse, too, will have many feelings about terminating with a patient with whom she worked so hard to build a relationship. Even the satisfaction of contributing to the growth of another person cannot erase the pain of severing the relationship. However, the experience of a well-handled termination can be the culmination of the therapeutic relationship by helping the patient learn to deal with a loss in a healthy, mature way.

■ Intervening in suspiciousness

■ **FOSTERING TRUST.** Nursing interventions with a suspicious patient are in many respects similar to those with the withdrawn patient. The primary long-term goal with the suspicious patient is that the patient will demonstrate trust in the nurse. The patient will then, hopefully, also develop the ability to trust others who are deserving of being trusted. People demonstrate trust by making themselves accessible to others, both physically and emotionally. Thus the trusting patient will not evade contact with the nurse and will also share thoughts and feelings with her. This process develops gradually in any relationship but may be particularly slow when the patient has difficulty trusting other people.

Reliability is one factor that helps to foster trust. The nurse must follow through on commitments made to the patient. When working with a suspicious or paranoid patient, the nurse can make a point of informing the patient of when they will be talking and then follow through with the schedule as a means of demonstrating reliability. Very suspicious people may not tolerate prolonged contacts, since this tends to raise the anxiety level as the person tries to defend himself from what he perceives as a potential attack from another person. In this instance the nurse may plan several brief contacts spaced throughout the day, thus also repeatedly reinforcing her reliability.

■ **MEETING BIOLOGICAL NEEDS.** Suspicious patients also at times may have difficulty in maintaining their physiological well-being. Fear may interfere with sleep. A light in the room at night may be helpful. Sleeping medication may be offered, but if the paranoid patient refuses to take it, insistence by the nurse will only increase the insomnia by further agitating the patient. Priority in this case should probably be given to persuading the patient to take prescribed antipsychotic medications, which will usually also cause some drowsiness. Refusal to eat and/or drink may be another problem encountered with the suspicious patient. Attempts to force oral intake usually meet with failure and are frustrating to both nurse and patient. Sometimes a suspicious patient will eat food brought by his family, food he prepares himself, or packaged food. Whenever possible these preferences should be respected. As the patient learns to trust the nurse and the hospital, he will begin to eat and drink. If the patient is in danger from dehydration or malnutrition, the physician may take drastic action and prescribe gavage feeding or intravenous therapy. If this does occur, careful explanations should be given as the treatment takes place. Treatment will be experienced by the patient as an intrusive assault on his physical being, and much supportive nursing care will be required.

■ **PACING THE RELATIONSHIP.** Since suspicious people do fear intrusion from others and question the motives of those who approach them, care must be taken to respect the patient's right to privacy. The patient may appreciate intervals of solitude that can be worked into the daily schedule. Warning should be given of the approach of another person so as to avoid startling the suspicious patient. The patient should be allowed to control the amount of self-revelation that takes place in the interaction with the nurse. A probing approach will only alienate the patient and retard the development of trust. As trust grows, anxiety will decrease and the patient will have less need of his suspicious defenses. The growth of the patient's ability to confide in the nurse is one way to measure the success of nursing intervention with the suspicious patient.

Most people interact with a variety of therapeutic team members, especially in the hospital setting. When the patient has difficulty establishing trust, it is best if one or two people are designated as those who will work consistently and closely with him. However, other staff members should be aware of the treatment plan, and their approach to the patient should be consistent with that of the primary caregivers. Significant others should also be made aware of the care plan and should be encouraged to participate in it. Consistency among those who have close contact with the patient also promotes the development of trust.

■ **TRUSTWORTHINESS OF THE NURSE.** Openness and honesty on the part of the nurse demonstrate to the patient that she can be trusted. For instance, if the nurse plans to meet with the patient's family, she should inform the patient of this plan. She should then discuss the issue of confidentiality of information with both the patient and family. Families of suspicious patients often abound with family secrets, and the nurse should not become involved in this communication pattern. The best way to avoid this problem is to include the patient in family meetings. If the patient refuses to attend or if the family attempts to exclude the patient by telephoning or intercepting the nurse during a visit, it is best to have a plan of action prepared. In most instances the nurse should inform the patient and the family that information shared between the nurse and family members will also be shared with the patient. This approach reinforces the value of openness in communication that is a characteristic of a trusting relationship. Families often try to keep information from the member who is the identified patient to protect him. In reality, the patient usually learns the hidden information and then feels justified in his lack of trust of those who did not include him.

■ **ADMINISTERING MEDICATIONS.** The nurse should also strive to be honest with the patient who asks questions about the plan of care. The patient has a right to participate in the care planning and should know the rationale for any treatment. For example, suspicious persons may believe that others are trying to control their behavior or are trying to do them harm. For either of these reasons, they may be reluctant to take medication. It is important that they have medication because it is usually being given to decrease the severe anxiety that is contributing to the patient's difficulty in trusting others.

Even though the nurse may be aware that a particular patient has been refusing medication, the initial approach to the patient should be confident and convey the expectation that the medication will be taken. A hesitant approach may arouse the patient's suspicion about the procedure. Verbalized directions should be clear and succinct, for example, "Here is your medication, Mr. Jones." If the patient hesitates, this can be followed by "Put it in your mouth and swallow it." Nonverbal communication should reinforce the verbalization. Also, to prevent confusion, the patient should be offered the same form of medication each time. For instance, if the order is for chlorpromazine, 150 mg, the nursing staff should agree to always give one 100 mg and one 50 mg tablet or three 50 mg tablets. If the liquid concentrate form of medication is used, it should be used consistently, and if it is mixed with fruit juice, it should be mixed with the same flavor each time. Attention to these details can save much time and discussion when medications are given. Another potential area of confusion for the patient occurs when the medication dosage is changed. If the patient can comprehend the information or if medication is being given in tablet form, the physician should inform the patient when a dosage change is made.

The nurse who is administering medicine to psychiatric patients should observe the patient's behavior carefully while the medicine is being taken. A suspicious patient may hide tablets or capsules in the cheek or under the tongue, removing these as soon as the nurse looks away. If the nurse suspects this behavior, a mouth check should be initiated. This involves directing the patient to open his mouth and using a tongue depressor to look thoroughly for hidden medication. If possible, a better solution to this problem is to give the medication in liquid form. Occasionally a patient will swallow medication when it is given and then immediately go into the bathroom and induce emesis. If a patient fails to respond to medication as expected, an initial nursing action should be to observe carefully the individual's behavior following medication administration. It may be necessary to provide one-to-one observation for the patient until enough time has passed for the medicine to be absorbed.

Sometimes patients absolutely refuse to take any medication by mouth. The nurse should never try to trick the patient to take medicine by putting it in food or fluids. Discovery of this by the patient will destroy any trust that he has in the staff and give his suspicions a basis in objective reality. In addition, the patient may then also refuse to eat or drink because of the possibility that medicine is concealed, thus compounding nursing care problems and jeopardizing his nutrition and hydration. For the suspicious patient, there should be a clear separation between medication and food.

Patients who adamantly refuse oral medications may at times need to be given an injection. This requires a physician's order. The nurse should also be aware of the laws in her area concerning the patient's right to refuse treatment. Generally, only life-saving treatments may be given without the patient's permission. The patient will sometimes take medication by mouth if given the alternative of "by mouth or by needle." However, the nurse should not become embroiled in a long debate trying to persuade the patient to take oral medicine. If the patient must have the medicine and refuses it by mouth, the injection should be given quickly with as much physical restraint as is necessary for the patient's safety. The procedure should also be carried out with regard for the patient's right to dignity. Injections should be discontinued promptly as soon as the patient accepts oral medication. When they are feeling better, patients rarely object to having been medicated when they were very disturbed.

As with a withdrawn patient, the nurse must help the suspicious person who has learned to trust her to be able to trust others as well. The nurse can help the patient identify behaviors that are characteristic of trusting and trustworthy people. The ultimate goal is for the patient to be able to differentiate trustworthy from untrustworthy people and to experience trust appropriately—not to trust everyone. Thomas[43] has described the trusting person as comfortable with growing self-awareness and able to share this awareness with others, accepting of others without needing to change them, open to new experiences, consistent in words and ac-

tions over time, and able to delay gratification. By sharing these characteristics with the patient, the nurse can teach a more rational basis for deciding who to trust. In addition, discussion of these criteria with reference to the patient will help to identify his progress toward the goal of becoming a trusting person.

■ Intervening in impaired communication

Good communication skills, empathy, and creativity are necessary for providing good nursing care to patients with impaired communication. In addition to the concepts presented here, the relationship principles discussed in Chapter 4 are also applicable. One effect that impaired communication has on interpersonal relationships is to maintain distance between the participants. This can be done by not revealing feelings or by transmitting unclear messages. In either case the receiver is allowed to perceive only a portion of the information that is available to the sender. At other times, inadequate or inaccurate perception and evaluation may interfere with clear communication.

■ **RESPONDING TO SYMBOLISM.** To understand the unclear messages of a schizophrenic patient, the nurse must listen carefully and observe the patient, in addition to being aware of the communication context. Much of the patient's speech may be symbolical. For example, a patient who was feeling pressured by a nurse's persistent efforts to persuade him to accept a visit from his wife remarked, "It sure looks hot outside." This was interpreted to mean that the patient was feeling "hot" (angry) because of the nurse's pressure. The nurse chose not to share the interpretation with the patient, who had difficulty handling anger, but responded to his message by easing the pressure she was placing on him. Interpretation to the patient of the meaning of symbolical communication must be done cautiously. The patient is speaking indirectly for a reason. The symbolism may screen thoughts and feelings that would be difficult to handle if stated directly. The patient is usually not consciously aware of the symbolical meaning of his speech. At best, the response to an ill-considered interpretation could be denial of the correctness of the interpretation. At worst, the patient could lose control of his behavior and enter a panic state because of the anxiety aroused by bringing unconscious material into awareness. The responsible nurse will try not to bring forth behavior that neither she nor the patient can handle.

■ **EXPRESSING FEELINGS.** A supportive approach often works well with patients who exhibit impaired communication. Many of these patients distrust the meaning of words because they have had past experi-

CLINICAL EXAMPLE 17-7

Ms. S was a nursing student who had been relating to Ms. A, a patient in a psychiatric unit, for 6 weeks. The relationship would terminate in 2 more weeks, when Ms. S's clinical experience in psychiatric nursing was to end. Ms. S arrived on time for her appointment with Ms. A and went to their usual meeting place. Ms. A was across the room watching television. Ms. S waited 10 minutes and then approached Ms. A, who agreed to talk with her. Ms. S was aware that she was annoyed because she had been looking forward to talking with Ms. A. She was also aware of the possible effect of the termination process on Ms. A's behavior.

ences with incongruent communications. They are very sensitive to nonverbal behavior and its meanings and immediately perceive whether the nonverbal behavior supports the verbal message. The nurse therefore needs to be self-aware and to use both verbal and nonverbal communication purposefully in the nursing intervention. Openness can be supportive to the patient. Real people become angry, sad, happy, contented, and fearful. The nurse can be a model for the patient of how to acknowledge feelings and, more important, how to express them appropriately. Feelings are part of human relationships. Consider Clinical example 17-7.

Contrast these two possible approaches that Ms. S could choose to take with Ms. A:

EXAMPLE 1

MS. S: **Ms. A, you seemed to be ignoring me.**

MS. A: **I was just interested in my story.**

MS. S: **Well, that's all right. I know your story's important to you—and we just have 2 weeks left.**

MS. A: **Uh-hum. I won't be here much longer myself.**

EXAMPLE 2

MS. S: **It seemed hard for us to get together today.**

MS. A: **I was just interested in my story.**

MS. S: **I know. I was feeling impatient with you because you seemed to be avoiding me. Then I realized that I'll be leaving in 2 weeks. That's really very frustrating to me.**

MS. A: **Every time I get so I can talk to somebody, they leave.**

MS. S: **Sounds like you're frustrated too.**

In the first example Ms. S maintains a you-me focus throughout the interaction sample. She implies her annoyance but does not validate this for Ms. A, who then indirectly expresses her annoyance. Ms. S also gives a double message when she says, "That's all right" and

then clearly indicates why it is not all right, "We just have 2 weeks left." Ms. A is likely to be confused at this point. In the second example Ms. S puts the interaction into an "us" context. She shared her analysis of the reason for her behavior and for the patient's behavior and shared her thoughts with the patient. She expressed her frustration in a nonthreatening way and indicated that she could understand that Ms. A might have similar feelings. She has set the stage for a productive discussion of termination.

Some patients, particularly schizophrenics, take time to reach a level of trust where they can tolerate feelings directed from the nurse toward them. The nurse can, however, model expression of feelings by interacting with other staff members in the presence of the patient and then discussing the situation with the patient. People who are frightened of feelings need to see that they can be verbalized without causing the devastation that the patient may have been fantasizing. When patients do take a risk and make a feeling statement to another person, they need feedback about how the other person was affected. The expression of caring can be even more difficult than anger because caring leaves one vulnerable to rejection. Patients often need to experience socially acceptable ways of giving and receiving both positive and negative feelings.

■ **MANAGING RESISTANCE TO CLOSENESS.** The threat of closeness can result in many behaviors that are indicative of the patient's resistance. Wildman[47] cites such behaviors of the schizophrenic patient as "physical withdrawal, psychological withdrawal, verbal threats or rejections, physical attack, symbolic derogations or gestures" as examples of resistance to closeness. She states that the nurse must be sensitive to the meaning of these communications and direct nursing intervention toward reducing the interpersonal anxiety, thereby reducing the patient's resistance to involvement. This means that the nurse may at times overlook behaviors that would, in another context, be unacceptable. For instance, a patient may use grossly obscene language in an effort to drive the nurse away. Inexperienced nurses may take the patient's remarks personally and respond with indignation or a moralistic lecture. To be successful, the nurse needs to respond at the level of the patient's anxiety and assure him that she will not demand more than he can tolerate. It is also important that the nurse continue to exhibit interest in the patient. If she is driven away, his negative self-concept will be reinforced, as will the antisocial behavior. When the patient has gained some trust in the nurse, feedback can be given about the effect of his behavior on other people, later coupled with the concept that the patient is responsible for his behavior and its consequences.

■ **USING TOUCH.** Because of the schizophrenic patient's fear of closeness, touch should be used judiciously. Touch is a powerful communicative tool. Patients who are sensitive to issues of closeness may experience a casual touch as an invasion or as an invitation to intimacy, which may be even more frightening. Physical contact with a person of the same sex may be experienced by the patient as a homosexual advance and may precipitate a panic reaction. If procedures requiring physical contact must be carried out, careful explanations should be given both before and during the procedure. An efficient impersonal approach to physical nursing care may be least threatening to a patient experiencing interpersonal anxiety.

Touch may also have significance for patients with poorly defined ego boundaries. Sometimes these patients touch other people to identify for themselves their separateness from the other. However, other patients, when touched, find it difficult to be aware of their individuality and experience a sense of fusion with the other. Very regressed patients may seek out cuddling and rocking as if they are trying to recreate the symbiosis of infancy. Some therapists, such as Laing, use this reparenting approach with schizophrenic patients who are severely interpersonally incapacitated. Ego boundaries may also be reinforced by clearly separating self from other in communication. Statements such as "It's time for us to take our bath" are extremely confusing to a patient who does not know where his self ends and the nurse's self begins. The use of "I" and "you" helps the patient clarify this issue.

■ **INTERVENING IN DELUSIONS.** Confusion about ego boundaries is one example of the problem that schizophrenic patients often have with reality orientation. The healthy ego can identify between fantasy and reality most of the time by using logical thinking, comparison with past experience, and consensual validation with other people. When the ego is overwhelmed with anxiety, the ability to reality test is seriously compromised. Another behavior representative of this problem is delusional thinking. The delusional patient is absolutely convinced of the reality of his beliefs even when they are contradicted by logical thought and by the perception of others. Nursing intervention with a delusional patient requires great sensitivity. Communication channels must be kept open while the nurse avoids supporting and reinforcing the delusion. Stripping the patient of his delusion is removing his desperate attempt to defend himself from overwhelming anxiety and could result in an outburst of uncontrolled assaultive behavior. A direct attack on the delusion usually results in an angry response and a feeling of alienation on the part of the patient. An expression of doubt,

tactfully phrased, is generally more acceptable. A patient who expresses fear that gangsters are planning to kill him may be able to accept the response, "You are safe here in the hospital and I would like to help you learn more about what makes you so afraid." This shifts the focus from the imaginary gangsters to the patient's fear, which is real. Consistent acceptance of the patient and supporting the growth of a therapeutic nurse-patient relationship will gradually alleviate the patient's anxiety, allowing him to relinquish his delusions. This is accomplished most easily when there is no loss of face involved. The nurse can help the patient explain the delusion and the purpose it served, saying, for example, "When you first came here you were very frightened and you did not understand what was happening to you. Your idea about the gangsters was a way of explaining your feelings. Now you are beginning to learn more about yourself and you are finding other explanations." Some patients have well-entrenched delusional systems and are not able to give them up. These patients are sometimes able to function well if they can learn not to talk about their delusions except in therapeutic sessions or with significant others who can tolerate such a discussion.

■ **INTERVENING IN HALLUCINATIONS.** Auditory hallucinations are another type of disruption in reality testing. Like delusions, they represent a high level of interpersonal anxiety and a projection of repressed ideation to objects outside of the self and originate at an unconscious level. Field and Ruelke[13] identify seven phases of hallucinatory behavior, the understanding of which can help to guide nursing intervention. The first phase is a recollection of interactions with a person who has been helpful to the patient in the past. This recollection results in a decrease of anxiety. The second phase is a repetition of the first-phase experience, establishing a pattern. During the third phase, the person begins to worry that the anxiety-relieving experience will not continue, which leads to more frequent repetition of the experience and a decreased ability to distinguish fantasy from reality. This requires withdrawal from interaction with real people. Other people notice and comment on the person's behavior at phase 4. This causes increased anxiety and more need for the hallucinated reassurance. At phase 5 the experience becomes less pleasant. Derogatory aspects of the person's self-system are introduced. As the voice (or voices) becomes accusatory and makes threats, the anxiety level begins to increase again. The person may be inclined to agree with the voice or may try to convince himself that it is wrong. Phase 6 is the point at which others usually intervene because interference with the patient's ability to function becomes severe, resulting in extreme withdrawal and preoccupation. At this point the patient also rejects responsibility for his behavior and feels under the control of outside forces. An attempt at compromise takes place at phase 7. The patient tries to bargain for a return to the earlier anxiety-relieving experience. According to this explanation of the hallucination process, the patient's objective is relief of anxiety. This principle must be kept in mind when nursing intervention is planned. As with the delusional patient, a vigorous effort at invalidating the hallucination could cause increased anxiety and result in an even greater need for the hallucination.

Schwartzman[37] has enumerated several principles for nursing intervention with the hallucinating patient. Before intervening, the nurse should assess the need that is being met by the hallucination. In the context of the process just described, the need would be related to the cause of the underlying anxiety. As the assessment proceeds, the nurse will also be establishing a trusting nurse-patient relationship. It is important to recognize and acknowledge the affective component of the hallucinated experience. Alertness to nonverbal communication can facilitate this recognition. Nonverbal cues can also help the nurse identify when the patient is hallucinating and thus be able to intervene. The nurse may then function as the patient's link with reality, telling the patient that the hallucination is not real to the nurse. The reality of the experience to the patient should not be negated; rather, the nurse tries to cast doubt on the experience by presenting her perception of reality. Encouraging the patient to talk about reality-based issues is also helpful. Many patients report that their auditory hallucinations are most bothersome when they are alone and there are no competing stimuli. Field[12] has conducted research regarding the incidence of hallucinatory experiences of hospitalized patients. He found that most of the patients did have auditory hallucinations, although they did not readily admit to this. He also validated that verbally dismissing the voices by saying "Go away" or "Be quiet" was effective for most patients. Of course, the patient needs to understand that this should take place in private or in the presence of a person who knows what he is doing. It may take some time before the patient is able to gain enough ego strength to reality test independently. Some patients continue to hallucinate indefinitely, but learn to live and function with the voices in the background.

■ **PROVIDING STRUCTURE.** In addition to reality testing, patients who have difficulty sorting out messages need help with organization. Schizophrenic patients are frequently disorganized. Sometimes behavior is so fragmented that nursing help is needed to accomplish even familiar tasks, such as eating and dressing.

Instructions should be given step by step and in clear simple language, such as "Put your right arm in the right sleeve; put your left arm in the left sleeve" until the person is fully dressed. It may be tempting to perform the task for the patient because structuring activity in this way can be time consuming. However, helping the patient to perform whatever activities he can helps to maintain his self-esteem. Another way of assisting the patient to structure his day is to provide him with a schedule of planned activities. He then knows what to expect and can prepare for events before they occur. Nursing contacts should be included in the schedule. Regular brief contacts are less threatening to the patient who fears closeness than a single long interaction with the nurse. The length of nurse-patient interactions can be increased as the patient is able to tolerate increased interpersonal intimacy.

■ **DECISION MAKING.** Decision making is another problem for patients who have difficulty processing complex messages, resulting in ambivalence. The nurse can be helpful by minimizing the need for the patient to make choices. Even filling out a selective menu can be overwhelming to a patient who is being bombarded by thoughts and feelings, as well as environmental stimuli. Family members can provide information about the patient's likes and dislikes and his usual routine so that nursing care can be individualized. As the patient's anxiety level decreases, choices can be offered, beginning with two alternatives such as "Do you want a ham sandwich or a roast beef sandwich?" As decision-making ability grows, the nurse can help the patient to identify and evaluate alternatives. Patients may try to persuade the nurse to make major life decisions for them. It should be kept in mind that decision making also entails responsibility for the outcome of the decision. A more appropriate role for the nurse is to assist the patient to assess all the facets of a decision and then to support the strength that he demonstrates by making his own choice.

Nursing intervention with a patient who is experiencing an impairment of his ability to communicate is challenging. The nurse must devise ways to circumvent the communication barriers erected by the patient. This requires alertness, keen observation, and openness to the subtle messages the patient transmits. The nurse's communication skills become her most important tools in engaging the patient in a helping relationship.

■ **Intervening in dependency**

At first the dependent patient may appear to be too trusting. However, this person also lacks confidence in the willingness of others to be available to him and to meet his needs. In addition, he lacks confidence in his own ability to be self-sufficient. Therefore he clings to others, fearing that if they are allowed any distance, they will not return.

■ **THERAPEUTIC GOALS.** Hill[18] has identified four therapeutic goals in her work with dependent women: (1) to express real feelings and ideas, (2) to make decisions comfortably, (3) to accept pleasurable experiences, and (4) to be able to control panic. She also points out that unless the patient has threatened or attempted suicide, it is best to help him remain out of the hospital, since the secondary gain of being cared for impedes progress toward these goals. Hill's goals have been in-

corporated into the mental health education plan presented in Table 17-3.

To help the patient express feelings and ideas and accept them as his own, the nurse first has to help the person identify feelings. Attention to nonverbal communication may provide clues as to the patient's feelings. It can be helpful to draw the patient's attention to gestures, body posture, and facial expression. The nurse should listen for undercurrents of thought and recurring themes in the patient's conversation and attempt to articulate these. Another approach is to consistently ask the patient, "What do you think

---

TABLE 17-3

MENTAL HEALTH EDUCATION PLAN FOR A DEPENDENT PATIENT

Content	Instructional activities	Evaluation
Identify common concerns related to open and honest expression of real feelings and ideas.	Identify a recent situation in which the patient had difficulty stating real feelings or ideas. List alternative ways to express thoughts and feelings. Role play each alternative. Select the one that was most effective.	The patient will identify feelings and ideas and express them directly to others.
Explain the decision-making process.	Describe the steps of decision making: Identify the problem. List alternatives. Evaluate alternatives. Test selected alternative.	The patient will apply the decision-making process when offered a choice.
Practice the decision-making process.	Offer the patient a choice. Guide the patient through the steps of the process.	
Explore the meaning of experiencing pleasure.	Discuss the difference between pleasurable and unpleasureable experiences. Identify one activity that has the potential for enjoyment. Participate in the activity together. Share feelings of pleasure at the time that they occur. Repeat on a regular basis. Assist the patient to identify and practice a solitary pleasant experience.	The patient will describe one activity that has been enjoyable. The patient will identify feelings of pleasure related to specific activities.
Describe behaviors that characterize anxiety.	List behaviors that indicate the various levels of anxiety.	The patient will identify behaviors and the related level of anxiety.
Explore situations that create anxiety.	Role play situations that require independence and monitor anxiety level.	The patient will identify anxiety related to specific situations.
Explain stress reduction techniques.	Describe the stress response. Demonstrate relaxation exercises (see Chapter 12). Assist the patient to return the demonstration. Role play anxiety provoking situation. Assist patient to use relaxation when early signs of anxiety appear.	The patient will perform relaxation exercises when signs of anxiety appear.

about . . .?" or "How do you feel about . . .?" thus conveying the expectation that the patient does have opinions and feelings to share. Role modeling can also help. The nurse can share her own feelings with the patient if they have had an experience that aroused an emotional response. For instance, the nurse might say, "I was annoyed when the head nurse called me away just as we were getting into a good discussion."

■ **ROLE CLARIFICATION.** Dependent people try to place the nurse in the parental role, which is also a comfortable role for most nurses to assume. Therefore the nurse must take care to relate to the patient as an adult, conveying the assumption that he is a mature person, perfectly capable of managing his own life. The patient will probably resist this and try to prove his helplessness to the nurse, who must resist the urge to act like a parent. This part of the nursing care of the dependent patient can be frustrating, since the patient becomes demanding and attention seeking. Reasonable requests should be consistently met, and limits of acceptable behavior should be discussed with the patient. Active involvement of the patient in developing the plan of care may greatly improve the chances for successful goal accomplishment.

■ **MEDICATIONS.** Contemporary culture is drug oriented. Pills and potions are promoted as the panacea for all ills. It is not surprising that many patients expect that a magical pill will be provided that will solve all life's problems and allay all anxieties. It is hard to convince these people that pills may ease pain but rarely take it all away and that hard work is necessary to resolve psychosocial problems. A pill will not mend a broken marriage or a broken heart, however much one longs for that to happen.

Dependent people are prone to be seekers of the perfect pill. Sometimes this search can lead to overdependency on medication, even to the point of addiction. The nursing problem presented by these patients is twofold. They persistently demand medication and, at the same time, resist being engaged in exploration of their behavior. The following interaction demonstrates this dilemma.

Mr. M is a 45-year-old man who is mildly depressed, anxious, and has multiple somatic complaints. A thorough medical workup has ruled out any physiological basis for his symptoms. He is receiving diazepam (Valium), 5 mg, PO, q4h, prn for anxiety. He approaches a staff nurse, Ms. J.

MS. J: **May I help you, Mr. M?**
MR. M: **I need my Valium.**
MS. J: **Tell me how you're feeling.**
MR. M: **I feel bad. Just get me my Valium.**
MS. J: **You feel bad?**
MR. M: **Look, I need my pill now!**

MS. J: **Your Valium is ordered to help you when you're anxious. I want to try to understand how you're feeling when you ask for the pill.**
MR. M: **Well, I'm anxious and I'm getting more anxious standing here talking to you about whether I'm anxious. Now, how about my pill?**
MS. J: **Well, it has been just 4 hours since your last one. Do you think you could try to hold out for a few minutes longer? Perhaps we could talk or play ping-pong to take your mind off your anxiety.**
MR. M: **Look, the doc says I can have Valium every 4 hours. For the last hour, I've been counting the minutes. My head aches, my stomach is in knots, and look how my hands are shaking. Please get me my pill.**
MS. J: **OK. If you can't wait, I'll get it for you. I'd like to talk to you later, though, to see if we can come up with some ideas of other ways you can handle your anxiety. Pills don't get to the root of the problem, you know.**
MR. M: **Sure, sure. I'll talk to you sometime when I'm calm. I'll wait right here while you get my pill.**

In this interaction the nurse and the patient were pursuing different goals, resulting in frustration for both. The nurse's concern about Mr. M's dependence on his medication was well founded. Her timing in approaching the idea of alternative coping mechanisms was not ideal. However, she was acting responsibly in asking Mr. M to describe his feelings before giving him medication. It can be tempting with dependent patients like Mr. M to automatically give medicine every 4 hours without question to avoid a hostile confrontation. Medication that is ordered "whenever necessary" can be withheld by the nurse if there is no objective evidence of need on the part of the patient. Of course, if the nurse is dealing with a patient whom she finds to be annoying, she must also evaluate whether her feelings are influencing her decision not to give medicine.

Close communication within the health team is helpful when working with patients like Mr. M. Frequency of medication should be reviewed regularly. All team members should be united in an effort to be supportive and to encourage the patient to confront his problems and to explore other coping mechanisms.

Placebos are sometimes given to dependent patients. This is, of course, done only with a physician's order. This plan of care should be thoroughly discussed and evaluated by the health care team before it is initiated. Deception of the patient is involved and could result in loss of trust in caregivers by the patient. It is imperative that this course of action not be undertaken as a retaliation against a frustrating patient. As a professional, the nurse should explore her own feelings about the use of a placebo and make her own decision about participating in this treatment.

Patients who are dependent on medication have great potential for addiction to medication. Nursing care of the addicted patient is addressed in Chapter 20. Nurses do have a role in combating addiction by discouraging indiscriminate use of medication and by helping patients explore healthier ways of meeting their needs.

■ **BEHAVIOR MODIFICATION.** The use of a type of behavior modification approach can be therapeutic when caring for a dependent patient. Appropriate behavior such as making decisions, helping others, or caring for the person's own needs is rewarded by attention and warm praise. Attention-seeking, dependent, or infantile behavior is ignored, and inappropriate requests meet with no response. In time, the incidence of mature behavior should increase as the patient realizes that dependent behavior results in little need gratification.

There is often a tendency on the part of nurses to avoid contact with dependent patients because of the expectation that they will be clinging and demanding. Unfortunately, this attitude tends to reinforce the patient's expectation that people will not seek him out and will not spontaneously meet his needs. His anxiety level then rises and he becomes even more demanding of attention, which reinforces the nurse's frustration with him. This cycle must be broken by the nurse. If the patient is given attention by the nurse without having to make demands, the anxiety level is alleviated and gradually the patient will begin to make fewer demands. If the nurse then begins to respond less to the patient's high anxiety level, the patient will also begin to learn to control his panic, thus beginning to learn to function as a mature adult. As this occurs, significant others must also be included so they can also learn new ways of interacting with the patient. This is another instance in which family therapy is often an important component of the overall therapeutic plan.

■ **Intervening in manipulation**

■ **FAMILY INVOLVEMENT.** Significant others must also be involved in the plan of care for the manipulative patient. This is particularly true because manipulative people frequently achieve their ends by setting others at odds. For instance, the patient may complain to his family about his treatment, encouraging the family to confront the staff about the poor nursing care their family member is receiving. At the same time the patient may be telling the staff about his mistreatment at the hands of his family. The staff therefore is tempted to interpret the family's complaint as an indication of guilt arising from past mistreatment of the patient. Staff and family are then in conflict, and attention is distracted from the patient, who thus can avoid the discomfort of

looking at his own behavior. When the staff finally realizes what is happening, the result is usually anger at the patient. There should be awareness of this tendency so that a punitive response can be avoided. Often when manipulative patients are hospitalized, this scenario is played out over and over until the patient is sent home still successfully relating to others as objects.

■ **INPATIENT TREATMENT.** Because of the great difficulty in promoting change in manipulative behavior and the long-term nature of its treatment, most of these patients are treated in community settings. However, it is necessary at times to hospitalize them. For instance, the person with a borderline personality disorder may be self-destructive or the antisocial person may require a structured environment with limit-setting. Kernberg and Haran[22] recommend the following nursing roles in caring for the hospitalized borderline patient:

1. Provide a structured environment.
2. Serve as an emotional sounding board.
3. Clarify and diagnose conflicts.

They emphasize the need for clinical supervision.

Countertransference is usually an issue when caring for these patients. Positive countertransference by some staff members, and negative by others, leads to staff dissension and splitting. Whenever these behavioral patterns emerge while there is a manipulative patient on the psychiatric unit, the staff need to examine their level of involvement with the patient.

Reid[34] addresses countertransference issues as they relate to the antisocial patient. Countertransference feelings may include, "impulses to rescue, support, hurt, admire, identify with, or accept compliments from, the patient."[34] The principles of inpatient treatment for these patients include

1. Establish control with no option to escape involvement.
2. Provide an experienced, consistent staff.
3. Implement a strict hierarchical structure, with rules that are firm, not necessarily fair, and rigidly interpreted.
4. Provide support while the patient learns to experience painful feelings.[34]

■ **LIMIT SETTING AND STRUCTURE.** Manipulative patients must be held responsible for their own behavior. They are adept at attributing responsibility to others. Staff members must communicate effectively with each other so that consistent messages are given. These patients alertly recognize any inconsistency and use it to again focus attention on others. They usually are resistive to rules and must have clear limits that are consistently enforced by all staff members and, whenever possible, by family members as well.

Masterson[29] describes guidelines for the treatment of borderline patients that incorporate several of these principles. He emphasizes the need for availability of staff attention combined with structured discipline. There must be an expectation that the patient will meet standards of healthy behavior. Failure to meet the standard is identified and acting out is confronted. Loss of control may be dealt with by room restriction, with the patient instructed to think about the episode so that it may be discussed in therapy. The length of the restriction should be related to the seriousness of the behavior. These approaches usually lead to the emergence of depression. The depressed feelings should be directed into formal psychotherapy sessions, but the staff can act as role models for appropriate behavior. A school program, occupational therapy, and the milieu may be used to teach age-appropriate social and achievement skills. Reality orientation may also be necessary.

■ **PROTECTION FROM SELF-HARM.** The deliberate self-destructive or self-mutilating behavior of the borderline patient is very difficult to treat. It frequently requires that the nursing staff provide constant observation of the patient to prevent serious physical harm. At the same time, the intense dependency needs of these patients, related to an unresolved separation-individuation developmental phase, makes it very difficult to wean them from this level of staff attention. Usually, the staff contact must be decreased very gradually, with the expectation that the level of observation may need to be increased if the patient seems out of control. Involvement of the patient in planning the decrease in constant observation may be helpful. In addition, reassurance must be provided that less contact does not equal no contact. Consistent, scheduled time with a staff member is recommended. Primary nursing is particularly effective with a patient who needs to work through these separation issues.

■ **FOCUS ON STRENGTHS.** These patients frequently have real strengths as leaders within the patient group. One constructive nursing approach is to encourage them to identify and capitalize on their strengths. They may be given responsibilities within the patient care unit and can be encouraged to help other patients with hygiene, eating, and other activities. They are often intelligent and respond well to being challenged to participate actively in planning their own care. However, they are extremely resistant to recognizing or dealing with feelings and need consistent encouragement to attempt this. Nurses become frustrated with manipulative patients because they seem to be so aware of what is happening and so in control of most situations, yet so unaware of the needs of others. It must be remembered that they have little tolerance for intimacy and that their maneuvering of others is an effective way of keeping them at a safe distance. Manipulative people are often charming, and it is easy to get involved with them. However, as soon as the other person begins to make demands or show signs of emotional closeness, the patient will dilute the relationship by withdrawing, by frustrating the other, or by distracting attention from himself.

■ **BEHAVIOR MODIFICATION.** Behavior modification techniques may be helpful in decreasing antisocial behavior. The patient is usually impatient with delays in gratification and relies on material, rather than emotional, means of gratification. Reinforcers used in a behavior modification program should therefore be concrete and readily available, such as points that may be accumulated to qualify for privileges, such as a weekend at home or a trip to the canteen. Other reinforcers might be a visit or a favorite food. Cigarettes are frequently used as reinforcers, but this should be weighed against the adverse effects of cigarette smoking and the seeming endorsement of the habit when cigarettes are provided by health professionals. Lack of response to undesirable behavior is the least reinforcing but is not always possible. If behavior is disruptive and there must be a response, it should be matter of fact and one that is not desired by the patient. For instance, removal from contact with others for a predetermined period of time may discourage undesirable behavior, whereas a lecture that entails a great deal of attention may in reality be a reinforcer.

Behavioral contracting is an approach that has been tried with borderline patients. McEnany and Tescher[27] describe the goals of behavioral contracting to be (1) to involve the patient in care planning, (2) to decrease regression, and (3) to assist the patient to maintain control. When a contract is negotiated, control is shared between the nurse and the patient. The nurse-patient contract is negotiated based on patient-identified strengths, learning needs, and goals. However, basic expectations are delineated, and the patient must agree to these. They include agreement to the length of the contract's effectiveness, and to refrain from behavior that would be harmful to the self or to others.

No matter what type of disruption in relatedness the patient is experiencing, the core concept on which nursing care is based is that of accessibility. The nurse must be physically accessible to the patient on a regular basis so that there is an opportunity for interaction. In addition, there must be psychological accessibility, meaning that the nurse exhibits interest in the patient and strives to understand him and to clarify communication and demonstrate an empathic attitude. If the nurse-patient relationship is a healthy one, the patient can learn how to find satisfaction in other human relationships. Table 17-4 summarizes some nursing interventions relevant to the care of the patient who is experiencing disruptions in relatedness.

 Evaluation

Evaluation of the degree of success or failure of nursing intervention when that intervention focuses on the therapeutic relationship can be a difficult process. Since the relationship is central to effective delivery of

TABLE 17-4

SUMMARY OF NURSING INTERVENTIONS WITH DISRUPTIONS IN RELATEDNESS

Goal—Growth toward achieving maximum interpersonal satisfaction by establishing and maintaining self-enhancing relationships with others

Principle	Rationale	Nursing interventions
Establish a trusting relationship	An atmosphere of trust facilitates open expression of thoughts and feelings; risk-taking is necessary when sharing thoughts and feelings; basic trust offers the patient the support needed to take interpersonal risks; support is also important when attempting new behaviors	Initiate a nurse-patient relationship contract that is mutually agreed on by nurse and patient Develop mutual, behaviorally stated goals for nursing intervention Maintain consistent behavior by all nursing staff members Demonstrate honest communication of responses to the patient's behavior Provide honest and immediate feedback to the patient concerning behavioral change Provide for privacy and comfort during interactions Maintain confidentiality Demonstrate accessibility
Identify and support the patient's strengths	Success in self-care, interpersonal relationships and activities promote enhanced self-esteem; recognition of strengths by trusted people helps the patient recognize his positive attributes; attention that is given to positive behavior is a reward and reinforces the behavioral pattern	Assess the patient's constructive coping behaviors Encourage the patient to perform self-care and make decisions to the extent of his ability Maintain the patient's dignity while providing needed assistance with activities of daily living Offer genuine praise for the patient's accomplishments Initiate activities that allow the patient to experience success Educate the patient and significant others about health care needs and treatment
Promote clear, consistent, and open communication	Healthy interpersonal relationships require open communication; patients with disordered thinking need assistance in identifying and understanding reality. Close relationships are often frightening at first and must be encouraged by a supportive environment; clear and consistent limits on behavior reduce the successful use of manipulative behavior	Individualize communication based on the patient's educational level, cultural background, and mental state Use congruent verbal and nonverbal communications Validate the meaning of communications with the patient Recognize the symbolic content of communication Act as a role model by sharing here-and-now feelings, perceptions, and reactions with the patient Give empathic encouragement of self-exploration by the patient Set limits as required in a clear and consistent manner

Continued.

TABLE 17-4—cont'd

SUMMARY OF NURSING INTERVENTIONS WITH DISRUPTIONS IN RELATEDNESS
Goal—Growth toward achieving maximum interpersonal satisfaction by establishing and maintaining self-enhancing relationships with others

Principle	Rationale	Nursing interventions
Alleviate high levels of interpersonal anxiety	Severe and panic levels of anxiety result in thought fragmentation, self-absorption, difficulty interpreting internal and external stimuli, impaired judgment, and a shortened attention span; these behaviors interfere with interpersonal relationships; a structured predictable environment and minimal interpersonal pressure alleviate anxiety	Whenever possible, respond to the patient's stated needs Maintain a calm supportive approach Minimize environmental stimuli Explain procedures and other events Recognize defensive behaviors utilized by the patient (e.g., delusions, hallucinations, and ego defense mechanisms) Assist the patient to use healthier coping responses, but avoid premature challenge of less healthy ways of coping Teach anxiety-relieving techniques (e.g., relaxation techniques and physical activities) Provide external controls when necessary Provide prescribed medications Promote structure by providing a schedule of activities, giving specific step-by-step instructions, minimizing the need to make choices, and having frequent brief contact with the patient Encourage self-control, but protect the patient from impulsive destructive behavior Respect the patient's need for control of his personal space
Maintain biological integrity	Use of the mechanisms of regression or projection may result in lack of attention to basic biological needs; lack of adequate rest and nutrients can endanger the patient; deficiencies in personal hygiene interfere with the development of interpersonal relationships; psychotropic medications may cause alterations in blood pressure and pulse, sometimes resulting in syncope; these medications also are associated with a number of side effects that are distressing, but usually reversible if appropriate intervention occurs	Assess the patient's eating, sleeping, elimination, and hygiene habits Ascertain food and fluid preferences If necessary, offer food and fluids at regular intervals Assist patient with eating and drinking if necessary Ascertain usual elimination patterns Assist to bathroom if necessary Record intake and output if a disruption is suspected or identified Record bowel movements and offer prescribed laxatives if needed Monitor vital signs Encourage bathing when needed; assist if necessary Ensure the availability of clean clothing; preferably the patient's own street clothing Ensure the availability of toiletries and cosmetics Encourage appropriate care of hair and teeth Facilitate shaving as desired Provide a restful environment for sleep Initiate sleep-promoting nursing measures Offer prescribed sedation if required Observe for medication side effects and initiate relevant health teaching

nursing care, it is threatening for many nurses to scrutinize their ability to relate to others. This kind of evaluation must take place at two levels. One level is directed toward the nurse and her participation in the relationship. Introspection may be of some value in accomplishing this, particularly if a nurse stops to review an interaction immediately after it takes place. Blind spots about one's own feelings that may be present while one is involved with the patient may become clearer in retrospect. However, self-evaluation is colored by one's self-perceptions. Supervision from an experienced nurse-therapist can be extremely helpful in identifying some of the nuances of the relationship that may be less obvious to the nurse herself. Constructive supervision can help the nurse to identify the dynamics of the relationship and can help her deal with the resistance to change that often occurs on the part of the patient. No matter how experienced a nurse becomes, her own perception of her participation in a relationship is affected by her self-concept, and the need for supervision is never lost.

At another level, evaluation of nursing care considers the patient's behavior and the behavioral changes that the nurse works to facilitate. Input about these changes is collected from several sources. The patient is the primary source. He should be encouraged to verbally explore experiences with relationships, past and present. Changes in behavior should be validated with the patient to determine if he is also aware of change. When the nurse and patient discuss their respective views of their relationship, the patient is again participating in an evaluation of the usefulness of the relationship to him. Sharing feelings and intimate thoughts denotes increased trust and a willingness to risk self-revelation. Nonverbally, the patient also reveals responses to the therapeutic relationship. Accessibility to the nurse for prearranged interactions indicates trust and involvement in the relationship. Eye contact usually takes place more often when one person is comfortable with another. Touching may communicate closeness. Initiation of activities with others indicates more openness to relatedness. Increased decision making and assumption of leadership roles imply an improved self-esteem and increasing self-confidence. Such behaviors can be observed and documented and also validated with other staff members. Therefore these are useful evaluation criteria.

Significant others may also contribute to the evaluation process. They have known the patient prior to the occurrence of any behavioral disruption and can provide information about the patient's behavioral norms. They can also assist in validating behavioral changes, particularly in terms of whether the changes continue in the patient's usual environment. For the hospitalized patient, change may be seen in the protected hospital setting, but the patient may have a great deal of difficulty in transferring this behavioral change to the community setting. Involving families in this kind of assessment helps to teach the family the behaviors that have been learned by the patient and gives them an idea of what is reasonable to expect from the patient. This may help to avoid some of the turmoil described by Leavitt[23] in her study of the families of discharged psychiatric patients. She found that most of the family members she surveyed found help and support outside the hospital and that they had little idea of what to expect of the patient after discharge. This emphasizes the need to involve families in the total nursing care plan, including evaluation of the results of the care that has been given.

Evaluation is, of course, continually taking place throughout the course of the relationship. The nurse must review the assessment and add more information as gaps become apparent. Knowledge of past relationship experiences can explain much about present behavior and should be progressively explored as the relationship grows. Observation of the patient's interaction with significant others may also reveal areas that require further exploration. As new behaviors are observed, the nursing diagnosis will be refined. Evaluation of the nursing diagnosis should lead the nurse to revision of the goals. Also, as the nurse and patient become more involved in a mutual relationship, the patient will become more active in participating in identification of nursing needs and goal setting. Nursing actions need constant revision based on feedback from the patient, the patient's family, peers, the clinical supervisor, and self. The nursing approach must be modified as the nurse-patient relationship grows and as the patient moves toward autonomy and the ability to establish and maintain mature interpersonal relationships.

■ SUGGESTED CROSS-REFERENCES ■

Therapeutic relationship skills are discussed in Chapter 4. The model of health-illness phenomena is presented in Chapter 3. The phases of the nursing process are discussed in Chapter 5. Nursing interventions related to severe and panic levels of anxiety are described in Chapter 12. Building social skills is described in Chapter 14. Working with dysfunctional families is discussed in Chapter 29.

DIRECTIONS FOR FUTURE RESEARCH

The following are some of the nursing research problems raised in Chapter 17 that merit further study by psychiatric nurses:

1. The relationship between various stressful life events, the individual's capacity for relatedness, and the individual's response to stress
2. Nursing interventions with children who are experiencing interpersonal stress that will assist them to continue to develop the capacity for relatedness
3. Investigation and validation of cross-cultural nursing interventions with schizophrenic patients based on the findings of the International Pilot Study of Schizophrenia
4. Determination of whether nurses recognize the need of patients to be alone and the extent to which this is taken into account in planning nursing care at either the individual or the program level
5. Nonverbal cues that can serve as indicators of a withdrawn patient's positive or negative response to a specific nursing intervention
6. Retrospective identification of the nursing interventions that recovered patients describe as having been helpful during a period of disruption in interpersonal relationships
7. Longitudinal outcome evaluation of the posthospital adjustment of psychotic patients who were involved in a consistent therapeutic nursing relationship during hospitalization
8. Nurses' sensitivity to and impact on the emotional climate of the inpatient unit
9. The personal space needs of individuals who have interpersonal relationship disruptions
10. Nursing interventions that will increase the schizophrenic person's tolerance for interpersonal closeness, including touch
11. Identification and validation of effective nursing approaches with delusional or hallucinating patients
12. Nurses' expectations of dependent or independent behavior by patients with various biological and psychosocial disorders
13. Description of the constructive use of manipulative behavior and nursing interventions that reinforce this aspect of functioning
14. Relationship between nurses' attitudes toward manipulative behavior, their own use of manipulation, and their ability to intervene effectively with manipulative patients
15. Characteristics of the therapeutic milieu that are effective in modifying manipulative behavior

■ SUMMARY ■

1. A healthy interpersonal relationship was defined as one in which the individuals involved experience intimacy with each other while maintaining separate identities. There should also be a balance between dependent and independent behavior, described as interdependence.

2. The capacity for relatedness develops throughout the life cycle. The normal process of the development of relatedness was described.

3. Possible disruptions that can occur in the process of relatedness included impaired communication, withdrawal, suspicion, dependency, and manipulation.

4. The concept of loneliness was presented as an existential experience involving profound emotional pain and a feeling of total alienation from human relationships. This was differentiated from aloneness and solitude, which may be sought out by those who also are able to relate to others.

5. Predisposing factors and precipitating stressors that lead to disruptions in relatedness were described. They include any disruption in the normal interpersonal developmental process; sociocultural factors, including value conflicts, isolation of certain societal groups, and fragmentation of family systems; biochemical formulations, particularly the dopamine hypothesis of schizophrenia; genetic theories; and psychodynamic processes, including the psychoanalytic, interpersonal, and family process models.

6. The behaviors associated with disruptions in relatedness were presented. Behavioral responses were identified as impaired communication, withdrawal, suspicion, dependency, and manipulation. These were related through presentation of case studies to the medical diagnoses of paranoid schizophrenia, catatonic schizophrenia, dependent personality disorder, panic disorder, antisocial personality disorder, and borderline personality disorder. An additional case example was provided of an isolated elderly man. Each of these behavioral disruptions involved an inability to establish and maintain healthy interpersonal relationships.

7. Examples of nursing diagnoses and descriptions of medical diagnostic criteria were presented.

8. Coping mechanisms were discussed as they apply to disruptions in the ability to maintain relatedness. It was emphasized that the behaviors of impaired communication, withdrawal, suspicion, dependency, and manipulation function as coping mechanisms.

9. Long- and short-term nurse-patient goals pertaining to relatedness were discussed. Emphasis was placed on the importance of patient involvement as soon as the nurse-patient relationship has matured to the level that the patient can trust the nurse with his goals. An example of a long-term and related short-term goals was presented.

10. The importance of the therapeutic nurse-patient relationship for a patient who has problems with relatedness was emphasized. Withdrawn patients require a consistent, patient approach with attention given to biological, psychological, and social needs. Each of these areas was discussed. Verbal

and nonverbal aspects of nurse and patient behavior were considered. Issues of intervention with significant others and termination of the relationship were also presented.

11. Trust was presented as the central issue in working with a suspicious patient. Reliability and consistency are essential for the growth of trust, as is respect for the patient's need for privacy. The nursing role in terms of the patient's biological integrity was also considered. Characteristics of a trusting person were described to be used as a means of assessing the patient's progress and as a possible topic for discussion with a recovering patient.

12. Nursing intervention with the dependent patient was focused on helping the patient to express feelings and ideas, make decisions, accept pleasure, and control panic. The nurse should treat the patient on an adult-to-adult basis, although there may be an attempt by the patient to put her in a parental role. A behavior modification approach was suggested as possibly helpful with a dependent person. A mental health education plan for the dependent patient was presented.

13. Consistency and limit setting were primary nursing interventions suggested with manipulative patients. Channels of communication between staff members must be open, since the patient may try to capitalize on any confusion. The patient must be held responsible for his behavior. Possible nursing approaches included involvement of the patient in care planning, protection from destructive behavior, and behavior modification.

14. Nursing interventions were suggested for patients who are unable to communicate clearly. The need to attend to both verbal and nonverbal levels of communication was discussed, as was the symbolical nature of psychotic communication. The role of the nurse in meeting the patient at his level and assisting him to feel secure enough to communicate directly was presented. Also included was the requirement that the nurse be aware of her own communications, verbal and nonverbal.

15. Accessibility of the nurse to the patient is of primary importance when the problem is one of relatedness.

16. Evaluation of nursing care was presented as a process that must involve the patient, the nurse, other staff, and significant others. The need for validation of observations was emphasized, as was the ongoing need for clinical supervision of nursing care by an experienced nurse therapist.

■ REFERENCES ■

1. American Psychiatric Association: Draft of the DSM-III-R in Development (subject to change), as proposed by the Work Group to Revise DSM-III. American Psychiatric Association, October 1985.
2. Bartko, J.J.: Statistical basis for exploring schizophrenia, Am. J. Psychiatry **138**:941, 1981.
3. Bateson, G.: Information and codification: a philosophical approach. In Ruesch, J., and Bateson, G.: Communication: the social matrix of psychiatry, New York, 1968, W.W. Norton & Co., Inc.
4. Bateson, G. et al.: Toward a theory of schizophrenia. In Howells, J.G., editor: Theory and practice of family psychiatry, New York, 1971, Brunner/Mazel, Inc.
5. Brown, M.M., Cornwell, J., and Weist, J.T.: Reducing the risks to the institutionalized elderly. Part I: Depersonalization, negative relocation effects and medical care deficiencies, J. Gerontol. Nurs. **7**:401, 1981.
6. Brown, R.P., and Mann, J.J.: A clinical perspective on the role of neurotransmitters in mental disorders, Hosp. Community Psychiatry **36**:141, Feb. 1985.
7. Burnham, D., Gladstone, A., and Gibson, R.: Schizophrenia and the need-fear dilemma, New York, 1969, International Universities Press.
8. Cancro, R.: The genetic studies of the schizophrenia syndrome: a review of their clinical implications. In Bellak, L., editor: Disorders of the schizophrenic syndrome, New York, 1979, Basic Books, Inc., Publishers.
9. Carpenter, W.T., Jr.: The phenomenology of schizophrenia, Am. J. Psychiatry **138**:948, 1981.
10. Carter, C., and Galliano, D.: Fear of loss and attachment: a major dynamic in the social isolation of the institutionalized aged, J. Gerontol. Nurs. **7**:342, 1981.
11. Danziger, S.: Major treatment issues and techniques in family therapy with the borderline adolescent, J. Psychosoc. Nurs. Ment. Health Serv. **20**:27, Jan. 1982.
12. Field, W.E.: Hearing voices, J. Psychosoc. Nurs. Ment. Health Serv. **23**:9, Jan. 1985.
13. Field, W.E., and Ruelke, W.: Hallucinations and how to deal with them, Am. J. Nurs. **73**:638, 1973.
14. Fromm-Reichmann, F.: On loneliness. In Bullard, D.M., editor: Psychoanalysis and psychotherapy, Chicago, 1960, University of Chicago Press.
15. Gordon, S.: Lonely in America, New York, 1976, Simon & Schuster, Inc.
16. Grosicki, J., and Harmonson, M.: Nursing action guide: hallucinations, J. Psychiatr. Nurs. **7**:134, May, 1979.
17. Gunderson, J.G.: Borderline personality disorder, Washington, D.C., 1984, American Psychiatric Press, Inc.
18. Hill, D.: Outpatient management of passive-dependent women, Hosp. Community Psychiatry **21**:402, 1970.
19. Hirschfeld, R.M.A.: Personality disorders: foreword. In Frances, A.J., and Hales, R.E., editors: Psychiatry update, vol. 5, Washington, D.C., 1986, American Psychiatric Press, Inc.
20. Kahn, E.M.: Psychotherapy with chronic schizophrenics: alliance, transference and countertransference, J. Psychosoc. Nurs. Ment. Health Serv. **22**:20, July 1984.
21. Kaplan, H.I., and Sadock, B.J.: Neurophysiology of behavior. In Kaplan, H.I., Freedman, A.M., and Sadock, B.J., editors: Comprehensive textbook of psychiatry, ed. 3, vol. 1, Baltimore, 1980, The Williams & Wilkins Co.
22. Kernberg, O., and Haran, C.: Milieu treatment with borderline patients, J. Psychosoc. Nurs. Ment. Health Serv. **22**:29, Apr. 1984.
23. Leavitt, M.: The discharge crisis: the experience of families of psychiatric patients, Nurs. Res. **24**:33, 1975.

24. Lehmann, H.E.: Schizophrenia: clinical features. In Kaplan, H.I., Freedman, A.M., and Sadock, B.J., editors: Comprehensive textbook of psychiatry, ed. 3, vol. 2, Baltimore, 1980, The Williams & Wilkins Co.

25. Lehmann, H.E.: Schizophrenia: history. In Kaplan, H.I., Freedman, A.M., and Sadock, B.J., editors: Comprehensive textbook of psychiatry, ed. 3, vol. 2, Baltimore, 1980, The Williams & Wilkins Co.

26. Liberman, R.P. et al.: The nature and problem of schizophrenia. In Bellack, A.S., editor: Schizophrenia: treatment, management and rehabilitation, New York, 1984, Grune & Stratton, Inc.

27. McEnany, G.W., and Tescher, B.E.: Contracting for care: one nursing approach to the hospitalized borderline patient, J. Psychosoc. Nurs. Ment. Health Serv. **23**:11, April 1985.

28. McGlashan, T.H.: Schizophrenia: psychosocial treatment and the role of psychosocial factors in its etiology and pathogenesis. In Frances, A.J., and Hales, R.E., editors: Psychiatry update, vol. 5, Washington, D.C., 1986, American Psychiatric Press, Inc.

29. Masterson, J.F.: Treatment of the borderline adolescent, New York, 1985, Brunner/Mazel, Inc.

30. Meltzer, H.Y.: Biochemical studies in schizophrenia. In Bellak, L., editor: Disorders of the schizophrenic syndrome, New York, 1979, Basic Books, Inc., Publishers.

31. Mullahy, P.: Psychoanalysis and interpersonal psychiatry: the contributions of Harry Stack Sullivan, New York, 1970, Science House, Inc.

32. Packard, V.: A nation of strangers, New York, 1972, The David McKay Co.

33. Pfohl, B., and Andreasen, N.C.: Schizophrenia: diagnosis and classification. In Frances, A.J., and Hales, R.E., editors: Psychiatry update, vol. 5, Washington, D.C., 1986, American Psychiatric Press, Inc.

34. Reid, W.H.: The antisocial personality: a review, Hosp. Community Psychiatry **36**:831, Aug. 1985.

35. Rogers, C.: On becoming a person, Boston, 1961, Houghton Mifflin Co.

36. Satir, V.M.: Symptomatology: a family production. In Howells, J.G., editor: Theory and practice of family psychiatry, New York, 1971, Brunner/Mazel, Inc.

37. Schwartzman, S.T.: The hallucinating patient and nursing intervention, J. Psychiatr. Nurs. **13**:23, Nov.-Dec. 1975.

38. Searles, H.F.: Collected papers on schizophrenia and related subjects, New York, 1965, International Universities Press, Inc.

39. Shostrom, E.: Man, the manipulator, Nashville, Tenn., 1967, Abingdon Press.

40. Siever, L.J., and Klar, H.: A review of DSM-III criteria for the personality disorders. In Frances, A.J., and Hales, R.E., editors: Psychiatry update, vol. 5, Washington, D.C., 1986, American Psychiatric Press, Inc.

41. Spitz, R.A.: The first year of life: a psychoanalytic study of normal and deviant development of object relations, New York, 1965, International Universities Press.

42. Sullivan, H.: The interpersonal theory of psychiatry, New York, 1953, W.W. Norton & Co., Inc.

43. Thomas, M.: Trust in the nurse-patient relationship. In Carlson, C., editor: Behavioral concepts and nursing intervention, Philadelphia, 1970, J.B. Lippincott Co.

44. Vaughn, C., and Leff, J.: The measurement of expressed emotion in the families of psychiatric patients, Part 2, Br. J. Soc. Clin. Psychol. **15**:157, June 1976.

45. Weinberger, D.R., and Kleinman, J.E.: Observations on the brain in schizophrenia. In Frances, A.J., and Hales, R.E., editors: Psychiatry update, vol. 5, Washington, D.C., 1986, American Psychiatric Press, Inc.

46. Weiner, H.: Schizophrenia: etiology. In Kaplan, H.I., Freedman, A.M., and Sadock, B.J.: Comprehensive textbook of psychiatry, ed. 3, vol. 2, Baltimore, 1980, The Williams & Wilkins Co.

47. Wildman, L.L.: Reducing the schizophrenic patient's resistance to involvement, Perspect. Psychiatr. Care **3**:26, 1965.

48. Will, G.T.: A sociopsychiatric nursing approach to intervention in a problem of mutual withdrawal on a mental hospital ward, Psychiatry **15**(2):193, 1952.

49. Will, O.A.: Human relatedness and the schizophrenic reaction. In Stein, M.I.: Contemporary psychotherapies, New York, 1961, The Free Press.

50. World Health Organization: Report of the international pilot study of schizophrenia. Vol. 1: Results of the initial evaluation phase, Geneva, 1973, The Organization.

51. World Health Organization: Schizophrenia: an international follow-up study, New York, 1979, John Wiley & Sons, Inc.

52. Wynne, L.C.: Current concepts about schizophrenics and family relationships, J. Nerv. Ment. Dis. **169**:82, Feb. 1981.

53. Wynne, L.C., Toohey, M.L., and Doane, J.: Family studies. In Bellak, L., editor: Disorders of the schizophrenic syndrome, New York, 1979, Basic Books, Inc., Publishers.

■ ANNOTATED SUGGESTED READINGS ■

Bateson, G. et al.: Toward a theory of schizophrenia. In Howells, J.G., editor: Theory and practice of family psychiatry, New York, 1971, Brunner/Mazel, Inc.

This classic paper on communicative patterns in the familiies of schizophrenic patients presents the "double-bind" theory.

Bellack, A.S., editor: Schizophrenia: treatment, management and rehabilitation, New York, 1984, Grune & Stratton, Inc.

This is an edited collection of papers on many aspects of schizophrenia. The contributors are experienced investigators and present the most recent findings of their research. This book is written at a level that requires understanding of more basic concepts. It is particularly recommended for advanced practitioners, faculty, and graduate students.

*Asterisk indicates nursing reference.

Bellak, L., editor: Disorders of the schizophrenic syndrome, New York, 1979, Basic Books, Inc., Publishers.

This is a collection of papers by authorities on the study of schizophrenia. The papers cover a broad spectrum of issues and provide the reader an opportunity to become aware of the multiple approaches that are being explored relative to this complex syndrome. Many of the papers are quite sophisticated and would probably be most meaningful to the graduate student or psychiatric nursing specialist.

Brown, R.P., and Mann, J.J.: A clinical perspective on the role of neurotransmitters in mental disorders, Hosp. Community Psychiatry **36**:141, Feb. 1985.

This informative article provides a complete overview of biological theories of etiology of schizophrenia and affective disorders. The charts linking pharmacological actions with neurotransmitter activity are particularly useful.

Bullard, D.M.: Psychoanalysis and psychotherapy: selected papers of Frieda Fromm-Reichmann, Chicago, 1959, The University of Chicago Press.

The collected papers of Frieda Fromm-Reichmann are fascinating reading as insight is provided into the philosophy of an outstanding psychotherapist. A section on schizophrenia is included that provides application of psychoanalytical theory to therapy with schizophrenic patients.

*Carser, D.L., and Doona, M.E.: Alienation: a nursing concept. J. Psychiatr. Nurs. **16**:33, Sept. 1978.

This thought-provoking article presents the existential concept of alienation and relates it to application by nursing students in the classroom situation.

*Carter, C., and Galliano, D.: Fear of loss and attachment: a major dynamic in the social isolation of the institutionalized aged, J. Gerontol. Nurs. **7**:342, 1981.

The authors describe group nursing interventions that were directed toward assisting elderly nursing home residents deal with fear of attachment. Social isolation was decreased by assisting the group members to recognize and express their feelings about the dangers inherent in close relationships. An excellent example of psychosocial nursing intervention at the primary prevention level directed toward improving the relatedness of a vulnerable group of people.

Cleckley, H.: The mask of sanity, ed. 5, St. Louis, 1976, The C.V. Mosby Co.

This text is a classical presentation of the characteristics of the antisocial personality. Detailed case histories are a rich source of graphic descriptive data on the behavior of these patients. The book does not focus to a great extent on treatment.

*Danziger, S.: Major treatment issues and techniques in family therapy with the borderline adolescent, J. Psychosoc. Nurs. Ment. Health Serv. **20**:27, Jan. 1982.

This article presents a clear description of the complex behaviors and defenses of the borderline patient. The author demonstrates, through the use of case-study vignettes, the interactive process between the adolescent and the family. Techniques for therapeutic intervention are suggested. The interventions are beyond the level of the generalist, but the explanation of the defenses would be very helpful to all psychiatric nurses.

*Doona, M.E., Annino, S.L., and Kelleher, M.J.D.: Professional affirmation in nursing care, J. Psychiatr. Nurs. **15**:16, 1977.

This article is written by a faculty member and two of her former students. It describes the students' experiences caring for a schizophrenic man in an inpatient setting. They describe the varied responses of students, patient, and staff through the course of the relationships. The focus is on the importance of a caring and accepting approach. This article should be very useful to beginning sutdents who are wondering what to expect in a psychiatric setting.

*Field, W.E., and Ruelke, W.: Hallucinations and how to deal with them, Am. J. Nurs. **73**:638, 1973.

The authors describe developmental phases related to auditory hallucinations and postulate nursing intervention based on this developmental process.

Fromm-Reichmann, F.: On loneliness. In Bullard, D.M., editor: Psychoanalysis and psychotherapy, Chicago, 1959, University of Chicago Press.

This is a classic presentation of loneliness as experienced by the psychotic person. It is written in a compassionate manner and includes thoughts about therapy with these patients.

*Gallop, R.: The patient is splitting: everyone knows and nothing changes, J. Psychosoc. Nurs. Ment. Health Serv. **23**:6, Apr. 1985.

The author describes the consultation/supervision process as it relates to nursing staff working with borderline patients. She uses a case study to illustrate the staff splitting that these patients often cause and discusses approaches to dealing with countertransference.

Gunderson, J.G.: Borderline personality disorder, Washington, D.C., 1984, American Psychiatric Press, Inc.

This book is written by a psychotherapist who has a wealth of experience in providing therapy to borderline personality disorder patients. The description of the etiology of the problem and suggestions regarding interventions are invaluable. This book is highly recommended as reading for any nurses who provide care to these difficult patients.

*Kroah, J.: Strategies for interviewing in language and thought disorders, J. Psychiatr. Nurs. **12**:3, Mar.-Apr. 1974.

Several disordered communication patterns are identified, and nursing approaches that are therapeutic for each identified pattern are explained. This article is particularly helpful for the neophyte.

*Lantz, J.E.: Adlerian community treatment with schizophrenic clients, J. Psychosoc. Nurs. Ment. Health Serv. **20**:25, Apr. 1982.

A case study helps to illustrate this author's application of the Adlerian model of psychotherapy to the treatment of a schizophrenic client. This is a good illustration of the usefulness of a conceptual model for planning and implementing patient care.

Lovejoy, M.: Recovery from schizophrenia: a personal odyssey, Hosp. Community Psychiatry **35**:809, Aug. 1985.

This account of a personal experience with mental illness not only describes the author's feelings, but also presents some techniques that she devised to deal with her symptoms. She calls on mental health professionals to be flexible and open to individualizing approaches according to patient needs.

*McEnany, G.W., and Tescher, B.E.: Contracting for care: one nursing approach to the hospitalized borderline patient, J. Psychosoc. Nurs. Ment. Health Serv. **23**:11, Apr. 1985.

Contracting with borderline patients provides structure and accountability in the treatment process. The author uses a case example to demonstrate the use of contracting and also describes a case in which the approach did not work.

Masterson, J.F.: Treatment of the borderline adolescent, New York, 1985, Brunner/Mazel, Inc.

This book is by a leading authority in the treatment of the patient with borderline personality disorder. His explanation of the disruption in the developmental process that leads to this disorder is particularly helpful. He also provides a thorough discussion of treatment in hospital and outpatient settings, including the identified patient and his parents.

*O'Brien, P., Caldwell, C., and Transeau, G.: Destroyers: written treatment contracts can help cure self destructive behaviors of the borderline patient, J. Psychosoc. Nurs. Ment. Health Serv. **23**:19, Apr. 1985.

This article describes the application of treatment contracting to nursing intervention with borderline patients. A case study illustrates the use of a contract with a patient who had been self-destructive.

*Pyke, J.: Nutrition and the chronic schizophrenic, Can. Nurse **75**:40, Nov. 1979.

In this article, the author demonstrates the value of careful nursing assessment, leading to identification of a problem of disrupted nutritional status that appeared to be common among chronic schizophrenic patients. The author describes her investigation of the problem and recommends several nursing interventions.

*Reid, L.: Approaches to the aftermath of schizophrenia, Perspect. Psychiatr. Care **17**:257, 1979.

The author presents a pragmatic approach to work with patients who are recovering from a schizophrenic episode. She advocates informing the individual about the problem, so events may be placed in the context of reality and the person may gain control of his life. A group approach is recommended.

*Rickelman, B.: Brain bio-amines and schizophrenia: a summary of research findings and implications for nursing, J. Psychiatr. Nurs. **17**:28, Sept. 1979.

The author summarizes the major biological theories of schizophrenia and describes implications for nurses. An extensive bibliography provides direction for the reader who wishes to explore this complex subject in greater depth.

Ruesch, J.: Disturbed communication, New York, 1972, W.W. Norton & Co., Inc.

In this work the author applies his classic work in communication theory to communication patterns associated with various psychiatric disorders. This book is helpful for conceptualizing communication problems and planning appropriate interventions.

Satir, V.: Peoplemaking, Palo Alto, Calif., 1972, Science & Behavior Books, Inc.

The focus of this book is on family development and role structure as it describes roles that facilitate or block healthy communication. How the use of blocking roles contributes to manipulative behavior is shown.

*Schwartzman, S.T.: The hallucinating patient and nursing intervention, J. Psychiatr. Nurs. **13**:23, Nov.-Dec. 1975.

The author discusses auditory hallucinations in the context of the interpersonal theory of psychiatry. Case study and good discussion of nursing intervention with a hallucinating patient are included.

Searles, H.F.: Collected papers on schizophrenia and related subjects, New York, 1965, International Universities Press, Inc.

A highly respected psychoanalyst presents his views on psychotherapy with schizophrenic patients in a readable manner. The book is impressive because of the empathy with his patients that the author has obviously experienced.

Shostrom, E.L.: Man, the manipulator, Nashville, Tenn., 1967, Abingdon Press.

This is a comprehensive analysis of manipulative behavior in terms of the development, manifestations, and implications of manipulation. It specifically relates theory to various interpersonal situations and describes the therapeutic approach.

*Topf, M., and Dambacher, B.: Teaching interpersonal skills: a model for facilitating optimal interpersonal relations, J. Psychosoc. Nurs. Ment. Health Serv. **19**:29, Dec. 1981.

These authors base an approach to interpersonal relationships on two dimensions: status and feelings. From these, they derive principles of effective social relations. These are interpersonal complementarity, interpersonal versatility, and interpersonal influence. They suggest that patients may benefit from being taught how to utilize these principles.

Torrey, E.F.: Surviving schizophrenia: a family manual, New York, 1983, Harper and Row, Publishers.

This excellent resource on schizophrenia was written for a lay audience, but is also worthwhile reading for professionals. The author is a physician who is also an advocate for high quality treatment for the seriously mentally disabled. He views schizophrenia as a brain disease and presents evidence supporting his belief.

Walsh, M.: Schizophrenia: straight talk for families and friends, New York, 1985, William Morrow and Co., Inc.

This book is an excellent presentation of the impact of schizophrenia on the family. The author is very frank in describing her experiences with the mental health care system and those of other families. Nurses should also recommend this book to families of patients. It contains much information and advice, including a list of rehabilitation resources.

*Will, G.T.: A sociopsychiatric nursing approach to intervention in a problem of mutual withdrawal on a mental hospital ward, Psychiatry **15**(2):193, 1952.

This article should be read and reread by every student of psychiatric nursing. It demonstrates the use of the nursing process to problem solve and provide therapeutic nursing care for withdrawn patients.

Will, O.A.: Human relatedness and the schizophrenic reaction. In Stein, M.I., editor: Contemporary psychotherapies, New York, 1961, The Free Press.

This absorbing account of psychotherapy with schizophrenic patients is based on the interpersonal theory of psychiatry; there are excellent descriptions of Sullivan's theory applied to the etiology and course of schizophrenia.

World Health Organization: Report of the international pilot study of schizophrenia. Vol. 1: Results of the initial evaluation phase, Geneva, 1973, The Organization.

World Health Organization: Schizophrenia: an international follow-up study, New York, 1979, John Wiley & Sons, Inc.

These two volumes present the results of a longitudinal epidemiological study of schizophrenia that took place in nine countries. These reports detail the construction of the study, as well as data collected and conclusions reached. These books are highly recommended for nurses who are interested in research, education, or advanced clinical practice.

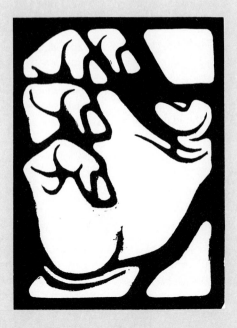

Healthy children raised in decent conditions among loving people in a gentle and just society where freedom and equality are valued will rarely commit violent acts toward others.

Ramsay Clark, A Few Modest Proposals to Reduce Individual Violence in America*

C H A P T E R   1 8

PROBLEMS WITH THE EXPRESSION OF ANGER

*Reprinted by permission from page 2 in *Violence and the Violent Individual* by J. Ray Hays, Thomm Kevin Roberts, and Kenneth S. Solway (eds.). Copyright 1981, Spectrum Publications, Inc., New York City.

LEARNING OBJECTIVES

After studying this chapter, the student should be able to:

- define anger in relationship to anxiety resulting from a threat.

- describe the continuum of behavior related to the feeling of anger.

- compare and contrast the biological/instinctual, frustration-aggression, and social learning theories concerning the predisposing factors related to anger.

- identify precipitating stressors related to the expression of anger.

- analyze biological responses to anger relative to high levels of anxiety and the fight-or-flight response.

- differentiate among passive, aggressive, and assertive behaviors.

- identify coping mechanisms relative to the experience of angry or aggressive feelings.

- formulate individualized nursing diagnoses for patients with problems with the expression of anger.

- assess the relationship between nursing diagnoses and medical diagnoses associated with anger.

- develop long- and short-term individualized nursing goals with patients who are experiencing problems with the expression of anger.

- examine one's own responses to anger.

- describe the process involved in developing assertive behavior.

- apply therapeutic nurse-patient relationship principles with appropriate rationale in planning the care of the angry patient.

- set appropriate limits on acting-out behavior.

- describe safe procedures for intervention in potential or actual violent behavior.

- develop a mental health education plan to assist the patient to express anger assertively.

- assess the importance of the evaluation of the nursing process when working with patients with problems with the expression of anger.

- identify directions for future nursing research.

- select appropriate readings for further study.

Anger is a feeling of resentment that occurs in response to heightened anxiety when the individual perceives a threat. It is characterized by a feeling of tension, and there is a need for the discharge of the tension. It is possible to suppress the overt expression of anger, but sooner or later, perhaps in a very different form, the tension will be released. The chronically angry person may develop a duodenal ulcer, become depressed, or explode inappropriately at a minor mishap. These are all signs that anger has not been expressed productively. Other persons may deal with anger by joining the army, kneading bread, or writing a symphony. These expressions are examples of sublimation and may be constructive for the individual. However, the basic issue is still avoided.

Direct expression of anger at the time that it occurs and toward the immediate cause is the healthiest and most satisfying way of releasing the tension. For most people this is also the most difficult response. Culturally, direct expression of anger is discouraged. Children are taught to "play nice" and to allow visitors to play with their toys, not even complaining if something is broken. Little boys who fight are chastised; little girls should never even think of fighting. Because of these attitudes, many people grow up fearing anger and viewing it as abnormal. This gives rise to the use of indirect means to express angry feelings.

Fear of expressing anger is related to fear of rejection. Parental disapproval is a powerful influence on the child's behavior. In adulthood similar disapproval is anticipated if one becomes angry at significant others. Yet it is hard not to become angry at those to whom one is close. When people are dependent or interdependent on each other, there is the expectation that needs will be anticipated and met. Sometimes there is even the irrational belief that needs will be recognized by the other without direct expression. When needs are not met, disappointment and, frequently, anger result. One then faces an inner conflict, because direct expression of anger to the other person may result in rejection, thus further reducing the possibility of gratification. On the other hand, failure to express the feeling leads to resentment and interferes with open participation in the relationship. Rothenberg[29] states that "when anger is accompanied by a clear communication, it is a sign of basic respect for a loved person."

People also become angry at life situations. If the car breaks down or the bank is closed or the taxes go up, an individual becomes angry. However, this anger seems to be much easier to express. In fact, the person may repeat the story several times, apparently becoming more emotionally aroused each time. This kind of experience can help the person express stored up anger and is a displacement of angry feelings from a threatening to a less threatening situation.

For some people, life situations become so unmanageable and overwhelming that anger builds up to the point of erupting explosively as violent behavior. It is known that poverty, unemployment, and family instability contribute to a higher incidence of family violence and violent crime.

Continuum of responses to anger

Anger may be described as on a continuum. Mild anger is an everyday part of life and is experienced as annoyance. Small annoyances may be forgotten almost immediately. For instance, most people have had the experience of undressing and discovering a small bruise, not remembering how it happened. Earlier in the day they probably bumped themselves, cried out, and promptly forgot the whole incident. Most people have no difficulty handling this level of anger.

At the next level there is interference with the accomplishment of a goal, resulting in frustration. For example, a sudden thunderstorm may cause the cancellation of a family picnic. There is temporary confusion as those affected share their feelings of angry disappointment. However, when feelings have been expressed, verbally or nonverbally, alternatives are considered and modified goals are set. The feelings associated with the experience will be remembered but are quickly resolved.

Further along the continuum, anger is more intense when frustration occurs and acceptable alternatives cannot be found. The person who has lost a job or has been told he has a terminal illness may feel anger related to impotence. This level of anger is more difficult to express and to resolve. Frequently the object of the anger is impervious to the person's feelings. This anger

may preoccupy much of the person's attention and interfere with his ability to function productively. Concerned support from significant others, and sometimes professional counseling, may be necessary to help the person reestablish equilibrium.

The extreme experience of anger is rage or fury. Rothenberg[29] differentiates anger from violence, hostility, and revenge, which involve destructiveness. At this level the person is totally consumed by angry feelings and unable to control their expression. It is at this point that violence may occur, and there is a danger to the angry person and to others who are nearby. Rage may result from a long series of frustrating experiences that have depleted the person's coping abilities. It is also seen in psychotic states when the person is completely unable to cope with frustration. It is a primitive response and is, in fact, seen in babies and small children who have not yet developed adaptive mechanisms. The fury of a 2-year-old having a temper tantrum would be difficult to control in an adult. This extreme degree of anger is frightening. Fear of losing control and becoming violent inhibits many people from overtly expressing anger.

Novaco[24] has identified the following positive functions of anger:

1. **Energizing function.** Anger energizes behavior.
2. **Expressive function.** Open expression of anger characterizes a healthy relationship.
3. **Self-promotional function.** Anger can be used to project a positive self-concept.
4. **Defensive function.** Anger serves as an ego defense in response to elevated anxiety by externalizing the conflict.
5. **Potentiating function.** Anger gives a sense of greater control over a situation.
6. **Discriminative function.** Anger can serve as an alerting mechanism and indicate a need for coping behavior.

Awareness of the positive aspects of anger is important to the implementation of a therapeutic nurse-patient relationship. Rather than discouraging the expression of anger, the nurse may help the patient to use its positive functions constructively. Figure 18-1 illustrates the continuum of responses to anger from constructive to destructive.

Nurses encounter anger frequently in the course of providing patient care. A disruption in health, no matter how minor it may appear, is a frustration, and frustration results in anger. In addition, the health care system is complex and may add to the patient's frustrations, leading to still more anger. It is therefore important for

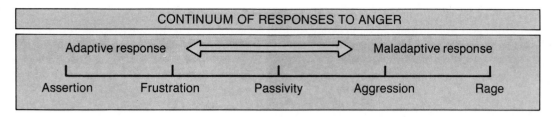

Fig. 18-1. Continuum of coping responses related to feelings of anger.

nurses to understand anger, to become aware of their own responses to angry feelings, and to help patients express anger in a healthy and productive way.

Unfortunately, nurses may also encounter instances in which the anger of a staff member is expressed inappropriately toward a patient. Patient abuse is a persistent problem in health care settings, particularly if staff are working under stressful conditions. Abuse may be physical, ranging from handling a patient roughly to actual physical assault. It may also be psychological, including speaking rudely, cursing, sarcasm, or ignoring a patient's needs. Whenever a nurse encounters this upsetting situation, there is a legal and ethical obligation to intervene directly if the patient is in immediate danger. If there is no immediate danger, the nurse may choose to report the incident to the appropriate supervisory nurse. Ignoring an incident of patient abuse only increases the likelihood that it will recur in the future. The principles discussed in Chapter 32 on the abusive family may also be applied to abuse that occurs in a health care setting.

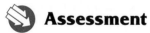 **Assessment**

There are several theories of the nature of the process of anger. In general, they may be categorized as biological, psychological, and social. There is no definitive evidence at present that gives one theory more validity than any other. There is a strong probability that anger really results from a combination of all these factors combined with the person's unique personality structure.

■ **Predisposing factors**

■ **BIOLOGICAL FACTORS**

Instinctual drive theory. Two major theorists, Sigmund Freud and Konrad Lorenz, have hypothesized that human aggression evolves from instinctual drives. Late in the development of his psychoanalytical theory, Freud came to believe that the person was under the influence of two basic drives. The first was the life drive, expressed through sexuality. This he called Eros. The second was the death drive, expressed through aggres-

sion. This he called Thanatos. Freud believed that life was a struggle to maintain a balance between the two drives. He hypothesized that destructive behavior such as suicide occurred when the death drive gained supremacy. Because of the strength of the drive, humans were always pressured to behave destructively, with the aim being either toward the self or toward others. This was described by Fromm as the "tragic alternative."[11:15] This particular theory of Freud's was not well received by many of his followers and was not thoroughly explored by him, since it was developed rather late in his career.[11]

Konrad Lorenz is a physician and naturalist. His theory of aggression is based on observations of animals, from fish and birds through the evolutionary ladder to humans. He believes that there is an instinctual aggressive drive that is common to all animals. Lorenz[19] acknowledges that this theory may be difficult for people to accept because of the comparison between human beings and other species. However, he maintains that human aggression derives from the same type of instinctual force as that of other species. He also states that modern man "suffers from insufficient discharge of his aggressive drive."[19:243] This inability to release aggression may result in various self-destructive behaviors, including neuroses and accidents.

An interesting and controversial aspect of the instinctive theories is that there is no allowance for the exercise of control by the individual. Essentially, they state that aggression will occur no matter what the person does. For some this idea is repugnant, since it implies that humans are simply the slaves of their drives. To others it is appealing because of the implication that the individual need not assume responsibility for his behavior. However, the hypothesis that aggression originates instinctively does not preclude the possibility of a variety of options for the discharge of aggressive feelings. The related behavior may be constructive or destructive according to the choices available to the individual.

Psychosomatic theory. Another biologically based theory views anger as a psychosomatic phenomenon. Stearns defines anger as a "combination of uneasiness, discomfort, tenseness, resentment (which is a response to selective stimuli) and frustration."[31:6] Anger may result from either environmental or internal stimuli and is characterized by an identifiable physiological response linked to activity of the sympathetic branch of the autonomic nervous system. Environmental stimuli have to do with the transmission of information, which, primarily through visual and/or auditory perception, provokes an angry response. Internal physiological stressors may include endocrine imbalance, such as hypothyroidism or hyperthyroidism, hypoglycemia, hunger, and fatigue,[31] as well as convulsive disorders and brain tumors. Ochitill[25] has identified additional factors that predispose the individual to violent behavior. Substance abusers are prone to violent outbursts, especially if deprived of their supply of drugs. The experience of pain results in irritability, sometimes progressing to violence. Also, some types of organic brain disorder may lead to violent behavior, particularly if there is a lesion in the part of the brain responsible for mediating anger.

Montague[22] describes the biological mechanisms that are believed to be associated with the experience of anger. She describes stimulus complexes that activate neural circuits, causing a tendency for the individual to behave aggressively toward environmental stimuli. The involved neurons are located in various areas of the brain and may be facilitated or inhibited by inputs from other neural systems. The limbic system plays a central role in both stimulating and inhibiting the aggressive responses. Research in this area is being pursued. This research is difficult because the affective areas tend to be buried deep in the primitive areas of the brain, and therefore much of the research so far has been performed on animals. Fromm[11] links this neural response to the "fight-or-flight" mechanism and views it as an innate method of self-preservation.

■ **PSYCHOLOGICAL FACTORS**

Frustration-aggression theory. One psychological approach to the evolution of aggressive behavior is the frustration-aggression theory developed by Dollard and co-workers.[8] According to this theory, all aggression results from an experience of frustration. Frustration occurs when the person is thwarted in an attempt to achieve a desired goal, whether this is because the goal is unrealistic or an obstacle is placed between the person and the goal. The sense of frustration, and thereby the degree of aggression, is increased if the goal is highly valued or if the person has made repeated attempts to achieve it. According to Fromm,[11] this theory has been criticized recently because there is no allowance for stressors other than frustration that might lead to aggression.

Frustration may be experienced as a threat. When people are threatened, they become anxious. The emotional response to the anxiety that results from a threat may be experienced as anger. In addition to frustration, there are other threats that lead to anger. One is the threatened loss of self-esteem. In this case the stressor may be real, as in the threatened loss of a job, or imagined, as when a mother interprets her child's leaving home for college as a rejection of herself. Conflict may also be viewed as threatening and lead to an aggressive response. An important element of a threatening situation is the person's perceived lack of control. Aggression can be an attempt to overcome the threat by taking control of the situation.

Coffey[5] relates the occurrence of violence to a feeling of impotence. Several potential sources of anger have been identified by Maynard and Chitty.[21] They support the frustration-aggression theory by stating that blocked progress toward a goal may lead to anger. Another cause is the failure by a valued person to live up to one's expectations. Anger may also arise when an individual is forced to confront his shortcomings and admit his weaknesses. Finally, a threat to authority frequently leads to an angry response. A common thread in this analysis of anger is disappointment in the achievement of established expectations whether of the self or of another person.

Behavioral theory. Another psychological approach to anger and aggression is that of the behaviorists. They view aggression as a learned response that has been reinforced by facilitating goal achievement. For instance, 4-year-old Johnny wants a cookie just before dinner. When his mother refuses, Johnny has a temper tantrum. If his mother then gives him a cookie, Johnny has learned that an aggressive outburst will be rewarded. If similar situations continue to occur in his life, Johnny will use an aggressive approach to need satisfaction. It is important to note that others learn that nonaggression is rewarded. Thus the behaviorists explain the range of aggressive behaviors that exist.

Existential theory. As an existential theorist, Erich Fromm[11] presents a different psychological theory. He believes that behavior is based on several existential needs. These include the needs for an object of devotion, relatedness, unity and rootedness, effectiveness, and stimulation and excitation. These needs must be met. For each need there are both positive and negative behavioral means to achieve satisfaction. The need for effectiveness may be met by loving productive behavior or by sadistic destructive behavior. When the person is not able to meet his needs through positive constructive behavior, he will resort to negative destructive behavior. Fromm describes the latter person as an "existential failure, a man who has failed to become what he could be according to the possibilities of his existence." The failure is a result of social conditions, combined with the individual's reason and will.

■ **SOCIOCULTURAL FACTORS.** Social and cultural factors may also have an influence on the occurrence of angry behavior. Cultural norms help to define acceptable and unacceptable means of expressing aggressive feelings. Sanctions are applied to violators of the norms through the legal system. By this means society controls violent behavior and attempts to maintain a safe existence for its members. Unfortunately, this prohibition against violent behavior is often extended to include any form of expression of anger. This inhibits people from healthy expression of angry feelings and thereby leads to behavior indicative of suppressed anger.

Social environment theory. The social environment in which the person lives influences his attitude toward expressing anger and the means he chooses to do so. A cultural norm supporting verbally assertive expressions of anger will assist persons to deal with anger in a healthy manner. A norm that reinforces violent behavior will result in physical expression of anger in destructive ways. Madden[20] notes that persons who have a history of being victimized are more likely to become violent. They have internalized a norm legitimizing aggressive acting out of anger. He also links a history of deprivation, inadequate social adjustment, and a lack of interpersonal relationship skills with increased incidence of violent behavior.

Urban life tends to foster increased aggressive behavior. In part, this may be related to the theory of personal space. Crowding is prevalent in cities. When people have little privacy or when they feel that their area of personal space has been invaded, there is frequently an aggressive response. In ghetto areas, where overcrowding is common, this anger becomes a smoldering resentment, which can erupt into violence, as was demonstrated in the riots of the late 1960s. Fast[9] reports on a study by Kinzel in which personal space needs of men who were imprisoned for violent behavior were compared to those of prisoners with no history of violent behavior. It was found that the violent group required twice the personal space of the nonviolent group. What would seem to most people to be a comfortable interpersonal difference would for these men be a provocation to a violent outburst. This tendency combined with alcohol use is particularly explosive, since usual social inhibitions are decreased as a result of drinking.

Issues related to personal space are also pertinent in a hospital setting. Nursing and medical care that involves touching is a direct invasion of intimate space. Patients may attempt to identify areas that belong to them, usually including the area immediately surrounding the bed, but sometimes extending to other areas, such as a particular chair in the day area or dining room. Intentional or accidental use of this space by another can lead to an angry outburst. Lathrop[16] has identified other characteristics of the hospital milieu that can lead to aggressive behavior, such as the following:

1. Staff disagreement concerning the treatment of a patient
2. Anger, distrust, and conflict among the staff
3. Staff inconsistency
4. A significant change in medication

She identifies the common element in these situations as the removal of a source of support for the patient. This is experienced as a threat, leading to a feeling of vulnerability. Aggression may result as the person tries to gain control of the situation. When aggressive behavior occurs in a hospital setting, it is important to analyze the characteristics of the milieu, as well as those of the patient. Intervention in staff behaviors sometimes results in positive behavioral change for patients.

Social learning theory. Social psychologists have formulated the social learning theory to explain the development of aggressive behavior. According to Roberts, this theory was originated by Miller and Dollard and later extended by first Rotter and then Bandura and Walters.[28] According to these theorists, aggressive behavior is learned as a part of the socialization process. This is essentially a behaviorist model of personality development. Children who grow up in violent settings learn to use aggression as an acceptable means of meeting their needs. Aggressive behavior may be learned by imitation or by direct experience.[28] Imitation may be related to the family, subculture, or symbolical models. It has been noted that parents who were victims of child abuse are more likely to abuse their own children. This is an example of imitation of a familial pattern. Subcultural patterns that lead to imitation of aggressive behavior involve the acceptance of violence as a means of achieving status. These include such diverse activities as violent crime, aggressive sports, and war. Symbolical modeling is best exemplified by the probable influence of television on the occurrence of violent behavior. There have been court cases in which the defense for a violent crime was the fact that the assailant had watched a similar act on television. It has also been observed that following a well-publicized act of violence, such as an assassination or mass murder, there is frequently a spate of similar assaults or threats of assaults. A cultural paradox in the United States is the contrast between the generally stated value that peace is good and the fascinated attention that is given to violence.

According to social learning theory, the other way of learning aggressive behavior is by direct experience.[28] This aspect of the theory draws heavily on behavioral theory: behavior that is rewarded will recur. This approach has been discussed as a psychological predisposing factor related to aggression. Social learning theorists also accept the premise that biological components of aggressive behavior interact with the psychosocial aspects. It is most likely that overt acts of aggression occur as a result of the interaction of the person's biological, psychological, and sociocultural characteristics, and each of these factors must be considered as components of the nursing assessment.

■ Precipitating stressors

The specific precipitants of angry behavior are individualized. The nurse needs to communicate with the patient in order to understand the events that he perceives as anger-provoking. In general, anger occurs in response to a perceived threat. This may be a threat of physical injury, or more common, a threat to the self-concept. When the self is threatened, the person may not be entirely aware of the source of his anger. In this case, the nurse and patient need to work together to identify the nature of the threat.

The threatening event may be external or internal. Examples of external stressors are physical attack, loss of a significant relationship, and criticism from others. Internal stressors might include a sense of failure at work, perceived loss of love, and fear of physical illness. Anger is but one of the possible emotional responses to these stressors. Some individuals might respond with depression or withdrawal. However, those reactions are usually accompanied by anger, which may be difficult for the person to express directly. Depression is sometimes viewed as anger directed toward the self, and withdrawal may also be a passive expression of anger.

Frequently, the event that appears to precipitate an outburst of anger does not seem proportionate to the intensity of the response. This is because people often have difficulty revealing their anger. The anger is stored and a relatively insignificant experience may be "the last straw" resulting in the release of a flood of feelings. Nurses need to be aware of this and to refrain from personalizing anger expressed by a patient. The nurse may seem to be a safer target than significant others with whom the patient may also be angry. If an angry experience is to be understood, stressors must be evaluated in terms of number, intensity, and meaning to the patient.

Violence or the threat of violent behavior may be the result of fear of loss of control and a search for external limits. Nigrosh[23] relates this to two factors. The first is a need to accomplish the developmental task of self-control. Lack of control is thus associated with infantile behavior. The second factor is the internalization of values opposing violence. Violation of this norm results in the experience of guilt. Patients who communicate imminent loss of control need prompt provision of external controls.

Other events may precipitate violent behavior in hospitalized patients. Conn and Lion[6] have documented that assaults on staff were most likely to occur during the process of seclusion of a patient, in the course of a verbal argument, or following denial of a privilege by a staff member. Depp[7] studied the occurrence of assaults in a public mental hospital and found that assaults were more common when there was a high level of demand for patients to increase their activity. This tended to happen between 6 and 8 A.M., on Mondays, and when there was a larger than usual number of staff working. Another finding was that the communication to the patient of low staff expectations for positive change and improvement appeared to lead to violent behavior. In planning care and in prevention of episodes of aggressive behavior, nurses need to consider these possible precipitants of the violent expression of anger.

■ Behaviors

■ **PHYSIOLOGICAL.** When a person becomes angry, the response is evident in both physiological and psychological behaviors. The physical feeling of anger is uncomfortable and, according to Stearns, results primarily from activity of the sympathetic fibers of the autonomic nervous system in response to secretion of epinephrine. In some instances there is also evidence of parasympathetic involvement. The cardiovascular response includes increased blood pressure and heart rate. It has been demonstrated that the tachycardia does not result from vagal stimulation. It is therefore believed to result from epinephrine secretion. Blood composition is also altered, with fewer lymphocytes and increased free fatty acids. Gastrointestinal behaviors reveal a combination of sympathetic and parasympathetic innervation. Behaviors include an increase in salivation, nausea, either increased or decreased secretion of hydrochloric acid, decreased gastric peristalsis, and, sometimes, constipation. The central nervous system responds to anger with increased alertness. Electroencephalographic changes have also been noted when anger is induced in experimental situations. There is an increase in muscle tension and heightened deep tendon reflexes. Frequency of urination is usually increased. Sensory alertness is enhanced and dilatation of the pupils is generally noted.[31]

■ **FIGHT-OR-FLIGHT RESPONSE.** These behaviors are usually labeled the "fight-or-flight" response. When the individual perceives a threat, there are two alternative reactions available. One is to confront the threat—to stand and fight. Many animals choose this response only when cornered. Because of social learning, humans may place a value on fighting and may choose this response even if it is not essential. The alternative is flight—to escape from the threat by removing oneself from its influence. Flight may involve leaving the scene of the threat or may be accomplished by emotional withdrawal. In the flight situation the individual's emotional response would probably be fear rather than anger.

Since the person responds to a threat by preparing to flee or to fight, the physiological response in fear and in anger is similar. Essentially, the person is prepared for the activity that is about to take place. Hyperalertness helps him to analyze the situation, including assessing the extent of the threat and scanning the environment for any additional threatening circumstances. Since the anxiety level is increased, mental activity is stimulated—at first productively—but the person's responses may become fragmented and confused if anxiety reaches panic levels (Chapter 12). Blood flow is diverted from the viscera to the skeletal muscle groups and the brain, since more activity will be required of these areas. In addition, the rate of blood flow is greater to speed nutrients to the cells. The respiratory rate increases in proportion to the body's increased need for oxygen. Subjectively, the person generally feels tense and flooded by feelings of resentment and hostility. When overwhelmed by intense anger, the person may act spontaneously without conscious planning of the behavioral response.

Penningroth[26] relates the fight-or-flight response to the situation of the hospitalized psychiatric patient who is feeling threatened by loss of control of his life. He points out that the opportunities for flight are limited, putting the patient in the situation of having to fight. This sequence of events may lead to episodes of violent behavior, as illustrated in Clinical example 18-1.

This patient demonstrates the following attributes of violence identified by Nigrosh[23]:

1. *A subjective threat to the self.* This person had felt threatened as a result of his delusional ideas about his neighbors. He was then threatened further by the demand that he remove his clothing.
2. *Loss of control.* The patient became overwhelmingly anxious and resorted to a fight-or-flight response, first fleeing and then, when cornered, fighting.

CLINICAL EXAMPLE 18-1

Mr. B was a 32-year-old man with a medical diagnosis of paranoid disorder who was admitted to the locked ward of a psychiatric hospital because he had been arrested after his neighbors complained that he was letting the air out of their tires. He said that he did this because the neighbors laughed at him and talked about him when he was out walking his dog. He was angry about being arrested and wanted to leave the hospital but was held under commitment because he also threatened to burn down the house of the neighbor who had called the police.

Mr. B resisted cooperating with the admission procedure. He belligerently demanded to be released, threatening to call the governor and "sue everybody in the place." When he was asked to undress for a physical examination, he ran down the hall and barricaded himself in the dining room. As staff forcibly entered the room, he began to lash out. Several staff members removed him to a seclusion room where he was given intramuscular medication and isolated until he regained control of his behavior. He paced the floor and pounded on the door for 30 minutes before he began to appear calmer.

Several days later, when Mr. B was used to the staff and felt more comfortable in the hospital, he related to a nurse, "I hope I didn't hurt you the other night, but I didn't know what you wanted to do to me. A man has to protect himself, you know."

---

3. *Levels of self control.* The range of violent actions extends from attacks on inanimate objects to homicide. This person's behavior escalated from letting air out of tires to attempting to assault staff.
4. *Diminished capacity to think and speak.* This patient was impaired in his ability to reason. This interfered with his capacity for reasoning out his anger and his alternatives for response to it. The use of cognitive processes can mediate violent behavior by allowing anticipation of consequences, prediction of the possible response of others, and devaluation of the importance of the antagonist.

Had the staff applied this approach to understanding violent behavior, the patient could have been given time to adjust to his new situation and to establish a degree of control before being confronted with a new threat.

> ## CLINICAL EXAMPLE 18-2
>
> Ms. J was a staff nurse on a busy surgical unit. She enjoyed her work and liked the patients. She also placed a high value on getting along with her co-workers. Other staff members always spoke positively of her. Ms. C, the head nurse, valued Ms. J as an employee, stating particularly, "She's not like the rest of them. She never complains."
>
> Ms. J made it a practice never to refuse a request made by a patient or another staff member. If a patient who was assigned to another nurse asked her to explain his diet or straighten his bed, she would do so, even if she was then behind in her own work. She never asked for help from others, since she felt that her assignment was her responsibility. If a co-worker asked to change days off with her, Ms. J always agreed, even if she had plans, rationalizing that the other person probably had more important plans.
>
> Ms. C began to sense a tenseness when she was around Ms. J. Since she could not think of any problem at work, she assumed that Ms. J must have been having a problem at home. She was concerned and asked Ms. J if she could help. To her amazement, Ms. J recited a long list of angry feelings related to the work situation. Ms. C then felt guilty when she realized that she and the other staff members had been taking advantage of Ms. J.

■ **ASSERTIVENESS.** Wolpe is one of the major behavioral theorists. He has provided the impetus for the development of the theory of assertiveness as a positive behavioral expression of one's rights. The basic assumption of assertiveness theory is that every individual has a right to behave in a way that meets his needs, as long as he does not impinge on the rights of another person. The primary obligation is to oneself. However, assertiveness theorists believe that this approach to need gratification also enhances the esteem of the other. The assertive person assumes that the other person also has the right and the ability to act in his own best interest.

Passive behavior. Assertiveness is at the midpoint of a continuum that runs from passive to aggressive behavior. The passive person consistently subordinates his own rights to his perception of the rights of others. When the passive person becomes angry, he tries to camouflage it, thereby creating increased tension in himself. In addition, if the other person becomes aware of the anger by observing nonverbal cues, he is deprived of the opportunity to confront the issue. This can in-

crease his tension as well. This pattern of interaction can seriously impair growth in an interpersonal relationship. Clinical example 18-2 illustrates passive behavior.

Although Ms. J had thought that she was acting in a healthy, mature way, she was actually negating her own needs and thereby diminishing her self-respect. Her co-workers, who superficially liked her, in reality felt uncomfortable with her because they were never allowed to reciprocate when she had been helpful to them. Ms. C's guilty response quickly changed to anger when she realized that she had been a victim of Ms. J's passivity. If Ms. J had informed Ms. C of her feelings, she would have treated her more equitably.

Chenevert[4] has listed ten basic rights for people in the health professions. They are the rights to

1. Be treated with respect
2. Have a reasonable workload
3. Be paid an equitable wage
4. Determine one's own priorities
5. Ask for what is wanted
6. Refuse without making excuses or feeling guilty
7. Make mistakes and assume responsibility for them
8. Give and receive information as a professional
9. Act in the best interest of the patient
10. Be human

Nurses like Ms. J tend to ignore these basic rights, which leads to passive, rather than direct, expression of anger.

A passive response to anger usually results in an indirect expression of the angry feelings. This was the source of the tension that Ms. C felt in this situation. Bach and Goldberg[3] have written about the "nice" people. They believe that a lack of aggression must cover up a great potential for violence. In their view, direct expression of aggressive feelings is healthy and desirable. "Nice" people are frequently passive-aggressive. At a superficial level they are concerned, interested, and sympathetic. However, there is an underlying tone of hostility that contradicts the superficial message. For example, a therapist may tell a patient in a condescending tone of voice, "You're doing very well—much better than I expected." Although the verbal message is overtly supportive and complimentary, the tone of voice conveys the hostile message "You're such a loser, I'm amazed that you get along as well as you do." The patient is at a real disadvantage in this situation. If he passively accepts the statement, he keeps peace with the therapist but decreases his own self-esteem. If he challenges the hostile undertone, he runs the risk of bringing the therapist's anger to the surface and of being labeled "paranoid." This is an example of a double-bind situation (Chapter 17), which involves a passive-aggressive message.

Passivity is also expressed nonverbally. The person may speak softly, frequently in a childlike manner. There is little eye contact from a passive person. Body language communicates diffidence and self-denial. The person may be slouched in posture and generally holds his arms close to his body. Fidgeting also communicates passivity. Gestures are seldom used, although the head may be nodded in agreement (even when the person really disagrees).

Sarcasm is another indirect expression of anger. This usually provokes anger in the person who is the target. It is differentiated from assertive behavior because it usually infringes on the rights of the other. A sarcastic remark generally conveys the message "You are not worthy of my respect." Sarcasm may be disguised as humor. Confrontation may then be responded to with a disclaimer such as "Can't you take a joke?" Humor that derogates another person is hostile and is indulged in for the purpose of self-enhancement. It tends to backfire because the joker is revealed as insecure and needing to downgrade others to bolster his own self-esteem.

Aggressive behavior. At the opposite end of the continuum from passivity is aggression. The aggressive person ignores the rights of others. He operates under the assumption that every person must fight for his own interests and he expects the same behavior from others. Life is a battle. An aggressive approach to life may lead to violence, either physical or verbal. The aggressive behavior frequently covers a basic lack of self-confidence. The person enhances his self-esteem by overpowering others and thereby proving his superiority. Clinical example 18-3 describes aggressive behavior.

Aggressive adults are not unlike Suzy. They try to cover up their insecurities and vulnerabilities by acting aggressive. The behavior is self-defeating because it drives people away, thus reinforcing the low self-esteem and vulnerability to rejection.

Aggressive behavior is also communicated nonverbally. The aggressive person usually speaks loudly with great emphasis. He may invade personal space and usually maintains eye contact over a prolonged period of time so that the other person experiences it as intrusive. Gestures may be emphatic and often seem threatening (e.g., the person may shake his fist, stamp his foot, or make slashing motions with his hands). Posture is erect and often the aggressive person leans foward slightly toward the other person. The overall impression is one of power and dominance.

Assertive behavior. In contrast to the passive and aggressive nonverbal behaviors, assertive behavior conveys a sense of self-assurance but also communicates respect for the other person. The assertive individual

---

CLINICAL EXAMPLE 18-3

Suzy was a 9-year-old girl brought to the child psychiatric clinic by her mother on referral from the school nurse. She was described as a "tomboy" who loved active play and hated school. She was the first girl to make the neighborhood Little League baseball team and had proved her right to be there by beating up several male team members. Suzy was sent to the clinic after the teacher caught her forcing younger children to give her their lunch money.

When Suzy came to the clinic, she presented a facade of toughness. She did not deny her behavior and explained it by saying that the "little kids don't need much to eat anyway. I let them keep some of the money." Suzy was saving money for a new baseball glove. When she was asked about school, she said angrily, "I'm not dumb. I could learn that junk, but who needs it. I just want to play ball."

Psychological testing revealed that Suzy's IQ was slightly below average. She attended school with a group of upper middle class college-bound children. Even in the fourth grade she was feeling insecure and unable to compete. She masked her insecurity with her bullying behavior, striving for acceptance in sports, where she did have ability. The medical diagnosis was conduct disorder, undersocialized, aggressive. When Suzy's problem was explained to her parents and the school, some of the pressure for academic achievement was alleviated. Her parents spent extra time helping her with her homework. Also, she was given genuine recognition for her athletic ability, demonstrated by the gift of a new baseball glove. Suzy gradually responded to the positive input from others by developing a sense of positive regard for herself. As she did so, she no longer needed to bully other children and began to grow into some real friendships.

---

speaks clearly and distinctly. He observes the norms of personal space appropriate to the situation. Eye contact is direct but not intrusive. Gestures are utilized to emphasize speech but are not distracting or threatening. Posture is erect and relaxed. The body language may be symmetrical with that of the other party. The overall impression is one of strength, but not threatening.

The content of assertive speech focuses on the individual's interpretation of his rights in the situation at hand. The assertive person feels free to refuse an unreasonable request. He will, however, share his rationale with the other person. He will also base the judgment about the reasonableness of the request on his own priorities. On the other hand, the assertive person does not hesitate to make a request of others, assuming that they will inform him if his request is unreasonable. If the other person is unable to refuse, the assertive individual will not feel guilty about making the request.

Assertiveness also implies communicating one's feelings directly to others. This applies to both negative and positive feelings. As a result, anger is not allowed to build up and the expression of feeling is more likely to be in proportion to the situation. If dissatisfaction is verbalized, the reason for the feeling is included. Assertive people also remember to express love to those to whom they are close. Compliments are given when deserved. Assertion also involves acceptance of positive input from others. Think about the real message in this brief interaction:

MARY: **That's a pretty dress, Jane. Is it new?**
JANE: **This old thing? I've had it for years. I couldn't find anything else to wear today.**

What did Jane really say to Mary? The implication is that Mary has poor taste to admire a dress that Jane thinks so little of. If Jane were assertive, she would thank Mary for the compliment and perhaps even agree with her that it really is a pretty dress.

Within each person lies the capacity for passive, assertive, and aggressive behavior. When one is confronted with a threat, therefore, there are options in terms of how to respond. These choices are to be passive, fearful, and to flee; to be aggressive, angry, and to fight; or to be assertive, self-confident, and to confront the situation directly. It is important that all these

choices do exist because none are inherently good or bad. Rather, the situation and the characteristics of the individuals involved define the appropriate response. When confronted by a mugger on a deserted street, one may assertively explain why the mugger should change his mind. However, if flight is available, it might be a better choice, or passive submission might be safer. Similarly, if the children are being persistently annoying and getting on mother's nerves, aggressively telling them to stop may be most effective. The problem related to assertiveness is not that people are sometimes passive or aggressive but that they do not have the option of being assertive because they have not learned how. Table 18-1 summarizes the major characteristics of passive, assertive, and aggressive behaviors.

■ **ACTING-OUT BEHAVIOR.** A variation on the indirect expression of angry feelings is acting-out behavior. Acting out may also convey such feelings as love, fear, or guilt, but frequently it involves anger. Acting out refers to behavior that attracts the attention of others and represents the feelings or conflicts the person is experiencing. Adolescents often use this behavior as they deal with the crises of that developmental stage, but acting out is by no means limited to teenagers. Loomis[18] points out that acting out is not a controllable behavior until the person understands the reason or learns alternative behaviors. In therapy it is frequently related to transference feelings. Clinical Example 18-4 illustrates this concept.

Peter's acting-out behavior was complex and in part unconsciously motivated. He was particularly frightened by feelings of caring, which made him vulnerable

---

TABLE 18-1

COMPARISON OF PASSIVE, ASSERTIVE, AND AGGRESSIVE BEHAVIORS

	Passive	Assertive	Aggressive
Content of speech	Negative Self-derogatory "Can I?" "Will you?"	Positive Self-enhancing "I can" "I will"	Exaggerated Other derogatory "You always" "You never"
Tone of voice	Quiet, weak, whining	Modulated	Loud, demanding
Posture	Drooping, bowed head	Erect, relaxed	Tense, leaning forward
Personal space	Allows invasion of space by others	Maintains a comfortable distance; claims right to own space	Invades space of others
Gestures	Minimal, weak gesturing, fidgeting	Demonstrative gestures	Threatening, expansive gestures
Eye contact	Little or none	Intermittent, appropriate to relationship	Constant stare

CLINICAL EXAMPLE 18-4

Peter was a 16-year-old boy who was referred to a halfway house for adolescents because he could not get along in a foster home setting. He refused to obey rules, used drugs, and constantly argued with the foster parents. He was consistently truant from school, where he had completed the eighth grade. He had been arrested once for stealing hubcaps, but the charges were dropped. Peter's family of origin had fallen apart when his parents divorced when he was 5 years old. His father left town and had no further contact with Peter. His mother was alcoholic and lost custody of her children to the city Department of Social Services when neighbors reported her for neglect. Although she never tried to regain custody of Peter, even after she remarried, she also never agreed to his adoption. Peter had spent 11 years moving from foster home to foster home—eight in all. At first, he had tried to get along, but he soon discovered that his behavior had little effect on how he was treated. He then began to use whatever means he could to meet his own needs.

When Peter entered the halfway house, he was initially agreeable, followed the rules, and seemed to be making a good adjustment. He was particularly close to a young male counselor and spent hours talking with him about his thoughts, feelings, and past experiences. However, after about 3 weeks, several small, mysterious fires were discovered in the house. They had obviously been set. After the group of residents were confronted with the situation, another boy approached a counselor and said he had seen Peter setting a fire. When presented with the evidence, Peter acknowledged that he had been the culprit and asked when he would have to leave. He seemed disbelieving when he was told that he could remain if he assumed responsibility for his behavior. He questioned why he was being trusted. Later, when talking with his counselor, he related that he had felt a need to get away from the house because he was beginning to like it. He feared that he would be hurt if he stayed and was later rejected. At a deeper level, his counselor believed that Peter was testing to see if the counselor really cared about him as he seemed to or if he would abandon him as his parents had when he was a small child. Unconsciously, Peter had always thought that he was responsible for his parents' divorce, since he had been told regularly that he was a bad person. Peter's medical diagnosis was conduct disorder, socialized, aggressive.

to hurt when the relationship ended. His response to this imagined threat of loss was to take the initiative and assume control of the situation by causing his dismissal from the home. If the sequence had gone as he expected, Peter would have also reinforced his beliefs about his own worthlessness and the vindictiveness of other people. When trust and concern were conveyed to Peter, he was able to begin to reassess some of his beliefs about himself and other people. Because the staff in this facility was used to working with acting-out behavior, Peter's experience became the beginning of a time of growth in self-awareness.

Misdirected anger also contributes to the development of other emotional problems. In particular, anger that is redirected toward the self and experienced as guilt is a prominent feature of depression, as described in Chapter 15. At other times internalized anger may be expressed physiologically as a psychosomatic illness. This mechanism has been considered in depth in Chapter 13.

■ Coping mechanisms

Many everyday activities serve to meet the demands of the aggressive drive. The competition that is so valued in Western cultures is fueled by aggression. Accomplishment of work often requires a degree of aggressiveness for success. People cope with aggressive feelings by using the energy they provide for productive accomplishments.

When aggression is uncontrolled, problems result. The anger that is then felt requires the implementation of psychological coping mechanisms. Since the anger is an expression of anxiety aroused by a threat, the ego defense mechanisms described in Chapter 12 are helpful. Angry feelings are frequently displaced. For instance, the man who was treated unfairly by his boss complains to his wife about the dinner she prepared. Sublimation also helps one to cope with angry feelings. Some great works of art reflect the anger that was felt by the composer or artist at the time the work was created. Music, in particular, can also help listeners to dispel some of their anger. This probably influences the popularity of musical fads such as "punk rock," whereby young people can ventilate some of their hostility toward the system in a nondestructive way.

A less healthy means of coping with anger is projection. In this case the angry feelings are attributed to someone or something else. As an example, the person who is flooded with unconscious hostile impulses may believe that others are plotting to kill him. This particular mechanism does not facilitate healthy functioning, since the person essentially trades his anger for fear. Repression may also apply to anger. However, the repression of anger contributes to what Rubin[30] refers to as the "slush fund," and later the anger reappears as hostility, explosiveness, bigotry, manipulation, and many other distorted expressions.

Madden[20] has identified denial as a prominent defense mechanism related to violent behavior. Denial is in operation when a person with a history of violent behavior asserts that he has no problem with violence. It is also apparent when an individual expresses lack of concern about the consequences of his behavior. This show of bravado is really protecting a very low self-esteem.

Reaction formation is the mechanism that underlies passive-aggressive behavior. Although the person presents an ingratiating facade, this is a defense against anger that the person is unable to express directly. Other defense mechanisms may also be used as an unconscious response to anger. The limitation inherent in any of them is that the real motivation for the observable behavior is outside of awareness. Thus the person is not able to examine his behavior and modify it.

There are also direct, conscious responses that may help to cope with anger. One is physical activity. Sometimes angry people need a time to work off the excess physical energy associated with the biological response. They can then deal more effectively with the interpersonal ramifications of the experience. Hitting a punching bag or taking a brisk walk is preferable to punching a friend and is also healthier than trying to set the feeling aside. An activity break also allows the person to review the situation and gain perspective before assertively confronting it.

Nurses also use coping mechanisms when they are confronted with angry behavior which has the potential for evoking their own anger. This is revealed in a countertransference response to the patient. Because it may not seem acceptable to express anger at a patient, the nurse may deny anger, which is then reflected indirectly in her relationships with the patient and others. Another mechanism that may be an attempt to cope with countertransference anger is projection.[10] In this case the nurse may provoke the patient to act out her own anger, resulting in scapegoating. Denial and projection may both lead to increased angry behavior by the patient who senses the nurse's inability to deal with this feeling. For this reason, it is critical for the nurse to be aware of her own response to anger and to use supervision to help understand her behavior.

Each person develops an individualized style for coping with anger. This results from past experiences, parental modeling, and cultural expectations. The key point to consider in assessing the person's coping ability is whether this personal style facilitates the expression of the angry feelings. If they are allowed to accumulate and fester or if they are expressed explosively, the person needs help in developing new, more satisfying coping mechanisms.

Nursing diagnosis

When formulating a nursing diagnosis relative to a patient's angry behavior, the nurse needs to consider the nature of the threat or physiological disruption to which the person is responding. This would include the predisposing factors and circumstances discussed as stressors. In addition, the observable response to the threat should be stated as the nursing care problem. The model in Fig. 18-2 summarizes the relationship between anger, anxiety, low self-esteem, and guilt. It indicates the two possible modes of expression of the anger—externally in either constructive or aggressive behavior, or internally in either nonassertive or self-destructive behavior. This model may be helpful to the nurse in formulating a nursing diagnosis.

The nursing diagnostic statement includes the identification of the nursing problem, the stressor that is responsible for the problem, and a statement of the behavior that provides evidence that the problem exists.

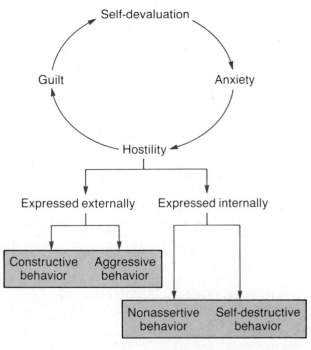

Fig. 18-2. Model representing the expression of anger.

Whenever possible, the patient should participate in the process of formulating the nursing diagnosis. However, a person who is experiencing a problem with the expression of anger may feel too threatened at first to be able to describe the problem clearly. Some patients who are using the coping mechanisms of denial and projection may actively resist identifying their problem as one involving anger.

Primary NANDA nursing diagnoses and examples of complete nursing diagnoses related to problems with the expression of anger are presented in the accompanying box. Since patients with this as their primary problem are likely to experience associated disruptions in behavior, other nursing diagnoses that are frequently applicable to these patients and relevant medical diagnoses from the Draft of DSM-III-R in Development[2] are presented in Table 18-2. These should not be interpreted as exhaustive, but should serve as a guide when conducting the assessment and formulating the diagnosis. The comprehensive plan of care will reflect the total range of the patient's biopsychosocial needs for nursing care.

There are multiple possible individualized nursing diagnoses related to anger. They will vary according to the source of anger, degree of anger, frequency of angry feelings, direction of anger, chosen mode of expression, and the person's physical condition. It can be challenging to recognize that a given behavior is a representation of anger and to identify the stressors involved. People often mask their anger and redirect it. Good communication among health team members can facilitate the successful accomplishment of this part of the assessment

process. Fig. 18-3 illustrates the nursing model of health-illness phenomena related to the expression of anger.

■ Related medical disorders

Several medical diagnostic categories include behaviors that may indicate problems with the expression of anger. These include the affective disorders, organic mental disorders, schizophrenic disorders, anxiety disorders, and personality disorders. These are discussed in other chapters of this book. The classifications of medical disorders that are primarily characterized by problems expressing anger are briefly described.

■ **OPPOSITIONAL DISORDER.** The essential features are argumentativeness, defiance, irritability, spitefulness, bullying, blaming others and frequent loss of temper for at least six months.[2]

■ **CONDUCT DISORDER.** Conduct disorders are associated with childhood and adolescence. The essential feature is a repetitive and persistent pattern of conduct characterized by a variety of antisocial behaviors such as lying, stealing, truancy, fighting, cruelty to others, destruction of property and substance abuse.[2]

■ **DELUSIONAL (PARANOID) DISORDER.** The essential feature is a nonbizarre delusion that focuses on everyday life experiences, such as a feeling of persecution, jealousy, a physical disorder (somatic), grandiosity or that a higher status person is in love with one (erotomanic).[2]

■ **ORGANIC PERSONALITY SYNDROME (EXPLOSIVE TYPE).** The essential feature includes recurrent outbursts of aggression without adequate provo-

---

Nursing Diagnoses Related to Problems with the Expression of Anger

Primary NANDA nursing diagnoses

Violence, potential for: directed at others
Coping, ineffective: individual

Examples of complete nursing diagnoses

Potential for violence directed at others related to the delusional perception that his life is in danger evidenced by verbal statements that the staff wants to kill him

Potential for violence directed at others related to need to control others evidenced by refusal to follow hospital rules

Potential for violence directed at others related to brain tumor evidenced by confusion and hypersensitivity to interpersonal stimuli

Ineffective coping related to inability to confront others directly with angry feelings evidenced by excessive use of sarcasm

Ineffective coping related to denial of angry feelings evidenced by statement, "I never get angry."

TABLE 18-2

MEDICAL AND NURSING DIAGNOSES RELATED TO PROBLEMS WITH THE EXPRESSION OF ANGER

Medical Diagnostic Class	Psychiatric Nursing Diagnostic Class
Disruptive behavior disorders	Problems with the expression of anger
Delusional disorder	
Related Medical Diagnoses (DSM-III-R*)	**Related Nursing Diagnoses (NANDA)**
Oppositional disorder	Anxiety
Conduct disorder	Communication, impaired: verbal
Delusional (Paranoid) disorders	†Coping, ineffective: individual
Organic personality syndrome (explosive type)	Grieving, dysfunctional
	Injury, potential for
	Posttrauma response
	Powerlessness
	Self-concept, disturbance in
	Social isolation
	†Violence, potential for: directed at others

*American Psychiatric Association: Draft of the DSM-III-R in Development (subject to change), as proposed by the Work Group to Revise DSM-III. American Psychiatric Association, October 1985.
†Indicates primary nursing diagnoses for problems with the expression of anger

---

cation and with evidence of abnormal brain function or structure.[2]

 ## Planning and implementation

■ Goal setting

Mutually set long- and short-term nurse-patient goals are essential to guide the intervention process. Long-term goals will be directed toward the constructive use of angry energy to accomplish tasks and to motivate self-growth. Short-term goals serve as guideposts along the way, helping the nurse and the patient to identify the progress of the therapeutic experience. If, for instance, the nursing diagnosis is job dissatisfaction resulting from inability to say no to the boss, a long-term goal would be "In 6 weeks the patient will assertively inform his boss when he is unable to accept a new responsibility that is offered to him." Related short-term goals might include the following:

1. In 1 week the patient will develop a list of present job responsibilities and time commitments.
2. In 2 weeks the patient will refuse a request from a salesperson whom he does not know.
3. In 3 weeks the patient will refuse a request from a neighbor.
4. In 4 weeks the patient will refuse a request from his wife.
5. In 5 weeks the patient will rehearse refusing a request from his boss that he take on more work.

This type of progression of behavioral goals gives the patient the sense of mastery and control that is sometimes the objective of aggressive behavior. It also makes a task that may at first appear overwhelming seem manageable. This is particularly important in working with a patient who becomes frustrated easily. It also meets the need for patient education, since the patient is a full participant in the therapeutic plan and should have input into devising the goal hierarchy.

■ Intervening in problems with the expression of anger

■ **SELF-AWARENESS.** Angry patients are frequently labeled as problem patients because of the responses of the nurses who are assigned to care for them. The attempt to provide nursing care may deteriorate into a power struggle as the nurse and the patient each strive to be the person in control. To avoid this outcome, the nurse should use the data collected about the patient to help identify the nature of his behavior and the reason for it.

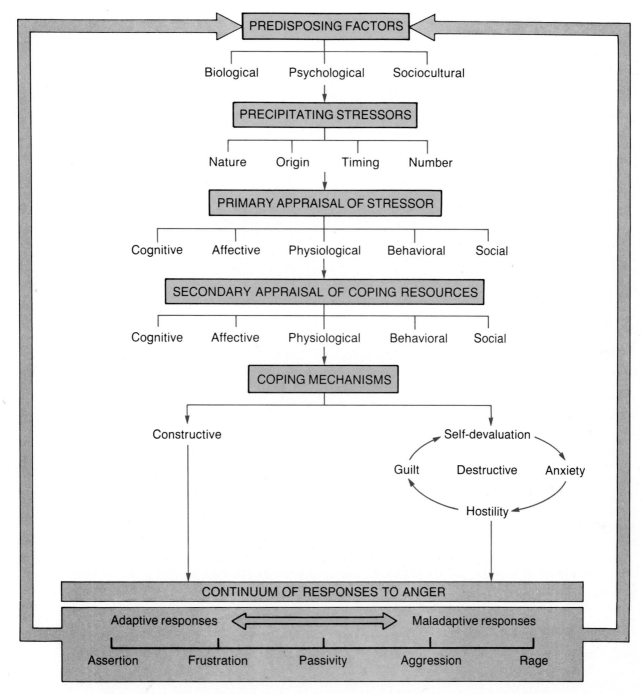

Fig. 18-3. Nursing model of health-illness phenomena related to the expression of anger.

If the person is experiencing anger for reasons that are primarily physiological (e.g., an endocrine imbalance, a brain lesion), the nurse may find it easier to accept outbursts of angry behavior. She can intellectually explain the reason for the patient's anger and may conclude that he "can't help it," thereby circumventing the power struggle aspect. This is particularly true if there is the expectation that medical intervention will soon bring the patient's behavior under control.

More often, the reason for the patient's behavior is hidden or not really related to the nurse. It is then harder to deal with the anger and more difficult not to take it personally, especially if it is expressed as an attack on the nurse's competency. Because it is threatening to be the recipient of anger, the nurse needs to develop an awareness of her own usual response to anxiety, threatening situations, and anger. There are several responses indicative of lack of self-awareness that are not therapeutic or productive.

Nontherapeutic responses. One nontherapeutic response to patient anger is **defensiveness.** The defensive nurse interprets the patient's anger as a personal attack and immediately tries to explain her actions to prove that the perceived attack is unjustified. For example, Ms. B, a nurse, awakened Ms. R, a patient who was hospitalized for control of her diabetes mellitus. When Ms. B told the patient that she had to give her an injection of insulin, Ms. R said, "You people here don't know anything. All you do is wake me up. I'm here for a rest, you know. Some rest!" Ms. B responded with a detailed explanation of why it was important for Ms. R to have her insulin at the correct time and also offered explanations for the possible reasons for the behavior of other staff members. The more she talked, the angrier Ms. R became. Following the interaction, the nurse described the interaction to her head nurse, who pointed out that Ms. R was probably responding to multiple feelings about hospitalization. That, combined with the interruption of her plan to withdraw for a while by sleeping, led to an attack that was not really directed toward Ms. B. The nurse's response was a result of her own insecurity and discomfort with anger.

A response by the nurse that is detrimental to the patient is one of **retaliation.** The nurse "pulls rank" or asserts herself as the one with the authority in the health care setting. For instance, Ms. T, an elderly patient, requested a bedpan. She had already called the nurse to her bedside several times with small requests that were not really urgent. The nurse labeled her behavior as indirectly aggressive. After she gave the patient the bedpan, she went to check on another patient at the other end of the hall. Fifteen minutes later she returned to Ms. T, who had finished with the bedpan long before her return. When Ms. T mentioned this fact, the nurse responded by saying, "I do have other patients. I can't spend all my time here with you." In reality, she could have removed the bedpan before looking in on the other patient. She, too, was responding to the superficial meaning of the patient's behavior. The nurse believed that the patient was irritable and deliberately seeking attention to annoy her. Actually the patient was frightened, lonely, and angry because she knew she would be going to a nursing home instead of her own house. The nurse's retaliatory behavior only reinforced the patient's feelings.

Somewhat related to retaliation is an attitude of **condescension.** The nurse assumes an attitude of superiority and discounts the patient's concerns. Mr. J was in the coronary care unit after a myocardial infarction. He was a hard-driving executive who was very frustrated because his physician had forbidden any contact at all with his business. When the nurse brought his lunch, he angrily refused to eat it and referred to the food as "garbage." The nurse replied, "Now really, Mr. J, you're acting like a child. Surely Dr. A has told you that it's important for you to eat. Let's have no more of this silliness." Mr. J then sat straight up in bed and shouted at the nurse, "Get out of my room! Right now!" After the nurse left, she told a co-worker, "He certainly is obnoxious. He'll kill himself unless he controls that bad temper." This nurse's approach only increased the patient's anxiety and ultimately his anger. He was already feeling impotent and did not need to hear himself compared to a child. Furthermore, he was given the message that his anger was unjustified and should not be expressed. On the other hand, the nurse later acknowledged that Mr. J's anger could be destructive but did not recognize that suppression of his feelings could be as harmful as explosive expression of them. Had she realized this, she would have spent some time helping him to explore his feelings and acquire some sense of mastery in the situation.

Another commonly noted nontherapeutic response to the patient's anger is **avoidance.** In avoidance, the nurse simply refuses to recognize or to deal with the patient's feelings. For instance, Mr. M said to his nurse as she changed his dressing, "You know, I think my doctor is botching my case. That infection is no better. I think he's a real quack." The nurse continued with the procedure and after a moment said, "Did your wife visit yesterday, Mr. M? She seems like such a nice person—so concerned about you." Mr. M sighed and closed his eyes as the nurse completed the procedure. Later she said to a friend, "That Mr. M is a strange one. He hardly responds at all when you talk to him." This nurse was prevented by her own defensive system from even acknowledging Mr. M's angry statement. He felt more frustrated and resorted to withdrawal when she did not acknowledge his statement. He also extended his assessment of the physician's ability to include the nurse.

■ **ASSERTIVENESS TRAINING.** The interactions described demonstrate the need for the nurse to be aware of her own response to anger in others. Otherwise the nurse's feelings may actually interfere with her ability to provide effective patient care. The nurse who responds to anger either passively or aggressively needs to take steps to modify her approach. Assertiveness training for the nurse can help to fulfill this need. Not only will she grow in self-awareness and be better able to respond therapeutically to her patients, but she will also be more likely to experience job satisfaction.

Alberti and Emmons[1] recommend to the nurse the following process for the development of assertiveness:

1. Observe your behavior.
2. Keep a record of assertive and nonassertive behavior.
3. Select one situation for examination.
4. Review your behavior in the selected situation.
5. Observe an effective person in action in a similar situation.
6. Identify alternative responses.
7. Put yourself in the place of the effective person; imagine how you would act.
8. Practice the new approach by role playing.
9. Provide yourself with feedback; repeat step 4. Get feedback from others if available.
10. "Behavior shaping"—practice the new response until you begin to feel comfortable.
11. Practice the new approach in a real situation.
12. Repeat training if necessary or apply to other problem areas where you wish to change.
13. Take note of social reinforcement—the positive response of others to your new assertive behavior.

A nurse who undertakes a self-growth program to develop assertive behavior is also learning a process that can be helpful to patients who experience difficulty in expressing anger. A healthy approach to the expression of anger is essentially a problem-solving approach. The steps to assertiveness just described are really components of a problem-solving process. They may be compared to the steps to dealing with anger recommended by Hays[12]:

1. Acceptance of the self as a person who experiences angry feelings
2. Exploration to find the reason for the anger
3. Constructive direction of the energy that is generated by the anger

Assertiveness training, in contrast, tends to deemphasize the reason for the response. This is consistent with its behavioral model origins. However, assertiveness theory provides a framework for the accomplishment of Hays' step 3.

Another model for intervention with an angry patient is described by Maynard and Chitty.[21] (This is represented in the mental health education plan presented in Table 18-3.)

These authors also advocate encouraging the patient to evaluate the experience and the feedback by the nurse.[21] This model includes most of the steps described

in the assertiveness training approach. However, it maintains a focus on the readiness of the patient for each step of the process. The role of the nurse is to guide the patient and to provide emotional support and honest feedback.

■ **LIMIT SETTING.** At times the nurse needs to intervene with a patient who is expressing his anger in ways that infringe on the rights of others. When this happens, it is necessary to set limits on the patient's behavior. Limit setting is not a punitive response to behavior, although the patient may experience it that way. It is a nonmanipulative confrontation in which the patient is informed what behavior is acceptable, what is not acceptable, and the consequences attached to behaving unacceptably. The nurse does not assume responsibility for the patient's behavior, positive or negative. It is recognized that the patient has the right to choose his preferred mode of behavior as long as the consequences are clear as well. Limits should be clarified before the negative consequences are applied. Otherwise the consequence is punitive and the patient may feel tricked.

Once a limit has been defined, the consequences must take place if the behavior occurs. Every staff member must be aware of the plan and carry it out. If this consistency is absent, the patient is likely to manipulate staff by acting out and then pointing out areas of inconsistency in limit setting. Firm, but not hostile, enforcement of limits is preferable. If the nurse responds angrily, she is less likely to see the situation clearly. This is also an indication that a power struggle is taking place. Power struggles are usually detrimental to the treatment plan.

Loomis[18] has identified three steps in the limit-setting process:

1. State expectations to the patient in a positive way.
2. Help the patient explore the reason for and meaning of his behavior.
3. Consider with the patient alternative ways to express his feelings.

This approach avoids rejection of the patient and conveys the attitude that the patient has the right to experience angry feelings and the ability to express them appropriately. Clinical example 18-5 shows acting-out behavior and constructive limit setting.

The nurse in this example applied the problem-solving process. She planned her nursing intervention and then approached Mary in a reasonable, adult-to-adult way. Ms. T was selected by the nursing staff to work with Mary because she did not have a punitive response toward marijuana use. This facilitated

TABLE 18-3

MENTAL HEALTH EDUCATION PLAN FOR THE PATIENT WHO HAS PROBLEMS WITH THE EXPRESSION OF ANGER

Content	Instructional activities	Evaluation
Assist the patient to identify anger	Focus on nonverbal behavior Role play nonverbal expression of anger Label the feeling using the patient's preferred words	The patient can demonstrate an angry body posture and facial expression
Give permission for angry feelings	Describe situations in which it is normal to feel angry	The patient describes a situation in which anger would be an appropriate response
Practice the expression of anger	Role play fantasized situations in which anger is an appropriate response	The patient participates in role play and identifies behaviors associated with expression of anger
Apply the expression of anger to a real situation	Assist the patient to identify a real situation which makes him angry Role play a confrontation with the object of the anger Provide positive feedback for successful expression of anger	The patient identifies a real situation which has made him angry He is able to role play expression of anger
Identify alternative ways to express anger	List several ways to express anger, with and without direct confrontation Role play alternative behaviors Discuss situations in which alternatives would be appropriate	The patient participates in identifying alternatives and plans when each might be useful
Confrontation with a person who is a source of anger	Provide support during confrontation if needed Discuss experience after confrontation takes place	The patient identifies the feeling of anger and appropriately confronts the object of the anger

Adapted from the model of intervention developed by Maynard, C.K., and Chitty, K.K.: Dealing with anger: guidelines for nursing intervention, J. Psychiatr. Nurs. 17:36, June 1979.

her being able to help Mary look at the reasons for her behavior and to select a constructive alternative. The interaction also served as the foundation for a therapeutic nurse-patient relationship between Mary and Ms. T.

■ **CONTROL OF VIOLENCE.** Unfortunately, some patients have more difficulty controlling their feelings and using angry energy constructively. A patient who loses control of his anger becomes violent. Violence refers to behavior that is physically assaultive and risks injury to the self, others, and the environment. The nurse in the psychiatric setting must develop the ability to deal with violent behavior in a way that minimizes the danger to all concerned.

Prevention of violence is preferable if it is possible. The intense anxiety associated with violent feelings is communicated interpersonally. By empathizing and carefully observing patients' behavior, the nurse may be

able to anticipate a violent outburst. Sometimes when a patient is on the verge of losing control, the atmosphere of the nursing unit becomes filled with tension. When the nurse becomes aware that tension is mounting, intervention may avoid an outburst. The nurse may isolate the disturbed patient from the rest of the patient group; may talk with the patient if he is receptive to this approach; and may give prescribed medication. Some patients respond to vigorous physical activity to express their anger, but this approach should be used with care, since it may also precipitate loss of control.

A patient who is on the verge of violent behavior is usually experiencing a panic level of anxiety. Nursing interventions related to patients who are in panic are described in Chapter 12. Kronberg[13] has recommended several interventions with the patient who is threatening to lose control. She suggests speaking softly, slowly, and with assurance. Directions should be given clearly and should be concise. It may be helpful to assist the patient to verbalize his feelings. The nurse should take care to protect the patient's self-esteem and dignity.

Felthous[10] suggests creating a social norm against violence. The norm needs to be clearly stated to the patient group and repeated periodically. Patients need to be involved in the establishment of the norm. This may be accomplished by such means as asking them to assist in writing an orientation manual for new patients, and by discussion of the norm in community meetings. Communication should focus on the creation of a comfortable, safe environment for everyone. Any episodes of violence that do occur should be discussed in a group meeting, and alternatives should be discussed with the patient group.

Self-protection is a concern when the nurse is working with a potentially violent patient. The nurse should never risk being hurt by failing to take adequate precautions for her own safety. Whitman[32] recommends the following precautions:

1. Never see a potentially violent person alone.
2. Call police or security staff if their help is needed.
3. Keep a comfortable distance away from the patient. Avoid intruding on his personal space.
4. Maintain a clear exit route for both the staff and patient.
5. Be prepared to move. Violent patients can strike out suddenly.
6. Be sure the patient has no weapons in his possession before approaching him.
7. If it is necessary to restrain a patient, have an adequate number of nursing staff on hand.
8. Give prescribed antianxiety or antipsychotic medication when it is needed.
9. Be supportive to the patient and intervene to increase his self-esteem.

If the patient does become violent, immediate response is essential. Penningroth[26] advises an initial assessment of the situation, followed by a plan for intervention, and then action. Enough people should be available to ensure the safety of the patient and staff. Staff members should be taught good body mechanics and methods of holding a struggling patient without causing injury. One person should direct the group action. Also, someone should talk with the patient, explaining what is happening and the reason for the intervention. Most violent patients are reassured if they see that they can be controlled and prevented from inflicting injury. Lenefsky, de Palma, and Locicero[17] recommend two to four people, depending on the situation. If the person is very disturbed, there should be one staff person assigned to restrain each limb and a fifth person to

direct the activity and communicate with the patient. Roles should be assigned prior to intervention, with the person who has the best relationship with the patient acting as communicator. It is also the responsibility of the nurse to be sure that there are staff available to stay with and support the other patients. They should be removed from the area if possible. Sometimes a "show of force" by the presence of several staff members will be enough to assist the patient to regain control and be able to talk about his feelings. The importance of a sense of confidence on the part of the staff has been emphasized.[17] They should be well-informed about the situation before taking action. All staff members in a psychiatric setting should receive training in the prevention and management of violent behavior, including an opportunity to discuss feelings and attitudes about this aspect of nursing care. It can be reassuring to a violent patient to see that his uncontrollable behavior can be

---

CLINICAL EXAMPLE 18-5

Mary was a 17-year-old girl who was admitted to the hospital for suspected hyperthyroidism. She quickly became bored with the hospital routine and phoned several of her friends to visit her. When the nursing staff was making rounds at the shift change, they found several teenagers in Mary's room. There was also a strong aroma of marijuana. Since there was a hospital limit of two visitors at a time, some were asked to leave. The group was also informed that marijuana smoking was not allowed in the hospital.

After visiting hours Ms. T, a young staff nurse, sat down to talk with Mary. She initiated a discussion of Mary's restlessness and irritability, which had led to the suspicion that she had a hyperthyroid condition. Mary readily shared her frustration with being in the hospital and her anxiety about her condition. Then she said, "I suppose you guys are mad at me for the pot, but that's a dumb rule. It's healthier than cigarettes, you know." Ms. T replied that she and the other nurses were not mad, but that they did expect Mary to obey the rule, now that she knew it. She also told Mary that she was responsible for telling her friends the rule. The consequence, if the behavior occurred again, would be restriction of visitors to her parents only. The nurse then initiated a discussion of what Mary might do to help out on the unit and thereby use some of her excess energy. Mary began to look excited and shared her love for plants. She proposed that she might visit other patients and help them care for their plants and flowers.

controlled and that he can be prevented from causing harm. The patient who has become violent may need medication or seclusion to help him gain control. These therapeutic techniques are discussed further in Chapters 22 and 23.

The last step in nursing intervention with a violent patient is to review the incident with the patient after he has achieved control. This helps the patient alleviate any guilt he might be feeling or fear that he might have harmed someone. The nurse can, in retrospect, review what happened and talk about alternatives should the patient become anxious and angry in the future.

Unfortunately, nurses are sometimes assaulted by patients. It is impossible to be totally successful in predicting and preventing all episodes of violent behavior in a psychiatric setting. If a staff member is assaulted, she or he needs the support and assistance of colleagues. Lanza[14,15] has studied the reactions of nursing staff to physical assault by a patient. The response is similar to that experienced during the post-traumatic stress syndrome. Surprisingly, she found that many staff members were reluctant to identify any response to the assault. The investigator thought that this might be related to a sense of guilt for not having prevented the episode and concern that others would not understand. Recently, there has been debate about whether staff should be encouraged to file legal charges against a patient who has assaulted them and did not appear to be unable to control his behavior. Phelan and associates[27] presented several points in support of filing charges. They included the creation of a public record of assaultive behavior, allowing a judge and jury to fulfill their duty of determining responsibility, possible deterrence of future attacks, and the potential for harsher penalties for repeat offenders. Phelan and associates attributed much of the difficulty that staff have in pursuing this course of action to the ethical dilemma of deciding whether the patient was actually responsible for his behavior. In addition, if care providers feel guilty for allowing the incident to occur, they are unlikely to take legal action against the patient. This is an issue that must be resolved by the nurse based on the situation. It would also be very helpful to seek the advice of a trusted professional mentor.

Dealing with anger is a challenge for both the nurse and the patient. Nursing interventions with patients who have problems with the expression of anger are summarized in Table 18-4. Anger is not inherently good or bad. Expression of anger is not always positive or negative. Effective dealing with anger implies that the person can accept his right to be angry and the reciprocal right of others to be angry. It is not therapeutic to encourage a patient to express angry feelings indiscrim-

inately. It is important that the patient feel free to choose whether to express anger and that, when he chooses to do so, he avoid abridging the rights of others. It is through this process that anger can facilitate growth.

 Evaluation

The evaluation of the nursing care provided to the patient who has problems with the healthy expression of anger should be based on observed behavioral change. The subjective response of the patient is also a helpful input. Maynard and Chitty[21] recommend that the following questions be asked of a patient who has had an experience of expressing anger:

- How do you feel about the experience?
- How did the other person behave in response to your anger?
- Was the confrontation well timed?
- Did the interaction take place in private?
- What would you change in the future?
- How would you change these aspects?

Evaluation should focus on the mode of expression of anger, the appropriateness of the object, the congruence between the degree of feeling expressed and the precipitating incident, and the patient's awareness of the process. If the patient does not change in the planned direction in one of these areas, the data base, goals, and nursing interventions should be reviewed and appropriate modifications made.

There should be a staff review of any episode of violent behavior. The focus of such a discussion is to dissipate any residual staff anxiety related to the incident and to objectively evaluate their performance. The situation should be analyzed to identify the precipitating stressors and the sequence of attempts to cope with the stress. Future prevention can be directed to alleviating stressors that seem to precipitate violent outbursts and to assisting the patient to develop more positive ways to deal with anger when it occurs. Feedback should be given to colleagues about the process of restraining the patient. Procedural modifications may be made as a result of this review.

If the patient is involved in learning techniques of assertiveness, the evaluation process is an integral part of the training program. Thus the patient should be involved in eliciting feedback about his behavior in selected situations. He should be encouraged to practice assertive behavior until he feels comfortable and consistently is perceived as behaving assertively. Patients in an assertiveness group may also participate in evaluating each other.

Successful problem solving in the area of assertively

TABLE 18-4

SUMMARY OF NURSING INTERVENTIONS WITH A PATIENT WHO HAS PROBLEMS WITH THE EXPRESSION OF ANGER

Goal: To recognize feelings of anger and, when appropriate, assertively communicate these feelings to other people

Principle	Rationale	Nursing intervention
Assertive expression of feelings	Passive behavior reinforces low self-esteem; anger builds up internally and may lead to depression; aggressive behavior also indicates insecurity and low self-esteem; the person may become isolated from others, leading to more hostility; violent behavior can result from pent-up anger; assertive behavior reinforces high self-esteem by protecting the individual's rights without violating the rights of others	Establish a trusting relationship Assist the patient to recognize and label anger Communicate that angry feelings are normal Identify usual means of coping with anger Support effective coping mechanisms Explore alternative behaviors Assist the patient to practice assertive expression Provide feedback
Promote respect for the rights of others	Adherence to reasonable limits on acting out behavior promotes socialization; expression of feelings is a reciprocal process and involves awareness of and respect for the rights of others; anger related to limit setting can be used to teach the person more effective coping behaviors	Inform the patient of acceptable limits for behavior, including rationale Clarify the patient's responsibility for his behavior Define the consequences for failure to observe rules Achieve staff agreement on definition of reasonable limits Enforce limits by implementing consequences if violations occur Explore reasons for acting out and identify alternative behaviors Give positive feedback for adherence to limits
Protection from harm to self or others	Violent behavior entails a high risk of physical injury to the patient and to others with whom he comes into contact, psychological damage may also occur as a result of guilt related to the patient's concern that he injured someone while out of control; outbreaks of violence decrease the sense of security that is important for people to feel while they are in the process of confronting their own disturbing behaviors, thoughts, and feelings	Maintain a calm, controlled, and consistent milieu Be alert to signs of tension If possible, remove an agitated patient from a stimulating situation Give antianxiety or antipsychotic medication for agitation Avoid challenges to the patient's self-esteem If restraining the patient is necessary: 1. Maintain the patient's dignity 2. Explain the procedure to the patient 3. Gather adequate trained staff to handle the situation 4. Avoid unnecessary force 5. Protect the patient and staff from injury 6. Review the situation with the patient and staff after calm has returned Discuss episodes of violent behavior with other patients who were present

expressing anger becomes a self-reinforcing process. As the patient successfully asserts himself, he experiences good feelings about himself and discovers that his needs are met more frequently. The assertive nurse experiences similar feelings and becomes increasingly effective professionally.

DIRECTIONS FOR FUTURE RESEARCH

The following are some of the nursing research problems raised in Chapter 18 that merit further study by psychiatric nurses:

1. The conditions that predispose to patient abuse
2. Primary prevention activities relative to patient abuse
3. Nurses' awareness of the presence of anger in others and their ability to label the feeling
4. Neural responses to anger-provoking, as compared to pleasure-provoking, stimuli
5. The occurrence of angry responses related to the amount of personal space allotted to the individual
6. The relationship between intrastaff dissension and episodes of angry behavior by patients
7. Nurse behaviors that promote or inhibit the expression of anger by patients
8. The relationship between intellectual understanding of assertive behavior and the incidence of assertive responses by nurses
9. The relationship between assertive behavior, perceived autonomy, and job satisfaction among nurses
10. The effectiveness of limit-setting interventions by nurses in response to selected acting-out behavior
11. The relationship between a nurse's comfort with assertive behavior and her effectiveness in setting limits with patients
12. Primary prevention nursing interventions relative to the occurrence of episodes of violent behavior by patients
13. Nursing interventions that will abort incipient episodes of violent behavior
14. Interventions with violent patients that minimize the risk of injury to the patient and to the involved staff members
15. Early identification of patients at risk for expressing anger through violent behavior
16. Interventions that assist staff members who have been assaulted by patients to recover from the experience
17. Validation of nursing diagnoses related to various modes and levels of expression of anger

---

■ SUGGESTED CROSS-REFERENCES ■

Therapeutic relationship skills and self-awareness of the nurse with respect to feelings are discussed in Chapter 4. The model of health-illness phenomena and the phases of the nursing process are discussed in Chapter 5. Nursing interventions to enhance self-esteem are discussed in Chapter 14. Facilitating a patient's expression of emotions and strengthening social skills are discussed in Chapter 15. Intervening with patients who have problems with interpersonal relationships is discussed in Chapters 15 and 17. Somatic therapies are discussed in Chapter 22. Nursing intervention in family abuse and violence is discussed in Chapter 32.

■ SUMMARY ■

1. Anger is a feeling of resentment that occurs in response to heightened anxiety when a person perceives a threat. Various overt and covert expressions of anger were described.

2. Anger is experienced on a continuum from mild annoyance to intense rage. Rage is destructive, but positive functions of anger were also described.

3. Biological predisposing factors include the instinctual drives postulated by Freud and Lorenz, as well as physiological disruptions such as endocrine imbalance, seizure disorders, and neoplasms.

4. Psychological predisposing factors were described, including the frustration-aggression theory of Dollard and co-workers, the behavioral theory, and the existential theory presented by Fromm.

5. Sociocultural predisposing factors include the imposition of social sanctions on behavior, crowding and intrusion on personal space, and role modeling by significant others and through the media. The social learning theory of anger was discussed.

6. Precipitating stressors that may result in anger were identified as a physical or psychological threat.

7. Physiological behaviors associated with anger result primarily from secretion of epinephrine and stimulation of the sympathetic nervous system. The behaviors resulting from this constitute preparation for fight or flight.

8. Assertive behavior was differentiated from passive and aggressive behavior as a constructive use of anger. Assertiveness theorists state that the individual has the right to pursue the gratification of his own needs so long as he does not infringe on the rights of others.

9. One may choose to be assertive or not. Assertiveness training enables the person to choose freely because he has the ability to act assertively if he wishes to accept the consequences of this behavior.

10. Acting-out behavior is often an indirect expression of anger. It attracts the attention of others and is a representation of the feelings the person is experiencing.

11. The coping mechanisms of goal-directed behavior and use of ego defense mechanisms were discussed.

12. Examples of nursing diagnoses relative to angry behavior were given and compared to selected medical diagnoses.

13. Long- and short-term goals for the development of healthy coping behaviors can guide the nurse and patient in their work together and provide a sense of accomplishment as progress is made.

14. The importance of self-awareness for the nurse was discussed. Nontherapeutic responses to a patient's expression of anger were identified as defensiveness, retaliation, condescension, and avoidance.

15. Assertiveness training is a problem-solving approach to dealing with anger that can help the nurse achieve self-awareness and improve her ability to cope with the angry patient. Steps to assertiveness were described.

16. Approaches to nursing intervention with the angry patient were introduced.

17. A mental health education plan for patients who experience problems expressing anger was illustrated.

18. Limit setting is a nursing intervention that may be employed with angry, acting-out patients. The patient is assumed to be responsible for his behavior and is informed of the consequences if the limited behavior occurs.

19. Intervention with the violent patient should focus on immediate control and safety, followed by discussion to alleviate guilt and identify alternative behaviors to help prevent future episodes of violence.

20. The legal and ethical dilemma of staff response to assault by a patient was presented.

21. Evaluation of the improved ability to express anger is based on objective and subjective feedback about the increased incidence of assertive behavior. The patient's increased self-esteem related to his improved communication skills tend to perpetuate assertive behavior once it has been learned.

■ REFERENCES ■

1. Alberti, R.E., and Emmons, M.L.: Your perfect right, ed. 2, San Luis Obispo, Calif., 1974, Impact Publishers.
2. American Psychiatric Association: Draft of the DSM-III-R in Development (subject to change), as proposed by the Work Group to Revise DSM-III. American Psychiatric Association, October 1985.
3. Bach, G.R., and Goldberg, H.: Creative aggression; the art of assertive living, New York, 1974, Avon Books.
4. Chenevert, M.: Special techniques in assertiveness training for women in the health professions, St. Louis, 1978, The C.V. Mosby Co.
5. Coffey, M.P.: The violent patient, J. Adv. Nurs. **1:**341, 1976.
6. Conn, L.M., and Lion, J.R.: Assaults in a university hospital. In Lion, J.R., and Reid, W.H., editors: Assaults within psychiatric facilities, New York, 1983, Grune & Stratton, Inc.
7. Depp, F.C.: Assaults in a public mental hospital. In Lion, J.R., and Reid, W.H., editors: Assaults within psychiatric facilities, New York, 1983, Grune & Stratton, Inc.
8. Dollard, J., et al.: Frustration and aggression, New Haven, Conn., 1939, Yale University Press.
9. Fast, J.: Body language, New York, 1970, Pocket Books.
10. Felthous, A.R.: Preventing assaults on a psychiatric in-
11. Fromm, E.: The anatomy of human destructiveness, New York, 1973, Holt, Rinehart & Winston, Inc.
12. Hays, E.: Anger: a clinical problem. In Burd, S., and Marshall, M., editors: Some clinical approaches to psychiatric nursing, New York, 1963, The Macmillan Co., Publishers.
13. Kronberg, M.E.: Nursing interventions in the management of the assaultive patient. In Lion, J.R., and Reid, W.H., editors: Assaults within psychiatric facilities, New York, 1983, Grune & Stratton, Inc.
14. Lanza, M.L.: The reactions of nursing staff to physical assault by a patient, Hosp. Community Psychiatry **34:**44, Jan. 1983.
15. Lanza, M.L.: A follow-up study of nurses' reactions to physical assault, Hosp. Community Psychiatry **35:**492, May 1984.
16. Lathrop, V.G.: Aggression as a response, Perspect. Psychiatr. Care **16:**202, Sept.-Dec. 1978.
17. Lenefsky, B., de Palma, T., and Locicero, D.: Management of violent behavior, Perspect. Psychiatr. Care **16:**212, Sept.-Dec. 1978.
18. Loomis, M.E.: Nursing management of acting-out behavior, Perspect. Psychiatr. Care **8:**169, 1970.
19. Lorenz, K.: On aggression, New York, 1966, Harcourt, Brace & World, Inc. (Translated by M.K. Wilson.)
20. Madden, D.J.: Recognition and prevention of violence. In Lion, J.R., and Reid, W.H., editors: Assaults within psychiatric facilities, New York, 1983, Grune & Stratton, Inc.
21. Maynard, C.K., and Chitty, K.K.: Dealing with anger: guidelines for nursing intervention, J. Psychiatr. Nurs. **17:**36, June 1979.
22. Montague, M.C.: Physiology of aggressive behavior, J. Neurosurg. Nurs. **11:**10, March 1979.
23. Nigrosh, B.J.: Physical contact skills in specialized training for the prevention and management of violence. In Lion, J.R., and Reid, W.H., editors: Assaults within psychiatric facilities, New York, 1983, Grune & Stratton, Inc.
24. Novaco, R.W.: The functions and regulation of the arousal of anger, Am. J. Psychiatry **133:**1124, 1976.
25. Ochitill, H.N.: Violence in a general hospital. In Lion, J.R., and Reid, W.H., editors: Assaults within psychiatric facilities, New York, 1983, Grune & Stratton, Inc.
26. Penningroth, P.E.: Control of violence in a mental health setting, Am. J. Nurs. **75:**606, 1975.
27. Phelan, L.A., Mills, M.J., and Ryan, J.A.: Prosecuting psychiatric patients for assault, Hosp. Community Psychiatry **36:**581, June 1985.
28. Roberts, T.K., Mock, L.A.T., and Johnstone, E.E.: Psychological aspects of the etiology of violence. In Hays, J.R., Roberts, T.K., and Solway, K.S., editors: Violence and the violent individual, Jamaica, N.Y., 1981, Spectrum Books.

29. Rothenberg, A.: On anger, Am. J. Psychiatry **128**:454, 1971.
30. Rubin, T.I.: The angry book, New York, 1969, Collier Books.
31. Stearns, F.R.: Anger: psychology, physiology, pathology, Springfield, Ill., 1972, Charles C Thomas, Publisher.
32. Whitman, J.: When a patient attacks: strategies for self-protection when violence looms, RN **42**:30, Sept. 1979.

■ ANNOTATED SUGGESTED READINGS ■

Alberti, R.D., and Emmons, M.L.: Your perfect right, ed. 2, San Luis Obispo, Calif., 1974, Impact Publishers.

This practical, straightforward presentation of assertiveness gives clear descriptions of assertive and nonassertive behavior and suggests ways to become more assertive. Part Two is directed toward the use of assertiveness training with patients and is recommended for readers who have advanced preparation in psychiatric nursing.

Bach, G.R., and Goldberg, J.: Creative aggression: the art of assertive living, New York, 1974, Avon Books.

The authors describe the many ramifications of misdirected anger. This book is particularly helpful in identifying family and cultural stressors leading to disruptions in the ability to express anger.

*Bowman, C., and Spadoni, A.J.: Assertion therapy: the nurse and the psychiatric patient in an acute, short-term psychiatric setting, J. Psychosoc. Nurs. **19**:7, June 1981.

This is an excellent presentation of assertiveness theory as applied in a short-term hospital setting. A detailed lesson plan outlines the six-session assertiveness therapy program that the authors have developed. They also discuss this therapeutic approach relative to behavioral therapy from which it was derived. This article is particularly recommended for nurses who have been trained to conduct assertiveness therapy and are planning to initiate a program.

*Campbell, W., and Mawson, D.: Violence in a psychiatric unit, J. Adv. Nurs. **3**:55, Jan. 1978.

The authors discuss the occurrence of violent behavior in an unlocked, architecturally open hospital. They raise a question as to whether there are patients who are unable to tolerate a high level of freedom, based on their observation of episodes of violence in this setting.

*Chenevert, M.: Special techniques in assertiveness training for women in the health professions, St. Louis, 1978, The C.V. Mosby Co.

This delightful book applies the principles of assertiveness theory to the experience of women, especially nurses, in health care settings. The author urges nurses to develop assertive skills for the sake of their patients as well as themselves. She identifies many difficult situations and gives practical suggestions for constructive behavior.

*DeFabio, S., and Ackerhalt, E.J.: Teaching the use of restraint through role-play, Perspect. Psychiatr. Care **16**:218, Sept.-Dec. 1978.

In this article, the authors describe a methodology that has been effective in teaching people to restrain violent patients. It contains a detailed presentation and discussion of the process that should be very helpful to in-service educators who are planning a class on this subject.

Engel, F., and Marsh, S.: Helping the employee victim of violence in hospitals, Hosp. Community Psychiatry **37**:159, Feb. 1986.

The authors recommend that staff victims of violence be provided with counseling. They point out the need to legitimize the staff member's need for assistance following an assault by a patient and present a model for the provision of such a service.

*Freeberg, S.: Anger in adolescence. J. Psychosoc. Nurs. **20**:29, Mar. 1982.

The author discusses anger in the context of normal adolescent development. Attention is also given to the many manifestations of anger when direct expression is blocked. Suggested nursing interventions are presented.

Fromm, E.: The anatomy of human destructiveness, New York, 1973, Holt, Rinehart & Winston, Inc.

This book develops an existential theory of the meaning and expression of anger and compares and contrasts the existential viewpoint with other basic theoretical frameworks.

Galassi, M.D., and Galassi, J.P.: Assert yourself: how to be your own person, New York, 1977, Human Sciences Press.

This is a workbook approach to learning assertive behavior. The presentation is very clear, and the directed practice exercises structure and enhance the learning process.

*Gluck, M.: Learning a therapeutic verbal response to anger, J. Psychosoc. Nurs. Ment. Health Serv. **19**:9, Mar. 1981.

This article is a description of a program developed by the author to teach nursing assistants to respond more therapeutically to angry patients. She advocates an understanding approach that focuses on the patient's stress and the means to relieve emotional tension.

Hays, J.R., Roberts, T.K., and Solway, K.S., editors: Violence and the violent individual, Jamaica, N.Y., 1981, Spectrum Books.

This collection of papers comprehensively views the problem of violence in the United States. Various theories are presented, and current research is examined. This book is recommended as a resource for someone who is interested in serious investigation of this subject.

*Lenefsky, B., de Palma, T., and Locicero, D.: Management of violent behavior, Perspect. Psychiatr. Care **16**:212, Sept.-Dec. 1978.

This article focuses on the procedure used for restraint of a person who is threatening violent behavior. Photographs illustrate the recommended techniques. The authors emphasize safety and the importance of a team approach by the staff.

Lion, J.R., and Reid, W.H., editors: Assaults within psychiatric facilities, New York, 1983, Grune & Stratton, Inc.

This book is an excellent resource regarding the phenomenon of violence in psychiatric settings. It includes data from current research and provides direction for further study. Of particular interest to the nurse is the attention given to legal perspectives on violent behavior and issues related to prevention and management of violence in the institutional setting.

---

*Asterisk indicates nursing reference.

*Loomis, M.E.: Nursing management of acting-out behavior, Perspect. Psychiatr. Care **8:**169, 1970.

This article presents theoretical concepts of the origins of acting-out behavior, including an excellent model of patient-staff interaction in the acting-out process. It also includes a helpful section on nursing intervention.

Lorenz, K.: On aggression, New York, 1966, Harcourt, Brace & World, Inc. (Translated by M.K. Wilson.)

This is a fascinating and readable presentation of the instinctual theory of aggressive behavior presented by a physician who is also a naturalist. This book is bound to stimulate reflection on the behavior of humankind as seen from the vantage point of the world of nature.

*Maynard, C.K., and Chitty, K.K.: Dealing with anger: guidelines for nursing intervention, J. Psychiatr. Nurs. **17:**36, June 1979.

This excellent article very clearly describes nursing interventions with patients who are having problems dealing with anger. The nursing process model is used. This is a very useful resource for nurses who are inexperienced and can benefit from a well-developed conceptual framework.

*Moritz, D.A.: Understanding anger, Am. J. Nurs. **78:**81, Jan. 1978.

The author describes anger as an expression of anxiety. She emphasizes the need for the nurse to analyze angry behavior in an effort to identify the cause. Nursing intervention is discussed in the context of two case examples.

Novaco, R.W.: The functions and regulations of the arousal of anger, Am. J. Psychiatry **133:**1124, 1976.

This author approaches anger from a positive standpoint and describes several useful functions. He then suggests a cognitive therapeutic approach to the patient who is having problems with anger.

Rothenberg, A.: On anger, Am. J. Psychiatry **128:**454, 1971.

This article differentiates anger and its growth-producing functions from the destructive emotions of hostility and vengefulness. It helps to clarify some of the hazy issues about defining aggression, anger, and other related terms.

*Rumpler, C.H., and Seigerman, C.: Violent behavior in an intensive care unit, Perspect. Psychiatr. Care **16:**206, Sept.-Dec. 1978.

The focus of this article is on the use of a behavior modification approach to intervene in aggressive behavior in an intensive care setting. The authors point out that aggression can be a particularly difficult problem in a general hospital. A case history is used to illustrate their creative and successful approach to the problem.

*Stewart, A.T.: Handling the aggressive patient, Perspect. Psychiatr. Care **16:**228, Sept.-Dec. 1978.

The author provides practical suggestions for physical restraint of a violent patient. Photographs are included that illustrate the text and clarify the suggested approaches.

Tavris, C.: Anger defused, Psychol. Today **16:**25, Nov. 1982.

This author challenges some of the traditional ways of viewing anger, claiming that ventilation may not always be the best way to handle this feeling. She points out that anger occurs in a social context and has meaning related to the transaction. She also addresses the sex role differences in acceptable expression of anger. This article would be useful in stimulating discussion.

*Whitman, J.: When a patient attacks: strategies for self-protection when violence looms, RN **42:**30, Sept. 1979.

This article presents some very practical information and guidelines concerning intervention in violent behavior. The focus is on protection of the patient and the nurse from harm. The author emphasizes the need to be alert to subtle clues and be prepared for unexpected violent behavior. She points out that it is unpleasant to think about this problem but ignoring it will not make it go away.

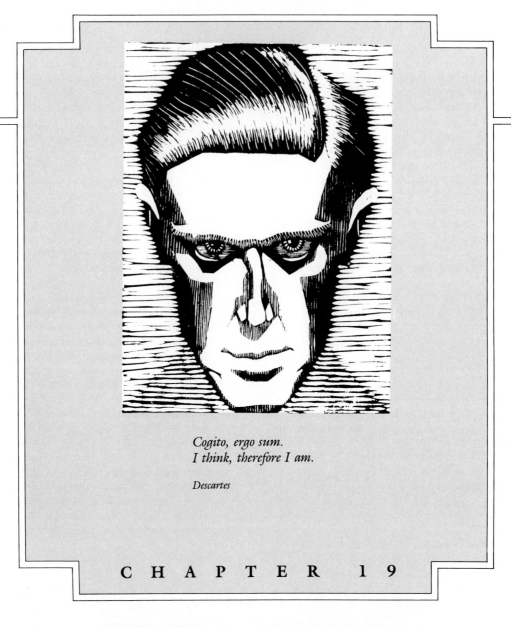

Cogito, ergo sum.
I think, therefore I am.

Descartes

IMPAIRED COGNITION

- define cognition in terms of its component processes.

- identify three models of cognitive functioning.

- describe Jean Piaget's three stages of cognitive development.

- discuss predisposing factors related to cognitive impairment.

- analyze precipitating stressors that contribute to cognitive impairment.

- identify the major categories of data that should be collected regarding an individual's level of cognitive functioning.

- compare and contrast the medical diagnoses of organic mental disease vs. organic brain syndrome and delirium vs. dementia.

- discriminate between the characteristic behaviors of an individual who is delirious and one with dementia.

- describe the purposes of psychological testing and several commonly administered tests.

- identify coping mechanisms that are used by individuals with cognitive impairment.

- formulate individualized nursing diagnoses for patients with cognitive impairments.

- assess the relationship between the nursing and medical diagnoses of individual patients with cognitive impairments.

- develop long-term and short-term individualized nursing goals for patients with cognitive impairments

- apply therapeutic nurse-patient relationship principles with appropriate rationale in planning the care of a patient with cognitive impairment characteristic of delirium or dementia.

- develop a mental health education plan for the families of cognitively impaired person

- assess the importance of evaluation of the nursing process when working with cognitively impaired people.

- identify directions for future nursing research.

- select appropriate readings for further study.

Continuum of cognitive responses

The ability to think and to reason is one of the distinguishing features of the human being. It is this ability that created civilization and allowed progress from the Stone Age to the Space Age. Knowledge is now proliferating at such a rapid rate that Toffler[26] coined the phrase "future shock" to describe the almost overwhelming impact on the individual of the need to assimilate new information. We have moved from the time when power was equated with physical strength to the use of money to acquire power to an era where there is little power without information. Although strength and money play a part in the use of power, they are most successfully wielded by the best informed. It is now anticipated that individual computers will be required to assist the person in effectively processing information.

Because of the importance of the ability to think rationally, intellectual functioning is highly valued by the individual. Most people are threatened at the prospect of losing their cognitive abilities, including reasoning, memory, judgment, orientation, perception, and attention. These processes allow the individual to make sense of experience and to interact productively with the environment. Impaired cognitive functioning leaves the affected person in a state of confusion, unable to understand experience, and unable to relate current to past events. Memory is a key cognitive process because to exercise judgment, make decisions, or even orient oneself to time and place, one must remember past experiences and points of reference. Therefore memory loss is a particularly frightening experience.

Cognitive impairment is so threatening that it has been difficult for others, even professionals, to confront those who suffer from this problem. As a result, these people have frequently been labeled as crazy or senile. Institutionalization has frequently been society's solution to meeting the basic needs of the person who is unable to adequately process information. Custodial care has been provided by caretakers who have had little knowledge of the needs of their patients. Only recently has there begun to emerge significant medical and nursing research into the needs of this patient population.

■ Associationist model of cognition

Psychology is the discipline that has historically been most involved in research on cognition. Experimental psychologists have been interested in defining the process of learning and developing models that will explain learned behavior. Bachrach[3] defines learning as "a change in behavior potential resulting from reinforced practice." This is an associationist model of learning theory. When the individual experiences a **stimulus,** a number of behavioral **responses** are available to him. He is most likely to select the response that has been **reinforced** in the past. In other words, he has learned a particular response to a given stimulus or set of stimuli. If the response is not reinforced on subsequent occasions, an alternative behavior may be substituted. If the new behavior is reinforced, the potential will be for the person to continue to behave in that way. Clinical example 19-1 illustrates this process.

By reinforcing Johnny's tantrums with cookies and cuddling, Ms. M had, in effect, taught him that this was an effective behavior. When she stopped reinforcing Johnny's negative behavior, he learned that another behavior was more effective in meeting his needs. Gradually, with continued reinforcement, the potential for

effective behavior increased. Learning theorists believe that this sequence is responsible for the development of much of human behavior and that behavior can be changed, or learning can take place, by altering the reinforcement.

This process is depicted in Fig. 19-1. Since response number 1 is not reinforced, it tends not to recur. Instead, the individual tries response number 2. It is reinforced and thus will tend to recur the next time the stimulus is produced. It is important to note that the reinforcement need not be a reward, although rewards are certainly powerful reinforcers. Punishment can also be a reinforcer of behavior if the alternative is lack of any response at all. Therefore, in the preceding examples, spanking Johnny would probably have been less effective than leaving him alone, since he would still be receiving his mother's attention. Also, a reinforcer need not be a material object. The cuddling may have been as effective in reinforcing Johnny's behavior as the cookie. The associationist model of learning theory was developed by such theorists as Pavlov, Skinner, and Wolfe. It is also referred to as a behavioral mode. Further information on the behavioral model and on the modification of behavior will be found in Chapters 2 and 27.

■ Cognitive model of cognition

Another major group of learning theorists, including Tolman and Bandura, ascribe to a cognitive model.[3] Their approach to learning is a broader one that focuses on "the acquisition of information about the environment rather than the attachment of particular responses to particular stimuli."[3] In this case, the stimulus is perceived as a **sign** that a desired resource may be available

---

CLINICAL EXAMPLE 19-1

Johnny M, age 3, asked his mother for a cookie. Ms. M told Johnny that he could have a cookie after he picked up his toys. Johnny began to kick and scream. Ms. M cuddled Johnny, gave him a cookie, and picked up the toys. When she discussed this experience with her neighbor, Ms. P, the mother of four children, Johnny's mother learned that he had had a temper tantrum and that the behavior was likely to continue if she gave in to Johnny's demands. The next time Johnny demanded a cookie, Ms. M again requested that he pick up his toys first. Johnny began his temper tantrum. His mother placed him in another room and informed him again that when he picked up his toys, he could have a cookie. After a few minutes, Johnny quieted, then came out and put away his toys. His mother responded with cuddling and a cookie. Over time, the temper tantrums disappeared.

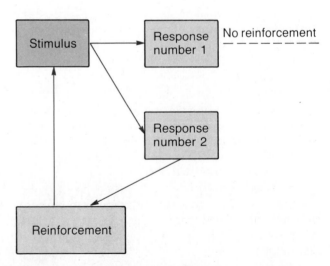

Fig. 19-1. The associationist, or behavioral, model of learning.

from the environment (for example, a cookie). This perception creates a **demand** that when combined with knowledge about the environment leads the individual to seek gratification. The individual's perception of the environment is referred to as a **cognitive map** that guides him in his quest to meet his need. Cognitive learning theorists would say that the change in Johnny's cookie-seeking behavior was due to a change in his perception of his mother's behavior as a part of his environment. Her changed behavior blocked the pathway that had previously led him to a cookie, so he had to find a new route.

Bachrach[3] believes that the cognitive learning theory model is closely related to the computer model of cognition. The computer also relies on stored information, or **memory,** about the environment in order to make decisions. The concept of reinforcement, be it reward or punishment, has no meaning to a computer. Decisions are based on an objective evaluation of the consequences of past actions. Consequences are evaluated in terms of their effectiveness in achieving the desired result.

■ Piaget developmental model of cognition

Human cognitive development has been described by Piaget[22] and is summarized in Table 19-1. His research revealed a three-stage process of the development of thought processes. The first developmental stage is "the period of sensorimotor intelligence." This phase lasts from birth until the development of language, usually about 2 years.[22] This stage is action oriented, with the actions first directed toward the self and then gradually incorporating more space and the ability to situate the self in space. There is also the beginning of memory for objects that are out of sight, a necessary precursor for the development of language using words to describe objects that are not present. The baby who plays "peek-a-boo" is practicing this ability.

The second stage is composed of two substages, which some theorists describe as separate stages. This is the "period of preparation and organization of concrete operations: of categories, relations, and numbers." This period lasts from 2 to 12 years of age and is divided into two substages. Early in this stage, during the preoperational substage, symbolism appears in language and in play. Objects are defined in terms of function, that is, a ball is "to throw."[8] This is also the period of magical thinking, in which thoughts and words are perceived as the equivalent of action. Preoperational behavior lasts from about 2 to 5 years of age. The child then enters the substage of concrete operations. At this point, he is "capable of relatability, i.e., combinations, associations, negations and reversibility."[9] Elkind[8] states that during this period, children develop the capacity for syllogistic reasoning, which enables them to make

TABLE 19-1

PIAGET'S LEVELS OF COGNITIVE DEVELOPMENT

Stage	Age (years)	Characteristics
Sensorimotor	Birth to 2	Action oriented No language Develops awareness of body in space Develops memory for missing objects
Preparation and organization of concrete operations		
Preoperational phase	2 to 5	Symbolism appears Objects defined by function Magical thinking
Concrete operations	5 to 12	Capable of relatability Syllogistic reasoning Makes and follows rules Quantifies experience
Formal operations	12 to 14 and older	Abstraction Development of ideals Criticism of others Self-criticism

and follow rules. They also develop the ability to quantify experience.

The third stage is "the period of formal operations."[22] This develops between the ages of 12 and 14, resulting in the ability to conceptualize at an adult level. It is only at this point that the person is "capable of abstract logic and has the ability to do manipulations in propositions, probabilities and permutations."[9] The period of formal operations enables individuals to explore idealistic concepts and to measure their own reality against their ideals.[8] This pertains to observations of significant others, such as parents, and of cultural institutions, such as government and religions. The same process is applied to the self in the form of self-criticism. This developmental process provides the foundation for continued cognitive growth as life experiences enrich and modify the individual's perception of the world.

In some individuals, cognitive processes may not develop fully or, once developed, may deteriorate. When cognitive deficiencies occur during childhood, they are generally referred to as mental retardation. The reader is referred to a textbook of pediatric nursing for a discussion of cognitive deficiencies. In this chapter, cognitive disruptions in the adult will be considered. In most cases, the individual will have developed to the level of formal operations. Although it may occur at any age, cognitive impairment is most common in the elderly. It is highly recommended that this chapter be read in conjunction with Chapter 35, because the content of the two chapters is complementary.

■ Continuum of cognitive responses

Cognitive impairments include impaired memory and judgment, disorientation, misperceptions, decreased attention span, and difficulties with logical reasoning. They may occur episodically or be present continuously. Depending on the stressor, the condition may be reversible or characterized by progressive deterioration in functioning. Fig. 19-2 illustrates cognitive functioning as it occurs on the continuum of health-illness coping responses.

 ## Assessment

■ Predisposing factors

Cognitive dysfunctions are generally the result of a biological disruption in the functioning of the central nervous system (CNS). The CNS requires a continous supply of nutrients to function. Any interference with the provision of supplies to the brain will be reflected in functional disruptions. For instance, the difficulties

in cognition experienced by some elderly people result from arteriosclerotic changes in cerebral blood vessels that deprive the brain of needed oxygen, glucose, and other essential basic chemicals. Other vascular abnormalities, such as transient ischemic episodes (small strokes), cerebral hemorrhage, and multiple small infarcts in brain tissue resulting from chronic hypertension, can also result in cognitive impairments.

Aging itself predisposes the individual to cognitive dysfunction. There is cumulative degeneration of brain tissue associated with aging. This is not extensive enough to be particularly noticeable in most people. However, if other stressors are added, the person may experience difficulty. Some toxins collect in brain tissue. A lifetime of exposure to a toxic chemical or a heavy metal may result in cognitive impairment.

Some metabolic disorders, such as chronic liver disease, chronic renal disease, and vitamin deficiencies, can result in disrupted information processing. Vitamin B-complex deficiency, particularly thiamine, is believed to be the cause of the Wernicke-Korsakoff syndrome found in chronic alcoholics who have a long-standing nutritional deficiency. One of the prominent features of this syndrome is a severe deficit in cognitive functioning. Malnutrition increases the individual's vulnerability to organic brain disease. This is frequently a problem in the elderly, who may lack the physical or financial resources to provide an adequate diet for themselves. However, young people with anorexia nervosa or bulimia are sometimes also at risk for cognitive impairment.

Genetic abnormalities may also cause this type of dysfunction. An example of a degenerative brain disease that is hereditary in nature is Huntington's chorea, which is inherited as an autosomal dominant trait. Although the specific genetic defect has not been identified, there is evidence that Alzheimer's disease occurs more commonly in first-degree relatives of victims. It is also more frequent in people with Down's syndrome, another hereditary brain disorder.

A degree of cognitive impairment may be found in conjunction with other disruptions in mental functioning. For instance, a delusional person may seem disoriented because he misidentifies the place he is in. People who are hyperactive related to a manic affective disturbance have short attention spans, as do depressed people. Depression may also result in memory disorders, although it is often difficult to determine whether the problem is related to memory loss or lack of motivation to try to remember or to communicate the memory. The factors related to these disorders of cognitive functioning would be those related to the primary problem.

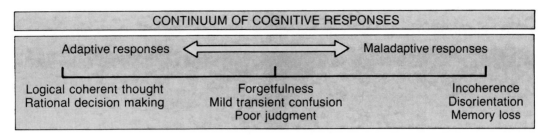

Fig. 19-2. Continuum of cognitive responses.

■ Precipitating stressors

Any major assault on the brain is likely to result in a disruption in cognitive functioning.

Wolanin[28] cites three major systemic problems that contribute to cognitive impairment: (1) hypoxia, (2) alterations in blood glucose content, and (3) toxicity. She further subdivides hypoxia into four types: anemic, histotoxic, that is, conditions that prevent cells from metabolizing oxygen; hypoxemic, that is, problems with ventilation; and ischemic.

■ **HYPOXIAS.** Anemic hypoxia may be insidious in onset. Possible stressors include aspirin ingestion, resulting in occult bleeding; other occult blood loss; or deficiencies of iron, folic acid, or vitamin B_{12}. Histotoxic hypoxia may be related to such stressors as dehydration, hyperthermia, or hypothermia. A possible stressor related to hypoxemic hypoxia is chronic obstructive lung disease. Others might include asthma or an acute respiratory tract infection. Ischemic hypoxia can result from congestive heart failure, atherosclerosis, hypotension, hypertension, or increased intracranial pressure resulting from a tumor, subdural hematoma, or normal pressure hydrocephalus.[28]

■ **METABOLIC DISORDERS.** Metabolic disorders frequently affect mental functioning, especially when severe or of long duration. Endocrine malfunctioning, whether it involves underproduction or overproduction of hormones, can adversely affect cognition. For example, the thyroid hormone is known to have a great influence on mental alertness. People with hypothyroidism are sluggish and retarded in their thinking. Those with severe hypothyroidism (myxedema) may develop psychotic behavior characterized by delusional thinking. People with hyperthyroidism, on the other hand, are frequently hyperalert and agitated, with acceleration of both thought and action. Other endocrine disorders that may cause cognitive disruptions include hypoglycemia, hypopituitarism, and adrenal disease.

■ **TOXIC AND INFECTIOUS AGENTS.** Toxic and infectious agents may also result in behavior typical of disturbed cerebral functioning. Toxins may originate either within the individual or in the external environment. An example of an internally generated toxin is the elevated blood level of urea found in a patient with renal failure. Environmental toxins would include various poisonous substances that might be ingested or animal venoms. Increased levels of aluminum have been found in the brains of people with Alzheimer's disease leading investigators to seek the source.[19] Acute viral and bacterial infections occur in the CNS, resulting in inflammation and impaired functioning. Chronic infections also affect the brain. One such condition is the neural manifestation of tertiary syphilis, general paresis. This is seldom seen any more, since early treatment of syphilis has become more prevalent. One of the stressors that is being considered in relationship to Alzheimer's disease is infection with a slow virus.[19] It has also been determined that individuals who are infected with human T-lymphotrophic virus (HTLV)-III almost always develop an organic brain syndrome.[21] This is apparently caused by direct invasion of brain tissue by the virus, which also causes acquired immune deficiency syndrome (AIDS). Infections in other body systems may also have a deleterious effect on the CNS if there is an extremely elevated temperature.

Wolanin[28] emphasizes the possible significance of prescription and over-the-counter drugs as toxic stressors. Thorough assessment of drug use is particularly critical with elderly patients, because of their increased sensitivity to drugs and because of the possibility that confusion could lead to difficulty in following directions for taking drugs. Drug-drug interactions or interactions between drugs and other substances, particularly alcohol, may also lead to disruptions in cognitive functioning.

■ **STRUCTURAL CHANGES.** Conditions that alter the structure of brain tissue are also reflected in impaired cognitive functioning. Tumors may cause proliferation or displacement of tissue, thus altering its function. Trauma, whether accidental or surgical, will result in a change in ability to process information. The specific effect will depend on the location of the lesion.

■ **SENSORY STIMULATION.** Sensory underload or overload can result in cognitive dysfunction. It has been found that people who are placed in environments with minimal stimuli seem to develop internally produced stimuli in the form of hallucinations. The proliferation of intensive care units (ICUs) in general hospitals has led to an interest in sensory overload. The constant light and activity in these areas has been noted to lead to disorientation, delusional thought, and hallucinations, sometimes referred to as "ICU psychosis." However, it is difficult to differentiate how much of the cognitive impairment results from the sensory experience as opposed to other concurrent stressors, such as the introduction of multiple drugs into the system and the result of massive assaults on physical integrity.

■ **NONSPECIFIC STRESSORS.** Unfortunately, there are many times when the specific stressor related to cognitive impairment cannot be identified. It must be noted that understanding of the biochemical processes of the brain and the response of brain and nervous tissue to stressors is still limited. As knowledge grows, it is conceivable that a specific biological component will be identified in the etiology of all disorders categorized as psychiatric. The fields of psychiatry and neurology may well merge at some time as knowledge grows more sophisticated. For example, deficiencies in neurotransmitters, including acetylcholine, somatostatin, substance P, and norepinephrine have been observed in patients with Alzheimer's disease.[19] It is not known whether this is a cause or effect of the illness. Also, it is known that some chemical substances can create hallucinatory experiences and are popular in the drug culture for that reason. As more is learned about the mechanism of action of the hallucinogens, such as LSD and PCP, more will also be understood about processes that may take place in the brains of psychotic people.

In general, physiological causes are ruled out first, then psychosocial stressors are considered in relationship to cognitive impairment. Even when physiological factors are present, psychosocial stress may further compromise the individual's thought process. Each patient must receive a complete assessment so that nursing care can be planned in a holistic manner.

■ **Behaviors**

Disruptions in cognitive functioning are most readily apparent in individuals who have a medical diagnosis of organic mental syndrome or disorder (DSM-III-R).[1] Conditions that are not definably organic may also be referred to as "functional." The distinction between organic and functional becomes blurred, since possible organic causes are found for medical conditions formerly considered to be the result of psychosocial stressors. Lipowski[14] defines organic mental disorders as conditions caused by permanent damage to or temporary dysfunction of the brain or a combination of permanent and temporary disruptions. The problem may originate in the brain or elsewhere in the system and may be diffuse or focal. In the Draft of the DSM-III-R in Development,[1] a distinction is made between **organic brain syndromes,** which are not differentiated in terms of etiology or are not listed in the International Classification of Disease, ninth edition, and **organic mental disorders,** in which a cause may be determined or are included in ICD-9. In other words, the organic mental disorder is a defined organic brain syndrome. For example, multi-infarct dementia is an organic mental disorder. Following are the eight categories of organic brain syndromes[1]:

1. Delirium
2. Dementia
3. Amnestic syndrome
4. Organic delusional syndrome
5. Organic hallucinosis
6. Organic affective syndrome
7. Organic personality syndrome
8. Organic anxiety syndrome

Discussions in this chapter will focus primarily on categories 1 and 2, delirium and dementia, because these are the medical diagnostic categories that will be encountered most frequently by nurses.

■ **ASSOCIATED WITH DELIRIUM.** In the recent past, delirium was also referred to as acute, or reversible, brain syndrome and dementia as chronic, or irreversible, brain syndrome. Acute vs. chronic referred to the rapidity of the onset of the disorder and to its duration. These terms are no longer recommended because they do not discriminate between delirium and dementia. Delirium is a diffuse disruption of the cognitive state that is characterized by a clouding of awareness manifested by a limited attention span, sensory misperception, and disordered thought.[1] There are also disturbances of activity patterns and of the sleep-wakefulness cycle. Generally, there is a rapid onset and a brief course of illness. Lipowski[14] describes the disordered thought process as including disturbed attention, memory, thinking, orientation, and perception. He further notes the tendency of the degree of impairment to fluctuate throughout the day, with periods of lucidity occurring intermittently. The disturbance is generally worse at night. Delirium usually occurs in response to a specific stressor, such as infection, trauma, a toxin or drug, or alcohol intoxication. However, the stressor may not be immediately apparent. Clinical example 19-2 will dem-

CLINICAL EXAMPLE 19-2

Ms. S was brought to the emergency room of a general hospital by her parents. She was a 22-year-old single woman who was described as having been in good health until 2 days prior to admission, when she complained of malaise and a sore throat and stayed home from work. She was employed as a typist in a small office and had a stable employment record. According to her parents, she had an active social life and there were no significant conflicts at home.

On admission, Ms. S was extremely restless and had a frightened facial expression. Her speech was garbled and incoherent. When she was approached by an unfamiliar person, she would become agitated, trying to climb out of bed and striking out aimlessly. Occasionally she would slip into a restless sleep. Her temperature on admission was 103.4° F (39.4° C) axillary, pulse was 108 per minute, and respirations were 28 per minute. Her skin was hot, dry, and flushed. Her mother said she had had only a few sips of water in the last 24 hours and had not urinated at all, although she had had several episodes of profuse diaphoresis.

Her ability to cooperate with a mental status examination was limited. She would respond to her own name by turning her head. When her mother asked her where she was, she said "home," but could not say where her home was. She would give only the month when asked for the date and said it was January, when the actual date was February 19. She also refused to give the day of the week. A neurological examination was negative for signs of increased intracranial pressure or for localizing signs of CNS disease.

The tentative medical diagnosis was that of delirium secondary to fever of unknown origin. Symptomatic treatment of the fever, including intravenous fluids, an aspirin suppository, and cool water mattress, was begun immediately while further diagnostic studies were carried out. Nurses caring for the patient noticed continued restlessness and disorientation. Her speech was still incoherent. In addition, they noticed that she was picking at the bedclothing. Suddenly she became extremely agitated, trying to get out of bed and crying out, "Bugs, get away, get bugs away." She was brushing and slapping at herself and the bed. As her mother and the nurse talked with her and held her, she gradually became calmer but periodically would continue to slap at "the bugs" and need reassurance and reorientation.

Later in the day additional laboratory results became available. A lumbar puncture was normal, as were skull x-ray films. Results of toxicological screening of blood were also negative. The electroencephalogram revealed diffuse slowing. There was an elevated white blood count and electrolyte imbalance consistent with severe dehydration. Cultures of her throat and blood were both positive for beta-hemolytic streptococci; so intravenous antibiotic therapy was begun at once while other supportive measures were continued.

As the infection gradually came under control and the fever decreased, Ms. S's mental state improved. A week later, when she was discharged from the hospital, her cognitive functioning was completely normal, with the exception of amnesia for the time during which she was delirious.

---

onstrate behaviors that are typical of a patient with delirium.

Ms. S demonstrates many characteristics that are frequently seen in patients with delirium. The behaviors are related to alterations in neurochemical and electrical responses in the brain as a result of the stressor that causes the disruption. **Disorientation** is generally present, sometimes in all three spheres of time, place, and person. Thought processes are usually disorganized. **Judgment is poor** and there is little decision-making ability. Stimuli may be misinterpreted, resulting in **illusions** or distortions of reality. An example of an illusion is the perception that a polka-dot drape is actually covered with cockroaches. Delirious patients may hallucinate. These **hallucinations** are most frequently visual and often take the form of animals, reptiles, or insects. They are real to the person and extremely frightening. Assaultive or destructive behavior on the part of the patient may be an attempt to strike back at a hallucinated image. At times, patients with delirium also exhibit a **labile affect,** changing abruptly from laughter to tearfulness and vice versa, with the affect unrelated to any environmental events. There may also be **loss of usual social behavior,** resulting in such acts as undressing, playing with food, and grabbing at others. Delirious patients tend to act on impulse.

Other behaviors may be specifically related to the causative agent of the behavioral syndrome. For example, the fever and dehydration experienced by Ms. S were a result of her systemic streptococcal infection, as was her brain syndrome. It is extremely important to differentiate behavioral manifestations, which help to identify the stressor. Treatment is usually conservative until a specific stressor has been isolated. Although most cases of delirium are reversed, with recovery of the patient, in about 12% of the cases[14] the person dies as a result of the severity of the stressor. If adequate intervention does not take place, delirium may become dementia.

■ **ASSOCIATED WITH DEMENTIA.** Dementia is a cognitive disruption that features a loss of intellectual abilities severe enough to interfere with usual social or occupational activities.[1] The loss of intellectual ability includes impairment of memory, judgment, and abstract thought. There are also frequently changes in personality. According to Lipowski,[14] the personality change may appear as either alteration or accentuation of the person's usual character traits. The onset of dementia is usually gradual. The course may be one of gradual deterioration or may be stable. It is also possible for the process of dementia to be reversed and for the person's intellectual functioning to improve if the underlying stressors are identified and treated.

Dementia can occur at any age but is most frequent in the elderly. According to Reisberg,[23] of the American population over 65 years old, 11% to 12% suffer from mild to moderate dementia, and 4% to 5% have severe dementia. Clark[5] stated that about 7% of the same age group are victims of Alzheimer's disease and more than 120,000 die of this illness each year. Dementia may be the result of trauma, either accidental or surgical; a chronic infection, such as tertiary syphilis; cerebrovascular disruptions, such as arteriosclerosis or chronic hypertension; or may be of indeterminate cause. "Senility" is a nonspecific term and usually applies to those who have degenerative brain disease of an unknown cause. Because of the pejorative connotation, use of the terms "senility" or "senile" is to be discouraged. Clinical example 19-3 will demonstrate behaviors associated with dementia.

The behaviors associated with dementia reflect the brain tissue alterations that are taking place. The cognitive changes are related to the actions of stressors that interfere with the functioning of the cerebral cortex. Other areas of the brain may be affected as well, which is one reason for being sure that the patient has a complete medical and neurological examination. Another reason for this is that although the condition may be irreversible, progression may be arrested by identification of the stressor and treatment of the underlying dysfunction. For instance, treatment of hypertension

may prevent further occurrence of small hemorrhages, which are a possible cause of irreversible brain syndrome. Recent research has demonstrated that many cases of dementia may be reversible. It has also been found that depression in the elderly is often misinterpreted as dementia and therefore not treated appropriately. This happens so often that the condition has been labeled **pseudodementia.** Depression differs from dementia in several ways.[1] A depressed person generally expresses concern about his perceived lack of cognitive ability, whereas a demented person will attempt to compensate for it and conceal it. If motivated, a depressed person is able to perform cognitive tests, and, if not, the deficits are less consistent than those found in dementia. In addition, the date of onset of depression can usually be more specifically identified than that of dementia. However, it is important to remember that the conditions can coexist, since a person who is to some extent aware of impaired cognitive ability may well experience depression.

Alzheimer's disease is one of the most prevalent causes of impaired cognitive functioning. Since it has now been accepted that the loss of mental abilities is not automatically associated with aging, intensive research efforts have been directed toward identifying the etiology, characteristics, and, ultimately, treatment for Alzheimer's. Investigators have found that there are characteristic alterations in brain tissue. Pajk[19] has summarized these as follows:

1. The presence of neurofibrillary tangles which are "pairs of filaments wrapped around each other in the cytoplasm of the neurons"[19]
2. Neuritic plaques which are "filamentous and granular deposits representing degeneration in the neuronal processes"[19]
3. Granulovascular degeneration in which "fluid pockets and granular material develop in the neurons"[19]

These phenomena are found throughout the cortex but are concentrated in the hippocampus, the structure that is the center for short-term memory. This is consistent with the short-term memory loss that is characteristic of Alzheimer's. Other behaviors associated with this disease are those found in most types of dementia.

Another organic brain disorder that results in the development of dementia is associated with infection with the human T-lymphotrophic virus (HTLV)-III which also causes the acquired immune deficiency syndrome (AIDS). Navia and Price[18] have described the course of the dementia. Early symptoms include memory impairment, decreased concentration, slowed mental responses, apathy, decreased socialization, and oc-

CLINICAL EXAMPLE 19-3

Mr. B is a 73-year-old widower who has resided in a nursing home for 3 years. He chose to move to the nursing home after the death of his wife, although his son encouraged him to live with him and his family. Mr. B stated that he did not want to burden his family and would be happier with others of the same age. He did well for the first 18 months. He was an active participant in social groups both in the home and in his church, where he continued to attend regularly. He also visited his son once a week and enjoyed seeing his grandchildren and puttering around his son's house.

About 18 months previously Mr. B began to seem forgetful. He would ask the same question several times and on occasion would prepare for church on a Friday or Saturday. He also became irritable and accused his son of not caring about him and abandoning him in "that place." Mr. B spent many hours taking papers from his desk and studying them. When asked what he was doing, he would say, "Attending to my business." He began to withdraw from activities, making flimsy excuses to avoid playing his favorite card game, gin rummy. When he was persuaded to play, he usually quit in frustration because he could not remember which cards had been played. At times Mr. B was quite anxious. He would periodically seem well oriented and expressed great concern about the changes he was experiencing, wondering if he was "going crazy."

Because of the concern of the nursing staff at the nursing home, Mr. B was scheduled for a complete physical examination by his family physician and a psychiatric evaluation by the geriatric psychiatric nurse consultant who came to the nursing home weekly. The physical examination revealed generally good health for a man of Mr. B's age. He suffered from a mild hearing loss and slight prostatic hypertrophy. Hypertension had been diagnosed 10 years prior to this examination but was well controlled by diuretics. Neurological examination revealed normal reflexes, normal muscle strength, a slight intention tremor, normal response to sensation, normal cranial nerves, and no disturbance of gait. An electroencephalogram was normal, as were a skull x-ray film and the results of laboratory studies of blood and urine. A brain scan and computerized axial tomography studies of the brain revealed some atrophy of the cerebral cortex.

The psychiatric examination confirmed the deficits in cognitive functioning that had been observed by the nursing home staff and by Mr. B's son. He was oriented to person and place but stated that the date was April 6, 1958. The real date was March 11, 1986. He also thought the day of the week was Friday, whereas it was actually Tuesday. He correctly identified the season of the year as spring. Mr. B was able to give correctly his birth date, the date of his son's birth, and the year he began to work at his first job. He spoke at length and with great detail about his exploits as a young man. However, he could not repeat the names of three objects after 5 minutes and could not remember what he had eaten for lunch or the last name of the man who shared his room. He became distressed when he was trying to answer these questions. His vocabulary was excellent, as was his fund of general information. However, he was unable to remember the names of the two most recent presidents. He could, however, recite the names of the eight presidents preceding them.

Mr. B's judgment was somewhat impaired. When asked what he would do if he found a stamped, addressed, sealed envelope, he said he would "read it, then mail it." His ability for abstract thinking was slightly concretized. His attention span and ability to concentrate were normal. His eye-hand coordination was disrupted, as demonstrated by his difficulty in copying simple figures. His tremor was evident both when he was drawing and when he signed his name.

He exhibited affect that was appropriate in quality and quantity to the content of the discussion. He appeared depressed when talking about his memory loss but cheerful and proud when describing his grandchildren. No abrupt mood swings were noted. The flow of speech was of a normal rate and volume. Content of speech was logical and coherent, except when Mr. B was trying to remember and describe recent events, when it became somewhat disjointed.

As a result of the data gathered in the physical and psychiatric examinations, a diagnosis was made of dementia of unknown cause.

Over the next several months, Mr. B's condition continued to deteriorate gradually. He became increasingly forgetful and began to confabulate. He was less conforming to social norms and needed reminding about hygiene and appropriate dress. He also became seductive with female residents and staff, making suggestive remarks and occasionally fondling someone. Visits to his son's home became impossible as his behavior deteriorated. His memory of the identity of family members sometimes was confused. He would misidentify his daughter-in-law as his wife and his grandson as his son. More and more, his conversation consisted of rambling reminiscences of his life in his youth. Because he is surrounded with caring people, Mr. B continues to live with dignity and respect in spite of his progressively limited ability to communicate.

casionally psychotic symptoms. Late symptoms include global cognitive impairment and psychomotor slowing. The person is alert, but not spontaneous in response to others. Sometimes there is agitation. At the end stage, the person is mute, immobile, and incontinent. A computerized tomographic scan reveals cortical atrophy and enlarged brain ventricles. Perry and Jacobsen[21] have identified two other behavioral patterns associated with HTLV-III. The first is a mild, chronic depression, with behaviors similar to those described for a major depressive episode. The second is an acute psychotic reaction, including behaviors of "grandiosity, suspiciousness, delusional thinking, hallucinations, psychomotor agitation, rambling and repetitive speech, confusion and blunted affect." They warn that it may be difficult to differentiate the organic and functional aspects of these behavioral patterns.

A common behavior related to dementia is **disorientation.** Usually time orientation is affected first, then place, and, finally, person. This behavior can be distressing to the patient, who may be aware of this difficulty and embarrassed and frightened by it. This is particularly true if the person's mental acuity is fluctuating, which sometimes happens. In these instances the individual is aware, during periods of lucidity, of the confusion and disorientation experienced at other times.

Memory loss is another prominent characteristic of dementia. Immediate recall and recent memory are generally most seriously affected. Remote memory may be intact, although it too deteriorates as the condition progresses. For example, Mr. B had difficulty remembering what he had eaten for lunch but gave accurate dates for significant events earlier in his life. Most aging people dwell on the past, but people with recent memory loss have difficulty shifting to the present and at advanced stages may seem to live in the past. This was exemplified by Mr. B's misidentification of his grandson and his daughter-in-law. Another behavior related to memory loss is **confabulation.** This is the tendency of a confused person to fabricate a response to a question when he cannot remember the answer. For instance, when Mr. B was asked if he knew one of the female residents of the home, he replied, "Of course I know her. I used to play gin with her husband." Actually, the woman's husband had been dead for many years and Mr. B had never met him. This behavior should not be viewed as lying or an attempt to deceive. Rather, it is the person's way of trying to save face in an embarrassing situation. He is aware that he should know the answer to the question and gives an answer that seems reasonable, not entirely disbelieving it himself. It is not unlike the situation in which one meets an acquaintance

and cannot recollect the person's name or where they met but acts as if these facts are remembered, hoping that the other person will offer clues about his identity.

Vocabulary and general information may be less affected by dementia, at least until its very late stages. This is influenced by how recently the information was learned. Facts learned early in life may be recalled well, whereas those learned recently may be quickly forgotten, as demonstrated by Mr. B's performance in listing the last ten presidents.

These patients may have **labile affective behavior,** particularly if the limbic system has been affected by the disease process. There may also be some **deterioration in social skills.** Impulsive sexual advances toward members of the opposite sex may occur. These reflect **decreased inhibition** and **impaired judgment.** Frequently this behavior is also an attempt to establish interpersonal contact and is a way of asking for caring from others. It is also a way of reinforcing an important part of the person's identity, which is becoming less secure as mental functioning declines.

Restlessness and **agitation** are other behaviors that occur with dementia. Extreme agitation may occur at night; this is sometimes referred to as the **sundown syndrome.** It is probably due to tiredness at the end of the day combined with fewer orienting stimuli, such as planned activities, meals, and contact with people.

Disorientation results in fear and agitation. Agitated behavior may also occur if the person is coerced to do something he does not understand or simply does not want to do. This may reflect an effort to keep control over the person's own life, thereby maintaining self-esteem. Change is not well accepted by these patients. Efforts to change behavior patterns will probably result in increased rigidity and, if efforts persist, agitated behavior. Routine is important, particularly a routine that is congruent with the person's previous life-style. Table 19-2 summarizes the characteristics of delirium and dementia.

A term that is frequently used when referring to the person with cognitive impairment is **confusion.** Although widely accepted as nursing and medical jargon, this term has not been specifically defined. Wolanin and Phillips[29] have focused their nursing research on this topic. They define confusion as "a condition characterized by the client's disorientation to time and place, incongruous conceptual boundaries, paranormal awareness, and seemingly inappropriate verbal statements that indicate memory defects."[29:8] The term should be used with caution, however, since Wolanin and Phillips discovered a wide array of meanings when they surveyed groups of physicians and nurses.

There is dissatisfaction among many mental health

TABLE 19-2

CHARACTERISTICS OF DELIRIUM AND DEMENTIA

	Delirium	Dementia
Onset	Usually sudden	Usually gradual
Course	Usually brief (under 1 month), with return to usual level of functioning	Usually long term and progressive; occasionally may be arrested or reversed
Age group	Any	Most common over age 65
Stressors	Toxins, infection, hyperthermia, space-occupying lesion, trauma, and sensory deprivation/overload	Hypertension, hypotension, anemia, normal pressure hydrocephalus, vitamin deficiencies, toxins, slow viruses, hypoglycemia, tumors, hyperthermia/hypothermia, and brain tissue atrophy
Behaviors	Fluctuating levels of awareness, disorientation, restlessness, agitation, illusions, hallucinations, disorganized thought, impaired judgment and decision making, affective lability, loss of inhibitions, and diffuse electroencephalogram (EEG) slowing	Memory loss, impaired judgment, decreased attention span, disorientation, inappropriate social behavior, labile affect, restlessness, agitation, and resistance to change

professionals with the terms delirium and dementia because of the stigma of the term dementia in particular and the lack of specificity of both terms. It has been suggested that "brain failure" would be a more accurate term and would connote a similarity with other organic conditions, such as heart failure and renal failure. Although this terminology is relatively new, it seems to be gaining acceptance.

■ **PSYCHOLOGICAL TESTING.** Frequently patients who have cognitive impairment are referred to a clinical psychologist for psychological testing. This referral should be made for a specific purpose, since the testing is time consuming, expensive, and tiring for the patient. Some reasons for psychological testing include identification of the stressor(s) causing the disruption, understanding of the dynamics of the problem, developing guidelines for therapeutic intervention, and obtaining a prognosis for recovery. DeCato and Wicks[7] present an excellent summary of indications for psychological referral and a description of the most common psychological tests administered to psychiatric patients. They divide the tests into three categories: intelligence, perceptual-motor, and projective tests.

Intelligence tests are used to assess the patient's general level of intellectual functioning. Those used most frequently are the **Wechsler Intelligence Scale for Children (WISC)** and the **Wechsler Adult Intelligence Scale (WAIS).** These tests must be evaluated by a skilled clinician, with consideration given to educational and sociocultural background of the patient. The result of the test is the individual's intelligence quotient (IQ), which can serve as a guideline for understanding the person's ability for intellectual performance. Some information about psychodynamics may also be obtained by analyzing the nature of the person's behavior in the testing situation.

Perceptual-motor testing is useful in determining whether an organic mental disorder is causing disturbed behavior. The **Bender-Gestalt** test requires that the patient copy a series of geometrical figures. The accuracy and facility with which the copying is done is significant in determining the presence of a biological stressor. Other factors, such as size and arrangement of the copied figures or the behavior of the patient in the testing situation, provide insight into the person's psychodynamic functioning. For example, a person who uses obsessive-compulsive behavior to cope with anxiety may try hard to make an exact copy of the stimulus figure.

Projective tests are directed specifically toward gaining information about psychodynamics. Probably the most widely known projective test is the **Rorschach test,** which consists of a standard series of inkblots. The patient is asked to respond to the inkblot, first generally and then in more detail. The response is then analyzed. Use and analysis of the Rorschach test is complex and must be done only by a qualified clinical psychologist. Another projective test that is commonly used is the **Thematic Apperception Test (TAT).** The patient is presented with a series of pictures of people engaged in nonspecific activities and asked to describe what might be happening in the situation. In both these situations the person's response is determined by his life experience as well as his current mental state. Valuable information may be gained about the person's anxiety level and the mechanisms used to cope with anxiety, which can have implications for therapy and prognosis.

There are many other psychological tests, some used for very specialized purposes. Clinical psychologists are good resource people both for explaining specific tests and for elaborating on the results of psychological testing. Frequently the psychologist is asked to determine whether or not the individual is experiencing a disruption that is organic. Further information about psychological testing may be found in Chapter 6.

■ Coping mechanisms

The way an individual copes emotionally with a disruption in his cognitive ability is greatly influenced by past life experience. A person who has developed an armamentarium of coping mechanisms that have been effective in the past is better able to handle the onset of a cognitive problem than is a person who already has coping problems.

The response of an individual to the onset of organic brain disease often mirrors that person's basic personality pattern. For instance, a person who has usually reacted to stress with anger directed toward other people and the environment will probably react similarly when he notices limitations in his intellectual abilities. A person who is more apt to direct anger inward and become depressed will be more likely to respond with depressive behaviors. A person who has relied on a mechanism such as intellectualization will be more threatened by loss of intellectual ability than a person who has used a mechanism such as reaction formation.

Regression is frequently used in an effort to cope with an advanced mental disorder. It may be caused in part by deterioration in mental function. It is probably also attributable to the behavioral manifestations of the problem, which result in the patient becoming more dependent on others for the fulfillment of basic needs such as nutrition and hygiene. Encouraging patients to perform self-care also supports their use of healthier coping mechanisms.

Because the basic behavioral disruption in delirium is altered awareness, which reflects the severe biological disturbance in the brain, psychological coping mechanisms are not generally used. For this reason, the nurse must protect the patient from harm and substitute for the person's own coping mechanisms by constantly reorienting him and reinforcing reality.

Early dementia is characterized by much use of the mechanism of denial. The person generally attempts to pursue his usual daily routine and makes light of memory lapses. He may be able to mobilize some environmental resources to help him cope. For instance, a businessman who is experiencing difficulty with recent memory might ask his secretary to remind him of all his appointments and provide him with a summary of the names of the people with whom he is meeting and the purpose of the meeting. As the impairment progresses, the individual may become very resistant to any limitations being placed on his independence. For instance, the family of a patient with a medical diagnosis of Alzheimer's disease might become very concerned about his ability to continue to drive a car safely. It is likely that the patient would be very reluctant to give up his driver's license and would deny that he was having any problem.

As the individual becomes more affected by decreasing cognitive ability, efforts to cope will be more obvious. The behaviors that become a concern to significant others and bring the person into contact with

---

Nursing Diagnoses Related to Impaired Cognition

Primary NANDA nursing diagnosis

Thought processes, alteration in

Examples of complete nursing diagnoses

Altered thought processes related to severe dehydration evidenced by hypervigilance; distractibility; disorientation to time, place, and person; and visual hallucinations

Altered thought processes related to barbiturate ingestion evidenced by altered sleep patterns, delusions, disorientation to time and place, and decreased ability to grasp ideas

Altered thought processes related to Alzheimer's disease evidenced by inaccurate interpretation of environment, deficit in recent memory, impaired ability to reason and confabulation

Altered thought processes related to HTLV-III infection evidenced by impaired ability to make decisions, to problem solve, to reason, to calculate and inappropriate social behavior

the health care system are frequently attempts to cope. For instance, a family member may complain that a relative has "always been irritable, but is now belligerent when he doesn't get his way." In other cases, the patient's behavior may be experienced by others as a personality change. Some behaviors that are probably attempts to cope with loss of cognitive ability include suspiciousness, hostility, jocularity, depression, seductiveness, and withdrawal. Because it is threatening to admit that a close relative has dementia, family members may also focus on the coping mechanism as the real problem, participating in the denial of the underlying cognitive impairment.

 ## Nursing diagnosis

The nursing diagnosis of the individual with cognitive impairment must take into consideration both the possible underlying stressors and the patient behaviors that have been observed by the nurse. Figure 19-3 summarizes the nursing model of health-illness phenomena as related to cognitive functioning.

Most disorders that result in some degree of cognitive impairment are physiological in origin. Therefore, the nurse must take into consideration the patient's physical needs as well as the psychosocial behavioral disruptions. For instance, the delirious patient may be reacting to an infection or an overdose of a drug. This problem and all its effects on the person must be reflected in a complete nursing diagnosis. Many people who are demented are also elderly. They will experience many effects of the aging process in addition to impaired cognitive functioning. A thorough nursing diagnosis will reflect all these influences on the patient's behavior. In addition, the nature of a cognitive impairment may inhibit the patient's ability to be an active participant in the care planning process. The nurse must rely on observational skills and on the input of significant others to arrive at an accurate and relevant diagnosis. If it is not possible to validate the nursing diagnosis with the patient, it is advisable to involve a family member who is familiar with the person's behavioral patterns. Primary NANDA nursing diagnoses and examples of complete nursing diagnoses related to impaired cognition are presented in the accompanying box. The range of frequently encountered NANDA nursing diagnoses and the Draft of the DSM-III-R in Development[1] medical diagnoses are included in Table 19-3.

■ Related medical diagnoses

There are several medical diagnostic categories related to impaired cognitive functioning. These differ according to the etiology of the disorder and the clinical manifestations. However, in all cases, the etiology is organic. Each one is described briefly.

■ DELIRIUM

The essential feature is clouded consciousness with impaired ability to perceive or respond to environmental stimuli. Other behaviors include hallucinations or illusions, incoherence, agitation or somnolence, disorientation and confusion. The onset is usually rapid.[1]

■ DEMENTIA

The essential feature is a loss of intellectual abilities that interferes with functional ability. Memory is impaired. Other behaviors may include problems with abstraction, judgment, higher cortical functioning and personality change. There is no clouding of consciousness.[1]

■ AMNESTIC SYNDROME

The essential feature is impairment in short- and long-term memory in the absence of clouding of consciousness or deterioration of intellectual ability.[1]

■ ORGANIC DELUSIONAL SYNDROME

The essential feature is the presence of delusions that occur in a normal state of consciousness in the absence of clouding of consciousness, deterioration of intellectual ability or hallucinations.[1]

■ ORGANIC HALLUCINOSIS

The essential feature is the presence of persistent or recurrent hallucinations that occur in a normal state of consciousness in the absence of clouding of consciousness, deterioration of intellectual ability, mood disorder, or delusions.[1]

■ ORGANIC AFFECTIVE SYNDROME

The essential feature is a disturbance in mood, resembling either a manic episode or a major depressive episode, in the absence of clouding of consciousness, deterioration of intellectual ability, hallucinations, or delusions.[1]

■ ORGANIC PERSONALITY SYNDROME

The essential feature is a behavioral pattern involving labile affect, aggressive outbursts, poor judgment in social situations, apathy, OR suspiciousness. These behaviors occur in the absence of clouding of consciousness, deterioration of intellectual ability, mood disorder hallucinations or delusions.[1]

■ ORGANIC ANXIETY SYNDROME

The essential feature is recurrent generalized anxiety or panic in the absence of clouding of consciousness, deterioration of intellectual ability, delusions or hallucinations.[1]

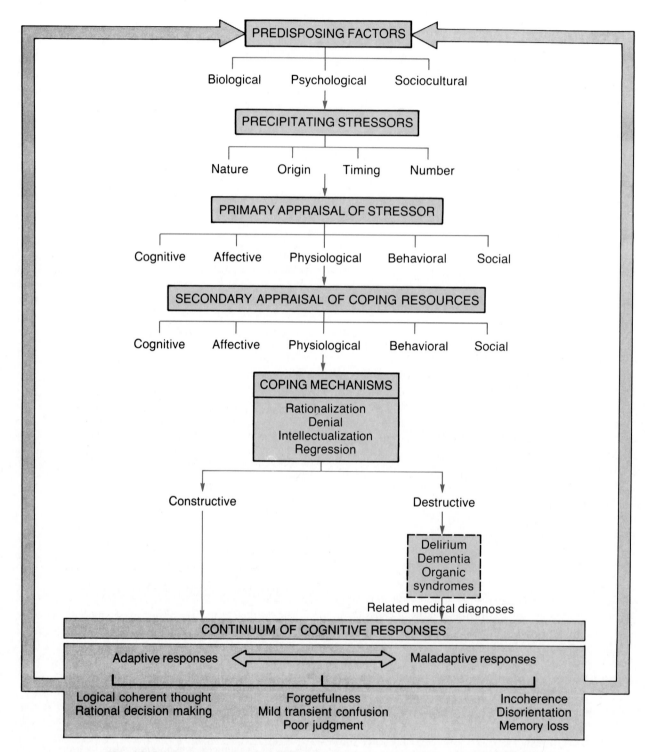

Fig. 19-3. Nursing model of health-illness phenomena related to cognitive functioning.

TABLE 19-3

MEDICAL AND NURSING DIAGNOSES RELATED TO IMPAIRED COGNITION

Medical Diagnostic Class
Organic mental disorders

Related Medical Diagnoses (DSM-III-R*)
Delirium
Dementia
Amnestic syndrome
Organic delusional syndrome
Organic hallucinosis
Organic affective syndrome
Organic personality syndrome
Organic anxiety syndrome

Psychiatric Nursing Diagnostic Class
Impaired cognition

Related Nursing Diagnoses (NANDA)
Anxiety
Bowel elimination, alteration in: incontinence
Communication, impaired: verbal
Coping, ineffective family: compromised
Fear
Fluid volume deficit: potential
Health maintenance, alteration in
Home maintenance management, impaired
Impaired social interaction
Injury, potential for: trauma
Mobility, impaired physical
Self-care deficit: feeding, bathing/hygiene,
    dressing/grooming, toileting
Self-concept, disturbance in: role performance
Sensory-perceptual alteration
Sleep pattern disturbance
Social isolation
†Thought processes, alteration in

*American Psychiatric Association: Draft of the DSM-III-R in Development (subject to change), as proposed by the Work Group to Revise DSM-III. American Psychiatric Association, October 1985.
†Indicates primary nursing diagnosis for impaired cognition

 Planning and implementation

◼ Goal setting

Goals that are related to cognitive impairment may be directed toward an improved ability to process information, if this is realistic, or toward optimal utilization of the abilities that the patient retains if the impairment is irreversible. For example, a goal for a patient who is disoriented because of drug withdrawal might be "The patient will verbalize the complete date within 3 days." In contrast, a goal for a patient who is disoriented because of chronic alcoholism and who is not in withdrawal might be "Within 1 month the patient will find his own bed every night without assistance." The latter patient may never be able to remember the exact date but may not need that information if he is to function in a protected setting. The first patient, however, will need that information. In addition, the nurse can use the assessment of the patient's orientation to time to assess the current status of his mental functioning. Goals should be realistic to avoid discouragement for

both the nurse and the patient. If the second person had been required to learn the date, it would result in a frequent confrontation with his deteriorated cognitive skills, leading to frustration, higher anxiety, and possibly less effective coping. Realistic long-term goals may be difficult to formulate while the evaluation process is taking place. During this time the nurse may elect to focus on short-term goals directed toward maintaining the patient's basic needs.

If there is an identified stressor that is causing the patient's behavioral disruption, goals should also be developed that focus on the stressor. For instance, if a person is delirious because of a fever, a goal might state, "The patient's temperature will be maintained below 100° F (37.8° C)." When the cause of the elevated temperature is identified, appropriate goals will be written to address that problem. For example, dehydration may be a stressor contributing to an elevated temperature. A related nursing goal would then be: "The patient's fluid intake will be at least 3000 ml in each 24-hour period." As the various elements of the person's behavior are explored and documented, nursing goals must be updated and modified; new goals must be added and accomplished goals deleted.

■ Intervening in delirium

■ **PHYSIOLOGICAL NEEDS.** In providing nursing care for a patient with delirium, highest priority is given to nursing interventions that will maintain life. If the individual is too disoriented or agitated to attend to basic physiological needs, nursing care must be planned to meet these needs. Nutrition and fluid balance may be maintained by intravenous therapy. If the patient is very agitated or restless, restraint may be necessary to keep the intravenous line open. Restraints should be applied only when absolutely necessary because the patient can become more agitated and frightened when restrained. A disoriented patient should never be restrained and left alone.

Sleep deprivation may be another problem with these patients. Intervention is important because lack of sleep can add to already existing cognitive dysfunction. If the stressor that is causing the disruption has not been identified, the physician may be reluctant to prescribe sedation for the patient, since sedative medication may confuse attempts to identify the original stressor. Nursing measures such as a back rub, a glass of warm milk, and soothing conversation may help a less agitated patient relax and fall asleep. The presence of a family member is also reassuring to the patient. Disoriented patients need to be in a lighted room. Shadows may be misinterpreted and add to the patient's fear. Also, it is less confusing to be able to use environmental objects to orient oneself to place and person.

■ **HALLUCINATIONS.** The disoriented patient may need to be protected from hurting himself or others, particularly if he is hallucinating. The visual hallucinations of delirium are often very frightening and the patient may try to escape by running away, even to the extent of jumping out of a window. The patient's room must be safe, with security screens and a minimum of extra furniture or other objects placed where he might hurt himself. Frequently these patients require one-to-one nursing observation and repetitive verbal reorientation.

It is tempting to respond to a patient who is experiencing frightening visual hallucinations by trying to eliminate the hallucinated object. For instance, the patient might request help in brushing the bugs off the sheets. Agreeing to do this is not usually therapeutic. By participating in this activity, the nurse is nonverbally communicating to the patient that the hallucinated objects are real and can be made to go away. In reality the hallucinations will continue until the underlying stressor

is eliminated. The nurse's reinforcement of the reality of the hallucination is likely to make the patient even more frightened. A more appropriate response would be to continually orient the patient to the reality situation of being sick and hospitalized. In addition, the patient can be assured that the nursing staff and physician are helping him and will keep him safe. Family members should also be helped to respond in a supportive way.

■ **COMMUNICATION.** Patients who are having difficulty processing information need clear messages and instructions from other people. Choices should be kept to a minimum because the patient will not be able to think of alternatives and decide priorities. Independent decision making can be introduced into the plan of nursing care as the patient's sensorium becomes clearer. Decisions related to orientation may be especially difficult for the patient. To respond appropriately to the question "What time would you like to take your bath?" one requires knowledge of the present time and some idea of the usual routine so that one does not decide to bathe during visiting hours or at mealtime.

Simple direct statements are reassuring to the patient and have the best potential for resulting in an appropriate response. Orienting phrases such as "here at the hospital" or "now that it's June" can be woven into a conversation. A patient who is having difficulty dressing or feeding himself needs matter-of-fact, specific direction from the nurse. A very confused patient will need to be fed or dressed, again in a manner that allows him to maintain his dignity. This is another nursing function with which families can often assist. It may alleviate the family member's anxiety to be able to do something helpful for the patient and the patient may be reassured by the family's physical closeness and concern.

■ **PATIENT EDUCATION.** As the patient recovers, he may be concerned about what happened to him. The health team needs to discuss this issue and arrive at a conclusion about the disruption in functioning that occurred. This should then be explained to the patient and family. The nurse should assess the patient's understanding of the nature of his problem, the stressors which were involved, any ongoing therapy that will be required, and preventive measures that will decrease the probability of a recurrence. Teaching may have to be repeated several times before the patient copes with the feelings the illness has aroused and then grasps the information that has been conveyed. If written materials are available, they can be helpful to patients who are having residual problems processing information. The teaching should include at least one responsible family member so that the information can continue to be

TABLE 19-4

MENTAL HEALTH EDUCATION PLAN FOR THE FAMILIES OF COGNITIVELY IMPAIRED PERSONS

Content	Instructional activities	Evaluation
Explain possible causes of cognitive impairment	Describe predisposing factors and precipitating stressors that may lead to impaired cognition; provide printed reference materials	The learner identifies possible causes of the patient's disorder
Define and describe orientation to time, place, and person	Define the three spheres of orientation; role play interpersonal responses to disorientation	The learner identifies disorientation and provides reorientation
Relationship of level of cognitive functioning to ability to communicate	Describe the impact of cognitive impairment on communication; demonstrate effective communication techniques; videotape and discuss return demonstration	The learner adjusts communication approaches to the patient's ability to interact
Effect of cognitive impairment on self-care behaviors	Describe the usual progression of gain or loss of self-care ability related to nature of disorder; encourage learner to assist in providing care to patient; provide written instructional materials	The learner assists with activities of daily living as required by the patient's level of biopsychosocial functioning
Referral to community resources	Provide a list of community resources; arrange to meet with staff members of selected community programs; visit meetings of selected programs	The learner will describe various programs that provide services relevant to the patient and family's needs; will contact appropriate programs when needed

reinforced when the patient goes home. A mental health education plan for families of cognitively impaired patients is presented in Table 19-4.

If the patient is discharged from the hospital with a residual deficit in cognitive functioning, a community health nursing referral may be helpful. The community health nurse can then continue to implement the nursing care plan and can validate the patient's compliance with the treatment plan.

■ **SUMMARY OF INTERVENTIONS WITH THE DELIRIOUS PATIENT.** Davidhizar, Gunden, and Wehlage[6] have recommended the following nursing interventions for the delirious patient:

1. Regulate lights and provide a window to show diurnal variation.
2. Verbalize orienting information which includes name and purpose of persons entering the room.
3. Provide proper functioning of eyeglasses and hearing aids.
4. Avoid rough excessive handling of patient during procedures or turning.
5. Minimize forced feeding.
6. Elevate the head of the patient or allow him to partially sit up, since *visual hallucinations are increased when the patient is confined to his back.*

7. Provide for presence of familiar personal objects in the room.
8. Encourage visits from family members and friends as indicated by condition.
9. Assign the same personnel to give care.
10. Convey warmth and reassurance. Physical presence can have a calming effect.
11. Maintain firmness when dealing with the agitated, hostile patient.
12. Encourage verbal and nonverbal expression.
13. Provide for diversional activities and meaningful use of time.
14. Protect from situations where judgment and intellectual capacity would be overtaxed.
15. Schedule medications, treatments, or other procedures at times that won't interrupt nighttime sleep.
16. Limit treatments and procedures and schedule them in a predictable way in order to avoid an overwhelming situation for the patient.
17. Provide clocks and calendars.
18. Inform patient of his condition and his progress during periods of lucidity.
19. Allow patient control over aspects of his environment as he is able.
20. Recognize cultural variables that affect patient's response to stimuli.

Intervening in dementia

Nursing care of the patient with dementia is similar in some respects to that of the patient with delirium. Usually the stressors involved do not present an immediate threat to life; so highest priority is given to providing nursing care that will help the patient to maintain an optimal level of functioning. This will differ for each individual. Frequently an attitude of hopelessness evolves in those who work with chronically ill people. This can lead to stereotyping and decreased ability to see and appreciate the uniqueness of each person. It is challenging to search for this uniqueness and rewarding to find it. Individualization of nursing care is probably most important for those who will be institutionalized for a long time.

Recently gerontological nursing has been receiving more recognition as a separate specialty area within the profession. Nursing research is beginning to focus on nursing intervention with the chronically ill person and with the aging person. One finding has been that individualized attention may stimulate enhanced functioning in people who appear to have severely limited cognitive abilities. Jones[13] has described the effect of social isolation and sensory deprivation on institutionalized elderly people. In her work with one such patient she was able to stimulate renewed interest in the environment by providing consistent social interaction. Peer[20] has developed a team approach to the geriatric patient that uses a number of group activities to assist the person in maintaining an optimal level of functioning. These include kinetic therapy, which focuses on body movement; reality orientation; sensory training, using restimulation of all the senses; activities of daily living; bowel and bladder retraining; occupational therapy; poetry therapy; recreational activities; and church services.

Gershowitz[10] recommends that therapeutic approaches with the elderly build on previous life experiences rather than requiring them to learn new skills. She describes the essence of remotivation therapy as helping the patient to "recapture the past and apply it to the present." She emphasizes that remotivation must be a continuous process, not confined to episodic group or individual interactions. This type of approach attends to the person as a complete individual with a many-faceted personality. It is a hopeful way of providing nursing care because it communicates to the patient that there is potential for activity and growth.

PHARMACOLOGICAL APPROACHES.
Attempts to find effective pharmacological approaches to the treatment of dementia are related to theories about the causation of the disorder. Much of the research is directed toward seeking a treatment for Alzheimer's disease. Pajk[19] described several approaches that are being explored. Substances that might promote the production of acetylcholine have not been effective. Arecoline has been tried as a substitute for acetylcholine but is too toxic. Physostigmine is being studied for its ability to decrease the breakdown of acetylcholine. Several agents that might stimulate neurotransmitter action are being investigated. Chelating substances that would decrease aluminum deposits are being tested, but have serious side effects. Vasodilators are sometimes used to increase cerebral circulation and maximize the functional level.

ORIENTATION.
Disorientation is a common problem of people with cognitive impairment. Nursing interventions should be directed toward assisting the patient to function in the environment. In an institution it is helpful to mark patient rooms with large, clearly printed signs indicating the occupant's name. This has the additional benefit of reminding forgetful people of others' names. Personal possessions can also be orienting devices. A favorite rocking chair, a handmade afghan, or a family picture gives the person a sense of identity and helps to identify a personal area of the institution. Everyone needs a personal space. A light in the room at night helps the person remain oriented if he awakens and helps decrease nighttime agitation. Some authorities recommend the use of small amounts of antipsychotic medications, such as phenothiazines and butyrophenones, to assist patients to rest, since barbiturate sedatives may cause paradoxical agitation in people with organic brain syndromes.[17]

Clocks with large faces assist with orientation to time. A digital clock is probably not a good idea, since the confused person may not identify it as a clock. Calendars with a separate page for each day and large writing also help with time orientation. Newspapers provide other orienting stimuli and also help to stimulate interest in current events. An institutional newspaper provides a creative outlet and focuses on patient strengths and also helps patients maintain awareness of the environment.

Reality orientation is a nursing approach that is generally helpful to patients with cognitive impairments. Orientation includes the dimensions of time, place, and person. Systematic reality orientation includes attention to each of these dimensions. Voelkel[27] compared a structural reality orientation approach to the use of a less structured group resocialization approach. She concluded that the most important factor in causing a positive behavioral change seemed to be the involvement in a caring group. Personal and physical contact was found to have a positive impact on group members. Hogstel[12] reported the results of a research project to study the effects of a reality orientation program. She also found that the most positive results were in the area of social interaction. Even if the level of confusion did not change significantly, patients who received reality orientation were noted to be happier and more involved with other people. Mulcahy and Rosa[16] used a reality orientation approach with a group of cognitively impaired patients in a general hospital. In addition to consistent orientation to person, place, and time, their nurse-patient goals included the following: awareness of the need to be hospitalized; cooperation with treatment; maintenance of self-esteem and development of self-confidence; relatedness to the environment through the use of sight, touch, and hearing; bowel and bladder continence; interpersonal interaction; accurate identification of others; and involvement in discharge planning. They developed a standardized nursing care plan and taught other nurses to use it.

■ **COMMUNICATION.** Recent memory loss is another frequently encountered behavior. It may be frustrating to the patient to be constantly confronted with evidence of his failing memory. Conversational focus can be directed toward topics that the patient initiates. Most patients will feel more comfortable talking about remote memories and may derive pleasure from discussing past experiences. Misperceptions of the present situation can be dealt with gently and diplomatically. As an example, if an elderly woman who has been widowed for 10 years says that she expects her husband to come home soon, the nurse might reply, "You must have loved your husband very much. Sometimes it seems to you that he's still here." Explicitly or implicitly agreeing that her husband will "come home" is fostering false hope, perhaps leading to a disappointment. Abrupt confrontation with the reality of her husband's death is cruel and will increase her anxiety.

Bartol and Storrie[4] have developed the following guidelines for communication with the demented patient:

I. Verbal
  A. Speech construction
    1. Short words.
    2. Simple sentences (not compound or complex).
    3. No pronouns; only nouns.
    4. Begin each conversation (particularly at night) by identifying yourself and calling the person by name.
  B. Speech style
    1. Speak slowly.
    2. Say individual words clearly.
    3. If you increase your speech volume, *lower* the tone, raise the volume *only for deafness,* not because you do not get a response you understand.
    4. If you ask a question, *wait* for a response.
    5. Ask only one question at a time.
    6. If you repeat a question, repeat it exactly.
    7. Utilize self-included humor whenever possible.
II. Nonverbal (facial motion, torso position, upper extremity gestures).
  A. General
    1. Convince yourself that your nonverbal style can be felt all the way across the room and by several people; not just the patient or staff person you are addressing.
    2. Every verbal communication is delivered by proper nonverbal gestures.
  B. Specific
    1. Stand in front (or directly in line of vision) of person.
    2. Maintain eye contact.
    3. Move slowly.
    4. If person starts or continues to walk while you are talking to him, do not try to stop him as your first move. Instead keep moving along in front of him and persevere.
    5. Use overemphasis and exaggerated facial expression to emphasize your point, particularly if vision and/or hearing is impaired.
III. General guidelines
  A. Listen actively. If you don't understand, say you don't understand and ask for a repeat of the statement. If this request precipitates a catastrophic reaction, offer your best guess. If you receive a "no," try another guess. Continue until resolution.
  B. Assume there is a capability for insight. If someone refuses to join an event he normally engages in, assume he has become sad, angry, frustrated, embarrassed, anxious about his condition. Your first job is to *check* and see if that is so—not just ask "are you okay" or some ritualistic expression.
  C. Chart all phrases and nonverbal techniques utilized that consistently "get through" for a particular person and a particular situation. Use each others' techniques. Compare notes on successes and failures.
  D. When encouraging participation in activities, regulate your exuberance on the following criteria: if you push hard enough to precipitate a catastrophic reaction you must have planned your time and energy so that you can now treat the reaction with verbal/nonverbal techniques.
  E. When possible utilize an observer to watch your exchange, make suggestions, and perhaps trade off with you. If you have not really "gotten anywhere" in 5 minutes or less, you will probably do better to leave and either return in 5 minutes or have a colleague try.
  F. Finally, if you say you are going to do something, *do it.* If you forget, find the person and

apologize. Assuming that the person has forgotten the episode insults both your intelligence and his/hers.

G. If you need to stop a patient-patient interchange do it firmly and quickly, get them out of each other's territory, wait 5 minutes then return and explain to each one why you acted as you did. Use *factual* explanations, not guilt induction.

■ **REINFORCEMENT OF COPING MECHANISMS.** Previously useful coping mechanisms are often emphasized by the patient with cognitive deficit. Sometimes these attempts to cope may be hard to understand unless placed in the appropriate context. An older man who pats and pinches the nurses and makes lewd remarks may have had past success dealing with his anxiety in heterosexual situations by behaving seductively. An elderly woman who hoards food in her room may equate food with security and may be hoarding because she feels insecure. An aging person who has been suspicious of others in the past may become more suspicious as time goes on. Because of the protective nature of these behaviors, they should not be actively confronted. Rather, the nurse should try to discover the source of the person's anxiety and attempt to alleviate that, thus allowing the person to behave less defensively.

■ **DECREASING AGITATION.** Patients may also become agitated when pushed to do something unfamiliar or unclear. Expectations should be explained simply and completely. If the patient can handle choices, they should be offered. An individual daily schedule of activities can help the person prepare for expectations and plan his day. If a patient refuses to participate in an activity, continued insistence usually leads to increased agitation, sometimes leading to loss of behavioral control. This has been called a "catastrophic response." The best approach may be to wait a few minutes and then return to see if the patient will agree to the request. In the interim the nurse can examine her approach to the patient to see if she might have contributed to the problem. Perhaps the nurse seemed to the patient to be too controlling and a power struggle developed, or perhaps the nurse initiated the request abruptly, not allowing the patient a time for transition from the activity in which he had been engaged.

Richardson[24] has described several approaches to demented patients that assist them to deal with stress and decrease the possibility of extreme agitation. Sincerity is important. The nurse should avoid infantilizing the patient and should offer real choices. Efforts should be made to eliminate unnecessary stress by maintaining environmental stability. Skills should be taught in the setting in which they will be used. It is important to encourage self care, utilizing the patient's strengths and abilities. If the patient becomes agitated and cannot be calmed, a change of the subject and a "sign of friendship," such as a smile or a handshake will often be effective.

■ **FAMILY AND COMMUNITY INTERVENTIONS.** Many individuals with dementia are maintained in community settings with their families. It is important to support these care providers, because the patient usually derives great benefit from being in a familiar setting with familiar and caring people. Mental health education is helpful to families of cognitively impaired people. Table 19-4 illustrates a mental health education plan that is directed toward significant others.

Teusink and Mahler[25] have identified a family reaction process in relatives of patients with Alzheimer's disease. It is likely that the same sequence of responses would also be characteristic of families of individuals with other dementing illnesses. This five-stage process closely parallels the grieving process identified in the significant others of dying persons. The stages are illustrated in Table 19-5.

Families may need assistance in providing 24-hour care for the patient. Home care agencies may be available to provide nursing and homemaking services to enable the person to remain in his or her own home. If family members are not available during the day, adult day-care centers are available in some communities. Mace[15] reports that these programs were first initiated in 1974. By 1984, there were 800 to 1000 of them operating in the United States. The services provided include help with activities of daily living, recreation, health supervision, rehabilitation, exercise, and nutrition. Families also receive support and assistance, particularly during the first few weeks of attendance, when the patient may be resistant because of difficulty adapting to a new experience.

■ **PRINCIPLES OF CONSERVATION.** Hirschfeld[11] recommends structuring the nursing care of the cognitively impaired older adult around Myra Levine's four principles of conservation:

1. Conservation of energy
2. Conservation of structural integrity
3. Conservation of personal integrity
4. Conservation of social integrity

Conservation of energy is related to the need to understand physiological disruptions that might deplete the person's energy supplies. Anxiety and depression are noted as other behaviors that use energy. Nursing intervention in these areas can free energy for other purposes, such as improving cognitive abilities. Conservation of structural integrity implies nursing attention to sensory and perceptual deficits that make it more

---

TABLE 19-5

PATTERN OF FAMILY MEMBERS' RESPONSES TO ALZHEIMER'S DISEASE

Stage	Family behavior	Intervention
Denial	May ignore severe memory loss; may use relatively intact remote memory as evidence of no problem; may interfere with treatment planning	Education Confrontation
Overinvolvement	Sacrifice of usual family activities; reluctance to seek help, often related to ethnicity	Determine cultural norms; help to see problems related to overinvolvement
Anger	Reaction to burden of care and feeling of abandonment by patient; often projected or displaced onto care provider	Assist to recognize and express feelings; be aware of countertransference
Guilt	Reaction to recognition of anger and wish that patient would die; may also be caused by past interpersonal experiences with the patient	Educate about the illness and what the family can and cannot control; assist to make decisions about care, even if patient objects
Acceptance	Resolution of other stages; realistic understanding of what to expect and what can be done	Provide support and knowledge as required

Adapted from Teusink, J.P., and Mahler, S.: Hosp. Community Psychiatry **35**:152, Feb. 1984

---

difficult for the person to comprehend the environment. Patients may need to be protected from injury, and medication use may need to be supervised. Conservation of personal integrity can be accomplished through sensitivity to the person's need to maintain self-esteem. This requires awareness of one's own feelings about organic mental disorders. The encouragement of self-care and the establishment of trust are essential. Reality orientation and listening are important nursing interventions, as are the provision of privacy and respect for personal space. Conservation of social integrity focuses on the maintenance of relationships with significant others. The nurse can help to interpret behavior and encourage frequent visits. Families need help to maintain healthy relationships with the cognitively impaired member, neither withdrawing nor fostering unnecessary dependency. These principles may be used as an organizing framework for planning the nursing care of the cognitively impaired patient (Table 19-6).

 Evaluation

Expectations of the patient who has cognitive difficulty must be realistic but not pessimistic. A brain-damaged person may never remember the correct date but may be able to find his own bedroom. However, if he is never asked to find his room, he has no opportunity to demonstrate his level of orientation. One evaluation criterion, then, is the appropriateness of the nursing goal

to the individual. The nurse should assess whether the expectation might have been either too high or too low. Levels of expectation can be increased until a level is reached where the patient is clearly unable to function and then lowered to the realistic level.

Improved performance on tests of orientation to time, place, and person are concrete measures of the person's level of orientation. The frequency of social interaction is another criterion that may be used to evaluate patient progress. The ability to assist with or perform self-care may also be measured and compared over time. For the person with a progressive disorder, these evaluation measures not only provide a way of assessing the effectiveness of nursing care, but also give a picture of the rate of progression over time, thus allowing the nurse to adjust interventions appropriately. Nurses in long-term care settings may wish to develop flow sheets identifying critical behaviors to facilitate this comparison over time. Anderson[2] developed a simple flow sheet relative to dementia for use by nurse practitioners (p. 611). A comparable flow sheet that she developed for use in evaluating delirious patients is given on p. 611.

If the disruption in behavior is reversible, it can be helpful to know the patient's usual life-style and level of functioning. A college professor is likely to have more highly developed cognitive skills than a laborer. A patient who is visited by numerous friends and relatives probably has different communication patterns than the person who is only visited by immediate family mem-

TABLE 19-6

SUMMARY OF NURSING INTERVENTIONS IN IMPAIRED COGNITION
Goal: Promotion of optimal cognitive functioning

Principle	Rationale	Nursing action
Conservation of energy	Physiological disruptions deplete energy; energy is used to ensure survival before supporting other functions; cognitive functioning is enhanced when adequate energy is available; patient survival and safety are always the highest priority nursing care activities	Maintain adequate nutrition Monitor fluid intake and output Monitor vital signs Provide opportunities for rest and stimulation Assist with ambulation if necessary Assist with hygiene activities if necessary Provide appropriate nursing care for identified physiological disruption Identify stressful situations to assist patient to avoid them Assess mood and intervene in identified disruptions (Chapter 15)
Conservation of structural integrity	Cognitive impairment usually involves sensory and perceptual disorders that can endanger the patient's safety	Assess sensory and perceptual functioning Provide access to eyeglasses, hearing aids, canes, walkers, etc., if needed Observe and remove safety hazards (e.g., obstacles, slippery floors, open flames, inadequate lighting) Supervise medications if necessary Protect from injury during periods of agitation with one-to-one nursing care; restraints only if absolutely necessary
Conservation of personal integrity	Cognitive impairment is a threat to self-esteem; a positive nurse-patient relationship can assist the patient to express his fears, and feel secure in his environment, recognition of accomplishments also raises self-esteem	Provide reality orientation Establish trusting relationship Encourage patient to be as independent as possible Identify patient's interests and skills; provide opportunities to utilize them Give honest praise for accomplishments Use therapeutic communication techniques to assist patient to communicate his thoughts and feelings
Conservation of social integrity	Caring relationships with others promote a positive self-concept; communication by significant others can often be understood more easily than that of strangers; family and friends can provide help in knowing patient's habits and preferences; involvement of significant others in caregiving often helps them cope with the stress of patient's health problem	Initiate contact with significant others Encourage patient to interact with others; involve him in group activities Teach family and patient about the nature of the problem and the recommended health care plan Allow significant others to assist in patient care if they wish Meet with significant others regularly and provide them with an opportunity to talk Involve patient and family in discharge planning

Chronic Organic Brain Syndrome Flow Sheet

If a majority of the following categories are marked "yes," the organic brain syndrome is probably chronic. *All or parts of these categories have changed insidiously.*

Yes	No	Behavior	Yes	No	Behavior
☐	☐	Memory impaired and immediate	☐	☐	Nocturnal restlessness
☐	☐	Difficulty in use of names and numbers	☐	☐	Disorientation to person, place, and time
☐	☐	Age greater than 70	☐	☐	Paranoia
☐	☐	Confabulation	☐	☐	Alert facade
☐	☐	Bowel or bladder incontinence	☐	☐	Decreased response to interviewer
☐	☐	Easily distracted			
☐	☐	Intellectual grasp reduced	☐	☐	Caution becomes suspiciousness
☐	☐	Rigidity of response	☐	☐	Compulsive orderliness
☐	☐	Wandering	☐	☐	Moodiness and depression
☐	☐	Confused by new places or situations	☐	☐	Poor judgment

From Anderson, D.J.: In Wolanin, M.O., and Phillips, L.R.F.: Confusion: prevention and care, St. Louis, 1981, The C.V. Mosby Co.

Acute Organic Brain Syndrome Flow Sheet

If a majority of the following categories are marked "yes," organic brain syndrome is probably acute (onset within 1 to 4 weeks). *All of these changes, or parts, occur rapidly.*

Yes	No	Behavior	Yes	No	Behavior
☐	☐	Fluctuating level of awareness	☐	☐	Delusional denial of illness
☐	☐	Recent medical, surgical, and neurological disease	☐	☐	Inappropriate sexual behavior
☐	☐	Recent change in alcohol/drug intake	☐	☐	Displacement, such as correct name and wrong address
☐	☐	Stupor progressing to delirium	☐	☐	Anxious when unable to find correct response
☐	☐	Visual hallucinations	☐	☐	Euphoria/blandness
☐	☐	Misidentification	☐	☐	Inappropriate joking
☐	☐	Great restlessness	☐	☐	Spatial inattention
☐	☐	Febrile, debilitating, or exhausting illness	☐	☐	Disorientation, but with ability to handle cognitive tasks
☐	☐	Dehydration	☐	☐	Paranoia/agitation
☐	☐	Delusional reduplication	☐	☐	Anxiety/depression
			☐	☐	Misnaming

From Anderson, D.J.: In Wolanin, M.O., and Phillips, L.R.F.: Confusion: prevention and care, St. Louis, 1981, The C.V. Mosby Co.

DIRECTIONS FOR FUTURE RESEARCH

The following are some of the nursing research problems raised in Chapter 19 that merit further study by psychiatric nurses:

1. Validation of nursing interventions that result in improved cognitive functioning when impairment results from hypoxia
2. Assessment of the ability of nurses who work with populations of elderly patients to identify changes in cognitive functioning
3. The ability of nurses who work with populations of elderly patients to assess the presence of physiological stressors related to identified cognitive impairments
4. Primary prevention measures that are effective in decreasing the incidence of dementia
5. The effects on cognitive functioning of commonly used prescription and over-the-counter medications
6. The relationship between dietary patterns and cognitive functioning
7. Specific stressors that lead to the occurrence of "intensive care unit psychosis"
8. Environmental modifications in intensive care units that would decrease the incidence of cognitive disorders
9. Interpersonal approaches that are effective in alleviating the anxiety of delirious patients
10. Characteristics that differentiate between delirium and dementia in the elderly
11. The process of confabulation, including its development and the need it fulfills for the individual
12. The relationship between the existence of a consistently identified area of personal space and the level of orientation of a patient with dementia
13. Validation of environmental manipulations that enhance the cognitive ability of individuals with dementia
14. Environmental characteristics of institutions that interfere with effective cognitive functioning
15. Interpersonal factors that interfere with effective cognitive functioning
16. Comparison of selected nursing interventions for cognitive impairment with objectively measured behavioral outcomes and patient satisfaction

bers. Knowledge of usual behavior serves as a gauge against which to measure progress. Friends and family are good judges of when the patient is "back to normal." However, this should also be validated with the patient. He may have different self-expectations and may use his therapeutic experience to progress beyond his pretherapy level of functioning.

Colleagues are also helpful in evaluating the nursing care plan. They may have suggestions of alternative interventions. They may also provide the nurse with feedback about transference-countertransference issues that may be occurring outside of her awareness. For instance, a nurse who is working with an aging patient with dementia may respond to concerns about her own aging or that of her parents and have difficulty seeing the patient as a unique person. Hallucinating patients frequently arouse anxiety in the nurse, who may then be responding under the influence of her own defense mechanisms. Regular supervision can help the nurse to develop enhanced self-awareness and to assess when a particularly anxiety-provoking situation has bothered her and why.

■ SUGGESTED CROSS-REFERENCES ■

The nursing process is discussed in Chapter 5. Therapeutic relationship skills are discussed in Chapter 4. The health-illness model is discussed in Chapter 3. Depression is discussed in Chapter 15. Substance abuse is discussed in Chapter 20. Psychological testing is discussed in Chapter 6. Behavior modification techniques are discussed in Chapter 27. Cognitive development of the child is discussed in Chapter 30. Gerontological psychiatric nursing is discussed in Chapter 35.

■ SUMMARY ■

1. Cognition is the ability to think and reason, including the processes of memory, judgment, orientation, perception, and attention.

2. Learning theorists have developed models of cognitive functioning, including the associationist model (Pavlov, Skinner, and Wolfe), the cognitive model (Tolman), and the computer model.

3. The developmental process of cognition was described by Piaget and is composed of three stages: the sensorimotor stage; the stage of preparation and organization of concrete operations, subdivided into the preoperational phase and the concrete operations phase; and the stage of formal operations.

4. Predisposing factors related to impaired cognition include interference with supply of nutrients to the brain, aging, metabolic disorders, genetic abnormalities, and co-existing mental disorders.

5. Biological stressors, such as impaired delivery of nutrients to brain cells, metabolic disorders, exposure to toxic and infectious agents, tumors, and trauma, can cause cognitive

impairment. In many instances the stressor cannot be identified.

6. Impairments in cognition are experienced by patients with the medical diagnoses of organic brain syndromes, including delirium and dementia.

7. Behaviors associated with delirium may include fluctuating levels of awareness, disorientation, disorganized thought processes, impaired judgment and decision making, illusions, visual hallucinations, affective lability, loss of inhibition, restlessness, agitation, diffuse EEG slowing, and behaviors directly attributable to the stressor.

8. Behaviors associated with dementia may include disorientation, memory loss, decreased attention span, labile affect, deteriorated social skills, impaired judgment and decision making, restlessness and agitation, and resistance to change.

9. Psychological testing is an assessment tool provided on consultation by a clinical psychologist. Examples of common psychological tests were presented.

10. Coping mechanisms used by patients with impaired cognition may be exaggerations of past methods of coping with anxiety.

11. Examples of nursing diagnoses of alteration in thought processes were presented and compared to the medical diagnostic criteria for delirium, dementia, and other organic mental disorders.

12. Nursing intervention with patients who have delirium includes life support, emotional support, and protection from impulsive behavior. Family members can provide valuable assistance.

13. Nursing intervention with patients who have dementia includes reality orientation, stimulation, encouragement of independent functioning, socialization, protection from accidental injury, maintenance of optimal biopsychosocial functioning, and encouragement of relatedness with significant others.

14. A mental health education plan for families of cognitively impaired patients was presented.

15. Evaluation of nursing care focuses on the appropriateness of the long- and short-term goals and the adequacy and effectiveness of the nursing interventions. Feedback can be obtained from the nurse's supervisor and colleagues, the nurse's self-assessment, the patient's significant others, and the patient. A flow sheet may be useful to record behavioral change over time.

■ REFERENCES ■

1. American Psychiatric Association: Draft of the DSM-III-R in Development (subject to change), as proposed by the Work Group to Revise DSM-III. American Psychiatric Association, October 1985.
2. Anderson, D.J.: Confusion in the elderly: a protocol to determine acute organic brain syndrome versus chronic organic brain syndrome. In Wolanin, M.O., and Phillips, L.R.F.: Confusion: prevention and care, St. Louis, 1981, The C.V. Mosby Co.
3. Bachrach, A.J.: Learning theory. In Kaplan, H.I., Freedman, A.M., and Sadock, B.J.: Comprehensive textbook of psychiatry, ed. 3, vol. 1, Baltimore, 1980, The Williams & Wilkins Co.
4. Bartol, M.A.: Nonverbal communication in patients with Alzheimer's disease, J. Gerontol. Nurs. **5:**21, July-Aug. 1979.
5. Clark, M. et al.: A slow death of the mind, Newsweek, p. 56, Dec. 3, 1984.
6. Davidhizar, R., Gunden, E., and Wehlage, D.: Recognizing and caring for the delirious patient, J. Psychiatr. Nurs. **16:**38, May 1978.
7. DeCato, C.M., and Wicks, R.J.: Psychological testing referrals: a guide for psychiatrists, psychiatric nurses, physicians in general practice and allied health personnel, J. Psychiatr. Nurs. **14:**24, June 1976.
8. Elkind, D.: Developmental structuralism of Jean Piaget. In Kaplan, H.S., Freedman, A.M., and Sadock, B.J.: Comprehensive textbook of psychiatry, ed. 3, vol. 1, Baltimore, 1980, The Williams & Wilkins Co.
9. Engelhardt, K.: Piaget: a prescriptive theory for parents, Maternal-Child Nurs. J. **3:**1, Spring 1974.
10. Gershowitz, S.Z.: Adding life to years: Remotivating elderly people in institutions, Nurs. Health Care **3:**141, Mar. 1982.
11. Hirschfeld, M.J.: The cognitively impaired older adult, Am. J. Nurs. **76:**1981, Dec. 1976.
12. Hogstel, M.O.: Use of reality orientation with aging confused patients, Nurs. Res. **28:**161, May-June 1979.
13. Jones, J.A.: Deprivation and existence or stimulation and life, J. Gerontol. Nurs. **2:**17, Mar.-Apr. 1976.
14. Lipowski, Z.J.: Organic mental disorders: introduction and review of syndromes. In Kaplan, H.I., Freedman, A.M., and Sadock, B.J.: Comprehensive textbook of psychiatry, ed. 3, vol. 2, Baltimore, 1980, The Williams & Wilkins Co.
15. Mace, N.: Day care for demented clients, Hosp. Community Psychiatry **35:**979, Oct. 1984.
16. Mulcahy, N., and Rosa, N.: Reality orientation in a general hospital, Geriatr. Nurs. **2:**264, 1981.
17. Mulder, D.W.: Organic brain syndromes associated with diseases of unknown cause. In Kaplan, H.I., Freedman, A.M., and Sadock, B.J., editors: Comprehensive textbook of psychiatry, ed. 3, vol. 2, Baltimore, 1980, The Williams & Wilkins Co.
18. Navia, B.A., and Price, R.W.: Dementia complicating AIDS, Psychiatric Annals **16:**158, Mar. 1986.
19. Pajk, M.: Alzheimer's disease inpatient care, Am. J. Nurs. **84:**216, Feb. 1984.
20. Peer, S.M.: Therapeutic programs for the long-term care geriatric patient, J. Gerontol. Nurs. **2:**24, Jan.-Feb. 1976.
21. Perry, S., and Jacobsen, P.: Neuropsychiatric manifestations of AIDS-spectrum disorders, Hosp. Community Psychiatry **37:**135, Feb. 1986.
22. Piaget, J.: The child and reality: problems of genetic psychology, New York, 1973, Grossman Publishers.

23. Reisberg, B.: Stages of cognitive decline, Am. J. Nurs. **84**:225, Feb. 1984.

24. Richardson, K.: Hope and flexibility: your keys to helping OBS patients, Nursing **12**:64, June 1982.

25. Teusink, J.P., and Mahler, S.: Helping families cope with Alzheimer's disease, Hosp. Community Psychiatry **35**:152, Feb. 1984.

26. Toffler, A.: Future shock, New York, 1970, Random House, Inc.

27. Voelkel, D.: A study of reality orientation and resocialization groups with the confused elderly, J. Gerontol. Nurs. **4**:13, May-June 1978.

28. Wolanin, M.O.: Physiologic aspects of confusion, J. Gerontol. Nurs. **7**:236, Apr. 1981.

29. Wolanin, M.O., and Phillips, L.R.F.: Confusion: prevention and care, St. Louis, 1981, The C.V. Mosby Co.

■ ANNOTATED SUGGESTED READINGS ■

*Adams, M. et al.: Psychological responses in critical care units, Am. J. Nurs. **78**:1504, 1978.

These authors relate concepts of nursing care for confused patients to critical care areas. The article includes a good example of the use of the mental status examination.

*Adams-Woodward, C.: Wernicke-Korsakoff syndrome: a case approach, J. Psychiatr. Nurs. **16**:38, Apr. 1978.

This discussion of a cognitive impairment disorder that is related to thiamine deficiency uses a case study to illustrate the behaviors. There is also a discussion of the pathophysiological processes involved.

*Bartol, M.A.: Nonverbal communication in patients with Alzheimer's disease, J. Gerontol. Nurs. **5**:21, July-Aug. 1979.

This author draws on her experience as a nurse working with a ward group of patients with Alzheimer's disease. She integrates communication theory as the rationale for nursing intervention, considering the nonverbal communication of the patient and the nurse. Descriptive case vignettes are used to clarify the theory.

*Burnside, I.M.: Alzheimer's disease: an overview, J. Gerontol. Nurs. **5**:14, July-Aug. 1979.

This is a companion article to Bartol's discussion. It is a comprehensive overview of the assessment of the patient with Alzheimer's disease. Of particular interest is a glossary of terms describing behaviors associated with the disease.

Butler, R.N., and Lewis, M.I.: Aging and mental health: positive psychosocial approaches, ed. 2, St. Louis, 1977, The C.V. Mosby Co.

The spectrum of problems inherent in aging is presented from a biopsychosocial framework. There is extensive information on the treatment of the aged in the community and in the institution. An excellent section on diagnostic evaluation is included.

*Davidhizar, B., Gunden, E., and Wehlage, D.: Recognizing and caring for the delirious patient, J. Psychiatr. Nurs. **16**:38, May 1978.

These authors concisely present the prominent features associated with delirium. The emphasis is on nursing care in relation to the observable behaviors that are commonly seen in these patients.

*DeCato, C.M., and Wicks, R.J.: Psychological testing referrals: a guide for psychiatrists, psychiatric nurses, physicians in general practice and allied health personnel, J. Psychiatr. Nurs. **14**:24, June 1976.

This article describes psychological evaluation, including descriptions of several tests and their purposes, and discusses reasons for psychological referral, when not to refer, and what to expect in a psychological testing report.

*Gershowitz, S.Z.: Adding life to years: remotivating elderly people in institutions, Nurs. Health Care **3**:141, Mar. 1982.

To be effective, nursing care of the elderly patient must be individualized. This author provides suggestions about how to accomplish this goal while working within a remotivational framework. Case studies are used to illustrate the theories that are discussed.

*Jarnagan, G.: Taking care of mama, Johns Hopkins Magazine **33**:37, Feb. 1982.

The author, who is a nurse, describes her own experience caring for her demented mother. She conveys an understanding of the decision-making process required and the psychological and life-style adjustments that were necessary for her.

*King, K.S.: Reminiscing psychotherapy with aging people, J. Psychosoc. Nurs. Ment. Health Serv. **20**:21, Feb. 1982.

The author discusses the value of reminiscence for elderly people. She includes a thorough review of relevant literature. Examples of the application of reminiscence approaches in group therapy are provided.

*Langston, N.F.: Reality orientation and effective reinforcement, J. Gerontol. Nurs. **7**:224, Apr. 1981.

This author identifies two aspects of reality orientation: a formal class providing specific information and 24-hour reality orientation using objects that are present in the environment. A helpful feature of the article is the comparison that is drawn between reality orientation and behavior modification.

Larson, E.B., et al.: Evaluating elderly outpatients with symptoms of dementia, Hosp. Community Psychiatry **35**:425, May 1984.

This article reports on a study of 107 elderly patients with a diagnosis of dementia. Fifteen were found to have a reversible problem with identifiable causes. Of these, only three returned to normal with treatment. The authors recommend a thorough physical workup for all cognitively impaired patients, because even truly demented patients may be assisted to improve their functioning if coexisting problems are corrected.

*Mulcahy, N., and Rosa, N.: Reality orientation in a general hospital, Geriatr. Nurs. **2**:264, 1981.

The authors describe a reality orientation program for confused patients that they introduced in a general hospital setting. They include an excellent example of a nursing care plan for use with a confused patient.

---

*Asterisk indicates nursing reference.

*Pajk, M.: Alzheimer's disease inpatient care, Am. J. Nurs. **84**:216, Feb. 1984.

This article contains a comprehensive review of the current neurophysiological research regarding Alzheimer's disease. A sample of a nursing care plan is included, focusing on the functional disabilities associated with this illness. A case study is also presented.

Rabins, P.V., and Mace, N.L.: The 36-hour day, Baltimore, 1981, The Johns Hopkins University Press.

This book is an indispensable guide for families and other care providers for individuals with dementia. The authors provide a wealth of practical information and explain behavioral changes in understandable terms. It would provide an excellent adjunct to health education.

*Trockman, G.: Caring for the confused or delirious patient, Am. J. Nurs. **78**:1495, 1978.

This article presents behaviors and nursing interventions relative to the delirious patient in a well-organized format. It should be particularly useful to the novice.

*Wolanin, M.O.: Physiologic aspects of confusion, J. Gerontol. Nurs. **7**:236, Apr. 1981.

This well-known authority in the field of geriatric nursing identifies the major physiological causes of confusion in the elderly. Nursing assessment is emphasized as a critical factor in determining the cause of confusion. Nursing interventions are described. The article is highly recommended for beginning students and nurses, including those in community settings who work with elderly individuals.

*Wolanin, M.O., and Phillips, L.R.F.: Confusion: prevention and care, St. Louis, 1981, The C.V. Mosby Co.

This book is an effort to clarify and operationalize the concept of confusion. Understanding this concept is central to the provision of effective nursing care to individuals with cognitive impairment. There is an emphasis throughout the book on nursing interventions as applied to various aspects of confusion.

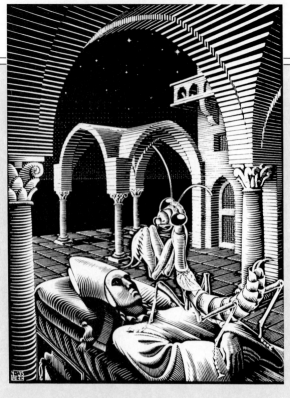

Sleepmonger,
deathmonger,
with capsules in my palms each night,
eight at a time from sweet pharmaceutical bottles
I make arrangements for a pint-sized journey.
I'm the queen of this condition.
I'm an expert on making the trip
and now they say I'm an addict.
Now they ask why.
Why!

Anne Sexton, The Addict*

CHAPTER 20

SUBSTANCE ABUSE

*Reprinted by permission from Quarterly Journal of Studies on Alcohol, vol. 13, pp. 673-684, 1952.
Copyright by Journal of Studies on Alcohol, Inc., Rutgers Center of Alcohol Studies, New Brunswick, NJ 08903.

LEARNING OBJECTIVES

After studying this chapter, the student should be able to:

- define substance abuse.

- discuss the role of cultural attitudes in determining the definition of substance abuse.

- describe statistically the seriousness of the substance abuse problem.

- compare and contrast the major categories of abused substances.

- discuss the occurrence of substance abuse among members of the nursing and medical professions.

- analyze the problem of substance abuse as it relates to the stress response and the health-illness continuum.

- describe various hypotheses concerning the predisposing factors that have been proposed as influencing the occurrence of substance abuse.

- analyze precipitating stressors that may lead to episodes of substance abuse.

- compare and contrast the major categories of abused substances in terms of usual route of administration, expected behavioral responses, behaviors related to overdose, and withdrawal syndromes.

- analyze substance abuse relative to the nursing model of health-illness behavior.

- formulate individualized nursing diagnoses that incorporate the substance abused, the relevant stressors, and the behaviors observed.

- assess the relationship between nursing diagnoses and medical diagnoses associated with substance abuse.

- develop long- and short-term individualized nursing goals with substance abuse patients.

- apply therapeutic nurse-patient relationship principles with appropriate rationale in planning the care of substance abuse patients.

- analyze the biological components of intervention with the substance abuser.

- compare and contrast interactive approaches to nursing intervention with substance abuse patients.

- describe common themes in the therapy of substance abuse patients and appropriate nursing interventions.

- discuss social support systems that may be engaged to assist the substance abuse patient.

- identify five components of substance abuse prevention programs.

- develop a mental health education plan for the substance abuse patient.

- assess the importance of the evaluation of the nursing process when working with substance abuse patients.

- identify directions for future nursing research.

- select appropriate readings for further study.

Continuum of chemically mediated coping responses

The use of mind-altering substances is widespread in the world today. A statement such as this usually brings to mind the use of narcotics, hallucinogens, and, perhaps, alcohol. However, one should also consider prescription drugs and materials containing nicotine or caffeine. To add to the complexity of the issue, some people believe that any substance use should be defined as abuse, whereas others maintain that abuse only exists within the norms of the culture and has no objective basis. For the purposes of this discussion, substance abuse will be defined as the use of any mind-altering agent to such an extent that it interferes with the individual's biological, psychological, or sociocultural integrity.

Interference with biological integrity might be exemplified by the heavy smoker who develops emphysema, the anxious politician who becomes physically dependent on diazepam, or the alcoholic who is in delirium tremens. Psychological consequences of substance abuse could include the acute psychosis of a teenager who has been taking PCP or the inability of an office worker to feel able to function without a morning cup of coffee. Sociocultural effects are experienced by the high school student who is expelled from school following arrest for the possession of marijuana or by the young woman who prostitutes herself to make money to buy narcotics.

Attitudes toward substance abuse

Volumes have been written about the various types of substance abuse and a great deal of research has been conducted. Still, definitive answers to questions about the origin and nature of these problems are yet to be found. Theories cover the gamut of conceptual models of psychology, psychiatry, sociology, and the other behavioral sciences. Some drugs, such as tobacco, alcohol, caffeine, and over-the-counter remedies are legal. Other drugs are illicit, including heroin, marijuana, cocaine, and hallucinogens. Others are legal only if obtained with a physician's prescription. The reason for these classifications is frequently unclear. Compounding the lack of clarity about the nature of substance abuse is a great deal of ambivalence present in society regarding acceptance or rejection of this behavior. This is perhaps best demonstrated by considering the issues that have arisen around the use of marijuana in the United States. There are those who believe very strongly that marijuana use is harmful to the individual and/or society and should be strictly prohibited by law. Others believe that marijuana is harmless and should be as freely available as tobacco and alcohol. Still others advocate little or no penalty for personal use of the drug but stiff penalties for its sale. Meanwhile, marijuana is widely used and in some settings, such as rock concerts, is used openly and generally ignored. However, it has been extremely difficult to obtain governmental approval for the medicinal use of marijuana, even though it has demonstrated effectiveness for problems such as the alleviation of the discomfort of people who are terminally ill with cancer and receiving chemotherapy. These various attitudes reflect the confused values that exist concerning the use of mind-altering substances.

In addition, abuse of substances is viewed differently, depending on the substance being abused, the person who is abusing it, and the setting in which abuse takes place. For instance, the upper middle class businessperson who has several martinis at lunch and is therefore unable to accomplish much work in the afternoon is not necessarily thought of as a substance abuser. However, if a secretary kept a bottle of wine in the desk drawer and sipped it during work, that person would probably be counseled to seek help for an alcoholism problem. Is there a real difference in the behavior of these two individuals? Tobacco abuse is so widely accepted in this country that there is serious debate about whether or not smokers have the right to inflict their habit on others even if it may cause them actual physical damage. Yet, a person who smoked opium would certainly be considered as deviant even if the behavior took place in private.

It is important for nurses to be aware of these cultural attitudes and to recognize their impact on the individual who abuses substances and on that person's significant others. Alcohol abuse may not be noticed because use of alcohol is generally acceptable. There is great stigma attached to alcohol abuse, thereby leading to reluctance on the part of the individual and the family to admit that there is a problem and seek help. Nurses must also take care that their own attitudes do not perpetuate the stigma and prevent them from providing help to the substance abuser. Self-awareness is especially critical when caring for these individuals. Substance abusers are very sensitive to the attitudes of others and may feel guilty because of their own basic acceptance of the culture's value system that has labeled their behavior as unacceptable. The nurse must be able to help them learn to accept themselves. This is difficult if the nurse is caught up in her own value judgments.

Incidence

ALCOHOL. Substance abuse is one of this country's major public health problems. In fact, alcoholism may be the single most important health problem at the present time if one considers morbidity rather than mortality.[27] It has been estimated that 10% of adult men who drink and as many as 3% of adult women drinkers are abusers of alcohol.[9] About 7% of the adult population (over 18) of the United States, or approximately 9.3 to 10 million persons, are alcoholics.[9] Alcohol abuse among adolescents has been increasing. By the age of 25, 95% of young people have tried alcohol at least once.[23] An estimated 3.3 million 14- to 17-year-olds are problem drinkers.[8] Alcohol abuse also affects people other than the drinker. Families of alcoholics experience increased stress and stress-related health problems as an indirect result of alcoholism. It has also been documented that alcohol is a factor in over 50% of traffic accidents, causing more than 28,000 fatalities per year.[8] Citizen pressure in several states to legislate stiffer penalties for driving under the influence of alcohol has been increasing recently.

OPIATES. Opiate use is much less widespread than alcohol use, but is still a serious problem. In 1978, 1.6% of high school seniors had used heroin at some time, and 9.9% had used other opiates, excluding those prescribed by a physician. This figure had decreased very slightly from that of a year earlier.[19] In 1984 less than 0.5% of 12- to 17-year-olds and 1.0% of 18- to 25-

year-olds had ever used heroin.[23] Opiate use is more prevalent in urban areas, among males and minority groups, although there has been a slight increase recently in use by white middle class adolescents and young adults.[11] Estimates of the total number of heroin users in the United States range from 1 to 3 million.[11] Accurate figures are difficult to determine because users can only be identified when they come to the attention of the legal or health care systems.

Opiate abuse is of great concern because it leads to severely deteriorated functioning on the part of the individual and frequently to criminal activity to raise money for purchasing drugs.

■ **PRESCRIPTION MEDICATIONS.** Another type of substance abuse that is of great concern is the habitual use of prescription medications, including sedatives and hypnotics, stimulants, and antianxiety agents. This problem frequently has an insidious pattern of onset. An individual may receive a prescription, like the feeling that the drug gives, and gradually take more pills at a time or take them more frequently. Next to alcohol, diazepam is probably the most frequently abused drug. Yet it is generally viewed as a relatively harmless substance and is freely prescribed for people who are anxious about problems of living. Categories of prescription drugs that are frequently abused include narcotics, barbiturates, amphetamines, benzodiazepines, meprobamate, methaqualone, and occasionally tricyclic antidepressants, particularly amitriptyline. Control of these drugs is difficult because of the many legitimate medical uses for them. There have been efforts to ban production of amphetamines based on the belief that medical uses of these drugs can be accomplished with other less dangerous medications, but so far, they remain on the market. Most of these substances have been placed under some degree of control by the Food and Drug Administration of the federal government, but the black market thrives. In addition, abuse is difficult to control because patients quickly learn that they can obtain prescriptions from several physicians and have them filled at different pharmacies, thus acquiring a large supply of drugs. Multiple addiction to prescription drugs in combination with each other and/or alcohol is becoming more prevalent.

Impaired Professionals. Among the groups with the highest incidence of abuse of alcohol and of prescription drugs are physicians and nurses. The narcotic addiction rate for physicians is estimated to be between 1% and 2%. This is contrasted to the national rate for the total population of 0.3%.[11] The National Institute on Alcoholism estimates that 18% of physicians are alcoholics, compared to 10% of the general population.[16] It has been estimated that 40,000 nurses are alcoholics.[17]

Known rates of substance abuse by nurses are probably artificially low. This is partially because the problem is hidden by the abuser. However, colleagues often work as enablers and fail to confront the nurse who has the problem. Whether this is due to the individual's ambivalence about substance abuse or the result of a misguided attempt to protect the addicted nurse, it is unfortunate, because it jeopardizes the well-being of the nurse and the safety of the patients for whom she is providing care. It is the absolute responsibility of any nurse to take whatever steps are necessary to intervene when a co-worker is practicing under the influence of alcohol or drugs. In recognition of the severity of this problem, in several states, state nurses' associations have established peer-assistance groups to work with addicted nurses. These groups are comprised of volunteer nurses, many of whom are recovered addicts. They offer support and referral services to addicted nurses. This helps them to avoid loss of licensure and ultimately assists them to return to work as effective and safe practitioners. At a national level, the Council on Psychiatric and Mental Health Nursing Practice of the American Nurses' Association has expressed concern about this serious problem.

■ **PSYCHOTOMIMETICS.** Since the early 1960s, another group of substances has been abused, particularly by adolescents and young adults. These substances induce a state similar to psychosis. They include hallucinogens, the most common of which has been LSD. Another substance that is unrelated to LSD, but also leads to an altered state of awareness is PCP. Other drugs included in this psychotomimetic group are tetrahydrocannabinol (THC), which is the active ingredient of marijuana, mescaline, psilocybin, and peyote. Discussion in this chapter will be limited to LSD and PCP, since they are most likely to be encountered by the nurse. In 1978, about 14% of high school seniors had used a hallucinogen at some time, and 10% had used at least one during the last year.[19] In 1984, 5% of 12- to 17-year-olds and 21% of 18- to 25-year-olds had ever used hallucinogens; 2% of 12- to 17-year-olds and 11% of 18- to 25-year-olds had used PCP at some time.[23] Use of these drugs is of concern to society because of the erratic and unpredictable behavior they produce. They are not generally addictive, but are inexpensive to produce and widely available. They may also be substituted by the seller for other more expensive drugs, thus making it difficult to determine exactly what the individual has taken.

■ **COCAINE.** The drug that is currently most popular and the use of which has the highest status in the United States is cocaine. According to a cover story in *Time Magazine,*[7] conservative estimates of cocaine use in the

United States were that 10 million people are regular users, and another 5 million have experimented with the drug. In 1984, 7% of 12- to 17-year-olds and 28% of 18- to 25-year-olds had used cocaine at least once.[13] Although classified as a narcotic, cocaine is really a stimulant, more similar in effect to the amphetamines than to the opiates. Habitual use can lead to deteriorated functioning, although users claim that they perform better under the influence of cocaine. It tends to be readily available in most cities, and its use continues to rise.

■ **MARIJUANA.** Marijuana use in the United States is pervasive. Although it is still illegal, marijuana is widely available and in some settings its use is acceptable and even expected. According to a study sponsored by the National Institute on Drug Abuse (NIDA), in 1978, 59.2% of high school seniors had used marijuana or its stronger derivative, hashish, at least once. In a 1984 study, 27% of 12- to 17-year-olds and 64% of 18- to 25-year-olds had ever used marijuana.[23] Twenty-eight percent reported that they used it at least once a week. These figures reveal an upward trend in the percentage of marijuana users in the high school population.[19] When marijuana use began to proliferate in the 1960s, the majority of users were young. However, years later, many of these people still use marijuana and are now beginning to struggle with the issue of how to advise their own children on the use of drugs. One serious concern about marijuana use is that it does seem to serve as a transition to the use of more harmful drugs. Most users of marijuana do not become heroin addicts. However, it is rare for a person who has never used marijuana to use opiates, hallucinogens, or cocaine.

■ **MULTIPLE SUBSTANCE USE.** A serious and increasing problem related to substance abuse is the rapidly increasing occurrence of the simultaneous or sequential use of more than one substance. For instance, barbiturates and amphetamines may be used alternately to achieve relaxation and then stimulation. Cocaine use is sometimes followed by heroin to moderate the stimulant effect. Such experimentation can be dangerous, particularly if synergistic drugs, such as barbiturates and alcohol, are used. It also complicates assessment of and intervention in substance abuse, since the individual may be experiencing withdrawal from several drugs at the same time.

■ **Natural opiates**

Some relate the high prevalence of substance use and abuse to the need to blunt or escape from the anxiety created by the stresses of life. It is interesting to note that there have been efforts to find means of achieving a "natural high" as an alternative to the use of chemicals to achieve euphoria or relaxation. Advocates of meditation, yoga, and self-hypnosis claim that they are able to find peace from within themselves. There has been an upsurge of interest in Eastern religions, which frequently teach followers to achieve states of altered awareness. Others have found that they can relieve tension through physical activity. Joggers report the occurrence of a "runner's high." Neurochemical research has begun to reveal possible biological explanations for these experiences. Snyder[28] has reported on the discovery of enkephalins and endorphins. These naturally occurring peptides bind with opiate receptors in the brain and pituitary gland. They have been described as natural opiates. It is hypothesized that experiences which result in a feeling of euphoria stimulate the release of these neurochemicals. Research in this area has great promise for increasing understanding of and the potential for treatment of the addictive phenomena.

An individual may achieve a state of relaxation, euphoria, stimulation, or altered awareness by a number of means. The range of these activities is illustrated in Fig. 20-1.

 Assessment

■ **Predisposing factors**

A great deal of research has been conducted concerning the factors that predispose a person to become

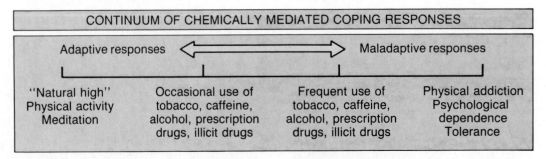

Fig. 20-1. Continuum of chemically mediated coping responses.

a substance abuser. This knowledge is essential to enable health care providers to focus on prevention. Although some information has been provided, much work remains to be done.

■ **BIOLOGICAL FACTORS.** Factors related to substance abuse may be biological, psychological, or sociocultural, but are most frequently a combination. Biological factors may include a familial tendency for substance abuse. This has been observed in the case of alcoholism. This problem tends to run in families and also tends to occur in families that have a concurrent high incidence of manic-depressive illness. About half of the children of alcoholics become alcoholics even though many are repelled by parental behavior while drinking. This is also suggestive of an inherited tendency for alcoholism. Another theory that has been proposed as a cause for alcoholism is that it is an allergic response to alcohol. This is an attempt to explain the fact that some people can control drinking behavior and others cannot. However, the only truly allergic response to alcohol that has been documented is an aversive one. A high percentage of Oriental people in particular have a physiological response to alcohol that includes flushing, tachycardia, and an intense feeling of discomfort.[13] This has been used to explain the low rate of alcoholism among people of Oriental descent.

■ **PSYCHOLOGICAL FACTORS.** A number of psychological theories have been proposed to explain substance abuse. For instance, it has been hypothesized that the person who comes to depend on drugs (including alcohol and tobacco)* is dependent and unable to rely on his own resources for gratification. Freudian psychoanalytical theory describes the oral-dependent personality type. This person is fixated at the oral stage of development and seeks need satisfaction through oral behaviors, including smoking or the ingestion of various substances. A related theory emphasizes the low self-esteem of the substance abuser. Gold[12] has described a cycle of behavior that is illustrated in Fig. 20-2. Substance use is reinforced because it gives the individual a sense of power regarding the area of conflict, thus reducing anxiety. Unfortunately, the substance use itself may create a new source of conflict and contribute to the individual's low self-esteem if guilt or fear of discovery are associated with the behavior. Eventually, the substance abuse itself perpetuates the need to continue taking the drug.

Family traits that predispose the individual to drug abuse have been identified. Chein[6] has described a family

that is too overwhelmed to treat children as persons, lacks a male role model, has no stability, distrusts society, and has no expectations of the child. Stanton[29] reports a higher than average number of deaths in the families of drug abusers. The usual family interaction picture is that of overinvolvement of the opposite-sex parent while the same-sex parent is "punitive, distant and/or absent."[29] The following characteristics are described as distinguishing the families of drug abusers from those with other types of disrupted behavior[29]:

1. A history of multigenerational addictive behaviors, including nonsubstance-related activities, such as gambling and television watching
2. More primitive and direct expression of conflict
3. Absence of schizophrenic behavior in parents
4. An illusion of independence of the drug abuser through peer group membership
5. Higher level of maternal symbiosis
6. The presence of death themes and untimely deaths
7. Immigrant parents, possibly resulting in cultural disparity between parents and children.

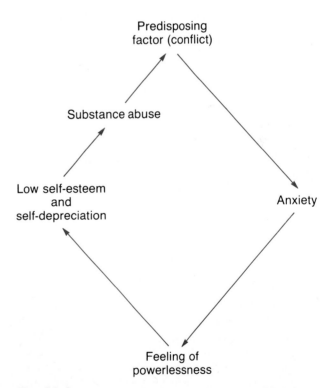

Fig. 20-2. The cycle of substance abuse. (Modified from Gold, S.R.: The CAP control theory of drug abuse. In Lettieri, D.J., Sayers, M., and Pearson, H.W., editors: Theories on drug abuse: selected contemporary perspectives, NIDA Research Monograph 30, Rockville, Md., 1980, National Institute on Drug Abuse.)

---

*The term "drug" will be used to refer to all abused substances, including alcohol, nicotine, and caffeine. Specific agents will be referred to by name or category when appropriate.

■ **SOCIOCULTURAL FACTORS.** Advertising bombards the average person with information on the relaxing properties of a variety of drugs. Even many illicit drugs are easily obtainable by those who are familiar with the drug culture. Marijuana and cocaine are frequently available at the social gatherings of all socioeconomic classes. A related predisposing factor is acceptance of drug use by the relevant sociocultural group.

Failure to assimilate a value system that opposes drug use is also a factor. The ambivalence of society in general about the use or abuse of various substances is perceived by the young and may be interpreted as permissiveness. Children of parents who use drugs, including alcohol and tobacco, grow up with attitudes of acceptance toward this behavior. It has been observed that members of religious groups with strong sanctions against the use of alcohol have much lower rates of alcohol use and alcoholism than members of religions that accept or encourage the use of alcohol. Cultural factors also play a role in alcohol use patterns. It has been found that Northern Europeans have higher alcoholism rates than those from Southern Europe. Of the major religious groups in the United States, Roman Catholics have the highest rate of alcoholism and Jews the lowest.

There are also sexual differences in the incidence of substance abuse. More men than women are abusers of alcohol and opiates. More women than men abuse prescription drugs such as diazepam. It must be noted, however, that the incidence of alcohol abuse by women may be higher than has been believed. Cultural attitudes toward drinking behavior differ for men and women. There is much less acceptance of female alcoholism. Therefore it is often hidden, and women tend to deny that they have a problem even longer than men do. Whereas the ability to drink large amounts is considered to be *macho* behavior for men, use of antianxiety drugs is viewed as weak and unmasculine. The latter behavior is acceptable for and even sometimes expected of women.

■ **Precipitating stressors**

The use or abuse of substances is often viewed as a way to shield the individual from the stressful events of life. Unfortunately, this attitude can lead rapidly to a spiral in which stress occurs, the substance is used, the effects wear off, more stress occurs, more substance is used, and so on. Eventually, the use of the substance becomes an additional stressor because of interference with the person's biopsychosocial functioning.

Substance abuse frequently arises during adolescence. Insecurity related to a poorly developed sense of identity may cause the young person to take drugs. In addition, adolescents are engaged in a conflict between the need to remain dependent on their parents and the need to assert their own independence. This conflict can erupt into rebellious behavior. The use or abuse of various drugs may be an expression of adolescent rebellion that is often reinforced by peer group approval.

The pleasure principle has been proposed as another explanation for substance abusing behavior. This theory suggests that organisms are motivated to seek pleasure and to avoid pain. The use of drugs induces a pleasurable state and reduces the experience of physical or psychological pain. Since the pain returns when the effect of the drug wears off, the individual is powerfully attracted to repeated drug use. This aspect of drug use is reflected in the use of the term "high" to describe the drug experience. A related factor is the described oversensitivity of substance abusers, suggesting that they might be particularly susceptible to the euphoria-inducing effects of drugs. Wurmser[31] has even described a relationship between various types of emotional pain and the type of drug that is abused. He states that narcotics and hypnotics combat rage, shame, and jealousy; stimulants alleviate depression and weakness; psychedelics ease boredom and disillusionment; and alcohol intervenes in guilt and loneliness. Some also relate the use of drugs to a mystical experience and claim that there is a drive to experience altered states of consciousness that is expressed through the use of drugs.[14] This is an existential approach to drug abuse and theorizes that drug use can lead to a spiritual experience which is achieved by most people without the use of drugs.

Sociocultural stressors are also generally present when substance abuse occurs. The complexity and tension of modern life often causes individuals to seek avenues of escape. Drugs are readily available and provide a tempting respite from pressure. The legal drugs, alcohol, caffeine, nicotine, and over-the-counter drugs, are readily available and are socially approved tension-reduction agents. Miller and Cisin[21] point out that illicit drugs are not usually sought by beginning users, but are offered by others. Ausubel[2] has identified ease of access as the primary precipitating factor for drug abuse.

Group influence and peer pressure frequently induce people to experiment with drugs. This is a particularly important factor for adolescents who are developmentally in a stage of concern about peer group acceptance. Peer influence is also reflected in the fact that fashions in drug use change as do fads in other areas. For instance, hallucinogen use had declined for several years, but recently has begun to increase again. Niven reports that young people rarely use true amphetamines now, but drugs called "legal stimulants" have become popular. These street drugs usually contain ephedrine, phenylpropanolamine, and caffeine. Cocaine is popular with older drug users as well as with the young, and its prevalence is increasing rapidly.

■ Behaviors associated with alcoholism

For the purpose of this discussion, the alcoholic will be defined as any person whose drinking behavior interferes with his ability to carry out his usual daily activities and/or adversely affects his interpersonal relationships. This encompasses the person who indulges in episodic excessive drinking as well as the one who is addicted to alcohol. Excessive alcohol use can result in both physical and psychological dependency. **Physical dependence** occurs when there is a biological need in the body for the abused substance. If the substance is not supplied, physical withdrawal symptoms result. **Psychological dependence** is the craving for the subjective effect of the substance on the user. The onset of alcoholism is often insidious. Many heavy drinkers fantasize that they are able to control their behavior when in reality they are addicted.

■ **IMPENDING ALCOHOLISM.** Several behaviors have been identified that are warning signs of impending alcoholism. These include sneaking drinks, morning drinking, blackouts, binge drinking, arguments about drinking, missing time at work, and an alcohol-related police record. The development of tolerance, so that more and more alcohol can be consumed without causing intoxication, is also a sign that alcoholism has developed. Intoxication has been defined as a blood alcohol level of 0.1% or more. Table 20-1 compares blood alcohol levels and behaviors.

■ **PROGRESSIVE ALCOHOLISM.** Seixas[26] has identified several other behaviors that are indicative of progressive alcoholism. One is an increased incidence of suicide in alcoholics. This may also be related to the losses that alcoholics usually experience. In other cases, people who are already depressed may begin to drink as an attempt at coping and may then become alcoholics. Since drinking usually reinforces depressed feelings, suicide may result. A second behavior is increased incidence of accidental injury to alcoholics. For example, about 50% of fatal automobile accidents are related to alcohol use.

Physically, there are a number of behaviors that are frequently related to alcoholism. Since the liver detoxifies alcohol, excessive ingestion eventually results in impaired liver functioning. Fatty liver, hepatitis, and cirrhosis of the liver are frequently complications of alcohol abuse. Other problems include esophagitis, gastritis, pancreatitis, cardiomyopathy, pulmonary function changes, myopathy, osteoporosis, various anemias, disruptions of the immune system, peripheral neuropathy,

TABLE 20-1

COMPARISON OF BLOOD ALCOHOL CONCENTRATIONS TO BEHAVIORAL MANIFESTATIONS OF INTOXICATION

Blood alcohol level	Behaviors
Up to 0.1% (100 mg/ 100 ml)	Loud speech, decreased inhibitions, silliness
0.1% to 0.2%	Slurred speech, moodiness, unsteady gait, decreased coordination shortened attention span, impaired memory
0.2% to 0.3%	Ataxia, tremor, irritability, stupor
0.3%	Unconsciousness

Modified from Butz, R.H.: Intoxication and withdrawal. In Estes, N.J., and Heinemann, M.E.: Alcoholism: development, consequences, and interventions, ed. 2, St. Louis, 1982, The C.V. Mosby Co.

and brain damage.[26] It is obvious that hardly any organ escapes adverse effects in the alcoholic.

Psychologically, the alcoholic may be depressed, hostile, and suspicious or exhibit many other painful emotions. Specific behaviors related to these types of disruptions may be observed. It is often debatable how much of the emotional response precedes and how much follows the development of alcoholism. Alcoholics are usually reluctant to confront or even admit to their problems. They may behave very dependently toward significant others and health care givers, expecting to be shielded from stress and using any conflict to justify drinking. An alcoholic patient once explained her drinking episode by saying, "It was Christmas Eve and I knew everybody in the world was drinking, so why shouldn't I?" Another person said, "If I stub my toe, it's a good enough reason to drink." This combination of dependency and rationalization can be difficult for significant others and often contributes to the breakdown of interpersonal relationships.

Socially, alcoholics may be inhibited people. Alcohol reduces the inhibitions enough to make them able to relate more comfortably to others. However, these relationships tend to be transient and superficial. The intoxicated person may also exhibit poor judgment in his selection of companions, making himself vulnerable to mugging and other forms of victimization.

Clinical example 20-1 illustrates many of the behaviors described. This person has the medical diagnoses of alcohol dependence and alcohol withdrawal delirium.

■ **WITHDRAWAL BEHAVIORS.** Alcohol withdrawal begins shortly after drinking has ended and lasts 5 to 7 days. It is characterized by a number of behaviors, some of which are dangerous. According to Butz,[4] the earliest and commonest behaviors are "anxiety, anorexia, insomnia, and tremor." In addition, there is hyperalertness and a feeling "often described as internal shaking." There may be a mild disorientation, which usually lasts a short time. If it persists, it may be a sign of impending delirium. Tachycardia (120 to 140 beats per minute) continues throughout withdrawal and may be used to monitor the patient's condition. Alcoholic hallucinosis is another withdrawal syndrome and is characterized by auditory hallucinations in a patient who has no other psychotic behavior. This condition generally lasts for just a few hours or days, although in rare instances, it becomes chronic.[1] These hallucinations may be distinguished from those of alcohol withdrawal delirium because they are auditory, whereas the latter are usually visual.

Delirium tremens, now called alcohol withdrawal delirium, is a very serious withdrawal syndrome also described by Butz.[4] Behaviors associated with it include "marked tremor, anxiety, insomnia, anorexia, paranoia, and disorientation." Frequently these patients have episodes of uncontrolled behavior. Delusions and visual hallucinations often occur. Other behaviors may include elevated temperature, tachycardia, tachypnea, hyperpnea, vomiting, diarrhea, and diaphoresis. Occasionally, delirium tremens may lead to death. Alcohol withdrawal delirium usually occurs on the second or third day after the last drink has been taken. It rarely occurs more than a week later. The episode is usually over within 48 to 72 hours after onset.[1]

Another serious behavioral manifestation of alcohol withdrawal is grand mal convulsions, sometimes called "rum fits." Other causes of seizure activity should be explored, including trauma and the use of other drugs. There is generally not any long-term problem related to these seizures.[4] Further information on alcohol withdrawal syndromes may be found in the suggested readings at the end of this chapter.

■ **PHYSICAL DISORDERS ASSOCIATED WITH CHRONIC ALCOHOLISM.** Alcoholics frequently are malnourished and have vitamin deficiencies. Shortage of the B vitamins contributes to the occurrence of peripheral neuropathies. Thiamine deficiency may result in the development of alcoholic amnestic syndrome,[1]

CLINICAL EXAMPLE 20-1

Mr. H was admitted to the detoxification center of a large metropolitan hospital in acute alcohol withdrawal. He was delirious and having visual hallucinations of bugs on crawling his body. He was extremely frightened, thrashing around in bed and mumbling incoherently. Since he had a long and well-documented history of alcohol abuse, family members were contacted and confirmed that he had recently stopped drinking after a 2-week binge.

The patient had been a successful lawyer with a large practice. He specialized in corporate law and conducted much business over lunch or dinner. He also kept a well-stocked bar in his office to offer clients a drink. Without his really being aware of it, Mr. H's drinking gradually increased. After a few years he was drinking almost nonstop from lunchtime to bedtime. He then began to have a Bloody Mary with breakfast "just to get myself going."

His wife reported that he had become irritable, particularly if she questioned his drinking. On two occasions he had hit her during their arguments. She was seriously considering divorce. He had also become alienated from his children, who appeared frightened of him. Infrequently he would feel guilty about his neglect of his family and plan a special outing. Most of the time he was too drunk to carry out his plans. The family had also become less involved in activities with friends. Mrs. H and the children felt embarrassed about his behavior and so did not invite anyone to their home. On two occasions, Mr. H had tried to stop drinking. The first time he went to a private hospital, where he was detoxified and remained abstinent for about a month after discharge. He then lost an important case and decided to have "just one drink" to carry him through the crisis. Soon his drinking was again out of control. His second hospitalization was at a general hospital with an active alcoholism rehabilitation program. He was introduced to Alcoholics Anonymous and started taking disulfiram (Antabuse). This program worked until he decided that he could manage without medication. A couple of weeks later his co-workers persuaded him to "help celebrate" at an office party. This was the start of a binge that ended when he had an automobile accident on the way home from a bar. A passenger in the other car was killed and Mr. H was charged with vehicular homicide and driving under the influence of alcohol. He stopped drinking abruptly, which resulted in his current hospital admission 3 days later.

also referred to as Korsakoff's disease. Individuals with this problem exhibit severe problems with memory. It frequently occurs following an episode of Wernicke's encephalopathy, which is manifested by neurological disturbances, such as confusion, ataxia, and abnormal eye movements. Wernicke's encephalopathy may be treated successfully with large doses of thiamine, but if it progresses to alcoholic amnestic syndrome, the prognosis for reversal of the memory loss is poor.[1]

■ Behaviors associated with drug abuse

Drug abuse refers to the use of any mind-altering substance (except alcohol, which has been considered separately) except as prescribed by a physician. Categories of drugs that are commonly abused include narcotics, stimulants, depressants, antianxiety agents, and hallucinogens. All the drugs mentioned except the hallucinogens can be addictive. Drug addiction may involve physical dependency, psychological dependency, or both. The combination of these two factors is a powerful incentive to continue using drugs. It should also be remembered that many drug abusers are simultaneously addicted to more than one substance.

■ **OPIATE ABUSE.** The opiates include opium, heroin, meperidine, morphine, codeine, and methadone. The first two drugs were used for medical and, in the case of opium, religious and recreational purposes in the past, but are generally no longer used. Meperidine, morphine, and codeine are frequently used analgesics that are found in any hospital medicine room. Methadone is a narcotic substance that is used as a treatment for addiction to other opiates, either to facilitate withdrawal or at a stable dose for maintenance purposes. Its usefulness lies in the fact that it does not interfere with the ability to function productively as other narcotics do. Individuals who are on a methadone maintenance regimen may work and carry on a normal life, although still addicted to narcotics. Opiates may be introduced into the body by ingestion; inhalation; smoking; or intravenous, intramuscular, or subcutaneous injection.

Narcotics addiction is a great social problem. People who are addicted to opiates generally deteriorate mentally and physically to the point that they are unable to function productively. Illegal behavior may be related to addiction as one steals or prostitutes oneself to acquire money for drugs. The obtaining and use of drugs becomes an all-consuming passion. Behaviors associated with addiction to narcotics include the development of **tolerance**. Tolerance refers to the increasing need for more and more of the drug to create the same effect. This, of course, also increases the expense of the habit.

Physiological effects of narcotics include decreased response to pain, respiratory depression, nausea, constriction of pupils, drowsiness, decreased response of the hypothalamus to external input, depressed pituitary functioning, decreased secretion of digestive juices, slower peristalsis, and constipation caused by increased intestinal absorption of water.[24] Psychological responses to opiate use include most importantly a sense of euphoria, referred to as feeling "high." It is this powerful pleasurable response that causes the individual to use the drug repeatedly, utlimately leading to addiction. Other psychological effects of narcotics include apathy, detachment from reality, and impaired judgment. The phrase "nodding out" is used to describe this complex of behaviors in combination with drowsiness. Clinical example 20-2 will demonstrate the behaviors associated with opiate abuse.

Withdrawal from narcotics is extremely uncomfortable, but not usually life threatening. It may be accomplished with the aid of methadone, which can be substituted for heroin or other opiates and then gradually decreased if total withdrawal is desired. When withdrawal is not mediated by the use of drugs, behaviors may include initially anxiety, yawning, diaphoresis, abdominal cramps, lacrimation, and rhinorrhea. These are followed by mydriasis, piloerection, achiness, muscular twitching, and anorexia, and later by insomnia, hypertension, elevated temperature, increased rate and depth of respirations, restlessness, nausea, vomiting, diarrhea, spontaneous ejaculation or orgasm, and blood chemistry alterations, including hemoconcentration, leukocytosis, eosinopenia, and hyperglycemia. Overdosage of narcotics can lead rapidly to coma, respiratory depression, and death. Accidental overdoses among narcotics addicts are not uncommon, particularly if the user is uncertain of the strength of the drug being used. Drugs are usually cut with inert substances before they are sold, thus resulting in the availability of varied strengths on the streets.

■ **BARBITURATE ABUSE.** The use of barbiturates results in a psychological experience that is very similar to that induced by alcohol. Barbiturate drugs include barbital, amobarbital (Amytal), phenobarbital, pentobarbital (Nembutal), secobarbital (Seconal), and butabarbital. These drugs are widely prescribed for their sedative and hypnotic properties. Like alcohol, they are basically depressants, but induce an initial response of euphoria. It is for this reason that barbiturates are popular street drugs. They do lead to both physical and psychological dependence. Behaviors that result from intake of barbiturates include euphoria followed by depression and sometimes hostility. Inhibitions are de-

---

CLINICAL EXAMPLE 20-2

Mr. C was a 35-year-old black man who had been jailed for auto theft. He was believed to be a member of a large ring of automobile thieves in a major metropolitan area. His previous arrest record included several episodes of armed robbery and breaking and entering. A few hours after he had been jailed, Mr. C complained of abdominal cramps and appeared very anxious. His nose and eyes were running, there were beads of perspiration on his brow, and he was rocking back and forth on his bunk. The guard called Ms. V, the correctional health nurse.

Ms. V observed Mr. C and performed a brief physical assessment. She noted that his pupils were dilated, his blood pressure was elevated, and he had "gooseflesh." In addition, there were multiple needle "tracks" on his arms. She asked him directly about drug use and he admitted that he had been addicted to heroin. He stated that his addiction began in 1967 while he was stationed with the army in Viet Nam. When he returned to the United States, he remained in the army for 18 months and was able to stop using drugs altogether. He planned to get a job and attend school after leaving the service. He related that he was disturbed by the attitude of people toward Viet Nam veterans. While he was still in the service, he was able to use peer support to cope with his feelings. However, after his discharge, he was reluctant to talk about his military experience. Others seemed disinterested, embarrassed, or hostile when he talked about it.

Mr. C had difficulty finding a civilian job. He was an artillery specialist in the army and found that it was difficult to apply this experience. He began to have nightmares and "flashbacks" of his combat experiences. Because of the anxiety associated with this, he finally returned to drugs. Without a job, he used illegal means to finance his habit and therefore repeatedly went to jail.

Ms. V discussed Mr. C's problem with the physician in the prison health department. They decided to assess Mr. C's eligibility for a methadone drug treatment program and to request consultation from a counselor at the local Viet Nam veterans counseling center. He was given the medical diagnoses of opioid dependence, opioid withdrawal, and posttraumatic stress disorder.

---

creased and judgment may be impaired. There is a lack of coordination and slurring of speech. The person may become quite drowsy, depending on the size of the dose taken and the individual's level of tolerance. Barbiturates are generally swallowed or injected. Tolerance occurs, resulting in the use of increasing amounts to achieve the desired effect. Because of the similarities in their actions, the use of barbiturates with alcohol is dangerous and may lead to accidental overdose.

Withdrawal from barbiturates can be dangerous and therefore is frequently conducted in the hospital. Withdrawal symptoms from barbiturates include postural hypotension accompanied by tachycardia, elevated temperature, insomnia, tremors, and agitation. If barbiturates are withdrawn abruptly, behaviors include apprehension, weakness, tremors, postural hypotension, twitching, anorexia, grand mal seizures, and psychosis.

■ **STIMULANT ABUSE: AMPHETAMINES AND COCAINE.** Stimulant use has been increasing rapidly in recent years. The alertness and feeling of extra energy that are the results of taking these drugs have resulted in widespread use. Caffeine is the most pervasive stimulant in current use. It is found in coffee, tea, chocolate, and many soft drinks. The wide acceptance of caffeine use may make the use of other stimulants seem more acceptable. The amphetamines are prescribed medically for the treatment of obesity and, rarely, narcolepsy. They are also given to hyperactive children because of a paradoxical calming effect. As other treatments for these conditions have been found, serious questions have been raised about whether there is any legitimate medical use for amphetamines, and serious consideration has been given to placing a ban on their production. Illicit users of these drugs include truck drivers on long trips; students who are cramming for examinations; and people, such as nurses, who work night shifts.

Addiction to barbiturates and stimulants, particularly the amphetamines, frequently occurs simultaneously. Sometimes, a patient who has been using "downers" finds he needs "uppers" to give him enough energy to function. Clinical example 20-3 illustrates this pattern.

Ms. W's pattern is not uncommon. Aside from street use, many people slip into drug abuse without being aware of the consequences of their behavior.

The amphetamine drugs include amphetamine, methamphetamine, dextroamphetamine, and benzphetamine. The effects of amphetamine use include euphoria, hyperactivity, irritability, hyperalertness, insomnia, anorexia, weight loss, tachycardia, and hypertension. It is not generally believed that these drugs cause physical dependence, but they do cause psychological dependence and tolerance occurs. Prolonged or

CLINICAL EXAMPLE 20-3

Ms. W was a 34-year-old woman who was moderately overweight. She had tried various diets on her own with little success. A friend told her about a "diet doctor" who had a reputation for helping his patients lose weight with minimal deprivation from eating their usual diet. Ms. W decided to see the physician and was accepted for treatment. She was given a diuretic and appetite depressant medication. The latter contained amphetamines. She began to lose weight as soon as she started the prescribed regimen and was delighted. She also liked the additional burst of energy she felt every time she took her medication. She completed projects that she had been planning to work on for months. However, her family began to complain because she was irritable and very restless. In addition, she developed insomnia and roamed about the house at night.

On the urging of her husband, she went to her family physician. She felt guilty about seeing another physician for her weight problem, so neglected to tell her regular physician about this. With the history of insomnia, irritability, and recent weight loss, her physician thought she might be depressed; so he ordered an antidepressant medication and a barbiturate sedative. Ms. W soon found that she was able to sleep well with her sedative. However, she felt slightly hung over in the morning and still wanted to lose more weight, so she continued with her diet pills as well. For a while she was able to function well. Gradually, however, she found that she needed two sedatives and then she also began to use extra stimulants. Her husband questioned her drug use. Ms. W had read about drug abuse and with her husband's help identified that she had a problem. She decided to see her family physician again and this time told him the whole story. He then advised a brief hospitalization so she could be withdrawn from both drugs under medical supervision. Ms. W was very embarrassed by her addiction. While in the hospital, she needed a great deal of nursing support to integrate this experience. The medical diagnoses that were applied to Ms. W included amphetamine dependence, amphetamine withdrawal, barbiturate dependence, and barbiturate withdrawal.[1]

(snort) cocaine through rolled up $100 bills. It may be inhaled, injected subcutaneously or intravenously, smoked, or applied topically to the genitals.[22] Those who want a more intense experience may smoke the drug after processing it chemically. This process is called "freebasing" and the result of the processing is called "crack." Use of cocaine has been glamorized by the publicity given to its use by movie stars, sports figures, and other well-known people. This makes it particularly inviting to adolescents who use famous people as role models. Historically, cocaine use was advocated for a time by Sigmund Freud. He later became disenchanted with it. The drug was also a part of the life-style of Sherlock Holmes as created by Sir Arthur Conan Doyle.

Cocaine is relatively short acting, with its effects lasting 20 to 30 minutes when it has been inhaled. The experience is very similar to that induced by the amphetamines. A cocaine high is also usually followed by a crash, leading to repeated use. Cocaine use has been known to result in sudden death. The most serious long-term effect of cocaine that has been identified so far is deterioration of the mucous membrane of the nose, eventually resulting in destruction of the nasal septum. Cocaine use does not seem to result in physical dependence.

■ **ABUSE OF HALLUCINOGENS AND PCP.** One behavior that became representative of the "drop-out" generation of the 1960s was the use of drugs that create experiences very similar to those which are typical of a psychotic state. These substances have been called hallucinogens, psychedelics, and psychotomimetics. LSD is representative of the hallucinogenic drugs. PCP use results in behaviors that are similar in many respects to those produced by hallucinogens. Because of the entirely different chemical structures, it is important to be able to compare and contrast these drugs.

LSD is generally swallowed. It is colorless and tasteless and is therefore often added to a drink or food, such as a sugar cube. It may also be given to a person without his being aware that he has taken a drug. Pleasurable effects of hallucinogen use include intensification of sensory experiences, with colors described as more brilliant, and sounds, smells, and tastes are heightened. Sometimes users of these drugs will report synesthesia, or a crossover of sensory experiences during which music may be seen or colors may be heard. Space and time become distorted.

The hallucinogens have not demonstrated addictive properties. They do, however, lead to self-destructive behavior because of the impairment of judgment that results from their use. LSD, peyote, mescaline, and psilocybin are commonly used hallucinogens. Vulnerable individuals who take these drugs may experience

excessive use may result in psychotic behavior. Withdrawal of the drugs usually results in a "crash," manifested by depression and lack of energy. This discomfort provides motivation to take more drugs.

Cocaine is a stimulant drug that is also becoming a symbol of sophistication. It is fashionable to inhale

"bad trips," which may deteriorate into psychotic episodes. The patient may experience paranoid, grandiose, or somatic delusions, usually accompanied by vivid hallucinations. The hallucinatory experience may be pleasant or frightening. The patient who is psychotic is not in contact with reality and frequently misinterprets environmental events. He may be unable to attend to any of his biological needs. He may also inadvertently hurt himself either in response to hallucinations or as an attempt to escape from the frightening experience. Since there is no physical dependence, withdrawal symptoms do not occur. Usually there is a gradual dissipation of psychotic behavior, although the patient may experience "flashbacks" for several months. These brief recurrences of the hallucinogenic experience can be frightening. Patients often express the fear that they are crazy and will never be free of the aftereffects of the drug.

PCP use has become more widespread than that of LSD and related drugs. It may be ingested and is frequently smoked in a mixture with another substance, such as marijuana or parsley flakes. PCP use may precipitate an intensely psychotic experience characterized by extreme agitation. The patient may become violent or exhibit other antisocial behaviors, such as insistence on removing his clothing or the use of profanity. Physical manifestations of PCP intoxication include hypertension, hypersalivation, diaphoresis, nausea and vomiting, ataxia, dysarthria, increased deep tendon reflexes, and decreased pain response. Nystagmus frequently occurs and may be lateral, vertical, or sometimes rotary. At high doses, serious physiological consequences can occur, including seizures, coma, and death.[15] PCP use may evoke the occurrence or exacerbation of an existing and previously controlled psychosis. The unpredictability of the reaction to PCP makes it an extremely dangerous drug.

■ **MARIJUANA USE.** Marijuana will be discussed briefly because it is an illicit drug. Nurses will rarely see anyone admitted to the health care system with a primary diagnosis of marijuana use. Use of marijuana generally produces an altered state of awareness accompanied by a feeling of relaxation and mild euphoria. Inhibitions are reduced and reflexes are slowed. Prolonged use may lead to a sense of apathy and loss of motivation, sometimes referred to as the amotivational syndrome. Psychosis may occur in individuals who are already at risk. The physiological effects of marijuana use are still being investigated, but do include drying of the oral and pharyngeal mucous membranes and reddening of the eyes. Pulmonary changes similar to those associated with tobacco use have also been found. Other long-term effects are yet to be identified.

■ **ABUSE OF ANTIANXIETY DRUGS.** Antianxiety agents, particularly the benzodiazepines, constitute a large part of legal drug abuse in the United States. Chlordiazepoxide (Librium) and diazepam (Valium) were welcomed by the medical profession and the public as the answer to the stresses of life. Because they were initially described as relatively safe drugs, the benzodiazepines were prescribed and used freely. However, it has now become apparent that these agents can be physically and psychologically addictive and that tolerance to their use does occur, resulting in the ingestion of gradually increasing amounts. Long-term abuse of benzodiazepines can be debilitating with psychological and social consequences very similar to those associated with alcohol abuse. The person who takes an antianxiety drug experiences a sense of relaxation and a feeling of confidence. As with most drugs, it is this pleasurable experience that leads to repeated use of the drug. This progression is illustrated in Clinical example 20-4.

The case of Ms. T demonstrates the seductive quality of the use of antianxiety drugs. Avoidance of anxiety is a powerful motivator of behavior. As with other drugs, as use escalates, guilt about drug taking develops, leading to anxiety that combines with the anxiety related to giving up the drug and results in increased intake. Antianxiety drugs have physiological as well as psychological effects. These may include drowsiness, hypotension, ataxia, and slurred speech. The withdrawal syndrome associated with abrupt cessation of benzodiazepines for patients who have taken the drugs for an extended period of time is similar to barbiturate withdrawal. Benzodiazepines have anticonvulsant properties, and withdrawal can lead to seizures, particularly in patients with a history of prior episodes of convulsive behavior.

Multiple drug abuse is becoming more common. The foregoing discussion reveals that many of the abused substances have similar effects. Abusers may use them interchangeably or simultaneously. Simultaneous use can lead to inadvertent overdose, since some of the substances are synergistic. It is extremely important that the exact nature of drug-abusing behaviors be identified, so that unanticipated occurrence of withdrawal symptoms can be avoided.

Table 20-2 summarizes the behaviors associated with substance abuse.

■ **Coping mechanisms**

The presence of substance abuse indicates that the person is experiencing serious difficulty coping. Healthier defense mechanisms and other adaptive behaviors are either inadequate or have not been developed.

CLINICAL EXAMPLE 20-4

Ms. T was a 28-year-old law student. She had always done well in school and had no difficulty with the theory portion of her law studies. However, she had always felt self-conscious and inadequate when she was required to speak before a group of people. She would become tremulous, her pulse and respiratory rate would increase, and her mouth would become dry. On occasion, she would lose track of her thoughts and be unable to continue speaking. This problem became a real handicap in her law classes. One of her professors gave her a failing grade for inadequate participation in class discussions. She went to her family physician and described her problem. He reassured her that he could give her medication that would help her overcome her "stress response." She was given diazepam, 5 mg, one tablet to be taken every 4 hours as needed for anxiety.

Ms. T was reluctant to take drugs because she recognized the danger inherent in the use of medication. However, she knew that she would never be able to stay in law school if she did not overcome her anxiety. Before her next class, she took a pill. She quickly felt relaxed and self-confident. She described the feeling as "like I had had a martini, only nicer." When the professor asked her a question, she was able to respond and was complimented for her answer. She felt a little drowsy after class but decided that she was probably tired because she had not been sleeping well.

Initially, Ms. T only took diazepam when she anticipated that she would need to speak in class. However, she was introduced to an attractive man by a friend and he asked her out for dinner. She felt anxious before the date and decided that it would do no harm to take a pill to help her relax. She was confident and charming on the date. Gradually, she began to use the drug more frequently. She rationalized that she needed the help to get through school and would stop during summer break. One day, she discovered that she had run out of pills just before she was scheduled to participate in a classroom debate. She went to the school health service, described her anxiety about the class and received another prescription for diazepam. She began to take more than one pill at a time and took them more frequently.

As her drug intake increased, Ms. T's performance in school deteriorated. She turned in papers late and missed classes. Her speech was slurred and she was uncoordinated. Her grades slipped. A year after she began to take pills to enable her to stay in school, she flunked out.

Therefore the person must resort to methods of coping that may provide temporary relief of anxiety but eventually involve even more anxiety as the person becomes aware that he is harming himself. Drug and alcohol addicts tend to resist this awareness by employing ego defense mechanisms and other behaviors that represent attempts to delude the self. Seixas[26] describes three such defensive maneuvers characteristically used by alcoholics: denial that there is a problem, projection that the drinking behavior is the result of outside experiences beyond the individual's control, and dissociation of the drinking behavior from its effects. Drug abusers also use denial. However, in contrast to alcoholics and users of prescription drugs who tend to isolate themselves from others, users of illicit drugs tend to band together into a drug culture. Although there may be little, if any, meaningful interaction while group members are high, there is the reinforcing effect of the group identity, which may be viewed as a justification for the behavior. A part of the group support is often an attitude of scorn and hostility toward "straight" people, which includes anyone who is not involved in drug abuse.

Nursing diagnosis

The nursing diagnosis of an individual who abuses substances must reflect the behavioral alteration, the substance used or abused, the degree to which it is used or abused, and the possible stressors involved. Jellinek[18] has proposed the following four phases of alcoholism that may assist the nurse in determining the degree to which alcohol is being used:

PHASE 1

Prealcoholic phase. This phase is characterized by social drinking, control over drinking behavior, and occasional alcohol use for stress reduction. At later stages of this phase there may be frequent drinking related to tension reduction.

PHASE 2

Early alcoholic phase. This phase begins with the first blackout. There is a slow increase in alcohol tolerance and progressive preoccupation with alcohol. The person may begin to drink alone and his behavior may be embarrassing to others. Guilt feelings lead to excuses for drinking. There may be periods of total abstinence, which are used as evidence of the person's control over his drinking behavior.

PHASE 3

True alcoholic phase. Everything revolves around alcohol. The person is avoided by significant others and resents this. It is impossible for the individual to stop after one drink.

PHASE 4

Complete alcohol dependence. Drinking begins in the morning and continues all day. Physical dependence is present.

TABLE 20-2

SUMMARY OF BEHAVIORS ASSOCIATED WITH SUBSTANCE ABUSE

Substance	Route (most common listed first)	Physical dependence	Psychological dependence	Expected behaviors
Alcohol	Ingestion	Yes	Yes	Euphoria, followed by depression and sometimes hostility; decreased inhibitions; impaired judgment; incoordination; slurred speech
Opiates Heroin	Injection Ingestion Inhalation	Yes	Yes	Euphoria, relaxation, relief from pain, lack of concern, detachment from reality, drowsiness, constricted pupils, nausea, constipation, slurred speech, impaired judgment
Morphine	Injection Ingestion	Yes	Yes	
Meperidine	Injection Ingestion	Yes	Yes	
Codeine	Ingestion Injection	Yes	Yes	
Opium	Smoking Ingestion			
Methadone	Ingestion	Yes	Yes	Relieves craving for drugs without causing impaired functioning
Barbiturates	Ingestion Injection	Yes	Yes	Euphoria, followed by depression and sometimes hostility; decreased inhibitions; impaired judgment; slurred speech; incoordination; drowsiness
Amphetamines	Ingestion Injection	No	Yes	Euphoria, hyperactivity, irritability, hyperalertness, insomnia, anorexia, weight loss, tachycardia, hypertension
Cocaine	Inhalation Smoking Injection Topical	No	Yes	Euphoria, elation, agitation, hyperactivity, irritability, grandiosity, pressured speech, tachycardia, hypertension, diaphoresis, anorexia, weight loss, insomnia

TABLE 20-2—cont'd

SUMMARY OF BEHAVIORS ASSOCIATED WITH SUBSTANCE ABUSE

Behaviors related to overdose	Withdrawal syndrome	Special considerations
Unconsciousness, coma, respiratory depression, death	Tremors, hallucinosis, seizure disorder, delirium tremens (alcohol withdrawal delirium)	Chronic use leads to serious disruptions in most organ systems; malnutrition and dehydration are common; vitamin deficiency may lead to Wernicke's encephalopathy and alcoholic amnestic syndrome; alcohol-dependent people are susceptible to other dependencies as well
Unconsciousness, coma, respiratory depression, circulatory depression, respiratory arrest, cardiac arrest, death	Watery eyes, dilated pupils, anxiety, abdominal cramps, piloerection, yawning, diaphoresis, rhinorrhea, achiness, anorexia, insomnia, fever, nausea, vomiting, diarrhea	Chronic use leads to lack of concern about physical well-being, resulting in malnutrition and dehydration; criminal behavior may take place to acquire money for drugs; injection sites may become infected; multiple drug use is common
Same	Same	
Respiratory depression, coma, death	Postural hypotension, tachycardia, fever, insomnia, tremors, agitation, anxiety; rapid withdrawal causes apprehension, weakness, tremors, postural hypotension, anorexia, grand mal seizures	Frequently used alternately with stimulants; combination with alcohol enhances effects and may lead to overdosage; paradoxical responses of hyperactivity may occur in children and the elderly
Restlessness, tremor, rapid respiration, confusion, assaultiveness, hallucinations, panic	Depression, fatigue	Prolonged use can result in psychotic behavior; a paradoxical depressant reaction occurs in children; frequently used alternately with depressant substances
Restlessness, tremor, rapid respiration, confusion, assaultiveness, hallucinations, panic	Depression, fatigue, anxiety	Psychotic behavior may occur following large doses; prolonged use by inhalation may result in destruction of the mucous membranes in the nose and deterioration of the nasal septum; use in combination with other substances is dangerous

Continued.

TABLE 20-2—cont-d

SUMMARY OF BEHAVIORS ASSOCIATED WITH SUBSTANCE ABUSE

Substance	Route (most common listed first)	Physical dependence	Psychological dependence	Expected behaviors
Hallucinogens (psychedelics)	Ingestion Smoking	No	No	Distorted perception, heightened sense of awareness, grandiosity, hallucinations, illusions, distortions of time and space, depersonalization, mystical experiences, dilated pupils, increased blood pressure, increased salivation
Phencyclidine (PCP)	Smoking Ingestion	No	No	Euphoria, perceptual distortion, agitation, violence, delusions, antisocial behavior, elevated blood pressure, increased salivation, diaphoresis, ataxia, increased DTRs, nystagmus, decreased pain response
Marijuana	Smoking Ingestion	No	Yes	Relaxation, mild euphoria, loss of inhibition, decreased motivation, red eyes, dry mouth
Antianxiety drugs (benzo-diazepines)	Ingestion Injection	Yes	Yes	Relaxation, increased self-confidence, relief of anxiety, drowsiness, ataxia, slurred speech, hypotension

Severe liver damage may occur. There is usually some brain damage. If drinking continues, death will occur. The person cannot stop drinking without help.

Similar phases may be identified for abuse of drugs other than alcohol. They are as follows:

PHASE 1

Experimentation. The person takes a drug to see what it is like or to conform with peers. No further use develops from the initial experience.

PHASE 2

Early drug abuse. A specific drug or various drugs are used with some degree of regularity for the pleasurable effects or to reduce anxiety. Drugs may be used socially.

PHASE 3

True drug addiction. Drugs are used regularly, several times a day. Physical dependence begins if it is a characteristic of the drug. Psychological dependence is present. The life-style is drug focused. Social functioning deteriorates.

PHASE 4

Severe drug addiction. The person does whatever is necessary to obtain drugs. Criminal behavior occurs. There is total alienation from the non–drug using culture. The physical condition deteriorates. Continued drug use will lead to death.

TABLE 20-2—cont'd

SUMMARY OF BEHAVIORS ASSOCIATED WITH SUBSTANCE ABUSE

Behaviors related to overdose	Withdrawal syndrome	Special considerations
Panic, psychosis	None	A "bad trip" may result in panic, unpredictable behavior, and psychotic behaviors; "flashbacks" may occur for several months after use; self-destructive behavior may occur while under the effect of the drug
Drowsiness, stupor, coma, grand mal seizures, death	None	Use may lead to psychotic behavior, irrationality, panic
Psychosis	None	Physiological consequences of use are under investigation
Drowsiness, confusion, hypotension, coma, death	Tremors, agitation, anxiety, grand mal seizures, abdominal cramps, vomiting, diaphoresis	Dependence may occur insidiously; users may underreport the actual amount taken because of guilt about multiple prescriptions and abuse

The nurse should also be aware that individuals who have substance abuse problems also tend to develop multiple physical problems, particularly if the substance abuse problem is severe. The involvement with the abused agent becomes all consuming, leading to self-neglect. The complete plan of nursing care would include diagnosis of all the patient's nursing care needs. For the purposes of this discussion, the presentation of nursing diagnoses will be limited to those more specifically related to substance abuse. The accompanying box presents primary NANDA nursing diagnoses and ex-amples of complete nursing diagnoses. In Table 20-3, nursing and medical diagnoses related to substance abuse are listed.

■ Related Medical Diagnoses

Medical diagnoses relative to substance abuse disorders reflect the organic brain syndrome that is produced by the abused substance. Those with unique characteristics will be listed and described separately. Syndromes with common characteristics will be described in general, with the agents associated with the behavior

Nursing Diagnoses Related to Substance Abuse

Primary NANDA nursing diagnoses

Thought processes, alteration in
Sensory-perceptual alteration: visual, auditory, tactile, kinesthetic, gustatory, olfactory

Examples of complete nursing diagnoses

Alteration in thought processes characteristic of true alcoholism related to pressures of a busy law practice and family demands evidenced by confusion and blackouts

Alteration in thought processes characteristic of severe drug addiction to amphetamines related to desire to lose weight evidenced by delusion that husband is having an affair with her mother

Sensory-perceptual alteration (visual) characteristic of complete alcohol dependence related to loss of job and rejection by family evidenced by asking staff to "get rid of these bugs" while brushing at his clothing

Sensory-perceptual alteration (auditory) characteristic of experimentation with hallucinogens related to peer pressure evidenced by covering ears and shouting, "Don't say those words to me," when alone in a room.

TABLE 20-3

MEDICAL AND NURSING DIAGNOSES RELATED TO SUBSTANCE ABUSE

Medical Diagnostic Class

Psychoactive substance use disorders

Related Medical Diagnoses (DSM-III-R*)

Alcohol intoxication
Alcohol withdrawal
Alcohol withdrawal delirium
Alcohol hallucinosis
Barbiturate or similarly acting sedative or hypnotic intoxication
Barbiturate or similarly acting sedative or hypnotic withdrawal
Opioid intoxication
Opioid withdrawal
Cocaine intoxication
Cocaine withdrawal
Amphetamine or similarly acting sympathomimetic intoxication
Amphetamine or similarly acting sympathomimetic withdrawal
Phencyclidine or similarly acting arylcyclohexylamine intoxication
Hallucinogen hallucinosis
Psychoactive substance dependence

Nursing Diagnostic Class

Substance abuse

Related Nursing Diagnoses (NANDA)

Anxiety
Ineffective individual coping
Impaired adjustment
Impaired social interaction
Injury, potential for
Self-concept, disturbances in
Sleep pattern disturbance
Violence, potential for
†Alteration in thought processes
†Sensory-perceptual alteration

*American Psychiatric Association: Draft of the DSM-III-R in Development (subject to change), as proposed by the Work Group to Revise DSM-III. American Psychiatric Association, October 1985.
†Indicates primary nursing diagnosis for nursing abuse.

listed. Table 20-2 also provides a reference to behaviors associated with these chemicals.

■ **ALCOHOL INTOXICATION.**[1] Essential features of alcohol intoxication include recent ingestion of alcohol combined with maladaptive behaviors, such as fighting or interference with usual functioning. Physiological signs include slurred speech, incoordination, unsteady gait, nystagmus, and flushed face. Psychological signs include mood change, irritability, loquacity, and impaired attention. At least one physiological and one psychological sign must be present.

■ **ALCOHOL WITHDRAWAL.** Essential features of alcohol withdrawal include recent cessation of prolonged heavy drinking followed by coarse tremor and at least one of the following: nausea and vomiting; malaise or weakness; autonomic hyperactivity; anxiety; depressed mood or irritability; orthostatic hypotension.

■ **ALCOHOL WITHDRAWAL DELIRIUM.**[1] Essential features of alcohol withdrawal delirium include delirium occurring within one week of ending or reducing heavy drinking, combined with autonomic hyperactivity.

■ **ALCOHOL HALLUCINOSIS.**[1] Essential features of alcohol hallucinosis include vivid auditory hallucinations following ending or reducing heavy drinking (usually within 48 hours) in an individual with apparent alcohol dependence. The response to the hallucinations is appropriate and there is no clouding of consciousness, as in delirium.

■ **BARBITURATE OR SIMILARLY ACTING SEDATIVE OR HYPNOTIC INTOXICATION.**[1] Essential features include recent use of a drug from this category with psychological signs including (at least one) mood lability, disinhibition of sexual and aggressive impulses, irritability, and loquacity. Neurological signs include (at least one) slurred speech, incoordination, unsteady gait, and impairment in attention or memory. Maladaptive behavior must also be present.

■ **BARBITURATE OR SIMILARLY ACTING SEDATIVE OR HYPNOTIC WITHDRAWAL.**[1] Essential features include prolonged heavy use of one of the drugs from this category or more prolonged use of smaller doses of a benzodiazepine. Following cessation or reduction at least three of the following must occur: nausea and vomiting; malaise or weakness; autonomic hyperactivity; anxiety; depressed mood or irritability; orthostatic hypotension; coarse tremor of hands, tongue and eyelids.

■ **OPIOID INTOXICATION.**[1] Essential features of opioid intoxication include recent use of an opioid with pupillary constriction and at least one of the following

psychological signs: euphoria, dysphoria, apathy, and psychomotor retardation. Neurological signs include at least one of drowsiness, slurred speech, and impairment in attention and memory. There are also maladaptive behavioral effects.

■ **OPIOID WITHDRAWAL.**[1] Essential features of opioid withdrawal include prolonged heavy use of an opioid drug, unless a narcotic antagonist has been given in which case withdrawal may occur after briefer use. At least four of the following symptoms will be present: lacrimation, rhinorrhea, pupillary dilation, piloerection, sweating, diarrhea, yawning, mild hypertension, tachycardia, fever, and insomnia.

■ **COCAINE INTOXICATION.**[1] Essential features of cocaine intoxication include recent use of cocaine with at least two of the following psychological signs within 1 hour: psychomotor agitation, elation, grandiosity, loquacity, hypervigilance. There are also at least two of the following group of symptoms: tachycardia, pupillary dilation, elevated blood pressure, perspiration or chills, nausea and vomiting. Maladaptive behaviors also occur.

■ **COCAINE WITHDRAWAL.**[1] Essential features of cocaine withdrawal include prolonged heavy use of cocaine followed by cessation or reduction. Signs include a depressed mood and at least two of the following: fatigue, disturbed sleep, and increased dreaming.

■ **AMPHETAMINE OR SIMILARLY ACTING SYMPATHOMIMETIC INTOXICATION.**[1] Essential features include recent use of a drug of this class and at least two of the following psychological symptoms within 1 hour of use: psychomotor agitation, elation, grandiosity, loquacity, hypervigilance. In addition, at least two of the following physical symptoms must also occur within 1 hour: tachycardia, pupillary dilation, elevated blood pressure, perspiration or chills, nausea or vomiting. Maladaptive behaviors also occur.

■ **AMPHETAMINE OR SIMILARLY ACTING SYMPATHOMIMETIC WITHDRAWAL.**[1] Essential features include cessation or reduction following prolonged heavy use of a drug of this class with depressed mood and at least two of the following: fatigue, disturbed sleep, and increased dreaming.

■ **PHENCYCLIDINE (PCP) OR SIMILARLY ACTING ARYLCYCLOHEXYLAMINE INTOXICATION.**[1] Essential features include recent use of a drug of this class followed within an hour by at least two of these physical symptoms: vertical or horizontal nystagmus, increased blood pressure and heart rate, numbness or diminished responsiveness to pain, ataxia, dysarthria. In addition, there should be at least two of the following psychological symptoms: euphoria, psychomotor agitation, marked anxiety, emotional lability, grandiosity, sensation of slowed time, synesthesias. Maladaptive behaviors also occur.

■ **HALLUCINOGEN HALLUCINOSIS.**[1] Essential features of hallucinogen hallucinosis include recent use of a drug of this class with perceptual changes occurring in a state of wakefulness and alertness. In addition, at least two of the following physical symptoms will occur: pupillary dilation, tachycardia, sweating, palpitations, blurring of vision, tremors, and incoordination. Maladaptive behavioral effects also occur.

■ **PSYCHOACTIVE SUBSTANCE DEPENDENCE.** The essential features include at least three of the following: preoccupation with taking the substance; larger amounts of the substance are taken over a longer period of time than intended; tolerance to the substance develops; characteristic withdrawal symptoms are evident; the substance is used to relieve withdrawal symptoms; there is the desire or effort to control the use of the substance; substance use impairs social or occupational obligations; important social, occupational or recreational activities are given up; or there is continued use of the substance despite a significant social, occupational, or legal problem or a physical disorder that is exacerbated by the use of the substance.

In addition to the above categories, there are several syndromes related to drug abuse that have similar characteristics related to the use of various agents.

Residual syndromes[1] are characterized by reduction in goal-directed behavior and deficits in cognitive functioning with a duration of at least 3 months.

Organic flashback syndromes[1] are characterized by reexperiencing one or more of the perceptual distortions that occurred while under the influence of the drug, and causing distress.

Organic mental syndromes that are not substance induced, such as delirium and dementia are described in detail in Chapter 19.

In summary, the model of health-illness phenomena may be applied to substance abuse as illustrated in Fig. 20-3.

❦ Planning and implementation

■ Goal setting

The establishment of nursing goals with a substance abusing patient must be done with recognition of the realities of the person's life-style and habits. The ideal long-term goal is frequently permanent total abstinence. However, the patient may be unable to face that level of commitment and is frequently very anxious at the thought of never again using the substance to which he is addicted. Recognition of this fact is reflected in the Alcoholics Anonymous (AA) approach to abstinence. AA members are advised to take 1 day, or sometimes 1 hour or 1 minute, at a time. The alcoholic is then able to take satisfaction in achieving short-term goals for sobriety. The thought of never drinking again is sometimes enough to send an alcoholic out to find a drink.

The nurse must also be aware that it is rare for an addicted person to suddenly stop substance use forever. Most addicts have to try at least once and usually several times to use the substance in a controlled way. Although some research indicates that this may be possible for some alcoholics, it is generally not a realistic goal. It should also be noted that people who tend to become addicted to one substance, such as antianxiety drugs, also have a tendency for other types of addictions. A new addiction that is substituted for the old one will only add new problems.

In general, the long-term goals for an individual who abuses substances are withdrawal from the drug if dependency is present and future abstinence. It is important that the patient participate in this decision-making process and agree about the approach to abstinence that will be tried. For instance, a heroin addict who is to be referred to a methadone program must decide whether to be on a maintenance or a withdrawal regimen and must agree to abide by the rules of the program. Goals for such a patient might be as follows:

Long-term goal

The patient will refrain from using narcotics other than methadone for 1 year, at which time the goal will be renegotiated.

Short-term goals

1. The patient will attend the methadone maintenance program daily for 3 months.
2. After 3 months, if there is no evidence of drug abuse, the patient will attend the methadone maintenance program three times a week, using take-home doses of methadone on the other days.
3. The patient will attend group discussions once a week and share his experiences with the group.
4. The patient will inform his counselor if he is unable to keep a scheduled clinic appointment.

It is very important that goals for a substance abusing patient be phrased so that it is clear that the patient has responsibility for his behavior. Displacement of responsibility onto others is a frequent behavior of dependent people. Writing the goals into a contract to be signed by the patient and the nurse and providing the patient with a copy of the contract will also help rein-

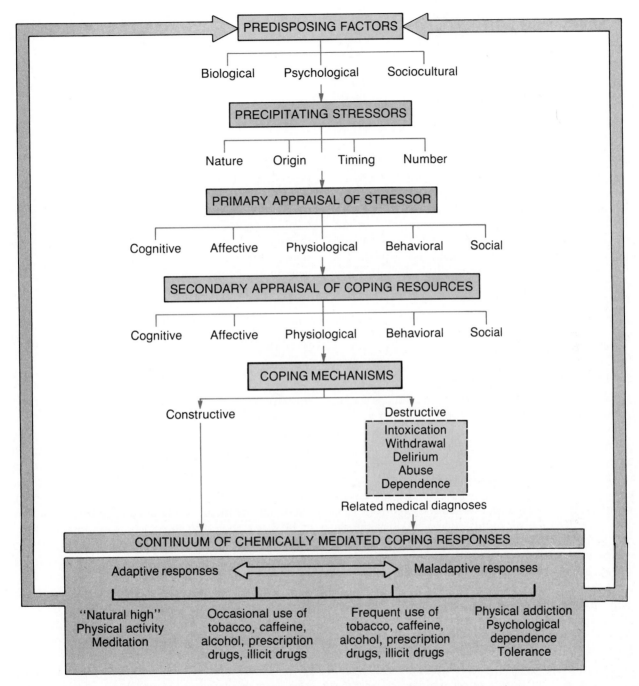

Fig. 20-3. Nursing model of health-illness phenomena related to substance abuse.

force the patient's responsibility for complying with the stated goals.

The nursing goals for patients who are experiencing drug withdrawal must attend to any life-threatening behaviors that are present. The highest priority will be given to stabilization of the patient's physiological status until the crisis of withdrawal is over. Emotional support will then be necessary as the person comes to terms with his behavior and begins to look to the future. The setting and constant modification of goals during this process convey to the patient the nurse's belief that there is hope for a more productive life in the future.

■ Intervening in substance abuse

Many theories have been described concerning the origin of substance abuse. There are also multiple theories about the effective treatment of this problem. The nurse will need to select the approach to intervention that seems most appropriate for each individual for whom she provides nursing care.

■ **BIOLOGICAL ASPECTS OF INTERVENTION.** Substance abusers frequently come into contact with the health care system because of a crisis in their physiological state. The crisis may be related to overdose, withdrawal, allergy, toxicity, or physical deterioration due to the deleterious effects of drugs, including such conditions as malnutrition, dehydration, and various infections. When an acute physical condition is present, it takes priority over the other health needs of the patient. It is particularly important with substance abuse patients to attend to the condition that they have identified as the problem. The nurse is then perceived as potentially helpful and will have added credibility when other aspects of the addictive problem are addressed.

Withdrawal. If the person is physically dependent on a drug, withdrawal must be accomplished with medical supervision. This process is referred to as **detoxification.** Gradual weaning from the substance may be instituted, especially if the person is addicted to prescription drugs, such as barbiturates, amphetamines, or benzodiazepines. Another approach is the use of alternative drugs to block the occurrence of withdrawal symptoms. For instance, chlordiazepoxide may be given to assist with alcohol withdrawal. The dose of the substituted drug is then tapered down and eventually discontinued. The danger in this approach is that the alcoholic can become dependent on the substitute drug or may even have been taking it in addition to alcohol. A variation on this approach is used when methadone is substituted for heroin. However, the treatment program may be aimed toward gradual withdrawal from methadone or toward indefinite maintenance on a stable dose of methadone. The decision between these two alternatives is based on assessment of the likelihood of recidivism if the person becomes drug free. This treatment approach has been controversial because methadone is a narcotic. However, addiction to methadone does not cause impairment in functioning, thus allowing the person to be productive while addicted. Proponents of methadone maintenance point out the benefits of avoiding the debilitating effects of narcotic addiction.

Withdrawal symptoms may occur even when efforts are made to prevent this. Substance abusers do not always give accurate drug-use histories, although it is extremely important for the nurse to obtain as specific an assessment as possible. If the amount of substance used has been understated or if multiple abuse is undetected, withdrawal symptoms may emerge. The possibility of seizures should always be anticipated and emergency equipment at hand. Drug abuse should always be considered as a possible condition when unexpected seizure activity occurs. If drug abuse is suspected, it is prudent to be sure that the physician is apprised of the situation so blood and urine specimens can be collected for laboratory analysis.

Overdose. Drug overdose is treated supportively, depending on the characteristics of the drug taken. It is, of course, important to identify the drug. In cases of narcotic overdose, narcotic antagonists, such as nalorphine may be given. After the person recovers from the acute illness, it is necessary to assess the circumstances of the overdose and particularly important to determine whether it was intentional or accidental. If the motivation is in doubt, it is best to assume that a suicide attempt has occurred until the nurse can obtain more information about the patient's mental state.

Toxic psychosis. Users of LSD and PCP often have an acute toxic psychosis. The behavior may be very similar to that of the schizophrenic patient. However, there may be no history of prior abnormal behavior. Careful assessment of an acute psychotic reaction, particularly in an adolescent or young adult, should include exploration of drug use. It may be necessary to interview friends of the patient to obtain this information. An attempt should be made to identify the specific drug used, although LSD and PCP may be taken without the knowledge of the person involved.* There is an important difference in the nursing approach to users of PCP as opposed to those who have an adverse reaction to LSD. Victims of PCP-induced psychosis do not respond well to attempts at interaction. They require an environment that has minimal stimuli and is safe. Agitated PCP users may strike out in response to their fear and panic and are potentially harmful to themselves and others.[30] LSD users experiencing a "bad trip" do respond to reassurance and may be "talked down." It seems to be most helpful if support is given by a friend or by someone who has experienced LSD. However, calm empathic reassurance and reorientation by the nurse will also help decrease the patient's panic. Provision must also be made for the safety of these individuals because they may act impulsively out of fear and harm themselves. Adequate staff should be present to control impulsive behavior of both PCP and LSD users. Vital signs should be monitored and other physiological needs met. Excretion of PCP is aided by acidifying the

---

*To assist in assessment of drug use, a glossary of drug terminology has been included in Appendix E.

urine by giving the patient cranberry juice or ascorbic acid. Gastric lavage may be necessary for persistent symptoms or if an overdose has been taken.[30]

Antabuse therapy. Another long-term biological approach to substance abuse is the prescription of disulfiram (Antabuse) for alcoholics. This drug sensitizes the person to alcohol, and an aversive physiological response occurs if the person uses alcohol in any form. The response consists of a severe headache, nausea and vomiting, flushing, hypotension, tachycardia, dyspnea, diaphoresis, chest pain, palpitations, dizziness, and confusion. It can also lead to respiratory and cardiac collapse, unconsciousness, convulsions, and death. It is therefore important that the patient agree to take disulfiram only after careful instruction about the potential consequences of drinking while on the drug. This educational process should include a written list of alcohol-containing preparations to be avoided, including cough medicines, rubbing compounds, vinegars, aftershave lotions, and some mouthwashes. Drinking must be avoided for 14 days after disulfiram has been taken. This medication cannot prevent drinking by someone who is determined to drink, because that person can wait until the disulfiram has been excreted. However, it helps to prevent impulsive drinking because the person does have to wait for a period of time to be able to drink safely. This treatment is used in conjunction with other supportive therapies.

Drugs in pregnancy. Since most of the drugs that are abused cross the placental barrier, women should be counseled about the possible effects of substance use during pregnancy. There have been incidents of congenital abnormalities in infants of mothers who have taken drugs. A fetal alcohol syndrome has been identified. In addition, use during pregnancy of drugs that cause physical dependency will result in the birth of an addicted baby who must then be withdrawn from the drug. The safest pregnancy is one in which the mother is totally drug free.

■ **INTERACTIVE INTERVENTIONS IN SUBSTANCE ABUSE.** Before attempting to initiate nursing intervention with a substance abusing patient, the nurse must develop an awareness of her own feelings and attitudes toward the problem. It is recommended that a values clarification approach be used, as described in Chapter 4. Most people have had personal contact with substance abuse by family, friends, or colleagues. This problem evokes many negative feelings. It is important that the nurse be able to differentiate feelings associated with past situations from those aroused by professional contacts with patients and their families. A supervisor, teacher, or senior clinical nurse can be of assistance when a nurse is having difficulty sorting out feelings.

Group support. The multiplicity of stressors relative to substance abuse have been discussed. It is very important that nursing intervention be directed toward alleviating the stressors that apply to each individual patient and identified in the nursing diagnosis. If the motivation for drug use has been peer pressure, the patient will need help in planning how to deal with the same kind of pressures in the future. This may be a particularly difficult problem for adolescents who rely very much on peer group approval to maintain their self-esteem. A group support approach to treatment is helpful to these patients. They also have a tendency to deny the potential for future problems. Peers in a group setting can confront the individual with the realities of social pressure. Alcoholics also need to learn how to refuse a drink, even when urged to indulge. Role playing can be a helpful approach by the nurse, especially in a group setting. Two patients can act out a social situation involving drinking and then receive feedback from the group about their behavior.

Patient education. Another nursing intervention that can be implemented effectively in a group setting is patient education. Substance abusers should be well informed about the drug they have used, its biological and psychosocial effects on the person, and community resources for future assistance. Films and other audiovisual materials reinforce important concepts. Handouts should be used for future reference.

Individual counseling. Individual counseling is frequently used as an approach with patients who are substance users. Liporati and Chychula[20] have described five guidelines for counseling the hospitalized drug abuser. They are

1. Define acceptable in-hospital behavior.
2. Make it clear that rules are set by the hospital, not the nurse.
3. Be honest about sharing information.
4. Document nursing interventions carefully.
5. Accept one's inability to cure the problem.

Niven[23] has also developed recommendations for intervention with adolescents who are substance abusers. He agrees that honesty is essential. The treatment team should be nonjudgmental and convey their concern for the patient's well-being. The diagnosis should be clearly stated and will probably need to be repeated periodically to confront the denial of the patient and the family. Treatment recommendations will also need repetition with supportive evidence of the substance abusing behavior. Commonly encountered problems include denial, dependency, low self-esteem, manipulation, and anger. Concepts related to these behaviors are discussed elsewhere in this book. However, it is necessary to address the special application of these concepts to substance abuse.

Intervening in denial. Denial must be dealt with because it is a potential obstacle to recovery from chemical dependency. Most patients deny that they are unable to control their substance abusing behavior even when drug-related problems have become serious. For instance, an intoxicated person who has caused an automobile accident may assert that he "just had a few beers." A barbiturate addict may claim that he can stop whenever he wants to do so. The denial is partially related to the stigma attached to drug abuse. It is difficult to apply the term "alcoholic" or "addict" to oneself. Denial also protects the person from admitting that he is unable to control his behavior. Self-control is a prized attribute that is central to the self-concept of most people. Admission of a problem is also the first step toward behavioral change. This commitment to change is very frightening to a substance dependent person. It involves a decision to stop using a substance that has become the major focus of the person's life. Anyone who has tried to stop smoking cigarettes or diet can understand to some extent the anxiety aroused by this decision.

It is essential that denial be overcome and that the patient make the commitment to behavioral change. Repeated confrontation with evidence of substance dependence may be necessary to evoke this response. However, this must be done carefully so the patient is not antagonized. Repeated contacts with the health care system may be necessary before the patient admits to the nature of the problem.

Behavioral contracts. Many therapists use behavioral contracts when working with substance abusers. The nurse and the patient discuss and agree on realistic behavioral objectives for the patient. These are written down, and the document is signed by both the nurse and the patient. Most therapists who work with substance abuse patients insist on a provision in the contract that the patient be drug and alcohol free when attending a therapy session. This communicates the therapist's belief that the patient is able to control his behavior and take positive action in his own behalf.

Intervening in dependency. Dependency is generally a personality characteristic of people who become involved in substance abusing behavior. This dependency may also be evident in the individual's interpersonal relationships. If the person is too dependent on others, it may drive them away, thus increasing the need to depend on alcohol or drugs. Clinical example 20-5 illustrates this problem.

Mr. B used alcohol to avoid responsibility for his actions and his life. He used his wife in a similar way. When she confronted him with her expectations, he responded in a childlike way and tried to place the nurse

---

CLINICAL EXAMPLE 20-5

Mr. B was a 45-year-old man who was admitted to the medical unit of a general hospital with a diagnosis of gastritis. He complained of abdominal pain, nausea, and vomiting. He had a slightly elevated temperature of 37.5° C (100° F). When the admitting nurse who was completing the nursing assessment asked Mr. B about alcohol use, he said he had "a couple of beers" after work every day. He also reported that his wife had left him the day before admission. He said he was not sure why she left, but he was sure she would be back. Ms. B did come to the hospital to visit her husband. His primary nurse met with them together and asked Ms. B why she left. She said she was tired of putting Mr. B to bed every night after he passed out from drinking and did not want to continue to call his employer saying he was sick when he was really hung over. She had threatened to leave before, but Mr. B had always begged her to stay and she had relented. She had married him because she felt sorry for him. He had been living alone and was not taking good care of himself. She revealed that her first husband was also an alcoholic. She would agree to try again to make the marriage a success if he would agree to stop drinking and seek counseling. Mr. B said to the nurse, "I'll be good and do what she says. You tell her I'll be good."

---

in the parental role. This avoidance of responsibility is one of the behaviors that is very difficult for the substance abuser to change. The nurse must be careful not to fall into the trap of making decisions for the patient. In Clinical example 20-5, the nurse suggested that Mr. B communicate directly with his wife about how he planned to change his behavior.

Ms. B represents another problem that is also encountered when working with a substance abusing patient. She is a woman who appears to be drawn to dependent men. She is probably a very maternal person who likes to take care of others. This increases the possibility that she will assume the role of **enabler.** The enabler perpetuates the substance abuse problem by not confronting the substance abuser and by helping to cover up the problem. When Ms. B called Mr. B's employer to say he was sick, she was being an enabler. When significant others play an enabling role, family counseling is necessary to help the family accept and support the changing behavior of the patient. Ms. B had left her husband, but he was her second alcoholic spouse, indicating that she was probably attracted to dependent men. Any increase in assertiveness by Mr. B would have further disrupted their relationship.

Increasing self-esteem. Assertiveness training can be very helpful in assisting both the dependent substance abuser and significant others to accomplish a behavioral change. This therapeutic technique is described in detail in Chapter 18. An increase in assertiveness may also have the added advantage of a positive effect on the person's self-esteem. Although some substance abusers present a facade of self-confidence, most basically have little regard for themselves. The relaxation, euphoria, or release of inhibitions imparted by the drug helps the person overcome this sense of inferiority. Another goal of nursing care must be to find ways of bolstering the person's self-esteem. This can be very difficult because many of these people have destroyed the relationships and activities that normally build self-esteem. They may have lost jobs, friends, and family. The nurse needs to help the person identify his remaining strengths and to build on them. Strengths may be related to overcoming the substance abuse problem itself. This was so in the case of Bobby F in Clinical example 20-6.

Mr. L used his relationship with Bobby to convey his belief that the patient could succeed in giving up drugs. This message had a core of positive regard for Bobby's potential strength. The staff of the drug treatment program added to this seed of self-esteem by encouraging Bobby to help others in the program and then to aim higher at becoming a counselor himself. This process taught Bobby that there were rewards in life other than those attached to drug use. Gradually, he learned to value the interpersonal rewards more than the drug rewards while making positive use of his past difficulties. Employment in drug programs has been a positive step for many ex-addicts who frequently become excellent counselors.

Intervening in manipulation. Manipulative behavior is another frequent characteristic of the substance abuser. This is often focused on obtaining access to drugs or alcohol. The hospitalized person may promise to give up the abused substance to get discharged, only to start using it again as soon as he returns home. Drug abusers sometimes manipulate the health care system by getting prescriptions from more than one physician or by forging prescriptions. This behavior must be confronted when it is discovered, and the patient should be helped to understand the self-defeating nature of this behavior. Although the behavior would appear to be directed toward others, the real victim is always the patient who perpetuates his self-destructive behavior.

Intervening in anger. When substance abusers are confronted with their behavior and are pressed to assume responsibility for it, they may become angry. The root of the anger is related to the pain that is felt when

---

CLINICAL EXAMPLE 20-6

Bobby was a 17-year-old who was admitted to the hospital acutely psychotic with a history of recent use of PCP. The emergency room nurse noted scarring of the veins in Bobby's arm and surmised that he was also a user of heroin. Blood and urine testing confirmed this suspicion. Bobby recovered from his psychotic episode in 24 hours but was then extremely uncomfortable due to opiate withdrawal. The decision was made to use titrated doses of methadone to assist with the withdrawal. Mr. L, a young nurse, established a close relationship with Bobby during this time. Bobby requested the nurse's help in planning for his future, but doubted that he had the strength to stay away from drugs. He was advised to take a day at a time. Mr. L took Bobby on a visit to a drug treatment program, and he agreed to try membership in one of the groups at this center. Bobby did well in the group and was very helpful to new members, describing his experiences and encouraging them to "take 1 day at a time." Bobby expressed an interest in finishing school and said he would like to become a drug counselor. The staff of the drug treatment program agreed that Bobby seemed to have an aptitude for that role and encouraged him to pursue his goal.

---

the person realizes he must give up a behavior that has been central to his existence. In addition, the patient is raging over the emerging understanding of the problems he has caused for himself. Carruth and Pugh have compared the loss of alcohol to the process of grieving.[5] This comparison seems particularly applicable to the anger experienced by the addict who is mourning the loss of the abused substance and the loss of life experience during the period of addiction.

The nurse must realize that the anger felt by the patient may be directed toward her but generally is not related to her behavior. The patient should be assisted to express this anger in nondestructive ways. Exercise may be helpful. Expression through art or music may also provide an outlet for rage. A danger associated with this anger is that the patient may use it as an excuse to return to using drugs or alcohol. The substance abuser needs to learn that human support can also be of help in confronting painful feelings. It is important that the person be helped to label the feelings he is experiencing. Drug users become so accustomed to avoiding feelings chemically that they have difficulty even recognizing what it is that they are feeling. Group counseling may also be helpful because individuals can see and identify feelings in others as well as themselves. Group support can help to decrease the sense of isolation that these patients often have.

Recidivism. Work with substance abusing patients can be frustrating. Behavioral change is very difficult for them so there is a high rate of recidivism. It may be very difficult for a nurse who has struggled to help someone overcome withdrawal symptoms and to rebuild his life to then see that person return to the health care agency readdicted. Rejection of the patient at this point is not helpful. These patients are very sensitive to rejection or criticism. They use such reactions to justify further substance abuse. They may make statements such as, "You're absolutely right. I'm not worth caring about. Nobody cares for me so why should I care for myself?" The nurse may communicate to the patient her disappointment that he did not continue to progress. However, the focus should be on beginning again, using the fact that the patient succeeded once to foster an optimistic attitude toward the future.

While the nurse is establishing a helping relationship with the patient, she should be alert to signs of other psychosocial disruptions. Some people become substance abusers because of their efforts to deal with underlying emotional problems. Alcohol and other drugs may be used in this way. Unfortunately, most of the substances which may be abused also have characteristics that tend to make problems worse, although there may be temporary relief. For instance, alcohol or barbiturates may be used to combat depression. There is an immediate sense of euphoria from these drugs. However, they are basically depressant substances and lead to later feelings of gloom. Amphetamines and cocaine bring about a "high," but there is also an inevitable "crash." People who use drugs to release inhibitions and relate more easily with others will find that they may develop a greater number of superficial relationships, but drive away the few people to whom they have been able to feel close. The nurse needs to explore these motivations for substance abuse and help the patient find other ways to alleviate his psychological pain.

■ **SOCIAL SUPPORT SYSTEMS.**

Family Counseling. Reliable support from caring people is crucial to the recovery of substance abusers. Families are often frustrated with the patient's behavior. Family counseling by a qualified health care provider is likely to be necessary to assist the family in adjusting to the patient's changing behavior. Family members may need sources of support so they can be supportive to the dependent member.

Self-help groups. Formal family counseling is one approach to providing support to the social system. Self-help groups are another way of helping the substance abuser and his significant others. AA is the prototype for self-help groups. AA is an organization that is composed entirely of recovering alcoholics. They believe that mutual support can give the alcoholic strength to abstain. AA aims for total abstinence. The member must admit to alcoholism openly and publicly by introducing himself at meetings, saying, "My name is John and I am an alcoholic." The other members promptly respond, "Hi John!" At each meeting, one or several members share their life histories with the group. This demonstrates that individual members are more alike than different, removing a resistance to involvement that is often cited by alcoholics. AA members also commit themselves to helping each other. As a member recovers, he is eventually assigned to be a sponsor for a new member. The sponsor role entails availability and accessibility to the other member whenever he feels the need to drink. This reciprocal relationship gives the new member caring support and the sponsor improved self-esteem. AA also involves a strong religious orientation that is experienced as supportive by some alcoholics. Most cities have many AA groups. These groups often differ from each other in the characteristics of the members. There may be groups that are mostly blue collar workers, homemakers, or physicians. A nurse who is referring an alcoholic patient to a group should become familiar enough with the characteristics of that specific group to know whether the patient is likely to feel comfortable with the other members. AA meetings are frequently open. It is highly recommended that every nurse arrange to attend an AA meeting to help her to understand the problem and to gain an appreciation for the work that is done by this organization.

Two other support groups have developed as extensions of AA. Alanon is a self-help group that was established to meet the needs of spouses and significant others of alcoholics. The alcoholic need not be involved in AA for the significant other to join Alanon. In fact, this organization is often very helpful to spouses of alcoholics who are actively drinking. The members support each other and offer advice to moving forward with their own lives without becoming totally absorbed in the alcoholic's problem. Alateen performs a similar function for adolescents who are involved with alcoholic family members. The message of both of these organizations is that the family member is not responsible for and cannot control the alcoholic's drinking. They can, however, still live meaningful lives. Bingham and Bargar[3] have decribed the importance of a peer support group for latency age children of alcoholics.

Transitional living programs. Many communities have transitional living programs, such as halfway houses, for alcoholics and drug abusers. These facilities serve as a transition between detoxification and complete return to the community. They usually have struc-

TABLE 20-4

SUMMARY OF NURSING INTERVENTIONS WITH THE SUBSTANCE ABUSING PATIENT

Principle	Rationale	Nursing actions
Goal—To substitute healthy coping responses for substance abusing behavior		
The nurse and patient should mutually define the problem and plan the nursing interventions	Motivation for change is related to recognition of a problem that is upsetting to the individual The patient must assume responsibility for his behavior Identification of predisposing and precipitating stressors must precede planning for more adaptive behavioral responses	Confront the patient with his substance abusing behavior and its consequences Assist the patient to identify his substance abuse problem Encourage the patient to agree to participate in a treatment program Involve the patient in describing situations that lead to substance abusing behavior Develop with the patient a written contract for behavioral change that is signed by the patient and nurse Assist the patient to identify and adopt healthier coping responses Consistently offer support and the expectation that the patient does have the strength to overcome his problem
Goal—To maintain safety and an optimum level of physical comfort		
Physical dependence must be managed in a safe environment with minimal withdrawal symptoms	Detoxification of the physically dependent person can be dangerous and is always uncomfortable The patient's physical safety must receive high priority for nursing intervention Withdrawal symptoms provide powerful motivation for continued substance abuse	Supportive physical care: vital signs, nutrition, hydration, seizure precautions Administer medication according to detoxification schedule Observe the patient carefully for withdrawal symptoms and report suspected withdrawal immediately
Goal—To engage social support systems in the patient's behalf		
Human support is to be substituted for dependence on chemicals Peer confrontation and support is often more acceptable than that of professionals	Substance abusers are often dependent and socially isolated people who use drugs to gain confidence in social situations Substance abusing behavior alienates significant others, thus increasing the person's isolation It is difficult to manipulate people who have participated in the same behaviors Social support systems must be readily available over time and acceptable to the patient	Identify and assess social support systems that are available to the patient Provide support to significant others Educate the patient and significant others about the substance abuse problem and available resources Refer the patient to appropriate resources and provide support until the patient is involved in the program.

TABLE 20-5

MENTAL HEALTH EDUCATION PLAN FOR PREVENTION OF SUBSTANCE ABUSE

Content	Instructional activities	Evaluation
Elicit perceptions of substance use	Lead group discussion regarding knowledge about chemical use and experience with it; correct misperceptions	Learner will describe accurate information about substance use
Demonstrate negative effects of substance abuse	Show films of physical and psychological effects of substance abuse; provide written materials	Learner will identify and describe physical and psychological effects of substance abuse
Interaction with peer who has abused chemicals	Small group discussion with peer group member who has abused substances and quit because of negative experiences	Learner will compare and contrast advantages and disadvantages of using mind-altering substances
Obtain agreement to abstain from use of mind altering substances	Discuss future plans for refusing abused chemicals if offered	Learner will verbally agree to abstain from using mind-altering substances.

---

tured programs that include individual and group counseling, education about the addictive problem, AA meetings, and vocational rehabilitation. It is believed that this intensive program helps the patient readjust slowly to the community. These facilities are especially helpful for people who are alienated from their families.

Community treatment programs. There are a variety of community programs that may be available for drug abusers. Drug treatment programs generally offer individual and group counseling, family counseling, vocational counseling, and drug and health education. Some also include methadone withdrawal or maintenance for opiate addicts. These programs must have special licensure to operate and have specific federal guidelines to follow. Peer group relationships are an important aspect of most drug treatment programs. The clientele of these programs may differ, but most are directed toward "street people."

The nurse is responsible to know about the treatment programs that are available in the community in terms of the services offered and the characteristics of the population that is generally served. Referral of a registered nurse who has been stealing narcotics to an inner city drug treatment program will not work. It is difficult to persuade a substance abuser to seek help at all. It is worthwhile to put forth the effort to find a treatment program that will meet the patient's needs as closely as possible.

Employee assistance programs. Another potential resource for the substance abusing patient is the employee assistance program that may be part of an employee health service. Many businesses and industries have found that it is profitable for them to help substance abusing employees. These programs generally offer counseling and health education. The employee is usually required to participate in the program to retain his job. Nurses are often key staff members in employee assistance programs. The health care system has been rather slow in developing these programs for health care providers. Since there is such a high prevalence of substance abuse among nurses and physicians, there is a great need for programs that can focus on their problems. Nurses can be advocates for the establishment of employee assistance programs in the agencies where they work. Nursing interventions with patients who abuse substances are summarized in Table 20-4.

■ **PREVENTION.** Prevention of substance abuse is an important public health problem. Nurses need to be aware of the need for primary prevention and incorporate this into their professional practice. Resnick[25] suggests several components for drug abuse prevention programs. The first is to work toward improvement of the social conditions that affect families. Strengthening of the family unit decreases the probability that a member will become involved in deviant behavior. The second component is to have an impact on the environment in which drug abuse takes place. There must be a focus on the schools, including their role in drug education. Table 20-5 illustrates a mental health education plan for substance abuse prevention. Legislative action may be needed. Another part of the prevention program is to strengthen the interpersonal and social skills of individuals. This leads to increased self-esteem and a positive self-concept, allowing the individual to resist peer pressure to use drugs. The fourth component is to create a strong network of interagency linkages. When different agencies work closely together, they can share resources and have a greater impact on the system. The final component is the sharing of resources between the federal and state governments.[25] This also helps to maximize the return on the investment of limited resources. Nurses can play an important part in developing and initiating policies that support the development of good substance abuse prevention programs.

 Evaluation

The evaluation of success in work with a substance abuse patient must be based on realistic expectations. Setting unreasonably high goals is discouraging to the nurse and the patient. For instance, it would be unrealistic to set a goal of total abstinence forever with a substance abuser. A more realistic goal is to lengthen periods of abstinence with the hope that the patient would eventually achieve control over his behavior.

Estes, Smith-DiJulio, and Heinemann[10] have identified evaluation criteria for the treatment of alcoholics. These criteria apply to abusers of other drugs as well:

1. Has the patient been able to progress significantly toward achieving the stated goals?
2. Can the patient usually communicate without being defensive?
3. Is the patient able to react appropriately, managing the demands of daily life without use of a drug?
4. Is the patient actively involved in a variety of activities, using external social and activity resources?
5. Does the patient use internal resources to be consistently productive at work and involved in meaningful interpersonal relationships?

The evaluation process should take place at regular intervals during the nurse-patient relationship.

■ SUGGESTED CROSS-REFERENCES ■

The model of health-illness phenomena is discussed in Chapter 3. The phases of the nursing process are discussed in Chapter 5. Therapeutic relationship skills are discussed in Chapter 4. Interventions in social support systems are discussed in Chapter 9. Alterations in self-concept are discussed in Chapter 14. Assertiveness training is discussed in Chapter 18. Group therapy is discussed in Chapter 28. Working with adolescents is discussed in Chapter 31.

SUMMARY

1. Substance abuse was defined as the use of any mind-altering agent to such an extent that it interferes with the individual's biological, psychological, or sociocultural integrity.

2. The importance of cultural attitudes in determining the response to substance use or abuse was discussed.

3. Statistics were presented to demonstrate the prevalence and seriousness of the problem of substance abuse.

4. Categories of drugs that are frequently abused were described.

5. Substance abuse is a very serious problem among nurses and physicians.

6. Substance abuse was illustrated in terms of the health-illness continuum.

7. Biological, psychological, and sociocultural predisposing factors and precipitating stressors relative to substance abuse were described. There is no agreement on the existence of a specific stressor or set of stressors that is always present when substance abuse occurs.

8. A comparison of the various categories of abused substances was done, including the usual route of administration, expected behavioral manifestations, behaviors related to overdose, and withdrawal syndromes.

9. Nursing diagnosis of the substance abusing patient was discussed relative to the stage of drug-using behavior, specific substance used, and relevant stressors. Relevant medical diagnoses were presented.

10. Goal setting must be realistic, taking into account the need for multiple short-term goals to enable the patient to experience success.

11. The biological aspects of nursing intervention include attending to physiological needs, detoxification, drug overdose, management of acute toxic psychosis, biofeedback, methadone treatment for opiate abusers, and disulfiram treatment for alcoholics.

12. Interactive interventions include peer group discussions, role play, patient education, and individual counseling.

13. Common themes in therapy with substance abuse patients include denial, dependency, low self-esteem, manipulation, and anger.

14. A mental health education plan for prevention of substance abuse was presented.

15. Social support systems for substance abusers include families, self-help groups, transitional living programs, drug treatment programs, and employee assistance programs.

16. Five components of drug abuse prevention programs were presented.

17. Evaluation of nursing care was described in terms of five questions to be asked about the behaviors of the patient.

REFERENCES

1. American Psychiatric Association: Draft of the DSM-III-R in Development (subject to change), as proposed by the Work Group to Revise DSM-III. American Psychiatric Association, October 1985.

2. Ausubel, D.P.: An interactional approach to narcotic addiction. In Lettieri, D.J., Sayers, M., and Pearson, H.W., editors: Theories on drug abuse: selected contemporary perspectives, NIDA Research Monograph 30, Rockville, Md., 1980, National Institute on Drug Abuse.

3. Bingham, A., and Barger, J.: Children of alcoholic families: a group treatment approach for latency age children, J. Psychosoc. Nurs. Ment. Health Serv. **23**:13, Dec. 1985.

4. Butz, R.H.: Intoxication and withdrawal. In Estes, N.J., and Heinemann, M.E., editor: Alcoholism: development, consequences, and interventions, ed. 2, St. Louis, 1982, The C.V. Mosby Co.

5. Carruth, G.R., and Pugh, J.B.: Grieving the loss of alcohol: a crisis in recovery, J. Psychosoc. Nurs. Ment. Health Serv. **20**:18, Mar, 1982.

6. Chein, I.: Psychological, social and epidemiological factors in juvenile drug abuse. In Lettieri, D.J., Sayers, M., and Pearson, H.W., editors: Theories on drug abuse: selected contemporary perspectives, NIDA Research Monograph 30, Rockville, Md., 1980, National Institute on Drug Abuse.

7. Demarest, M.: Cocaine: middle class high, Time **118**:56, July 6, 1981.

8. Dusek, D., and Girdano, D.A.: Drugs: a factual account, Reading, Mass., 1980, Addison-Wesley Publishing Co., Inc.

9. Estes, N.J., and Heinemann, M.E.: Alcoholism, development, consequences, and interventions, ed. 2, St. Louis, 1982, The C.V. Mosby Co.

10. Estes, N.J., Smith-DiJulio, K., and Heinemann, M.E.: Nursing diagnosis of the alcoholic person, St. Louis, 1980, The C.V. Mosby Co.

11. Freedman, A.M.: Opiate dependence. In Kaplan, H.I., Freedman, A.M., and Sadock, B.J., editors: Comprehensive textbook of psychiatry, ed. 3, Baltimore, 1980, The Williams & Wilkins Co.

12. Gold, S.R.: The CAP control theory of drug abuse. In Lettieri, D.J., Sayers, M., and Pearson, H.W., editors: Theories on drug abuse: selected contemporary perspectives, NIDA Research Monograph 30, Rockville, Md., 1980, National Institute on Drug Abuse.

13. Goodwin, D.W.: The bad-habit theory of drug abuse. In Lettieri, D.J., Sayers, M., and Pearson, H.W., editors: Theories on drug abuse: selected contemporary perspectives, NIDA Research Monograph 30, Rockville, Md., 1980, National Institute on Drug Abuse.

14. Greaves, G.B.: An existential theory of drug dependence. In Lettieri, D.J., Sayers, M., and Pearson, H.W., editors: Theories on drug abuse: selected contemporary perspectives, NIDA Research Monograph 30, Rockville, Md., 1980, National Institute on Drug Abuse.

15. Grinspoon, L., and Bakalar, J.B.: Drug dependence: non-narcotic agents. In Kaplan, H.I., Freedman, A.M., and Sadock, B.J., editors: Comprehensive textbook of psychiatry, ed. 3, Baltimore, 1980, The Williams & Wilkins Co.

16. Hughes, R., and Brewin, R.: The tranquilizing of America: pill popping and the American way of life, New York, 1979, Harcourt, Brace, Jovanovich, Inc.

17. Isler, C.: The alcoholic nurse: what we try to deny, R.N. **41**:48, July 1978.

18. Jellinek, E.M.: Phases of alcohol addiction, Q.J. Stud. Alcohol **13**:672, 1952.

19. Johnston, L.D., Backman, J.G., and O'Malley, P.M.: Drugs and the class of '78: behaviors, attitudes and recent national trends, Rockville, Md., 1979, National Institute on Drug Abuse.

20. Liporati, N.C., and Chychula, L.H.: How you can really help the drug-abusing patient, Nursing '82 **12**:46, June 1982.

21. Miller, J.D., and Cisin, I.H.: Highlights from the national survey on drug abuse: 1979, Rockville, Md., 1980, Department of Health and Human Services.

22. Mittleman, H.S., Mittleman, R.E., and Elser, B.: Cocaine, Am. J. Nurs. **84**:1092, Sept. 1984.

23. Niven, R.G.: Adolescent drug abuse, Hosp. Community Psychiatry **37**:596, June 1986.

24. Ray, O.S.: Drugs, society, and human behavior, ed. 3, St. Louis, 1982, The C.V. Mosby Co.

25. Resnick, H.S.: It starts with people: experience in drug abuse prevention, Rockville, Md., 1978, Department of Health, Education, and Welfare.

26. Seixas, F.A.: The course of alcoholism. In Estes, N.J., and Heinemann, M.E., editors: Alcoholism: development, consequences, and interventions, ed. 2, St. Louis, 1982, The C.V. Mosby Co.

27. Selzer, M.L.: Alcoholism and alcoholic psychoses. In Kaplan, H.I., Freedman, A.M., and Sadock, B.J., editors: Comprehensive textbook of psychiatry, ed. 3, Baltimore, 1980, The Williams & Wilkins Co.

28. Snyder, S.H.: Opiate receptors and internal opiates, Sci. Am. **236**(3):44, 1977.

29. Stanton, M.D.: A family theory of drug abuse. In Lettieri, D.J., Sayers, M., and Pearson, H.W., editors: Theories on drug abuse: selected contemporary perspectives, NIDA Research Monograph 30, Rockville, Md., 1980, National Institute on Drug Abuse.

30. Vourakis, C., and Bennett, G.: Angel dust: not heaven sent, Am. J. Nurs. **79**:649, 1979.

31. Wurmser, L.: Drug use as a protective system. In Lettieri, D.J., Sayers, M., and Pearson, H.W., editors: Theories on drug abuse: selected contemporary perspectives, NIDA Research Monograph 30, Rockville, Md., 1980, National Institute on Drug Abuse.

■ ANNOTATED SUGGESTED READINGS ■

*Anonymous: Interview: life with an alcoholic husband, J. Psychosoc. Nurs. Ment. Health Serv. **23**:30, Mar. 1985.

Two women describe their experiences living with and leaving alcoholic husbands. Of particular interest are their observations about their experiences in psychotherapy. Their candid remarks would be helpful to nurses as they work with families of alcoholics.

*Betemps, E.: Management of the withdrawal syndrome of barbiturates and other central nervous system depressants, J. Psychiatr. Nurs. **17**:31, Sept. 1981.

This excellent article provides information on recognition and nursing management of withdrawal from CNS depressant drugs, including a system for judging the seriousness of impending withdrawal. The detoxification process is discussed in detail.

Celentano, D.D., McQueen, D.V., and Chee, E.: Substance abuse by women: a review of the epidemiologic literature, J. Chron. Dis. **33**(6):383, 1980.

These authors reviewed the research literature pertaining to substance abuse by women. They found that very little research has been done on "substance abuse" as opposed to drug or alcohol abuse and still less explores the problem in the female population. Several areas for research are identified. This article would be very useful to the graduate student or the nurse researcher who is interested in investigating substance abuse.

Dusek, D., and Girdano, D.A.: Drugs: a factual account, Reading, Mass., 1980, Addison-Wesley Publishing Co., Inc.

This book provides a wealth of information about the use and abuse of alcohol and other drugs. It provides a good overview of the scope of the problem, including information on risk factors and epidemiological data.

*Estes, N.J., and Heinemann, M.E., editors: Alcoholism: development, consequences, and interventions, ed. 2, St. Louis, 1982, The C.V. Mosby Co.

This edited volume provides an extremely comprehensive survey of current literature on alcoholism. The broad spectrum of topics make this an interesting and useful resource book.

*Estes, N.J., Smith-DiJulio, K., and Heinemann, M.E.: Nursing diagnosis of the alcoholic person, St. Louis, 1980, The C.V. Mosby Co.

This book is highly recommended as a nursing reference on alcoholism. The authors are experienced in providing nursing care to alcoholic patients. They have used a nursing process framework to discuss nursing care. Of particular interest is the inclusion of interviewing guides and tools that may be used in the assessment of the alcoholic patient.

*Fultz, J.M., Jr., et al.: When a narcotic addict is hospitalized, Am. J. Nurs. **80**:478, 1980.

The authors pay particular attention to the legal ramifications of treating a patient who is addicted to narcotics. Methadone maintenance and withdrawal are clearly discussed. Signs and symptoms of opiate withdrawal and opiate overdose are described.

*Gareri, E.: Assertiveness training for alcoholics, J. Psychiatr. Nurs. **17**:31, Jan. 1979.

This article discusses the relationship between lack of assertiveness and alcohol abuse and describes an assertiveness training group specifically for alcoholics.

*Huberty, D.J., and Malmquist, J.D.: Adolescent chemical dependency, Perspect. Psychiatr. Care **16**:21, Jan-Feb. 1978.

This article relates the development tasks of adolescence to drug-abusing behavior. It includes a discussion of recovery as well. The authors compare the family process when a teenage member abuses drugs to Kübler-Ross' stages of death and dying.

---

*Asterisk indicates nursing reference.

*Jaffe, S.: First-hand views of recovery, Am. J. Nurs. **82**:578, 1982.

The author describes her experience in treating a group of nurses who were alcoholics. She addresses issues that concern substance-abusing nurses in particular. This article is recommended as a means of sensitizing nurses to the needs of their addicted colleagues.

*Jefferson, L.V., and Ensor, B.E.: Confronting a chemically impaired colleague, Am. J. Nurs. **82**:574, 1982.

This article applies concepts related to substance abuse to the addicted nurse. Case studies are used to illustrate the characteristics of drug- and alcohol-abusing nurses. The authors describe clues that should lead one to suspect the presence of substance abuse. Of particular importance is the section on intervention, including advice concerning confrontation of a nurse colleague who may be alcoholic or abusing drugs. This is highly recommended reading for all nurses.

Lettieri, D.J., Sayers, M., and Pearson, H.W., editors: Theories on drug abuse: selected contemporary perspectives, NIDA Research Monograph 30, Rockville, Md., 1980, National Institute on Drug Abuse.

This publication includes reports of a number of research studies exploring the causes of substance abuse. It is recommended for a reader who wishes to explore theories about predisposing factors and stressors in greater depth. An ability to critique research is also helpful.

*Liporati, N.C., and Chychula, L.H.: How you can really help the drug-abusing patient, Nursing '82 **12**:46, June 1982.

The authors present practical suggestions for interacting with patients who are substance abusers. The article is directed toward nurses who work in general hospitals, but the information is pertinent to all settings. Particularly valuable are the examples of how to approach a patient when drug abuse is suspected.

*McCoy, S., Rice, M.J., and McFadden, K.: PCP intoxication: psychiatric issues of nursing care, J. Psychiatr. Nurs. **19**:17, July 1981.

This is an excellent article that provides a wealth of information relative to PCP intoxication. Patient behaviors and related nursing interventions are presented in depth and with clarity. This would be a worthwhile reference in any setting providing health care services to adolescents and young adults.

*Michael, M.M., and Sewall, K.S.: Use of the adolescent peer group to increase the self-care agency of adolescent alcohol abusers, Nurs. Clin. North Am. **15**:157, Mar. 1980.

This publication provides a good example of the application of a particular conceptual model to a specific therapeutic modality. They used a reality therapy approach in a group setting with adolescent drug abusing patients. This article is especially recommended for experienced nurse therapists who are interested in exploring an innovative therapeutic approach.

*Mittleman, H.S., Mittleman, R.E., and Elser, B.: Cocaine, Am. J. Nurs. **84**:1092, Sept. 1984.

This article provides a good summary of basic information about cocaine, including methods of administration, expected response, toxic reactions and nursing interventions. The descriptions of treatments for toxic reactions are especially good.

*Morgan, A.J., and Moreno, J.W.: Attitudes toward addiction, Am. J. Nurs. **73**:497, 1973.

This article should be particularly helpful to the inexperienced nurse who needs help in analyzing her own feelings about working with addicted patients. It presents many of the realities of drug addiction that may be hard to handle emotionally.

Niven, R.G.: Adolescent drug abuse, Hosp. Community Psychiatry **37**:596, June 1986.

The author provides a comprehensive analysis of the assessment and care of drug abusing adolescents. The suggestions are practical. The author is realistic but hopeful in his approach. An appendix includes information about self-help groups and sources of educational materials.

*Personatt, J.D.: Couples therapy: treatment of choice with the drug addict, J. Psychiatr. Nurs. **16**:18, Jan. 1978.

The author reviews several group treatment modalities and assesses the appropriateness of each for the drug abuser. She then describes a couples group which she co-led and states her belief that the family can provide the best support for a drug abuser who is trying to become drug free. This is a good example of the role of a clinical nurse specialist in a drug abuse program.

*Pisarcik, G.: Management of phencyclidine toxicity, J. Emerg. Nurs. **4**:35, Sept.-Oct. 1978.

This article is recommended for nurses who are likely to have contact with patients experiencing toxic reactions to PCP. It includes a very clear description of the behaviors characteristic of this condition. There is also a practical discussion of nursing intervention.

Ray, O.S.: Drugs, society, and human behavior, ed. 3, St. Louis, 1982, The C.V. Mosby Co.

This book is highly recommended as a basic resource on all aspects of chemical dependency. In addition to discussion of the relevant psychosocial factors, there is also presentation of the pharmacological aspects.

Szasz, T.: Ceremonial chemistry, New York, 1974, Doubleday & Co., Inc.

In this provocative book, the author looks at drug use from a cultural point of view. He presents the case that drug "abuse" is culturally defined and serves the purpose of providing society with a group of scapegoats. He views the use of drugs as a type of religious observance in terms of its significance to the user. This is a thought-provoking work that forces one to reassess attitudes about drug use and abuse.

*Van Gee, S.J.: Alcoholism and the family: a psychodrama approach, J. Psychiatr. Nurs. **17**:9, Aug. 1979.

This article describes the enabler role of the wives of alcoholics. Intervention into the spouse's behavior can have impact on the alcoholic. Wives frequently overcompensate, becoming dominant and making all the decisions. Psychodrama can assist her to refuse to be an enabler.

*Vourakis, C., and Bennett, G.: Angel dust: not heaven sent, Am. J. Nurs. **79**:649, 1979.

This excellent article presents a thorough overview of the manifestations of PCP use and related nursing care. The authors organize the presentation of theory around a primary, secondary, and tertiary prevention model. There is also a discussion of the pharmacological characteristics of the drug.

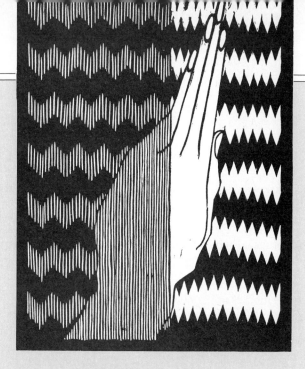

I locked myself away from you
Too long,
Tossing aside my feelings
For you.
Looking for a way out, an excuse
Not to touch you;
Because I want to,
Inciting a riot within me.

To reach out for you
Is difficult,
But less difficult
Than turning away.

Leslie Bertel

C H A P T E R   2 1

VARIATIONS IN SEXUAL RESPONSE

Susan G. Poorman

After studying this chapter, the student should be able to:

- discuss why nurses need knowledge of human sexuality, the kind of knowledge needed, and problems encountered in obtaining it.

- describe the dimensions of sexual behavior and the continuum of adaptive and maladaptive sexual responses.

- identify two major responsibilities of the nurse in assessing variations in sexual response.

- analyze the four phases of the nurse's growth in developing self-awareness of human sexuality.

- analyze the predisposing factors and precipitating stressors that are associated with variations in sexual response.

- identify and describe behaviors and coping mechanisms associated with variations in sexual response.

- formulate individualized nursing diagnoses for patients with variations in sexual response.

- assess the relationship between nursing diagnoses and medical diagnoses associated with variations in sexual response.

- develop long- and short-term individualized nursing goals with patients who are experiencing variations in sexual response.

- apply therapeutic nurse-patient relationship principles with appropriate rationale in planning the care of a patient who is experiencing a variation in sexual response.

- describe nursing interventions appropriate to the needs of the patient who is experiencing variation in sexual response.

- critique some commonly held myths regarding human sexuality.

- develop a mental health education plan to promote a patient's adaptive sexual responses.

- assess the importance of the evaluation of the nursing process when working with patients with variations in sexual response.

- identify directions for future nursing research.

- select appropriate readings for further study.

As nursing moves toward a holistic approach to patient care, nurses are often called on to intervene in situations regarding patients' sexuality. As a profession, nursing has historically fallen short of its responsibility to counsel individuals in this area. Nurses have a wide variety of reactions to patients' concerns regarding sexuality. For example, some nurses claim that "nurses are not sex therapists and therefore do not understand sexual issues." Other nurses ignore or deny sexual issues that patients raise and "pass the buck" to physicians, social workers, or other health professionals. Nurses tell patients to ask their physician about sexuality questions, but physicians may not necessarily be more open or prepared to address these issues. Nurses may feel embarrassed when a man talks about his fear of impotence during chemotherapy. Or they may be repelled or shocked by patients who "come out" and disclose their gay identity. More than a few nurses may be hesitant to talk with a woman after her mastectomy who is worried that her husband will no longer find her sexually appealing.

Sexuality cannot be separated from the condition of being human; therefore it is imperative that nurses develop skill and confidence in addressing sexual issues with their patients if holistic health care is to be provided. Education regarding sexuality will provide professional nurses with the theoretical knowledge necessary for clinical application in nursing practice.

Since nurses confront difficult issues on a daily basis with patients, such as death, family problems, and crisis situations, the question can be raised as to why nurses are unable to intervene appropriately in patient issues regarding sexuality. Several factors contribute to nurses' difficulty in providing sexual counseling or health teaching:

1. Nurses often do not obtain adequate theoretical knowledge in their nursing education. Sexuality is addressed basically in terms of the anatomical and physiological functions of the male and female bodies. Nurses often do not address their feelings and thoughts about sexual issues, and

in many cases nurses do not think of themselves as sexual beings. It seems that to view oneself as a professional, many nurses behave as if they believe themselves to be asexual beings. Nurses tend to deny the fact that they are human beings with needs and feelings that include sexual desires.

2. Many nursing educators are improperly prepared to address the issue of sexuality with students because of deficiencies in their own education. The effect of inadequate preparation is ignorance, which breeds ignorance and results in inadequate assessment and intervention with patients regarding issues of human sexuality.

3. Nurses often believe that physicians are more knowledgeable regarding sexuality; therefore nurses refer any sexual concern raised by patients to the physician. Several important issues arise for consideration from this assumption. First, physicians often have no more sexual education and knowledge than nurses. Second, nurses spend more time with patients on a daily basis, and therefore many patients are more comfortable talking about sexual issues with the nurse than with their physician. Most important, nurses fail to treat the "whole person" if they fail to include sexuality as a component of nursing care.[18]

Most nursing textbooks address sexuality from the viewpoint of the medical model, that is, the content primarily includes charts of the anatomy and physiology of male and female reproductive organs and graphs of hormonal levels in the adult male and female bodies. Anatomical and physiological information is of vital importance in understanding human sexuality; however, such information is available and best described in anatomy and physiology nursing texts. This chapter will depart from the traditional approach by integrating concepts of sexual counseling in a nursing process model.

Continuum of sexual responses

Not all nurses will become experts in the area of sexuality; however, if nurses are aware of basic principles of human behavior, they will have a better understanding of a patient's sexual needs and problems. Nurses come in contact with sexual issues on a daily basis, regardless of their field of nursing practice. If nurses are comfortable with sexual issues, they will convey that comfort to the patient, which in turn gives the patient permission to discuss sexual issues with the nurse. The nurse-patient relationship is an intimate relationship in many ways. Nurses care for patients who are often experiencing painful and changing events in their lives.

Thus it is appropriate that the nurse-patient relationship allow for open honest discussion of sexuality. In answering the question "What do nurses need to know about sexuality?" several factors need to be considered.

First, nurses need to know themselves, to be aware of their own feelings and values regarding sexuality. If nurses are not aware of their feelings, they cannot adequately or competently help patients meet their needs. For example, nurses may become distressed when they find patients masturbating. Many people have been raised to feel that there is something innately wrong with masturbating, even though they know intellectually that masturbation is a normal healthy expression of sexual behavior. Thus a nurse who is distressed by a patient who is masturbating will have difficulty in talking with the patient about his or her sexual needs.

Second, nurses need to understand that everyone's feelings and values regarding sexuality are not going to match their own feelings and values. Anytime the topic of sex or any issue that vaguely hints at a sexual connotation comes up, nurses frequently feel threatened and tend to lose objectivity. This may occur because of a difference of values between the nurse, patient, or norms of society. For example, the nurse who is staunchly opposed to abortion may have a difficult time caring for a patient who has just aborted a pregnancy. Nurses may ignore patients with different beliefs and values or may become passively or even actively hostile toward them. Nurses have been known to dehumanize patients with value systems that differ from their own or detach themselves from their care and then feel guilty for doing so. In such cases a vicious cycle results in which the nurse and patient both lose.

When nurses have different beliefs and values from their patients, a common response is to misunderstand, feel scared and confused, and judge others' values as wrong. Although nursing textbooks tell nurses to be nonjudgmental, the ideal attitude is much easier to instruct than implement. It is critically important, if sensitive competent nursing care is to be provided to patients, that nurses get in touch with what it is they feel and believe about sexuality and about themselves as sexual beings.

Nurses also need to develop basic skills in helping patients approach their sexual concerns. Although all nurses will not become sex therapists, all nurses can become educated and enlightened about the sexual health of patients and can use practical sound counseling methods with patients. Specifically, nurses can:

1. Learn interviewing skills for sexual assessment and history taking
2. Develop confidence in their ability to approach or allow patients to approach sexual issues

3. Effectively counsel or refer patients for appropriate counseling regarding sexual issues

■ Dimensions of sexual behavior

Sexuality is broadly defined as a desire for contact, warmth, tenderness, or love.[1] It incorporates far more than genital sex. Sexuality includes looking and talking, poetry and long walks, hand holding, kissing, self-pleasuring, and the production of mutual orgasms through various means.[11] Sexuality also includes one's total sense of self. Kirkendall and Rubin[17] believe people must concern themselves with sexual feelings and behaviors throughout the life cycle. Sexuality is an integral part of every human being and every day of one's life. It is evident in the way one looks, believes, behaves, and relates to other human beings. Accepting a broad concept of sexuality allows the nurse to explore ways in which people are sexual beings, and understand more fully one's own feelings, beliefs, and actions related to human sexuality.

It is difficult, if not impossible, to define "normal" sexual behavior without making value judgments. One's parents, relatives, friends, and society are all likely to have different views on normal sexuality. Goldstein[9] defines normal sexual behavior as any sexual act between adults that is consensual, lacks force, and is performed in private, away from unwilling observers. If one accepts Goldstein's definition of normal behavior, then homosexuality, the act of obtaining sexual pleasure from a member of the same sex, would be considered normal because the behavior meets the requirements of consent, adult, lacking force, and privacy. Conversely, pedophilia, the act of obtaining sexual pleasure by molesting a child, would not meet Goldstein's requirements of normal sexual behavior, since the action is not performed by consenting adults.

Experts in the area of sexuality and sexual behavior do not agree on what types of sexual behavior are normal. For years, many people believed that any deviation from sexual relations between married partners for procreative purposes was problematic or abnormal. Today more people are beginning to view sexual behavior with a wider range of attitudes and values. It is possible to view expressions of sexuality on a continuum ranging from adaptive to maladaptive (see Fig. 21-1). The most adaptive sexual responses are seen as sexual behaviors that meet the following criteria: between two consenting adults, mutually satisfying to the individuals involved, not psychologically or physically harmful to either party, lacking in force or coercion, and conducted in private.

In some instances, however, sexual behavior can meet the criteria for adaptive responses but include variables that may interfere with the overall satisfaction of the relationship. Sexual responses that may otherwise be considered adaptive might be altered by the impact of what society dictates as acceptable and unacceptable behavior. Unfortunately, society often makes these decisions based on fear, prejudices, and lack of information, rather than on data and facts. For example, the homosexual person may have the potential for healthy adaptive sexual responses but his or her sexual responses may be impaired because of anxiety from responses to societal disapproval of sexual preference.

Maladaptive sexual responses include sexual behaviors that do not meet one or more of the criteria for adaptive responses. The degree to which these behaviors are maladaptive will vary. Some sexual behaviors may not meet any of the above mentioned criteria. For example, incest may include force and is often psychologically harmful if a child is involved. However, other sexual responses may meet four out of five of the criteria for adaptive responses but still have a maladaptive element involved. For example, a couple experiencing a sexual dysfunction (e.g., premature ejaculation) may meet Goldstein's criteria for normal behavior, but their sexual behavior may be unsatisfactory or even psychologically harmful to one or both members of the relationship.

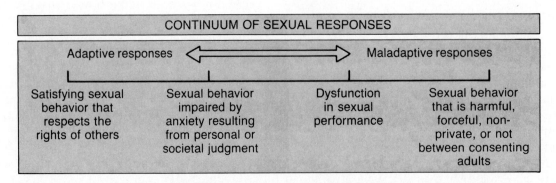

CONTINUUM OF SEXUAL RESPONSES

Adaptive responses	⟵⟶		Maladaptive responses
Satisfying sexual behavior that respects the rights of others	Sexual behavior impaired by anxiety resulting from personal or societal judgment	Dysfunction in sexual performance	Sexual behavior that is harmful, forceful, non-private, or not between consenting adults

Fig. 21-1. Continuum of sexual responses.

Caution must be used when attempting to label sexual behaviors as adaptive or maladaptive. There will never be total agreement on what should be considered adaptive or maladaptive sexual responses; there will always be exceptions to the rule. The continuum shown in Fig. 21-1 is intended to be free of moral judgment and was developed to aid the nurse in understanding the range of possible sexual responses.

 ## Assessment

Some people who experience stress in the area of their sexuality may be reluctant to accept their need for help in this area. Others seek help indirectly in that a diffuse symptom often masks an underlying sexual problem. The nurse is often the health professional who first comes in contact with these patients. The nursing process will assist her in working with patients as they develop a collaborative relationship and assess problems, assign priorities to needs, and mutually arrive at a plan of intervention.

Assessment, the first phase of the nursing process, includes two clearly defined responsibilities in the sexual counseling of patients: (1) the development of self-awareness in relation to sexuality and (2) the assessment of the patient. The most critical element in being able to competently counsel patients about sexuality is for the nurse to be aware of her own feelings and values. The nurse's level of self-awareness has a direct impact on her ability to intervene effectively with patients. In developing self-awareness, nurses may progress through four phases of a predictable growth experience: cognitive dissonance, anxiety, anger, and action. In assessing a patient, the nurse assesses the individual's situation and presenting problem.

■ Self-awareness of the nurse

The first step in developing self-awareness preparatory to sexual counseling is for the nurse to clarify values in response to her own sexuality. Foley and Davies[7] identified patterns of growth experiences developed around the nursing care of rape victims. Their model is applicable in the sexual counseling of patients as well and has been adapted accordingly.

■ **COGNITIVE DISSONANCE.** The first phase of the growth experience in developing sexual self-awareness is characterized by cognitive dissonance. This is defined as a state that exists when two opposing beliefs exist simultaneously.[30] For example, nurses grow up learning what society, family, and friends believe about sexual issues. If a nurse is raised in an environment that teaches her that nice girls do not talk about sex, the nurse will carry that belief into nursing practice. When the nurse

encounters a patient who wants to discuss an issue of sexual concern with her, she may experience the following two opposing reactions simultaneously:

1. As a professional, I should be able to discuss any problem, including sexual problems, with my patient.
2. Nice girls do not discuss sex.

Experiencing both of these conflicting thoughts at the same time makes the nurse uncomfortable. This feeling of discomfort eventually forces the nurse to examine her feelings and values about discussing the sexual problems of patients as part of nursing care. The nurse will resolve the cognitive dissonance in one of two ways: (1) denying professional responsibilities to the patient and continuing to ascribe to personal beliefs, such as nice girls do not talk about sex, or (2) examining values and feelings about sexuality, including the fact that sexuality is an integral part of the human condition which seeks expression.

If the nurse continues to believe the myth that nice girls do not talk about sex, she may make excuses for unprofessional behavior by projecting blame onto the patient for introducing sexual topics or rationalizing that she cannot be expected to be knowledgeable about sexuality, since she is "just a nurse, and can't know everything." Rationalization encourages such behaviors as avoidance of or denial of a patient's sexual concerns. Rationalization and blaming the patient also allow the nurse to ignore her discomfort in viewing herself as a sexual human being. However, ignoring or denying one's discomfort does not allow one to move toward understanding personal feelings and values about sexuality.

Nurses need to examine what they believe about sexual issues and why they hold those beliefs. It is impossible to deny that environment and family background influence one's beliefs. In regard to sexual issues the professional nurse needs to ask: "Do I believe this because I am knowledgeable in this area and have researched the facts, or do I believe this because my parents or peers believe it?" Only when the nurse can say that the available information has been examined and an informed choice on values has been made, will the nurse have truly examined personal values and clarified them.

■ **ANXIETY.** If one's cognitive dissonance leads to a self-examination of values, a second phase of growth occurs. In the second phase anxiety, shock, and fear are experienced. Anxiety is a state of "apprehension cued off by a threat to some value which the individual holds essential to his existence as a personality.[22] Fear is a subjective feeling state arising from life and limb being

---

CLINICAL EXAMPLE 21-1

Ms. G works as a staff nurse at an outpatient psychiatric clinic. One day at an interdisciplinary team meeting, Ms. G presented a new case to the treatment team for review. Her case was a 29-year-old female patient who came to the clinic because she thought she was transsexual. Ms. G began to explain the patient's history to the treatment team when one of the team members interrupted, stating "If this isn't the sickest thing I've ever heard of. . . . I hope you don't expect us to treat this woman, or should I say man!" The other members of the treatment team began to snicker and continued to make jokes about the transsexual patient.

After the team meeting, Ms. G felt very confused. She usually respected her co-workers' clinical judgment and considered them to be good clinicians. But her new patient was obviously experiencing problems with her sexuality and was really serious about wanting treatment for sexual reassignment. Ms. G was also anxious because of her lack of facts and knowledge about transsexuality. She decided to do some research that evening at the library.

The next day at the office, one of the other nurse clinicians teased Ms. G about the new "half and half" patient. Another co-worker cautioned Ms. G not to see this patient in the back treatment room alone because "you never know about those perverts, they might grab you." Ms. G became irritable with her co-workers and called them ignorant bigots. Despite the problems with her co-workers she continued to research the nature of transsexualism to help her patient. Finally, she found a psychologist in the city who worked with transsexual patients and made an appointment to talk about transsexuality.

Ms. G explained the reaction of her co-workers to the psychologist, her own difficulties in understanding transsexuality and in finding an appropriate referral for the patient. "This isn't the first time this has happened at our clinic," Ms. G told the psychologist. "Anytime we get a patient with sexual problems everybody makes jokes and nothing is ever really done for them."

After the consultation appointment, the psychologist offered to do an inservice program on sexuality for the staff. Ms. G returned to the clinic, fearful that the staff would refuse the inservice program and laugh at her for suggesting the program.

The next day Ms. G told the staff at the team meeting of the psychologist's offer to talk with them about providing care to patients expressing sexual preferences that differ from their own. One of the team members responded by laughing, "We don't need anyone to teach us about sex—I think we know everything we need to know." Everyone laughed and agreed. Ms. G, although anxious, spoke up stating, "If we all know so much, why all this nervous laughter? Look, I know it's hard to talk about sex and sexual issues but we have got to admit that we do not do a very good job addressing some of the sexual issues or problems that patients present us with here. And many patients do. We just can't go on laughing and making judgments about people—Let's face it, that doesn't help anyone."

After Ms. G spoke up there was a long silence in the room until another nurse spoke up. "You know, I think Ms. G is right. There are lots of times I just don't know what to say or do for people who come in here with sexual concerns. What could it hurt to have an inservice?" After some discussion, the staff agreed to let Ms. G call the psychologist and set up the inservice program.

---

in danger due to a specific stimulus that is external to the person.[30] Shock is a severe "disturbance in the equilibrium or permanence of something characterized by feelings of surprise, terror, horror, or disgust."[30]

In the second phase, the nurse realizes that uncertainty, insecurity, questions, and problems regarding sexuality are experienced by everyone. Often the nurse experiences anxiety because of the realization that everyone is capable of a variety of sexual feelings and behaviors and that anyone can experience a sexual dysfunction or question one's sexual identity. The nurse who is experiencing anxiety may exhibit behaviors that are ineffective in discussing sexual issues with a patient, such as talking too much (not allowing patients to verbalize their feelings), failing to listen (failing to pick up on patient cues or messages), and diagnosing and analyzing (becoming preoccupied with facts rather than eliciting feelings from the patient).

■ **ANGER.** Because anxiety is an uncomfortable feeling, the nurse strives to eliminate the discomfort. The process of learning facts about sexuality and facing the ignorance of society or one's colleagues brings the nurse to a third phase of the growth experience. Anger characterizes phase three of the growth experience and generally arises after anxiety and shock subside. Anger is directed at oneself, one's patients, and society. The nurse begins to recognize that issues associated with sex or sexuality are highly volatile and emotionally charged. Rape, abortion, birth control, the equal rights amendment, child abuse, pornography, and religious issues all have an obvious or subtle connection with sexuality and give rise to vehement debates. Similarly, attempts to formulate legislation relating to sexual matters is often ineffective because these issues are emotion laden. The realization of society's emotionality and irrationality in relation to issues having a sexual element often breeds anger and contempt in the nurse. For example, a nurse may become angry at what she perceives to be the ignorance, bigotry, or unprofessional attitude of a colleague or friend who judges homosexuals to be perverted deviants.

During this phase of anger nurses may begin to get on a "soapbox" and lecture others about the need for sex education to rid society of ignorance about sex and sexual issues. The nurse may develop an impatient hostile attitude toward a patient or co-worker who is not educated in the area of sexuality. For instance, a nurse may critically judge a patient who becomes pregnant because of ignorance about simple birth control methods. Furthermore the nurse is often angry with society for perpetuating ignorance about sexuality and may not understand when others do not share her enthusiasm for wanting to change society's beliefs.

The nurse may also be angry with herself for her own ignorance and feel guilty and embarrassed for her lack of sexual knowledge. It is essential that the nurse be able to admit her negative feelings and lack of knowledge without fear of disapproval from colleagues or friends. Openness to one's feelings and limitations within a trusting relationship is a key step in beginning to be able to seek out and ask for information basic to understanding human sexuality.

■ ACTION. The final step in the growth experience is the action phase in which the nurse experiences a decrease in anger and an increased ability to understand that blaming herself or society for ignorance and prejudice does not aid in self-understanding and helping patients with sexual concerns. During the action phase nurses often wonder, "Why didn't anyone ever teach me what I really needed to know about sexuality?" "Why aren't people educated properly?" "Where should sex education start?" "How can I gain more knowledge for myself and others?"

Several behaviors characterize the final action phase of the growth experience: data inquiry, choosing values, and prizing values. Data inquiry is demonstrated when the nurse obtains information about sexuality and sexual issues so that, properly informed, values about sexuality can be freely chosen. After choosing a value position, the final behavior is one of prizing the valued position. Prizing consists of an awareness and cherishing of one's feelings and values and being willing to share them publicly. Although prizing values is considered the final step in a positive growth experience, prizing does not mean that what one values now will not change. Values are never static, but evolve and shift as a person changes, grows, and acquires new life experiences. Thus a person who once ascribed to pro-life values may later become understanding and empathetic toward women who seek an abortion. Clinical example 21-1 illustrates a nurse who prizes values enough to share them publicly.

Clinical example 21-1 illustrates the phases of growth health professionals experience while increasing self-awareness in the area of sexuality. These phases are represented in Fig. 21-2. Ms. G experienced cognitive dissonance when the staff called the transsexual patient sick, and she was faced with conflicting feelings. She agreed with the staff because she respected them as expert clinicians, but she also believed the patient was not sick, weird, or perverted and had a very real problem that needed professional help. Ms. G experienced anxiety when she realized that she did not know anything about transsexuality. Her anxiety also stemmed from being faced with the reality that people express their sexuality in different ways, some of which were very different from anything she had been exposed to before. Ms. G experienced anger at herself and the staff for ignorance and judgmental attitudes and lashed out at the staff by calling them bigots. Her anger finally motivated her into action. She decided to explore her feelings, educate herself through reading and talking with a knowledgeable professional, and finally spoke up in a conflictual staff meeting to facilitate a needed staff inservice program on sexuality.

■ **Assessment of the patient**

Any basic health history needs to include questions regarding sexual history. Nurses are often involved in history gathering and assessments of patients. Because of the possible anxiety and embarrassment associated with sexual issues, nurses react in a variety of ways when obtaining this assessment data. One common reaction is for nurses to ignore the sexual questions or to look at the floor and stutter while asking interview questions. Another common reaction is for the nurse to blurt out rapidly, "You don't have any sex problems, do you?" or "How's your sex life?" Patients usually respond to these statements with embarrassment and feel that these questions are intrusive. Each of these interview questions, when asked by the nurse, gives the patient a clear message that it is not appropriate to talk about sex. When

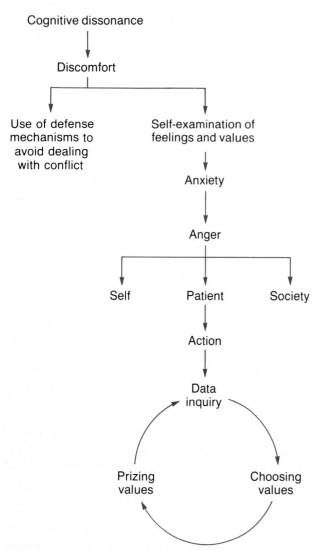

Fig. 21-2. Phases of the nurse's growth in developing self-awareness of human sexuality.

the nurse is uncomfortable, the patient will be uncomfortable, often to the point that no sexual concerns will be discussed with the nurse.

Comfort in discussing sexual issues is the first requirement for the nurse who wishes to successfully assess a patient's sexuality. A nurse who is comfortable in discussing sexuality conveys the message that it is normal to talk about sexual health as a part of a health assessment interview. If nurses are able to remove the attitude that "sex is dirty and should not be discussed" by presenting a calm and professional manner, questions about patients' sexual health can be asked in a factual manner, and the patient is allowed the freedom to discuss sexual matters without guilt or embarrassment.

The second requirement for a nurse to successfully assess a patient's sexuality is effective interviewing skills.

Many nurses who demonstrate excellent interviewing skills become uncomfortable asking questions about sex. However, concepts of effective interviewing are the same for sexual issues as for any presenting problem. For example, open-ended questions are often most helpful to initiate a discussion on sexuality. The question must be at the patient's level of understanding, because each person is a unique individual. The amount of time and depth needed to complete an interview will vary with each patient and problem. Often one or two questions may be sufficient to assess a person's sexual health. Other times, when patients have specific sexual problems, a detailed and specific assessment needs to be done. A sexual health assessment form that may be used by the nurse is given in the accompanying box.

Another important factor to convey in assessing a patient's sexual health is to inform the person that information gathered during the interview is strictly confidential and that the patient's medical chart cannot be given out without the patient's written permission. Assurance of confidentiality is important in the care of all people. Many sexual minority patients are especially sensitive about confidentiality, since they often fear losing their jobs or family rejection if their sexual minority status was accidentally discovered by employers or relatives.

■ Predisposing factors

At present, there is no one theory that can adequately explain the process of sexual development or the factors predisposing a person to maladaptive sexual responses. A number of theories have been postulated, however, and some of these theoretical perspectives will now be briefly described.

■ **BIOLOGICAL FACTORS.** Biological factors are initially responsible for the development of gender—that is, whether one is genetically male or female. One's somatotype therefore includes chromosomes, hormones, internal and external genitalia, and gonads. The process of sex differentiation is set off by the Y chromosome. Research in humans confirms the general rule that maleness and masculinity depend on fetal and paranatal androgens.

A biological female typically has XX chromosomes, with estrogen as the predominant hormone, appropriate internal and external genitalia, and ovaries. A biological male typically has XY chromosomes, with androgen as the predominant hormone, appropriate internal and external genitalia, and testicles. However, each of these typical configurations may be subject to variation. A person may have triple chromosomes, such as XXX, XXY, or XYY, or a single chromosome, XO. There is no YO chromosomal pattern. The triple pattern XXX

Sexual Health Assessment Form

1. When you were a child, how were your questions about sex answered? Where did your sexual information come from? (Appropriate for adolescents.) When you were a teenager, how were your questions about sex answered? (Appropriate for adults.)
2. How did you first find out about sexual intercourse (how babies are made)? (Appropriate for adolescents and young adults.)
3. How would you describe your current sexual activity?
4. What, if anything, would you change about your current sexual activity?
5. At this time in your life, how important is a sexual relationship to you?
6. Do you have any concerns about birth control?
7. Do you have any health problems that, in your opinion, affect your sexual health or happiness?
8. Are you taking any medicines that, in your opinion, affect your sexual health or happiness?
9. Is there anything about these questions that you would like clarified or explained?

From Sexuality: a nursing perspective by F.H. Mims and M. Swenson. Copyright © 1980, McGraw-Hill Book Company. Used with the permission of McGraw-Hill Book Company.

and the single pattern XO (Turner's syndrome) will develop into a female body, while the triple patterns XXY (Kleinfelter's syndrome) and XYY will develop male bodies. Assuming no variation occurs, the biological factors result in a single, fully developed gender, either male or female.

■ **PSYCHOANALYTIC VIEW.** Sigmund Freud's influence on society is ever present. His psychoanalytic theory has served as the basis for contemporary psychiatry all over the world. Freud saw sexuality as one of the key forces of human life. In *Three Essays of the Theory of Sexuality*,[8] he theorized extensively about the nature of sexuality and sexual development. He was the first theorist to believe that sexuality was developed before the onset of puberty and believed that a person's choice of sexual expression depended on an interplay of heredity, biology, and social factors. He wrote extensively about childhood sexuality and believed infantile sexuality was central to personality development. He further believed that the development of sexuality in individuals was specifically related to the development of object relations during the psychosexual stages of development.

Freud termed the sex drive *libido* and viewed it as one of the two major drives necessary for life (the other being aggression). He believed the libido was focused in various regions of the body that were extremely sensitive to stimulation (erogenous zones). The child, according to Freud, passes through a series of developmental stages in which a different erogenous zone is dominant. The first developmental stage is the oral stage (birth to 12 or 18 months) where the infant's chief sense of pleasure is derived from the stimulation of the lips and mouth, that is, sucking. The second stage is the anal stage (ages 1 to 3 years) where the child's attention is focused on elimination functions and control over body sphincters. The third stage is the phallic stage (ages 3 to 5 years) in which the erotic focus is on the genitals. A very important occurrence in this stage is the development of the Oedipus complex for boys and the Electra complex for girls.

In the Oedipus/Electra complex, the child experiences sexual feelings for the parent of the opposite sex and has feelings of resentment for the parent of the same sex. According to Freud, the boy fears retaliation from his father for desiring his mother and fantasizes that the father will cut off his penis (castration anxiety). This fear is the impetus for the young boy's eventually giving up the resentment of the father and identifying with him and the male gender role. The girl, on the other hand, has no penis to fear losing. She believes that at one time she had a penis but it was cut off, and she blames her mother for this occurrence. Since she has no penis to fear losing, her motivation for resolving the Electra complex is not as strong, and her resolution remains incomplete. Thus, according to Freud, the female remains somewhat less mature than her male counterpart.[12]

After the resolution of the Oedipus or Electra complex, the child enters a prolonged stage where sexual impulses are repressed—latency. This stage lasts until adolescence when the child enters the genital stage in which sexual urges reawaken. This genital phase is triggered by the biologic focus that activates puberty. The reemergence of oedipal/electra feelings and the need to assert themselves with parents also occur during this phase of development. The adolescent then makes the final transition into mature adult genital sexuality. If fixation occurred at any of the earlier stages of development, object cathexis would be incomplete and the individual may have a narcissistic object choice as a result.

In recent years, there has been criticism of Freud's theory of psychosexual development. Feminists argue that psychoanalytic theory is male centered and views women as anatomically inferior to men (because they have no penis). Freud also made judgments about the quality of vaginal versus clitoral orgasms. He believed that young girls explored their clitoris in play because it was more accessible, but would give up interest in the clitoris as they matured and would move their sexual interest to the vagina. He believed the mature woman was vaginally responsive and that sexual orgasm from clitoral stimulation was immature.[27] However, recent research has found no evidence to support this viewpoint.

Lack of scientific evidence is one of the major problems with Freud's theory. Most of Freud's concepts cannot be studied and thus verified in any of the usual scientific methods. Other criticisms include that Freud was a victim of the Victorian era, a time of sexual repression, and that his thoughts and writings were bound by the times in which he lived. Finally, Freud's data were collected from observations of his patients who were probably not representative of the total population but who were to some degree emotionally disturbed.

■ **BEHAVIORAL VIEW.** From the perspective of a behaviorist, the most legitimate data for understanding sexual reactions are observable responses to overt, quantifiable stimuli. Behaviorists are not concerned with the complex childhood and intrapsychic processes that represent one's early childhood and adolescent experiences. Rather, they view sexual behavior as a measurable response with both physiological and psychological components to a learned stimulus or reinforcement event. For example, behaviorists would consider the sexual behavior of adults caring for children to be important in their later sexual development.

In a similar fashion, treatment of sexual problems involves processes to change behavior through direct intervention without the need to identify underlying etiology and psychodynamics. Aversive therapy has also been used to treat persons who exhibit socially stigmatized sexual behavior.

■ Precipitating stressors

Feelings about oneself as a sexual being change throughout the life cycle. Sexual identity cannot be separated from one's self-concept or body image. Therefore when changes occur in one's body or emotions, they will effect a change in one's sexual response as well.

■ **ILLNESS AND INJURY.** Physical and emotional illness may precipitate alterations in sexuality. The patient who needs to be hospitalized for these illnesses may find that the hospitalization alone may cause changes in sexual feelings and behavior. Nurses usually provide care to patients who experience alterations in sexuality, and they need to discuss and therapeutically intervene in a patient's response to changes in sexual functioning. A person experiencing rheumatoid arthritis may experience body disfiguration and a change in body image because of swollen areas around joints. The same patient may experience decreased sexual interest because of fear of joint and muscle pain during intercourse. Patients who suffer from depressive episodes often experience a decrease in libido as a symptom. People who have had a myocardial infarction in the past may have a decreased sexual interest because of fear of a heart attack from becoming sexually aroused. Psychotic patients may experience hallucinations and delusions in which they become sexually preoccupied.

Some medications contribute to sexual dysfunction, failure to reach orgasm in women, and impotence or failure to ejaculate in men. Nurses are responsible for being knowledgeable about the medications they administer and educating patients regarding possible side effects, informing them to notify a health professional when side effects occur. For example, a patient may not be aware that his medication can be the cause of his impotence, yet he may be extremely embarrassed and hesitant to talk with the physician or nurse about the problem. Abuse of alcohol or nontherapeutic drugs may also have a debilitating effect on sexuality. Although many people believe that alcohol is a sexual stimulant, prolonged use can cause erectile difficulty and other sexual dysfunctions.

Patients who become disfigured because of injury or surgery may also experience alterations in sexuality. Sudden injury leaves patients with little or no time to prepare for the loss. People who experience spinal cord injuries may lose sexual functioning because of full or partial paralysis.

Some sexual problems that arise from injury or surgery are organic in origin; others are psychological. The most common types of surgical procedures that present the potential for postsurgical difficulty with sexual responses include the following[24]:

1. Loss of an external body part, such as with a mastectomy or penectomy
2. Loss of internal organs, such as with a prostatectomy or hysterectomy
3. Loss of body function, such as surgery that would result in impotence
4. Relocation of a body orifice, such as a colostomy or ileostomy

Changes in sexuality, regardless of the precipitating factor, may mean changes in sexual patterns and behaviors. The role of the professional nurse includes assistance and counseling to aid patients with changes as a result of illness or injury understand their feelings and explore their options, and then to facilitate their adaptive adjustment.

■ **THE AGING PROCESS.** Although many researchers have documented decreased sexual activity with aging, sexuality remains an important part of expressing oneself throughout the life cycle. The aging process causes some changes in sexual anatomy and responsiveness for both men and women. Physiological changes in women are related to depleting estrogen supplies (after menopause) and include atrophy of the vaginal mucosa and decreased vaginal lubrication; actual shrinkage in size and loss of elasticity in the vaginal canal, especially in sexually inactive women; and a decrease in actual breast size.[18] In a study of 34 women from the ages of 51 to 78, Masters and Johnson[20] noted a number of alterations in sexual response patterns as compared to premenopausal women: (1) a vasocongestive increase in breast size usually seen during sexual excitement was decreased or nonexistent, (2) generalized myotonia was decreased, (3) there is less expansion of the vagina during sexual stimulation, and (4) vaginal lubrication decreased and required a longer time to develop. Masters and Johnson also noted that some aging women begin to experience painful uterine contractions during orgasm.

Physiological changes in the male include a gradual decrease in circulating levels of testosterone from approximately age 60 on. However, decreased testosterone levels in men are usually not as pronounced as the estrogen deficiency in postmenopausal women. Spermatogenesis does decrease with age; however, men often remain fertile until death. Aging alters the sexual response pattern of the male in that (1) longer time and more direct genital stimulation is requried to achieve erection, (2) there is a decrease in the firmness of the erection, (3) a less intense ejaculation is experienced, and (4) the time interval after ejaculation when the male is physiologically unable to ejaculate again also tends to lengthen.[18]

In Western culture the myth of the older adult as an asexual being still prevails. Westerners tend to regard the older adult as one who has no interest in sexual feelings or behavior. Many personality theorists have participated in and encouraged the myth of the older adult as an asexual or childlike being. Psychoanalytical theory describes the sexuality of the aging person as a regression to oral and anal levels of gratification. Since many theories about development have had their roots in psychoanalytical theory, it is not surprising that the stereotypical myth of sexless old age is perpetuated.

Not only have people been taught that older adults have little interest in sex, but also that it is normal for the older person to have no interest in sex. Therefore when health professionals encounter older individuals who do indicate an interest in sex or who are sexually active, the professional often judges the older adult as perverted or "oversexed." Older adults themselves are not exempt from society's false beliefs about sexuality and aging. Many older adults deny sexual attractions and feelings because they also have been socialized to believe that sexual behavior in older people is abnormal or perverted. Older adults are influenced by cultural values of Western society that currently prize youth and vitality and often look with disgust at an elderly person doing anything other than sitting in a rocking chair.

Sexual capability can be maintained throughout a person's life. There are, however, several reasons for decreased sexual activity among older adults. Kolodny and co-workers[18] identified five categories of altered sexuality related to the aging process: general sexual disinterest, sexual boredom, impaired physical sexuality, cultural inhibition, and attrition by disuse. General sexual disinterest included people who, with advancing years, viewed sex as an unnecessary indulgence. Sexual boredom occurred in couples who realized that boredom may be a factor in the sexual relationship but failed to experiment with changing sexual habits developed over the years. Boredom may be associated with decreased self-esteem, cultural inhibitions, or changes in the health status of the aging individual.

An extremely important variable affecting altered sexuality because of aging is attrition by disuse: "use it or lose it." Prolonged abstinence from sexual activity caused more physiological problems in the older adult. For example, the older female who abstains from sexual activity will have a greater degree of shrinkage in the size of her vagina than a female of the same age who is sexually active. The older male who abstains from sexual activity may experience difficulty having erections when attempting to return to sexual activity. In general, the effects of disuse or lack of sexual activity magnify physical problems of sexuality in the older adult.[18] Most researchers at present agree with the original Kinsey studies, which indicated that persons who enjoy an active sex life as young adults will probably continue their usual pattern in older adulthood with some modifications, rather than experiencing a sudden decrease or cessation of sexual activity and interest in older adulthood.[16]

■ **Behaviors**

There are many modes of sexual expression. In 1948, Kinsey used a seven-point rating scale in examining sexual preference (see Fig. 21-3) in which a 0 represented exclusively heterosexual experiences, a 6

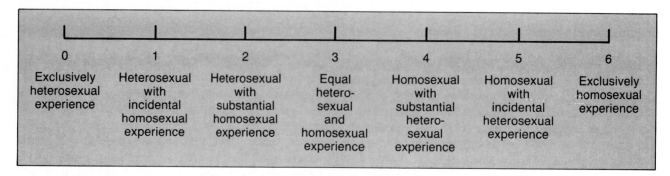

Fig. 21-3. Kinsey's rating scale of sexual preference.

represented exclusively homosexual experiences, and a bisexual would rate a 2, 3, or 4 on the scale. He suggested that most individuals are not exclusively heterosexual or homosexual. His studies indicated that a substantial percentage of men and women had experienced both heterosexual and homosexual activity. Specifically, the Kinsey study reported that 25% of United States males and 6% to 14% of females have had more than incidental homosexual experiences.[16] More recent work suggests that the incidence of homosexuality is significantly higher than that reported by Kinsey's early work.[15]

■ **HOMOSEXUALITY.** Marmor defined the homosexual person as "one who is motivated in adult life by a definite preferential erotic attraction to members of the same sex and who usually (but not necessarily) engages in overt sexual relations with them."[19] Marmor's definition excludes transitory incidental homosexual activity in adolescence and in primarily heterosexual persons. Persons who believe in or participate in sexual practices that differ from society's norm are often termed sexual minorities. Homosexuals are the largest sexual minority. The incidence of homosexuality in the United States today has been conservatively estimated at 10% to 15% of the population.[2]

For many years the medical profession, including psychiatry, has searched for causes of homosexuality. The message in looking for the cause of a condition is that it is a maladaptive state that can be treated or cured. Many theories of the cause of homosexuality have been formulated; however, no cause has ever been established. Today emphasis is placed on learning more about homosexuality and viewing it as a sexual preference or mode of sexual expression. Recent research findings indicate that gay men and lesbian women generally function at least as well psychologically, emotionally, and sexually as nongays do, and in some cases may even function better.[4]

If current estimates of the incidence of homosexuality are accurate, nurses come into contact with homosexuals on a daily basis. Despite this high incidence of homosexuality, nurses generally know very little about homosexuality and almost always assume that all patients are heterosexual.

■ **BISEXUALITY.** Bisexuality, sometimes called ambisexuality, is defined as sexual attraction to persons of both sexes and engagement in both homosexual and heterosexual activity.[28] Determining the precise points on the Kinsey scale that would indicate bisexual behavior is a controversial issue. It can be argued that only individuals who are rated as 3 (equal homosexual and heterosexual experiences) are considered bisexual. However, a more flexible interpretation of bisexual behavior could include all the individuals who are rated from the scores of 1 through 5, suggesting that bisexuals constitute a large segment of the population.[23] The actual number of adult bisexuals in society today has not been documented.

Despite suspected large numbers of bisexuals, there has been very little research on this sexual orientation. Often bisexual individuals are included in research samples with homosexual populations which makes it difficult to examine the bisexual person specifically. Society often labels anyone who has had a homosexual experience as a homosexual; however, the few studies that have been done on bisexuality indicate that bisexuals differ significantly from both the homosexual and the heterosexual populations. It therefore seems important to conduct further research on bisexuals alone, and the practice of combining bisexuals in samples with homosexuals should be discontinued if we are to learn more about this sexual orientation.[4]

■ **TRANSVESTISM.** Transvestism is defined as crossdressing or dressing in the clothes of the opposite sex. Clinically defined, "transvestism is a condition in which a male has a sexual obsession for or addiction to women's clothes, such that he periodically experiences intolerable psychic stress if he does not dress up."[25] Most often the transvestite that seeks treatment is a male; very little is known about female transvestism. No reliable statistics concerning the incidence of transvestism are available; however, many professionals believe the condition is more common than generally assumed.

Transvestites tend to be married men who report heterosexual behavior, and, although they occasionally or frequently dress in female garb, they do not wish hormonal or surgical sex change, as does the transsexual. Many transvestites try to find willing partners and typically their activities of cross-dressing do not prevent sexual relationships with others.[15]

■ **TRANSSEXUALISM.** The word transsexual simply implies going from one sex to another. A more specific definition specifies a transsexual to be a person who is anatomically a male or female but who expresses, with strong conviction, that he or she has the mind of the opposite sex, lives as a member of the opposite sex part time or full time, and seeks to change his or her original sex legally and through hormonal and surgical sex reassignment.[25] Many times the transsexual client will describe himself as "feeling trapped in the wrong body." Transsexuals genuinely feel they belong to the other sex. Many transsexuals experience intense emotional turmoil because of the stigma from society. There are no accurate estimates of the incidence of transsexualism. However, postoperative transsexuals in the United States now number in the thousands.[25]

Transsexuality is very different from homosexuality in that homosexuals are comfortable with their anatomical identity and do not want to change their sex. Many transsexuals are heterosexual and express some distaste for homosexual activity. Transsexuals are essentially heterosexual, not homosexual, but are commonly mistaken by others or themselves as being homosexual.

In Clinical example 21-2, the transsexual's attraction to others of the same sex is understood in the context of his inner identification with the opposite sex. The transsexual does not want a sexual relationship with a person of the same sex, but wishes to have his or her own genitals changed to that of the opposite sex. Thus the attraction is heterosexual.[15]

■ **THE SEXUAL RESPONSE CYCLE.** In addition to modes of sexual expression or sexual preference, it is also possible to describe the physiological and psychological behaviors that characterize a person's response to sexual stimulation. Masters and Johnson were the first to describe the physiological changes that actually occur when men and women engage in sexual activity. According to Masters and Johnson, the sexual response cycle consists of the following four phases[18]:

CLINICAL EXAMPLE 21-2

Mr. L is a 21-year-old biological male who was admitted to the psychiatric unit for evaluation after a serious suicide attempt. Mr. L was interviewed by Mr. W, the charge nurse on the unit. Mr. L told the nurse that he tried to kill himself because he has been "sexually mixed up for years" and is tired of feeling like a freak of nature. He said that his friends make fun of him and tell him he is a homosexual, but that he does feel sexually attracted to other men and does not see himself as a homosexual. "I guess I don't feel like a man, I feel like a woman inside a man's body, and as a woman I am attracted to men."

---

1. **Excitement Phase**

   This phase occurs as a result of sexual stimulation (either physical or psychic).

   The excitement phase in the female is characterized by vaginal lubrication, expansion of the inner two thirds of the vaginal barrel, elevation of the cervix and the body of the uterus, and flattening and elevation of the labia majora. The clitoris increases in size, and erection of the nipples occurs.

   The excitement phase in the male is characterized by penile erection. Skin ridges on the scrotal sac smooth out, and the scrotum flattens. The testes are partially elevated toward the perineum. In some but not all men, nipple erection occurs during the excitement phase.

2. **Plateau Phase**

   This phase describes a high state of sexual arousal that occurs prior to reaching orgasm. The duration of the plateau may vary greatly with different individuals.

   In the female, prominent vasocongestion occurs in the outer third of the vagina (orgasmic platform), and the opening of the vagina narrows. The inner two thirds of the vagina undergoes minimal expansion, and there is an increase in the elevation of the uterus. Vaginal lubrication usually decreases in this phase. The shaft and the glans of the clitoris retract against the pubic bone.

   In males, there is a minimal increase in the diameter of the proximal portion of the glans penis and a deepening in color due to venostatis. Testes increase in size. Small amounts of fluid from the urethra may appear.

3. **Orgasm**

   The orgasm phase is a total body response.
   In females, rhythmic contractions of the uterus, orgasmic platform and rectal sphincter occur. In males, there are rhythmic contractions of the prostate, perineal muscles, and the shaft of the penis which combine to assist the propulsion process of ejaculation.

4. **Resolution Phase**

   In the resolution phase, the anatomic and physiologic changes that occurred in the excitement and plateau phase are reversed.
   In females, the orgasmic platform disappears, the uterus moves back in to the true pelvis, the vagina shortens, and the clitoris returns to its normal position.
   In males, the erection diminishes and the testes decrease in size and descend into the scrotum.

Helen Singer Kaplan has proposed an alternative way of viewing the sexual response cycle. Along with the physiological, Kaplan addresses the psychological responses as well. According to Kaplan, the sexual response cycle consists of a complex series of autonomically mediated visceral reflexes, which can work successfully only if the person is in a calm state, and if the process is not impaired by the conscious monitoring processes. To function well sexually, the person must be able to abandon oneself to the erotic experience. One must be able to temporarily give up control and, to some degree, decrease one's contact with the environment.

Kaplan identifies three categories or stages of the sexual response cycle: **desire, excitement,** and **orgasm.** One of the most significant features of Kaplan's model is her inclusion of desire as a separate and distinct phase of the sexual response cycle. She describes desire as the prelude to the physical sexual response. Sexual desire is defined as an appetite or drive which is produced by the activation of the brain, while the excitement and orgasm phases involve genital orgasms.

Impairment in one's sexual response may occur in any one of these three phases or stages. For example, when the orgasm phase of the human sexual response cycle is disrupted, clinical syndromes such as premature or retarded ejaculation in males and orgastic inhibition in females may result. If the excitement phase of the sexual response cycle is inhibited, it may produce erectile dysfunction in males and a general sexual dysfunction in females. If there is inhibition in the desire phase of sexual response, it may be evidenced by low libido in both the male and the female.[14]

■ Coping mechanisms

Numerous coping mechanisms may be utilized in the expression of one's sexual response. These coping mechanisms may be adaptive or maladaptive, depending on how and why they are being employed. **Fantasy** is a coping mechanism that is used by individuals who wish to enhance their sexual experiences. Men and women may escape to erotic fantasies with unknown lovers during sex with their husband or wife. Although many people fear that fantasies about individuals other than their specific sexual partner indicate that they are unsatisfied or unattracted to their partner, this is typically not the case. Fantasies are often a creative way to increase sexual excitement and enjoyment and are not usually indicative of dissatisfaction with one's current partner. However, excessive fantasy can be maladaptive when it is used as a replacement for actual sexual expression or the development of intimate relationships with others.

Nursing Diagnoses Related to Variations in Sexual Response

Primary NANDA diagnoses

Altered sexuality patterns
Sexual dysfunction

Examples of complete nursing diagnoses

Altered sexuality patterns related to embarrassment about one's body after a mastectomy evidenced by lack of desire for sex
Altered sexuality patterns related to inability to achieve orgasm evidenced by lack of sexual satisfaction

Altered sexuality patterns related to marital conflict evidenced by lack of arousal during foreplay/intercourse
Sexual dysfunction related to excessive alcohol ingestion evidenced by inability to attain an erection
Sexual dysfunction related to fear of penetration evidenced by pain with intercourse

Maladaptive coping mechanisms may result from problems with self-concept. Often one member of a sexually dysfunctional couple may use **projection** in blaming his partner for the total problem, absolving himself of any participation, "I never had a sex problem with any of my previous lovers. I think you are the problem." Projection is also the coping mechanism utilized when a person's thoughts and feelings are unacceptable and anxiety producing. For example, a wife constantly accuses her husband of wanting to have an affair when in actuality it is the wife who is contemplating an affair. Because her feelings are unacceptable to her, she projects them on to her husband and accuses him of having the feelings she cannot accept in herself.

Denial and **rationalization** are also commonly utilized coping mechanisms. The following are maladaptive examples of denial and rationalization. Both allow the individual to avoid dealing with sexual issues:

Denial: "I don't have a problem with sex" or "I never feel sexual."

Rationalization: "I don't need sex, I'm fine without it, besides a good marriage is a lot more than just sex."

To cope with unacceptable feelings about becoming vulnerable and the resulting ambivalent feelings about intimacy, some individuals **withdraw** from any form of sexual behavior. Others may engage in increased sexual behavior with multiple partners to protect themselves from the threat of one intimate relationship.

 Nursing diagnosis

When developing a nursing diagnosis for variations in sexual response, the nurse should consider all the information gathered in the assessment phase and the components of the nursing model of health-illness phenomena (see Fig. 21-4). The identified nursing diagnosis serves as a foundation for future problem-solving activities. The primary nursing diagnoses according to NANDA are those of altered sexuality patterns, which includes lack of sexual satisfaction, alterations in perceived sex role, and conflicts involving values, and sexual dysfunction, which includes actual physical limitations. The primary NANDA diagnoses and examples of complete nursing diagnoses are presented in the accompanying box.

Other related nursing diagnoses that address additional behavioral problems related to variations in sexual response may also need to be included. For example, a patient may experience confusion regarding his sexual identity while remaining sexually functional. Nursing diagnoses related to the range of possible maladaptive responses of the patient and related medical diagnoses are identified in Table 21-1.

■ **Related medical diagnoses**

Many people who experience transient variations in sexual response will have no medically diagnosed health problem. Those individuals with more severe or persistent problems will be classified into one of four basic categories of variations in sexual response according to the Draft of the DSM-III-R in Development[2]—gender identity disorders, paraphilias, sexual dysfunctions, and other gender and sexual disorders. The specific medical diagnoses that fall under each of these diagnostic classes according to the Draft of the DSM-III-R in Development[2] will now be briefly described.

■ **TRANSSEXUALISM.** The essential features of transsexualism are persistent discomfort and sense of inappropriateness about one's assigned sex, and persistent preoccupation for at least 2 years with getting rid of one's primary and secondary sex characteristics and acquiring the sex characteristics of the other sex.

■ **NONTRANSSEXUAL CROSS-GENDER DISORDER.** The essential features of this disorder are persistent or recurrent discomfort and sense of inappropriateness about one's assigned sex, and cross-dressing in the role of the other sex, either in fantasy or actuality. There is no persistent preoccupation with getting rid of one's primary and secondary sex characteristics and acquiring the sex characteristics of the other sex. This individual has reached puberty.

■ **GENDER IDENTITY DISORDER OF CHILDHOOD** (Individuals have not reached puberty).

Females. The essential features are persistent and intense distress about being a girl and a stated desire to be a boy (not merely a desire for any perceived cultural advantages from being a boy), or insistence that she is a boy. There is either a persistent marked aversion to normative feminine clothing and insistence on wearing stereotypic masculine clothing, for example, boy's underwear and other accessories, or a persistent repudiation of her female anatomic structures as manifested by at least one of the following:

1. An assertion that she has, or will grow, a penis
2. Rejection of urinating in a sitting position
3. Assertion that she does not want to grow breasts or menstruate

Males. The essential features are persistent and intense distress about being a boy and an intense desire to be a girl. There is either a preoccupation with female stereotypic activities (as manifested by a preference for either cross-dressing or simulating female attire, or by a compelling desire to participate in the games and pastimes of girls) and rejection of male stereotypic toys, games, and activities or persistent repudiation of his male anatomic structures, as manifested by at least one of the following repeated assertions:

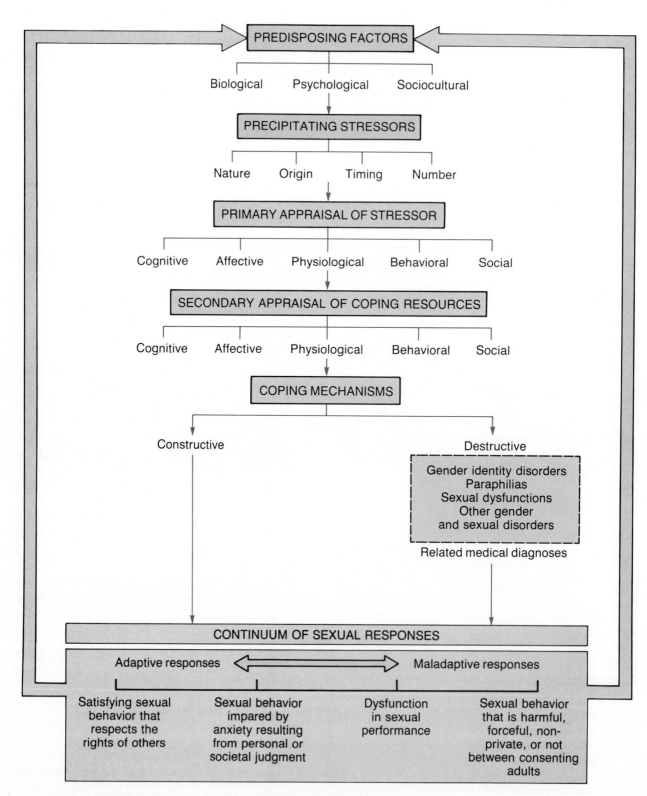

Fig. 21-4. Nursing model of health-illness phenomena related to variations in sexual response.

┌───┐

TABLE 21-1

MEDICAL AND NURSING DIAGNOSES RELATED TO VARIATIONS IN SEXUAL RESPONSE

Medical Diagnostic Class

Gender identity disorders
Paraphilias
Sexual dysfunctions
Other gender and sexual disorders

Psychiatric Nursing Diagnostic Class

Variations in sexual response

Related Medical Diagnoses (DSM-III-R*)

Transsexualism
Nontranssexual cross-gender disorder
Gender identity disorder of childhood
Pedophilia
Exhibitionism
Sexual sadism
Sexual masochism
Voyeurism
Fetishism
Transvestic fetishism
Zoophilia
Frotteurism
Paraphilia NOS
Hypoactive sexual desire disorder
Sexual aversion disorder
Female/male sexual arousal disorder
Inhibited female/male orgasm
Premature ejaculation
Functional dyspareunia
Functional vaginismus
Sexual dysfunction NOS
Ego-dystonic homosexuality
Sexual disorder NOS

Related Nursing Diagnoses (NANDA)

†Altered Sexuality Patterns
Anxiety
Comfort, alteration in: pain
Fear
Grieving, dysfunctional
Health maintenance, alteration in
Knowledge deficit
Mobility, impaired physical
Powerlessness
Self-care deficit
Self-concept, disturbance in
Sensory-perceptual alteration
†Sexual dysfunction
Sleep pattern disturbance
Social isolation
Spiritual distress
Violence, potential for

*From American Psychiatric Association: Draft of the DSM-III-R in Development (subject to change), as proposed by the Work Group to Revise DSM-III. American Psychiatric Association, October 1985.
†Indicates primary nursing diagnosis for variations in sexual response.

1. That he will grow up to become a woman (not merely in role)
2. That his penis or testes are disgusting or will disappear
3. That it would be better not to have a penis or testes

■ **PEDOPHILIA.** The essential feature of pedophilia is a persistent association, lasting at least 6 months, between intense sexual arousal or desire, and acts, fantasies, or other stimuli involving one or more children age 13 or younger. The individual is 16 years old or older and at least 5 years older than the involved child or children. This does not include a late adolescent in an ongoing sexual relation with a 12- or 13-year-old.

■ **EXHIBITIONISM.** The essential feature of exhibitionism is a persistent association, lasting a total of at least 6 months, between intense sexual arousal or desire, and acts, fantasies, or other stimuli involving exposing one's genitals to an unsuspecting stranger.

■ **SEXUAL SADISM.** The essential feature of sexual sadism is a persistent association, lasting a total of at least 6 months, between intense sexual arousal or desire, and acts, fantasies, or other stimuli involving the infliction of real or simulated psychological or physical suffering (including humiliation).

■ **SEXUAL MASOCHISM.** The essential feature of sexual masochism is a persistent association, lasting a total of at least 6 months, between intense sexual arousal or desire, and acts, fantasies, or other stimuli involving being humiliated, beaten, bound, or otherwise made to suffer (real or simulated).

■ **VOYEURISM.** The essential feature of voyeurism is a persistent association, lasting a total of at least 6 months, between intense sexual arousal or desire, and acts, fantasies, or other stimuli involving observing unsuspecting people who are either naked, in the act of disrobing, or engaging in sexual activity.

■ **FETISHISM.** The essential feature of fetishism is a persistent association, lasting a total of at least 6 months, between intense sexual arousal or desire, and acts, fantasies, or other stimuli involving nonliving objects by themselves (e.g., female undergarments). Fetishes are not limited to articles of female clothing used in cross-dressing (transvestic fetishism) or to objects used for the purpose of sexual stimulation (e.g., vibrator).

■ **TRANSVESTIC FETISHISM.** The essential feature of transvestic fetishism is a persistent association in a heterosexual male, lasting a total of at least 6 months, between intense sexual arousal or desire, and acts, fantasies, or other stimuli involving cross-dressing (does not meet the criteria for transsexualism).

■ **ZOOPHILIA.** The essential feature of zoophilia is a persistent association, lasting a total of at least 6 months, between intense sexual arousal or desire, and acts, fantasies, or other stimuli involving animals.

■ **FROTTEURISM.** The essential feature of frotteurism is a persistent association, lasting a total of at least 6 months, between intense sexual arousal or desire, and acts, fantasies, or other stimuli involving rubbing against a nonconsenting person.

■ **PARAPHILIA NOS.** This is a residual category for individuals with a sexual disturbance that meets the general criteria for a paraphilia that does not meet the criteria for any of the other specific categories. Examples of paraphilias NOS include: hypoxyphilia (oxygen deprivation), paraphilic assault other than rapism or frotteurism (e.g., toucherism), necrophilia (corpse), telephone scatologia (lewdness), and partialism (exclusive focus on part of body).

■ **HYPOACTIVE SEXUAL DESIRE DISORDER.** The essential feature of this disorder is a persistent or recurrent deficit or absence of sexual fantasies and desire for sexual activity. The judgment of deficiency or absence is made by the clinician taking into account factors that affect sexual functioning such as age, sex, and the context of the individual's life.

■ **SEXUAL AVERSION DISORDER.** The essential features are persistent or recurrent extreme aversion to and avoidance of all or almost all genital sexual contact with a sexual partner.

■ **SEXUAL AROUSAL DISORDER**
Female. The essential feature is either a persistent or recurrent partial or complete failure to attain or maintain the lubrication-swelling response of sexual activity or a persistent or recurrent lack of a subjective sense of sexual excitement and pleasure in a female during sexual activity.

Male. The essential feature is either a persistent or recurrent partial or complete failure in a male to attain or maintain erection until completion of the sexual activity or a persistent or recurrent lack of a subjective sense of sexual excitement and pleasure in a male during sexual activity.

■ **INHIBITED FEMALE ORGASM.** The essential features are persistent or recurrent delay in or absence of orgasm in a female following a normal sexual excitement phase during sexual activity that is judged by the clinician to be adequate in focus, intensity, and duration. Some women are able to experience orgasm during noncoital clitoral stimulation, but are unable to experience it during coitus in the absence of manual clitoral stimulation. In most of these women this represents a normal variation of the female sexual response and does not justify this diagnosis. However, in some of these women this does represent a psychological inhibition that does justify the diagnosis. This difficult judgment is assisted by a thorough sexual evaluation, which may even require a trial of treatment.

■ **INHIBITED MALE ORGASM.** The essential features are persistent or recurrent delay in or absence of ejaculation in a male following a normal sexual excitement phase during sexual activity that is judged by the clinician to be adequate in focus, intensity, and duration, taking into account the individual's age.

■ **PREMATURE EJACULATION.** In this disorder, persistently or recurrently, ejaculation occurs with minimal sexual stimulation, or before, upon, or shortly after penetration, and before the individual wishes it. The clinician must take into account factors that affect duration of the excitement phase, such as age, novelty of the sexual partner or situation, and frequency.

■ **FUNCTIONAL DYSPAREUNIA.** The essential feature is a recurrent or persistent genital pain in either a male or a female, occurring before, during, or after sexual intercourse. This disturbance is not caused exclusively by lack of lubrication or vaginismus.

■ **FUNCTIONAL VAGINISMUS.** The essential feature is recurrent or persistent involuntary spasm of the musculature of the outer third of the vagina, which interferes with coitus. This disturbance is not caused exclusively by a physical disorder.

■ **SEXUAL DYSFUNCTION NOS.** This is a residual category for disorders in sexual functioning that do not meet the criteria for any of the specific sexual dysfunctions. Examples of this dysfunction include no erotic sensation, or even complete anesthesia despite normal physiologic component of orgasm, the female analogue of premature ejaculation, postcoital headache, and genital pain occurring during masturbation.

■ **EGO-DYSTONIC HOMOSEXUALITY.** The essential feature is persistently absent or weak heterosexual arousal, which significantly interferes with initiating or maintaining wanted heterosexual relationships. There is a sustained pattern of homosexual arousal that the individual explicitly states has been unwanted and a persistent source of distress.

■ **SEXUAL DISORDERS NOS.** This is a residual category for disorders in sexual functioning that are not classifiable in any of the previous categories. Examples of this disorder include marked feelings of inadequacy related to self-imposed standards of masculinity or femininity, such as body habitus, size and shape of sex organs, or sexual performance, distress about having a pattern of repeated sexual conquests with a succession of individuals who exist only as things to be used (Don Juanism, nymphomania), and confusion about preferred sexual orientation.

❦ Planning and implementation

■ Goal setting

After obtaining assessment data regarding the sexual problem, which often includes a complete physical examination, the nurse implements the planning stage of the nursing process. It is at this point that the nurse and patient review the assessment data, define problems, and work together to establish goals that the patient wants to achieve. It is important that the nurse does not identify goals that she wants the patient to achieve, but rather helps the patient identify his own goals and develop a realistic plan to achieve these goals.

The planning phase could simply involve reviewing assessment data with the patient, exploring options, and making referral sources known and available. The nurse's level of expertise determines the amount and degree of planning done with a patient. The planning phase could also include developing a plan of sexual teaching for the patient or for the patient and partner together. After reviewing the assessment data, the nurse and patient can discuss what needs to be known about a specific sexual issue and plan approaches that will give the patient the needed information. A mental health education plan for a patient recovering from an organic illness is presented in Table 21-2.

Goals must be formulated within a realistic framework, taking into consideration the uniqueness of each person. The nurse and the patient will need to prioritize goals and the motivation for achieving them. Goals should be written in behavioral terms so that changes in the patient's behavior can be measured.

■ Intervening with health education

Primary prevention strives to promote health and prevent problems from occurring through specific methods, such as teaching and preplanning. Before being able to engage in either health education or counseling, however, the nurse must examine her own values and beliefs about patients who practice sexual behavior that may be different. This can be facilitated by exploring the myths commonly held by society regarding human sexuality.[21] Table 21-3 presents a list of some of these sexual myths, the result of believing the myth, and the corresponding facts.

Education is the most frequent method of primary prevention for sexual problems and issues. The controversial question of where sex education belongs stimulates much debate among different educational and religious groups throughout the country.[26] Some groups believe that sex education should be censored in public schools and that sexuality should never be publicly discussed. However, if a professional nurse believes in the principles of primary prevention, sex education is a vitally important component of a comprehensive education in today's society.[29]

According to Hacker[11] sex education needs to be incorporated into education from kindergarten throughout one's entire educational career. When individuals are not properly educated in the area of human sexuality, they are denied the opportunity to explore their own values and beliefs about sexuality and to know themselves as sexual beings. Lack of knowledge breeds ignorance that can adversely affect the sexual counseling of patients. When individuals are not aware of facts about sexuality and do not understand their own feelings, important decisions are made on limited information that they may later regret. Sex education can help people know themselves better when the curriculum allows for expression of thoughts, feelings, and examination of behavior, while learning factual information.

Basic concepts that must underlie effective sex education include the following: (1) we are sexual from birth and sexuality is an inseparable part of our identity and (2) all sexual thoughts and feelings are considered normal, but it is our behavior that needs to be monitored in terms of its appropriateness. The key principle in effective sex education is teaching individuals when

TABLE 21-2

MENTAL HEALTH EDUCATION PLAN—SEXUAL RESPONSE FOLLOWING AN ORGANIC ILLNESS

Content	Instructional activities	Evaluation
Describe the variety of human sexual response patterns	Discuss the range of sexual desires, modes of expression, and techniques	Patient identifies his preferences and typical level of sexual functioning
Define the primary organic problem experienced by the patient	Provide accurate information regarding the disruption caused by the organic impairment	Patient understands the nature of his organic illness
Clarify relationship between the organic problem and one's level of sexual functioning	Reframe distorted or confused perceptions regarding the impact of the illness on one's sexual functioning	Patient accurately describes the impact of the illness on his sexual functioning
Identify ways to enhance one's sexual functioning and improve interpersonal communication	Describe additional experiences that would add to the sexual satisfaction and the relationship between the patient and one's partner	Patient and partner report reduced anxiety and greater satisfaction with their sexual responses

TABLE 21-3

MYTHS AND FACTS ON HUMAN SEXUALITY

Myth	Result of myth	Fact
Most individuals who suffer from sexual dysfunctions are deeply psychologically disturbed	Individuals who experience sexual dysfunctions are embarrassed and ashamed, often try to hide their problem, and do not seek professional help	According to Masters and Johnson, "sociocultural deprivation and ignorance constitute the etiologic background for most sexual dysfunctions, not psychiatric illness"[19]
Excessive masturbation is harmful	Individuals often feel guilty or ashamed about masturbating; some individuals deny themselves this experience because of uncomfortable feelings society perpetuates	No physical harms have been reported; no medical definition for excessive masturbation exists; masturbation seems to be a self-limiting practice; when sexually satiated, the individual will then lose interest in being sexually aroused[13]
Women can be excessively amorous (nymphomania)	Women are ashamed (and guilt ridden) of sexual desires and fantasies; in marital relationship responsibility for initiating sex is always on husband, which can cause feelings of resentment from both partners	According to Masters and Johnson classic nymphomania is statistically nonexistent; nymphomania in our culture does not refer to objectively measured states of female excitation, but rather to what males perceive as excessive[20]
Sex during menstruation is unclean and harmful	Women often view their bodies as unclean and even unfit or inferior during menstruation; women use menstruation as an excuse to avoid intercourse rather than simply saying no without a "good reason"	Medically, menstrual flow is in no way harmful or dirty; if women desire, there is no reason to abstain from intercourse during menstrual flow[20]

TABLE 21-3—cont'd

MYTHS AND FACTS ON HUMAN SEXUALITY

Myth	Result of myth	Fact
Oral and anal intercourse are perverted and dangerous	Many individuals refrain from these behaviors or indulge in them only to feel ashamed and guilty afterward	According to Masters and Johnson, "nothing could be further from the truth"; they suggest certain precautions when performing anal intercourse, such as avoiding contamination of vaginal tract and wearing a condom to prevent bacteria from entering penile passage[20]
Teenagers are sexually promiscuous because they all learn sex education in school	Parents who believe this myth fight against comprehensive sex education programs in public education; many parents believe their children have sex education in school, when in fact, the majority do not	Recent estimates indicate that only 10% of today's youth receive comprehensive sex education[10]; existing sex education programs vary greatly in content and quality
Most homosexuals molest children	Known homosexuals are often fired from teaching jobs, and many parents will not allow their children to spend any time with anyone who is homosexual; children learn from an early age that homosexuals are "bad people," that they should stay away from them	Of all reported cases of molestations, 90% are heterosexual, adult male with minor female[29]
Homosexuals are sick and cannot control their sexual behavior	Homosexuals are denied jobs and are sometimes jailed for their homosexuality; homosexual parents may have their children taken away by courts	According to Bell and Weinberg, who studied 979 homosexual men and women in a study conducted by the Institute for Sex Research in 1978: (1) most homosexuals' social and psychological adjustment is indistinguishable from the heterosexual majority and (2) objectionable sexual advances are far more likely to be made by a heterosexual (usually male to female) than a homosexual[4]
All homosexuals are alike; men, limp wristed, speak with lisp; women, unattractive, masculine, "butch," short hair, deep voice	Society considers any individual who does not conform to the correct "macho male" and "fluffy female" stereotypes to be homosexual	Bell and Weinberg's study indicates that relatively few homosexual men and women conform to hideous stereotypes[4]
Advancing age means end of sex	Many older adults become victims of this myth not because their bodies have lost the ability to perform, but because *they* believe that they have lost the ability to perform	Sexually men and women can function effectively into their 80's if they understand the physiological changes that occur with aging and do not let these changes frighten them[20]
Alcohol ingestion reduces inhibitions and therefore enhances sexual enjoyment	Many individuals use alcohol in the hope that it will increase their sexual pleasure and performance; alcohol ingestion can also provide an excuse for engaging in sexual behaviors—"I would never have gone to bed with him if I hadn't had all that wine."	According to Wilsnack, there is a lack of empirical data to support the belief that alcohol ingestion reduces inhibitions and enhances sexual enjoyment[31]

and where to act on feelings, as well as when and where not to act on them. Finally, sexuality needs to be viewed as more than genital sex. It encompasses one's total sense of self.[11]

Nurses have a professional responsibility to become educated in the field of human sexuality so that holistic health care becomes a reality. The educational process can be accomplished in nursing curricula and continuing education programs. However, some nurses elect additional education and clinical practice in the field of human sexuality. These nurses may become sex educators in schools and the community in such facilities as outpatient clinics and planned parenthood agencies. Nurses prepared at the master and doctoral levels may choose to become sex therapists through postgraduate work in the field of human sexuality and through extensive clinical supervision from qualified sex therapists.

■ Intervening in sexual responses within the nurse-patient relationship

■ **SEXUAL RESPONSES OF NURSES TO PATIENTS.** A clinical situation in which a nurse experiences feelings of sexual attraction to a patient for whom she is caring can be a problem. Although this is not an uncommon experience, it has received little attention in the nursing literature. One of the major reasons for this is that nurses often deny any sexual feelings they may have for their patients. However, feelings of sexual attaction and sexual fantasies are part of the human experience, and these feelings should be attended to by the nurse. If the nurse does not explore the feelings of sexual attraction for a patient, it can interfere with the quality of nursing care given by focusing the relationship on meeting the needs of the nurse rather than meeting the needs of the patient.

The first thing the nurse needs to do when this situation occurs is to acknowledge his or her own feelings without evaluating them as negative or wrong. Often nurses try to ignore or deny these feelings because they are uncomfortable and frightening. Nurses make judgments about themselves such as, "What's wrong with me—I shouldn't feel this way about my patients. I must be really weird." "I'm sure I'm the only nurse who ever had these feelings!" The nurse who admits these feelings without judging them is then able to deal with them appropriately. Eldwich and Brodsky[6] offer several suggestions to help resolve feelings of sexual attraction for patients:

1. Don't share personal information about oneself with patients
2. Don't get overly involved in patient's problems

3. Don't discuss one's feelings of sexual attraction with the patient
4. Seek consultation

Asking for consultation from a more experienced nurse or a supervisor on how to handle these feelings often helps the nurse to sort out feelings and most importantly maintain a professional therapeutic relationship with the patient. These interventions are summarized in Table 21-4.

■ **SEXUAL RESPONSES OF PATIENTS TO NURSES.** One of the most commonly occurring sexual behaviors of hospitalized patients is sexual acting out or displaying seductive behaviors toward the nurse. Nurses are often extremely uncomfortable when they are the recipients of sexual acting out behavior and are unsure of how to respond. Patients making passes at nurses, making suggestive sexual comments, asking nurses for their phone numbers, requesting a date are common examples of sexual acting out behavior.

The first step in intervening with these behaviors is to let the patient know that his behavior is unacceptable to the nurse. The nurse needs to respond in a firm, matter-of-fact manner that clearly states what limits are being set. For example, "Mr. Moore, I am uncomfortable when you suggest that I get into bed with you. Please stop saying that." or "Mr. Dean, Take your hand off my breast."

Nurses are sometimes embarrassed or afraid to confront patients who are sexually acting out in this way, and as a result, attempt to laugh it off or ignore it with a "boys will be boys" attitude. Providing health care to patients does not give them permission to be verbally offensive nor touch nurses' bodies without permission. As health care providers, nurses are taught to always be accepting of patients' behavior, and this principle is difficult to dispute. However, when the patient's behavior does not respect the rights of the nurse as a human being, then the nurse needs to set limits on that behavior.

Although nurses must confront and set limits on patients' sexual behaviors, they also have a responsibility as professionals to attempt to understand it. It is important to examine the sexual behaviors displayed by patients and try to analyze the variety of possible meanings of such behavior. Patients may show seductive behaviors for various reasons. These may or may not include an intention for their behaviors to lead to sexual activities with the nurse. The seductive behavior is often a way of getting the nurse's attention, which the nurse may attempt to ignore or deny. Hospitalized patients can also feel unattractive or insecure about themselves

TABLE 21-4

SUMMARY OF NURSING INTERVENTIONS IN SEXUAL RESPONSES OF NURSES TO PATIENTS

Goal: Maintain a professional nurse–patient relationship that will enable the nurse to provide therapeutic nursing care

Principle	Rationale	Nursing intervention
Acknowledge nurse's own sexual feelings	The nurse needs to acknowledge sexual feelings toward the patient, remembering that feelings cannot be judged as right or wrong, but behavior can be evaluated as therapeutic or nontherapeutic for the patient.	Openness to one's own feelings. Acceptance of one's feelings. Explore the course of feelings.
Examine nurse's behavior with patient	If the nurse works toward increasing awareness of feelings and thoughts he or she will be able to more effectively change any nontherapeutic behavior to a more therapeutic approach.	Keep the relationship patient-focused. Don't get overly involved in patients' problems (to the point it would impair one's clinical judgment). Don't share personal information about oneself with the patient. Do not discuss feelings of sexual attraction with the patient.
Seek consultation	After the nurse has acknowledged feelings and examined behavior, consultation from a more experienced nurse may prove helpful in developing ways to appropriately resolve this issue and feel more comfortable in approaching the patient.	Confide in a nurse, experienced colleague, or supervisor. Request help in exploring this issue in terms of gaining insight into the factors influencing one's feelings. Explore possible ways to resolve one's feelings and maintain a professional relationship with the patient.

sexually, thus seductive behaviors may be a request for reassurance that others continue to view them as sexual human beings.[3] Sometimes patients confuse their feelings of gratitude and appreciation for the nurse with feelings of sexual attraction. These feelings may then in turn generate thoughts such as, "Wouldn't my nurse make a wonderful wife. She's so giving and understanding all the time." In this case, the patient views the nurse's professional behavior and concern as self-sacrificing and altruistic.

Finally, patients may have difficulty understanding the difference between the professional and social relationship. In many ways, the nurse-patient relationship is idealized for the patient. All the attention and caring is given to him by the nurse, and he is not expected to give anything back in return. It is easy to see how the patient could possibly be confused about his relationship with the nurse.

Clinical example 21-3 illustrates this point.

In Clinical example 21-3 the nurse helps the patient clear up his confusion regarding his relationship with the nurse. She defines the purpose of the professional therapeutic relationship to aid the patient in understanding why it is impossible to compare his relationship with the nurse to his relationship with his wife. As stated previously, there are many reasons why the patient might behave in a sexual or romantic manner with the nurse (manipulation, altered self-concept, attention seeking, anxiety related to altered health status). Nursing intervention should be determined by the underlying needs that the patient is expressing. Table 21-5 summarizes the nursing interventions appropriate to dealing with the sexual responses of patients to nurses.

■ Intervening in maladaptive homosexual and bisexual responses

Many people accept their homosexual or bisexual orientations as an adaptive mode of sexual expression, whereas others have difficulties and seek professional help. Because of the homosexual element of bisexuality, bisexuals often encounter much of the same difficulties stemming from societal attitudes as homosexuals do.

CLINICAL EXAMPLE 21-3

Mr. P has been hospitalized for an exacerbation of a chronic illness for the past 3 weeks. Ms. S has been his primary nurse during this hospitalization. The following is a conversation between the nurse and patient the day prior to his discharge.

MR. P: **I wish my wife were more like you, Ms. S.**

MS. S: **Mr. P, I'm not sure I understand what you are saying.**

MR. P: **Well, it's just that you are always so concerned about me. You always try to make me feel good and want to help me all the time. Sometimes my wife's a grouch, she's so wrapped up in her job and the kids she doesn't always pay as much attention to me as you do.**

MS. S: **I'm glad you feel taken care of, Mr. P, but I think it's impossible to compare my role as your nurse with your wife's role.**

MR. P: **I'm not sure I follow you . . .**

MS. S: **They are very different types of relationships. It's nice to have someone take care of us when we can't take care of ourselves, but when we are healthy, we don't need someone to take care of us all the time. Your relationship with your wife is more of a sharing one with mutual benefits. You take care of her needs, and she takes care of your needs in return.**

CLINICAL EXAMPLE 21-4

Ms. A, a 25-year-old single female, came to the mental health clinic with the complaint of a "sexual problem." Her history revealed that she had been sexually inactive for the past 5 years. At the age of 20, Ms. A had a brief sexual encounter with a man she had been dating for 2 years. She ended the relationship shortly afterward because she had no interest in maintaining a sexual relationship with the man. Recently, she became involved in a relationship with a woman that was very satisfying to her. She felt she had to end the relationship because she would not tolerate thinking of herself as a homosexual. During one of the initial counseling sessions Ms. A told the nurse that she must end the relationship before "it" happens again.

NURSE: **What are you afraid will happen?**

MS. A: **I'm afraid I'll feel attracted to her again.**

NURSE: **What about that frightens you?**

MS. A: (becoming upset) **That will mean I'm homosexual!**

NURSE: **What does being homosexual mean for you?**

MS. A: **It means I'm sick. It's a sin, I couldn't go to church anymore.**

NURSE: **Are all homosexuals sick?**

MS. A: **Yes.**

NURSE: **How do you know this?**

MS. A: **Everybody knows that homosexuals hang out in sleazy bars and don't work and are on welfare. They all have emotional problems, need therapy, and eventually wind up in mental institutions.**

NURSE: **Do you know any homosexual people?**

MS. A: **Well, not exactly. . . .**

NURSE: **What have you read about homosexuality?**

MS. A: **Nothing.**

NURSE: **Then it looks to me like you are basing all of your conclusions on hearsay and not real knowledge. I think that you and I need to explore your beliefs in more detail, then you can do some reading to find out the facts.**

Another factor that may present a problem for the bisexual is that of isolation from a support group. Because bisexuals are frequently accused of "fence sitting," they can be rejected by both heterosexual and homosexual groups. Bisexuals may complain of lack of support, and are pressured by friends and family to decide on one sexual orientation (usually they are encouraged to be heterosexual), so they will fit into society.

The first step in counseling the homosexual or bisexual person who views his or her sexual response as maladaptive and a source of distress is the nurse's acceptance of the patient. Most patients are extremely perceptive of their therapist's values and attitudes toward them. The nurse who believes she is hiding her prejudices from the patient is only fooling herself. Because the nurse has grown up in a society that believes homosexuals are sick and perverted, it is often difficult to examine myths and search for facts. The patient has grown up in the same society and, although experiencing homosexual feelings or behaviors, still goes through the same growth experience about homosexuality as anyone else.

Often an important step in counseling the homosexual individual is to aid him or her in exploring values

TABLE 21-5

SUMMARY OF NURSING INTERVENTIONS IN SEXUAL RESPONSES OF PATIENTS TO NURSES

Goal: Maintain a professional nurse-patient relationship that will enable the nurse to provide therapeutic nursing care

Principle	Rationale	Nursing intervention
Establish a trusting relationship	An atmosphere of trust allows for open, honest communication between patient and nurse; when this occurs the nurse can aid the patient in discovering the underlying issues related to his sexual feelings and behavior.	Express nonsexual caring and concern for the patient. Be a responsive listener especially to feelings and needs that the patient may not be able to directly express. Reinforce the purpose of the professional, therapeutic nurse-patient relationship.
Awareness of nurse's own feelings and thoughts	When the nurse is aware of her feelings and thoughts she will begin to understand how they influence her behavior. With increased self-awareness the nurse will be able to increase the effectiveness of her interactions with patients.	Recognize own feelings and thoughts. Identify any specific patient interaction or behavior that influences the nurse's feelings and thoughts. Identify the influence of the nurse's feelings and thoughts on one's behavior in an attempt to increase the effectiveness of nursing interventions.
Decrease patient's expressions of sexual feelings and behavior	If the nurse is able to help the patient see that his sexual interactions and behavior are being expressed to an inappropriate partner (the nurse) the sexual acting out will usually decrease. This then opens the door for the nurse to help the patient begin to identify the reasons for his behavior.	Set limits on patient's sexual behavior. Use a calm matter-of-fact approach without implying judgment. Reaffirm nonsexual caring for the patient. Explore the meaning of the patient's feelings and behaviors.
Expand patient's insight into his sexual feelings and behavior	Once the patient begins to identify the reasons for his sexual feelings and behaviors, he is able to see that the nurse is not an appropriate outlet for these feelings and behaviors and can move toward a more appropriate and therapeutic relationship with the nurse.	Clarify misconceptions regarding any feeling patient may have about the nurse as a possible sexual partner. Point out the futile nature of his romantic or sexual interest in the nurse. Redirect patient's energies toward appropriate health care issues.

and beliefs about homosexual people. It is possible that the person has internalized some of society's prejudices about homosexuals, such as, "homosexuals are sick, evil people who should not be allowed to live homosexual life-styles." Therefore "because I am homosexual, I am sick and should not act on my sexual feelings because they are evil and bad." Common responses evidenced by patients who attempt to cope with society's prejudices include denial, confusion, and sexual promiscuity, which is especially prominent among those who are trying to prove to themselves that they are not gay.

It is helpful to have patients discuss and specifically list beliefs they hold about homosexuality and bisex-

uality and for the therapist and patient to review and discuss each one. A review of beliefs about homosexuality may not be sufficient because, although the nurse and patient work to dispel the myths, society consistently and very powerfully reinforces them. Having the person read appropriate materials about homosexuality and bisexuality will also be helpful in discriminating myths from facts. Throughout this review process the patient will be extremely sensitive to the therapist and will test the therapist's acceptance or rejection.

In Clinical example 21-4, the nurse and Ms. A developed a plan commonly used in sexual counseling to explore the issue of homosexuality over the next several sessions. Two goals that were identified by the patient and the nurse included the following:

1. Understand the facts vs. myths about homosexuals and their life-styles
2. Understand the patient's feelings about herself in regard to her sexual identity

Some of the actions taken to implement the plan included:

1. Ms. A listed all her beliefs about homosexuality and homosexuals.
2. The nurse encouraged Ms. A to explore the literature on homosexuality and suggested readings to help dispel the myths.
3. The nurse then discussed these with Ms. A and suggested that Ms. A attend a social gathering for gay people to test out her new-found knowledge. (The nurse suggested the social gathering because many people struggling with a homosexual identity are frightened to test out situations that would dispel the myths.)

■ Intervening in transsexual responses

Treatment of the person who is a transsexual has been the topic of heated debate in recent years. The debate ranges from recommending long-term psychotherapy to surgical reassignment. Recently standards of care were developed by the Harry Benjamin International Gender Dysphoria Association.[5] These standards set guidelines for individuals who are to receive hormonal therapy, psychotherapy (including qualifications of therapists), and surgical reassignment. The standards help professionals who treat transsexual patients give quality care.

Briefly, treatment advocated by the Harry Benjamin International Gender Dysphoria Association includes thorough assessment of the patient by a trained professional, hormonal therapy, and finally surgical reassignment (not all transsexuals choose surgical reassignment). Phases of treatment include the following steps:

1. The person must demonstrate a sense of discomfort with self and the wish to live in the genetically opposite sex role.
2. The person must be known to a professional therapist (who is an expert in the field of sexuality) for a period of 3 to 6 months and demonstrate a sense of discomfort with self and the desire to live in the genetically opposite sex role.

If the person meets these criteria, the therapist then endorses him or her for hormonal therapy. A male

changing to a female receives estrogen; a female changing to a male receives testosterone. Before starting hormonal therapy, the patient receives a complete physical examination with specific blood work (serum glutamic pyruvic transaminase levels in females changing to males and serum glutamic pyruvic transaminase, bilirubin, triglyceride, and fasting glucose levels in males changing to females). If the person desires surgical reassignment (a penectomy, castration, or vaginaplasty for a male changing to a female; a hysterectomy, vaginectomy, or phalloplasty for a female changing to a male), they must be known to the professional therapist for at least 6 months. The individual must have been successful in living in the genetically opposite sex role for at least 1 year and up to 2 years. Before the transsexual receives the surgical alteration, the original therapist's endorsement must be agreed on by a second therapist who has evaluated the person.

It is imperative that professionals who provide care for transsexual patients be educated in the field of human sexuality. The assessment phase of the treatment process is especially important. The patient and therapist must be certain that implementing the treatment plan is the best approach because the surgery is not reversible.

■ Intervening in dysfunctions of the sexual response cycle

Conducting sexual therapy is beyond the scope of the nurse generalist. However, the nurse should be aware of the basic principles involved and should also be aware of creditable sex therapists in the community in which she works so that she will be able to refer patients appropriately.

Although patients with dysfunctions of the sexual response cycle are treated from many different treatment modalities, two brief treatment models of sex therapy commonly implemented are discussed here: the Masters and Johnson and the Helen Singer Kaplan models.

■ **MASTERS AND JOHNSON MODEL.** Masters and Johnson began pioneering research in the area of sexuality in the 1950s. Their book, *Human Sexual Inadequacy*,[20] describes their research in specific detail and their counseling methods for sexual dysfunctions.

Before the work of William Masters and Virginia Johnson, patients who experienced problems in the area of sexuality were generally referred to a psychiatrist for psychotherapy or psychoanalysis. Health professionals assumed that anyone who had a problem with sexuality was emotionally disturbed. Problems with dysfunction of the sexual response cycle are usually not psychiatric problems, but the result of sociocultural deprivation and ignorance of sexual physiology.[20] Masters' and Johnson's treatment for sexual dysfunctions includes short-term education with step-by-step instructions regarding the physical aspects of sexual activity and supportive psychotherapy. The researchers believe that attitudes and ignorance are responsible for most sexual dysfunctions, contrary to the belief by the general populace that dysfunctions of the sexual response cycle indicate a severe psychiatric illness.

Masters' and Johnson's therapeutic approach to patients begins by obtaining a detailed sexual and background history. They recommend a male-female therapeutic team, a dual therapist approach. On day one of the treatment program, therapists meet with the couple to review and clarify their histories taken the previous day. Meeting with the couple is called a round table discussion. After this discussion, the couple is instructed to carry out the sensate focus exercise. This exercise requires each partner to instruct the other in specific ways of caressing for the purpose of sensual pleasure without involving the breasts or genitals. The activity is done first by one partner and then the other partner. The next day the exercise is repeated, including breasts and genital areas, but without performing coitus. The purpose of the exercise is to alleviate performance anxiety and to enhance warm comfortable feelings between partners. The exercises are done in comfortable private surroundings with both partners in the nude. After the sensate focus exercises are completed, the attention of therapy is directed to the presenting sexual dysfunction.

Some of the specific behavioral approaches used by Masters and Johnson are briefly described in Table 21-6. The Masters and Johnson model emphasizes education, communication, and cooperation between partners in their treatment plan.

■ **HELEN SINGER KAPLAN MODEL.** Kaplan's method[13] of treating sexual dysfunctions integrates psychodynamic behavioral principles into conjoint therapeutic sessions. Kaplan combines specific behavioral tasks with psychodynamic insights, dyadic approaches, dream interpretations, and gestalt and transactional techniques, Kaplan differs from Masters and Johnson in that she believes the single therapist is as effective as co-therapists of opposite sexes. According to her, the primary objective of sex therapy is symptomatic relief, which can be achieved by treating the patient without a partner in some cases.

Kaplan's treatment process begins with an extensive evaluation that includes marital, psychiatric, sexual, medical, and family history from both partners. If profound intrapsychic or interpersonal difficulties are found, the couple may be referred to appropriate individual or conjoint therapy and are not accepted for sex therapy at that time. According to Kaplan, sex therapy is usually contraindicated in couples who are severely disturbed.

Like Masters and Johnson, Kaplan employs the sensate focus exercises and variations of the exercises, such as showering together, to begin sex therapy or further

---

TABLE 21-6

SUMMARY OF TWO MODELS OF TREATMENT TECHNIQUES FOR DYSFUNCTIONS OF THE SEXUAL RESPONSE CYCLE

Sexual dysfunction	Masters and Johnson	Helen Singer Kaplan
Premature ejaculation	*Squeeze technique:* As soon as full erection is achieved, woman's thumb is placed on frenulum, located on ventral surface of penis, and first and second fingers on dorsal surface of penis immediately adjacent to one another on either side of coronal ridge; pressure is applied by woman squeezing thumb and first two fingers together for 3 or 4 seconds; pressure makes man lose urge to ejaculate; procedure is repeated so couple can enjoy 15 to 20 minutes of continuous sex play without ejaculation	*Stop-start technique.* Woman masturbates man until he feels urge to ejaculate; he then tells woman to stop; after ejaculation urge abates, he will then tell woman to begin stimulating him again and when he feels the urge to ejaculate, instructs her to stop; this is repeated four times, with final time allowing ejaculation; it is important with this technique for man to focus sharply on his erotic sensations and not allow himself to be distracted; this exercise is repeated with petroleum jelly several times and then with penis inserted in vagina with man controlling woman's hip movements

Continued.

TABLE 21-6—cont-d

SUMMARY OF TWO MODELS OF TREATMENT TECHNIQUES FOR DYSFUNCTIONS OF THE SEXUAL RESPONSE CYCLE

Sexual dysfunction	Masters and Johnson	Helen Singer Kaplan
Inhibited male orgasm	Woman stimulates man demandingly, specifically asking him for verbal direction in stimulative techniques that are pleasurable; by doing this, woman forces ejaculation manually; hopefully when this occurs, man will identify this pleasure with her rather than regard her as threat or contaminated sexual object; after establishing competence in ejaculatory function with masturbation techniques, next step is intravaginal ejaculation; after manual stimulation of penis by woman she inserts penis into vagina (female superior position) and begins pelvic thrusting; if man does not ejaculate, shortly after thrusting, woman returns to manual stimulation	Two principles of treatment: 1. Progressive in vivo desensitization to intravaginal ejaculation; treatment goal is to gradually shape ejaculatory response toward ejaculation on coitus; specific behavioral prescriptions will vary with each individual case but will be structured with the above stated goal in mind, e.g., man who can only ejaculate if woman has left house and he is alone might have behavior prescription to masturbate behind locked doors in his bedroom with her downstairs; if successful, next step is to bring her close, e.g., next room, until couple reaches goal 2. Stimulation and distraction. Person is physically stimulated intensely, while at the same time mentally distracted; mental absorption in erotic fantasy while genital stimulation is being experienced is an ideal method of releasing orgasm reflex
Male sexual arousal disorder (Erectile dysfunction)	Couple instructed not to have intercourse; progression from nongenital caressing and pleasuring exercises to genital pleasuring exercises; each member of couple instructs the other in specifics of their own pleasure; when intercourse is attempted, woman assumes superior position and inserts male's penis into her vagina; couple is continuously reassured in nonpressure, no hurry environment; at no time in this treatment is couple instructed to have intercourse	Client and partner are gradually led through the following sequence of events: 1. Erotic pleasures without erection 2. Erection without orgasm 3. Extravaginal orgasm 4. Intromission without orgasm 5. Coitus
Inhibited female orgasm	After sensate focus and lowering hostile environment between couple, controlled genital play is initiated with woman showing man what her actual preferences are; gradually penis is inserted (female superior position) without thrusting; gentle movements are made by woman and finally penile insertion with male thrusting	First step is orgasm alone by digital stimulation plus distraction by fantasy (sometimes vibrator is suggested here); this gradually moves to orgasm with partner, either by masturbation or by man stimulating woman's clitoris; when this is successful couple moves to orgasm with intercourse; if orgasm with intercourse does not occur, bridge maneuver is employed; *bridge maneuver:* either partner manually stimulates clitoris while penis is contained in vagina up to point of, but not actually to, orgasm and then let coital thrusting trigger orgasmic reflex
Functional vaginismus	First vaginal constriction is shown to both partners during physical examination; then dilators in graduated sizes are employed in privacy of couple's bedroom; gradually size of dilation is increased until woman can tolerate man's penis	Couple is instructed to observe vaginal entrance with mirror and woman gradually inserts finger into vaginal canal, then inserts two fingers; after woman can tolerate insertion of two full fingers, man is included; he repeats procedure, gradually couple moves to penile insertion without thrusting and finally penile insertion with thrusting

Modified from: Kaplan, H.S.: The illustrated manual of sex therapy, New York, 1975, The New York Times Book Co.; and Masters, W.H., and Johnson, V.E.: Human sexual inadequacy, Boston, 1970, Little, Brown & Co.

evaluate a client's suitability for sex therapy. The therapy process itself consists of erotic tasks, performed at home, plus weekly or semiweekly meetings with the therapist. At the therapy sessions, clients and the therapist explore feelings experienced during the erotic exercises. The Kaplan method prescribes a unique series of home or private exercises for the couple and the dysfunction that take into account the motivations and dynamics of the relationship. The integration of experiential and dynamic modes is a major feature of Kaplan's approach. The role of the therapist includes education, clarification, and support.

Table 21-6 describes a number of commonly used behavioral techniques specific to dysfunctions of the sexual response cycle. The techniques in no way indicate the total comprehensive treatment for sexual dysfunctions, but give a baseline description of exercises that are implemented in sex therapy. Both Kaplan and Masters and Johnson emphasize communication between partners and the exploring of the relationship and emotional concerns during therapy. The reader is referred to original works of these sex therapists for more specific information.

Evaluation

In the evaluation phase of the nursing process, the nurse works with the patient to evaluate the effectiveness of the sexual counseling or intervention used. Factors to consider in evaluating the process of treatment include the following:

1. **Sense of well-being.** How does the person feel about himself or herself as a person? Have his or her feelings about self improved during the treatment?
2. **Functioning ability.** If the individual was dysfunctional, is functional ability restored? Somewhat improved? What about the person's ability to function within primary relations at work? with friends?
3. **Satisfaction with treatment.** Does the patient feel that treatment was helpful? Were his or her goals adequately met?

Evaluation of any form of sexual counseling or intervention should be an ongoing process in which the nurse and the patient work together in evaluating goals, problems, and alternatives. Clinical example 21-5 illustrates the evaluation process in a nurse-patient situation.

CLINICAL EXAMPLE 21-5

Mr. and Mrs. S sought sex therapy because they had been experiencing sexual difficulties since their marriage 2 years ago. Mr. S had been suffering from premature ejaculation and Mrs. S claimed that she had lost any interest in a sexual relationship with her husband and refused to discuss the problem of premature ejaculation with him.

The couple was seen by a nurse clinician who was an experienced sex therapist. At the onset of the therapy both the couple and therapist established the following goals:

1. Improve communication between the couple
2. Discuss the premature ejaculation problem and explore options of improving the sexual relationship that would prove satisfying to both partners

During the therapy, the nurse worked with the couple to openly discuss important issues with each other and improve the patterns of communication. Behavioral sex therapy techniques were employed for Mr. S's problem with premature ejaculation. After ten weekly sessions the couple and the therapist evaluated the course of treatment together. The following factors for evaluating treatment effectiveness were explored:

1. *Sense of well-being.* Both Mr. and Mrs. S felt better about themselves as individuals and their relationship. They were better able to discuss and solve issues of concern. They felt a renewed affection for each other and a desire to problem solve rather than ignore problematic issues.
2. *Functioning ability.* With the use of behavioral sex therapy techniques, Mr. S's premature ejaculation problem had significantly decreased and both members began to enjoy a satisfying sexual relationship.
3. *Satisfaction with treatment.* Both Mr. and Mrs. S felt that the goals of treatment had been accomplished and that there was a general improvement in the quality of their relationship.

After the evaluation, the couple, with the therapist's agreement, decided to terminate therapy, since the presenting problem was resolved and the goals of treatment were accomplished. By maintaining a facilitative position, the nurse helped the couple make their own choices in problem solving, and the responsibility for their choices remained solely with the couple. Thus their autonomy and sense of self were affirmed by the nurse and the goals of high-level wellness and holistic health care were promoted.

DIRECTIONS FOR FUTURE RESEARCH

The following are some of the nursing research problems raised in Chapter 21 that merit further study by psychiatric nurses:

1. The degree to which nursing educational programs are successful in teaching students to adopt nonjudgmental attitudes in relating to patients with sexual concerns
2. The amount of time nursing curricula devote to sex education in undergraduate and graduate nursing programs
3. The possible stressors that predispose patients to maladaptive sexual responses
4. The specific nursing behaviors that promote or inhibit the expression of sexual concerns by patients
5. The long-term success of brief-treatment sex therapy
6. The effectiveness of nursing interventions in the sexual acting out behaviors of patients
7. The validity of various sexual assessment tools in sexual history taking
8. The effects of nurses' feelings, attitudes and values on therapeutic interventions with patients with sexual concerns
9. Patient satisfaction after sex reassignment surgery
10. The ability of psychiatric nurses to diagnose maladaptive sexual responses in physical and emotional illness
11. The long-term effects of alcohol abuse on male and female sexual functioning
12. The relationship between levels of self-esteem and healthy sexual behavior
13. Effective strategies for sensitizing nurses to the sexual needs of the institutionalized elderly
14. The effectiveness of sexual education programs in discussing maladaptive sexual responses
15. Variations in sexual responses in patients experiencing illness or surgery

■ SUGGESTED CROSS-REFERENCES ■

Therapeutic relationship skills and self-awareness of the nurse are discussed in Chapter 4. Alterations in self-concept and personal identity are discussed in Chapter 14. Nursing interventions with sexual assault and rape victims are discussed in Chapter 33.

■ SUMMARY ■

1. The need for knowledge of human sexuality in nursing was discussed. Information important for implementing the nursing role was identified and included self-awareness, value clarification, and effective counseling and communication skills.

2. Sexuality was broadly defined as a desire for contact, warmth, tenderness, and love. Criteria for adaptive sexual behavior were identified as sexual behavior that (1) is consensual, (2) lacks force, (3) is performed in private, (4) is not physically or psychologically harmful, and (5) is mutually satisfying to the individuals involved.

3. The assessment phase of the nursing process includes two major responsibilities for the nurse: (1) self-awareness in relation to sexuality and (2) assessment of the patient according to situation and presenting problem. Phases of a positive growth experience in working with patients who have sexual concerns were identified and discussed as cognitive dissonance, anxiety, anger, and action. Patient assessment was described in terms of interviewing and history taking.

4. Predisposing factors were described from biological, psychoanalytical, and behavioral perspectives. Precipitating stressors that may affect changes in sexuality include physical and emotional illness, therapeutic and nontherapeutic drugs, surgical intervention, hospitalization, and the aging process.

5. Data collection includes behavioral responses such as homosexuality, bisexuality, transvestism, and transsexualism. Two models of the human sexual response cycle were presented: (1) Masters and Johnson's four phases: excitement, plateau, orgasm, and resolution; (2) Kaplan's three phase model: desire, excitement, and orgasm.

6. A variety of coping mechanisms are utilized with expressions of sexuality: fantasy, projection, denial, and rationalization. Coping mechanisms may be adaptive or maladaptive depending on how and why they are used. To cope with ambivalent feelings regarding intimacy individuals may withdraw from any form of sexual expression or engage in sexual behavior with multiple sexual partners to avoid sexual closeness.

7. Related nursing and medical diagnoses according to NANDA and the Draft of the DSM-III-R in Development[2] were described.

8. The planning of the nursing process requires active involvement on the part of the patient. The nurse must be careful not to develop a plan and establish goals that she feels the patient should follow, but to help individuals identify their own goals and develop a plan to work toward achieving them. A mental health education plan was presented.

9. Interventions with patients would depend on the person's situation and specific individualized needs. Primary prevention, which includes sex education and preventive counseling, as discussed along with interventions for: (1) expressions of sexual feelings and behaviors within the nurse-patient relationship, (2) various modes of sexual expression if they

are maladaptive (homosexuality, bisexuality, etc.), and (3) dysfunctions of the sexual response cycle.

10. In the evaluation process, the nurse and patient need to consider the following factors in assessing the effectiveness of the nursing care: the patient's sense of well-being, functioning ability, and satisfaction with treatment.

■ REFERENCES ■

1. Aletkey, P.J.: Sexuality of the nursing home resident, Top. Clin. Nurs. **1**:60, 1980.
2. American Psychiatric Association: Draft of the DSM-III-R in Development (subject to change), as proposed by the Work Group to Revise DSM-III. American Psychiatric Association 1985.
3. Assey, J.L., and Herbert, J.M.: Who is the seductive patient? Am. J. Nurs. **83**(4):531, 1983.
4. Bell, A.P., and Weinberg, M.S.: Homosexualities: a study of diversity among men and women, New York, 1978, Simon & Schuster, Inc.
5. Berger, et al.: Standard of care, 1981, The Harry Benjamin International Gender Dysphoria Association, Inc.
6. Edelwich, J., and Brodsky, A.: Sexual dilemmas for the helping professional, New York, 1982, Brunner/Mazel Publishers.
7. Foley, T., and Davies, M.: Rape: nursing care of victims, St. Louis, 1982, The C.V. Mosby Co.
8. Freud, S.: Three Essays of the Theory of Sexuality, ed. 3, London, 1962, Hogarth Press (originally published 1905).
9. Goldstein, B.: Human sexuality, New York, 1976, McGraw-Hill, Inc.
10. Graves, H., and Thompson, E.: Anxiety: a mental health vital sign. In Longo, C., and Williams, R., editors: Clinical practice in psychosocial nursing: assessment and intervention, New York, 1978, Appleton-Century-Crofts.
11. Hacker, S.S.: It isn't sex education unless. . . . J. Sch. Health **5**:209, Apr. 1981.
12. Hyde, J.S.: Understanding Human Sexuality, ed. 3, New York, 1986, McGraw-Hill, Inc.
13. Kaplan, H.S.: The illustrated manual of sex therapy, New York, 1975, The New York Times Book Co.
14. Kaplan, H.S.: Disorders of sexual desire and other new concepts and techniques in sex therapy, New York, 1979, Brunner/Mazel Publishers.
15. Kelly, G.F.: Sexuality: the human perspective, New York, 1980, Barron's Educational Series, Inc.
16. Kinsey, A.C., Pomeroy, W.B., and Martin, E.C.: Sexual behavior in the human female, Philadelphia, 1953, W.B. Saunders Co.
17. Kirkendall, L.A., and Rubin, I.: Sexuality and the life cycle. In Barbour, J.R., editor: Human sexuality 79/80, Guilford, Conn., 1979, The Dushkin Publishing Group, Inc.
18. Kolodny, R.C., et al.: Textbook of human sexuality for nurses, Boston, 1979, Little, Brown & Co.
19. Marmor, J., editor: Homosexual behavior: a modern reappraisal, New York, 1980, Basic Books, Inc., Publishers.
20. Masters, W.H., and Johnson, V.E.: Human sexual inadequacy, Boston, 1970, Little, Brown & Co.
21. Masters, W.H., and Johnson, V.E.: Ten sex myths exploded. In Barbour, J.R., editor: Human sexuality 79/80, Guilford, Conn., 1979, The Dushkin Publishing Group, Inc.
22. May, R.: The meanings of anxiety, New York, 1950, Ronald Press.
23. McDonald, A.P.: A little bit of lavender goes a long way: a critique of research on sexual orientation. J. Sex Research **19**:95, Apr. 1983.
24. Mims, F.H., and Swenson, M.: Sexuality: a nursing perspective, New York, 1980, McGraw-Hill, Inc.
25. Money, J., and Wiedeking, C.: Gender identity role: normal differentiation and its transpositions. In Wolman, B.B., and Money, J., editors: Handbook of human sexuality, Englewood Cliffs, N.J., 1980, Prentice-Hall, Inc.
26. Scales, P.: Barriers to sex education, J. Sch. Health **50**(6):337, 1980.
27. Sherfey, M.J.: The nature and evaluation of female sexuality, New York, 1972, Random House.
28. Thomas, S.P.: Bisexuality: a sexual orientation of great diversity. J. Psychosoc. Nurs. Ment. Health Serv. **18**(4):19, Apr. 1980.
29. U.S. Dept. of Health, Education, and Welfare, National Center on Child Abuse and Neglect: Child abuse and neglect: the problem and its management, Pub. no. (OHD) 75-30073, U.S. Government Printing Office.
30. Webster's new collegiate dictionary, Springfield, Mass. 1977, G. & C. Merriam Co.
31. Wilsnack, S.C.: Alcohol abuse and alcoholism in women. In Pattison, E.M., and Kaufman, E., editors: Encyclopedia handbook of alcoholism, New York, 1982, Gardner Press.

■ ANNOTATED SUGGESTED READINGS ■

*Adams, G.: The sexual history as an integral part of the patient history, Am. J. Maternal Child Nurs. **1**:170, May-June 1976.

The author convincingly and thoroughly presents the importance of the sexual history in the patient's total health history. The article gives the what, why, and how of sexual history taking. It is highly recommended reading for all nurses.

*Anderson, M.L.: Talking about sex with less anxiety, J. Psychosoc. Nurs. Ment. Health Serv. **18**(6):10, June 1980.

This article helps the professional nurse examine the anxiety that is often involved in discussing clients' sexual concerns with them. Anxiety is discussed from both the client's and the nurse's perspective. First the client's anxiety, what causes it, and how

---

*Asterisk indicates nursing reference.

the nurse can help to decrease client's anxiety is discussed; secondly, the author examines anxiety of the nurse, causes for it, and what can be done to reduce it.

Barbach, L.: For each other: sharing sexual intimacy, New York, 1982, Signet Books: New American Library.

The author provides women with important knowledge about complex aspects of a relationship that affect satisfaction. She has included basic exercises to help women explore communication patterns within their relationships and enhance sexual pleasure. This self-help book would be useful to the client involved in sexual counseling.

Bell, A.P., and Weinberg, M.J.: Homosexualities: a study of diversity among men and women, New York, 1978, Simon and Schuster.

This official publication of the Institute for Sex Research reports on a survey of 1,456 homosexual and heterosexual men and women living in the San Francisco area. The study examines the variety of homosexual life-styles and demonstrates that homosexuality encompasses much more than people's sexual activities.

Bell, A., Weinberg, M., and Hammersmith, S.: Sexual preference, Bloomington, Ind., 1981, Indiana University Press.

This book asks why some people become homosexuals, while others become heterosexuals. It retires many cherished ideas and suggests that sexual identity is impervious to the influence of parents and psychotherapy. Controversial and important research based on data from interviews with approximately 1,500 individuals.

Clark, D.: Loving someone gay, New York, 1978, Signet Books: New American Library.

This book examines the myths and mysteries surrounding "gay" (homosexual) people. It includes an excellent chapter written to help professional counselors who work with gay clients.

Crooks, R., and Baur, K.: Our sexuality, ed. 2, Menlo Park, Calif., 1983, The Benjamin/Cummings Publishing Co.

This current and comprehensive text on the topic of human sexuality contains well researched and complete chapters on issues such as: communication in sexual behavior, sex research, methods and problems and sex and the law. The authors do an excellent job of reviewing current literature in every chapter and presenting all viewpoints with a nonjudgmental attitude.

*deChesnay, M.: Father-daughter incest: issues in treatment and research, J. Psychosoc. Nurs. Ment. Health Serv. **22**(9): 8–16, Sept. 1984.

This article discusses the practical and legal definitions of incest. It presents the incestuous family as a system that acts to maintain the status quo. The author suggests that family therapy can be an effective mode of treatment for this problem.

Edelwich, J., and Brodsky, A.: Sexual dilemmas for the helping professional, New York, 1982, Brunner/Mazel Publishers.

This text provides nurses with many helpful suggestions for intervening in sexual situations with clients. It presents a comprehensive analysis of the sexual feelings between client and therapist. The book covers such rarely discussed topics as: client seduction of therapist, therapist seduction of client, referring out clients who arouse sexual feelings in the therapist, and ethical responses to feelings of attraction and seductive behavior. Important reading for any health professional.

Fromer, M.J.: Ethical issues in sexuality and reproduction, St. Louis, 1983, The C.V. Mosby Co.

This text examines important ethical issues in sexuality and reproduction. The author begins with a discussion of ethical theory and includes chapters on such controversial issues as: abortion, fetal research, homosexuality, and contraception.

*Hacker, S.S.: Students' questions about sexuality: implications for nurse educators, Nurse Educator **10**(4):28–31, Winter 1984.

The author identifies major areas of concern for graduate and student nurses in regard to human sexuality. Based on the responses of 350 nurses, the most commonly voiced concerns are identified and discussed in detail. The critical need for sex education in the nursing curriculum is also addressed in this article.

Kaplan, H.S.: The new sex therapy, New York, 1974, Brunner/Mazel, Inc.

This book describes Kaplan's method of brief treatment for sexual dysfunctions. It clarifies basic underlying concepts by relating technical material to the theory of psychopathology.

Kaplan, H.S.: Disorders of sexual desires and other new concepts and techniques in sex therapy, New York, 1979, Brunner/Mazel Publishers.

This book addresses the dysfunction of inhibition of sexual desire, which occurs when one or both members of a couple have no desire for sex or find sex distasteful. Kaplan presents cases throughout the book of couples with this disorder and explains her treatment approach.

Kaplan, H.S.: The evaluation of sexual disorders, New York, 1983, Brunner/Mazel Inc.

The emphasis of this text is placed on assessment and diagnosis of sexual disorder. It aids the clinician in differentiating between psychological and medical causes of sexual dysfunctions. Data-gathering procedures used in sexual assessment are described, and case studies are included.

*Krozy, R.: Becoming comfortable with sexual assessment, Am. J. Nurs. **78**(4):1036–1038, June 1980.

The author offers some practical suggestions for initiating a sexual assessment with clients. She discusses the need for the nurse to be comfortable with human sexuality and gives specific characteristics of the "sexuality comfortable person."

Levine, S.B., and Lothstein, L.: Transsexualism or the gender dysphoria syndromes, J. Sex Marital Ther. **7**(2):85, 1981.

This comprehensive article summarizes the existing knowledge about gender dysphoric clients and presents a clinically useful diagnostic approach to patients requesting sex reassignment surgery. It also discusses the ethical dilemmas associated with the treatment of gender dysphoric clients.

*Lion, E., editor: Human sexuality in nursing processes, New York, 1982, A Wiley Medical Publication.

This text written for nurses in a nursing process format provides concise case examples demonstrating common clinical issues and problems that nurses must face. Comprehensive chapters on sexual development throughout the life cycle are included.

Masters, W.H., and Johnson, V.E.: Human sexual response, Boston, 1966, Little, Brown & Co.

This book is Masters' and Johnson's first effort to explore the physiology of sexual response. It discusses the anatomy and phys-

iology of the male and female sex organs. The authors describe their research findings regarding sexual response and orgasm.

Masters, W.H., and Johnson, V.E.: Human sexual inadequacies, Boston, 1970, Little, Brown and Co.

This book identifies and describes sexual dysfunction and specific treatment methods for those dysfunctions. Masters' and Johnson's dual therapy treatment approach is explained, and case samples are included.

*Moses, A.E., and Hawkins, R.: Counseling lesbian women and gay men, St. Louis, 1982, The C.V. Mosby Co.

This innovative textbook is one of the first to discuss counseling the homosexual client. It addresses issues such as attitudes toward gay people, coming out, and the development of sexual identity. Numerous personal accounts of "gay" clients add increased understanding to the reader of the special concerns of this population.

Nass, G.D., Libby, R.W., and Fisher, M.P.: Sexual choices: an introduction to human sexuality, ed. 2, Monterey, Calif., 1984, Wadsworth Health Science Division.

This is a current comprehensive textbook on the subject of sexuality. It includes chapters on sexual identity, pregnancy choices, and three excellent chapters on sexual development: Early Sexual Learning, Adult Sexual Lifestyles, and Sex and Older People. A unique feature of this book is a section entitled "Yellow Pages for Informed Sexual Choices," which is a resource list for students who want to pursue a special interest in specific sexual issues or services.

*Satterfield, S., and Stayton, R.: Understanding sexual function and dysfunction, Topics in Clinical Nursing 1:4, 1980.

This article discusses the similarities and differences of sexual dysfunction in the male and female. The article helps the reader to understand the etiology of sexual dysfunction, the disorders of response and the treatment options open to the clinician specializing in sex therapy.

Sgroi, S.: Handbook of clinical intervention in child sexual abuse, Lexington, Mass. 1982, Lexington Books.

This handbook discusses a variety of topics that professionals working with sexually abused children face, ranging from reporting, interviewing, and investigating to various forms of therapy that have proven effective. Excellent chapters are included on the evaluation of child sexual abuse programs.

*Thomas, S.: Bisexuality: a sexual orientation of great diversity, J. Psychosoc. Nurs. Ment. Health Serv. **18**(4):19–27, Apr. 1980.

This article presents one of the few readings devoted to exploring the sexual orientation of bisexuality. It is a very good introductory reading with a reference list for further study of the topic.

Zilbergeld, B.: Male sexuality, New York, 1981, Bantam Books, Inc.

This book is a practical guide to understanding male sexuality. The author carefully explores common myths about male sexuality and male sexual performance. It includes exercises designed to enhance sexual awareness and pleasure for both partners. It is helpful reading for the client involved in sexual counseling.

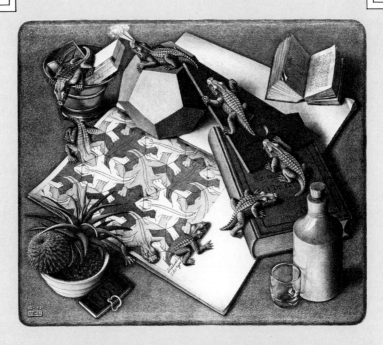

Canst thou not minister to a mind diseas'd,
Pluck from the memory a rooted sorrow,
Raze out the written troubles of the brain,
And with some sweet oblivious antidote
Cleanse the stuff'd bosom of the perilous stuff
Which weighs upon the heart?

William Shakespeare, Macbeth, Act V

C H A P T E R   2 2

SOMATIC THERAPIES AND PSYCHIATRIC NURSING

LEARNING OBJECTIVES

After studying this chapter, the student should be able to:

- state reasons for the use of physical restraint of patients, including mechanical restraints and seclusion.

- discuss the nursing care of a patient who is in restraints or seclusion.

- identify issues associated with psychosurgical treatment.

- describe the nursing care of a patient receiving electroconvulsive therapy, including patient

education, patient care during the treatment and recovery period, and assessment of the patient's response to the treatment.

- analyze legal and ethical issues related to the use of restraint, seclusion, psychosurgery, and electroconvulsive therapy.

- identify directions for future nursing research.

- select appropriate readings for further study.

I n the past, many somatic treatments have been used in psychiatric settings. As research into the pathophysiology of mental illness continues, it is likely that more and increasingly sophisticated somatic treatment modalities will be developed. At the same time, treatment modalities such as restraint, which was among the earliest means of providing nursing care for psychiatric patients, are still used. Psychiatric nursing therapy, like psychiatry, is in a time of transition. Old therapies are being reassessed and reconsidered. New therapies are being discovered and investigated. Nurses will be important contributors to the growth of knowledge in this area and need to scientifically study the effectiveness of the various somatic therapies.

The treatment modalities described in this chapter are presented in a way that should also provide some historical perspective regarding the progression of knowledge in this area of psychiatric care. Although several treatment forms may have been used by clinicians at a given time, generally one form was more frequently used than others. Few therapies of the past have been totally abandoned. There also seems to be a tendency for relatively unused treatments to be repopularized. Therefore some treatments that are rarely used today, such as insulin coma therapy, are presented briefly. The emphasis in all cases will be on the nursing implications applicable to the treatment described. However, since some treatments are viewed as specific to certain psychiatric diagnostic categories, there will be reference to these diagnoses, and parts of the chapter will incorporate the medical model more heavily than do other portions of this book. Psychopharmacology, also a somatic therapy, is discussed in Chapter 23.

Use of physical restraints

Physical restraint was one of the earliest means used to try to cope with people who were unable to control their behavior. Prior to the early nineteenth century, shackles and fetters were used to control the "insane" in "asylums." Some persons spent years bound hand and foot or chained to the wall. Small wonder that families tried to keep disturbed members at home. Modifications in these practices took place after Philippe Pinel campaigned for humane treatment of the mentally ill in France. Similar objectives were pursued in England by Tuke, and in this country by Benjamin Rush and Dorothea Lynde Dix. Gradually the chains fell into disuse. However, other forms of physical restraint, including camisoles ("straitjackets"), sheet restraints, wrist and ankle restraints, sheet packs, and seclusion were commonly used until the advent of the convulsive therapies and psychopharmacotherapy. Good psychiatric nursing care was essential to humanize what could be a dehumanizing experience.

It is still necessary at times to physically restrain patients. In this era of increasing sensitivity to civil liberties and the rights of the individual, restraint should be used with great discretion. Two court decisions have been influential in clarifying this issue. *Rogers v. Okin*,[16] 1975, prohibited the use of seclusion or restraint for treatment purposes. It was the court's opinion that these measures could be used only for control of a behavioral emergency. The 1982 Supreme Court decision in *Youngberg v. Romeo*[23] supported the exercise of professional judgment in the use of seclusion or restraint. The standard to be applied is that of usual and customary professional practice. Wexler[21] notes that "professional" was defined very broadly in this case and could really apply to any direct care provider. Soloff, Gutheil, and Wexler[19] point out that there are issues still unresolved by this decision. For instance, it is unclear whether the use of physical restraint to protect property or to preserve a therapeutic environment would be acceptable. Likewise, the decision did not address the use of seclusion or mechanical restraints as consequences in behavior modification programs. Study of the discussion of legal and ethical aspects of psychiatric care presented in Chapter 7 will assist the nurse to analyze the ramifications of the use of restrictive or intrusive approaches to patient care.

■ Related research

Although the use of physical restraint has led to controversy in psychiatry, there is a lack of research that provides guidance to the practitioner. Recent literature reviews have revealed thirteen reports of research studies of physical restraint between 1976 and 1983. These were difficult to compare because of variation in treatment programs and patient characteristics. Soloff, Gutheil, and Wexler[19] were able to make several generalizations. In acute settings, schizophrenic and manic patients were secluded most frequently; in chronic settings, mentally retarded and nonpsychotic patients were secluded or restrained more often. Physically restrained patients were also younger, more chronically ill, and involuntarily hospitalized. An interesting finding was that in most cases seclusion or restraint was initiated based on nonviolent behavior patterns. The length of time spent in restraints or seclusion was related to age, sex, and diagnosis, but not to the precipitating behavior. Males who were under 35 years old and not psychotic were restricted for a longer period of time.

Okin[14] reported on a study of the frequency and rationale for the use of seclusion and restraint in seven public mental hospitals in the same state. The purpose of the study was to determine if there were differences in the use of these procedures given that all the hospitals were operating within the same set of policies and regulations. Differences were found. The investigator concluded that this was influenced by such hospital-related factors as the following:

1. Differences in staff perceptions of patient behaviors
2. More frequent use of alternative interventions in some settings
3. Failure to prevent violence and sometimes even promotion of violent behavior at some hospitals
4. Variation in quality and quantity of staff
5. Different levels of staff competence in prevention and management of violent behavior
6. Varying approaches to the medication of disturbed patients

---

Factors Related to Increased Rates of Seclusion and Restraint

Increase in:

- Violence of patient population
- Number/proportion of involuntary patients, perpetrators of violent crimes
- Attack on the facility from legal, political, professional, economic quarters
- Inter-staff tensions, resentments, disagreements
- Legal or departmental intrusiveness, regulation, undermining of on-site decisions

Decrease in:

- Number of staff
- Number of senior, experienced staff
- Number of male staff
- Public support of facility
- Staff morale and sense of security
- Available alternatives through regulation, policy, change, legal interdiction

Increase in rates of seclusion, restraint, forced medication, administrative discharge, transfer to security setting
(*Note:* Prohibition of one of these interventions may lead to increases in rates of the others.)

From Gutheil, T.G.: Review of individual quantitative studies. In Tardiff, K., editor: *The psychiatric uses of seclusion and restraint*, Washington, D.C., 1984, American Psychiatric Press, Inc.

7. Differences in the characteristics of the milieu
8. More clarity and firmness in limit setting at some of the hospitals
9. Variations in ward organization and physical characteristics[14]

Studies such as this provide useful clues about factors that may enable nurses to avoid unnecessary use of restrictive treatment approaches. The box on page 684 illustrates Gutheil's[7] analysis of factors related to increased rates of seclusion and restraint. When it is necessary to limit a patient's freedom and mobility, good nursing care is a necessity and a great challenge. Nursing interventions with the mechanically restrained or the secluded patient are summarized in Table 22-1.

■ Mechanical restraints

Mechanical restraints include camisoles, wrist restraints, ankle restraints, sheet restraints, and sheet packs. Any of these measures should be applied only with a physician's order. The patient should be released from restraints as soon as any dangerous behavior has subsided or other less drastic means of restraint such as medication become effective. Nursing care of patients with restraints other than sheet packs will be discussed first. Care of patients in packs differs slightly and will be discussed separately.

Prevention of restraint is the emphasis of Rosen and DiGiacomo.[17] They recommend that informed consent for the use of restraints be obtained from the patient and family at the time of admission to the psychiatric

TABLE 22-1

NURSING INTERVENTIONS WITH THE SECLUDED OR MECHANICALLY RESTRAINED PATIENT

Principle	Rationale	Nursing intervention
Right to least restrictive treatment	Constitutional right of all patients	Identify precipitating events; observe patient for agitated behavior; attempt alternative interventions; document patient behavior and nursing interventions
Protect patient from physical injury	An individual who is not in control of his behavior is at risk of injury and needs external limits, safely applied	Provide adequate staff resources to control the patient; be sure staff is trained to manage violent behavior; plan the approach to the patient; use safe physical restraint techniques
Provide a safe environment	An individual who is not in control of his behavior may have impaired judgment and may harm himself accidentally or purposefully	Observe the patient constantly or very frequently, depending on his condition; remove dangerous objects from the area
Maintain biological integrity	Physically restrained patients are not able to attend to their own biological needs and are at risk for complications related to immobility	Check vital signs; bathe the patient and provide skin care; take to the bathroom or provide a bedpan or urinal; regulate the room temperature; position the patient anatomically; pad restraints; offer food and fluids; release restraints at least every 2 hours
Maintain dignity and self-esteem	Loss of control and the imposition of physical restraint may be embarrassing to the patient	Provide privacy; explain the situation to other patients without revealing confidential patient information; maintain verbal contact with the patient at regular intervals while awake; assign a consistent staff member to work with the patient; assign a staff member of the same sex to provide personal care; involve the patient in plans to terminate physical restraint; wean the patient from the protected setting

unit. Verbal intervention and medication should be attempted before physical restraints are introduced. They have found that failure to respond to alternative approaches is generally related to one of several factors, including failure by the staff to respond soon enough, failure to explain what is planned or expected, ambivalent or hostile staff attitudes, and approaches by staff who are unfamiliar to the patient. They also describe several reasons for using physical restraint with psychiatric patients: violence directed toward the self or others; agitated behavior when medication is contraindicated, for example, a delirious patient; hyperactivity accompanied by regressed socially unacceptable behavior that alienates others; refusal to meet basic biological needs for rest and nutrition, resulting in the threat of physical collapse; the need for decreased stimuli, mutually determined by the patient and the therapist; and the patient's request if it does not represent an untherapeutic need for dependency and regression.

The patient in mechanical restraint may be confused or delirious and will probably be frightened at the limitation of movement. The nurse should not assume that the patient understands the need for restraint. Support and reassurance are essential. Restraints should be applied efficiently and with care not to injure a combative patient. Adequate personnel need to be assembled before the patient is approached and should be assigned responsibility for controlling specific body parts. Restraints should be available and in working order. Padding of cuff restraints helps to prevent skin breakdown. For the same reason, the patient should be positioned in anatomical alignment. Provision of privacy is important. If visitors are allowed, an explanation of the treatment and the reason for it before they see the patient may help them accept the situation. Physical needs must be included in the nursing care plan. Vital signs should be checked. Regular observation of circulation in the extremities is necessary. Fluids should be offered regularly and opportunities for elimination provided. Skin care is also essential. Restraints must be released at least every 2 hours to allow exercise of the extremities. Good nursing care and the communication of concern for the patient will contribute to better behavioral control. Immobilization for any reason is physically hazardous and should be avoided whenever possible.

Whaley and Ramirez[22] recommend that restraints or seclusion be terminated when a therapeutic alliance with the patient has been established and violent behavior has subsided. Release should be gradual with intervals out of restraints increased over time.

Cold, wet sheet packs may be ordered occasionally for extremely disturbed patients who are refractory to treatment with medication. In this procedure the patient is immobilized by being wrapped mummy fashion in several layers of linens. The innermost layer of sheets is soaked in ice water. The patient is in a bed with a waterproof mattress and dressed in a hospital nightgown. The sheets are wrapped so that no skin surfaces are in contact, since this could cause chafing and perhaps skin breakdown. The wet sheets are covered by layers of blankets, preferably wool. Although the pack is initially experienced as very cold, it quickly becomes warmed by the patient's body heat, which is retained in the pack. The combination of the warmth, wetness, and swaddling are very soothing and can have a calming effect on even extremely agitated patients. A patient in a pack needs constant nursing observation. Temperature, pulse, and respirations should be monitored, and the pack should be discontinued with any significant change in vital signs. The patient will perspire, and fluids should be offered frequently. Soothing verbal contact may be helpful, but the environment should be quiet and conducive to rest. In general, the patient should remain in the pack for about 2 hours. Maximum calming does not usually occur in less than this time, but hazards of immobility increase as the duration of restraint increases. When the pack is removed, the skin should be thoroughly towel dried and skin care given. Privacy should, of course, be provided throughout the procedure.

■ Seclusion or isolation

A patient who is restrained by the use of seclusion is confined alone in a single room. Degrees of seclusion may range from confinement in a room with a closed but unlocked door to a locked room with a mattress without linens on the floor, limited opportunity for communication, and with the patient dressed in a hospital nightgown or a heavy canvas coverall. The latter are minimally acceptable conditions for seclusion, which is to be used only when essential for the protection of the patient or others.

Seclusion is prescribed for a number of reasons. It may be used as a means of controlling the behavior of a patient who has been acting destructively and cannot be controlled by interpersonal contact, either physical or verbal. Seclusion is often helpful to patients who are hyperactive and extremely responsive to environmental stimuli. Sometimes these patients will ask to be isolated for a period of time and this should be allowed. Behavior modification protocols sometimes include seclusion as a negative reinforcer. This use of seclusion borders on punishment and should be used judiciously.

■ **THEORETICAL BASES.** Gutheil[6] has identified three theoretical bases for the use of seclusion. The first is containment. This implies that the patient is at immediate risk for causing harm to himself or others. Seclusion protects him from this danger until his internal behavioral controls have been reestablished. He is also protected from the guilt that would potentially be experienced as a result of loss of control. Another theoretical base concerns isolation. The patient is relieved of the burden of needing to relate interpersonally. There is a limitation on the amount of space available to the patient, allowing him to master a reasonable area before being confronted with the need to relate appropriately in the setting of the whole ward. The last concept is that of a decrease in sensory input. Seclusion may be calming to a person who is hyperalert and feeling bombarded by the many sensory stimuli that occur in the hospital environment.[6]

Gutheil and Tardiff[8] have described several contraindications for the use of seclusion. A patient who is medically unstable may not be observed closely enough while isolated in a seclusion room. Mechanical restraints may be more appropriate for such a patient. If there is high potential for self-harm, the patient also requires close observation and must be readily accessible to the staff. No seclusion room is totally safe. A self-destructive patient can hurt himself in a totally empty room by banging his head against the wall. If the seclusion room environment does not meet minimal safety standards, other means of restraint must be used. For instance, if the temperature is too high, the conditions may be dangerous for agitated patients whose temperature-regulating mechanisms have been impaired by phenothiazine medications. Lion and Soloff[12] caution that secluded patients may become exhausted if agitated behavior continues in seclusion. They also warn that sensory deprivation may actually result in an intensification of psychosis. Socially deviant behavior, such as fecal smearing, may lead to reluctance by staff to have contact with the patient. The nurse, as the leader of the direct care staff, must be aware of these potential risks. Continuous nursing assessment and revision of the patient care plan will assist the nurse to anticipate hazardous conditions and take appropriate preventive nursing actions.

Several negative effects of the injudicious use of seclusion have been identified.[6] One is the jealousy other patients might feel over the attention given to the patient who has needed seclusion. This has been termed *seclusion envy*. Another potential problem is the creation of a lasting rift between the staff and the patient who was secluded. This will occur if the patient does not understand or agree with the reason for the procedure. The use of seclusion for the wrong reasons can also lead to negative consequences. Seclusion should not be used as a punishment or as a way to relieve the staff of the care of a demanding patient. Secluded patients require frequent and intensive nursing care.

■ **PROCEDURE.** When the decision has been made to place a patient in isolation, the procedure should be carried out quickly and in a manner that demonstrates concern for the patient's dignity. The room should be prepared before the patient is approached.

Lion and Soloff[12] have described the following specific techniques to implement when secluding an agitated patient:

1. Designate a staff member to be the leader.
2. Amass enough staff to provide a "show of force."
3. Assign a monitor to clear the area, observe the implementation of the procedure, and provide feedback after it is completed.
4. Communicate clearly and unambiguously with the patient.
5. Proceed without hesitation.
6. Control aggressive behavior in a safe manner, avoiding pain or injury.
7. Move the patient to the seclusion room.
8. Remove clothing and dangerous objects.
9. Staff should leave the room in a planned and organized way.
10. A debriefing session should be held.

Legal requirements for the care of the secluded patient vary from state to state and are minimal at best. Good nursing care should always provide for optimal fulfillment of basic human needs and concern for the dignity of the person. The nurse must assist the patient to meet biological needs by providing food and fluids, a comfortable environment, and opportunity for use of the bathroom. Frequent observation is essential, and the room must be constructed so the patient can be observed without being unnecessarily exposed to those who are not involved in his care. There should also be a means provided to allow communication with the patient. Careful records should be kept of all nursing care and observation of the isolated patient. The need for continued isolation should be assessed on a regular basis. It may be necessary for the nurse to initiate this review of the patient's condition with other health team members.

Whenever the use of seclusion has been required, the nursing staff should review the events that led up to the decision to undertake this means of treatment. In particular, staff should be encouraged to give each other feedback about observations of interpersonal relationships involving the secluded patient. An effort should be made to identify preventive measures that may assist the patient to gain control in the future without requiring seclusion. It is also useful for staff to have an opportunity to ventilate their own feelings following an episode of seclusion. Management of violent behavior is physically and emotionally stressful.

Timely nursing intervention before loss of control occurs can often avert the need for seclusion of an agitated patient. Spending time with the patient may be helpful. Sometimes the energy of agitation can be channeled into nondestructive physical activity. If a patient is angry and feels misunderstood, an effort to understand may avoid an explosion. Medication may also be useful in calming a patient if it is given in time. Allowing a patient to be alone without being forcibly isolated may also be helpful at times. Careful nursing assessment and the establishment of a trusting nurse-patient relationship are a good foundation for deciding on an effective plan of action when a patient becomes upset. Any form of physical restraint should be used as a last resort when other nursing interventions have failed.

Psychosurgery

The American Psychiatric Association[3] has defined psychosurgery as:

> . . . surgical intervention to sever fibers connecting one part of the brain with another, or to remove, destroy or stimulate brain tissue with the intent of modifying or altering disturbances of behavior, thought content, or mood for which no organic pathological cause can be demonstrated by established tests and techniques. Such surgery may also be undertaken for the relief of intractable pain.[3:251]

It does not include surgery to treat an organic brain disease.

First introduced in 1936, the early operations were referred to as lobotomies because the focus of the surgical intervention was the pathway from the thalamus to the frontal lobes of the cerebral cortex. These surgical procedures were nonspecific because of the limited knowledge at that time of brain functioning. Extensive personality change was almost inevitably a result of surgery. A nursing article from that era describes vividly the deterioration in social skills that resulted from psychosurgery and the retraining which became an integral part of the nursing care for these patients.[4] Because of the pervasive influence on the individual's ability to function adequately, the procedure was most often done as a last resort and fell into relative disuse following the introduction of new psychopharmacological agents.

Recently, however, there has been a resurgence of interest in psychosurgery as knowledge of neuroanatomy and physiology has become increasingly more sophisticated. Progress has been made in "mapping" the cortex, which has led to the possibility of the surgeon being more able to isolate and sever tracts that relate more directly to the patient's individual behavioral problem. Technology has also contributed sophisticated surgical tools, such as lasers, which cause far less generalized tissue damage. Proponents of this approach now claim that psychosurgery can be beneficial to patients who are unresponsive to other forms of therapy with minimized damage to the personality and to social functioning. Patients who benefit from various types of psychosurgery are those with chronic neurotic and chronic depressive behaviors. Contrary to the practice of the past, schizophrenic patients are not good candidates because of their basically inadequate personality structure.[2]

The nursing care of the psychosurgical patient will not be discussed in detail here, since it is more pertinent to the specialty of neurosurgical nursing. However, the nurse should be aware that the major effect of surgery is on the *emotional* component of the patient's behavior. Intelligence is not affected. Also, the patient may continue to have some preoperative symptoms, such as hallucinations, but will not have the same emotional response, thus facilitating improved functioning in activities of daily living.

The renewal of interest in this form of therapy has raised moral and ethical questions for many professionals relative to the issue of mind control. Although other somatic therapies, such as pharmacotherapy and the convulsive therapies, undoubtedly exert some degree of control over the person's thought process, psychosurgery seems to many to be more drastic because it is permanent and irreversible. Nervous tissue, once damaged, does not regenerate. These questions arise particularly when psychosurgery is suggested as a possible treatment for antisocial and violent behavior, such as murder and rape. The responsible professional nurse must form independent opinions about such issues, collecting facts and objective data. Knowledge about the functioning of the brain is in a period of rapid growth. Therefore forms of therapy such as psychosurgery will also be changing and improving. An open mind is an asset in evaluating varied approaches to the treatment of psychiatric disorders.

Electroconvulsive therapy

Electroconvulsive therapy (ECT), also referred to as electric shock therapy (EST), was first described by Cerletti and Bini in 1938 as a treatment for schizophrenia. At that time it was believed that epileptics were rarely schizophrenic and hypothesized that convulsions would cure schizophrenia. Later research did not support this hypothesis. Further experience with ECT demonstrated that it is much more effective as a treatment for affective disturbances than it is for schizophrenia. It has also been noted that epilepsy and schizophrenia do occur concurrently. ECT is now most frequently used as a treatment for severe depression.

ECT is a treatment in which a grand mal seizure is artificially induced by passing an electrical current through electrodes applied to the temples. The electrodes are generally applied bilaterally, although some therapists have used unilateral electrodes and claim that patients treated in this way experience less confusion. For the treatment to be effective, a grand mal seizure must occur. The voltage is generally adjusted to the minimum level that will produce the therapeutic effect. The number of treatments given in a series varies according to the patient's presenting problem and therapeutic response as assessed during the course of treatment. The most common range for affective disorders is from 6 to 10 treatments, whereas as many as 20 to 30 may be given for schizophrenia. ECT is most commonly given three times a week on alternate days, although it can be given daily or more than once a day. Some therapists have used multiple ECT in which several convulsions are induced immediately following each other. The proponents of this approach claim greater therapeutic effectiveness with no increase in confusion or untoward responses seen in the patient. However, the American Psychiatric Association has refused to endorse this practice.[1]

■ Nursing intervention

Nursing intervention with a patient who is to receive ECT begins as soon as the individual and family are presented with this treatment alternative. Most people respond emotionally when told that they or a loved one needs "shock therapy." When discussing the subject with them, one should talk about "treatment" and avoid unnecessary use of the term "shock." This places the emphasis on the therapeutic value of the procedure. However, people also need an opportunity to express their feelings about ECT. Fear is usually present. Many people have heard or read about or seen movies portraying ECT. Many of these are done in a sensationalistic manner, emphasizing the frightening aspect of the experience. Also, the very idea of an electric current passing through their head causes fear in most people. The nurse must assess the patient's response and provide opportunity for communication. As the patient reveals feelings and concerns, the nurse can listen for misconceptions and clarify information about which the patient is confused. The very act of discussing ECT openly and directly communicates the attitude that it is a usual method of treatment, without undue risk. However, as with any procedure requiring general anesthesia, there

is a degree of risk. Therefore the patient is asked to sign a consent form indicating that he has been fully informed about the procedure and the risks involved.

When the patient has had an opportunity to express feelings to a receptive person, teaching about the procedure of ECT should take place. Learning will be facilitated when the patient's anxiety is slightly increased but not overwhelming. Some information will probably have been given to the patient by the physician at the time informed consent was obtained. However, a thorough review by the nurse is recommended to reinforce what the patient already knows, remind him of what was forgotten, and provide an opportunity for questions. Enough time should be provided to create a relaxed atmosphere conducive to a free exchange of communication. The nurse should also be observant for nonverbal cues of the patient's response to the teaching. Asking the patient to repeat what has been explained also helps identify areas of confusion.

Much of the nursing procedure related to ECT is similar to that which is needed when a patient undergoes surgery. The patient is not given anything orally after midnight when ECT is scheduled for the morning. One exception to this may be to give prescribed sedation with a small amount of water to a patient who has difficulty sleeping. Prior to the treatment the patient is asked to remove jewelry, hairpins, eyeglasses, and hearing aids. Full dentures may be removed. Partial plates should be left in the mouth to provide even pressure on the teeth and jaw during the tonic phase of the convulsion. Dress should be loose and comfortable, usually bed clothing. The bladder should be emptied. The patient awaiting ECT should also be accompanied by a trusted, understanding nurse staff member. Under no circumstances should a patient waiting for ECT see another patient during or right after a treatment.

In the early days of ECT no medication was given prior to the administration of the shock. Therefore the individual experienced a full-blown, and frequently violent, grand mal convulsion. Although the patient was amnesic for the convulsive episode, it was a frightening experience. Some complications, particularly fractures and dislocations, were also associated with the unmedicated procedure. Current American Psychiatric Association standards unequivocally state that ECT should be given under general anesthesia with the use of a muscle relaxant drug.[1] The patient therefore has no memory of the procedure and the convulsion occurs in an attenuated form. This change has also resulted in the involvement of an anesthesiologist as a member of the treatment team.

■ MEDICATIONS. The following medications are commonly given prior to ECT:

1. Methscopolamine or atropine sulfate is administered for its vagolytic effect.[5] It is frequently given subcutaneously or intramuscularly 30 minutes prior to treatment but is most effective when given intravenously with the other premedications. To avert the bradycardia that occurs with the onset of the seizure activity, the anticholinergic drug is given intravenously immediately prior to the treatment. The pulse rate is monitored and enough medication is given to increase it by about 10%. This titration is not possible if the medication is given subcutaneously or intramuscularly.[5]

2. A short-acting barbiturate such as sodium methohexital (Brevital Sodium) is administered intravenously to induce anesthesia.

3. Succinylcholine chloride (Anectine), a muscle relaxant, is administered intravenously after the anesthetic. If it is given prior to the anesthetic, the patient will feel paralyzed. The inability to breathe resulting from paralysis of the respiratory muscles can be very frightening and may be remembered after the treatment. The face and extremities are observed for muscle fasciculations, which indicate that the muscle relaxant has taken effect. Some authorities recommend isolating one extremity from the general circulation by the use of a tourniquet or blood pressure cuff before administration of the muscle relaxant. This limb can then be observed for unmodified seizure activity when the ECT is given.[5]

These medications may be injected directly into the vein or through the tubing of a previously started intravenous (IV) infusion. The advantage of the latter route is that the IV line is in place should complications arise during the procedure.

O'Connell[13] recommends discontinuation of psychotropic medications prior to beginning ECT. Lithium may prolong the effect of the succinylcholine. Many psychotropic drugs act synergistically with anticholinergics.

ECT may be given in the operating room or in an especially equipped room in the inpatient or outpatient psychiatric setting. It is a nursing responsibility to check all emergency equipment, including oxygen, suction, and cardiac resuscitation equipment prior to ECT. The ECT machine and IV equipment, if used, should also be in readiness.

Frankel[5] has recommended that specific drugs and equipment be available when ECT is given. These are listed in the box on page 691.

■ **ADMINISTRATION.** The patient lies supine on a bed or cot. Usually, 100% oxygen is administered for 1 to 2 minutes while an IV infusion is being started. This hyperoxygenation prepares the patient for the period of apnea that will result from the muscle relaxant and the convulsion. The patient will also need reassurance while these preparations take place. The medications are then administered. As soon as muscle paralysis has occurred, the treatment is given. Electrodes are placed on the temples or on the nondominant side temple for unilateral ECT. A mouth gag is inserted between the teeth, and the jaw is gently supported. There is no need to restrain the limbs. The shock is administered. The fingers and toes are watched carefully for a rhythmic twitching, which is the only visible evidence that a grand mal convulsion has occurred. When the twitching has stopped, oxygen is given by bag-breathing the patient through a mask until spontaneous respiration resumes.

During the period immediately after ECT the patient requires close nursing observation in a recovery area. Emergency equipment should be readily available, although adverse reactions are rare. While unconscious, the patient should receive the same nursing care as is required by any comatose patient. A patent airway must be maintained. Occasionally, suctioning may be required to remove excessive secretions from the mouth and throat. Positioning should be on the side to prevent aspiration of secretions or in the event of vomiting. Blood pressure, pulse, and respirations should be monitored closely until the patient has fully reacted.

The patient will generally begin to respond after 10 to 15 minutes. Some drowsiness will be experienced even after the anesthesia wears off. When the patient responds to his name, the nurse should provide orientation to time, place, and situation. Most patients are confused immediately following a treatment and become frightened if they are not oriented. Since ECT is frequently given in the morning, the patient may not remember getting out of bed and preparing for the treatment and may assume that something happened to him during the night while he was asleep. Following is an example of this type of disorientation:

One patient, who was receiving ECT in the operating room, began to talk about people "cutting on" him and suspected that one of his fingers had been removed and another sewn on in its place. This was viewed as his attempt to make sense of a situation about which he was confused. He responded well to an explanation that he did indeed go to the operating room but received a treatment other than surgery when he was there. It was further explained that the treatment was for his depression.

Drugs and Equipment to Accompany ECT

Drugs

It is recommended that the following drugs and solutions be available with dose instructions for immediate administration:

1. Atropine sulfate - 0.4 mg/ml
2. Calcium chloride - 10% solution - 10% ml vial (emergency syringe)
3. Dexamethasone (Decadron) - 4 mg/ml and/or 24 mg/ml
4. Dextrose - 5% in water - 250 ml units
5. Diazepam 5 mg/ml - 2 and 10 ml (emergency syringe)
6. Epinephrine - 1:10,000 solution - 10 ml vials
7. Lidocaine (Xylocaine): special preparation for use in cardiac dysrhythmias - 2% solution = 5 ml = 100 mg in emergency syringe
8. Metaraminol (Aramine) - 1% solution - 10 ml vial
9. Methylprednisolone (Solu-Medrol) - 125 and 1,000 mg/vial
10. Sodium bicarbonate - 7.5% solution = 44.6 mEq. - 50 ml (emergency syringe)
11. L-norepinephrine (Levophed) - 2 mg/ml-4ml ampuls.

Equipment

Equipment to be available for immediate use:

1. Suction—tested for proper function
2. Needles
3. Infusion sets
4. Electrocardiograph
5. Defibrillator. While rare cases of cardiac arrest occurring with ECT can usually be managed by a blow to the precordium, the adjunctive use of a defibrillator may occasionally be necessary. This apparatus should be reasonably accessible for this contingency.

When ECT is administered in a hospital, the emergency (crash) cart should be readily available. In other facilities, a comparably equipped unit should be available.

From the American Psychiatric Association Commission of Psychiatric Therapies: THE PSYCHIATRIC THERAPIES: PART I, THE SOMATIC THERAPIES. Chaired by Karasu, T.B., Washington, D.C., The American Psychiatric Association, 1984, p. 218. Used by permission.

Orientation may need to be repeated several times following ECT. It must also be repeated every time the patient has a treatment because confusion may occur each time and for some persons becomes more severe as they have more treatments. This is particularly true for older persons, who may already have some organic brain changes associated with aging.

When vital signs are stable, the patient should be assisted to ambulate. Postural hypotension sometimes occurs, and it is wise to check the blood pressure and pulse in sitting and standing positions before allowing the patient to walk.

On occasion, a patient may become quite agitated as consciousness returns. These persons should be restrained gently to prevent injury. Forceful restraint increases the agitation by frightening the patient. The period of agitation is usually brief. However, it does tend to recur after each treatment. An injection of an antianxiety agent such as hydroxyzine hydrochloride (Vistaril) 30 minutes prior to ECT may alleviate this problem. There is no way to predict prior to the first treatment how a patient will respond during the recovery phase.

When the patient is ambulatory, he may be returned to his own bed and allowed to sleep for about an hour if he wishes. A light breakfast with others who have had ECT is often reassuring and helps orient the patient to the beginning of the day. Patients should then be included in the usual hospital routine. Resumption of normal activity soon after treatment places it in proper perspective as one part of the patient's therapy and not incapacitating.

As stated, confusion may persist to varying extents following the treatment. Nurses must be sensitive to this and provide needed orientation. There may also be some amnesia for the period of time just prior to beginning ECT, which usually subsides gradually after the course of treatment is completed. This may also be frightening to the patient who may fear that he is "losing his mind." Reassurance can be very helpful to these people. Observations about the degree of confusion the patient exhibits should also be reported to the physician, who can sometimes minimize the problem by decreasing the frequency or modifying the technique of administering the ECT.

Some physical discomfort is frequently experienced after ECT. Most patients have a headache ranging from mild to severe. An analgesic should be included in routine ECT orders. Nursing assessment of the patient should include an inquiry about headache, since the patient may be confused about who to ask for medication. There is no need to be concerned about creating a headache when there is none, since the majority of patients do develop one. Analgesia after ECT also helps relieve any muscle soreness. Occasionally, patients also complain of nausea, which is readily relieved by the administration of an antiemetic medication such as trimethobenzamide (Tigan) or prochlorperazine (Compazine).

■　**PATIENT TEACHING.** The amount of information about the actual treatment that is shared with the patient by the nurse should be individualized, based on the patient's ability to understand, his anxiety level, and coping mechanisms. Some people become less anxious when they know and understand a great deal about an anxiety-provoking situation. Others want to know only generalities. It is the nurse's responsibility to assess this prior to initiating patient teaching.

The family should also be included in teaching. At times, when the patient is incapable of decision making, they may be asked to give informed consent for ECT. This is an extremely difficult decision to make for someone else, particularly when the treatment is frightening and surrounded by myth, as is ECT. The nurse can be helpful to the family by providing time for them to discuss their concerns and answering their questions honestly and directly. Frequently the family can be helped to be supportive to the patient, which can alleviate the patient's anxiety. Family members also need to be informed about what to expect of the patient after ECT. Confusion, particularly, may be distressing to them unless they understand that it is expected and temporary. Hospitalized patients are usually completely recovered from the treatment, dressed, and engaged in their usual activities by the time the family visits. This is reassuring to the family. Family members should never be left alone to watch a patient who is recovering from ECT. Predischarge teaching should include both the patient and the family. They need to know that some lingering confusion may exist. For this reason it is helpful to explain medication dosages and schedules to both

the patient and a responsible family member. Outpatient appointments should also be communicated to both the patient and a significant other person. The nursing care of the person who is receiving ECT is summarized in Table 22-2.

If a patient is receiving ECT on an outpatient basis, it is important that the family understand the expected posttreatment behavior. Usually, these patients arrive at the treatment facility in the morning, receive ECT, and remain there until fully awake and ambulatory. They may receive a light breakfast before leaving. The patient must be accompanied by someone who can escort him home after ECT. This is necessary because of the probable presence of confusion and because there will probably be some aftereffects of the anesthesia. The accompanying person should be instructed in how to orient the patient and what to do for headache or nausea, if present. A telephone number should be provided in case any questions arise after the patient has returned home. Outpatient ECT is generally done about once a month as a maintenance treatment for a person who has recovered from a severe depression. The procedure usually goes smoothly, without complications. Outpatient ECT is less frequently given to patients who are acutely ill or who have not had this treatment previously. These patients are usually hospitalized because of the severity of their conditions.

■　**Indications**

Although ECT was originally considered as a treatment for schizophrenia, it did not prove to be particularly helpful to most schizophrenic patients. Affective disturbances, however, were frequently alleviated by treatment with ECT. Until the development of antidepressant medications and the discovery of lithium therapy, ECT was a treatment of choice for affective disorders. It is still useful for patients who cannot tolerate or who fail to respond to treatment with medication. ECT may also be used as an emergency therapy for a patient who is extremely suicidal or so hyperactive that he is in danger physically. ECT is given in these cases to avoid the lag time between initiation of pharmacotherapy and the establishment of a therapeutic level of medication for the individual. For some older persons who tend to be very sensitive to side effects from medication, ECT may be a safer therapeutic modality.[11]

On occasion, ECT may be used for conditions other than affective disorders. It has been effective in the treatment of catatonic stupor or catatonic excitement. It is sometimes still given to paranoid schizophrenic patients but generally with little success. A recent survey conducted by the American Psychiatric Association revealed that most psychiatrists who use ECT recommend it for

TABLE 22-2

NURSING INTERVENTIONS FOR THE PATIENT RECEIVING ELECTROCONVULSIVE THERAPY

Principle	Rationale	Nursing intervention
Informed participation in the procedure	A patient who understands his treatment plan will be more cooperative and experience less stress than one who does not; an informed family is able to provide the patient with emotional support	Educate regarding ECT, including the procedure and expected effects; teach family about the treatment; encourage expression of feelings by patient and family; reinforce teaching after each treatment
Maintain biological integrity	General anesthesia and an electrically induced seizure are physiological stressors and require supportive nursing care	Check emergency equipment prior to procedure; keep NPO several hours before treatment; remove potentially harmful objects, such as jewelry, dentures; check vital signs; maintain patient airway; position on side until reactive; assist to ambulate; offer analgesia or antiemetic as needed
Maintain dignity and self-esteem	Patients are usually fearful preceding the treatment; amnesia and confusion may lead to fear of becoming insane; patient will need assistance to function appropriately in the milieu	Remain with the patient and offer support before and during treatment; maintain the patient's privacy during and following the treatment; reorient the patient; assist family members and other patients to understand behavior related to amnesia and confusion

patients with diagnoses of affective disorders or schizophrenia. A few practitioners use it with other patients, including neurotics and those with organic mental disorders, and a very few use it with children and adolescents. The American Psychiatric Association strongly recommends that research be conducted to validate these less common applications of ECT. It does endorse the helpfulness of ECT for affective disorders and some schizophrenic disorders, particularly those with an affective component.[1] Although some patients may view ECT as punishment, it should certainly never be used for this purpose, nor should a patient be threatened with punishment by ECT.

■ Mechanism of action

The specific way in which ECT works is the subject of a great deal of research, but it has not yet been identified. It used to be believed that ECT alleviated depression because the patient viewed it as punishment. The depressed person was supposed to feel better because the self-directed anger that was at the root of the depression was expressed through the electric shock and the frightening experience of the treatment. This point of view is no longer widely accepted.

It is now believed that there is a biochemical response within the brain to the passage of the electric current in ECT. The observable behavior that indicates that this response has occurred is the convulsion. Several possible mechanisms of action have been identified. The most promising of these is that the seizure activity in the brain produces biochemical changes similar to those induced by antidepressant medications. This and other hypotheses require further research. It is also believed that the mechanism of action which is effective with schizophrenia differs from that which occurs with depression.[1]

The American Psychiatric Association Task Force on ECT[1] ruled out several possible modes of action. Stress or fear induced by anticipation of the procedure has been disproven as a therapeutic effect because simulated ECT is not as effective as actual induction of a convulsion. Because patients are now usually well oxygenated during the procedure, anoxia does not seem to be involved in ECT's effectiveness. Amount of memory loss is unrelated to success of the treatment. Unilateral ECT resulting in less amnesia seems as effective as bilateral, although it may take longer for the therapeutic effect to occur.

Systemic effects of ECT have been identified and may provide clues as to the mechanism of action, as well as providing guidance for safe administration of the treatment. Following the administration of the shock, there is a transient drop in blood pressure and sinus tachycardia. This is followed by sympathetic hyperactivity resulting in increased blood pressure, increased intracranial pressure, and, less frequently, cardiac arrhythmias.[5]

■ Complications

Complications associated with the administration of ECT are infrequent.[11] The only real contraindication to ECT is the presence of a brain tumor, which would cause dangerously increased intracranial pressure during ECT. Prior to the use of muscle relaxants, spontaneous fractures, especially of the spine, occasionally occurred. Cardiac complications, when they do occur, are more likely to be a result of the anesthesia than the ECT. In fact, some authorities believe that it is better not to anesthetize patients with cardiac problems when they receive ECT.[11] Since anesthesia is generally given and since tonic and clonic seizure activity may occur even with the use of muscle relaxants, the pre-ECT workup usually includes an EKG and x-ray films of the spine, skull, and chest. Potential problems can then be prevented.

■ Ethical considerations

The legitimacy of ECT as a form of treatment continues to be debated in psychiatric circles. Many professionals believe that it is a punishment rather than a treatment and that administering a shock to a person is inhumane. Others feel that it is more inhumane to allow a person to suffer the pain of a severe emotional disturbance when ECT frequently provides relief in a short time. Some are concerned that permanent brain damage could result. Others say that it should be given prophylactically to prevent recurrence of problems. It is up to each professional to reach a personal resolution of this debate. These decisions should be based on objective data, including experience with patients who have been treated with and without the use of ECT. Kalayam and Steinhart[10] conducted an attitude survey of a group of patients, professionals, and members of the general public concerning their perceptions of ECT. There was general agreement by all these groups that ECT is an appropriate treatment for certain conditions and that it does cause clinical improvement.

Janicak and colleagues[9] have reported a study of the knowledge and attitudes of mental health professionals regarding ECT. They found that for physicians and nurses knowledge increased with professional experi-ence. As knowledge increased, there was a significant positive change in attitude about ECT. This trend was less pronounced with social workers and not characteristic of psychologists. The investigators concluded that education about ECT should lead to higher levels of acceptance by professionals. If there is an opportunity to observe ECT being administered, the nurse should take advantage of this. Fantasy is usually much different from the reality of the treatment experience. Also, nurses who are unable to accept the use of ECT should try not to communicate negative attitudes to the patient who will have this treatment. ECT continues to be used because it has been found to be helpful to many patients.

Insulin shock therapy

Prior to the use of medication as a treatment for serious emotional disorders, insulin shock therapy was a frequently used treatment modality. Use of insulin therapy was first reported by Sakel in 1933. It is rarely used in contemporary psychiatric facilities.[20] This is primarily because equally good results can be achieved by pharmacotherapy. Insulin shock therapy required a large, specialized nursing staff who could provide intensive nursing care to a small group of patients for several hours. The usual course of therapy was 50 treatments, given at a rate of one per day 5 days a week. Both of these factors made insulin coma an expensive form of therapy. It was also dangerous. If a coma was allowed to continue too long, it became irreversible.[15]

Insulin therapy was induced by the administration of a large dose of insulin intramuscularly. The exact dose needed to cause a coma was individual and was found by starting with a low dose and increasing it over several days until coma resulted. The patient would usually begin to have hypoglycemic symptoms about an hour after the injection, progressing through a stage of disorientation and restlessness to coma after about 3 hours. The length of the coma was then gradually increased to a maximum of an hour. The coma was terminated by administration of glucose solution by nasogastric tube or intravenously or glucagon intramuscularly or intravenously. Close observation of the patient was required for the rest of the day because repeat comas sometimes occurred during the afternoon of the treatment day. Contraindications to insulin coma therapy included serious medical illness, such as cardiovascular, renal, liver, or respiratory disease, untreated hyperthyroidism, and pregnancy.[20]

Future directions

Somatic therapies have always had an important place in the psychiatric nurse's repertoire of skills and will undoubtedly continue to do so. The rate of the growth of knowledge at the present time makes it mandatory that nurses maintain their awareness of current practice through continuing education. Public education is also essential as more and more information is disseminated to the community at large. The consumerism movement has stimulated interest in mental health and psychiatric treatment. Because abuses have occurred in the past, professionals are being held accountable for their actions. Consumer education will be a more and more important priority for the nurse.

At the same time, nurses must examine and resolve their own feelings about the treatments that have been presented in this chapter. Many are intrusive to some extent on the person's exercise of free will and personal decision making. Some seem barbaric and unscientific because the reason for effectiveness is vaguely understood, if at all. Yet the consequences of treatment may be vastly preferable to the continuing pain and disability of a serious mental illness. Each nurse must arrive at a personal answer to the questions raised through experience with these treatment modalities. Each nurse has a contribution to make in adding to the growing store of knowledge about the biological aspects of psychiatric disorders. As knowledge grows, so will satisfaction with the treatment that is given.

■ SUMMARY ■

1. Physical restraint has been used for centuries and is still appropriate at times for treatment of psychiatric patients. Civil liberties must be considered when physical restraint is used.
   a. Mechanical restraints include camisoles, wrist and ankle restraints, sheet restraints, and cold wet sheet packs. The nurse should be familiar with the procedure of applying restraints. Good nursing care includes attention to the patient's biological integrity, interpersonal needs, and right to dignity.
   b. Seclusion or isolation involves the confinement of a patient alone in a room. This procedure should be used infrequently for a short time and with a specific rationale. Good nursing care includes frequent observation of the patient, provision for biological needs, and concern for the patient's dignity and privacy. An open channel of communication with the patient must be maintained.
2. Psychosurgery refers to the surgical interruption of selected neural pathways that govern transmission of emotion between the frontal lobes of the cerebral cortex and the thalamus. Nursing care focuses on postoperative needs plus whatever retraining might be necessary for the patient to function in the usual social setting.
3. Electroconvulsive therapy is the passage of an electrical current through the brain to induce a grand mal seizure. On the average, six to ten treatments are given in a series. Nurses must be supportive to patients who are receiving this frightening treatment. Patient teaching and reassurance are helpful.

DIRECTIONS FOR FUTURE RESEARCH

The following are some of the nursing research problems raised in Chapter 22 that merit further study by psychiatric nurses:
1. Nursing interventions that are effective alternatives to the use of mechanical restraints or seclusion
2. Exploration of the physiological effects of use of the cold, wet sheet pack
3. Correlation of the relationship between nurse attitudes concerning the use of restraints and the effective use of this therapeutic intervention
4. Indicator behaviors that can be used as guidelines for terminating the use of mechanical restraints, cold wet sheet packs, or seclusion
5. Description of the awareness of nurses of the legal and ethical issues related to the use of somatic therapies
6. Elements of the decision-making process that are most effective in determining the need for seclusion
7. The reactions of agitated patients to approaches by individuals or groups of the same, opposite, or both sexes
8. Correlations between characteristics of the milieu and the use of seclusion or restraint
9. Outcome evaluation relative to the psychosocial functioning of patients who have had psychosurgery
10. Nurses' perceptions of the effectiveness of ECT
11. Information concerning ECT that is helpful to patients who are deciding whether to agree to this treatment
12. Identification of patterns of cognitive responses to ECT and exploration of pretreatment predictors of cognitive response
13. Factors that discriminate between depressed patients who will respond better to ECT and those who respond best to medication
14. Predictors of the occurrence of agitation after ECT during the early recovery period
15. Description of patient responses to memory loss and identification of therapeutic nursing interventions

■ SUGGESTED CROSS-REFERENCES ■

Legal issues and ethical decision making are discussed in Chapter 7. Care of suicidal and noncompliant patients is discussed in Chapter 16. Legal issues in psychiatric care are addressed in Chapter 7. Psychopharmacology is presented in Chapter 23. Interventions with violent patients are discussed in Chapter 18.

Later, orientation and supervision are necessary if confusion occurs. The patient may also need help meeting physiological needs.

4. Insulin shock therapy is infrequently used at the present time. A state of physiological shock is induced by injection of high doses of insulin. The patient is gradually brought to the point of coma. Intensive nursing care is required to monitor the patient's condition both during and following the treatment.

■ **REFERENCES** ■

1. American Psychiatric Association: Task force report 14: electroconvulsive therapy, Washington, D.C., 1978, The Association.
2. Donnelly, J.: Psychosurgery. In Kaplan, H.I., Freedman, A.M., and Sadock, B.J., editors: Comprehensive textbook of psychiatry, ed. 3, vol. 3, Baltimore, 1980, The Williams & Wilkins Co.
3. Donnelly, J.: Psychosurgery. In Karasu, T.B., editor: The somatic therapies, Washington, D.C., 1984, American Psychiatric Association.
4. Ewald, F.R., Freeman, W., and Watts, J.W.: Psychosurgery: the nursing problem, Am. J. Nurs. **47**:210, 1947.
5. Frankel, F.H.: Electroconvulsive therapy. In Karasu, T.B., editor: The somatic therapies, Washington, D.C., 1984, American Psychiatric Association.
6. Gutheil, T.G.: Observations on the theoretical bases for seclusion of the psychiatric inpatient, Am. J. Psychiatry **135**:325, 1978.
7. Gutheil, T.G.: Review of individual quantitative studies. In Tardiff, K., editor: The psychiatric uses of seclusion and restraint, Washington, D.C., 1984, American Psychiatric Press, Inc.
8. Gutheil, T.G., and Tardiff, K.: Indications and contraindications for seclusion and restraint. In Tardiff, K., editor: The psychiatric uses of seclusion and restraint, Washington, D.C., 1984, American Psychiatric Press, Inc.
9. Janicak, P.G., et al.: ECT: An assessment of mental health professionals' knowledge and attitudes, J. Clin. Psychiatry, **46**:262, July 1985.
10. Kalayam, B., and Steinhart, M.J.: A survey of attitudes on the use of electroconvulsive therapy, Hosp. Community Psychiatry **32**:185, Mar. 1981.
11. Kalinowsky, L.B.: Convulsive therapies. In Kaplan, H.I., Freedman, A.M., and Sadock, B.J., editors: Comprehensive textbook of psychiatry, ed. 3, vol. 3, Baltimore, 1980, The Williams & Wilkins Co.
12. Lion, J.R., and Soloff, P.H.: Implementation of seclusion and restraint. In Tardiff, K., editor: The psychiatric uses of seclusion and restraint, Washington, D.C., 1984, American Psychiatric Press, Inc.
13. O'Connell, R.A.: A review of the use of electroconvulsive therapy, Hosp. Community Psychiatry **33**:469, June 1982.
14. Okin, R.L.: Variation among state hospitals in use of seclusion and restraint, Hosp. Community Psychiatry, **36**:649, June 1985.
15. Peasley, E.L.: The patient having coma shock treatment, Am. J. Nurs. **49**:623, 1949.
16. *Rogers v. Okin*, 478, Fed. Supp. 1342, 1979.
17. Rosen, H., and DiGiacomo, J.N.: The role of physical restraint in the treatment of psychiatric illness, J. Clin. Psychiatry **39**:228, March 1978.
18. Runck, B.: Consensus panel backs cautious use of ECT for severe disorders, Hosp. Community Psychiatry **36**:943, Sept. 1985.
19. Soloff, P.H., Gutheil, T.G., and Wexler, D.B.: Seclusion and restraint in 1985: a review and update, Hosp. Community Psychiatry **36**:652, June 1985.
20. Surawicz, F.G., and Ludwig, A.M.: Miscellaneous organic therapies. In Kaplan, H.I., Freedman, A.M., and Sadock, B.J., editors: Comprehensive textbook of psychiatry, ed. 3, vol. 3, Baltimore, 1980, The Williams & Wilkins Co.
21. Wexler, D.B.: Legal aspects of seclusion and restraint. In Tardiff, K., editor: The psychiatric uses of seclusion and restraint, Washington, D.C., 1984, American Psychiatric Press, Inc.
22. Whaley, M.S., and Ramirez, L.F.: The use of seclusion rooms and physical restraints in the treatment of psychiatric patients, J. Psychiatr. Nurs. **18**:13, Jan. 1980.
23. *Youngberg v. Romeo*, 102 Supreme Ct 2452 (1982).

■ **ANNOTATED SUGGESTED READINGS** ■

American Psychiatric Association: Task force report 14: electroconvulsive therapy, Washington, D.C., 1978, The Association.

This is a comprehensive report of a task force that was formed by the APA to study the use of ECT. The report is based on an extensive survey of psychiatrists and a thorough review of the literature. It is an excellent source of current information, including recommendations for policies and procedures relative to ECT. There is also a good model for obtaining informed consent.

*Bridges, P., and Williamson, C.: Psychosurgery today, Nurs. Times **73**:1363, 1977.

This article provides a good update on current use of psychosurgery, including indications, evaluation of candidates and preoperative and postoperative care. The authors address the ethical issues related to this procedure and offer suggestions about conducting a psychosurgery unit in an ethical manner. This is a thorough article that is of interest to nurses in neurosurgical and psychiatric settings.

Crowe, R.R.: Electroconvulsive therapy: a current perspective, N. Engl. J. Med. **311**:163, July 1984.

An excellent survey of research on ECT is presented in this article. The author addresses indications and effectiveness, contraindications, mortality, adverse effects, modifications in procedure, and patient acceptance. The conclusion is that this is a safe, effective treatment for mental disorders with an affective component with relatively few complications and side effects.

Asterisk indicates nursing reference.

*Grigson, J.W.: Beyond patient management: the therapeutic use of seclusion and restraint, Perspect. Psychiatr. Care **22**:137, Oct.-Dec. 1984.

The author demonstrates the use of theoretical constructs as a basis for nursing care planning. She describes her theoretical framework, based on psychodynamic theories of behavior. Case examples are provided to demonstrate the model.

Gutheil, T.G.: Observations on the theoretical bases for seclusion of the psychiatric inpatient, Am. J. Psychiatry **135**:325, 1978.

The author has identified conditions under which it is appropriate and inappropriate to seclude a patient. He conveys the belief that this can be a helpful treatment for some patients. However, he also presents drawbacks and contraindications for its use. This is a good overview of some of the debatable issues relative to seclusion.

Karasu, T.B., editor: The somatic therapies, Washington, D.C., 1984, American Psychiatric Association.

This book provides an excellent review of current theory and research in somatic approaches to psychiatric care. It is the somatic therapy component of the report of the American Psychiatric Association Commission on Psychiatric Therapies.

Laitinen, L.V., and Livingston, K.E.: Surgical approaches in psychiatry, Baltimore, 1973, University Park Press.

This highly technical description of the various procedures being developed in the area of psychosurgery is recommended only for the nurse who is directly involved in care of these patients and who has extensive knowledge of neuroanatomy, neurology, and neurosurgery.

*Mulaik, J.S.: Nurses' questions about electroconvulsive therapy, J. Psychiatr. Nurs. **17**:15, Feb. 1979.

This author has comprehensively and concisely described the nursing considerations related to ECT. This article would be an excellent resource for nurses who are about to have their first experience with patients who are receiving ECT. It would also be very helpful to nurses who are planning nursing care with ECT patients.

O'Connell, R.A.: A review of the use of electroconvulsive therapy, Hosp. Community Psychiatry **33**:469, June 1982.

This is an excellent article that presents a complete overview of the use of ECT. The author addresses the major issues of indications, contraindications, risks, procedure, and legal/ethical considerations. Recent research is cited.

*Pilette, P.C.: The tyranny of seclusion: a brief essay, J. Psychiatr. Nurs. **16**:19, Oct. 1978.

This is an admittedly emotional essay opposed to the use of seclusion. It can be a stimulus to thought, leading to discussion and, hopefully, more scientific approaches to this issue.

Runck, B.: Consensus panel backs cautious use of ECT for severe disorders, Hosp. Community Psychiatry **36**:943, Sept. 1985.

This article summarizes the findings of an NIMH consensus panel on ECT. The panel members received testimony from health care providers and consumers, and reviewed research. This summary of their findings provides a complete overview of current information about ECT.

Tardiff, K., editor: The psychiatric uses of seclusion and restraint, Washington, D.C., 1984, American Psychiatric Press, Inc.

This book provides a collection of articles written by many of the most knowledgeable authorities on the uses of seclusion and restraint in psychiatric settings. The contents are comprehensive and include references to research.

*Thomas, S.P.: Uses and abuses of electric convulsive shock therapy, J. Psychiatr. Nurs. **16**:17, Nov. 1978.

The author has thoroughly reviewed the literature pertaining to ECT and has presented the major controversial issues concerning this treatment. The material is presented objectively. A good bibliography is included.

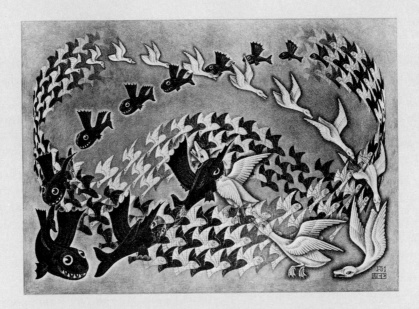

We must recollect that all our provisional ideas in psychology will some day be based on an organic substructure. This makes it probable that special substances and special chemical processes control the operation. . . .

Sigmund Freud

C H A P T E R   2 3

PSYCHOPHARMACOLOGY

MICHELE T. LARAIA

LEARNING OBJECTIVES

After studying this chapter, the student should be able to:

- Identify the role of the nurse in psychopharmacological treatment regimes.

- Describe various aspects of patient assessment prior to the initiation of pharmacotherapy.

- Relate various brain visual imaging techniques being explored in psychiatry.

- Define the concept and implications of polypharmacy and drug interactions.

- Identify reasons for patient noncompliance with pharmacotherapy and related needs for patient education.

- Describe "neurotransmission," including three possible effects of psychotrophic drugs on neurotransmission.

- For each of the four major classes of psychotrophic drugs described in this chapter, explain the mechanism of action.

- For each of the four major classes of psychotrophic drugs described in this chapter, list the clinical indications and target symptoms.

- For each of the four major classes of psychotrophic drugs described in this chapter, identify the related side effects and nursing considerations.

- Discuss guidelines for the administration of drugs from each psychotrophic category including acute and long-term use.

- Identify directions for future nursing research.

- Select appropriate readings for further study.

The past 30 years have produced a revolution in the treatment of psychiatric disorders and in the hypotheses formulated about the pathogenesis of these disorders. This has been due to the introduction of neuropsychopharmacology: drugs that treat the symptoms of mental illness, and whose actions in the brain provide us with models to better understand the mechanisms of mental disorders. This sense of "revolution" continues as new theories are controversially received by experts in the field of drug research, and more centers around the world are funded for clinical research drug studies.

Amidst the growth and controversies of new and sophisticated scientific information, the nurse is frequently the pivotal professional to integrate these treatment drugs with the wide range of non-pharmacologic treatments in a manner that is knowledgeable, safe, effective, and acceptable to the patient. Regardless of the theoretical framework of the nurse, the upheaval in psychiatric treatment will not soon stabilize, and the reality of drug treatment of psychiatric illness must be recognized. Nurses should progress with scientific advancements and incorporate psychopharmacology within the knowledge base of nursing theory, the arena of nursing research, and the art and science of nursing care. Nurses should continue to do what nurses do best—lead the patient through the maze of medical care possibilities

in a holistic manner, incorporating these possibilities into an individualized and effective treatment plan.

This chapter is designed to introduce the nurse to psychopharmacology in a basic way, and to describe some of the important principles of drug treatment in psychiatry. The theoretical framework suggested here is one of integration: drug therapy can complement problem-solving procedures and the wide range of psychodynamic, psychosocial, and interpersonal interventions. Drug therapy should never be viewed as "an easy way out," "a quick fix," or "a miracle pill." At this time, drug therapy treats symptoms of mental illness with some success, but drugs do not treat the personal, social, or environmental responses of the patient to the mental illness. In addition, drug therapy side effects and adverse reactions add another level of concern and need for expertise and judgment in the care of people receiving these treatments. Thus this is a very exciting and optimistic time in psychiatric treatment, and nurses are in an excellent position to add new dimensions to their professional role in this expanding area of patient care.

Role of the nurse

The focus of this chapter on psychopharmacologic drugs used in psychiatry is intended to be integrated with the principles of psychiatric nursing practice presented throughout this text. While it is important that the nurse be knowledgeable about the psychopharmacologic strategies available, this tool must be put in the proper context of a holistic approach to patient care. The psychiatric nurse clinician possesses a wealth of integrated knowledge and techniques that make this role unique in the care of people with psychiatric disorders. The rich potentials of this role continue to be expanded in an all-encompassing and progressive frame of reference. The following are some examples of the role of the nurse in psychopharmacologic treatment regimes.

■ **Collection of pretreatment data.** The nurse is well equipped for the important task of establishing a baseline view of each patient. The nurse brings to this role a rich background in the biological and behavioral sciences, an understanding of the impact of mental illness on the life of the patient, and the ability to integrate an interdisciplinary approach to data collection in a manner which maintains the patient's sense of integrity. These are necessary elements in designing a psychopharmacologic drug trial and treatment plan.

■ **Coordination of treatment modalities.** The nurse has an important role, based on his or her knowledge and relationship with the patient, in designing a viable treatment program for the patient. The most appropriate treatment choices, integrated in a holistic manner and individualized for each patient, should be reflected in the care plan designed by the nurse. The strength of the therapeutic alliance is the single most important factor in a successful treatment program, particularly when psychopharmacology is a component of that program.

■ **Patient education.** Due to the nature of mental illness and the special needs that psychopharmacology brings to the treatment plan, the nurse is in a pivotal position to help integrate complex and varied information for the patient in a manner that is understandable, acceptable, achievable, and often critical for his health and safety.

■ **Monitoring drug effects.** The nurse, usually the most accessible professional to the patient, has the critical role of consistent and knowledgeable monitoring of the effects of psychopharmacologic drugs including their effects on target symptoms of illness, side effects and adverse reactions, and the overall, yet often subtle, effects on the patient's self-concept and sense of trust.

■ **Psychopharmacologic drug administration principles.** No one on the health care team is as able as the nurse is to have daily impact on the patient's experience with psychopharmacologic agents. The nurse administers each medication dose, works out a dosing schedule based on drug requirements and the patient's prefer-

ences, and is continually alert for drug effects. This role defines the nurse as a key professional in the administration of appropriate measures to maximize therapeutic effects of drug treatment, and to minimize drug side effects in such a manner as to include the patient as a true collaborator in his medication regimen.

■ **Viable drug maintenance program.** The nurse is in a position to be the patient's contact with the mental health care system during maintenance drug treatment. For some patients the maintenance program could last many years. Whether the nurse is engaged with the patient in a formal therapeutic contract, or is the designated contact for the patient regarding maintenance pharmacotherapy, the nurse can assume the important role of maintaining a therapeutic alliance with a patient on drug maintenance in the after-care setting.

■ **Concommitant nonpharmacologic treatments.** With advanced clinical preparation, the role of the nurse can extend to clinical therapist. The nurse would then choose from a wide range of therapeutic options for the patient, integrate the treatment plan with the patient's pharmacotherapy regimen, and work with the patient in a formalized, ongoing, psychotherapeutic alliance.

■ **Interdisciplinary clinical research drug trials.** As a member of the interdisciplinary research team, the nurse is in an invaluable position to contribute to the body of scientific knowledge on a large scale, often contributing a nursing perspective to team research efforts. The nurse can be included on several levels, from data collector, to co-investigator, to principal investigator. The roles of the nurse in interdisciplinary clinical research drug trials in the clinical setting are just beginning to be adequately appreciated and defined.

Patient assessment

Psychoactive drugs treat symptoms of mental disorders. However, not all behaviors are treated by drug therapy, and not every identified personality trait is a symptom of illness targeted for treatment with drugs. It thus becomes an important component of patient care to obtain baseline or predrug treatment information about each patient. This information helps describe components of the patient's psychiatric illness as compared to one's premorbid personality. As a result, a list of psychiatric symptoms can be identified as appropriate targets for drug treatment. Residual symptoms of the illness and nonillness-related personality characteristics then become components of nonpharmacological treatments. In addition, drug side effects can be effectively identified and appropriately treated as they emerge. Symptoms indicative of organ system dysfunction caused by drug treatment can be identified and treated.

Finally, careful assessment of each patient can help identify medical illnesses that the patient may have, which are either concurrent with psychiatric illness or possibly causing psychiatric symptomatology. Before initiation of psychopharmacologic treatment, thorough psychiatric evaluation must be completed. Such an evaluation needs to include the following:

1. Thorough physical examination
2. Laboratory studies
3. Mental status evaluation
4. Medical and psychiatric history
5. Medication and drug history
6. Family history

Various tools can be used to assist in the evaluation process. Specifically, the clinician may use a variety of psychological assessment tools and behavioral rating, scales[15] (see Appendix F) that can help not only to define current pretreatment components of the patient's illness but can also be valuable in ongoing assessment to document the patient's progress over time and the efficacy of a treatment regimen. These tools are also useful to compare a patient to the average test results of groups of people within the same diagnostic population. This information can help formulate treatment plans and expectations based on each patient's relationship to the norm of others with the same illness. Behavioral rating scales are also used as objective data-gathering tools in psychopharmacological research studies and are heavily relied upon as objective outcome measures to document efficacy of psychoactive drugs. It is always useful to complement clinical notes with standardized objective measurements. Rating scales are also useful prior to discharge or discontinuation of medication as post-treatment assessments.

In addition, specialized diagnostic procedures, such as electroencephalograms (EEGs) and neurological studies, can provide important information relative to effective treatment agents. More recently, techniques of brain visual imaging are showing great promise for in-

---

Medication and Drug Assessment Tool

1. **Psychiatric medications** (for each medication ever taken by the patient obtain the following information):
   A. Name of drug
   B. Why prescribed?
   C. Date started
   D. Length of time taken
   E. Highest daily dose
   F. Who prescribed it
   G. Was it effective?
   H. Side effects or adverse reactions
   I. Was it taken as prescribed? If not, explain.
   J. Has anyone else in family been prescribed this drug?
   K. If so, why prescribed and was it effective?
2. **Prescription (nonpsychiatric) medications** (for each medication taken by the patient in the past 6 months and for major medical illnesses if more than 6 months ago obtain the following information):
   A. Name of drug
   B. Why prescribed
   C. Date started
   D. Highest daily dose
   E. Who prescribed it?
   F. Was it effective?
   G. Side effects or adverse reactions
   H. Was it taken as prescribed? If not, explain.
3. **Over-the-counter (non prescribed) medications** (for each medication taken by the patient in the past 6 months obtain the following information):
   A. Name of drug
   B. Reason taken
   C. Date started
   D. Frequency of use?
   E. Was it effective?
   F. Side effects or adverse reactions
4. **Alcohol and street drugs** (see Appendix E for common street names of abused substances)
   A. Name of substance
   B. Date of first use
   C. Frequency of use?
   D. Summarize effects
   E. Adverse reactions

creasing knowledge of the pathophysiology of mental illness, enhancing diagnostic assessment, and choosing more specific treatments for individual patients.[8,11] A thorough discussion of the range of psychiatric evaluation procedures is presented in Chapter 6. A firm knowledge of them is necessary for both prescribing and evaluating psychopharmacologic interventions.

Further elements of baseline patient assessment include a longitudinal description of major illnesses, particularly psychiatric illness. These data should include: when the illness began, symptoms, progression, treatments, and treatment outcomes. Family history of illness, particularly psychiatric illness, is also important information. Psychiatric illnesses have been correlated in biological family members, and drug treatments tend to have similar outcomes in family members. For example, if schizophrenia has occurred in a patient's genetic family member, he or she is more likely to get schizophrenia than a person who has no history of this illness in one's genetic line; and he or she is also more likely to get schizophrenia rather than an affective disorder. Furthermore, a drug which successfully treated a family member with the same illness is frequently the first drug of choice to treat the patient. The box on page 702 provides a medication and drug assessment tool for the nurse to use in taking a drug history.

The family history should also include a social support assessment. The family should be integrated into the ongoing treatment process and in the aftercare planning. Family support contributes to patient compliance with treatment regimens and is an important component of holistic nursing care. Family and support system status is essential information in helping the nurse organize the patient's resources and adjunct treatment considerations.

In the initial period of assessing the patient, the nurse should remember that the hospitalization itself, by removing the patient from the stresses in his environment, often results in decreased symptomatology. If the person's behavior is not overtly disruptive, he can be carefully observed during the diagnostic, psychological, and psychosocial evaluation period. A drug-free evaluation period can be particularly useful. One must be certain to determine if the patient had been taking drugs prior to hospitalization which cannot be precipitately withdrawn. If the clinician determines that acute occur, if the symptoms or the patient's behavior are severe enough to preclude a drug-free trial, if the patient has a long history of exacerbations of psychiatric illness, or if the patient is a threat to himself or others, then treatment with psychoactive drugs should be instituted without delay. Hollister[20] provides a succinct guide describing when to use psychopharmacologic drugs.

Pharmacokinetics

Drugs are chemicals that have specific properties that affect treatment. For example, it is often useful to know a drug's half-life. The half-life determines how long it takes to achieve a "steady-state" concentration. Steady-state means that the amount of drug excreted equals the amount ingested, and it occurs in approximately four to six half-lives. Until steady-state is reached, the drug level continues to accumulate, and it fluctuates after each dosing. This accounts for some acute side effects in some patients. It also means that until steady-state is reached the optimal dose for a given patient cannot be determined, nor is a blood level accurate in determining a proper dose range. It may take longer to reach steady-state in the elderly due to slower gastrointestinal activity and liver metabolism.

Another significance of half-life is in frequency of dosing. Usually, a drug with a 24 hour or more half-life can be administered once a day when steady-state is reached and a drug with a shorter half-life should be administered more frequently to achieve constant clinical effects. Termination of drug treatment is also affected by half-life. In general, drugs with long half-lives have inherent tapering, and their effects can last a long time (sometimes weeks) after the last dose. Drugs with a short half-life usually must be tapered (discontinued gradually over several days or weeks). In general, all psychoactive drugs should be discontinued by a tapering period.

The focus of this chapter is on the adult patient, although children and the elderly are frequently administered psychoactive drugs. Generally, adults and children metabolize drugs similarly, although children exhibit a variable response to these drugs. Children must receive lower drug doses because of their lower body weight. Refer to Chapter 30 of this text, and Koplan[22] and Rapoport[31] for further discussion. The elderly and the newborn are particularly sensitive to psychotropic drugs. For the elderly, drug distribution, hepatic metabolism, and renal clearance are all affected by age.[33] If a pregnant woman takes psychoactive drugs prior to delivery, the infant may experience withdrawal symptoms unless the baby is detoxified from the drug. The infant whose mother takes psychoactive drugs generally should not be breast fed.[13,23] Patients with liver disease are extremely sensitive to most psychoactive drugs, and patients with renal impairment are particularly sensitive to lithium.

Guidelines for Polypharmacy

1. Identify specific target symptoms for each drug.
2. If possible, start with one drug and evaluate effectiveness and side effects before adding a second drug.
3. Be alert for adverse drug interactions.
4. Consider the effects of a second drug on the absorption and metabolism of the first drug.
5. Consider the possibility of additive side effects.
6. Change the dose of only one drug at a time and evaluate results.
7. Be aware of increased risk of medication errors.
8. Be aware of increased cost of treatment.
9. Be aware of decreased patient compliance in the aftercare setting when medication regimen is complex.
10. In follow-up treatment, eliminate as many drugs as possible and establish the minimum effective dose of the drugs utilized.
11. Patient education programs regarding concomitant drug regimens must be particularly clear, organized, and effective.
12. Patient follow-up contacts should be more frequent.

Increased Risk Factors for Development of Drug Interactions

Polypharmacy
High doses
Geriatric patients
Debilitated/dehydrated patients
Concurrent illness

Compromised organ system function
Inadequate patient education
History of noncompliance
Failure to include patient in treatment planning

■ Drug interactions

Drugs can interact with each other on two levels.

1. *Pharmacokinetic*—one drug interferes with the absorption, metabolism, distribution, and excretion of another drug, thus raising or lowering its blood and tissue levels
2. *Pharmacodynamic*—one drug combines with another to increase or decrease effects in an organ system

Concurrent use of drugs, or polypharmacy, can enhance a specific therapeutic action, can be necessary to treat concurrent illnesses, and can counteract unwanted effects of the first drug. Unfortunately, there are a number of problems associated with concurrent drug use; confusion over therapeutic efficacy and side effects and development of drug interactions are just a few. In general, polypharmacy in psychiatry should be used only when necessary and with caution. The accompanying boxes list guidelines for polypharmacy and alert the nurse to patients at a higher risk for drug interactions. Table 23-1 is a reference list of the more common drug interactions of psychotropic drugs.

This chapter refers to drugs by their generic names. There is a strong movement in practice to use generic names to be more accurate, to take advantage of price differences, and to avoid confusion when a drug becomes generic (when the patent runs out and the drug can be made by any company). A patent secures a drug for the company that owns it for 18 years from the time the drug is discovered. After the patent expires, other companies can market it, and the price decreases, sometimes drastically. Many drugs which have been in regular use in psychiatry are becoming generic in the 1980s. Once a drug becomes generic, the patient should be educated to use the same brand of a drug, as the bioavailability of psychoactive drugs may vary significantly from one brand to another, thus affecting drug dose and steady-state. The patient can use one pharmacy regularly and can ask the pharmacist to use the same company when filling generic prescriptions of a particular drug.

TABLE 23-1

INTERACTIONS OF PSYCHOTROPIC DRUGS AND OTHER SUBSTANCES

Drug/category	Interacting drug/class	Possible consequences
Antipsychotic agents		
	Antacids, oral	Antacids may inhibit absorption of orally administered phenothiazines
	Central nervous system depressants: alcohol barbiturates antianxiety agents antihistamines narcotic analgesics	Additive central nervous system depression increasing the risk of mental or physical impairment of performance
	Anticholinergic agents: levodopa* (Bendopa, Larodopa, Levopa)	Additive atropinelike side effects; antiparkinson effects of levodopa may be antagonized by antipsychotic agents
Antianxiety agents		
Benzodiazepines	Central nervous system depressants: alcohol barbiturates antipsychotics antihistamines	Potential additive central nervous system effects, especially sedation and decreased daytime performance
	cimetidine	Interferes with metabolism of long-acting benzodiazepines
Antidepressant agents		
Tricyclics	MAO inhibitors*	May cause hypertensive crisis if tricyclic is added to MAO inhibitors
	Alcohol, other central nervous system depressants	*Acute:* additive CNS depression. *Chronic:* may increase tricyclic metabolism.
	Antihypertensives* guanethidine (Ismelin) methyldopa (Aldomet) clonidine (Catapres)	Antagonism of antihypertensive effects with loss of control of blood pressure
	Antipsychotics Anticholinergics	Additive atropinelike effects
	Antiarrhythmics quinidine procainamide	Additive antiarrhythmic effects, prolongation of QRS complex
Mood stabilizer		
Lithium	Diuretics* hydrochlorothiazide	Diuretic-induced sodium depletion can increase lithium levels; may cause toxicity
	Nonsteroidal anti-inflammatory agents* ibuprofen indomethacin phenylbutarone	Increases lithium blood levels; may cause toxicity
Sedative hypnotic agents		
	Alcohol—acutely Analgesics—narcotics Antihistamines Antidepressants Antipsychotics	Combined use of sedative-hypnotics with other central nervous system depressants may impair mental and physical performance (e.g., motor vehicle operation) and result in lethargy, respiratory depression, coma, or death. These drugs may enhance the sedative effects of barbiturates and nonbarbiturates.
	Anticoagulants*—oral	Increased rate of coumarin anticoagulant metabolism, decreasing plasma levels of coumarin and reducing its ability to prevent blood coagulations; higher dose of coumarin required; when barbiturate withdrawn and dose of courmarin not reduced, bleeding episode may occur.

*Potentially clinically significant.

Increased Risk Factors for Patient Noncompliance

Failure to form a therapeutic alliance with the patient
Devaluation of pharmacotherapy by treatment staff
Inadequate patient and family education regarding treatment
Poorly controlled side effects
Insensitivity to patient complaints or wishes
Multiple daily dosing schedule
Polypharmacy
History of noncompliance
Social isolation
Expense of drugs
Failure to appreciate patient's role in drug treatment plan

Lack of continuity of care
Increased restrictions on patient's life-style
Unsupportive significant others
Remission of target symptoms
Increased suicidal ideation
Increased suspiciousness
Unrealistic expectations of drug effects
Failure to target residual symptoms for nonbiological therapies
Relapse or exacerbation of clinical syndrome
Failure to alleviate intrafamiliar and environmental stressors that precipitate symptoms

---

■ Patient education

The importance of taking psychotropic drugs knowledgeably cannot be overemphasized. It is sobering to consider the serious consequences of what can seem to be minor changes in some of the instructions for drug use, such as skipping medication one day, eating cheese, or failing to recognize certain side effects. Patients and their families need thorough and ongoing instruction in the art and science of psychotropic drug treatment. Patient education programs run by nurses have been shown to be effective adjuncts to drug treatment programs for psychiatric patients.[25,35,41]

In addition to normal charting practice, the nurse should be sensitive to the importance of documenting the following issues in the pharmacologic treatment of mental illness:

1. Drugs administered above daily recommended levels
2. Rationale for medication changes
3. Drugs used for other than the indications approved by the Food and Drug Administration
4. Continued use of a drug that is causing clinically significant side effects
5. Polypharmacy rationale

Patients who do not take their drugs as prescribed, or who do not recognize warning signs of drug problems, are at risk for unsuccessful therapeutic results. The box shown above lists common risk factors for patient noncompliance with drug treatment regimens. Youssef[43] found patient eduction to have a positive effect on patient adherence to psychopharmacology.

Based on current trends in psychoactive drug research, the nurse can expect to see new drugs approved for use in mental disorders on a regular basis. It is important to evaluate new drugs as they come into clinical use with a great deal of scrutiny. The nurse should determine the advantages and disadvantages of a new drug as compared to the standard drugs in that class, and in relationship to patient reactions and preferences. The following list is a partial guide to help evaluate a new drug and separate the pertinent facts from a drug company's merchandising descriptions. The nurse should be able to answer questions concerning whether the new drug has:

1. A different mechanism of action more specific to desired biological actions
2. Quicker onset of action
3. Fewer drug interactions
4. A lower side effect profile
5. No addictive or abuse potential
6. No long-term adverse effects
7. No suicide potential
8. Effects on neurotransmitter regulation in a permanent, or curative manner
9. Several routes of administration, at least PO and IM
10. A wide therapeutic index
11. Fewer discontinuation problems
12. Cost effectiveness

Finally, the administration of psychotherapeutic drugs is an empowering experience. It is essential for the nurse to explore the many implications of this. The

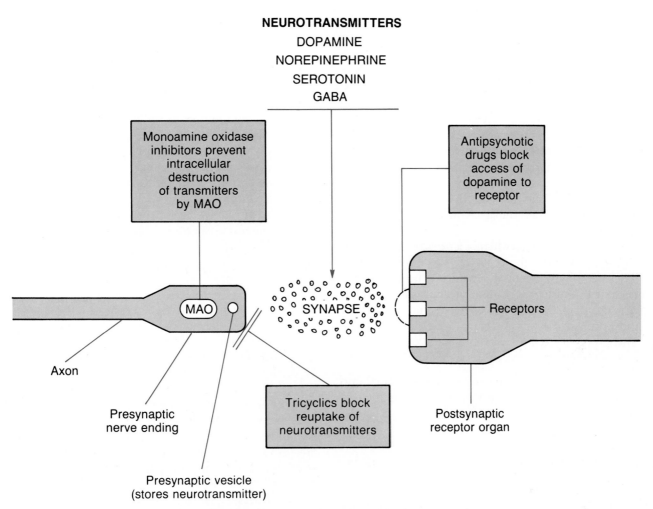

NEUROTRANSMITTERS

DOPAMINE

NOREPINEPHRINE

SEROTONIN

GABA

Monoamine oxidase inhibitors prevent intracellular destruction of transmitters by MAO

Antipsychotic drugs block access of dopamine to receptor

MAO

SYNAPSE

Receptors

Axon

Presynaptic nerve ending

Tricyclics block reuptake of neurotransmitters

Postsynaptic receptor organ

Presynaptic vesicle (stores neurotransmitter)

Fig. 23-1. Neurotransmission at the synapse.

nurse should never withhold a drug that a patient needs. It is also the nurse's obligation to be aware of counter-transference issues and personal attitudes toward the individual patient, the prescribing physician, the patient's diagnosis, and his psychotropic drug treatment regimen. Effective and safe drug treatment in psychiatry is dependent on many factors, not the least of which is the impact of the nurse.

■ **Biological basis for psychopharmacology**

All communication in the brain involves neurons "talking" to each other at synapses. These nerve cells are the basic functional unit of the nervous system. The study of this communication process forms the basis of much of the neurosciences.[38] The following description is simplified to present a very basic frame of reference from which to view the rather overwhelming complexity of neuropharmacological mechanisms.

The synapse is a narrow gap separating two neurons (the presynaptic cell and the postsynaptic cell) at a transmission site (see Figure 23-1). During neurotransmission, there is a release of the chemical neurotransmitter from a storage vesicle in the presynaptic cell, and the neurotransmitter then crosses the synapse. The receptor on the postsynaptic cell membrane recognizes the chemical (this is called binding). Receptors are the cellular recognition sites for specific molecular structures, like neurotransmitters, hormones, and many drugs. Thus their action is selective for specific chemicals. Neurotransmitters, the "chemical messengers" which travel from one brain cell to another, are synthesized by enzymes from certain dietary amino acids, or precursors. At the synapse, neurotransmitters act as receptor activators (agonists) or inhibitors (antagonists) and trigger complex biological responses within the cell. The chemical remaining in the synapse is either reabsorbed and stored by the presynaptic cell or is metabolized (inactivated) by synaptic enzymes, one of which is monoamine oxidase.

Many of the psychiatric disorders are thought to be caused by an overresponse or an underresponse somewhere along the complex process of neurotransmission. For instance, psychosis is thought to involve excessive dopamine neurotransmission. Depression and mania are thought to result from disruption of normal patterns of neurotransmission of norepinephrine, serotonin, and other neurotransmitters. Anxiety, poorly understood at this time, is thought to be a dysregulation of gamma-aminobutyric acid (GABA) and endogenous antianxiety chemicals, the first of which was discovered in 1985.

If one understands whether a particular psychiatric illness seems to be the result of "too much" or "too little" neurotransmission in a particular neurotransmitter system, and the mechanism of action of the psychiatric drugs, one begins to recognize some order in the various pharmacological strategies used in psychiatry. This process of cell-to-cell communication at the synapse can be affected by drugs in several important ways:

1. Release: More neurotransmitter is released into the synapse from the storage vesicles in the presynaptic cell.
2. Blockade: The neurotransmitter is prevented from binding to the postsynaptic receptor.
3. Receptor sensitivity changes: The receptor becomes more or less responsive to the neurotransmitter.
4. Blocked re-uptake: The presynaptic cell does not reabsorb the neurotransmitter well, leaving more neurotransmitter in the synapse and therefore enhancing or prolonging its action.
5. Interference with storage vesicles: The neurotransmitter is either released again into the synapse (more neurotransmitter) or is released to metabolizing enzymes (less neurotransmitter).
6. Precursor chain interference: The process which "makes" the neurotransmitter is either facilitated (more neurotransmitter is synthesized) or disrupted (less neurotransmitter).
7. Synaptic enzyme interference: Less neurotransmitter is metabolized, so more remains available in the synapse.

Not all the above strategies have yielded clinically relevant treatments. Several have, however, and will be emphasized in this chapter (see Figure 23-1): antipsychotic drugs block dopamine from the receptor site; tricyclic antidepressants block the reuptake of norepinephrine and serotonin; monoamine oxidase inhibitors prevent enzymatic metabolism of norepinephrine

and serotonin; and benzodiazepines potentiate GABA.

Understanding this process has led to the variety of treatment approaches in pharmacotherapy that attempt to change or modify one or more of the steps in neurotransmission. Unfortunately, to date, the actions of psychopharmacologic drugs are not confined to the specific brain areas that are thought to be associated with psychiatric symptoms. These drugs spread out in the body, causing unwanted drug reactions or side effects, and undesirable drug interactions during concomitant drug therapy. Current psychopharmacologic research attempts to better understand the etiology of psychiatric illness at the neurotransmission level, and the increased specificity of psychopharmacologic drugs.[9,24,37]

Antianxiety and sedative-hypnotic drugs

The diagnosis of anxiety is based on the patient's description and the nurse's observation of behaviors, and the process of elimination of alternative diagnoses. The possibility of a medical etiology must be considered. Hyperthyroidism, hypoglycemia, and severe pulmonary disease are characteristic illnesses associated with high levels of anxiety. In addition to a careful review of systems and standard baseline laboratory tests, the patient should be asked about use of over-the-counter drugs, "recreational" substances, alcohol, and caffeine. Anxiety also accompanies many psychiatric disorders. In general, the primary disorder should be treated with the appropriate medication. Anxiety may be associated with psychosis or an affective disorder and often goes away when the target symptoms for the primary disorder subside with appropriate treatment.

This section divides antianxiety and sedative-hypnotic drugs into two categories: the benzodiazepines and non-benzodiazepines, which includes several classes of drugs. The benzodiazepines are the most widely prescribed drugs in the world, and within the last two decades they have almost entirely replaced the barbiturates in the treatment of anxiety and sleep disorders. Their popularity is related to their effectiveness and wide margin of safety and they are the principal drugs used in the treatment of anxiety and insomnia.

■ Benzodiazepines

■ **MECHANISM OF ACTION.** The benzodiazepines are thought to exert their antianxiety effects because they are powerful potentiators of the inhibitory neurotransmitter gamma-aminobutyric acid (GABA), although the role of GABA in anxiety is not yet clear. A postsynaptic receptor site specific for the exogenous benzodiazepine molecule has been discovered. The search for the naturally occurring "anti-anxiety" chemical has recently resulted in the discovery of an endogenous benzodiazepine-binding inhibitor (DBI). It is interesting to note that the benzodiazepine molecule and GABA do not compete for the same receptor site. However, the benzodiazepines do compete with DBI for a role in neurotransmission indicating that DBI may be the antianxiety neurotransmitter. Ongoing research in this field promises to give us a great deal of information in the near future.

■ **CLINICAL USE.** The benzodiazepines are the drug treatment of choice in the management of anxiety, insomnia, and stress-related conditions. The target symptoms for the use of these drugs are listed in the accompanying box. The major indications for their use are generalized anxiety disorder, anxiety associated with depression, sleep disorders, anxiety associated with phobic disorders, post-traumatic stress disorder, alcohol and drug withdrawal, anxiety associated with medical disease, skeletal muscle relaxation, seizure disorders, and the anxiety and apprehension experienced preoperatively. Major studies are beginning to show that higher dose benzodiazepines, particularly alprazolam, a triazolobenzodiazepine, appear to have specific antipanic effects in the treatment of agoraphobia.

The specific types of benzodiazepines in general have no significant clinical advantages over each other. Some rational prescribing decisions can be made based on whether or not they break down into active metabolites which extend drug half-life (Table 23-2). Duration of action after a single dose can be relatively brief, depending on how rapidly the drug is metabolized and how extensively it is distributed to body tissues (in turn, this is based on lipid solubility). Duration of action at steady-state can be much longer. Differences in half-life can be clinically useful. For example, patients with persistent high levels of anxiety should take a drug with a long half-life. Patients with fluctuating anxiety might be better off with short-acting drugs. The benzodiazepines used as hypnotics ideally should induce sleep rapidly, and their effect should be gone by morning. The rate of absorption of the different benzodiazepines from the gastrointestinal tract varies considerably, thus affecting the rapidity and intensity of onset of their acute effects. Diazepam and chlorazepate are absorbed fastest, while prazepam and oxazepam are slowest. Antacids or food in the stomach slow this process.

Because the benzodiazepines are in the same pharmacological class as alcohol, they can be used to suppress the alcohol withdrawal syndrome. The concomitant use of these two substances can be dangerous by producing extreme sedation. Some of the differences suggested for the use of these drugs can be attributed more to marketing strategies than clinical efficacy. Any of the benzodiazepines can be effective sedative-hypnotics when administered at bedtime.[42]

Although some patients may need to take antianxiety drugs for extended periods of time, the drugs are not without their drawbacks and should always be used concomitantly with nonpharmacological treatments for the patient who experiences anxiety more chronically. Psychotherapy, behavioral techniques, environmental manipulations, and an ongoing therapeutic relationship continue to have an important place in treatment of anxiety disorders.

Most experts feel that medication treatment with benzodiazepines should be brief, during a time of specific stress. Those with a long half-life (greater than 18–24 hours) can be given once a day. Those with a short half-life (8–15 hours) need to be given more frequently. They can be taken as needed for increased symptoms of anxiety that are intermittent. The patient should be observed frequently during the early days of treatment to assess target symptom response and monitor side effects so that the dose can be titrated. Some patients, however, require long-term antianxiety medication treatment. Plasma concentrations of benzodiazepine drugs

---

Target Symptoms for Antianxiety and Sedative-Hypnotic Benzodiazepines

Psychological

Vague sense of irritability and uneasiness
Sense of impending doom or panic
Insomnia

Physical

Flushed skin
Hot or cold flashes
Sweating
Dilated pupils
Dry mouth
Nausea or vomiting
Diarrhea
Tachycardia, palpitations
Dizziness, light-headedness
Shortness of breath
Hyperventilation, with paresthesias
Tremor
Restlessness
Headache
Urinary frequency

TABLE 23-2

ANTIANXIETY AND SEDATIVE-HYPNOTIC DRUGS: THE BENZODIAZEPINE CLASS

Drug family				Drug dosage		
Chemical class generic name (Trade name)	Active metabolites	Half-life (hr)	Days to steady state	Equivalence (mg)	Usual dosage range (mg/day)	Available forms (mg)
Antianxiety drugs						
Benzodiazepines						
alprazolam (Xanax)	Yes (Not signifi-cant)	6–20	3	0.5	0.5–4	tabs: 0.25, 0.5, 1.0
chlordiazepoxide (Librium)	Yes	5–200	1–3	10	20–100	tabs: 5, 10, 25 inj: 100
chlorazepate (Tranxene)	Yes	30–200	5–16	7.5	7.5–60	tabs: 3.75, 7.50, 15
diazepam (Valium)	Yes	20–200	4–8	5	10–40	tabs: 2, 5, 10, sus-tained release 15 inj: 5/ml
halazepam (Paxipam)	Yes	20–100	4	20	80–160	tabs: 20, 40
lorazepam (Ativan)	No	10–20	2–3	1	2–6	tabs: 0.5, 1, 2 inj: 2/ml, 4/ml
oxazepam (Serax)	No	5–15	1–2	15	15–90	tabs: 10, 15, 30
prazepam (Centrax)	Yes	30–200	5–32	10	10–60	tabs: 5, 10, 20
Sedative-hypnotic drugs						
Benzodiazepines						
flurazepam (Dalmane)	Yes	30–250	4–8	15	15–60	caps: 15, 30
temazepam (Restoril)	No	10–20	2–3	15	15–30	caps: 15, 30
triazolam (Halcion)	No	1.5–4	1	0.25	0.25–0.5	tabs: 0.25, 0.50

have not yet been firmly correlated to clinical effects, although they may be ready for general clinical use in the near future. All the benzodiazepines are rapidly absorbed by mouth. The injectable benzodiazepines have been proven reliable when administered in the deltoid muscle and lead to rapid and predictable rises in the blood level when used IV. When utilized intravenously, administration should be slow (over 1 minute) and direct, not mixed in an IV infusion, because plastic tubing absorbs the drug and the drug can precipitate when mixed with saline or dextrose.

Another clinical indication for the use of benzodiazepines is as sedative-hypnotics to improve sleep. Insomnia (poor sleep) is characterized by either difficulty

falling asleep, difficulty staying asleep, or awakening too early. It is a symptom with many etiologies and often responds to creative nonpharmacologic strategies, such as talking about problems, increased daytime exercise, and physical comfort measures at night. Drugs to induce sleep have their place, but should be used with discretion and are never a substitute for good nursing care.

■ **ADVERSE REACTIONS.** The benzodiazepines have a very high therapeutic index, thus overdoses of benzodiazepines alone almost never cause fatalities. Side effects are common, dose related, and almost always harmless. Table 23-3 summarizes these reactions and nursing considerations. The benzodiazepines generally

TABLE 23-3

BENZODIAZEPINE SIDE EFFECTS AND NURSING CONSIDERATIONS

Side effects	Nursing considerations
Acute/Common	
Drowsiness, sedation	Activity helps; caution when using machinery
Ataxia, dizziness	Caution with activity, prevent falls
Feelings of detachment	Discourage social isolation
Increased irritability or hostility	Observe carefully, offer support, be alert for disinhibition of control over socially unacceptable impulses
Anterograde amnesia	Inability to recall events that occur while the drug is active; desirable in preoperative use
Long Term/Common	
Minor tolerance to some effects	Short-term use if possible; discontinue, utilizing a slow taper; not recommended for use with people with history of drug or alcohol abuse
Dependency	
Rebound insomnia/anxiety	
Rare (causal relationship uncertain)	
Increased appetite and weight gain	Weight control measures
Cutaneous reactions	Usually not clinically significant
Nausea	Dose with meals, decrease dose
Headache	Usually responds to mild analgesic
Confusion	Decrease dose
Gross psychomotor impairment	Dose related, decrease dose
Depression	Decrease dose; may require antidepressant treatment
Paradoxical rage reaction	Discontinue drug

do not live up to their reputation of being strongly addictive if their discontinuation is accomplished by gradual tapering, if they have been used for appropriate purposes, and if their use has not been complicated by other substances, like chronic use of barbiturates or alcohol.

Tolerance does develop to the sedative effects of benzodiazepines, but it is unclear whether sleep maintenance or antianxiety effects develop tolerance. Taper should be relatively slow to minimize withdrawal symptoms and to minimize rebound symptoms of insomnia or anxiety. The general rule is a decrease by 5% of the dose each 1 to 3 days, although this varies. All benzodiazepines, regardless of half-life, should be discontinued by tapering. When these drugs are discontinued too rapidly, or precipitously stopped, especially with prolonged use of high doses, a benzodiazepine withdrawal syndrome can occur as described in the accompanying box. If this occurs, it is necessary to raise the dose until symptoms are gone and then resume a slower taper.[36]

The geriatric patient is more vulnerable to side effects because the aging brain is more sensitive to sedatives. The benzodiazepines with no active metabolites

Benzodiazepine Withdrawal Syndrome

Usually worsens several days after taper begins, and increases over several weeks, then subsides. Minimize by slowing taper.

Mild Symptoms	Severe Symptoms
Tremulousness	Diarrhea
Insomnia	Hypotension
Dizziness	Hyperthermia
Headaches	Neuromuscular irritability
Tinnitus	Psychosis
Anorexia	Seizures
Vertigo	
Blurred vision	
Agitation	
Anxiety	

are less affected by liver disease, age of the patient, or drug interactions. Use of benzodiazepines during pregnancy has been associated with infant cleft lip/cleft palate, multiple congenital deformities and intrauterine growth retardation, especially when used during the first trimester. When used late in pregnancy or during breast feeding, these drugs have been associated with "floppy infant syndrome," neonatal withdrawal symptoms, poor sucking, and hypotonia. More detailed description of the benzodiazepines can be found in reviews by Ballenger[4] and Greenblatt and co-workers.[14]

■ Non-benzodiazepines

The advantages of the benzodiazepines when compared to most other antianxiety and sedative-hypnotic agents have led to greatly decreased use of these drugs. Non-benzodiazepine anxiolytics and sedative-hypnotics, listed in Table 23-4, are used when alternatives to benzodiazepines are sought, or when preferred by physicians or patients.

The barbiturates have been largely replaced by the benzodiazepines, although they are used occasionally. There are numerous disadvantages to their use: tolerance develops to the antianxiety effects of barbiturates; they are more addictive; they cause serious, and even lethal withdrawal reactions; they are dangerous in overdose, and cause CNS depression; and they have a variety of dangerous drug interactions.

The propranediol, meprobamate, has also dropped in popularity. Adverse effects, drug interactions, liability to abuse, and withdrawal syndromes resemble those observed with barbiturates. Also, many studies show meprobamate to be no more effective than placebo.

The quinazoline, methaqualone (Quaalude), has

TABLE 23-4

THE ANTIANXIETY, SEDATIVE-HYPNOTIC DRUGS: NON-BENZODIAZEPINES

Chemical class generic name (Trade name)	Hypnotic dose (mg)	Half-life (hr)
Barbiturates		
secobarbital (Seconal)	100–200	19–34
pentobarbital (Nembutal)	100–200	15–48
amobarbital (Amytal)	100–200	8–42
butabarbital (Butisol)	100–200	34–42
phenobarbital (Luminal)	100–200	24–140
Propanediols		
meprobamate (Equanil, Miltown)	800	10
Acetylinic alcohols		
ethychlorvynol (Placidyl)	500–1000	10–25
Piperidinediones		
glutethimide (Doriden)	250–500	5–22
methyprylon (Noludar)	200–400	4
Chloral derivatives		
chloral hydrate (Noctec, Somnos)	500–2000	4–10
chloral betaine (Beta-Chlor)	870–1740	4–10
triclofos sodium (Triclos)	750–1500	4–10
Monoureides		
paraldehyde (Paral)	3000–8000 (liquid)	brief
Antihistamines		
diphenhydramine (Benadryl)	50	unknown
hydroxyzine (Atarax)	100 tid	unknown
Serotonin precursor		
tryptophan	250–1500	unknown
Beta-adrenergic blocker		
propranolol (Inderal)	10 qid	3
Anxiolytic		
buspirone (Buspar)	10–40	2–5

been popular intermittently since the 1970s and has a high abuse history. Due to this and the other usual CNS problems observed with practically all hypnotics, this drug has been taken off the market.

Ethychlorvynol, an acetylinic alcohol, has a variety of side effects: confusion, hangover, ataxia, hypotension, and GI distress. Physical dependence occurs, tolerance develops, abuse is possible, and discontinuation can cause withdrawal reactions.

The piperidinedione derivatives have all the drawbacks of the barbiturates without any added advantages. They have remained in use despite their low therapeutic index, high lethality, and addiction potential because they produce relatively few unwanted effects at therapeutic doses.

Chloral derivatives can cause gastrointestinal irritations and have a variety of drug interactions. Tolerance, physical dependence, addiction, and a withdrawal syndrome are all problems with these drugs. In general, these agents are best avoided.

Paraldehyde, a foul-smelling liquid which is extremely irritating to the body's tissues, produces tolerance, dependence, and withdrawal syndromes. It is difficult to handle and affords no benefits over safer, more pleasant drugs.

Antihistamines, especially hydroxyzine, are usually not as effective as the benzodiazepines, cause sedation, but do not cause physical dependence or abuse. A disadvantage of the antihistamines is that they lower the seizure threshold.

Tryptophan is an essential amino acid present in various foods and is a precursor of serotonin. Serotonin is believed to play an important role in sleep. Because tryptophan is a natural food substance, it is not patentable, has been poorly studied, is not FDA regulated; thus, its composition is variable. Supplies contaminated with toxic matter have been found in some health food stores. In general, tryptophan has few unwanted effects and does not seem to cause long-term toxicity, acute intoxication, dependence, or withdrawal reactions.

Propranolol blocks beta-noradrenergic receptors centrally and in the peripheral cardiac and pulmonary systems. This drug probably decreases certain physiological symptoms of anxiety, especially tachycardia, rather than centrally acting on anxiety. Defining a proper role for propranolol in the treatment of anxiety requires more research.[19]

Buspirone, a non-benzodiazepine anxiolytic drug, has been the subject of much discussion. It appears to be a potent antianxiety agent with no addictive potential. It has become available as Buspar in late 1986 and, like all new drugs, will require careful clinical scrutiny.[2]

Antidepressant drugs

The 1950s were a pivotal time in the history of psychopharmacology with the discovery of drugs that were effective in treating depression. Early in the 1950s, dramatic improvements in mood and well-being were noted in tuberculosis patients being treated with iproniazid before improvement in the tuberculosis lesion was noted. This led to the use of monoamine oxidase inhibitors (MAOIs) as primary drug treatments for depression. The first tricyclic antidepressant (TCA), imipramine, was initially tested for potential antipsychotic activity. It was found to be an ineffective antipsychotic, but depression improved. It was marketed in 1958 for its significant antidepressant properties. These two types of drugs, the MAO inhibitors and the tricyclics, remain the major antidepressant medications at present.

Research on the biology of depression has been intense and rewarding, although many new discoveries have led to even more questions. It has been proposed that both serotonin and/or norepinephrine are relatively reduced in depression, and norepinephrine is in excess in mania. The biological understanding of antidepressant drugs supports this theory: monoamine oxidase inhibitors "inhibit" the metabolism of these neurotransmitters, and tricyclic antidepressants block their re-uptake at the presynaptic neuron. Both these mechanisms result in allowing more neurotransmitter to remain in the synapse, therefore solving the functional "deficit" in depression. Several problems challenge the simplicity of this theory: 25% to 30% of people who are depressed do not respond to antidepressant drugs, and several new drugs that seem to be effective antidepressants do not appear to affect norepinephrine or serotonin levels. There is also evidence that antidepressants regulate the locus ceruleus, the part of the brain that makes most of the norepinephrine.

The integrative model of depression proposed by Akiskal and co-workers[1] more than 10 years ago continues to support the holistic approach to patient care so important to psychiatric nursing (see Chapter 15). This model suggests that many factors contribute in varying degrees to a functional impairment of central nervous system centers that help to maintain mood, motor activity, appetite, sleep, and libido. Among the list of predisposing and precipitating stressors for depression are biological vulnerability, developmental deficits, and physiological, psychological, and social factors.

The primary clinical indication for the use of antidepressant drugs is major depressive illness. They are also useful in the treatment of panic disorder, and enuresis in children. A variety of preliminary research stud-

TABLE 23-5

PREDICTORS OF ANTIDEPRESSANT RESPONSE

Tricyclics	MAOI
Positive predictors	
Anorexia	Hypochondriasis
Weight loss	Somatic anxiety
Insomnia (middle and late)	Irritability
Diurnal mood swing	Agoraphobia
Psychomotor retardation	Social phobias
Agitation	Anergia
Decreased functioning	Hysterical traits
Acute onset	Bipolar disorder
Family history of depression	Unresponsive to other antidepressants
Self and family history of drug responsiveness	
Therapeutic blood levels of antidepressants	
Agoraphobia (imipramine)	
Negative predictors	
Presence of other psychiatric disturbances	Depressed mood
Chronic symptoms	Guilt
Psychotic features	Ideas of reference
Predominant somatic symptoms	Nihilistic delusions
Previous unsuccessful drug trials	Affective personality disorders
Previous sensitivity or adverse reactions	

Modified from Schoonover, S.C.: In Bassuk, E.L., Schoonover, S.C., and Gelenberg, A.J., editors: The practitioner's guide to psychoactive drugs, ed. 2. New York & London, 1984, Plenum Medical Books Co. and Nardil: Parke-Davis Product Monograph, ed. 4. Morris Plains, N.J., 1982, Park-Davis, Medical Affairs Department.

ies suggest their usefulness in attention deficit disorders in children, bulimia, obsessive-compulsive disorder, and narcolepsy. Table 23-5 lists predictors of antidepressant response to guide the clinician in the appropriate choice of the type of antidepressant drug.

The treatment of depression today is greatly enhanced by a variety of therapeutically effective drugs, yet depressive illness remains frequently misdiagnosed and often undertreated. It is estimated that 20 million Americans suffer from a serious depressive disorder each year, and suicide is the most frequent complication of depression. Suicide is the tenth greatest cause of death for all ages and the leading cause of death in adults under 25 and young adolescents. The suicide rate in people with unrecognized or inadequately treated depression is 60 times the rate of suicide in nondepressed patients. These statistics are alarming and make vigorous and thorough treatment of depressive illness a mandate for ethical care. When pharmacotherapy is a component of the treatment regimen for a depressed patient, the nurse can help minimize side effects, assess drug effectiveness, and maximize patient safety and drug efficacy. Stimmel[39] and Hayes and Bloom[18] provide guides for nurses treating patients with antidepressants.

■ Biological markers

Perhaps more than in any other diagnostic category investigators have identified biological markers of clinical usefulness in the diagnosis and treatment of depression. These tests, however, are not 100% accurate, research results are often contradictory, they are new and expensive, and they uphold the biological psychiatry frame of reference. Thus, they are controversial. They merit recognition by nurses because of their increasing popularity, and because biological markers are an important research endeavor with implications for the future understanding of exogenous "chemical" treatments in mental illness.

■ **URINARY MHPG.** Norepinephrine, when metabolized, is broken down into several other chemicals. A main metabolite of norepinephrine is 3-methoxy-4-hydroxy-phenylglycol (MHPG). This metabolite crosses the blood–brain barrier, thus its CNS activity can be estimated by measuring MHPG elimination in urine. This measurement is complicated by the fact that peripheral MHPG is also excreted in the urine, although urinary MHPG is felt by many investigators to give us accurate clues about levels of brain norepinephrine. An aliquot is taken from a 24-hour urine collection, on a day (it is hoped) that is average for the individual patient in terms of activity, anxiety, and dietary tyramine ingestion. Serotonin, on the other hand, can be validly measured only in cerebrospinal fluid, since its main metabolite, 5-HIAA, does not cross the blood–brain barrier. Investigators have proposed that patients with low MHPG have less norepinephrine to metabolize, and thus theoretically would respond to an antidepressant which blocks the re-uptake of norepinephrine. Some evidence suggests patients with normal or high MHPG have a serotonin-deficient depression (since their norepinephrine levels are not low) and would respond to a drug that better blocks serotonin re-uptake.

Table 23-6 lists the degree to which each of the antidepressant drugs is thought to potentiate these neurotransmitters. The clinical implication here is that if an adequate trial of desipramine (4+ norepinephrine) is unsuccessful, the next antidepressant of choice should be a serotonin potentiator, like amitriptyline, or tra-

TABLE 23-6

PHARMACOLOGIC PROFILES OF THE ANTIDEPRESSANTS

Antidepressant drug	Acute side effects			Potentiation of neurotransmitter			Antianxiety effect
	Anti-cholinergic	Cardio-vascular	Sedative	5-HT	NE	DA	
Tricyclic agents							
amitriptyline	4	4	4	3	1	0	4
amoxapine	3	2	3	1	4	0	2
desipramine	1	2	1	0	4	0	1
doxepin	4	2	4	2	1	0	3
imipramine	4	3	3	2	3	0	2
nortriptyline	3	3	2	2	3	0	1
protriptyline	2	3	1	2	4	0	0
trimipramine	4	3	4	2	3	0	3
Nontricyclic agents							
bupropion	1	1	0	0	0	0	0
maprotiline	3	2	3	0	4	0	3
trazodone	0	1	4	4	0	0	4

4 = high   3 = moderate   2 = low   1 = slight   0 = none
5-HT = serotonin   NE = norepinephrine   DA = dopamine

zodone. If this drug is also unsuccessful, the third drug trial might be with a monoamine oxidase inhibitor, which has a completely different mechanism of action. Although it is still highly theoretical, this type of system takes the choice of antidepressant drugs from a "grab-bag" to a scientifically based decision-making process. The hope for the future is that a simple urine or blood test will reliably indicate which antidepressant drug to use for each individual patient, saving what could be several months of frustrating, not to mention expensive and dangerous (if the patient is suicidal) unsuccessful drug trials.

■ **DEXAMETHASONE SUPPRESSION TEST.** Another biological marker for depression in current use is the dexamethasone suppression test, or DST. Researchers have established that a majority of depressed people have cortisol secretion that does not follow the usual biological rhythm documented in nondepressed people. Normal cortisol levels are relatively flat from late afternoon until about 3 A.M., when they begin to spike at regular intervals until about noon. They then begin to level out again. Biologically depressed people have been found to have erratic spikes over a 24-hour period. The DST involves giving a small dose of the synthetic steroid, dexamethasone, at 11 P.M., and drawing plasma cortisol at 4 P.M. the next day. The dexamethasone usu-

ally suppresses pituitary ACTH and circulating adrenal steroids for at least 24 hours with no ill effects to the patient. Researchers report that between 40% and 70% of depressed people "escape" the cortisol suppression. That is, at some time in the next 24 hours, their cortisol levels return to erratic, above normal spikes. If the post-dexamethasone cortisol level is ≥ 5 ng/ml, then it "escaped" suppression, and support is added for a diagnosis of biological depression.

The most consistent and currently helpful use for the DST is to repeat this test after depressive symptoms have remitted. If the DST was abnormal previously and has not yet normalized, continued antidepressant drug treatment is indicated. If a depressed patient's initial DST is normal, assuming it is accurate, it means the DST is not helpful in confirming a diagnosis of biological depression. In either case, it is important to include nonpharmacologic assessments and interventions when treating most people with depression, considering the impact this illness has on the well-being of the individual person and society as a whole.

■ **REM LATENCY MEASUREMENT.** Using electro-encephalographic tracings during sleep, researchers have identified five patterns, or stages, of sleep. The sleep cycle begins with stage one, the lightest sleep stage, which is followed by successively deeper stages two, three, and four. Stages three and four are characterized by increasing quantities of slow (delta) waves and probably have a restorative effect on body metabolic functions. After this initial cycle of the four stages of sleep, about 60 to 90 minutes in the normal person, the fifth cycle, or rapid eye movement (REM) sleep begins. REM is associated with dreaming, decreased muscle tone, and fast-frequency, low-amplitude EEG waves. This sleep cycle repeats itself approximately four to six times each night, at intervals of approximately 90 minutes. Depressed patients have been shown to spend less time in the more refreshing slow-wave phases of sleep, may have increased periods of REM sleep, and typically have a shorter than normal period before their first REM phase; this is called decreased REM latency, and it provides us with another biological marker for depression. When sleep studies are done on depressed patients, they frequently attain REM sleep within minutes to a half hour after falling asleep, rather than the normal 90 minutes, thus adding another indication for a diagnosis of depression.

■ Tricyclic antidepressants

■ **MECHANISM OF ACTION.** As new antidepressants were discovered and researched, their varied actions at the synapse went far beyond the simple reuptake blockade theory. Most experts now feel that depressions can have several different biological mechanisms. It remains the task of future research to expand current knowledge and to further refine drugs with specific mechanisms of action to treat depressions with specific biological abnormalities.

Although the class of tricyclic antidepressants includes some drugs which are structurally dissimilar, they are quite similar to one another in their clinical effects and adverse reactions. They are divided into several categories: tertiary tricyclics (or parent drugs), secondary tricyclics (or metabolites), and a newer or nontricyclic (or heterocyclic) group of drugs which are included in the discussion of tricyclic antidepressants in this chapter.

■ **CLINICAL USE.** The antidepressant drugs are listed in Table 23-7. Elderly patients and patients with a concomitant medical illness may require lower doses of these drugs than healthy adults and require careful assessments for side effects while they are taking these drugs. With an acceptable cardiac history and an EKG within normal limits, particularly for people over 40 years old, tricyclic antidepressants are safe and effective in the treatment of acute and long-term depressive illness.

Two of the tricyclic antidepressants (imipramine, ≅ 225 ng/ml, and nortriptyline, 50–150 ng/ml) have plasma levels which have been correlated with clinical response. This is helpful since each individual patient metabolizes drugs at somewhat different rates. A plasma level can help keep the dose within the therapeutic range and can help assure the adequacy of a drug trial with each of these drugs. Some drugs, particularly nortriptyline, have a "therapeutic window," and a plasma level above the upper range limit results in a decrease in antidepressant effectiveness. Blood for a plasma level should be drawn 8 to 12 hours after a single (usually bedtime) dose. Measuring the level soon after drug ingestion results in an artificially high level, representing the peak of the drug metabolism rather than the steady-state level.

It is estimated that at least 15% to 20% of patients with depressive illness have chronic or recurrent symptoms. These patients may benefit from a maintenance regimen of antidepressant drugs.[34] A tricyclic that has been successful in the past for a particular patient may be continued indefinitely, usually at a much lower dose than was successful during an acute episode. These patients need to be followed and assessed regularly, and the drug gradually discontinued after a long period of stability to determine the need for continued maintenance pharmacotherapy.

■ **ADVERSE REACTIONS.** The nurse should know the common side effects of the antidepressants and should be aware of toxic effects and their treatment as described in Table 23-8. Most of these side effects cause minor discomfort, but some can produce serious morbidity. There are no known long-term adverse effects with these drugs, tolerance to therapeutic effects does not develop, and persistent side effects can often be minimized by a small decrease in dose. Antidepressants do not cause either physical addiction or psychological dependence, and cause no euphoria, thus they have no abuse potential. Because of their long half-life (24 hours or more), antidepressants can be conveniently administered once a day, usually at night for most people. If they cause some activation immediately after dosing, or nightmares, the dose should be given in the morning, or divided into several doses throughout the day. Patients with bipolar illness may be switched into mania by these drugs; they should be watched closely for increased activation and eating, and decreased sleeping patterns.

It is unfortunate that all antidepressants have a three to four or more week lagtime before therapeutic response is evident. Table 23-9 describes the target symptoms for these drugs in the approximate order of the time it takes for each symptom to begin to resolve. It is important to remember when caring for suicidally depressed patients that they become more motivated and begin to look better long before their subjective

TABLE 23-7

ANTIDEPRESSANT DRUGS

Chemical class generic name (Trade name)	Usual dosage range (mg/day)	Available forms (mg)
Tricyclic drugs		
Tertiary (parent drug)		
amitriptyline (Elavil, Endep)	50–300	tabs: 10, 25, 50, 75, 100, 150 inj: 10/ml
amoxapine (Asendin)	50–600	tabs: 25, 50, 100, 150
doxepin (Adapin, Sinequan)	50–300	caps: 10, 25, 50, 75, 100, 125, 150 oral conc: 10/ml
imipramine (SK-Pramine, Tofranil)	50–300	tabs: 10, 25, 50 caps: 75, 100, 125, 150 inj. 25/2 ml
trimipramine (Surmontil)	50–300	caps: 25, 50, 100
Secondary (metabolite)		
desipramine (Norpramin, Pertofrane)	50–300	tabs: 25, 50, 75, 100, 150
nortriptyline (Aventyl, Pamelor)	50–150	caps: 10, 25, 75 solution: 10/5 ml
protriptyline (Vivactil)	15–60	tabs: 5, 10
Nontricyclic drugs		
maprotiline (Ludiomil)	50–225*	tabs: 25, 50, 75
trazodone (Desyrel)	50–600	tabs: 50, 100, 150
buproprion (Wellbutrin)	50–600*	tabs: 50
Monoamine oxidase inhibitors		
isocarboxazid (Marplan)	30–70	tabs: 10
phenelzine (Nardil)	45–90	tabs: 15
tranylcypromine (Parnate)	20–60	tabs: 10

*Antidepressants with a ceiling dose due to dose-related seizures.

depressive feelings and suicidal thoughts are relieved. The nursing care plan must include suicide assessments and suicide precautions for these patients weeks after they begin to look less depressed.

Because these drugs are among the most dangerous substances available when taken in excessive amounts, overdoses and suicide attempts using antidepressants are extremely serious and require emergency medical attention. Ingestion from 1000 to 3000 mg can be lethal. This may represent barely a 1-week supply of medication. For inpatients, mouth checks may be necessary. Even for outpatients who are not suicidal, supplies of antidepressants should be prescribed in small amounts and frequent assessments made. Accidental overdoses in children whose parents are taking an antidepressant are unfortunately common and often lethal. Part of the health teaching and care of these patients should include an assessment of household members, cautioning patients to leave these drugs in their childproof bottles received from the pharmacy and out of the reach of children, and to discard leftover drugs when pharmacotherapy is completed.

Most patients develop tolerance to side effects, and most side effects are dose related, thus they can be minimized by increasing the dose gradually when first prescribed. This gives the patient time to physiologically adjust to the drug. This is especially true when these drugs are used to treat panic disorder. Patients with panic disorder are particularly sensitized to any drug side effects which remind them of symptoms of anxiety or panic attacks (e.g., rapid heart beat, dizziness, nausea, blurred vision). In the case of severely depressed patients

TABLE 23-8

TRICYCLIC ANTIDEPRESSANT SIDE EFFECTS AND NURSING CONSIDERATIONS

Side effects	Nursing considerations
Gastrointestinal	
Heartburn, nausea, vomiting	Administer drug with meals or at bedtime
Decrease in intestinal motility, paralytic ileus	Occurs in half of all patients; elderly are particularly susceptible; bran, bulk laxatives, high-fiber foods, stool softeners, decrease dose, change to a less anticholinergic drug
Dry mouth	Common, tolerance can develop; encourage adequate hydration, sugar-free products, mouth lubricants, try bethanecol (cholinergic agent—25 mg tid), lower dose, change to a less anticholinergic drug
Hematological	
Leukopenia and thrombocytopenia	Monitor; rarely clinically significant
Agranulocytosis: Allergic response of sudden onset; appears 40 to 70 days after initiation of drug (low WBC, normal RBC, infection of the pharynx, fatigue, malaise)	Very rare; discontinue drug and place patient in reverse isolation immediately; never administer drug again; try antidepressant with a different chemical structure and follow patient closely
Hepatic	
Liver toxicity within first 8 weeks of treatment: abdominal pain, anorexia, fever, mild transient jaundice, abnormal liver function tests	Rare hypersensitivity response; discontinue drug; switch to another type of antidepressant
Endocrine	
Amenorrhea, galactorrhea	Due to increased prolactin caused by amoxapine; rare with other tricyclics
Menstrual irregularities	Rare and reversible; decrease dose; change to a different tricyclic
Opthalmologic	
Blurred vision due to ciliary muscle relaxation	Tolerance can develop over the first few weeks of treatment; distant vision is usually intact; do not use with patients with narrow-angle glaucoma
Cardiovascular	
Postural hypotension: lightheadedness or dizziness on rising due to decrease in blood pressure on rising	Occurs frequently; take vital signs sitting and then standing ½ hour after dose; rise slowly, dangle feet, tolerance can develop in first few weeks; not dose related, can continue to raise dose
Tachycardia: rapid heart beat	Occurs frequently; tolerance usually develops; can increase symptoms of angina in patients with coronary artery disease; very frightening to panic disorder patients; in other patients, not clinically significant
EKG changes	QRS and QT interval prolongation; worsening of intraventricular conduction problems; take a careful cardiac history and do a pretreatment EKG, especially with patients over 40 years old
Sudden death	Rare; patients at risk for cardiac heart block: over age 50, family history of heart disease, pre-existing cardiac disease or recent myocardial infarction, or bundle-branch block

TABLE 23-8—cont'd

TRICYCLIC ANTIDEPRESSANT SIDE EFFECTS AND NURSING CONSIDERATIONS

Side effects	Nursing considerations
Neurological Sedation, psychomotor slowing, difficulty concentrating and planning Muscle weakness, fatigue, nervousness, headaches, vertigo, neuropathies, tremors, ataxia, paresthesias, twitching Lowered seizure threshold Extrapyramidal side effects (EPS): acute dystonic reactions, akathisia, Parkinson's syndrome, tardive dyskinesia Psychiatric symptoms: increased anxiety, depression, insomnia, nightmares, psychotic reactions, or confusional states with delusions, hallucinations, and disorientation; mania	Inform the patient, especially if he or she operates machinery or must perform mental tasks; tolerance can develop Not common; tolerance can develop; lower dose Start drugs at lower dose and increase more gradually with seizure disorder patients Rare, since they do not block dopamine; *amoxapine,* the exception, can cause all the common EPS reactions, possibly tardive dyskinesia with long-term use Uncommon, may have to discontinue drug; mania may be precipitated if patient has prior history of mania in self or family (avoid tricyclics if possible in patients predisposed to mania)
Cutaneous Maculopapular rashes, petechiae, photosensitivity	Rare; can give an antihistamine; may have to discontinue antidepressant
Genitourinary Increased or decreased sexual desire, delayed ejaculation Urinary retention	Decrease dose, change to a less anticholinergic drug; take daily dose after sexual intercourse, not immediately before, for delayed ejaculation Lower dose, change to a less anticholinergic drug, try bethanecol; rare: acute renal failure following an atonic bladder
Miscellaneous Tinnitus, weight loss, increased appetite and weight gain, psychomotor stimulation, parotid swelling, alopecia, allergic response: edema, generalized on face, tongue, and orbits Pathological sweating	Very rare; weight control; decrease dose; may have to discontinue drug and try on antidepressant that is structurally different Occurs in 25% of patients; head, neck, and upper extremities; episodic, or occurs only at night
Withdrawal Syndrome Mild withdrawal after sudden discontinuation: malaise, muscle aches, coryzia, chills, nausea, dizziness, anxiety	Taper patient off drug gradually (one to several weeks)
Intoxication Syndromes Poisoning: usually seen in overdose with CNS depression and/or cardiotoxicity: hallucinations, delirium, agitation, sensitivity to sounds, dilated pupils, hypothermia, hyperpyrexia, seizures, coma, arrhythmias, respiratory arrest	Treat aggressively; recovery can be slow; induce emesis, gastric lavage, cardiac monitoring, respiratory support, blood chemistry, arterial blood gases, tricyclic plasma levels monitored, carefully administer physostigmine, valium, mannitol, lidocaine, and other symptomatic treatments
Anticholinergic Syndromes Confusion, delirium, disorientation, agitation, hallucinations, anxiety, motor restlessness, seizures, delusions, constipation, urinary retention, decreased sweating, increased pupillary size, dry mouth, increased temperature, motor incoordination, flushing, tachycardia	Usually occurs with high doses of several psychoactive drugs with anticholinergic effects; physostigmine, cardiac monitoring, respiratory support; in sensitive or aged patients, may occur at normal, therapeutic levels

TABLE 23-9

ANTIDEPRESSANT DRUG TARGET SYMPTOMS

Onset of drug effect	Symptom
Week 1	Middle and terminal insomnia
	Appetite disturbances
	Anxiety
Week 2	Fatigue
	Poor motivation
	Somatic complaints
	Agitation
	Retardation
Week 3	Dysphoric mood
	Subjective depressive feelings (anhedonia, poor self-esteem, pessimism, hopelessness, self-reproach, guilt, helplessness, sadness)
	Suicidal thoughts

Signs and Treatment of Hypertensive Crisis on MAOI

Warning signs

Increased blood pressure, palpitations, frequent headaches

Symptoms of hypertensive crisis

Sudden elevation of blood pressure
Explosive headache, occipital that may radiate frontally
Head and face are flushed and feel "full"
Palpitations, chest pain
Sweating, fever
Nausea, vomiting
Dilated pupils
Photophobia
Intracranial bleeding

Treatment

Hold next MAOI dose
Do not lie patient down (elevates blood pressure in head)
IM chlorpromazine 100 mg, repeat if necessary (*Mechanism of action:* blocks norepinephrine)
IV phentolamine, administered slowly in doses of 5 mg (*Mechanism of action:* binds with norepinephrine receptor sites, blocking norepinephrine)
Fever: Manage by external cooling techniques

or those who are suicidal, doses are generally increased more rapidly to minimize the time it takes to reach steady-state and therapeutic effectiveness.

Tricyclic antidepressants, like all psychiatric drugs, should be avoided if possible during pregnancy, especially in the first trimester. However, these drugs have been given throughout pregnancy without harmful effects on the fetus, and should be considered if a pregnant woman is severely depressed, especially if suicide is a risk.

■ Monoamine oxidase inhibitors (MAOIs)

The monoamine oxidase inhibitors are very effective antidepressant/antipanic drugs that have been underutilized and overly feared. The MAOIs currently used in psychiatry are listed in Table 23-7.[44] Because of the potential for a hypertensive crisis when tyramine-containing foods and certain medicines are taken concomitantly with these drugs, careful health teaching of a reliable patient is quite important. The patient must avoid certain foods, drinks, and medicines (Table 23-10), must know the warning signs, symptoms, and even the treatment of a hypertensive crisis (box), and must be taught the more common side effects of MAOIs (Table 23-11). For various indications (Table 23-5) these drugs are effective, and are safe when used as prescribed.[27,28] They are nonaddicting, and tolerance

does not develop toward therapeutic effects; however, safety in pregnancy has not been established. The patient should be on the restricted diet several days prior to beginning the medication, while on the medication, and for 2 weeks after discontinuing the medication. MAOIs should not be given concomitantly with each other, and their concomitant use with tricyclics is controversial and contraindicated except in limited cases and under expert supervision.

Tyramine is an amino acid released from proteins when they undergo hydrolysis by fermenting, aging, pickling, smoking, and spoiling. It is deactivated by MAO in the gut wall and liver. When MAO is inhibited, tyramine may reach adrenergic nerve endings, causing the release of large amounts of norepinephrine, producing a hypertensive reaction. Also, sympathomimetic drugs act on the neurotransmission process by releasing norepinephrine from the storage vesicles in the presynaptic nerve ends. Because MAO has been inhibited when MAOIs are used, large amounts of norepinephrine are released and a severe hypertensive reaction can occur. Thorazine, an antipsychotic drug, and the alpha-

TABLE 23-10

DIETARY RESTRICTIONS ONE DAY BEFORE, DURING, AND TWO WEEKS AFTER TAKING MAOIs

Food and beverages to avoid

Cheese, especially aged or matured
Fermented or age protein
Pickled or smoked fish
Beer, red wine, sherry, liqueurs, cognac
Yeast or protein extracts
Fava or broad bean pods
Beef or chicken liver
Spoiled or overripe fruit
Banana peel
Yogurt

Food and beverages to be consumed in moderation

Chocolate
Yogurt and sour cream
Clear spirits and white wine
Avocado
New Zealand spinach
Soy sauce
Caffeine drinks

Medications to avoid

Cold medications
Nasal and sinus decongestants
Allergy and hay fever remedies
Narcotics, especially meperidine
Inhalants for asthma
Local anesthetics with epinephrine
Weight-reducing pills, pep pills, stimulants
Other medications without first checking with a physician

Illicit drugs to avoid

Cocaine
Amphetamine

Safe food and beverages

Fresh cottage cheese
Cream cheese
Fresh fruits
Bread products raised with yeast (bread)

Safe medications

Aspirin, Tylenol
Pure steroid asthma inhalants
Codeine
Plain Robitusin or terpin-hydrate with codeine
Local anesthetics without epinephrine
All laxatives
All antibiotics
Antihistamines

Medications that may need dose decreased

Insulin and oral hypoglycemics
Oral anticoagulants
Thiazide diuretics
Anticholinergic agent
Muscle relaxants

Modified from Zisook, S.: Psychosomatics **26**(3):240–251, March 1985 and Moreines, R., and Gold, M.S.: In Gold, M.S, Lydiard, R.B., and Carman, J.S., editors: Advances in psychopharmacology: predicting and improving treatment response, pp. 157–177. Boca Raton, Fla., 1984, CRC Press.

adrenergic blocking agent, phentolamine, bind to the norepinephrine receptor sites, thus preventing norepinephrine stimulation and resolving the hypertensive crisis. It remains to be seen if the monoamine oxidase inhibitors will continue to be used for certain patient populations, or if they recede further from the front line drug treatment of depression and other disorders.

Lithium drug therapy

Lithium, a naturally occurring salt, was noted to have medicinal properties during the nineteenth century when it was found to be present in the waters of some European mineral springs. It was described as having antimanic properties in 1949, but was not accepted for use in the United States until 1970 because of reports of its toxic effects. Today it is readily and safely admin-

TABLE 23-11

MAOI SIDE EFFECTS AND NURSING CONSIDERATIONS

Side effects	Nursing considerations
Postural lightheadedness	Get up slowly, dangle feet, wear elastic hose, increase salt intake, reduce dose
Constipation	Bran, bulk laxatives, stool softeners, fiber, exercise, reduce dose
Delay in ejaculation or orgasm	Separate last dose and sexual intercourse by as many hours as possible (i.e., 8 A.M. and 12 noon dose, evening sexual intercourse), reduce dose
Muscle twitching	300 mg/day vitamin B_6 often helps; reduce dose
Drowsiness	Encourage activity, avoid using machinery, take short daytime naps
Dry mouth	Lemon/glycerin swabs, sugarless gum and candies, fluids
Fluid retention	Low dose thiazide diuretics
Insomnia	Last dose should be as early in the day as possible; encourage patient not to remain physically active all evening, but to start relaxing several hours before bedtime; reduce dose
Urinary hesitancy	Urecholine may help; reduce dose

istered under careful clinical guidelines and has an important clinical role as a mood stabilizer in the treatment of cyclical affective disorders.

■ **MECHANISM OF ACTION.** The exact mechanism of action of lithium is not fully understood, but many neurotransmitter functions are altered by the drug. It has been postulated that lithium corrects an ion exchange abnormality; alters sodium transport in nerves and muscle cells; normalizes synaptic neurotransmission of norepinephrine, serotonin, and dopamine; increases the re-uptake and metabolism of norepinephrine; and changes receptor sensitivity for serotonin. Its clinical effectiveness, more than likely, is due to several of these complex actions.

■ **CLINICAL USE.** Acute episodes of mania and hypomania, and recurrent bipolar illness are the most frequent indications for lithium treatment. Other disorders with an affective component, like recurrent unipolar depressions, schizoaffective disorder, catatonia, and alcoholism, are sometimes effectively treated with lithium, especially when they are periodic or cyclical. In general, lithium is not as helpful in the initial treatment of an acute depressive episode, but can be coadministered with antidepressant drug treatment. Table 23-12 lists the target symptoms of mania and depression for lithium therapy.

Prior to treatment with lithium, a complete history and physical examination are required, with special attention to the kidney (lithium is excreted by the kidneys) and the thyroid. Regular medical checkups (see accompanying box) while on maintenance lithium treatment are essential.

Pre-Lithium Work-up

Renal: Urinalysis, BUN, creatinine, electrolytes, 24-hour creatinine clearance; history of renal disease in self or family; diabetes mellitus, hypertension, diuretic use, analgesic abuse

Thyroid: TSH (thyroid-stimulating hormone), T_4 (thyroxine), T_3 RU (resin uptake), T_4 I (free thyroxine index); history of thyroid disease in self or family

Other: Complete physical, history; EKG, fasting blood sugar, CBC

Maintenance lithium considerations

Every 3 months: Li level (for the first 6 months)

Every 6 months: reassess renal status, lithium level, TSH

Every 12 months: reassess thyroid function, EKG

Assess more often if patient is symptomatic

TABLE 23-12

TARGET SYMPTOMS FOR LITHIUM THERAPY

Mania	Depression
Irritable	Irritable
Expansive	Sadness
Euphoric	Pessimistic
Manipulative	Anhedonia
Labile with depression	Self-reproach
Sleep disturbance (decreased sleep)	Guilt
Pressured speech	Hopelessness
Flight of ideas	Somatic complaints
Motor hyperactivity	Suicidal ideation
Assaultive/threatening	Motor retardation
Distractibility	Slowed thinking
Hypergraphia	Poor concentration and memory
Hypersexual	Fatigue
Persecutory and religious delusions	Constipation
Grandiose	Decreased libido
Hallucinations	Anorexia or increased appetite
Ideas of reference	Weight change
Catatonia	Helplessness
	Sleep disturbance (insomnia or hypersomia)

Factors Predicting Lithium Responsiveness

Positive response

Family history of mania or bipolar illness
Positive response of family member to lithium
Prior manic episode
Onset of illness with mania
Alcohol abuse
Cyclothymic personality features (numerous periods of mood disturbances but lack symptom severity and duration to meet DMS-III-R bipolar diagnostic criteria)
Euphoria and grandiosity
Diagnosis of primary affective disorder
History of treatment compliance with pharmacotherapy

Negative response

Rapid cycling (more than 2 episodes/year)
Thought disorder with depression and paranoia
Anxiety
Obsessive features
Onset after age 40

In acute episodes, lithium is effective in 1 to 2 weeks but may take up to 4 weeks or even a few months to contain the affective episode fully. Sometimes an antipsychotic agent is used during the first few days or weeks of an acute episode to manage severe behavioral excitement and acute psychotic symptoms. In a maintenance regimen, lithium decreases the number of affective episodes, their severity, and the frequency of occurrence. However, mild mood swings or the recurrence of affective symptoms are not uncommon while on lithium maintenance. These usually respond to a temporary increase in lithium dose or short-term psychotherapeutic support. The maintenance dose for each patient must be individualized and may vary from time to time. The accompanying box lists factors predictive of a lithium response.

Lithium therapy is usually initiated with 300 mg t.i.d. until steady state is reached, usually in 7 days. Then a blood level is drawn in the morning, 12 hours after the last dose. Even though the half-life of lithium is 18 to 36 hours, it cannot be given in a single daily dose because of toxic effects of high doses at its peak (3 hours after dosing). Thus b.i.d. or t.i.d. dosing is necessary. Lithium maintenance can be switched to sustained release capsules for once daily dosing. Table 23-13 lists lithium preparations. Because of the low therapeutic index of lithium, toxic blood levels can be reached rapidly. Also, because lithium is a salt, the sodium and fluid balance of the body affects lithium regulation. It is essential clinical practice to monitor serum blood levels at appropriate intervals (every week for first month, then every 3 to 6 months), to regulate the dose based on these levels, and to educate the patient regarding lithium toxicity symptoms and issues regarding salt and fluid intake.

The dose is increased until bipolar symptoms are reduced, until side effects are prohibitive, or until the upper limit of the therapeutic blood level is reached. The therapeutic range is considered to be between 0.6 and 1.4 mEq/l for adults. After a clinical response has occurred, the maintenance lithium dose is usually much lower to maintain a therapeutic blood level. Raising a

TABLE 23-13

LITHIUM PREPARATIONS

Lithium salts (Trade name)	Available forms (mg)
Lithium carbonate (Eskalith) (PFI-Lith) (Lithotabs) (Lithane) (Lithonate)	300 mg
Lithium carbonate sustained release (Eskalith C-R) (Lithobid)	450 mg 300 mg
Lithium citrate concentrate (Ciba-Lith) (Lithonate-S)	5 ml/300 mg

Lithium Side Effects

Acute/common/usually harmless

CNS: Fine hand tremor (50% of patients), fatigue, headache, mental dullness, lethargy

Renal: Polyuria (60% of patients), polydipsia, edema

Gastrointestinal: Gastric irritation, anorexia, abdominal cramps, mild nausea, vomiting, diarrhea (dose with food or milk; further divide dose)

Dermatologic: Acne, pruritic maculopapular rash

Cardiac: EKG changes, usually not clinically significant, may be persistent

Body image: Weight gain (60% of patients); can be persistent

Long-term/adverse/usually not dose related (patient usually can remain on lithium)

Endocrine: a) Thyroid dysfunction—hypothyroidism (5% of patients); replacement hormone may be necessary

b) Mild diabetes mellitus—may need diet control or insulin therapy

Renal: a) Nephrogenic diabetes insipidus—decreasing dose can help; patient must drink plently of fluids; thiazide diuretics paradoxically reduce polyuria and may be helpful

b) Microscopic structural kidney changes: (10%–20%) of patients on lithium for 1 year); usually does not cause significant clinical morbidity

Lithium toxicity/usually dose related

Prodrome of intoxication (lithium level ≥2.0 mEq/l)

Anorexia, nausea, vomiting, diarrhea, coarse hand tremor, muscle fasciculations, twitching, lethargy, dysarthria, hyperactive deep tendon reflexes, ataxia, tinnitus, vertigo, weakness, drowsiness

Lithium intoxication (lithium level ≥2.5 mEq/l)

Fever, decreased urine output, decreased BP, irregular pulse, EKG changes, impaired consciousness, seizures, coma, death

daily dose by 300 mg usually increases the level by 0.2 mEq/l.

In geriatric patients, or those with intercurrent medical illness, a serum lithium level of 0.6 to 0.8 mEq/l is recommended. Use of lithium in pregnancy is not recommended. Various congenital abnormalities have been reported in babies exposed to lithium in utero, particularly during the first trimester.

■ **ADVERSE REACTIONS.** Although lithium is frequently used, it presents a challenge to patient education for nurses and other clinicians. Usually patients are on lithium therapy for several years, and various physiological and environmental factors can rapidly pull their blood levels of lithium above the therapeutic limit. Patients must be taught to differentiate between acute and long-term side effects and signs of lithium toxicity (see accompanying box). Patients must also be taught the common causes for an increase in lithium level and ways to stabilize a therapeutic level as described in the first box on page 725. Lithium toxicity is an emergency. Management of serious toxic states is outlined in the second box on page 725. Bohn[7] and Prien[30] provide educational pamphlets about lithium for patients.

Treatment failures are unfortunately not uncommon, even at therapeutic blood levels of lithium. Several reasonable alternatives to lithium alone include the addition of carbamazepine for manic breakthroughs[29] or the addition of antidepressant drugs for depression breakthroughs. ECT for either mania or depression is

Stabilizing Lithium Levels

Common causes for an increase in lithium levels

1. Decreased sodium intake
2. Diuretic therapy
3. Decreased renal functioning
4. Fluid and electrolyte loss: sweating, diarrhea, dehydration
5. Medical illness
6. Overdose

Ways to maintain a stable lithium level

1. Stable dosing schedule by dividing doses or use of sustained-release capsules
2. Adequate dietary sodium and fluid intake (2 to 3 quarts/day)
3. Replace fluid and electrolytes during exercise or GI illness
4. Monitor signs and symptoms of lithium side effects and toxicity
5. If patient forgets a dose, he may take it if he missed dosing time by 2 hours; if longer than 2 hours, skip that dose and take the next dose; never double up on doses

Management of Serious Lithium Toxicity

1. Rapid assessment of clinical signs and symptoms of lithium toxicity; if possible, obtain rapid history of incident, especially dosing, from patient; explain procedures to patient and offer support throughout
2. Hold all lithium doses
3. Check blood pressure, pulse, rectal temperature, respirations, level of consciousness. Be prepared to: initiate stabilization procedures, protect airway, provide supplemental oxygen
4. Obtain lithium blood level immediately; obtain electrolytes, BUN, creatinine, urinalysis, CBC when possible
5. Electrocardiogram; monitor cardiac status
6. Limit lithium absorption; if acute overdose, provide an emetic; nasogastric suctioning may help since lithium levels in gastric fluid may remain high for days
7. Vigorously hydrate: 5 to 6 liters/day; keep electrolytes balanced; IV line and indwelling urinary catheter
8. Patient will be bedridden: range of motion, frequent turning, pulmonary toilet
9. In moderately severe cases:
   a. Implement osmotic diuresis with urea, 20 g IV two to five times per day, or mannitol, 50 to 100 g IV per day
   b. Increase lithium clearance with aminophylline, 0.5 g up to every 6 hr and alkalinize the urine with IV sodium lactate
   c. Ensure adequate intake of NaCl to promote excretion of lithium
   d. Implement peritoneal or hemodialysis in the most severe cases. These are characterized by serum levels between 2.0 and 4.0 mEq/liter with severe clinical signs and symptoms (particularly decreasing urinary output and deepening CNS depression).
10. When appropriate: interview patient; ascertain reasons for lithium toxicity; increase health teaching efforts; mobilize post-discharge support system; arrange for more frequent clinical visits and blood levels; assess for depression and/or suicidal intent; consider concomitant antidepressant drug treatment and supportive nonpharmacologic therapy

also effective and should be considered particularly when suicide risk seems high. Most importantly, there is no psychopharmacologic substitute for a strong therapeutic relationship, patient education, psychodynamic intervention, and regular maintenance evaluations. A more thorough discussion of lithium treatment can be found in Lydiard,[26] Harris,[16] and Beeber.[5]

Antipsychotic drugs

This pharmacological family has become a mainstay in the treatment of the psychotic disorders and some nonpsychotic conditions. While not offering a cure for psychosis, the effectiveness of these drugs in reducing psychotic symptoms is well established. The discovery in 1952 that chlorpromazine produced significant behavioral changes in psychiatric patients revolutionized psychiatric care and introduced psychopharmacology as a viable treatment modality and research focus. In spite of the potential for almost untenable side effects, antipsychotic drugs are extensively prescribed and can offer an alternative for some patient populations who might otherwise face a lifetime of institutionalization. In light of these issues, the administration of drugs from this family requires careful considerations, skill, and patient education.

■ **MECHANISM OF ACTION.** The antipsychotic drugs are dopamine antagonists and block dopamine receptors in various pathways in the brain. Their effectiveness is thought to be related to their ability to block dopamine receptors in the limbic system, which is the emotional part of the brain. Unfortunately, they also block dopamine receptors in other parts of the brain. This accounts for their side effects and for the differences in tolerance to desired and undesired drug effects. A thorough discussion of the biology of the antipsychotic drugs can be found in Richelson.[32]

■ **CLINICAL USE.** The most frequently prescribed antipsychotic drugs are listed in Table 23-14. Despite the variety of chemical classes, these drugs are not different from each other in terms of overall clinical efficacy at equivalent doses: they all have an equal chance of treating the target of psychosis. What notably distinguishes the chemical classes of the antipsychotic drugs is the extent, type, and severity of side effects produced. Thus an understanding of the side effect profile of each class of drug becomes a major nursing focus when caring for patients receiving antipsychotic medications. Black and co-workers[6] provide a succinct discussion of choice of drug according to anticipated side effects.

Past success with a psychiatric drug in a patient or his first degree relative may be the first indication for the choice of a particular antipsychotic drug. The most common cause of treatment failure in acute psychosis is an inadequate dose. The most common cause of relapse seems to be patient noncompliance with maintenance drug therapy.

The major uses for antipsychotic drugs are in the management of schizophrenia, organic brain syndrome with psychosis, and the manic phase of manic-depressive illness. Their occasional use may be indicated in severe depression with psychotic features, or in severe anxiety, particularly when the patient may have a tendency toward drug or alcohol dependency. Several nonpsychiatric uses for the antipsychotic drugs are in the treatment of vomiting, vertigo, and the potentiation of analgesics for pain relief.

The clinical symptoms of psychosis that are considered to be the major target symptoms for pharmacotherapy with the antipsychotic drugs are listed in the accompanying box. The initial nursing care plan should address drug dose, target symptom response, emergence of side effects and their treatment, along with patient safety, education, and reassurance. Although the relationship the nurse establishes with the patient who is

---

Antipsychotic Drug Target Symptoms

Appearance
    Bizarre or disheveled
    Poor hygiene, poor nutrition
Behavior
    Hyperactivity
    Bizarre actions
    Hostility, assaultiveness
    Insomnia
    *Motivation—poor
    *Social functioning—poor
Mood and affect
    Flat affect
    Agitation
    Anxiety and tension
Intellectual functioning—poor
    *Unrealistic planning
    *Lack of insight
    *Poor judgment
Thought processes
    Loose associations
    Delusional ideas
    Hallucinations
    Suspiciousness
    Negativism

---

*Residual symptoms: Not highly responsive to pharmacotherapy

---

very psychotic forms the basis for an ongoing therapeutic alliance, active nonpharmacological treatment of the more residual symptoms of psychosis is more successful when elements of the patient's behavior, mood, and thought processes begin to show improvement with pharmacotherapy. Ereshefsky and Stimmel[10] provide a good review of psychoses, using a case presentation format.

General Pharmacological Principles Dosage requirements for individual patients are highly variable and must be titrated as the target symptom changes and side effects are monitored. Initially, the patient is dosed several times a day, and the daily dose can be raised every 1 to 4 days until symptom improvement occurs. Some patients respond in 2 to 3 days, some take as long as 2 weeks. Full benefits may take 6 weeks or more. Parenteral high doses can be used initially to control a highly excited or dangerous patient.

TABLE 23-14

DRUG FAMILY (CATEGORY): ANTIPSYCHOTIC DRUGS

Chemical class Subtype generic name (Trade name)	Drug dosage: Equivalence (mg)	Usual maintenance dosage range (mg/day)	Available forms (mg)
Phenothiazines			
Aliphatic type chlorpromazine (thorazine)	100	300–1400	tabs: 10, 25, 50, 100, 200 time released: 30, 75, 150, 200 caps: 300 syrup: 10/5 ml conc: 30/ml; 100/ml supp: 25, 100 inj: 25/ml
Piperidine type thioridazine (Mellaril)	100	300–800*	tabs: 10, 15, 25, 50, 100, 150, 200 conc: 30/ml, 100/ml susp: 25/5 ml, 100/5 ml
mesoridazine (Serentil)	50	100–500	tabs: 10, 25, 50, 100 conc: 25/ml inj: 25/ml
Piperazine type perphenazine (Trilafon)	10	8–64	tabs: 2, 4, 8, 16 conc: 16/5 ml inj: 5/ml
trifluoperazine (Stelazine)	5	10–80	tabs: 1, 2, 5, 10 conc: 10/ml inj: 2/ ml
fluphenazine (Prolixin)	2	5–40	tabs: 0.25, 1, 2.5, 5, 10 conc: 5/ml elix: 0.5/5 ml
Thioxanthene			
thiothixene (Navane)	4–5	10–60	caps: 1, 2, 5, 10, 20 conc: 5/ml inj: 2/ml, powder 5/ml
Butyrophenone			
haloperidol (Haldol)	2	5–100	tabs: 0.5, 1, 2, 5, 10, 20 conc: 2/ml inj: 50/ml
Dibenzoxazepine			
loxapine (loxitane)	15	50–250	caps: 5, 10, 25, 50 conc: 25/ml inj: 50/ml
Dihydroindolone			
molindone (Moban)	10–15	25–250	tabs: 5, 10, 25, 50, 100 conc: 20/ml

*Upper limit to avoid retinopathy.

When the patient has been stabilized for several weeks, the daily dose can be lowered to the lowest effective dose. The half-life of these drugs is over 24 hours, so the patient can be dosed once a day after steady-state is reached (approximately 4 days). Bedtime dosing allows the patient to sleep through side effects when they are at their peak. After approximately 6 to 12 months of stable maintenance drug therapy, the patient can be slowly tapered from medication to ascertain the need for continued drug treatment. Some schizophrenic patients require a lifetime of continuous medication management. A patient who is unresponsive to an adequate trial (6 weeks at a proper dose), will frequently respond to another chemical class of antipsychotic drug, so a second drug trial is usually warranted.

Most of these drugs can be administered by oral and intramuscular routes. Fluphenazine comes in two depot injectible forms which can be given every 7 to 28 days. Haloperidol decanote is an injectible form of haloperidol that has a 4-week duration of action. It is not appropriate to treat an acute psychotic episode with haloperidol decanote alone because it takes 3 months to reach steady-state drug levels. Thus, it is more of a long-term maintenance medication. Acute psychotic episodes require a shorter-acting drug. Test the patient's ability to take these drugs by first administering the oral form for several days. Long-acting injectibles have been important in treating the outpatient who requires supervision of medication intake because of noncompliance. With the exception of thioridazine, antipsychotic drugs also have anti-emetic effects. Hayes,[17] Kessler,[21]

and Towery[40] provide excellent guidelines for the use of antipsychotic drugs.

Contrary to package inserts, there are no ceiling doses for these medicines, with the firm exception of thioridazine, which can cause pigmentary retinopathy when given over 800 mg/day. Abrupt discontinuation of the antipsychotic drugs can cause dyskinetic reactions and some rebound side effects. The drugs should be tapered slowly over several days to weeks.

The antipsychotic drugs do not cause chemical dependency, nor is there tolerance to their antipsychotic effects over time. Due to their wide therapeutic index, overdoses of these drugs ordinarily do not result in death, thus they have a very low suicide potential. They do not produce euphoria, therefore they also have a very low abuse potential. Antipsychotic drugs are not respiratory depressants but produce an additive depressant effect when combined with drugs which produce respiratory depression. Therefore, carefully observe patients on concomitant therapy with drugs like benzodiazepines. The effects of antipsychotics on the fetus are inconclusive. It is always best to avoid administration of any drug during the first trimester, although what is best for a psychotic pregnant mother must be carefully considered.

■　**ADVERSE REACTIONS.** The side effects of antipsychotic drugs are many and varied and demand a great deal of clinical attention from the nurse for optimal care. Table 23-15 is a comprehensive list that includes risk factors and treatment considerations. Some side effects are merely uncomfortable for the patient and most are

TABLE 23-15

SIDE EFFECTS AND ADVERSE REACTIONS OF ANTIPSYCHOTIC DRUGS

Side effects/adverse reactions	Mechanism of action	Risk factors	Treatment and nursing considerations
Acute/Common/Side Effects			
Neurological	Dopamine blockade: Acetylcholine/dopamine balance is disturbed	Extra Pyramidal Symptoms: 40% of all patients get EPS; differs between neuroleptics, highest with high potency drugs	*General EPS Treatment Principles* 1. Tolerance usually develops by the third month 2. Decrease dose of antipsychotic drug if possible 3. Add an anticholinergic drug for 3 months then taper 4. Change to an antipsychotic with lower EPS profile 5. Patient education and supportive care

Continued.

TABLE 23-15—cont'd

SIDE EFFECTS AND ADVERSE REACTIONS OF ANTIPSYCHOTIC DRUGS

Side effects/ adverse reactions	Mechanism of action	Risk factors	Treatment and nursing considerations

Extrapyramidal Symptoms (EPS)
1. Acute Dystonic Reactions: Occur suddenly and are very frightening to the patient; spasms of major muscle groups of the neck, back, and eyes; catatonia; respiratory compromise.
 	
2. Akathisia
Patient cannot remain still; pacing, inner restlessness; leg aches which are relieved by movement
3. Parkinson's Syndrome
  a. Akinesia—absence or slowness of motion; patient turns like one solid block of wood; gait is inclined forward with small, rapid steps; masklike facies
  b. Cogwheel rigidity and muscle stiffness on physical exam
  c. Bilateral fine tremor, anywhere in body; "pill-rolling" motion of the fingers
		1. 10% of all EPS; occurs within the first 5 days; non-geriatric patients, especially children; males twice as often as females; high potency antipsychotics
		
		2. 50% of all EPS; high potency antipsychotic drugs
		
		3. 40% of all EPS; females twice as often as males; geriatric patients; occurs within weeks to several months or longer after drug treatment begins
			Acute dystonic reactions
			Administer a drug from Table 23-17; parenteral routes work more rapidly than PO; have respiratory support equipment available.
			
			Akathisia
			Rule out anxiety or agitation (difficult but important distinction)
			Parkinson's Syndrome
			Tolerance does not develop in all patients; the dopamine agonist, amantadine, is sometimes effective (patient must have good renal function to avoid amantadine toxicity); use step 3 (above) early and vigorously.

Behavioral *Sedation* Sleepy, groggy, fatigued		Peaks 2 to 3 hours after dosing	Tolerance occurs within days to several weeks; rule out over-medication; dose once daily at h.s.; change to an antipsychotic drug with a lower sedation profile
Autonomic *Anticholinergic Side Effects* Blurred vision, constipation, tachycardia, urinary retention, decreased gastric secretion, decreased sweating and salivation (dry mouth), heat stroke, nasal congestion, decreased pulmonary secretion; *"atropine psychosis"* in geriatric patients: hyperactivity, agitation, confusion, flushed skin, dilated pupils which are slow to react, bowel hypomotility, dysarthria, tachycardia	Cholinergic receptor blockade at some central and peripheral sites	Concurrent use of anticholinergic drugs; geriatric patients; patients with tachycardia; low-potency antipsychotic drugs; can return as rebound symptoms during antipsychotic drug withdrawal; men with prostatic hypertrophy may have particular difficulty with urinary retention	Tolerance develops in days to weeks; change to drug with a lower anticholinergic profile; treat symptomatically: frequently moisten dry mouth, use sugarless candy and gum; bulk diets, stool softeners, fluids, and exercise for constipation; avoid operating machinery if vision is blurred; cholinergic agonist (bethanecol) for urinary retention; IM physostigmine for severe atropine psychosis; avoid polypharmacy if possible; avoid getting overheated
Cardiac (autonomic) *Orthostatic Hypotension* Dizziness, tachycardia, drop in diastolic BP by >40 mm/H with a change of position from lying to sitting or sitting to standing	α-adrenergic blockade producing vascular dilation and pooling of blood	Concurrent administration of antihypertensives, diuretics, antidepressants; geriatric patients; worse with injectable low-potency drugs	Tolerance develops in several weeks; lower dose; change to an antipsychotic with a lower hypotension profile, monitor BP; increase fluid intake to expand vascular volume; have patient rise slowly and dangle feet while sitting; have patient wear support hose; use a pure α-adrenergic pressor agent (metaraminol) for hypotensive crisis

Continued.

TABLE 23-15—cont'd

SIDE EFFECTS AND ADVERSE REACTIONS OF ANTIPSYCHOTIC DRUGS

Side effects/adverse reactions	Mechanism of action	Risk factors	Treatment and nursing considerations
Acute/Rare Adverse Reactions			
Allergic Reactions	Hypersensitivity reaction		
Hematologic Agranulocytosis: develops abruptly; fever, malaise, ulcerative sore throat, leukopenia (WBC below 500)		Occurs within 3 to 8 weeks of treatment; very rare; phenothiazines, especially chlorpromazine; thiothixene; geriatric females; 30% mortality rate	This is an *extreme emergency;* be alert for high fever and ulcerative sore throat with patients on these drugs, particularly geriatric females; monitor WBC with this risk group; if this occurs, discontinue drug immediately and initiate reverse isolation; antibiotics when appropriate
Dermatologic 1. Systemic Dermatosis: maculopapular, erythematous, itchy rash on face, neck, chest, extremities; contact dermatitis when touching drug		Occurs 2 to 8 weeks after treatment; chlorpromazine	Non-dose related; discontinue drug and start again cautiously when rash disappears; change to a drug in another chemical class; topical steroids if necessary
2. Photosensitivity: severe sunburn		Low-potency drugs; brief exposure to direct sunlight	Lower dose; change to a high-potency drug; use sunscreen and wear clothing over exposed areas; topical relief of sunburn
Hepatic Jaundice: fever, nausea, abdominal pain, malaise, pruritus, jaundice; abnormal liver function tests		Rare; was more common in the 1950s and 1960s due to impurities in the drugs; phenothiazines, especially chlorpromazine; occurs in first month of treatment	Discontinue drug, reversible and self-limiting; bedrest; high-protein/carbohydrate diet
Cardiovascular *EKG abnormalities*	Effects in the hypothalamus and the heart	Pre-existing cardiac conditions; geriatric patients; low-potency drugs, especially when combined with tricyclic antidepressants (thioridazine and amitriptyline are worst)	Baseline and follow-up EKG and vital sign monitoring for patients with pre-existing cardiac disease; change to high-potency drug
Neurological *Seizures* Usually grand mal, no warning aura	These drugs lower the seizure threshold	Patients with pre-existing seizure disorder; patients who are poorly controlled psychiatrically; low-potency drugs; during sedative-hypnotic or alcohol withdrawal	Decrease dose; change to a high-potency drug; anticonvulsants don't protect non-seizure disorder patients.
Long-Term/Common Adverse Reactions			
Neurological *Extrapyramidal Symptom (EPS)* Tardive Dyskinesia: tongue protrusion, lip smacking, puckering, sucking, chewing, blinking, lateral jaw movements, grimacing; choreiform movements of the limbs and trunk, shoulder shrugging, pelvic thrusting, wrist and ankle flexion or rotation, foot tapping, toe movements	After prolonged blockade from dopamine, postsynaptic receptor site becomes overactive, supersensitive	Estimated that between 15% and 50% of all people receiving antipsychotics, particularly high doses for long-term use (occurs usually after years, but can occur as early as 4 months); geriatric patients; especially females; brain-damaged patients; anti-cholinergic drugs given for EPS may increase risk	These are stereotyped, involuntary movements which may be mild or become severely crippling; employ primary preventive measures (see Figure 23-2); patients with severe tardive dyskinesia can become very distressed; may need soft foods, and soft shoes for feet movements. There is no treatment for tardive dyskinesia, though several drugs are in the experimental stages; may be irreversible, especially if not discovered early and if antipsychotic drugs cannot be stopped.

Continued.

TABLE 23-15—cont'd

SIDE EFFECTS AND ADVERSE REACTIONS OF ANTIPSYCHOTIC DRUGS

Side effects/adverse reactions	Mechanism of action	Risk factors	Treatment and nursing considerations
Endocrine Galactorrhea, amenorrhea, breast enlargement and engorgement, decreased libido, ejaculatory incompetence, appetite increase and weight gain, hypo- or hyperthermia, false positive pregnancy test	Effects on the hypothalmus and pituitary causing an increase in prolactin and leuteotropic hormone secretion	Low-potency drugs, especially thioridazine	Partial tolerance over many months or years may develop; decrease dose or change to high-potency drug, especially with persistent symptoms; be sure that female patients are not actually pregnant; for weight gain—diet and exercise regimen (molindone has less appetite stimulant effects); women should have periodic breast exams especially with a personal or family history of breast cancer, although there is no clear evidence that the risk of breast cancer is increased
Long Term/Rare/Adverse Reactions			
Opthalmologic Problems *Toxic Pigmentary Retinopathy* Patient notices brownish discoloration of vision, loss of visual accuity, possible blindness		Doses of thioridazine above 800 mg/day, even for brief periods of time	Degenerative and irreversible; completely avoidable; never give thioridazine above 800 mg/day; change to another drug if 800 mg/day of thioridazine does not treat target symptoms of psychosis
Skin/Eye Syndrome Sunlight-exposed skin turns slate gray to metallic blue or purple in color. Color changes are also noted in eyes, without vision impairment.	Deposits of drug substance and pigment in the cornea, lens, and the skin	Prolonged use of chlorpromazine or thiothixene and exposure to sunlight	Change to another drug class; deposits will disappear over many months after drug is discontinued
Short- or Long-Term/Rare/Life Threatening			
Neuroleptic Malignant Syndrome High fever, tachycardia, muscle rigidity, stupor, tremor, incontinence, leukocytosis, elevated serum CPK, hyperkalemia, renal failure, increased pulse, respirations, and sweating	Presumably extreme dopamine receptor blockade is at least part of mechanism	50 cases have been reported in the literature between 1980 and 1985. This develops explosively over 1 to 3 days, from hours to many months after drug treatment begins; high-potency drugs are worse, but other psychiatric drugs have been implicated also; patients with marked dehydration; patients with organic brain disease; 20% mortality rate *Speculative:* young adult men, polypharmacy, haloperidol, fluphenazine, parenteral, long-term drug use	This is an *extreme emergency*—early recognition is critical; avoid marked dehydration in all patients; discontinue all drugs immediately; supportive symptomatic care: nutrition, hydration, renal dialysis for renal failure, ventilation for acute respiratory failure, reduction of fever *Speculative:* dantrolene, bromocriptine. Antipsychotic drugs can be cautiously reintroduced.

TABLE 23-16

ACUTE SIDE EFFECTS PROFILE: ANTIPSYCHOTIC DRUGS

Drugs	Sedation	EPS	Anticholinergic	Postural hypotension
Low potency				
chlorpromazine	4	2	3	4
thioridazine	4	1	4	4
High potency				
trifluoperazine	2	3	2	2
thiothixene	2	3	2	1
loxapine	2	3	2	2
molindone	2	3	2	2
mesoridazine	3	2	3	3
perphenazine	2	3	2	2
fluphenazine	1	4	2	1
haloperidol	1	4	1	1

1 = lowest incidence; 4 = highest incidence.

TABLE 23-17

DRUGS TO TREAT EPS (EXTRAPYRAMIDAL SIDE EFFECTS): NEUROTRANSMITTER SPECIFICITY

Chemical class generic name (Trade name)	Equivalence (mg)	Usual dosage range (mg/day)	Available forms (mg)
Anticholinergic			
benztropin (Cogentin)	2	1–6	tabs: 0.5, 1,2 inj: 1/ml
trihexyphenidyl (Artane)	5	1–10	tabs: 2, 5; 5 sustained release; elix: 2/5 ml
biperiden (Akineton)	4	2–6	tabs: 2 inj: 5/ml
procyclidine (Kemadrin)	5	6–20	tabs: 5
diphenhydramine (benadryl)	50	25–150	tabs: 50 caps: 25, 50 elix: 12.5/5 ml; inj: 10/ml, 50/ml
Dopaminergic			
amantadine (Symmetrel)	100	100–300	caps: 100 mg syrup: 50/5ml
Gabaminergic			
diazepam (Valium)	10		(See Table 23-2.)
lorazepam (Ativan)	2		

Treatment considerations of anticholinergic drug therapy

1. Geriatric patients are particularly sensitive to these drugs.
2. They can produce a euphoria and have abuse potential.

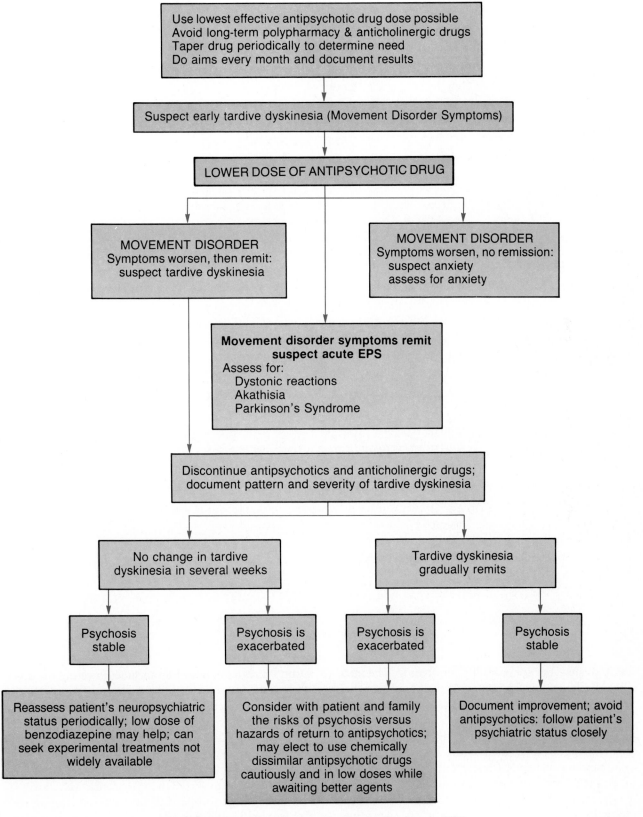

Fig. 23-2. Preventive measures for Tardive Dyskinesia (TD).

Abnormal Involuntary Movement Scale: AIMS

A Simple Method to Determine Tardive Dyskinesia Symptoms—
Total Score Equals the Sum of the Items

Patient Identification: _____ Date: _____

Rated by: _____ Treatment period: _____

Either before or after completing the examination procedure observe the patient unobtrusively at rest (e.g., in waiting room).

The chair to be used in this examination should be a hard firm one without arms.

After observing the patient he may be rated on a scale of 0 (none), 1 (minimal), 2 (mild), 3 (moderate), and 4 (severe) according to the severity of symptoms at time of interview.

Ask the patient whether there is anything in his/her mouth (i.e., gum, candy, etc.) and if there is to remove it.

Ask patient about the *current* condition of his/her teeth. Ask patient if he/she wears dentures. Do teeth or dentures bother patient *now*?

Ask patient whether he/she notices any movement in mouth, face, hands, or feet. If yes, ask to describe and to what extent they *currently* bother patient or interfere with his/her activities.

0	1	2	3	4	Have patient sit in chair with hands on knees, legs slightly apart and feet flat on floor. (Look at entire body for movements while in this position.)
0	1	2	3	4	Ask patient to sit with hands hanging unsupported. If male between legs, if female and wearing a dress, hanging over knees. (Observe hands and other body areas.)
0	1	2	3	4	Ask patient to open mouth. (Observe tongue at rest within mouth.) Do this twice.
0	1	2	3	4	Ask patient to protrude tongue. (Observe abnormalities of tongue movement.) Do this twice.
0	1	2	3	4	Ask the patient to tap thumb with each finger as rapidly as possible for 10–15 seconds separately with right hand then with left hand. (Observe facial and leg movements.)
0	1	2	3	4	Flex and extend patient's left and right arms (one at a time).
0	1	2	3	4	Ask patient to stand up. (Observe in profile. Observe all body areas again, hips included.)
0	1	2	3	4	*Ask patient to extend both arms outstretched in front with palms down. (Observe trunk legs and mouth.)
0	1	2	3	4	*Have patient walk a few paces turn and walk back to chair. (Observe hands and gait.) Do this twice.

*Activated movements

easily treated, but some are life threatening. The nurse should refer to this list frequently but should pay particular attention to the extrapyramidal syndromes (EPS), both short- and long-term. These are discussed in detail in Gelenberg[12] and the APA Task Force report on tardive dyskinesia, Baldessarini.[3] It is important to minimize the patient's fears, increased sense of stigmatization, and potential noncompliance with drug treatment by effective patient education and support. Some EPS side effects are common, effectively treated, and not dangerous consequences of drug treatment.

Drug strategies to treat EPS include: lowering the dose of the antipsychotic drug; changing to an antipsychotic drug with a lower profile for that side effect (Table 23-16); or administering one of the drugs listed in Table 23-17 to treat acute EPS. These drugs are administered concomitantly with antipsychotic drugs if acute symptoms of EPS occur. Since tolerance to these symptoms usually occurs in the first 3 months of antipsychotic drug treatment, drugs to treat EPS are used only during the first 3 months and then discontinued. Their long-term use is usually not necessary.

Unfortunately, the long-term common extra-pyramidal syndrome, tardive dyskinesia, has no effective treatment to date. Thus, primary preventive measures are important (see Figure 23-2). The Abnormal Involuntary Movement Scale (AIMS) should be an ongoing component of every patient's treatment (see the box on the opposite page). Most patients and their families consider the potential side effects of antipsychotic drugs preferable to an alternative of a life dominated by psychosis, but they should be presented with the choices available to them in an appropriate manner.

At this time, the correlation between plasma blood levels of antipsychotic drugs or serum dopamine receptor binding, and clinical response, has yet to be determined, but these tests hold future promise for refining drug selection and dosing regimens. Psychopharmacologic research has yet to discover a chemical class of antipsychotic drugs whose mechanisms of action are highly specific for the target symptoms of psychosis, without incurring a variety of unwanted side effects.

■ SUGGESTED CROSS-REFERENCES ■

Elements of a psychiatric evaluation are discussed in Chapter 6. Legal and ethical issues in psychiatric care are discussed in Chapter 7. Care of suicidal and noncompliant patients is discussed in Chapter 16. Nursing interventions with suspicious and dependent patients are discussed in Chapter 17. Supplemental somatic therapies are discussed in Chapter 22. Psychopharmacology with children is discussed in Chapter 30.

■ SUMMARY ■

1. Psychopharmacology is the fastest growing treatment in the present practice of psychiatry. Psychopharmacological research is widely funded, and results can be confusing, controversial, and dramatically effective.

2. Nursing care of patients with psychiatric illnesses includes assisting the patient with what can be complex, uncomfortable, and dangerous, as well as helpful pharmacological components of their treatment regimen. Data gathering, patient education, and knowledge of drug administration and treatment are essential aspects of psychiatric nursing care.

3. Patient assessment includes evaluation of one's physical status, mental status, medical and psychiatric history, medication and drug history, and family history.

4. Various aspects of pharmacokinetics were presented including half-life, steady state, polypharmacy, drug interactions, and aspects of patient noncompliance with related implications for patient education. The biological basis for psychopharmacology was also briefly described.

5. Benzodiazepines, the most widely prescribed class of drugs in the world, have almost completely replaced other classes of antianxiety and sedative-hypnotic agents. They are therapeutically effective and have a wide margin of safety when taken alone. They can be mildly addictive, especially when

DIRECTIONS FOR FUTURE RESEARCH

The following are some of the nursing research problems raised in Chapter 23 that merit further study by psychiatric nurses.
1. Identification of people at risk for particular side effects and adverse reactions to psychopharmacological drugs
2. Predictors of factors related to patient noncompliance with medication treatment regimens
3. Effective nursing interventions that maximize patient compliance with medication treatment regimens
4. Non-pharmacologic interventions that enhance drug effectiveness and treat residual target symptoms
5. Development of behavioral rating scales that are specific in assessing nursing care effectiveness in the psychopharmacologic treatment of mental disorders
6. Descriptive studies of the various roles assumed by nurses in psychopharmacology
7. Outcomes associated with the role of the nurse clinician in the long-term psychiatric treatment of patients on drug maintenance regimens
8. Patient education strategies associated with drug therapy effectiveness, compliance, and safety
9. Ways to maximize nurse-patient collaboration in medication treatment regimens and related outcomes
10. Evaluation of the effectiveness of involving the patient's social support system in short- and long-term medication regimens
11. Characteristics of the expanded role of the nurse, role satisfaction, and multidisciplinary team approaches to medication effectiveness
12. Knowledge level of nurses of the biological basis, mechanisms of action, clinical uses, and adverse effects of psychopharmacological drugs and its correlation with the effectiveness of nursing care

used in high doses over long periods of time, or when used concomitantly with other addictive agents such as barbiturates or alcohol. The most common side effects include drowsiness, dizziness, slurred speech, and blurred vision.

6. Antidepressant drugs are frequently used, usually effective, nonaddicting, and can be lethal in overdose. Tricyclic (and several other nontricyclic) antidepressants are more commonly used than are monoamine oxidase inhibitors because they are safer in combination with other substances. MAOIs, although generally more effective than tricyclics, are not commonly used because they require restrictions on tyramine-containing foods and a variety of other medications. Side effects of antidepressants are usually mild.

7. The mood stabilizer, lithium, is fairly effective in the treatment of bipolar illness in acute phases and in long-term maintenance regimens when cyclical exacerbations of the illness tend to be frequent. Lithium is nonaddictive but can be toxic. The therapeutic dosage range is narrow and must be monitored by regularly assessing serum lithium levels. Patients must be taught the differences between common side effects and signs of toxicity, and ways to stabilize lithium levels.

8. Antipsychotic agents have made a major differences in the treatment of people with psychotic disorders. The various classes have similar therapeutic effects, but are dissimilar in side effect profiles. Side effects are varied and can be disabling and life-threatening. Thus, a major focus in learning about antipsychotic drugs is learning to prevent, recognize, and treat their related side effects.

■ REFERENCES ■

1. Akiskal, H.S., McKinney, W.I., Jr.: Overview of recent research in depression; integration of ten conceptual models into a comprehensive clinical frame. Arch. Gen. Psychiatry **32**:285–305, 1975.
2. Ayd, F.J., Jr.: Buspirone update: comparison with the benzodiazepines. International Drug Therapy Newsletter, Baltimore, MD., Ayd Medical Communications.
3. Baldessarini, R.J. et al.: Tardive dyskinesia: summary of a task force report of the American Psychiatric Association. Am. J. Psychiatry **137**(10): 1163–1172, Oct. 1980.
4. Ballenger, J.C.: Psychologpharmacology of anxiety disorders. Psychiatr. Clin. North Am. 7(4): 757–771, Dec. 1984.
5. Beeber, L.: Psychopharmacotherapy. In D. Critchley, and Maruin J., editors: The Clinical Specialist in Psychiatric Mental Health Nursing, pp. 295–343. New York, 1985, John Wiley and Sons.
6. Black, J.L., Richelson, E., and Richardson, J.W.: Antipsychotic agents: a clinical update. Mayo Clin. Proc. **60**:777–789, 1985.
7. Bohn, J., Jefferson, J.W.: Lithium and manic depression: A guide, pp. 7–29. Madison, Wisc. 1982, Publishing Board of Regents, University of Wisconsin System, Lithium Information Center.
8. Brown, R.P., and Kneeland, B.: Visual imaging in psychiatry. Hosp. Community Psychiatry **36**: 489–495, May 1985.
9. Brown, R.P., Mann, J.J.: A clinical perspective on the role of neurotransmitters in mental disorders. Hosp. Community Psychiatry **36**(2): 141–149, Feb. 1985.
10. Ereshefsky, L., and Stimmel, G.L.: Psychoses. In Katcher, B.S., Young, L.Y., Koda-Kimble, M.A., editors: Applied therapeutics: The clinical use of drugs, ed. 3, pp. 985–1016. Spokane, Wash. 1983, Applied Therapeutics, Inc.
11. Friedel, R.O., et al.: Changing colors in psychiatry. Proceedings of a symposium: Changing colors in psychiatry:

advances in brain imaging techniques, pp. 1–51. Pfizer Inc. New York, 1984.
12. Gelenberg, A.J.: Psychoses. In Bassuk, E.L., Schoonover, S.C., Gelenberg, A.J., editors: The practitioner's guide to psychoactive drugs, ed. 2, pp. 115–165. New York and London, 1984, Plenum Medical Books Co.
13. Goldberg, H.L., and DiMascio, A.: Toxicology and side effects: psychotropic drugs in pregnancy. Psychopharmacology: a generation of progress, pp. 1047–1055, New York, Jan. 1981. Raven Press.
14. Greenblatt, D.J., Shader, R., and Abernethy, D.R.: Medical intelligence; drug therapy, current status of benzodiazepines. N. Engl. J. Med. **309**:354–356, 410–416, 1983.
15. Guy, W.: ECDEU assessment manual for psychopharmacology, revised. Rockville, Md, 1976, U.S. Department of Health, Education, and Welfare, National Institute of Mental Health, Psychopharmacology Research Branch, Division of Extramural Research Program.
16. Harris, E.: Lithium. Am. J. Nurs. **81**:1329–1365, July 1981.
17. Hayes, P.E.: Rational prescribing guidelines for antipsychotic drugs. Family and Community Health 1–12, Nov. 1983.
18. Hayes, P.E., and Bloom V.L.: A nurse's guide to psychotherapeutic drugs: Recognition and treatment of depressive illness. P.R.N. learning systems, pharmacology for nurses by home study **2**(5): 1–14, 1982.
19. Hayes, P.E., and Schulz, S.C.: Beta blockers in anxiety disorders. Psychiatr. Med. **3**: 41–60, 1985.
20. Hollister, L.E.: When to use psychotherapeutic agents. Drug Ther. 213–223, April 1982.
21. Kessler, K.A., and Waletzky, J.P.: Therapy review: clinical use of the antipsychotics. Am. J. Psychiatry **138**(2): 142–148, Feb. 1981.
22. Koplan, C.R.: Pediatric psychopharmacology. In Bassuk, E.L., Schoonover, S.C., and Gelenberg, A.J., editors: The practitioner's guide to psychoactive drugs, ed. 2, pp. 313–352. New York and London, 1984, Plenum Medical Books Co.
23. Koplan, C.R.: The use of psychotropic drugs during pregnancy and nursing. In Bassuk, E.L., Schoonover, S.C., and Gelenberg, A.J., editors: The practitioner's guide to psychoactive drugs, ed. 2, pp. 353–369. New York and London, 1984. Plenum Medical Books Co.
24. Lader, M.: Introduction to psychopharmacology. Kalamazoo, Mich., 1983, Scope Publication, the Upjohn Company.
25. Larkin, A.R.: What's a medication group? J. Psychiatric Nurs. Ment. Health Serv. **20**(2): 35–37, Feb. 1982.
26. Lydiard, R.B., and Pearsall, R.: Lithium: predicting response/maximizing efficacy. In Gold, M.S., Lydiard, R.B., and Carman, J.S., editors: Advances in psychopharmacology: predicting and improving treatment response, pp. 121–155. Boca Raton, Fla., 1984, CRC Press.

27. Moreines, R., and Gold, M.S.: MAO inhibitors: predicting response/maximizing efficacy. In Gold, M.S., Lydiard, R.B., and Carman, J.S., editors: Advances in psychopharmacology: predicting and improving treatment response, pp. 157–177. Boca Raton, Fla., 1984, CRC Press.

28. Nardil: Parke-Davis Product Monograph, ed. 4. Morris Plains, N.J., 1982, Parke-Davis, Medical Affairs Department.

29. Post, R.M., and Uhde, T.W.: Carbamazepine in psychiatric disorders: carbamazepine in bipolar illness. Psychopharmacol. Bull. **21**:10–17, 1985.

30. Prien, R.F.: Information on . . . Lithium (DHHS Pub. No. (ADM) 81-1078). National Institute of Mental Health, U.S. Department of Health and Human Services, 1981.

31. Rapoport, J.L.: Pedatric psychopharmacology: clinical assessment for pediatric psychopharmacology. Psychopharmacology: A generation of progress, 1481–1488, Jan. 1981.

32. Richelson, E.: Pharmacology of neuroleptics in use in the United States J. Clin. Psychiatry **46**(8): 8–14 (sec. 2), Aug. 1985.

33. Salzman, C., Hoffman, S.A., and Schoonover, S.C.: Geriatric psychopharmacology. In Bassuk, E.L., Schoonover, S.C., and Gelenberg, A.J., editors: The practitioner's guide to psychoactive drugs, ed. 2, pp. 353–369. New York and London, 1984, Plenum Medical Books Co.

34. Schoonover, S.C.: Depression. In Bassuk, E.L., Schoonover, S.C., and Gelenberg, A.J., editors: The practitioner's guide to psychoactive drugs, ed. 2, pp. 19–74. New York and London, 1984, Plenum Medical Books Co.

35. Selander, J.J., and Miller, W.C.: Prolixin group. J. Psychosoc. Nurs. **23**(11): 17–20, 1985.

36. Smith, D.E., and Wesson, D.R.: Benzodiazepine dependency syndromes. J. Psychoactive Drugs **15**(1–2): 85–95, 1983.

37. Snyder, S.H.: Biological aspects of mental disorder, 3–253, Oxford, 1980, Oxford University Press.

38. Snyder, S.H.: Neurosciences: an integrative discipline. Science **225**(4668):1255–1257, Sept. 1984.

39. Stimmel, G.L.: Affective disorders. In Herfindal, E.T., and Hirschman, J.L., editors: Clinical pharmacy and therapeutics, ed. 3, pp. 727-743. Baltimore, 1984, Williams & Wilkins.

40. Towery, O.B., and Brands, A.B.: Psychotropic drugs: Approaches to psychopharmacologic drug use (DHHS Pub. No. (ADM), 80-758). U.S. Department of Health and Human Services, May 1980.

41. Whiteside, S.E.: Patient education: effectiveness of medication programs for psychiatric patients. J. Psychiatr. Nurs. Ment. Health Serv. **21**(10): 17–21, Oct. 1983.

42. Wincor, M.A.: Benzodiazepines drug review: insomnia and the new benzodiazepines. Clin. Pharm. **1**: 425–432, 1982.

43. Youssef, F.A.: Adherence to therapy in psychiatric patients: An empirical investigation. Int. J. Nurs. Stud. **21**(1): 51–57, 1984.

44. Zisook, S.: A clinical overview of monoamine oxidase inhibitors. Psychosomatics **26**(3): 240–251, March 1985.

■ ANNOTATED SUGGESTED READINGS ■

American Psychiatric Association Task Force: The current status of lithium therapy: report of the APA task force, Am. J. Psychiatry **132**:997, 1975.

This is a comprehensive review of issues relevant to lithium therapy, including indications for use, contraindications, biochemistry, side effects, and research needs. It is an excellent resource for those who are involved with patients receiving lithium.

*Backinsky, M.: Geriatric medications: how psychotropic drugs can go astray, R.N. **41**:50, Feb. 1978.

The author describes the effects of psychotropic medications on elderly patients. Changes in metabolism and biological responses after the reactions of the elderly to drugs. This reference will be useful to nurses who work with this age group. A summary chart of drugs and adverse effects is included.

Gelenberg, A.J., et. al: Treating Extrapyramidal Reaction, *Massachusetts General Hospital Newsletter,* Biological Therapies in Psychiatry **6**(4):13–15, April 1983. PSG Inc., 545 Great Road, Littleton, Mass. 01460

This article discusses the treatment of acute dystonic reactions, akathisia, drug-induced Parkinson's syndrome, and tardive dyskinesia. It states that, since treatment is far from perfect, future research must find antipsychotic drugs without neuroleptic properties. Until then, attention to diagnosis and to optimal use of available therapies is necessary for greater patient comfort, enhanced clinical effectiveness, and improved compliance.

*O'Brien, J.: Teaching psychiatric inpatients about their medications. J. Psychiatr. Nurs. **17**:17–30, Oct. 1979.

This article describes the development and implementation of medication classes for patients as a result of a nursing staff's concern about readmissions related to noncompliance. It describes the teaching approaches used and specifies the areas in which nurses can and cannot actively educate the patient.

O'Hare, T. F., J.D.: Legal issues in prescribing psychoactive medications. In Bassuk, E.L., Schoonover, S.C., and Gelenberg, A.J., editors: The practitioner's guide to psychoactive drugs, ed. 2, pp. 399–409. New York and London, 1984, Plenum Medical Book Co.

The conflicts in psychiatry and patient advocacy regarding the legal issues that must be considered when prescribing and administering psychoactive medications are focused on in this chapter. It covers the areas of torts, civil rights, informed consent, right to withdraw consent, and lists suggestions for avoiding litigation.

*Pliette, W.L.: What is an adequate trial of psychotropic medication? *Perspect. Psychiatr. Care* **15**:170, Oct.-Dec. 1977.

---

*Asterisk indicates nursing reference.

The author reviewed the literature regarding the dosage, range, and length of time recommended for a therapeutic trial of antipsychotic and antidepressant medications. He found that there were no generally accepted guidelines incorporating both of these factors. He strongly recommends that research be conducted to establish reliable guidelines.

Pillard R. C., and Fisher, S.: Human models and behavioral pharmacology, normal humans as models for psychophармacologic therapy, Psychopharmacology: A generation of progress, 783–790, Jan. 1981.

This article discusses the selection of non-psychiatric persons as normal volunteers for research studies designed to learn about psychopharmacologic drug effects. The volunteers used in drug research to date have been 1) nonpsychiatric persons given drugs in a relaxed laboratory setting: generally there is no psychotropic medication effect; 2) persons selected for traits that approximate patient symptoms: this group does show drug effects; 3) persons in whom a state has been induced approximating patient symptoms: this research is growing in popularity and seems promising to future psychopharmacologic studies. The use of nonpsychiatric, normal volunteers as subjects in psychiatric drug research will most likely be increasing in centers around the country.

Sloboda, W. and Currier, C. Free Communications-Session B, FDA's Monitoring of Clinical Trials, Psychopharmacol. Bull. **21**(1):105–109, 1985.

As part of the FDA's Bioresearch Monitoring Program, clinical studies are inspected to monitor the conduct of research involving investigational drugs. Inspections generally focus on which team member did what, where the study was performed, and how the drug was accounted for. These inspections also include an audit for the study performance by comparing data submitted to FDA with supporting records on-site. An interview is held with the clinical investigator, and the results are presented and discussed.

Stanley, B. et al.: Psychopharmacologic treatment and informed consent: empirical research. Psychopharmacol. Bull. **21**(1)110–113, 1985.

Informed consent of research participants is required by federal regulation for psychopharmacologic research. Yet there are few studies regarding the informed consent process and the mentally ill. Timing of the informed consent has been the subject of much controversy. This study investigated the effect of psychotropic medication on the ability to give informed consent to research. The results indicate that medication status does not substantially alter competency, that comprehension of consent information improves over the course of the hospitalization, and schizophrenics tend to have more difficulty in the consent process than patients with major affective disorders.

White, J.H.: Pediatric psychopharmacology: a practical guide to clinical application, Baltimore, 1977, The Williams & Wilkins Co.

This book is recommended for nurses specializing in pediatric or child psychiatric nursing. It is a thorough consideration of the use of psychopharmacological agents with children. The material is illustrated with selected case histories.

Wittenborn, J.R.: Psychotrophic drug assessment: guidelines for clinical trials in psychopharmacology. Psychopharmacology: a generation of progress, 833–840, Jan. 1981.

The American College of Neuropsychopharmacology has begun to produce guidelines to be used for evaluating international psychopharmacologic research and for guiding investigators. This article summarizes results to date. The guidelines specify each phase of drug development for use in humans, once appropriate pharmacological and toxicological studies have been completed in lower animals. Phase I: provides evidence of dose-related pharmacologic effects and side effects in normal volunteers and/or psychiatric patients. Early phase II: knowledge of effective dose, probable side effects and therapeutic potential are established, and comparison groups are not requiring; remaining phase II studies required comparison groups and are designed to provide reasonable evidence of clinical efficacy in defined patient populations. Phase III involves extensive controlled studies; seeks evidence of efficacy in a wide range of patient groups and settings, and also in specific symptoms; common and rare adverse reactions are documented.

PART TWO

PRACTICE
OF PSYCHIATRIC NURSING

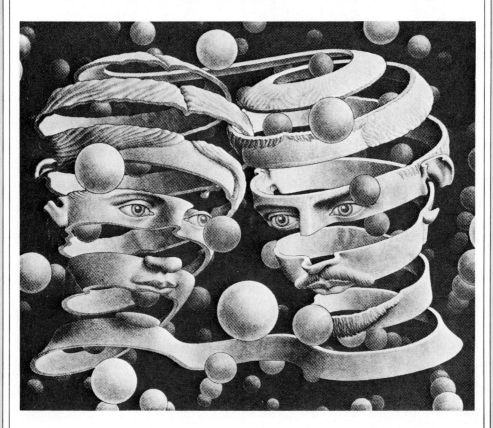

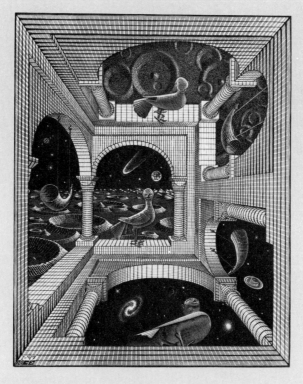

"We're all mad here. I'm mad. You're mad."
"How do you know I'm mad?" said Alice.
"You must be," said the Cat, "or you wouldn't
have come here."
Alice didn't think that proved it at all.

Lewis Carroll, *Alice's Adventures in Wonderland*

C H A P T E R   2 4

EVOLUTION OF INPATIENT PSYCHIATRIC NURSING

KAY SIENKILEWSKI

LEARNING OBJECTIVES

After studying this chapter, the student should be able to:

- describe the historical events that have influenced the role of the psychiatric nurse in an inpatient setting.

- discuss the advantages and disadvantages of the utilization of a primary nursing model for the delivery of psychiatric nursing care.

- discuss the role of the clinical nurse specialist on an inpatient unit.

- identify the two levels of patient education and discuss the nursing implications.

- analyze and compare the concepts of milieu therapy as described by Cumming and Cumming and the therapeutic community as described by Jones.

- identify the role of individual, group, and family therapy programs in the inpatient setting.

- describe psychodrama in terms of major concepts and the therapeutic process.

- discuss the utilization of the various occupational and activity therapies in the inpatient setting.

- compare the characteristics of acute intensive and long-term custodial inpatient psychiatric units and discuss the nursing implications of the differences in the settings.

- identify directions for future nursing research.

- select appropriate readings for further study.

The practice of inpatient psychiatric nursing is rich in history and tradition. It would be impossible to separate the evolution of modern psychiatric nursing from the developmental stages of medical practices in psychiatry, mental health concepts, and the growth of nursing as a profession. Years of progress and successful attainment of knowledge and skills in the areas of psychiatric treatment and nursing care delivery systems have given rise to inpatient psychiatric nursing practice that is exciting, innovative, and challenging. No longer is the inpatient nurse the "keeper of the key." Inpatient psychiatry offers the nurse an opportunity to use the nursing process and employ a variety of skills in responding directly to the needs of the patient and significant others.

Inpatient psychiatric nurse as a caretaker

Early inpatient psychiatric nursing was characterized by custodial care, which ranged from humanistic to neglectful and cruel. In the early Middle Ages the mentally ill were admitted into general hospitals and treated with kindness. Seventh century writings reveal that treatment of the "insane," particularly those "subject to melancholy," bore close resemblance to some practices followed in the mental hospital of the late 1930s and early 1940s.[20] Frequent baths, a wholesome

diet, and "suitable exhilaration" of the mind were the primary modes of treatment for the depressed patient. The more severely disturbed were also provided these forms of therapy but were restrained in their beds to prevent them from injuring themselves or others. It was in the three centuries following the Reformation that the system of "appalling neglect and revolting cruelty" developed in the treatment of the mentally ill. This lasted until the drastic reforms of the nineteenth century.

The nurse's role was primarily to oversee the care given to the patients and to ensure the smooth operation of the ward. It was not uncommon that tasks of housekeeping, dietary management, and laundry care became the responsibility of the nurse. Thus the early inpatient psychiatric nurse was more a manager of a unit than a provider of direct patient care.[9]

The reforms of the nineteenth century had great impact on inpatient psychiatric nursing. The care of patients once again became humane, and the scientific understanding of the nature, causes, and treatment of mental illness was of primary concern. As this scientific body of knowledge increased, there was great demand for advancement in psychiatric nursing to ensure that psychiatric treatment kept pace with the rapid growth in other branches of medicine and nursing.

Despite this "new era," the role of the inpatient nurse remained primarily custodial in nature. Much of the emphasis was placed on performing tasks and administering somatic therapies. However, the seed had been planted, and the future of psychiatric nursing as a viable specialty was taking root.

Inpatient psychiatric nurse as a member of the team

With the development of social psychiatry, the role of the inpatient psychiatric nurse began to change. Nurses became key figures in milieu therapy and therapeutic communities. The nurse was used as a role model for the patients and their families. There was a dramatic shift in emphasis from the importance of performing tasks to the importance of establishing interpersonal relationships. Nursing was given "almost free rein" to involve the patient in activities of daily living. Together the nurse and the patient would problem solve important issues centered around self-care and interactions with others within the community.

As early as 1949 nursing was to enter yet another "hallowed hall."[23] For the most part, individual psychotherapy had been limited to physicians. Nurses were often instructed to observe and record the patients' behavior but not to make any type of interpretation. With the advent of the health team concept, nurses were encouraged to learn more about the psychodynamics of mental illness and to engage in individual nursing therapy. It was not infrequent that a physician would supervise a "promising nurse therapist" who was providing individual therapy to a patient.

By the mid-1950s nurses were recognized as being capable of functioning as group leaders and therapists. This was a major breakthrough, since no longer was nursing limited to custodial care and unit management. Nurses were finally participating in collegial relationships with psychiatric social workers, occupational and recreational therapists, psychologists, and physicians.

In 1949 Dr. Robert H. Felix, Director of the National Institute of Mental Health, U.S. Public Health Service, spoke of the importance of a team approach to psychiatric care. At this time teamwork was still in an early experimental stage, and in some institutions even the concept of the team approach was not yet accepted, let alone practiced.[21]

In these early days of the team concept the psychiatric team was defined as consisting of the psychiatrist, clinical psychologist, psychiatric social worker, and psychiatric nurse. According to Robinson,[21] professional rivalries were often evident, and territoriality became a block to progress. The psychiatrist continued to view himself as "the sole dispenser of psychotherapy rather than the captain of a therapeutic team." Psychiatric so-

cial workers and psychiatric nurses were often more concerned about "delineating their separate areas of professional responsibility than about cooperating for the total welfare of the patient."[21] To overcome these early stumbling blocks, advocates of the team concept in psychiatric treatment were pressed to clarify the purpose and to demonstrate the desirability of this approach.

The definition of a clinical team comprises several explicit and implicit characteristics. The purpose of the psychiatric team is to provide a forum in which the psychiatrist, psychiatric social worker, clinical psychologist, and psychiatric nurse democratically share professional knowledge and together evolve a therapeutic plan of action.[18]

There are many implications that arise from this definition of the psychiatric team. It implies that all members have an equal opportunity to share what they have learned about the patient and that these inputs will be welcomed when it is time to develop a definite goal-directed plan of action. Implicit to the concept of a clinical team approach is the need for a team leader. It is the psychiatrist who most frequently functions in this capacity. According to Mereness, it is the responsibility of the leader to "help mold into an understandable unity the specialized information which is brought to the group by other team members." A final implication is the presence of mutual respect and understanding of the contributions that each team member brings to the situation.[18]

In the early stages of the team approach most nurses were receptive to the concept and grateful for the opportunity to contribute to patient care. However, old stereotypes of the subordinate role that nurses usually played and inadequate communication skills placed nurses at a disadvantage. It became apparent that "the nurse's academic and professional background must be equivalent to that of her colleagues if she is to feel secure and be accepted as a fully participating member of the team."[18]

Nursing educators responded to the challenge and began to make needed changes in their educational systems. Curriculum changes included the addition of scientific psychiatric nursing education, with special emphasis on psychodynamics and interpersonal theory, communication skills, and skills in understanding and working with other disciplines. Thus there began to develop a new breed of psychiatric nurses who viewed themselves as professionally and academically competent to be fully participating members of the psychiatric clinical team.

There is little doubt that the joint endeavor of a team approach promoted mutual respect among the various disciplines, and nursing was a definite benefactor of this new-found mutuality. However, what ground nursing may have gained in collegiality may have been lost in its search for autonomy. Thus the nagging doubts about nursing being a "true profession" continued to remain as many nurses adopted a compensatory role of "junior psychiatrist."

Inpatient psychiatric nursing and the nursing process

Once nurses had been accepted as members of the mental health team and had developed sophistication, skills, and knowledge in the specialty of psychiatry and psychiatric treatment, there came a need for reassessment and clarification of purpose and identity. Psychiatric nursing returned to the nursing process.

If there is anything that is unique to nursing, it is the nursing process. Sundeen and co-workers[24] describe the nursing process as an "interactive, problem-solving process used by the nurse as a systematic and individualized way to fulfill the goal of nursing care." They distinguish problem solving, which is used by many disciplines, and the nursing process as follows:

Many disciplines incorporate aspects of the problem-solving process. The nursing process, however, is distinguished from the problem-solving process in its purpose and method. The purpose of the problem-solving process is the development of new knowledge. The purpose of the nursing process is to maximize a client's positive interactions with his environment, his level of wellness, and his degree of self-actualization. The methods also differ. With the scientific process one can problem-solve in isolation, manipulating objects and ideas without interacting with other people. The nursing process, however, is founded on the helping, interpersonal relationship; the nurse interacts with a client to analyze and meet his biopsychosocial needs.[24:5]

Today's inpatient psychiatric nurses use the nursing process to provide care to individuals, families, and groups. Through this process the nurse strives to assist the patient to establish more effective ways of handling those stresses which led to his immobilization. It is the goal of the nurse to participate with the patient in planning the nursing care. By capitalizing on the patient's strengths, the nurse may help him to establish more harmonious interpersonal relationships and function more independently. These successful accomplishments will lead to a more positive self-concept and a sense of well-being.

The manner in which inpatient psychiatric nurses implement the nursing process may vary from institution to institution or from nurse to nurse. However, there are several factors that remain constant. The col-lection of a data base is the initial step in the process. This is usually accomplished in an individual interview, which is conducted by the nurse within 24 to 48 hours after the patient's admission to the unit. Depending on the patient's ability to be an accurate historian, the nurse may choose to use family members or friends as sources of information. Once a data base is gathered, the nurse develops a diagnostic impression and plans the appropriate nursing actions to be implemented. The results of these nursing actions are evaluated as frequently as necessary, and changes and modifications are made when appropriate. (See Chapter 5 and Appendices B, C, and D for tools of assessment.)

■ **TEAM RELATIONSHIPS.** It is important to stress that the nursing process does not exist in a vacuum. It is essential to the patient that each discipline on the health team work toward common goals and objectives. However, within these common goals and objectives, each discipline has a variety of dependent, independent, and interdependent functions. The most familiar dependent nursing functions are those of carrying out the physician's orders. It is the responsibility of the nurse to give treatments and medications accurately and on time. The nurse must facilitate the process by which the patient is assured of receiving all the prescribed laboratory tests, psychological tests, and other appropriate consultations. Despite the fact that these are truly dependent fuctions, the nurse has the right and the obligation to question any physician's orders that are unclear or possibly unsafe. Interdependent functions of the inpatient psychiatric nurse may range from the mutual sharing of information with the health team to acting as cotherapist with physicians or social workers in family or group therapy, providing she has appropriate preparation for these roles.

It is those independent functions of nursing which often give rise to the greatest sense of job satisfaction for the inpatient psychiatric nurse. It is within the realm of the nurse to implement nursing action ranging from the taking of vital signs to carrying out special types of nursing observations and supervision. Together the nurse and the patient develop goals and determine the course that seems most likely to lead to the accomplishment of those goals. Along the way the nurse must decide what teaching is necessary to provide for the patient, his family, and significant others. The nurse must answer the questions of how much can be learned from the patient's milieu and what needs must be met within the patient's home environment, community, or employment situation. It is the inpatient psychiatric nurse who often provides the vital link in bridging the gap between inpatient hospitalization and successful reintegration into the community.

■ **PATIENT INVOLVEMENT.** It is difficult, if not impossible, to accomplish these objectives without the active participation of the patient. One method of encouraging the patient's participation is the use of nursing rounds. In nursing rounds the patient is interviewed by a "nurse consultant" in front of members of the nursing staff who are working directly with him. The nurse consultant encourages the patient to discuss both those experiences in his hospitalization which are useful and those which are nonproductive. The patient is requested to say how he believes the nursing staff can best help him reach his goals. He is urged to identify his internal and external resources and to capitalize on these strengths during the period of his hospitalization as well as when he returns to the community.

Patient response to this particular format of nursing rounds has been favorable. Many patients have articulated that in nursing rounds they have experienced being treated as "intelligent adults." They believe that they are given the right, as consumers of health care, to demand to be informed participants in that care.

Clinical example 24-1 demonstrates the implementation of the nursing process on an inpatient psychiatric unit.

Thus today's psychiatric nursing practice is characterized by a body of knowledge that is founded in behavioral science theories, biopsychological aspects of stress, and sound effective interpersonal relationships. This body of knowledge is translated into action by way of the nursing process. The question now becomes, What modality of care delivery is best suited for the implementation of the nursing process?

■ Primary nursing and the nursing process

This portion of the chapter will be devoted to a discussion of primary nursing as a modality of care delivery on an inpatient psychiatric unit and the experiences of inpatient psychiatric nurses who, in becoming primary nurses, "rediscovered" the nursing process.

■ **CHARACTERISTICS.** Primary nursing is a modality of care delivery that is characterized by the assignment of one nurse to coordinate the total nursing care of a patient from the time of admission to discharge. This care delivery system provides highly individualized, comprehensive care with a degree of continuity that other nursing modalities have failed to provide. It is the assumption of 24-hour responsibility that sets the primary nurse apart from other nurses. It is the primary nurse who assesses the patient's nursing needs, develops a plan of care to be implemented around the clock, and evaluates the results of that care. Primary nurses may delegate the responsibility of implementing the care plan

> ## CLINICAL EXAMPLE 24-1
>
> Ms. R was a 17-year-old, single, high school student who was admitted to an inpatient psychiatric unit with the diagnosis of bipolar disorder. She was admitted for uncontrollable behavior (i.e., sexual promiscuity, running away from home, hyperverbalization, extreme irritability).
>
> The initial nursing assessment provided a data base that revealed a chaotic family system with a long history of mental illness on both sides of the family, a social and cultural environment in which drug and alcohol abuse were prevalent, and a community that, because of its low socioeconomic status, possessed limited mental health resources. However, the patient was very bright, cooperative, and motivated to benefit from her hospitalization.
>
> The initial nursing actions were to carry out the dependent functions of administering the prescribed medications including lithium carbonate, and assuring that blood levels were checked three times a week until a therapeutic level was reached. The nurse assessed that there was an immediate need to protect the patient from her impulsive uncontrollable behavior. The patient was placed under close nursing observation at all times until she was able to be in control of her own behavior.
>
> Once the patient's mood had stabilized, she was presented in nursing rounds. During this time the patient was able to identify a great need for the nurse to teach her and her family about bipolar disorder and the importance of continued lithium treatment. The patient and staff agreed that a home visit would reveal the pressures that the family placed on the patient to function as surrogate mother to her eight siblings. The patient also believed that it was important that her illness not be viewed in exactly the same manner as that of her sister, who was diagnosed as schizophrenic. The patient viewed her intellectual ability and the "love" that existed in her family system as her best resources. She thought that, with the assistance of the nursing staff, she and her family could develop more understanding of her illness and decrease the chaos within the family system.
>
> After discharge the patient was treated in outpatient therapy by a nurse therapist. The family was being seen by a psychiatric social worker.

in their absence, but it is they who are accountable for providing the directions through written and verbal communications. Marram, Barrett, and Bevis[17] view the primary nurse as a "triple A" nurse who has "three basic characteristics: autonomy, authority, and accountability."

These three characteristics, more than any other, differentiate between a nursing practice that is professionally oriented and one that is task oriented. A primary nurse who has autonomy functions in a collaborative manner with other disciplines. Other health professionals are used by the primary nurse as resources and consultants. However, the nursing care plan is developed by the primary nurse and the patient. In a professionally oriented practice, the person who is providing direct care must have the authority to make decisions concerning that care. Primary nurses have the authority to develop and implement a total comprehensive nursing care plan on a 24-hour basis. A true test of a professional is the demonstration of a willingness to stand accountable for all his decisions and actions. The primary nurse is accountable for all decisions made and actions taken in the nursing care of her patients.

The department of nursing of several inpatient psychiatric facilities across the United States have chosen to use primary nursing as their care delivery system. Many have reported that primary nursing has led to increased job satisfaction among the professional nursing staff and increased satisfaction among the patient population. On the surface it appears that a transition to primary nursing in an inpatient psychiatric setting could be accomplished with ease. The nature of psychiatric nursing lends itself to the establishment of one-to-one relationships. For years psychiatric nurses have been engaging in individual nurse-patient interactions. Despite this past experience, many institutions have encountered numerous difficulties in implementing primary nursing.

■ **PROBLEMS.** Two types of problems are likely to be encountered during the transitional period. First are those problems that are internal to nursing. Second are the problems that result from the impact that implementing change in one discipline has on other disciplines. Internal problems center around the redefinition of all nursing positions from the director of psychiatric nursing to the psychiatric aides and unit clerks. How to include the nonprofessional nursing staff in primary nursing remains an unsolved problem in need of further exploration. The primary nurses themselves seem to encounter the most difficulty in accepting accountability for their decision making and practice.

To successfully implement primary nursing, there must be support and acceptance of this care delivery system from both the administrative and staff levels. Unfortunately, hierarchical authority and bureaucracy continue to be predominant characteristics of the nursing culture. Hospital and nursing administrators are reluctant to provide the adequate staffing pattern and the decentralization of decision making that is imperative to the success of primary nursing.[17]

Thus nursing administrators must view themselves as facilitators of change and must be willing to delegate certain authority to make decisions about patient care to the nurses at the clinical levels. Administrators must also be committed to providing adequate staffing patterns and resource people for clinical supervision, staff development, and inservice education. Once nursing administration has made this commitment, it must realize that organizational change alone will not lead to successful implementation of primary nursing.[14] However, by lending support and leadership through active participation, nursing administration can provide an environment that fosters an enthusiam toward viewing change as a challenge and as an opportunity for personal and professional growth.

Can all psychiatric nurses be primary nurses? This is perhaps the most difficult of the internal problems encountered in the transitional period of implementing this system. In their study on the use of psychiatric nurses, Anderson and Apostoles[2] found that all 26 nurses in their research program were able to successfully complete their rotation through the 18-month project. It was only after the completion of the program that two of the 26 nurses resigned.

A closer look at this project reveals that in this study population associate degree and baccalaureate graduates were overrepresented, and diploma and master's degree graduates were underrepresented. The project nurses generally agreed (75%) that "any new graduate has the basic skills to function as a primary care nurse." However, these nurses added a qualifier to this statement by making the provision that the guidance of a clinical specialist, support from the physician, and team cooperation were essential.[2]

In their study on primary nursing Coates, Falck, and Sienkilewski[3] observed that the essential ingredients to being a successful primary nurse on an inpatient psychiatric unit were innovation, motivation, and a patient-centered orientation. They further observed that, with few exceptions, those primary nurses possessing these characteristics who did not already have their baccalaureate degrees soon began working toward them.

It is obvious that not all psychiatric nurses can be primary nurses. No one care delivery system is able to satisfy the needs of all. There is some evidence that, given a supportive nursing administration, most nurses who are willing to stand accountable and are motivated to accept the challenge will experience some success as primary nurses.

The transition to primary nursing has an impact on

other health care providers, and the responses to this impact may vary from humorous to serious. An initial response from the resident physician group is often to become territorial about their patients. This phase may be referred to as the "not with my patients, you don't" phase. In a similar manner, psychiatric social workers may respond to the threat of boundary encroachment by countering, "Not with my families, you don't." Occupational and recreational therapists, who are often involved in their own search for autonomy, may be heard to say, "Here we go again."

Once the initial impact is over and resolutions to many of the internal and external problems are found, the multidisciplinary team enters into the second phase of transition. This phase is frequently characterized by the beginning development of mutual sharing, respect, and trust. "Not with my patient" becomes "What can nursing offer the patient?" "Not with my family" is replaced by "Would you like to sit in on a family assessment?" or "Shall we do a joint home visit?" It is at this stage that the "here we go again" truth tellers may ask, "Have we really made it this time?"

The benefactor of a collaborative approach to care is the patient. When the psychiatric team works in a collegial fashion, there is little need for energy to be wasted on protecting boundaries and territories. Thus the team's attention is focused on the needs of the patient. Clinical example 24-2 is an actual patient's account of her experience as a primary patient in an inpatient psychiatric unit.*

Problems related to psychiatric settings. The three major characteristics of the primary nursing modality (autonomy, authority, and accountability) are the same in inpatient psychiatric nursing as in any other clinical specialty. However, unique complications do arise because of the nature of the specialty of psychiatry. More than in other areas of medicine, psychiatric care providers share an almost universal ingredient—the therapeutic use of self. Frequently, clinical territory is shared and skills are equalized, and "gender and character style rather than strict professional discipline lines are drawn."[26] Psychiatric nurses are often asked to expand their roles to include psychotherapy and social work. If this occurs too frequently, and if primary nurses are supervised exclusively by other disciplines, the nurse can lose her identity with her own profession. At this point she can no longer be considered a primary nurse.

Thus primary nursing in psychiatric settings must be clearly defined in relation to other professionals and paraprofessionals. Primary nurses must maintain their

---

*Excerpt from an interview I conducted for nursing rounds.

> ## CLINICAL EXAMPLE 24-2
>
> When I came here I was completely immobilized. I was afraid of everything. The fears started as small silly things that my family and I tried to laugh off. But soon the little fears became bigger and bigger, and soon I wasn't able to function as a wife, a mother, or a human being.
>
> Do you know that I hadn't been able to do any shopping for 2 years. I hadn't been out of my house at all for the past 6 months—except to come to the hospital. I had often thought of killing myself, but I was even too afraid to do that.
>
> I can't tell you what being here has meant to me. Everyone has been understanding and supportive. My psychiatrist saw me three times a week in therapy and helped me learn about my illness and what caused my fears. The more I understood, the less frightening things seemed.
>
> But I give most of the credit for my recovery to my primary nurse. She was the person who helped me to function again. She made me feel less ashamed and helped me to realize that I wasn't a total, no good weakling.
>
> Together we planned strategies of how to get me moving. We started very slowly with short trips off the ward. The next step was to go to the market to buy cake mix for the ward bake sale. The big step happened just a few weeks ago when my nurse and I went all the way downtown to Christmas shop for my family. My family and I cried together when I gave them their gifts on Christmas Day. It was the first time in 2 years that I was able to buy them anything. I'm preparing for discharge with my primary nurse. Last weekend I went home, and I was able to shop alone. I am still apprehensive, but my nurse says that this is not unusual.
>
> I'm being discharged next week and the plans are for me to see my doctor on an outpatient basis for awhile. My primary nurse is going to make a follow-up home visit in 2 weeks to see how things are going. I really feel comfortable with this arrangement.
>
> Are all the other wards going to start primary nursing? I think that all the patients here should have the opportunity to have a primary nurse.

involvement in the milieu. They must participate in experiences with patients "because they are part of patients' everyday lives."[26] The primary nurse teaches the patient how to use all his social, interpersonal, and environmental experiences within the hospital system. It is from these experiences that the patient can often learn more effective ways of dealing with those real-life stresses which can lead to the need for hospitalization.

It is this involvement in the patient's everyday life that places the primary nurse in the position of being able to provide and integrate data from many sources. It is also this involvement that best differentiates the role of the primary nurse from other psychiatric professionals.

Recent legislative changes and budgetary constraints have had great impact on mental health care and the utilization of professional personnel. As previously mentioned, psychiatric nurses are being asked to expand their roles to include such functions as psychotherapist and case manager. Nursing administrators must be responsive to these current trends and creative in their approaches in meeting these additional service demands. The consequences of a lack of responsiveness could re-

sult in a professional loss of identity for psychiatric nurses and a decrease in the quality of nursing care provided to psychiatric patients.

■ **MODELS OF PRIMARY NURSING.** It is possible to combine the concepts of primary nursing and primary care in psychiatric settings. This combination provides a system in which nurses are encouraged to expand their roles and are expected and supported to continue their primary nursing activities and milieu involvement. The amalgamation of these two concepts should be tailored to meet the organizational, treatment, and fiscal policies of the institution. However, the integrity of the modalities must be maintained. Two models of a primary nursing–primary care system are given in Table 24-1.

Model A was developed for a small psychiatric department in a general hospital. The department housed one 20-bed inpatient unit and an active outpatient clinic.

TABLE 24-1

COMPARISON OF TWO MODELS FOR THE IMPLEMENTATION OF PRIMARY NURSING

Models	Primary nurses	Outpatient therapists
Model A		
Who assigns patients?	Head nurse	Treatment team
Who provides supervision?	Clinical nurse specialist	Clinical nurse specialist
	Peer group	Psychiatrist
Specific role functions	Nursing assessments	Individual psychotherapy
	Nursing care plans	Group therapy
	Direct nursing care, that is, activities of daily living, giving and monitoring medications and treatment	Family therapy
		Coordinating activities, such as agency referrals, housing arrangements, vocational placement, monitoring medication
	Milieu involvement	
	Nursing discharge planning	
	Home visits	
	Family and patient teaching	
Model B		
Who assigns patients?	Head nurse	Psychiatrist
Who provides supervision?	Clinical nurse specialist	Psychiatrist
		Clinical nurse specialist
Specific role functions	Nursing assessments	Psychiatric history
	Nursing care plans	Mental status examination
	Direct nursing care, that is, activities of daily living, giving and monitoring medications and treatment	Social assessment and history
		Family contacts
		Medical and psychiatric coordination
	Milieu involvement	Community resource coordination
	Nursing discharge planning	Discharge planning
	Home visits	Therapist: individual, family, group
	Family and patient teaching	

In this model, the nurses functioned exclusively as primary nurses on the inpatient unit. Each primary nurse spent approximately half a day in the outpatient clinic functioning as a psychotherapist. Thus the primary nurse's case load consisted of three or four primary nursing patients and two or three psychotherapy outpatients.

In this model, the head nurse was responsible for assigning the nursing case loads. Supervision for nursing care was provided by clinical nurse specialists with graduate education in psychiatric nursing and in peer groups with other primary nurses. The assignment of outpatients was made by the treatment team responsible for planning the follow-up care of the patients on the inpatient unit. The supervision for outpatients was provided by the same clinical specialists (who were also qualified therapists) with regular consultations from assigned medical-psychiatric backups. The primary nurses had direct input into the selection process of both the inpatient and outpatient case loads.

Model B was developed for a large state psychiatric hospital. In this model the primary nurse functioned as both case manager and primary nurse on an inpatient admissions unit. As in Model A, the head nurse was responsible for assigning the primary nursing patient case load, and supervision for these patients was provided by clinical nurse specialists with graduate education.

The patients for whom the nurse functioned as case manager and therapist were assigned by the psychiatrist in charge of the treatment team. Supervision for these patients was provided by the psychiatrists and the clinical specialists. The average case load for these nurses was approximately five or six primary nursing patients and two or three case management patients. The primary nurses maintained direct input into the selection process of both case loads.

Essential to the success of both models was a comprehensive inservice educational program and qualified clinical nurse specialists. If primary nurses are to expand their roles, they must have an adequate theoretical and clinical base. Participation in an in-depth inservice program that is balanced in didactic theory and related clinical experience should be a required activity for all primary nurses who are expanding their roles. These program models should be designed, implemented, evaluated, and controlled by nursing. In this way, primary nurses are given the support they need to maintain the integrity of the nursing model and of their professional identity.

The immediate future of primary nursing in inpatient psychiatric settings will more likely be influenced by political, legislative, and financial factors than by therapeutic objectives or philosophies. Cost containment has become a major focus of public and private hospitals. Hospitals must utilize their financial resources and personnel to provide timely patient evaluations, family involvement, relevant treatment modalities, and appropriate dispositions. The long-term future of primary nursing will depend on psychiatric nurses' ability to demonstrate that this modality of care provides quality therapeutic interventions in a cost-effective manner.

The clinical nurse specialist in the inpatient setting

The concept of a "specialist" who provides nursing care to a patient or a group of clients took root early in the nursing profession in the form of the private duty nurse. However, it was not until the mid-1960s that the master's level clinical nurse specialist (CNS) role was developed for the purpose of improving the quality of nursing care. Those first nursing visionaries realized that they would need to justify having master's prepared nurses at the patient's bedside. Consequently, early writings were characterized by broad definitions of educational qualifications and role functions.[7]

Although the role of the CNS may differ from one inpatient facility to another, Clinical example 24-1 and Table 24-2 suggest a model that may be modified to meet many inpatient settings.

It is an unhappy fact that the utilization of the CNS has not lived up to the high expectations of the nursing leaders who conceived and developed the role. Nursing now more than ever needs research to identify ways to demonstrate that quality care and cost containment are not mutually exclusive. If this cannot be accomplished in the near future, the survival of the CNS may well be endangered.

Patient education on an inpatient unit

The consumer movement in mental health has led to requests for information by patients and their families. Mental health care providers are recognizing that informed patients are more likely to participate actively and productively in the treatment process. Families who are knowledgeable about the patient's illness are able to act in partnership with nurses to assist the patient toward wellness.

Because of their frequent and intimate contact with patients, nurses should be actively involved in formal and informal patient education. The education process begins with the orientation of the patient and significant others to the inpatient setting. Frequently, this includes

CASE EXAMPLE 24-1

In 1980, the nursing department of a large state psychiatric hospital made a commitment to the introduction of the role of the clinical nurse specialist as a vital part of its integrated organizational structure. These nursing leaders believed that quality nursing care can be accomplished only when nursing administrators, clinical nurse experts, nursing educators, and nursing researchers work in unison toward a common goal of excellence. The director of nursing, along with the three associate directors, designed an organizational plan based on ANA standards of practice (see Chapter 5 and Appendix A) and current Joint Commission on Accreditation of Hospitals (JCAH) standards which required that hospitals develop an internal mechanism to privilege all core clinicians.[10] The plan called for

1. Nursing administration to appoint a task force to develop a protocol for all registered nurses to be privileged in basic nursing care and expanded role functions

2. Nursing inservice to develop the appropriate educational modules to provide the didactic and theoretical basis needed by staff nurses for expanded role functions

3. Clinical nurse specialists to provide formal clinical supervision, role modeling, and consultation to staff nurses

4. Nursing researchers to provide program evaluation to identify quality and cost issues

Fourteen clinical nurse specialists were recruited and placed strategically in the clinical areas. Their job descriptions called for them to

1. Provide direct patient care

2. Provide formal clinical supervision to staff nurses

3. Act as expert nursing consultant to the interdisciplinary team

4. Provide formal and informal inservice education to nursing staff

5. Participate in nursing research

The clinical nurse specialists were given the autonomy to determine which aspect of their job needed to take priority. Along with this autonomy, they were given the authority to arrange their work schedules to meet patient and staff needs. After 6 years, the CNS has been accepted and has become a valued member of the nursing team. The impact of their efforts on the organization has not been limited to direct patient care. Much of the success in recruiting professional nurses and much of the credibility the department of nursing has gained are a result of the presence of these nursing experts. This experience has convinced the nursing leaders of this hospital that the risks they took and the initial resistance they had to face were well worth their efforts. They believe that the CNS is a necessity in an inpatient psychiatric setting.

the use of written materials to describe the policies, procedures, and activities that take place in the hospital. Of course, the nurse must validate the learner's reading ability and level of comprehension and plan the educational approach accordingly. Important points should always be presented verbally as well as in writing.

Although the physician may initiate the education of the patient about the medical diagnosis, the nurse needs to reinforce the teaching. In addition, nurses are usually the best sources of information about practical management of illness-related behaviors, including symptoms as well as expected responses to treatment approaches. The basic services that are provided to the patient by the nurse in the hospital may need to be continued by the family at home. Therefore, it is important that the family be informed of pertinent aspects of the treatment plan. Both the patient and the family must be aware of such information as side effects of medications and signs of a relapse.

Aside from personalized, individual, or family-oriented patient education, nurses frequently initiate group education programs for patients and/or significant others. Some types of groups that might be led by nurses include medication groups, assertiveness training groups, sexuality groups, community living skills groups, health education groups and stress management groups. Education in a group setting may be enhanced by the feedback and peer support received from other members. Further information on patient education in groups may be found in Chapter 28.

Aside from the primary goal of developing an informed consumer, there are also legal implications related to patient education. Consumers are beginning to bring suit against providers who have not given them adequate information to practice self-care safely. It is the obligation of the nurse to provide necessary information in a manner that is understandable to the patient. Careful documentation of the material presented and the method of evaluation of patient comprehension that was used is also required. Of course, it is important for the nurse to coordinate all patient education activities with the rest of the health care team.

In addition to health-related educational programs, many long-term hospitals also provide academic and pre-vocational education programs for patients. These are usually under the auspices of the vocational rehabilitation department frequently in conjunction with the local school system. Patients who are enrolled in this type of program need the support and encouragement of nurses. Successful mastery of vocationally useful training may make the difference in a patient's ability to survive in the community.

TABLE 24-2

MODEL FOR INPATIENT PSYCHIATRIC CLINICAL NURSE SPECIALIST ROLE FUNCTIONING

Direct patient care	Clinical supervision	Consultation	Education	Research
Individual therapy	Individual supervision of staff	Serve as nurse expert to treatment team	Assist inservice faculty in developing and teaching education modules	Conduct clinical studies to identify effective nursing intervention for specific diagnostic groups
Family therapy	Group supervision of staff	Provide link between hospital and community (e.g., follow patients to community mental outpatient program; consult to nursing homes; consult to public health nurse)	Serve as guest speakers at schools of nursing	Participate in program evaluation to determine the impact and cost-effectiveness of the CNS
Group therapy	Conduct staff meetings	Conduct transition groups in placement homes	Serve as guest speakers to community and patient advocacy groups	Identify effective methods for clinical supervision
Patient education groups a) Medication b) Sex education c) Activities of daily living group	Peer supervision			Identify effective intervention for the chronically mentally ill
Milieu group meetings	Cross-discipline supervision (e.g., may supervise a member of another discipline for family therapy)			
Community living transitional groups Nursing rounds Case management Program coordinator (e.g., design and implement behavior modification program for an individual patient or group of patients) Home visiting				

Design of an inpatient psychiatric unit

The design of an inpatient psychiatric unit is important to the patients, families and friends, and the members of the health care team. The design of the facility should reflect the philosophy of the department, the methods of care provided, and the types of patients to be served. It should make the statement that patients are "worthy of an attractive facility" and that the facility's environment should "correspond as much as possible" to the environment to which he will soon return.[8]

Despite changing tastes in architectural and interior design, there are several principles that seem to continue to hold true. Adequate space is of utmost importance. Patients must be provided with an environment that promotes socialization but allows room for privacy. The unit should have flexibility. Day areas and dining rooms can be designed to easily convert into group meeting rooms. Adequate storage space should be provided to prevent a cluttered unkempt look.

There should be offices provided for individual sessions, charting, and dictating functions. An adequate treatment room facility is essential to the provision of quality medical treatment for the patient. In the more modern inpatient units there is no nurses station per se. Instead there is likely to be a reception desk with work areas that are open and accessible to patients.

In addition to a day area, dining room, and lounge facilities, space should be provided for kitchen and laundry and linen area. The bedrooms should be furnished with comfortable, attractive, sturdy beds and chairs. There should be a combination of single and semiprivate rooms. Small dormitory rooms of three or four patients may be desirable in some hospital settings.

Room for occupational and recreational activities is provided either on the unit or in a separate activities wing adjacent to the inpatient wing. These activities wings may include an arts and crafts room, and music room, and areas for indoor exercise and sports such as yoga, table tennis, and basketball.

Occasionally psychiatric patients need to be secluded or isolated. Isolation rooms can be designed to maintain the privacy and dignity of the isolated patient but still allow for free flow of traffic. This is accomplished by constructing a vestibule between the door of the isolation room and a door that opens onto the main corridor. Often private bathrooms are located in these vestibules. Provision for patient-safety is of primary importance in the design of isolation rooms.

The use of color, furniture, plants, paintings, graphics, and decorator pieces is of great importance. The walls of the rooms are usually painted with subtle quiet hues. Colorful accents are added with graphics, paintings, and furniture. The development of new materials that withstand long-term use and maintenance, as well as meet safety requirements, has enabled architects and interior designers to create noninstitutionalized inpatient units at reasonable costs.

Modalities of therapy on an inpatient psychiatric unit

Many inpatient psychiatric facilities for acutely ill patients offer a variety of therapies in the treatment of psychiatric and behavioral disorders. The inpatient psychiatric nurse is involved to some extent with all therapeutic modalities. The extent of involvement depends on the nurse's relationship with the patient and the philosophy of the institution.

■ Milieu therapy

Milieu therapy is a "scientific manipulation of the environment aimed at producing changes in the personality of the patient."[4] The actual use of the word "milieu" to mean a scientifically planned environment came into being in the work of Bettleheim and Sylvester in the late 1930s and early 1940s.

■ **CONCEPTS.** Early research and experiments in milieu therapy almost exclusively used psychological or psychiatric theories of illness and from these theories attempted to determine the kinds of environments that would be most therapeutic. There were attempts to "prescribe" minutely detailed interpersonal environments based on the psychodynamic needs of a "carefully diagnosed" patient. This ambitious undertaking included attempts to prescribe and program staff attitudes and responses as well as patient activities.

In 1954 Stanton and Schwartz introduced the concept that the environment can be the primary treatment as well as a supporting or complementary influence to other forms of treatment. They presented the fact that the environment may frequently have components that are irrelevant to the psychodynamics of the patient but may be important to his general welfare. Later Caudell described the effect that culture, organized values, norms, and customs have on patient care. In 1958 Freeman, Cameron, and McGhie developed the relationship between ego psychology and specific characteristics of the environment. Despite all this accumulated information, until the work of Cumming and Cumming in 1962 there had been a reluctance to consider the possibility that "the milieu might itself bring about specific changes in the behavior of patients and thus specific changes in their personalities."[4]

Milieu programs may differ widely from system to

system. Despite these differences there appear to be several basic assumptions that are common to all therapeutic milieu approaches to inpatient psychiatric treatment. The first assumption is that patients have strengths and conflict-free portions of their personalities. It is these strengths which are optimally used by the scientific manipulation of the institutional environment. Second, patients have abilities to constructively influence their own treatment, the treatment of others, and to some degree the organizational structure of the hospital. The third assumption is that successful treatment of seriously disturbed patients is extremely dependent on a pervasive, therapeutic staff involvement. The final assumption is that all levels of hospital personnel have the potential for exercising a therapeutic influence.[25]

■ **ROLE OF THE NURSE.** There is little question that the advent of milieu therapy helped to change the course of psychiatric nursing. Before 1946, psychiatric nursing literature stressed the importance of the management of a safe and secure environment. With milieu therapy the role of the nurse in the environment began to change from custodial to therapeutic and rehabilitative. Sills recommends a "social learning model" as an appropriate guide for nurses to use for their interventions in a therapeutic milieu. This would shift the emphasis away from "caring for the patient" to teaching the patient social skills. This would complement and support the basic goals of milieu therapy. These two basic goals are limit setting and learning the basic social skills of orientation, assertion, occupation, and recreation.[25]

Cumming and Cumming[4] view the nurse as a "facilitator and a helper to the patients rather than a therapist." In a therapeutic milieu the nurse keeps the focus on action and problem solving. Discussions of interpersonal relationships are kept in the context of a goal-directed activity. The following nurse-patient interaction may help to distinguish between a nursing intervention in a milieu therapy setting and one in a psychoanalytical setting.

PATIENT: **I can't stand the sight of you. You are always getting in my way.**

NURSE: **We are supposed to go look at the halfway house today. I wonder how your being angry with me is going to affect our plans?**

In this intervention the nurse has attempted to bring the interpersonal discussion back to the social task at hand. On a unit where the approach is more psychoanalytical, the nurse may respond in the following manner:

PATIENT: **I can't stand the sight of you. You are always getting in my way.**

NURSE: **Can we talk more about your anger? We may be able to learn what it is that is making you so unhappy with our relationship.**

This approach is an invitation to the patient to explore his feelings and the possible transference phenomena in the nurse-patient relationship.

What is the outcome of milieu therapy? Because of the lack of standard assessment tools and techniques, studies related to treatment environment and treatment outcome have been limited. However, some consistent findings have been discernible. It appears that a treatment environment which emphasizes involvement, a practical orientation, order and organization, and a reasonable degree of staff control is most successful in keeping patients out of the hospital.[25] Therefore staff and patients should work together to provide an environment that is physically safe and secure; in which expectations, norms, rules, and standards are clear and concise; and where staff and patients have the freedom to communicate openly.

■ Therapeutic community

According to Kraft, "The therapeutic community is a very special kind of milieu therapy in which the total social structure of the treatment unit is involved as part of the helping process."[13:543] How does this differ from the concept of milieu therapy and what are the implications of those differences? Perhaps the clearest distinction is that in the therapeutic community it is believed that all social and interpersonal interactions in the hospital are the main therapeutic tools used to bring about specific changes in the patient. As previously mentioned, in milieu therapy the emphasis is on the manipulation of the environment to bring about changes in patient behavior, with effort being invested in keeping all interpersonal discussions in the context of a goal-directed activity.[4]

■ **CONCEPTS.** It is impossible to discuss the treatment modality of therapeutic community without exploring the original concept as set forth by Maxwell Jones. According to Jones,[11] what most distinguishes a therapeutic community from other comparable treatment programs is the way in which the total resources of the staff, the patients, their relatives, and the institution are pooled for the purpose of treatment. Thus the patient must undergo a change in status. The staff must encourage his active participation in his care planning. This would be a marked contrast to the conventional passive recipient role.[12]

In the structuring of a therapeutic community, Jones suggested that the emphasis should be placed on free communication both within and between staff and patient groups. The end results of free communication were hoped to be the examination of roles, the clarification of what behavior is regarded as appropriate, some loss of apparent distinctiveness of particular roles, and attempts to modify some overall cultural attitudes and beliefs that are antitherapeutic. Thus the therapeutic community would be democratic as opposed to hierarchical, rehabilitative rather than custodial, permissive instead of limited and controlled, and, finally, communal as opposed to emphasizing the specialized therapeutic role of the physician. In the early Maxwell Jones models of a therapeutic community, the environment was essentially permissive and flexible.

Roles of the participants were purposely unspecified, the patients' activities were highly individualized, and participation was completely voluntary. The one exception was a daily community meeting that all staff had to attend and all patients were encouraged to attend. Group responsibility was emphasized, and opportunities for corrective learning experiences were deliberately provided. The primary role of the staff was to assist the patients to gain new insights and to test new behavioral patterns.

Jones believed that each treatment unit should ideally be free to operate in the manner which was best suited to its own particular style and approach. However, he offered several components that he believed were characteristic of a therapeutic community. The daily community meeting was used as a format for discussing day-to-day life on the unit. Since these gatherings were often composed of 80 or 90 patients, many of the tensions and concerns of the individual patients were "worked through" in small group therapy sessions that followed the community meeting.

Another component of the therapeutic community is patient government. The purpose of the patient government or ward council is to deal with practical unit details such as privileges and housekeeping rosters. Jones suggested that a staff member be available to the patient government and that all decisions be fed back to the community through the community meetings.

Jones viewed the staff meeting or review as essential to on-the-ward training. He saw these as taking place for at least 30 minutes following each community meeting. In this meeting the staff would examine their own responses, expectations, and prejudices. Another important characteristic of the therapeutic community is the living-learning opportunities provided to the patient within the social milieu. Thus the therapeutic community is like a "school for living" in which the patients learn to meet the demands of everyday life.

According to Jones, "Feedback is one of the fundamental concepts in therapeutic community practice."[12] It is of great importance that all decisions, disputes, progress, and accomplishments be conveyed to the community as a whole. There is very little, if anything, that is purely confidential in a therapeutic community. The staff must be sensitive in their role of demonstrating how and when to feed back information to the community.

Although there have been additions and modifications of Jones' original concept of the therapeutic community, it is still considered as a viable model. The Marlborough Hospital in London has used the Maxwell Jones model of therapeutic community and has added some creative and innovative activities. Included in this program are the typical community meetings, staff meetings, small psychotherapy groups, work groups, admission meetings, badminton groups, and pottery groups. In addition, this therapeutic community offers individual reviews, encounter groups, projective art sessions, gestalt groups, occupational therapy workshop sessions, patient meetings, and a dream group. There are three other groups that have been created for this particular community. The "Leavers Group" is designed to look at the feelings and problems related to leaving the community. It is in this group that the need for further treatment is discussed. The "Concern Group" is composed of patients who the community believes are not able to make use of their therapy. The purpose of this group is to clarify the aim and purpose of the hospital and the individual's role within it. "The Committee" is composed of five patients, one from each small psychotherapy group, and a number of staff. It functions as a feedback source to the community meetings and to the business and patients' meetings.[15]

■ **ROLE OF THE NURSE.** As in milieu therapy, the nurse's role in the therapeutic community requires maturity and a willingness to have one's own behavior the subject for discussion. Holmes and Werner suggested that nursing interventions in a therapeutic community reflect three features: patients are included in almost all information-sharing processes, patients' opinions are included in decisions about other patients, and the democratic community process is considered treatment. The social learning model is another appropriate guide to nursing interventions in a therapeutic community as well as in milieu therapy.[25]

Nurses are involved in the various group activities within the therapeutic community. Therefore it is essential that the nurse be skilled in group behavior and dynamics. It is interesting to note that a basic assumption in Jones' concept of therapeutic community is that patients have strengths and should be active participants in their care planning. This is exactly the basic assumption of primary nursing and the nursing process.

There are many problems related to the concept of

the therapeutic community. Some concerns are that patients are taught patterns of behavior that are basically inappropriate outside the hospital. Therefore they cannot generalize these newly learned skills to the community environment.[25]

Other problems include staff anxiety because of the threat of loss of professional identity, the fact that "group responsibility" can easily be distorted to mean "no responsibility," and the possibility that the individual patient may become lost in the concern for the group.[13]

If these problems can be resolved, the future of the therapeutic community will be more assured. It will be interesting and challenging to be part of that future.

■ Individual psychotherapy

Traditionally, individual inpatient psychotherapy is conducted by the psychiatrist, who sees the patient on the average of one to three times weekly. The purpose of individual psychotherapy is to offer the patient an opportunity to develop insights into the sources of his thoughts, feelings, perceptions, and behavior. By developing these insights, the patient is able to improve his skills in establishing and maintaining interpersonal relationships and use more effective behaviors in dealing with stress. Despite the fact that it has recently come under attack as an effective modality of treatment, most acute psychiatric facilities continue to view individual psychotherapy as a viable and desirable practice.[5]

In a multidisciplinary approach to patient care other health care providers may function as psychotherapists. In this type of setting it is possible for the nurse to function as primary nurse for a selected number of patients and as psychotherapist for others. It is important that the "expanded role" of the nurse as a psychotherapist not be confused with primary nursing. Although primary nursing is purely a modality of nursing care delivery, the expanded role of psychotherapist requires additional training in the fields of human growth and development, psychodynamics of human behavior, and the art and science of psychotherapy.

■ Family therapy

The focus of family therapy is to treat as the primary unit a social system, rather than an individual member who has been defined as a "patient." A variety of techniques and practices may be used in the process of family therapy. There may be any combination of pairing or grouping in each session or a series of sessions. For example, Ackerman recommends that the entire family unit be seen for therapy, but for the diagnostic phase he conducts sessions with various individuals, pairs, or triads. Wynne varies the member composition to dis-

cover which family members should be included in treatment. Bowen will see the entire family in what he calls "family group therapy" for brief periods. He views the optimum approach as starting with the husband and wife together and continuing with both for the entire period of family therapy. Bowen will often see a single family member to assist that person to achieve a higher level of differentiation.[22]

The goals of family therapy are to reduce conflict and anxiety, to make the family members more aware of each other's needs, to increase the family's ability to deal with external and internal crises, to develop more appropriate role relationships, to help individual family members to cope with destructive forces within and without the family, and to promote health and growth.

The psychiatric nurse should have special training in family systems and conjoint family therapy before attempting to function as a family therapist. The role of the therapist is to penetrate family secrets and myths, to counteract the process of scapegoating, and to pick up nonverbal communication and make it explicit. At other times the therapist may serve as a parent figure or a personal instrument for reality testing. The family therapist must be sensitive to the needs of the individual members and the family unit as a whole and respond appropriately.

A more comprehensive discussion of family therapy is presented in Chapter 29.

■ Group therapy

There are various types of group therapy. Traditionally the term "group therapy" is used to describe a form of psychiatric treatment in which six to eight patients attend a specified number of meetings that are conducted by a therapist. The advantages of group therapy lie in the fact that most people's problems involve their feelings and behavior toward others. In a group setting the patient is able to develop an awareness of how his thoughts, feelings, and behavior affect others. Through group feedback and support the patient will be able to change his behavior and establish more effective interpersonal relationships.

Too frequently groups are established as a "time-saving" device or because there are not enough therapists to care for individual patients. There are times when unskilled personnel are made "group leaders." This is a grave misuse of an effective therapeutic modality. Nurses who become group leaders or therapists should ensure that their group is being offered because for those patients involved it is the most appropriate form of treatment. The nurse should be skilled in group dynamics and behavior as well as have a thorough understanding of individual psychodynamics and psychopathology.

The types of group psychotherapy used on inpatient psychiatric units vary in aim, purpose, and intensity. The selection of specific groups will be determined by the philosophy of the unit, the skills of the staff, and the capacities of the patient population. Some of the more common inpatient group therapies are personality reconstruction groups, insight without reconstruction groups, problem-solving groups, remotivation and reeducation groups, and supportive groups.[16]

Recently, assertiveness training has become a popular form of group therapy. The goal of assertiveness training is to help the patient differentiate between passive, assertive, and aggressive behavior. Opportunities are provided for the patient to practice using assertive behavior. The result is that the patient has a choice of how he will approach a situation. The payoff is that he develops more self-confidence and is able to make his views and needs known without infringing on the rights of others.

"Specialty groups" are used on many inpatient psychiatric units. These groups are often composed of patients within a specific age range (e.g., young adult groups), patients with common problems or needs (e.g., predischarge groups), or patients of the same sex (e.g., women's sex education groups). These groups may be open-ended discussion groups or highly structured didactic groups. They may be offered on a continuing basis or be time limited. The important factors are that all groups should serve some purpose and meet some therapeutic need and the therapist should be skilled in group process and group dynamics.

The role of the psychiatric nurse in group therapy is explored in Chapter 28.

■ Psychodrama

Psychodrama is a modality of therapy that uses structured and directed dramatizations of a patient's emotional problems and experiences. The purpose of these "dramas" is to provide the opportunity for the patient to develop greater awareness of his thoughts, feelings, and actions and how they impact on others. Psychodrama was devised by Dr. Jacob L. Moreno in 1914.

Moreno established psychodrama on several theoretical principles. The **action principle** simply stated is that just as life is not limited to a single verbal dimension, so psychodramatic action overcomes the linguistic restrictions placed on understanding oneself. Moreno believed that action is "the most integrative vehicle for social learning and has the most cathartic impact."[22]

The principle of the **social atom** states that each person is the center of his "structure of primary interpersonal relationships." This interpersonal network is filled with incomplete perceptions and distortions. Psychodrama allows for the recreation of the social atom and the exploration of role function in an immediate feedback system that is conducive to learning.[19]

An important goal or outcome of psychodrama is spontaneity. Moreno[19] defined spontaneity as an ability to respond to a new situation with some "degree of adequacy" and to an old situation with a "degree of novelty."

Moreno believed that the human being was not overdetermined by his past. He thought that at any moment in time the human is in "a state of great growth-potential."[19] In psychodrama, **catharsis** is used to mean a bursting through of a personal or cultural conserve. **Tele** is a word that is used to describe a two-way feeling that cements and holds a relationship together. **Surplus reality** refers to the act of going beyond reality. An example of this may be having a dead person, as represented by a group member, speak.

There are several important elements of psychodrama. Although a stage is not an absolute necessity for psychodrama, it provides a flexible, multidimensional living space. The stage should be round and should have two or three steplike levels. Since psychodrama is primarily a group process, the psychodramatist's effort is to mobilize the group to work together. It is not uncommon that the response to the action on the stage is greater in the group than it is with the people on the stage. The protagonist is the star. It is he who at the moment best typifies the concern of the group. The auxiliary egos are people in the group who take roles on stage in relationship to the protagonist and his action. Psychodramatic techniques are used to help the star and the group achieve spontaneity. Two important techniques are role reversal, in which the star exchanges his role for that of a significant other, and the use of the double, which is an auxiliary ego who gets behind the protagonist and attempts to express thoughts and feelings with which the protagonist is having difficulty.

There are three phases of psychodrama. The first phase is the warm-up. During the warm-up the psychodramatist involves the group in a discussion of issues deemed important to explore for that session. Once a group concern emerges, a protagonist is supported and encouraged to come forth. The second phase is composed of the shaping and presentation of the drama. If this stage is done properly, the entire group may benefit from the action. The final phase is the postaction group sharing. In this phase the group members express what events in their own lives were touched on by the action.

The psychodramatist attempts to draw from the group some identification with the protagonist.

What are the indications for psychodrama? Advocates of this modality of therapy have reported success with treating individual patients, groups of patients with marital discord, and groups of alcoholics. Psychodrama is used in milieu therapy as a form of group therapy and as a diagnostic tool in the dealing with problems within the social system of the therapeutic community.

Psychodrama seems to have a valid place among the group treatments on an inpatient psychiatric unit, as shown in Clinical example 24-3, which is an account of an actual psychodrama.

■ Activities therapy

Under the general classification of activities therapy may be found a number of vital programs that are used on an active inpatient psychiatric unit either as adjunctive or primary treatment modalities. Occupational therapy, recreational therapy, art therapy, plant therapy, and dance and music therapy comprise this general classification while being specialties in and of themselves.

Occupational therapy was formally established on March 15, 1917. From a modest beginning this profession has grown into a highly complex specialty with a specific body of knowledge and several conceptual frameworks of its own. Occupational therapy is defined as the art and science of directing a person's participation in selected activity to diminish or correct pathological problems and promote and maintain health.[6]

On an inpatient unit the occupational therapy program usually consists of a wide range of both individual and group experiences that are constructed to meet the social, emotional, and occupational needs of the patients. After an initial assessment, the occupational therapist helps the patient to select group and individual activities depending on the patient's skill levels. Occupational therapy programs usually offer the traditional crafts groups in which patients learn to sew, make leather projects, work in ceramics and wood, and weave. Beyond this, these programs offer assertiveness training, daily living skills groups, and current events groups. It is the occupational therapist who is most frequently involved in adjunctive treatments, such as plant therapy and pet therapy. In the absence of an educational therapist, occupational therapists will often work with psychiatric nurses in a joint endeavor to provide patients with needed tutoring or intellectual stimulation.

Recreational therapy may be offered by a certified recreational therapist or by an occupational therapist who has special training in this area. These programs

---

> ### CLINICAL EXAMPLE 24-3
>
> A member of a psychodrama group came to each session with his mattress strapped on his back. He would enter a closet, close the door behind him, and remain there until the session was finished.
>
> During one session the group decided during the warm-up phase that they wanted to deal with rejection. They believed that the group member in the closet best typified rejection. The patient was invited to be the star and to everyone's astonishment he accepted.
>
> The psychodramatic action centered on the death of the patient's father. During the drama the patient was able to express all the anger that he had kept inside. He screamed and yelled at his father (who was described as being in hell but could hear him) for abandoning his family. Finally, he was able to say good-bye without anger.
>
> During the group sharing phase many of the group members were in tears. Many shared their own experiences of the loss of someone close to them. The patient from that time on came to the sessions without his mattress and was able to sit on the fringe of the group.

---

are usually geared toward those activities which are more physical or gamelike in nature. The theory behind this modality of therapy incorporates the concepts that the relationship of one's physical self to the immediate environment is important to the total health of an individual. Movement or dance therapy is a specific example of how the body can be used as a medium for change. Since body and mind cannot be separated, the dance therapist works toward integrating the muscular and cognitive expressions of the patient's feelings and thoughts. On a more traditional level, organized tournaments in volleyball, basketball, table tennis, cards, dominoes, or checkers provide the patients with useful leisure activities and assist them to develop skills in engaging in healthy, competitive interactions. Recreational therapists may also develop programs using community resources to help patients identify socialization activities that they can become involved with after discharge from the hospital.

Art therapy is used as both a diagnostic tool and a treatment modality. The art therapist's goals are to assist the patient to express through his drawings his thoughts and emotions, to help the patient gain relief from anxiety by graphically representing conflicts and aggressive and traumatic material without guilt, to provide a socially acceptable outlet for fantasy and wish fulfillment, and to assist the patient to develop more dexterity.

The general goal of pet and plant therapy is to allow the patient to express tender, loving, and nurturing feelings without great fear of rejection. Plants and pets respond well to care but make fewer demands than families and friends usually make on the care provider. Through this form of therapy patients become alerted to the needs of other living organisms and may develop a sensitivity and sense of responsibility to respond to these needs in an appropriate manner.

Thus activities therapies are used to assist patients to develop occupational and leisure skills that will help to provide a smoother transition back into their communities. These programs have become an important and highly respected part of active treatment facilities throughout the country.

■ Somatic therapies and psychopharmacology

The somatic therapies and psychopharmacology are discussed in detail in Chapters 22 and 23. However, it is important to emphasize the role of the nurse in these vital modalities of treatment.

On the modern inpatient psychiatric unit for acutely ill patients, chemotherapy and ECT are the most frequently used of all the somatic treatments. It is imperative that the inpatient psychiatric nurse develop an in-depth knowledge of these therapies. This knowledge is essential to providing quality nursing care. The two most important functions of the nurse in relationship to these somatic therapies are the observing of the patient's responses to his treatment and teaching and preparing the patient and his family.

Other forms of somatic therapies are used infrequently on an inpatient unit. Psychosurgery is used so rarely that a nurse may never encounter this particular treatment. However, recent research indicates that new and innovative technologies may lead to safe and effective procedures which may be used as a "last resort" method of treatment. Insulin shock has all but become a treatment of the past. Cold, wet sheet packs are more frequently used but are still more of historical interest, since their use is diminishing.

Long-term custodial facilities

Although the purpose of this chapter is to present what inpatient psychiatric nursing can be when it is practiced in an environment that promotes professional, innovative, creative patient care, it must be recognized that many long-term custodial care facilities still exist. These are the institutions in which are housed patients who (1) have not responded to treatment in an acute treatment facility, (2) will not seek treatment on a voluntary basis, (3) have been committed by the courts, (4) do not have the financial resources to seek treatment elsewhere, (5) are chronically ill and cannot function in society, or (6) are homeless and forgotten.

These facilities generally share several common characteristics. There is usually a severe shortage of staff, particularly qualified registered nurses. Conditions are often crowded, and the physical environment is frequently drab and depressing. Patients are likely to be required to wear clothing provided by the institution. Their personal possessions may be kept under lock, and access to them may be limited to rigid routine schedules created for staff convenience. The design of the units is routinely stark. Beds are most likely to be lined up in dormitory fashion, with little or no provisions made for privacy. It is not uncommon for each unit to have a large sparsely furnished day area in which the patients watch television, play games, or congregate to have a cigarette whenever the smoking lamp is lit.

The quality of care provided by these long-term facilities is extremely inconsistent. Federal, state, and local legislation has made some attempts to ensure improvements and standardization. Some of the dedicated and caring staff of these institutions have made heroic efforts to develop quality programs of treatment and rehabilitation. However, lack of funding and incredible bureaucratic snags and snarls make it painfully difficult, if not impossible, to implement change in a system that is invested in maintaining a status quo.

Consequently, patients in chronic long-term custodial care facilities are more often subjected to a program of therapeutic routine than of therapeutic design. Some of the modalities of therapy most commonly offered in long-term custodial facilities are group therapy, occupational and recreational therapy, chemotherapy, and work therapy. Most of the group therapies are remotivational groups. Since long-term hospitalization often produces apathy and social isolation, detachment, and impoverishment, activities may be used to stimulate group interactions. Activities such as games, sports, artwork, and music can be used to prepare the patients for verbal interaction. Once the patients are ready to talk, the activities are gradually decreased.[16]

Work therapy is used to describe various employment situations. In some institutions patients are used as part of the work force in housekeeping, food preparation, and maintenance of the grounds. Most institutions pay the patients for this work; others offer no monetary compensation. In a few institutions patients are involved in a planned vocational rehabilitation program, including sheltered workshops, and may be employed in the community.

Chemotherapy is frequently the primary modality of treatment prescribed for patients in a long-term custodial care facility. The reasons for this are numerous. The nature of the patient's illness often dictates an aggressive, long-term drug regimen. Shortage of staff and limited psychotherapy programs greatly influence the physician's decision about the types of chemotherapy programs to implement for his patients. In many of these institutions, one of the most noticeable elements is the staff's need to be in control. Thus chemotherapy may be used to control patient behavior that is viewed as antagonistic, rebellious, or disruptive to the system.

We have now come full circle from the early days when psychiatric nursing was custodial in nature and the nurse's role was to ensure control and the smooth operation of the unit to the present where many of these practices still exist. This is the skeleton in our closet. Nurses cannot expect that all psychiatric patients will respond to active treatment, but they can strive to provide the best possible care they are capable of giving.

In recent years, deinstitutionalization programs have been established to assist chronically hospitalized patients to move back to community settings. Case management and community support programs provide the services that are necessary to effect this change. The nursing care of the chronically mentally ill patient is discussed in greater depth in Chapter 34.

Future of inpatient psychiatric nursing

The treatment of hospitalized psychiatric patients is continually undergoing change. At present there appear to be two major directions psychiatry may follow in the future. The first direction is the familiar interpersonal, psychodynamically oriented approach. The second is the psychobiochemical orientation that has been adopted by many of the leading research and treatment facilities throughout the country.

The role of the inpatient psychiatric nurse will certainly reflect the philosophy and direction of the treatment within the institution. With the biochemical approach, the institution is likely to stress research and the medical model. This will have an impact on the nurse in terms of specific priorities, functions, and care delivery systems. Thus the need for nursing research in this area is vital. Nurses must continue to define nursing.

Even within the interpersonal, psychodynamically oriented approach, there will be need for change and the development of new knowledge and skills. The nurse must be prepared for a reevaluation of roles and functions. It is possible that the psychiatric nurse of tomorrow will be involved in primary care. The function of this psychiatric nurse practitioner will be to coordinate the care of the patient's mental health problems. There is also likely to be increasing use of day care, partial hospitalizations, and short-term hospitalizations.

The role of the mental health team in a primary care system was a topic of animated discussion at a recent American Psychiatric Association annual convention. Leaders in the mental health field view involvement in primary care as an absolute necessity, and they frequently include psychiatric nurses as a vital part of the mental health team of tomorrow.

Despite changes in the future, one may assume that nursing care will be delivered through the application of the nursing process. Individual assessment, nursing diagnosis, planning, implementation, and evaluation are

---

DIRECTIONS FOR FUTURE RESEARCH

The following are some of the nursing research problems raised in Chapter 24 that merit further study by psychiatric nurses:

1. Description of effective nursing interventions that increase patient compliance with medication regimens
2. Description of patient outcomes that are directly related to nursing intervention
3. Evaluation of the role of the CNS in cost containment
4. Effective methods of clinical supervision to enhance role expansion of psychiatric nurses
5. Patient education techniques that result in greater patient participation in treatment
6. Description of factors that influence the nurse's effective participation as a member of the treatment team
7. The nurse's role in the deinstitutionalization of the chronically mentally ill
8. The effectiveness of nurse-led transitional groups in keeping chronic mental patients out of hospitals longer
9. The impact of primary nursing on the "revolving door" syndrome
10. Comparison of various staffing patterns and methods of utilization of nursing resources in an inpatient psychiatric setting
11. Components of nursing care that require the services of a professional registered nurse as opposed to those which may be delegated
12. Marketing strategies to increase consumer awareness, consumer demand, and consumer support for psychiatric nursing services

the vehicles by which any mode of treatment may be delivered. Nursing will probably continue to emphasize the importance of using the patient's strengths to assist him in reaching an optimum level of functioning. Hopefully, nursing will never lose sight of the patient as an individual with the need of respect for his privacy and human dignity.

A health care provider once said with great disgust that the problem with "all this individual assessment" is that it "makes a person a snowflake." How sad that he cannot see that just as the beauty of a snowflake lies in the uniqueness of its pattern, so does the key to wellness and recovery lie in the uniqueness of the individual's strengths and desires. That is the beauty of the human spirit.

■ SUGGESTED CROSS-REFERENCES ■

The roles and functions of the psychiatric nurse and the mental health team are discussed in Chapter 1. The phases of the nursing process are discussed in Chapter 5. Rehabilitation of psychiatric patients is discussed in Chapter 11. Somatic therapies are discussed in Chapter 22. Family therapy is discussed in Chapter 29. Deinstitutionalization of the chronically mentally ill is discussed in Chapter 34.

■ SUMMARY ■

1. The history of inpatient psychiatric nursing practice reflects an evolutionary process from that of custodial caretaker to active member of the mental health team. The reforms of the nineteenth century were the first major influences to have an impact on the role of the psychiatric nurse.

2. The development of social psychiatry opened the door for nursing involvement in the areas of group and milieu therapy. By 1949 nurses were functioning as individual therapists, and by the mid-1950s the role of group therapist had become a recognized and accepted part of nursing practice.

3. The concept of the health team led to needed changes in the educational preparation of psychiatric nurses. This new breed of psychiatric nurses viewed themselves as professionally and academically competent to be fully participating members of the health team.

4. The implementation of the nursing process is vital to inpatient psychiatric nursing. The steps of the nursing process include the collection of a data base, development of a diagnostic impression, planning and implementation of appropriate nursing actions, and evaluation and modification of those actions.

5. There are various modalities of nursing care delivery that may be used on an inpatient psychiatric unit. Primary nursing is a care delivery system that has recently gained much support and recognition from many professional nurses throughout the country. Advocates of this modality of care delivery report that primary nursing leads to increased job satisfaction among the professional nursing staff and increased satisfaction among the patient population.

6. The necessity of the CNS in inpatient psychiatric nursing may be debated. Budgets, fiscal constraints, and pressures for cost containment make it difficult for nursing administrators to justify a role that was originally developed solely to improve the quality of nursing care. However, when given the opportunity, the CNS can demonstrate that quality care is worth the investment.

7. Inpatient psychiatric units should be designed to reflect the philosophy of the department, methods of care provided, and types of patients to be served.

8. Many active psychiatric treatment facilities use concepts of milieu therapy in their inpatient programs. According to Cumming and Cumming, milieu therapy is a planned manipulation of the environment to produce changes in the personality of the patient.

9. Maxwell Jones coined the term "therapeutic community." He believed that all social and interpersonal interactions in the hospital are therapeutic tools that should be used to bring about specific changes in the patient. Jones stressed that the patient must be an active participant in his care planning.

10. The focus of family therapy is to treat a primary social system, rather than one individual who has been defined as a "patient." The goals of family therapy are to reduce conflict and anxiety, make the family more aware of each other's needs, increase the family's ability to deal with internal and external crisis, develop more appropriate role relationships, help individual family members cope with destructive forces within and without the family, and promote health and growth.

11. Individual psychotherapy continues to be the most common modality of treatment offered on active inpatient psychiatric units. The purpose of individual therapy is to offer the patient an opportunity to develop insights into the sources of his thoughts, feelings, perceptions, and behavior.

12. Many active treatment facilities offer group therapy either as a primary treatment modality or as an adjunctive treatment to individual psychotherapy. Group therapy should never be used as a "time-saving" device. Some of the more common inpatient groups are the supportive groups, remotivation groups, personality reconstruction groups, problem-solving groups, and insight groups.

13. Psychodrama was devised by Dr. Jacob L. Moreno in 1914. The purpose of psychodrama is to allow the patient to express himself in both words and action. Psychodrama is considered to be a special form of group therapy. It is frequently used in milieu therapy to deal with problems within the social system of the therapeutic community.

14. Activities therapies are used on inpatient units to assist patients to develop occupational and leisure skills that will help to provide a smoother transition back into the community. Occupational, recreational, art, dance, pet and plant therapies are all highly respected parts of active treatment facilities throughout the country.

15. Somatic therapies play a vital role in psychiatric treat-

ment. Some of the common somatic therapies are chemotherapy, ECT, and psychosurgery.

16. To this day, there still exist psychiatric facilities that offer little more than custodial care. Some patients do not respond to active treatment and must be hospitalized for long-term care. Others, because of the nature of their illness, will not voluntarily admit themselves to active treatment facilities. Efforts are being made to improve the treatment provided by these long-term hospitals.

17. The future of psychiatric nursing appears bright for those willing to accept the challenge. Primary care, day care, partial hospitalizations, and community support for chronically mentally ill patients appear to be the subjects of many future-oriented discussions.

■ REFERENCES ■

1. American Nurses' Association, Congress of Nursing Practice, Description of practice. Clinical nurse specialist: The scope of nursing practice, Kansas City, Mo., 1976, The Association.
2. Anderson, C., and Apostoles, F.: Primary care nursing: an exploratory project in psychiatric nurse utilization. In Kneisl, C., and Wilson, H., editors: Current perspectives in psychiatric nursing: issues and trends, vol. 2, St. Louis, 1978, The C.V. Mosby Co.
3. Coates, D., Falck, A., and Sienkilewski, K.: Primary nursing: one giant step toward professionalism, 1974. (Unpublished; available from K. Sienkilewski, Springfield Hospital Center, Sykesville, Md. 21784)
4. Cumming, J., and Cumming, E.: Ego and milieu, Chicago, 1962, Atherton Press.
5. Detre, T., and Jarecki, H.: Modern psychiatric treatment, Philadelphia, 1971, J.B. Lippincott Co.
6. Engelhardt, H.T.: Defining occupational therapy: the meaning of therapy and the virtues of occupation, Am. J. Occup. Ther. **31:**666, 1977.
7. Hamric, A., and Spross, J.: The clinical nurse specialist in theory and practice, Orlando, Fla., 1983, Grune & Stratton Inc.
8. Ingenious design meets budget, space constraints for hospital's community mental health center, Hospitals **52:**41, Apr. 16, 1978.
9. Jamieson, E., and Sewall, M.: Trends in nursing history, Philadelphia, 1941, W.B. Saunders Co.
10. Joint Commission on Accreditation of Hospitals: Consolidated standards manual for child, adolescent and adult psychiatric alcoholism and Drug Abuse Facilities, Chicago, Ill., 1981 JCAH.
11. Jones, M.: Towards a clarification of the therapeutic community concept, Br. J. Med. Psychol. **32:**200, 1959.
12. Jones, M.: Social psychiatry in practice, Harmondsworth, England, 1968, Penguin Books, Ltd.
13. Kraft, A.: The therapeutic community. In Arieti, S., editor: American handbook of psychiatry, vol. 2, New York, 1966, Basic Books, Inc.
14. Manthey, M.: Primary nursing is alive and well in the hospital, Am. J. Nurs. **73:**83, Jan. 1973.
15. Marlborough Hospital: Therapeutic community, 1976. (Unpublished; available from Marlborough Hospital, 38 Marlborough Place, St. John's Wood, London, England.)
16. Marram, G.: The group approach in nursing practice, ed. 2, St. Louis, 1978, The C.V. Mosby Co.
17. Marram, G., Barrett, M.W., and Bevis, E.: Primary nursing: a model for individualized care, ed. 2, St. Louis, 1979, The C.V. Mosby Co.
18. Mereness, D.: Preparation of the nurse for the psychiatric team, Am. J. Nurs. **51:**320, 1951.
19. Moreno, J.: Psychodrama, New York, 1959, Beacon House.
20. Pavey, A.: The story of the growth of nursing, Philadelphia, 1937, J.B. Lippincott Co.
21. Robinson, A.: Changing of the guard, Am. J. Nurs. **50:**152, Mar. 1950.
22. Saklas, C.: Psychosocial group therapies, The Practice of Medicine and Psychotherapy **10:**41.
23. Santos, E., and Stanbrook E.: Nursing and modern psychiatry, Am. J. Nurs. **49:**107, Feb. 1949.
24. Sundeen S., et al.: Nurse-client interaction: implementing the nursing process, ed. 3, St. Louis, 1985, The C.V. Mosby Co.
25. Wolf, M.S.: A review of literature on milieu therapy, J. Psychiatr. Nurs. **15:**7, May 1977.
26. Zander, K.: Primary nursing: development and management, Germantown, Md., 1980, Aspen Systems Corp.

■ ANNOTATED SUGGESTED READINGS ■

*Carser, D.L.: Primary nursing in the milieu, J. Psychiatr. Nurs. **19:**35, Feb. 1978.

In this article, the author examines the interaction between primary nursing and the therapeutic milieu. She uses case examples to illustrate the impact at the individual patient level. She also discusses the effect of the introduction of primary nursing on the treatment team and recommends interventions with the staff that are helpful during the transitional period.

Cumming, J., and Cumming, E.: Ego and milieu, Chicago, 1962, Atherton Press.

This book is considered a classic. It represents one of the first major undertakings to theoretically describe the relationship between ego and milieu. Until this time no advocate of milieu therapy had risked making the direct statement that scientific manipulation of the environment could lead to changes in behavior and personality.

Engelhardt, H.T.: Defining occupational therapy: the meaning of therapy and the virtues of occupation, Am. J. Occup. Ther. **31:**666, 1979.

This volume marks the sixtieth anniversary of the occupational therapy journal. Each article presents an informative historical overview as well as current conceptual frameworks. It will give the nurse an appreciation of the struggles that another discipline has encountered in its search for professional recognition and autonomy.

---

*Asterisk indicates nursing reference.

*Hegyvary, S., guest editor: Symposium on primary nursing, Nurs. Clin. North Am. **12**:185, June 1977.

This symposium on primary nursing will give the reader an overview of the joys and pains of primary nursing. It provides a theoretical and empirical base for primary nursing, discusses patient and staff perceptions, elaborates on the structural and organizational supports needed for the implementation of primary nursing, and discusses some experimental outcomes of implementing this modality of care delivery.

Jones, M.: Social psychiatry in practice, Harmondsworth, England, 1968, Penguin Books, Ltd.

This little book is packed full of information. A large section is devoted to the concept of therapeutic community, but Jones also elaborates on the concept of social psychiatry in general. The author is outspoken in his opinions about the preparation and participation of nurses and other health team members.

Kraft, A.: The therapeutic community. In Arieti, S., editor: American handbook of psychiatry, vol. 3, New York, 1966, Basic Books, Inc., Publishers.

This is a frequently quoted reference on the concept of therapeutic community. The author attempts to pull together the thoughts, ideas, and beliefs of the leading authorities in the fields of therapeutic community and milieu therapy.

*Marram, G., Barrett, M.W., and Bevis, E.: Primary nursing: a model for individualized care, ed. 2, St. Louis, 1979, The C.V. Mosby Co.

Although there is no discussion of primary nursing as it relates to inpatient psychiatric nursing, this book should be considered a must. It was the only text in this field for a long time. The reader may enjoy the introductory comparison of the growth of the women's movement and the growth of nursing as a profession.

*Mereness, D.: Preparation of the nurse for the psychiatric team, Am. J. Nurs. **51**:320, 1951.

Despite the era in which it was written, this article continues to be ageless. There will always be a need for changes in educational curricula as the role of the professional nurse continues to grow and expand.

*Sundeen, S., et al.: Nurse-client interaction: implementing the nursing process, ed. 3, St. Louis, 1985, The C.V. Mosby Co.

This is a consistently excellent text. The use of clinical illustrations is of particular value both to experienced nurses as well as beginners. While much of the literature "talks" about the nursing process, this work puts it into "action."

*Templin, H.: The system and the patient, Am. J. Nurs. **82**:108, Jan. 1982

This thought-provoking article looks at three aspects of psychiatric hospitals from both the patient's view and the view from organizational theory—the hospital as a hierarchical system, mutual adaptation and modes of transaction. It demonstrates the benefits of viewing these hospitals as social systems.

*Wolf, M.S.: A review of literature on milieu therapy, J. Psychiatr. Nurs. **15**:27, May 1977.

This article is a comprehensive overview of the development of milieu therapy. What makes this work of particular value is the presentation of several studies on the effectiveness of milieu therapy, the discussion of the nurses' role, and the all-inclusive bibliography.

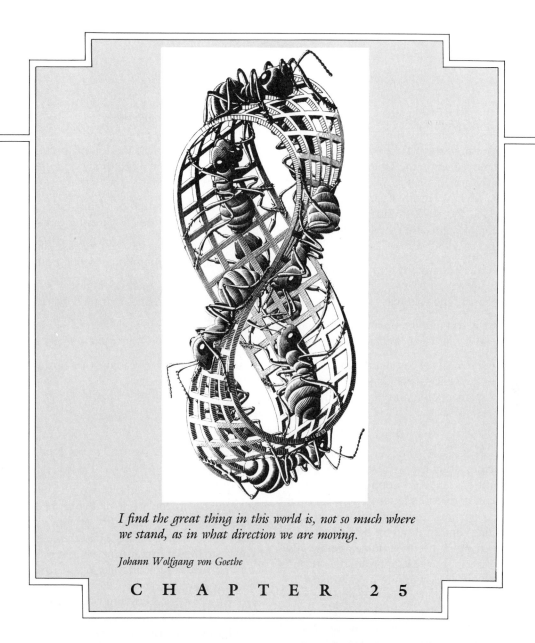

I find the great thing in this world is, not so much where we stand, as in what direction we are moving.

Johann Wolfgang von Goethe

C H A P T E R   2 5

THE PSYCHIATRIC NURSE'S ROLE IN COMMUNITY MENTAL HEALTH

JEANETTE LANCASTER
WADE LANCASTER

LEARNING OBJECTIVES

After studying this chapter, the student should be able to:

- describe the history of the community mental health movement in the United States and the role of the government as reflected in the Community Mental Health Center Acts of 1963 and 1975, the 1978 President's Commission on Mental Health, and the Mental Health Systems Act of 1980.

- critique the community mental health movement with regard to its goals, staff, services, effectiveness, and clientele.

- contrast a community orientation to mental health with that of an individual orientation.

- relate the role of the community mental health nurse in assessment, including the strategies of market segmentation and target marketing.

- discuss the implementation of the role of the community mental health nurse in the areas of primary, secondary, and tertiary prevention.

- analyze the impact of deinstitutionalization and its implications for nursing care.

- assess the importance of interdisciplinary collaboration in community mental health.

- describe three methodologies for program evaluation and issues that must be considered in their use.

- identify directions for future nursing research.

- select appropriate readings for further study.

The twentieth century has witnessed many American social institutions undergo continuous introspection, reassessment, and reorientation. The pressure for responsiveness, openness, and humaneness revolves around a deepening concern about the human condition and the rapidly changing needs of human beings. Psychiatric nursing has not been exempt from the pressures of societal change. Nurses working in psychiatric settings have been at the forefront of change. The scope of psychiatric nursing has changed dramatically, moving from its infant state of custodial care to the present community mental health orientation. Not only has the orientation changed, but also the work environment of the psychiatric nurse has expanded from the confines of mental institutions to the everchanging boundaries of the community. To better appreciate the current role of the psychiatric nurse in community mental health, it is helpful to briefly examine the historical motivators of the community mental health movement.

Historical development of community mental health nursing

Before 1840 people diagnosed as mentally ill were housed in jails and county homes. The environmental conditions barely allowed existence and certainly offered no treatment, since mental illness was considered a permanent affliction. For the affluent and more fortunate a scarce few private and public hospitals were available.

■ Humanitarian reforms in mental health

Humanitarian methods in psychiatry were first seen in America in the work of Benjamin Rush, who has since been called "the father of American psychiatry." Rush is considered a transitional figure in that he encouraged humane treatment while at the same time continuing to use remedies like blood letting, purgatives, and a torturelike device called "the tranquilizer."

An energetic New England school teacher, Dorothea Dix, carried on the pioneering work of Rush. In 1841 Miss Dix appointed herself inspector of institutions for the mentally ill and began crusading for more humane treatment. She recommended that each state assume responsibility for its mentally ill. The result of her effort was the establishment of 32 mental hospitals in the United States. During this period most mental hospitals were built in rural areas, which offered inexpensive land, the removal of troublesome people from the mainstream of society, fresh air, and a quiet atmosphere for the patients.

As the population in the United States increased, the number of state hospitals grew steadily until 1900. However, in the years following 1900 the patient population grew more rapidly than the construction of hospitals. This trend led to overcrowding and deplorable living conditions. To further complicate the situation, the hospitals operated on meager budgets and were inadequately staffed. The hopes and plans of Dorothea

Dix were not realized at this time. Although Dorothea Dix's crusade was not oriented toward community mental health, it certainly had an impact on the trend toward humane treatment for the mentally ill.

The care and treatment of mentally ill individuals continued on a downhill swing until Adolf Meyer took up the banner that Dorothea Dix had once waved. Meyer was actually the first person to espouse the basic concept of community mental health. He proposed that a clinic for mental diseases be responsible for a certain segment of the population so that studies of the social situation and the factors leading to the onset of mental derangement could be pursued. The accompanying box chronicles the development of the community mental health movement.

■ Governmental involvement in mental health

The federal government first entered the health field in 1935 with the passage of the Social Security Act. During the depression the view was held that if the community could not care for its sick, then the government should assume this responsibility. World War II had a significant impact on the community mental health movement when an estimated 875,000 draftees out of 15 million were rejected from military service on the basis of mental or neurological impairment.[36] At the conclusion of the war the federal government assumed an active role in funding endeavors for mental health. In 1946 the United States Congress enacted the National Mental Health Act, which made grants available to states to develop mental health programs outside of state hospitals.

This act, signed into law by President Harry S Truman, radically altered the care of mentally ill Americans. Shocked at the number of young men rejected from military service for reasons of mental illness, embarrassed by the inhumane custodial treatment, and tempted by the vision of a new enlightened system, citizens, professionals, and legislators banded together to support a broad-based national program. The intent behind these efforts was to apply a public health approach to the problem of mental illness.[31] Although the intent was to focus on prevention, in actuality individual psychotherapy was supported.

Under the provisions of the act, the National Institute of Mental Health (NIMH) was organized in 1949 to serve as headquarters for the new federal mental health program. Initially the function of NIMH emphasized research into the cause and treatment of mental illness. The institute also assumed responsibility for training programs and providing assistance to individual states as they attempted to develop treatment programs.

The 1940s saw the widespread development of two important types of treatment facilities: outpatient clinics and psychiatric units in general hospitals. In contrast, advances in research had little effect on state hospitals. Meanwhile, psychiatry continued its preference for providing private care to those who could afford it, with subsequent serious inequities between private and public provisions for treatment.

In 1955 Congress enacted the Mental Health Study

Milestones in the Development of the Community Mental Health Movement

1841 Dorothea Dix appointed herself inspector of institutions for the mentally ill
1935 Passage of Social Security Act
1946 Enactment of the Mental Health Act
1949 Creation of NIMH under the Mental Health Act
1955 Congress enacted the Mental Health Study Act creating the Joint Commission on Mental Illness and Health
1960 Joint Commission on Mental Illness and Health submitted its report to Congress
1961 Report of the Joint Commission on Mental Illness and Health published as *Action for Mental Health*

1963 First Presidential message on behalf of the mentally ill; Enactment of Public Law 88-164, the Mental Retardation Facilities and Community Mental Health Centers Construction Act
1975 The Community Mental Health Centers Amendments of 1975, Title III of Public Law 94-63 was enacted
1977 President Jimmy Carter organized the President's Commission on Mental Health
1978 Report of the President's Commission published
1980 Mental Health Systems Act

Act, creating the Joint Commission on Mental Illness and Health, which consisted of representatives from 36 organizations and agencies selected by the NIMH. The agencies represented were largely medical and allied medical in character.[36] In the latter part of 1960 the Joint Commission submitted its report to Congress. Published in 1961 as *Action for Mental Health,* the 338-page report emphasized the need for training personnel, supporting education in the field, providing early and intensive treatment for acutely disturbed patients, and carrying out research activities. The report further recommended that additional clinics and psychiatric units in general hospitals be established and that regional state hospitals of not more than 1000 beds be supported. The report suggested the creation of aftercare, rehabilitation programs, and mental health education.[16]

After the publication of this report, President John F. Kennedy appointed a cabinet-level committee to review the report and to make recommendations regarding federal action. This report and that of a presidential panel on mental retardation formed the basis for President Kennedy's message to Congress in 1963 on mental illness and retardation. This first presidential message on behalf of the mentally ill called for a "bold new approach to bring psychiatry back into the mainstream of medicine and community life."[32] The president further stated that a new facility to be known as a community mental health center was needed to provide a complete range of care in the community, including a strong emphasis on prevention.

■ **COMMUNITY MENTAL HEALTH CENTERS ACT.** Eight months later, on October 31, 1963, the Eighty-eighth Congress enacted Public Law 88-164, the Mental Retardation Facilities and Community Mental Health Centers Construction Act of 1963, which authorized federal matching funds of $150 million over a 3-year period for use by the states in constructing comprehensive community mental health centers. The intent of the act was to provide comprehensive mental health services to meet the needs of all residents in a specific area. Each center was to serve a catchment area or population base ranging from 75,000 to 200,000 residents. Geographically each catchment area ranged from a circumscribed section of a large city to an area covering several counties with a sparse population. In addition to providing new and renovated buildings, each center was also to provide a program of mental health services to the community.

To qualify for federal funds, a program had to offer the five following services[20]:

1. Inpatient care for patients requiring short-term hospitalization

2. Partial hospitalization, which included day hospital care for those patients who could return to their own homes at night and night hospital care for patients who were able to work but needed some care each day

3. Outpatient treatment, which allowed patients to live at home and go to the center at regular intervals

4. Emergency care with services available around the clock

5. Consultation and education for members of the community

Full comprehensive services in the original community mental health legislation included five additional services. Centers applying for federal support were looked on favorably if they documented a plan for the following additional services:

1. Diagnostic services, including treatment recommendations whenever possible

2. Rehabilitative services and vocational counseling

3. Precare and aftercare with screening prior to admission and follow-up evaluation in the home after discharge

4. Training for all kinds of mental health personnel

5. Research and evaluation

The original legislation provided federal funding for a center for 8 years on a decreasing percentage formula. During the 8 years, the federal proportion of the funding decreased in nonpoverty areas from 80% the first year to 25% in the seventh and eighth years. In poverty areas the federal proportion decreased from 90% in the first year to 30% in the eighth year. At the end of the eighth year the federal grants ceased, and each center was to operate on state and local funds as well as revenue collectd from services.[20]

This fiscal arrangement did not work effectively because many centers were unable to secure sufficient revenue to meet operational costs. State and local funds were not consistently available and often centers were forced to terminate services, especially those which did not produce revenue, such as consultation and educational services, in an effort to increase revenue through direct treatment services. Centers in urban areas and medical centers were often able to generate funds to support their range of services through fee-for-service or research activities. In contrast, rural centers had a difficult time sustaining themselves financially.

The seed money provided through the 1963 enactment of the Mental Health Centers Act was to encourage states to develop new or to expand community-based mental health centers. This aim to promote deinstitutionalization was congruent with the social and political tone of the 1960s as reflected in President Kennedy's "bold new approach." However, the MHC Act along with the Medicare/Medicaid Bill of 1965 led to a 75% reduction in the populations of state hospitals.[25] Although the reduction achieved the goal of limiting the size of institutions, it, in effect, "dumped" mentally ill people into the community before systematic, comprehensive strategies and facilities were developed. Deinstitutionalization, while a victory in theory, fell far short of its actual goal: humanistic care and treatment in the least restrictive alternative. In essence, the outcome of the early community mental health legislation has been to create a "revolving door" syndrome for the chronically mentally ill.

By 1970 deinstitutionalization and community mental health was a disaster. To deal with the crisis, the federal government provided nominal fiscal support to develop community support systems. Concurrently, mentally ill patients began to file lawsuits stating they were not provided with humane care or given adequate treatment while hospitalized. Between 1972 and 1977, a series of judicial decisions were made that led to revolutionary changes in community mental care. These decisions revolved around assuring that patients were held in the least restrictive alternative, protected from harm, provided with protection and safeguards in the civil commitment process, and that the use of restraint, excessive psychotropic drugs, electroconvulsive therapy, and psychosurgery were increasingly monitored.

This movement to avoid hospitalization came at a time when a variety of other changes were occurring in the United States. Advances in health care were allowing people to live longer, thereby causing additional financial drains on health care funds. Health care costs began to escalate dramatically, and the average age of the chronically mentally ill began to decrease. Indeed, a new breed of chronically ill young adults between 18 and 35 years old began to consume a disproportionate amount of mental health funds.

■ **COMMUNITY MENTAL HEALTH CENTERS AMENDMENTS OF 1975.** The Community Mental Health Centers Amendments of 1975, Title III of Public Law 94-63, was enacted by the Ninety-fourth Congress on July 22, 1975. This amendment extended the flow of funds to community mental health centers and in doing so set forth specific guidelines for services.[27] Congress reiterated the original intent of the Community Mental Health Centers Act to provide construction and operation funds to centers on a declining basis with the ultimate goal of independence from federal support. Specific requirements included providing accessible

comprehensive care to people living in a designated geographical area, regardless of their ability to pay or their past or current health conditions. The amendments also urged that services in a community be coordinated between centers and other agencies and be provided 24 hours a day, 7 days a week, in a humane manner to all who seek care. Centers were to be governed by a community board and have an ongoing quality assurance program, an integrated medical records system, a professional advisory board, and an identifiable administration unit to provide consultation and education services.[7]

Additionally, the 1975 amendments emphasized that the original required services should continue to be provided and also that services for children and the elderly must include diagnosis, treatment, liaison, and follow-up care.[7] Screening services were required for residents of the catchment area who were being discharged from a psychiatric hospital. Other required areas included transitional services for residents of the community as well as treatment for alcohol and drug abuse problems.

The impact of the 1975 amendments was to legally define a community mental health center program and explicitly document the list of services required. However, the amendments were severely criticized because they limited the flexibility that centers could exercise in determining services based on the needs of the catchment area. Furthermore, the complexity of the grant process and the timetable for reduction of federal funds were criticized.

■ **REPORT OF THE PRESIDENT'S COMMISSION ON MENTAL HEALTH, 1978.** Early in 1977 President Jimmy Carter organized the President's Commission on Mental Health; of the five professionals on the commission, one was a nurse. The president's general charge to the group was "to identify the mental health needs of the nation."[8] Specific attention was directed toward the extent to which the mentally ill were served, projected needs for dealing with stress, governmental support for mental illness, including research activities and agency coordination essential in a unified program to support mental health and intervene in mental illness.

After a 1-year study period the 20-member commission released its final report containing 117 recommendations. The commission's recommendations were divided into eight sections: community support systems, service delivery, financing, personnel, patients' rights, research, prevention, and public understanding.[24] The principal recommendation called for the establishment of a "new federal grant program for community mental health services to encourage the creation of necessary services where they are inadequate and increase the flexibility of communities in planning a comprehensive network of services."[24]

In general, the report spoke to the components of the original presidential charge. Specifically the commission recommended that community networks be strengthened between existing service components and that new ways of meeting the mental health needs of underserved populations be studied, including increased flexibility in defining the parameters of a catchment area. A call was made for attention to focus on high-risk populations, such as minorities and the chronically mentally ill. An advocacy program for the chronically mentally ill was advised, since an increasing number of state hospitals were being closed.

The commission gave serious attention to evaluation, suggesting that governmental agencies consolidate their evaluation efforts into a centralized, organized approach. Furthermore, a plea was made for mental health coverage in all insurance plans with flexibility in outpatient coverage, which would support an individual who chose to be maintained in the community yet needed ongoing or periodic mental health follow-up care. Recruitment and personnel use were addressed particularly in regard to high-risk populations. Training support was given high priority for personnel choosing to work with children, the elderly, and cultural minorities.

The commission recommended increased support for research according to the following target areas: incidence of mental health problems, use of research, public knowledge related to mental health, and investigation into the major mental illnesses. Preventive measures paid special attention to the mental health needs of children. Although the report did not cover each area in the original charge, it indicated target areas for mental health intervention and suggested ways in which goal attainment could be accomplished.

The 1980 mental health legislation continued the trend toward flexibility in planning services to meet the needs of a designated community.[29] This legislation gave states greater authority over mental health grants, allowed more flexible and innovative program planning and development, and emphasized prevention and planning of treatment approaches for priority populations. In addition, it provided linkages between mental health and other types of providers to avoid duplication of services and to foster greater coordination of resources and programs offered. Furthermore, provisions were made for funding innovative projects for retraining mental health workers whose positions were eliminated by program restructuring as more states emphasized community-oriented vs. institutional care for the mentally ill population.[29]

■ Community mental health in the 1980s

Despite the promise of a reorientation toward community mental health as evidenced in the 1980 legislation, the troubles of the 1970s were redoubled when the 1980 elections made it clear that a conservative trend had begun in the United States. By the late 1970s, many of the operating community mental health centers were plagued with financial problems. These financial woes were compounded by the progressive decline of federal support and the general ravaging of the economy by inflation and growing unemployment.[6] Before the decrease in financial support, many centers had extended their range of services into the community to attract new populations. Now they were trying to serve more populations with less money.

In the 1980s, the community mental health center program was modified by the Mental Health Systems Act's reaffirmation of community care and its designation of the state as the program coordinator. Monies were thereafter given to states in the form of block grants. Unfortunately, mental health programs historically have not fared well in capturing block grant funds.

Criticism of the community mental health movement

The enthusiasm of the 1960s for community mental health has been overshadowed by a wide range of criticism. Former enthusiasts are dissatisfied, since the original goals and mandates are unmet. Critics contend that the most obvious shortcoming of community mental health has been a tendency to move treatment into the community without concomitant changes in treatment techniques. There has been a reluctance to view the community itself—the macrosystem—as the client. Instead, the focus continues to be on the individual within the community—the microsystem.[42]

In addition, the professional staff required to operate a community mental health program are generally recruited from traditional delivery systems. The leadership for centers is provided by staff who have been trained and educated in isolation from each other, yet the approach in community mental health calls for collaboration and team functioning. Also, the use of paraprofessionals has aroused controversy. One point of view holds that these health care providers are highly effective in that they are not hindered by a medical model or disease orientation. The counterview is that paraprofessionals have an inadequate knowledge base for providing psychiatric services.

Criticisms related to community mental health have dealt not only with the lack of collaboration and the educational background of providers but also with the type of services provided, the balance between direct and indirect services, and the lack of responsiveness to the needs of the individual community. Prevention, a mandated service for community mental health, is viewed by some as an unmeasurable activity that serves to distract from more urgent treatment approaches.

■ Discharged patients

Themes of dissatisfaction with community mental health also relate to the failure to provide well-thought-out and carefully planned aftercare programs for discharged patients. As state hospitals rapidly discharged patients in the late 1960s, few communities were able to plan and implement follow-up treatment services for their chronically ill discharged patients. In many communities merely the setting changed for a large number of patients; they were moved from an impersonal state hospital to an often equally impersonal group home.

Arnhoff[1] cites studies which indicate that community treatment is no more effective than hospital care for acutely psychotic patients. He maintains that deinstitutionalization places an unnecessary burden on the family as well as the community. He further emphasizes the long-range implications of discharging psychotic patients when follow-up care is lacking or inadequate. The prematurely discharged patient has increased opportunities to procreate, provides ineffective parenting, and requires public assistance because of unemployment.

The inability to develop a comprehensive community mental health system has led to the "revolving door" syndrome, whereby patients discharged from psychiatric hospitals continue to need well-planned and individually designed follow-up services that few communities are able to provide. Hence, patients decompensate on discharge because of lack of aftercare, thus necessitating reentry into the hospital. There is mounting evidence that many chronically mentally ill patients do not require continuous hospitalization but can be maintained in the community if they are provided with appropriate medication and a variety of therapeutic services, including individual, group, and/or family therapy, as well as assistance in finding and maintaining jobs, schooling, housing, and social support.[34]

A major criticism of community mental health is that limited coordination has been achieved, and services have continued to be fragmented and specialized with no one system actually offering an integrated program of services. Tarail[39] contends that each segment of the mental health system has survival as a goal. Such a priority discounts the possibility of collaboration and organization of a comprehensive system of services. All too often patients are discharged from the hospital be-

fore community programs are developed to receive them, thereby reducing their existence to run-down hotels, inadequate boarding homes, or nursing homes supported by Medicare and Medicaid. Essentially, it is contended that the only change has been who pays the bill.[21]

Further, Langsley[21] purports that the most detrimental feature of community mental health centers has been their abandonment of treating mentally ill patients in preference to focusing on counseling and crisis intervention. He says that the initial goal of treating people with major mental health disruptions has been forgotten in favor of a focus on social action programs. He also believes that the large decrease in psychiatrists has affected treatment because in many instances, they are so few in centers that they primarily sign prescriptions.

Community mental health centers also suffered from the strain of serving two masters—the federal regulations regarding funding guided programs and a local citizen board often inexperienced in mental health and frequently pressured by local political groups.[6]

Initially, most state mental hospitals served three primary purposes: (1) to protect the public from insane people, (2) to provide an asylum and humane care for mentally ill people, and (3) to provide a place for "deviant" members of society who were not candidates for jails.[15] In the enthusiasm to overcome the syndrome characterized as "institutionalism" or a lack of initiative, apathy, withdrawal, and submissiveness to authority, mental health providers forgot that these characteristics might well be attributed to the schizophrenic process itself, not just to the length of tenure in a hospital. The needs of chronic mentally ill patients to have structure provided for them, to receive medical care, and to have a social network was forgotten in the rush to provide patients with freedom from the "shackles of hospitalization." The pressure during the earliest days of deinstitutionalization to provide patients with the least restrictive alternative (LRA) led to hasty actions. The LRA means providing patients with the greatest freedom from restrictions, especially freedom from long-term hospitalization.

■ Dysfunctional characteristics

Tarail[39] summarized the problems of the mental health delivery system by describing 24 dysfunctional characteristics. The first 12 of these pertain to the community mental health system. They are

1. The mental health care delivery systems are fragmented and specialized.
2. Not only is there no one single system of service, but there is no comprehensive, integrated,

or coordinated system of service among the several systems that exist.

3. Each of these mental health systems have a built-in self-maintenance and self-survival goal with different characteristics.
4. Special emphasis is placed on the preservation of proprietory private systems instead of the creation of a network of public and voluntary nonprofit special care facilities.
5. There is no reimbursement and very limited funds for outreach, prevention, and community mental health education programs.
6. The various third-party reimbursement agencies, upon which the mental health facilities depend for financial support, have different and limited benefits.
7. Mental health is not a right in the value system or social policy system in this country.
8. A conservative finding is that 20% of the population need professional intervention for mental health needs.
9. Mental health services are low on the scale of priorities in this country.
10. Mental illness has a special stigma.
11. The schizophrenic patients who live in local communities are very visible in relation to their sometimes bizarre behavior.
12. State mental health facilities often are the largest employers in the local communities in which they are located.

Benefits of community mental health

Although many criticisms have been leveled against community mental health, supporters have acknowledged the benefits. Community mental health centers have been correlated with increased use by new clients as well as a change in the type of clientele. More children and adolescents are receiving psychiatric treatment in community mental health centers than received treatment previously.[2] Moreover, there has been a documented diminution of sociodemographic bias toward the consumers of mental health services since the expansion of community mental health services.[41]

The acknowledged benefits of community mental health, its criticisms and shortcomings, as well as the commission's report provide stimuli for new directions. Once again a "bold new approach" is being called for, emphasizing the community as client and using a holistic approach to the delivery of services. This approach is to be based on a thorough assessment of community needs, awareness of existing resources, and comprehensive informed planning procedure.

■ Successful centers

In thinking about the flaws in the community mental health system, it is important to acknowledge that some centers have worked well. These are centers located in communities having populations and resources compatible with the community mental health movement's view of the community and the prevalent model of mental health care. Other centers have developed slowly and progressively, continually responding to the needs of the community and in concert with available funds. Successful centers have tended to construct strong community linkages and to focus on local needs rather than solely rely on federal guidelines.[6]

The Committee on Psychiatry and Community of the Group for Advancement of Psychiatry lists thirteen ingredients of successful centers.[6] These ingredients synthesized from a comprehensive review of centers include:

- Consistent and adequate funding
- Assignment of top priority to the needs of the most seriously ill
- Accessibility of services
- Availability of a full range of treatment and rehabilitation measures for individual patient needs
- Responsiveness to expressed local needs as opposed to categorical needs
- Effective interagency communication and planning
- Maximum use of existing community resources and the development of new resources for demonstrated service gaps
- Active involvement of psychiatrists as caregivers and planners
- Use of well-trained professionals for providing both services and supervision
- Internal harmony among the staff
- Pursuit of staff development and "anti-burnout" strategies
- Encouragement of active participation of the private psychiatric sector in patient care
- Objective assessments of needs and well-designed program evaluations

Community orientation to mental health

A community orientation requires an alteration in focus. A premise basic to community mental health is that all people experience stress and have problems coping but some have fewer support systems available to them and react in a dysfunctional way to stress.[26] The community approach to mental illness focuses on prevention by identifying high-risk populations and providing services before mental health is disrupted. The aim is to strike a balance between the level of stressors and the available supports. Innumerable ways exist to actuate a community approach to mental health. Intervening in poverty, crowding, discrimination, and crime serves to decrease stressors, whereas effective health care, police, social service, and educational resources increase community supports. On a personal or small-group level, crisis intervention, anticipatory guidance, consultation, and mental health education decrease stressors and provide supports.

The treatment area is the local community within which the client is experiencing his stress. It is insufficient to deal only with the client's internal dysfunction, but, rather, treatment implies attention to sociocultural background, adaptive ability, support systems, and family interaction.[42] Community mental health identifies the root of most emotional disorders as occurring within a network of interacting systems.[23] Although it is beyond the scope of this chapter to provide a detailed systems theory framework, selected principles are incorporated in a description of the human-environment relationship. A systems approach to mental health states that a person's health status results from the dynamic interaction between his internal environment and the external multienvironments in which he exists. A systems approach is used in community mental health nursing to provide a holistic view of a person as he relates to both his intrinsic and extrinsic environments. Each person's reactions to his multienvironments are never static but rather are dynamic and ever changing. One's responses comprise ongoing attempts to maintain homeostasis. The human system, like all living systems, is an open one in continuous interaction with the environment. Each individual's personality develops out of this interaction with the subsystems comprising his daily life. For example, interactions with family, significant groups, and the school and work environment play a crucial part in psychological development and coping. Problems or stresses in an interacting system have an effect on other systems.

The complexity of adaptive efforts is accentuated by the fact that one responds to the total environmental insult. One cannot sort out selected environmental components; adaptive responses attend to the total environmental impact. Furthermore, each human system strives to achieve a steady state or homeostasis. Symptoms of emotional disturbance signal system distress and subsequent disequilibrium. In regard to prevention, community mental health assumes that relieving stress in one component of the system will affect other components. Factors such as poor housing, lack of sanita-

tion, unemployment, crowding, and other manifestations of economic deprivation affect mental health.

The assessment process

One of the major criticisms of the community mental health movement, as mentioned earlier, was the inability of health care professionals to focus their attention on the community as the client. The challenge for a "bold new approach" to mental health still exists; whether it is found will be determined not only by a holistic approach to the delivery of services but also by the very ways in which services are planned and delivered.

To view the community as the client is to recognize a dynamic rather than a static entity. It is inevitable that change will occur within the community. Not only will the physical environment of the community change, but also there will be changes within the health care delivery system as well as changes in health needs. Consequently, one of the most important tasks of the community mental health nurse is to plan for change. Unfortunately, good planning does not just happen; it requires a continuous monitoring and assessment of the mental health needs and status of the community.[33]

Before the development of a community mental health plan it is necessary to diagnose and assess the health needs and resources of the community. A carefully planned and implemented assessment should yield data that reveal early warning signs of trouble, such as current mental health problems that are in the greatest need of attention and the extent to which problems at various stages are unattended and unprevented. An assessment should tell what is "right" as well as what is "wrong" and suggest how the community's resources ought to be allocated.

■ Nursing strategies

A community mental health nurse faced with the task of performing a comprehensive community assessment may tend to be overwhelmed by the potential scope and magnitude of the chore. This would certainly be a natural, perhaps even an expected, reaction. However, if the assessment is approached in a scientific fashion, much of the needed data can be obtained with relative ease and a minimum of effort. This is especially true for nurses who are intimately involved in the community.

Community mental health nurses possess a wealth of knowledge about their communities. Not only do they work with the families who make up the community, but they also interact with various individuals, groups, and organizations both within and outside the community. This information about the community, which all too frequently is neither reported, assembled, nor documented, together with recorded data provides the basis for a community assessment. Thus the important thing for the nurse to keep in mind is that the key to a successful meaningful assessment lies not so much in what data to gather but, more important, in where to gather the data.

A variety of strategies are available for assessing a community. Although each of these strategies certainly has its merits, a newer, more innovative approach to community assessment is needed. This new approach should include traditional assessment data but should also recognize the importance of consumers. It should focus on their special needs and wants rather than the perceptions of health care providers as to what consumers ought to have. To be truly consumer-oriented, nurses should acquaint themselves with contemporary health care marketing tools and concepts that hold to the philosophy that health care providers have an obligation to determine market needs and to meet these needs in a cost-effective way.[19]

Identifying consumer needs is extremely important to both health care marketers and community health nurses. Two interrelated concepts have been useful to marketers in their attempts to become more responsive to both present and potential consumers. The first concept is known as market segmentation; the second is called target marketing.

Community Assessment Tool

Market Analysis

Environmental Analysis: describes major demographic, economic, technological, governmental, and cultural trends or developments affecting the community

Demographic developments will affect the ultimate size of the community and its needs. The main demographic factors are:
Size of the population
Age distribution
Birth and death rate trends
Geographic distribution
- What major demographic developments and trends pose opportunities or threats for this community?
- What actions have been taken in response to these developments?
- What effect will the forecasted trends have on the community?

Economic developments have a strong effect on the demand for products and services and the cost of providing them.
- What major developments and trends in income, prices, savings, and credit have an impact on the community?
- What actions have been taken in response to these developments and trends?

Technological developments have a great significance for possible new products and services and cost savings.
- What major changes are occurring in product technology?

Resource Analysis

Competitor Identification: enumerates the community's major competitive professional resources.
Forms of Competition includes generic, service form, and enterprise professional resources.
Generic: other broad service categories that might satisfy the same need
Service form: specific versions of the service that may be competitive
Enterprise: specific organizations that are competitive purveyors of the same services
- Who are the community's major competitive professional resources?
- How are these competitive professional resources defined? Generic, service form, or enterprise?
- What types of competitors?
- How many in each category?
- What trends can be foreseen in the competitive environment?

Attitude and Image Analysis: profiles the attitudes and images held by various constituencies within the community
- What are the attitudes of those professionals who work with mental health clients?
- What are the attitudes and images of special interest groups regarding community mental health issues?
- What are the attitudes and images of clients regarding community mental health issues?
- What are the attitudes and images of nonclients regarding community mental health issues?

Continued.

■ **MARKET SEGMENTATION.** In marketing terminology, markets tend to be heterogeneous and need to be segmented into several smaller homogeneous groups. Once this has been accomplished, segments or target markets become the focus of specialized programs tailored to the needs of the market. Applying these concepts to the community is an acknowledgment on the part of the nurse that the community is heterogeneous and therefore requires specialized programs that cater to the specific needs of its members.

If usable market segments are to be developed, three conditions must be considered. The first condition is **measurability.** This is the degree to which information exists or is obtainable about particular characteristics of the consumer. Unfortunately, many useful characteristics such as values and attitudes are not easy to measure. Likewise, many mental health stressors may not be easily identified. The second condition is **accessibility.** Frequently, measurable differences in consumer attributes do exist, but it is not feasible to reach them. The third condition is **substantiality,** which refers to the degree to which segments are large enough to be worth subdividing for separate programs.

There is no unique way to divide a community into segments. However, several segmentation variables might be useful to the community mental health nurse (see the accompanying box).

One approach, for instance, might be to segment

Community Assessment Tool—cont'd

■ What major changes are occurring in service technology?

■ What major changes are occurring in process technology?

Governmental developments are difficult to predict but can have a profound effect on the community.

■ What new legislation could affect this community?

■ What laws are being proposed that may affect this community?

■ What federal, state, and local agency actions should be watched?

■ What actions has the community taken in response to these developments?

Social-cultural developments have an effect on values and life-styles in the community.

■ What changes are occurring in life-styles and values that might affect this community.

■ What actions have been taken in response to these developments?

Market Definition: defines the characteristics of the community's major mental health care markets

■ Who are the primary (actual and potential) markets for mental health care in this community?

Market Segmentation: divides a market into groups of people who have relatively similar needs

Bases for segments:
Geographic
Demographic
Psychographic (life-style)

Service usage
Benefits sought
High-risk groups
Readiness or predisposition to respond

■ What are the major market segments in this community?

■ What are the characteristics of each market segment?

Criteria for segments:
substantiality—must be large enough to justify effort
measurability—information can be obtained
accessibility—they can be reached

■ What is the present size of each market segment?

■ What is the expected future size of each market segment?

Needs Assessment: identifies needs unique to each segment

■ What is the present state of needs of each market segment?

■ What is the expected future state of needs of each market segment?

Satisfaction Assessment: identifies level of needs satisfaction within each market segment

■ How satisfied are the needs of each market segment?

Identifying Target Markets: focuses on unsatisfied or undersatisfied needs

■ Which market segments have needs requiring attention?

■ On which market segments are our resources best directed?

the community according to demographic variables, such as age, education, income, occupation, race, religion, and sex. A note of caution is appropriate at this point to emphasize that demographic variables are only the foundation for more detailed segmentation strategies and are rarely effective by themselves. However, even such broad segments as children and adults could be tremendously helpful. It should also be noted that the needs of the segment determine the health services needed, rather than the other way around.

Additional possibilities are to segment the community by socioeconomic variables, stages in the family life cycle, or psychographic variables such as activities, values, interests, attitudes, opinions, and life-styles. The number of different ways in which a community might be meaningfully segmented is limited only be the creative abilities of the nurse. Still another possibility is to segment in terms of identified mental health problems. Since the emphasis in community mental health focuses on prevention, one way to segment a community while maintaining an orientation toward prevention is to identify populations that are "at risk" for disruption in psychological equilibrium or mental health. For example, families under stress, victims of aggression, and discharged mentally ill persons are all strong candidates for market segmentation.

■ **TARGET MARKETING** After the community has been segmented into target markets requiring mental health programs, the following information should be gathered. First, a geographical area of the community should be defined, thereby limiting the target market to those individuals who reside within a certain geographically limited area. Boundaries that result may be appropriate geographically but questionable by other standards because some people may live outside one catchment area yet be closer to its health facilities than their own. Consequently, strictly enforced boundaries tend to create time and travel problems. The solution is cooperation between communities with common boundaries.

After the establishment of geographical boundaries, there is the need to determine the size of the various target markets. Obviously the larger the target market, the more important it becomes to the health of the community. Consideration should also be given to the location of a target within the community. For example, a target group with a widely dispersed population may require an entirely different program approach compared with a target group that is clustered in a small pocket of the community.

Once the community has been assessed in terms of its problems and needs, the community mental health nurse can then turn attention to assessing the community's resources. Information should be gathered to determine the availability of professionals who have training in the traditional mental health disciplines, such as psychiatrists, clinical psychologists, social workers, and nurses. In addition, the availability of professionals outside the traditional mental health area, such as physicians, clergy, and schoolteachers, should be considered. Other resources such as hospitals, halfway homes, and nursing homes should be included in the assessment, as well as existing mental health facilities and service organizations. In many communities, existing services are often fragmented and clients are frequently forced to obtain services from several different agencies, none of which is aware of the work being performed by the others.

A final input to the community assessment is identifying the community's attitudes toward mental health. Specific attitudinal information should be gathered from these groups and individuals currently working with clients, such as private practitioners, public and private hospital administrators and staff, and social workers. In addition, the attitudes of special interest and power groups as well as the attitudes of the general population should be considered in the community assessment.

Stewart[38] describes a three-phase community needs assessment approach that is similar to the marketing framework used here. He defines the three steps as problem description, desire for services, and solutions needed to solve the problems. The problem area includes (1) a description of the size and nature of the problem (number of people, where they live, and what they are like), (2) a description of the community, and (3) identification of available services that help to meet the needs identified in the problem statement.

Desire refers to the attitudes held about both the problem and the services. This step also sets priorities as to the relative importance of the identified problems. A solution is arrived at based on the previous two steps. When more than one choice of solution is suggested, then the alternatives are arranged by priority.

In summary, any assessment of the community should take into account an analysis of the existing mental health programs and facilities, an audit of the resources available, an evaluation of the attitudes toward mental health, and, most important, an identification of the specific needs of the community. Any comprehensive community analysis requires a certain depth and breadth of awareness of community needs to optimize program effectiveness.

Implementing the role

Community mental health nursing is defined as a broad continuum of activities ranging from health maintenance and promotion to curative and rehabilitative functions. Community mental health nursing is differentiated from psychiatric nursing in that in the broadest sense the community rather than the individual is the client. Psychiatry refers to a medical specialty concerned with the identification and treatment of mental disorders. Mental health refers to the maintenance and enhancement of functioning, including the prevention of disorder. Similarly, psychiatric nursing seeks to provide care to individuals who evidence psychological dysfunction, whereas community mental health nursing applies a public approach to mental health by focusing on the macrosystem or community as client. Nursing attention is directed toward factors within the community that impede the maintenance of mental health. Nursing intervention at this level focuses on such factors as the effects of poor housing, crowding, and unemployment on the mental health of residents. The nurse often serves as a catalyst in bringing stress factors to the attention of concerned groups, who then work to ameliorate the situation.

A major component of the community mental health nursing role is directed toward identifying populations at risk and seeking interventions that decrease stress and reduce the incidence of mental disorder. For example, a nurse might provide counseling for a group of divorced women to support and guide them during a crisis. Although the clients are not emotionally disturbed, the family crisis makes them "at risk" for psychological dysfunction. Activities to promote and enhance mental health can be described in accordance with Caplan's levels of primary, secondary, and tertiary prevention.[5] This schema is used to identify selected high-risk populations and describe nursing interventions designed to reduce stress and promote mental health.

■ Primary prevention

Primary prevention of mental disorders is described as biological, social, or psychological intervention that promotes emotional well-being or reduces the incidence of mental illness in populations. Primary prevention attempts to lower the new cases of mental disorder over a period of time. According to Caplans' model of primary prevention,[5] the rate of mental disorder in a community is related to the interaction of both long- and short-term factors influencing the adaptive capacities of its members. Thus mental illness occurs in a community context and the resources for helping are provided in the community.

Primary prevention in mental health is an elusive concept in that it is often difficult to document its success. DeWild[10] identified two models of primary prevention in mental health. The first provides services to

". . . increase health and reduce stress for an identified population of people who are presumed at risk, under stress, or in crisis." Such groups served by this model include single parents, expectant parents, families with preschool children or older adults in the home, those with physical handicaps, and so on. Such programs are designed to support people in working out their life stresses. The second model deals with groups who are not yet mentally ill, but who do have an educational, occupational, or social problem. For example, one program of this type works with children who were unable to adjust in school. This model seeks to reduce the vulnerability to mental illness of a group of people who are at risk because of a defined social dysfunction.

Bloom[4] points out an interesting perspective on prevention when he suggests that the previous public health paradigm used in the prevention of infectious diseases is not effective in mental illness. In the classic public health paradigm, a disease is identified, its natural history of development and progression is traced, and a program of intervention is developed. In contrast, he recommends a new paradigm for mental illness that is directed toward identifying a stressful life event which has undesirable mental health consequences. This would include identifying people at risk, studying the effects of the event, and implementing and evaluating intervention programs (see Chapter 9). The basic difference is that the specific cause or manifestation of disease or disability is not important; the focus is on preventing any form of disability from identification of known stressors.

Consistent with both the models of DeWild and Bloom, activities for primary prevention include teaching mental health principles to a variety of community groups, including the PTA, church groups, and youth organizations. Conducting interactional groups in schools, day-care centers, or children's homes also provides a medium for preventive activities. Referral constitutes a preventive approach if persons undergoing stress are directed to mental health resources before mental disorder occurs. Thus, consultation and education are major tools of community mental health nursing.

■ Secondary prevention

Secondary prevention seeks to reduce the prevalence of mental disorder by providing interventions that decrease the stressors and shorten the duration of disequilibrium. New directions in techniques for providing secondary prevention are being sought in the area of short-term interventions such as crisis intervention designed to lessen discomfort and return the individual to effective functioning (see Chapter 10). Treatment developments include a wide variety of group therapies, marital and family therapy, and intervention strategies combining psychotherapy with environmental manipulation, such as psychodrama, dance therapy, poetry, art, or activity therapy. Each type of therapy is aimed at helping the individual gain self-awareness and thereby learn new ways of responding to stressors.

Specific techniques for secondary prevention include home visits designed to help individuals cope with high levels of stress without being removed from their home setting, suicide prevention counseling, and preadmission services, which frequently include home visits. The aim of community mental health in regard to secondary prevention is to treat the acute phase as early as possible and to use inpatient psychiatric care only when essential and when outpatient care or partial hospitalization is inadequate for the patient's needs.

■ Tertiary prevention

Tertiary prevention refers to measures designed to reduce the level of mental disorder in a community through rehabilitation. Implicit in rehabilitation is early planning for care on discharge from the hospital, follow-up care to reduce stressors and promote coping ability, and use of a wide range of supportive activities such as transitional or halfway homes, foster homes, home visits, and partial hospitalization (see Chapter 11). A specific plan for tertiary prevention is described in the following discussion of a plan for discharged psychiatric patients.

Deinstitutionalization: impact on long-term psychiatric patients

With the Community Mental Health Centers Act of 1963 and the 1978 report of the Joint Commission on Mental Illness and Health come mandates for providing decentralized community care for long-term psychiatric patients. During the 15 years between these two significant mental health documents there was a dramatic decrease in the populations of state hospitals. The question arises as to whether the patients are sufficiently well to negotiate the community system or whether many have been discharged without adequate preparation and subsequent follow-up care relative to community living.

■ Judicial decisions

The paradoxical nature of the *Wyatt v Stickney* decision of 1972 affects the goal of decentralization. Essentially the U.S. Supreme Court ordered the State of Alabama to draw up within 6 months a comprehensive plan for providing relevant treatment for all patients in mental health facilities. The court order required (1) a humane psychological and physical environment, (2) qualified staff in sufficient numbers to provide adequate treatment, and (3) individualized treatment plans.[17] The significance of this court order is that funds mandated for community mental health were reallocated for inpatient care, thereby seriously altering any attempts to plan new approaches for discharged mentally ill persons. In particular this court action emphasizes the pressure community mental health experiences from legal and, especially, federal and state funding decisions. The majority of mental health programs depend largely on external funding sources, which often limit creativity and innovation.

In a further judicial decision, *O'Connor v Donaldson,* the Supreme Court ruled unanimously that mentally ill patients who pose no threat to society and who are able to survive outside the hospital cannot be confined against their will and without treatment.[17] A key point relates to the definition of "ability to survive"; the whole question of quality of life can be raised. The majority of long-term psychiatrically hospitalized patients pose no societal threat; many, though, are incapable of meeting the barest needs for survival. For example, for the patient who has been hospitalized for 15 years, the reality shock resulting from spontaneous hospital discharge and the immediate need for survival can be overwhelming. Merely securing a place to live, purchasing food, and arranging for household utilities is a task compounded by gross lack of familiarity with each system involved.

Another issue that must be at the forefront of planning for a community approach is that the majority of individuals who are hospitalized for an extended period are diagnosed as schizophrenic. These individuals often lack the self-concept and confidence required to demand quality services. Furthermore, lengthy hospitalization tends to prepare individuals for a subservient role that hinders the ability to meet their needs in a societal context.

■ Community ideology

One of the basic principles of community mental health ideology refers to continuity of care. If programs are to be effective, some member of the staff must maintain contact with and responsibility for each discharged patient as he moves from one system to another.[33] Although this belief is widely held, it is infrequently practiced. Few community mental health approaches provide systematic assistance in locating housing, obtaining employment, managing finances, developing a social system for interaction, and, of primary importance, teaching basic coping skills essential to functioning outside the hospital.[36] A large number of patients discharged from public mental hospitals lack problem-solving abilities to meet the goals and demands of life outside the hospital.

Rachlin[30] contends that the major reasons why deinstitutionalization has not been successful is that the needs of patients and the directions of programs have been disjointed. In many instances, deinstitutionalization has served only to decrease the population in mental hospitals. Substitute domiciles and coordinated integrated program planning for discharged patients has been lacking in both quality and quantity. Additionally, even when unique model programs have been successfully developed, it has been a challenge to sustain enthusiasm for the goal because dealing with chronically ill patients is difficult and does not always provide visible and immediate treatment results.

Dickey and co-workers[11] documented the success of a deinstitutionalization program by studying 27 patients 4 years after discharge. These patients had been hospitalized for an average of 24 years. Using interviews with both patients and caretakers, data were gathered regarding the place of residence, mental status, time spent in the hospital since discharge, level of functioning, and quality of life. The authors found that rehospitalization decreased significantly once patients moved from the hospital to the community. They also found that the best predictor of success at remaining in the community was age of hospital admission. Those who entered the hospital at an early age had increased difficulty readjusting to community life. They also found that all but two preferred their present living situation to that of the hospital. Also, patients living in the community had a better average mental status score and level of functioning than patients who were currently hospitalized. This study supported the belief that organized and systematic aftercare is a prerequisite for maintaining chronically ill patients in the community.

Personnel deployment poses a serious consideration when large numbers of patients are discharged into community-care programs. The dilemma in deployment planning is whether personnel familiar with one role can focus their attention on a new concept of mental health care. Inpatient psychiatric care has been accused of rigidity, lack of interest in the individual, and limited creativity. Each of these criticisms must be reversed if community care is to enhance mental health. For a community to establish a comprehensive program for discharged patients, inpatient services must be available. It can be anticipated that some patients will experience an exacerbation of symptoms and require short-term hospitalization.

■ Patient placement

Perhaps the greatest criticism of community mental health programming lies in the failure of tertiary prevention through deinstitutionalization. The era of deinstitutionalization was ushered in with "much naiveté and many simplistic notions about what would become of the chronically and severely mentally ill."[18] Several of the factors leading to deinstitutionalization have been discussed. These include the advent of psychotropic medications in the 1960s which successfully controlled the behaviors of many patients, especially those diagnosed with schizophrenia or manic depressive illness; a new philosophy of social treatment which advocated attention to patient's rights, particularly civil rights; and a wish to reduce the federal financial burden for mental health care.

Two significant pieces of legislation, the funding of community mental health centers and categorical Aid to the Disabled (ATD) in 1963, accelerated the thrust toward deinstitutionalization. The latter made the mentally ill eligible for federal financial support in the community for the first time. This funding enabled patients to either support themselves or be supported in homes or facilities like board and care homes or hotels at little cost to the state. Aid to the Disabled is now called Supplemental Security Income (SSI) and is administered by the Social Security Administration.

Concurrently, sweeping changes in commitment laws in some states made the involuntary commitment of psychiatric patients a difficult process. In 1955, there were approximately 559,000 patients in state and county psychiatric hospitals; there were 475,202 in 1965, 215,573 in 1974, and 138,000 in 1983.[14] More than 400,000 patients have been discharged with a large number failing to find supportive, community-based care. The money simply did not follow the patients into the community. Although state hospitals discharged large numbers of patients, many still required a substantial portion of available mental health funds because of union contracts and other regulations. This left community services chronically short of funds.

In the initial years of deinstitutionalization approximately two thirds of the discharged patients returned to their families. Countless others went to nursing homes and group homes with varying degrees of care. The latter, often called board and care homes, typically provide a shared room, three meals a day, the dispensing of medication, and minimal staff supervision. Another alternative, single room occupancy (SRO) homes provide even less supervision and structure.

Thousands of discharged patients live on the streets, on beaches, in parks, under bridges, and in doorways. These homeless people frequent city shelters in such numbers that these facilities are becoming mini-institutions for the chronically mentally ill. Other mentally ill patients have found shelter in the criminal justice system. Society has a limited tolerance for dealing with mentally disordered behavior.[18] Rather than being hospitalized in a psychiatric hospital many mentally ill people are subjected to inappropriate arrest and incarceration. Finally, deinstitutionalized patients are appearing at urban general hospitals. The emergency department is the first place these patients turn when anything goes wrong in their unstructured and unsupervised lives.

■ Proposal for nursing intervention

A comprehensive community-based program for discharged mentally ill patients encompasses community acceptance, client advocacy, teaching basic skills of everyday living, and ongoing support in the form of individual or group supervision.[40] Although a collaborative interdisciplinary approach is required to implement the community follow-up plan, the nursing component is emphasized. While a variety of professionals could serve as coordinators of the program, the community mental health nurse is used in the following proposal. Public health nurses are described as the actual client advocates in that they possess knowledge, skill, and an entrée in regard to community care. Ideally a plan should be developed prior to the discharge of psychiatric patients; in reality, a large number of patients already reside in the community despite lack of coping skills. Therefore a community program could begin with patients already in need of supervision or start with newly discharged persons.

Prior to the onset of a continuity-of-care program for discharged patients some degree of community responsibility should be assured. Interaction should occur in advance of purchasing or leasing any property for a transition home or similar group residence. The purpose of staff and community dialogue is to discuss plans, elicit fears from residents, and assess the degree of support available in a given community. Community residents often cite fears of physical assault, bizarre behavior, or a decrease in property values. In truth, communities may profit from a group home in that housing in poor repair is often secured because of limited funds. Residents and staff frequently renovate with zeal and soon increase property values.

Clients must be taught basic skills of daily living before they are discharged from the hospital. Activities such as meal preparation, budgeting, doing laundry, and use of public transportation and telephones are often foreign to individuals hospitalized for many years. They may need to practice social skills, such as job seeking, shopping, and requesting services. Teaching strategies include instruction, demonstration, and practice either through simulations, such as role playing, or actual performance of an activity, such as meal planning, shopping, and food preparation. The community mental health nurse often coordinates activities designed to facilitate reentry into society. Hospital staff provide the actual teaching with coordination and supervision from the consultant.

■ CLIENT ADVOCACY.

The concept of client advocacy has long been discussed, but there has been little comprehensive use. Public health nurses are used as client advocates, since they have ready access to both clients and the mental health system. In essence, each client has a public health nurse who monitors his functioning and progress much as in hospital rounds. Each nurse is assigned a certain number of clients; the nursing role is to help clients interact more effectively with the multitude of community systems supportive to daily living. Not only does the nurse make home visits and coordinate client activities, but also includes each client in a small group that meets regularly to discuss common problems.

Each group session focuses on a specific topic. Lack of structure proves threatening for many. Topics such as side effects of medication, rehabilitation plans, or problems in getting along with others are discussed.[12] The objectives of the group session include (1) helping clients function outside the institution through support and medication monitoring, (2) reinforcing strengths, and (3) assisting clients to learn more effective ways to interact with others.[22] The community mental health nurse serves as consultant and coordinator by meeting regularly with each public health nurse or group of nurses to discuss common case load difficulties. The community mental health nurse consultant supports other public health nurses just as they support the clients.

Davies[9] describes a Continuing Care Program at Western Psychiatric Institute and Clinic in Pennsylvania that implements many of the concepts noted in the model presented. In the Pennsylvania program a model approach was designed to meet the needs of chronically ill psychiatric patients. In this program each client is provided with a continuum of care that meets individual needs. Each is assessed as to physical and psychological status, sociocultural variables, and community support network. Services are offered in three categories: direct, community, and case management.

Direct services include individual, group, or family counseling based on a crisis intervention framework. Community coping skills are also assessed, and structured activities are arranged where needed to teach basic skills. Also, outreach services include home visits or telephone calls when patients cannot come to the unit. Educational opportunities teach skills, medication maintenance, and so forth. The second set of services includes the community network, which provides consultation and education to the community to strengthen resources available to chronically ill patients. The third set of services refers to case management, including coordination of services and active involvement in the treatment program.

In community mental health, case management has taken varied forms. The goals, however, consistently include "providing a client with an individual who is responsible for helping coordinate the client's care and treatment within a complex human service system."[35] The Joint Commission on Accreditation of Hospitals lists five functions of case management: (1) assessment, (2) planning, (3) linking, (4) monitoring, and (5) advocacy. These functions are consistent with the nursing process and are activities typically associated with psychiatric nursing. The objective of case management is to make certain that clients receive the services they need to function effectively in the setting least restrictive for them. Case management is not easy. To be effective, resources must be available, communication among provider systems must be clear and direct, and the numerous barriers to cooperation must be eliminated.[35]

Interdisciplinary collaboration in community mental health

Interdisciplinary interaction is a basic tenet of community mental health. In the community mental health movement, professionals increasingly seem to perform tasks using strikingly similar skills. Further rapid societal change has demanded new services to meet the mental health needs of consumers. Health professionals are attempting to adapt, change, and expand skills to provide a relevant service to consumers. The subsequent "identity crisis" in what belongs uniquely to each profession has added stress to the effectiveness of service delivery.[3] Nursing is changing rapidly, as is every other health profession. Each nurse should have a clear concept of nursing's unique role and contribution to the team. To interpret one's role and maintain accountability, one must know what is implicit in the role as well as where one's area of responsibility ends.

Interprofessional teamwork is subject to the same rules of group process as any other organized group. Considerable time and energy must be expended to facilitate team communication to define and delegate responsibilities and thus avoid infringing on each other's sense of territoriality. A major team goal is to determine comfortable and mutually satisfactory modes of inter-

action and relationship negotiation. Teamwork is a problem-solving approach both to providing services and determining ways in which members can work together. It is essential that the team be clear about the purposes, goals, and individual member responsibilities and that a mechanism be established for renegotiation of roles. Just stating the goals of the team in no way ensures consensus. Dialogue is continuous in an interdisciplinary team, with modification of goals and strategies integral to functioning.

Interprofessional teams typically go through a series of interactional stages: (1) early enthusiasm and lively interest in each other's contributions, (2) insecurity and sense of role threat combined with guarding of one's territory, and (3) role negotiation and effective functioning or abandonment of the team concept. Teams in community mental health are described as more democratic than those in other settings. Also, the leader is likely to be elected rather than designated by job title. Decisions regarding the tasks of team members are made on the basis of competence, interest, availability, and match between client or family needs and provider ability and preference.

Evaluation in community mental health

Community mental health is a new concept in a field that is defined by lack of agreement about values, modes of treatment, and standards of practice. Evaluation, although exceedingly difficult because of the intangible nature of community mental health services, is essential as a system for quality control and a catalyst for accountability. Program evaluation must answer questions about both the quantity and quality of services.

■ Quality assessment methodologies

In general, three quality assessment methodologies—structure, process, and outcome—used either singly or in combination, comprise the foundation of current health care standards' procedures. In the **structural** approach to quality assessment, standards and criteria are designed to determine the impact of organizational patterns on the delivery of quality health care services. Two basic assumptions underlie the use of a structural approach: it is possible to assess what is "good" by identifying staff, physical, and organizational structure, and care is improved as staff qualifications are upgraded, physical facilities are improved, and sounder fiscal and administration procedures are applied.[28] Structural standards are widely used in assessment because they provide a means to assess quantifiable data. This method is traditionally undertaken by the government, since it is the easiest to apply.

In the **process** approach to assessing quality care the activities of health professionals are evaluated in terms of what is determined to be "good care." The assumption underlying process assessment is that health care providers can agree on what constitutes quality care. Process standards are of two types: "normative," which are derived from the formulations of recognized leaders, and "empirical," which are based on actual patterns of care. Both approaches entail observation and experimentation and change over time. This approach is largely used by the providers to pinpoint problem areas.

The **outcome** approach assesses care on the basis of the result of treatment. These standards measure survival, recovery, and the patient's satisfaction with his treatment. Outcome measures can be used by both government and the providers and are considered by many to be the most useful forms of evaluation, albeit the most difficult to obtain.

■ National standards

The National Standards for Community Mental Health Centers developed by the NIMH describe three major areas for evaluation. Attention is focused on administration and direction of the center, which includes organizational patterns, staffing, facilities, use review, and provision for requested information. The second category of evaluation calls attention to accessibility and specifically focuses on community orientation, visibility, prevention, including consultation and education, and coordination and collaboration with other agencies. The third area relates to specific service activities and includes the five major modes of treatment: inpatient, outpatient, partial hospitalization, emergency care, consultation and education, and individualized treatment plans, a range of treatment modalities, and continuity of care. As a public agency NIMH evaluates programs to ensure that grant recipients are using their funds according to stipulated guidelines. The governmental monitoring process is carried out through site visits, applications for future support, and an annual inventory completed by each center.[13]

■ Issues in evaluation

Within each community mental health program a decision must be reached as to the mode of evaluation. The major decision includes selecting between a structural approach, which relies largely on enumeration, and an outcome methodology, which is more difficult to complete but may be more useful in terms of program change to provide more relevant services to consumers. Although quantity of services, that is, the number of individuals who partake of any service, is far easier to measure than quality, relevant evaluation demands attention to effectiveness of services delivered. Client outcomes after treatment constitute a major criterion for evaluation. Outcome is measured against predetermined goals often stated in the form of behavioral objectives. A current disadvantage to this method of evaluation is that little outcome or follow-up data are collected in community mental health programs. Evaluation is one segment of a total monitoring package that focuses on how services affect the clients who receive them.[37] Follow-up examination is a component of evaluation that examines long-range effects of treatment approaches.

An outcome evaluation program begins with stated goals determined at the onset of treatment. Essentially the client and the nurse decide what they expect to accomplish in the treatment relationship. Many call this delineation of goals a contract. The items on the contract are stated in behavioral terms, such as "the patient will return to work with less than a 10% absentee rate due to 'nervousness.'" The major problem in outcome evaluation relates to determining the measurements to be assessed. What kinds of information or change constitute effective treatment? Outcome measures should be simple, concrete, readily observable or measurable, and open to minimal interpretation based on opinion. Both client self-reports and nurse observation comprise a component of evaluation. Although indicators, such as number of hours expended in services, number of patients seen, and scope of services offered constitute data for evaluation, these measures are no longer sufficient. Outcome and service effectiveness measures must be included despite the difficulty in establishing such criteria.

■ SUGGESTED CROSS-REFERENCES ■

Evolutionary perspectives of psychiatric nursing are discussed in Chapter 1. A nursing model of health-illness phenomena is discussed in Chapter 3. Evaluation of the nursing process is discussed in Chapter 5. Defining mental health, high-risk populations, and primary prevention activities are discussed in Chapter 9. Crisis intervention is discussed in Chapter 10. Tertiary prevention and rehabilitation activities are discussed in Chapter 11. Liaison psychiatric nursing and consultation are discussed in Chapter 26. Care of the chronic mentally ill patient is discussed in Chapter 34.

DIRECTIONS FOR FUTURE RESEARCH

The following are some of the nursing research problems raised in Chapter 25 that merit further study by psychiatric nurses:

1. Exploration of factors present in successful community mental health programs
2. The role of nurses in community mental health
3. Specific benefits associated with patients' use of community mental health services
4. Identification of successful primary prevention programs
5. The cost-effectiveness of treatment of specific patient target groups in the community versus the cost of hospitalization
6. Systematic analysis of the role of case manager in terms of efficiency, effectiveness of coordination, and aspects of cost
7. The differential characteristics of patients who do and do not respond to coordinated social treatment in the community
8. Predictor variables related to patients who do not follow-up and benefit from community mental health care
9. The specific effects of primary preventive programs on reducing the incidence of mental illness in the community
10. Development of an accurate evaluation method for use in community mental health
11. The relationship between early discharge planning and aftercare and readmission of psychiatric patients
12. The effects of the changing family structure on individuals in the community

SUMMARY

1. A brief overview of the history of mental health care in the United States was presented, including the work of Benjamin Rush, Dorothea Dix, and Adolf Meyer. A summary was provided of governmental involvement in the mental health field leading up to the legislation enabling the development of community mental health centers.

2. The five essential services described in the 1963 legislation—inpatient, partial hospitalization, outpatient, emergency care, and consultation and education services—were described as were the additional services of diagnosis, rehabilitation, precare and aftercare, training and research, and evaluation. Modifications of the law included in the 1975 amendments, the 1978 report of the President's Commission

on Mental Health, and the 1980 legislation were also described.

3. Several criticisms and benefits of community mental health programs were compared.

4. A brief presentation of systems theory and a holistic view of human beings was included to provide a philosophical foundation for understanding community mental health.

5. The nurse's role in community assessment was addressed. It was emphasized that attention must be given to the needs of the consumer as well as those of the community. Therefore concepts of market segmentation and target marketing were presented as they are applicable to community and consumer assessment.

6. The role of the community mental health nurse in implementation is directed toward the community rather than the individual. This role was further elaborated on according to Caplan's formulations of primary, secondary, and tertiary prevention. Consultation and education are major tools used by the nurse in community mental health.

7. The impact of deinstitutionalization and a proposal for nursing intervention was described.

8. The concept of the mental health team was described as it pertains to the role of the community mental health nurse.

9. Evaluation is an extremely important facet of community mental health and was presented in terms of both quantity and quality of services. Methods of evaluation are applied to structure, process, or outcome of services.

■ REFERENCES ■

1. Arnhoff, F.N.: Social consequences of policy toward mental illness, Science **188:**1277, 1975.
2. Babigian, H.: The impact of community mental health centers on the utilization of services, Arch. Gen. Psychiatry **34:**385, 1977.
3. Bandler, B.: Interprofessional collaboration in training in mental health, Am. J. Orthopsychiatry **43:**97, Jan. 1973.
4. Bloom, B.L.: Prevention of mental disorders: recent advances in theory and practice, Community Ment. Health J. **15**(3):179, 1979.
5. Caplan, G.: Principles of preventive psychiatry, New York, 1964, Basic Books, Inc.
6. Committee on Psychiatry and Community, Group for the Advancement of Psychiatry: Community psychiatry: a reappraisal. New York, 1983, Mental Health Materials Center.
7. Community Mental Health Services Support Branch: A citizens guide to the community mental health centers amendments of 1975, Washington, D.C., 1977, U.S. Government Printing Office.
8. Council of Advanced Practitioners in Psychiatric and Mental Health Nursing: Pacesetter **2:**2, Spring 1977.
9. Davies, M.A.: Continuing care unit: a model of services for chronic psychiatric patients, J. Psychiatr. Nurs. **19**(2):42, 1981.

10. DeWild, D.W.: Toward a clarification of primary prevention, Community Ment. Health J. **16**:306, 1981.

11. Dickey, B., et al.: A follow-up of deinstitutionalized chronic patients four years after discharge, Hosp. Community Psychiatry **32**:326, 1981.

12. Donlon, P., and Rada, R.: Issues in developing quality aftercare clinics for the chronic mentally ill, Community Ment. Health J. **12**:29, Spring 1976.

13. Feldman, S., and Windle, C.: The NIMH approach to evaluating the community mental health centers program, Health Services Report **88**:174, Feb. 1973.

14. Friedman, E.: The light that failed, Hospitals **57**(16):88, 1983.

15. Hager, L., and Kincheloe, M.: The disintegration of a community mental health outpatient program, or off the back wards into the streets, Perspect. Psychiatr. Care **113**:102, 1983.

16. Joint Commission for Accreditation of Hospitals: Principles for accreditation of community mental health service program, Chicago, 1979, p. 19.

17. Kaplan, H.A.: Institutions and community mental health: the paradox in *Wyatt v. Stickney*, Community Ment. Health J. **9**:34, Spring 1973.

18. Lamb, H.R.: Deinstitutionalization and the homeless mentally ill. Hosp. Community Psychiatry **35**:899, 1984.

19. Lancaster, W.: Health care marketing: a model for planned change. In Lancaster, J., and Lancaster, W., editors: Concepts for advanced nursing practice: the nurse as a change agent, St. Louis, 1982, The C.V. Mosby Co.

20. Landsberg, G., and Hammer, R.: Possible programmatic consequences of Community Mental Health Center funding arrangements: illustrations based on inpatient utilization data, Community Ment. Health J. **13**:63, Spring 1977.

21. Langsley, D.G.: The community mental health center: does it treat patients? Hosp. Community Psychiatry **31**:815, 1980.

22. Lindberg, H., and Braach, C.H.: Community health nursing in the changing mental health scene, J. Nurs. Admin. **3**:41, Nov. 1973.

23. Marmor, J.: The relationship between systems theory and community psychiatry, Hosp. Community Psychiatry **26**:807, 1975.

24. MH-MR Report: A Morris Associates report from Washington, D.C. **15**:1, May 5, 1978.

25. Morrissey, J.P., and Goldman H.H.: Cycles of reform in the care of the chronically mentally ill, Hosp. Community Psychiatry **35**(89):785, 1984.

26. Murray, J.: Failure of the community mental health movement, Am. J. Nurs. **75**:2034, 1975.

27. National Council of Community Mental Health Centers: Renewal of CMHC Act: amendments to PL 94-63, Washington, D.C., 1977.

28. National Institute of Mental Health: National standards for community mental health centers: report to Congress, Rockville, Md., 1977, The Institute.

29. Nation's health. Mental health bill signed into law, Washington, D.C., Am. Public Health Assoc. **10**(11):1, 1980.

30. Rachlin, S.: When schizophrenia comes marching home, Psychiatric Q. **50**(3): 202, 1978.

31. Ramshorn, M.T.: The major thrust in American psychiatry: past, present, and future, Perspect. Psychiatr. Care **9**(4):144, 1971.

32. Rubins, J.: The community mental health movement in the United States circa 1970, Am. J. Psychoanal. **31**:68, Jan. 1971.

33. Ruybal, S.: Community health planning. Fam. Commun. Health **1**:9, Spring 1978.

34. Schulberg, H., Becker, A., and McGrath, M.: Planning the phasedown of mental hospitals, Community Ment. Health J. **12**:3, Spring 1976.

35. Schwartz, S.R., Goldman, H.H., and Churgin, S.: Case management for the chronic mentally ill: models and dimensions, Hosp. Community Psychiatry **33**(12):1006, 1982.

36. Snow, D., and Newton, P.: Task, social structure, and social process in the community mental health center movement, Am. J. Psychol. **31**:582, 1976.

37. Speer, D., and Tapp, J.: Evaluation of mental health service effectiveness: a start up model for established programs, Am. J. Orthopsychiatry **46**:217, 1976.

38. Stewart, E.: The nature of needs assessment in community mental health, Community Ment. Health J. **15**:287, 1979.

39. Tarail, M.: Current and future issues in community mental health, Psychiatric Q. **52**(1):27, 1980.

40. Test, M.A., and Stein, L.: Practical guidelines for the community treatment of markedly impaired patients, Community Ment. Health J. **12**:72, Spring 1976.

41. Tischler, G.L., Henisz, J., Myers, J., and Garrison, V.: Catchmenting and the use of mental health services, Arch. Gen. Psychiatry **27**:389, 1972.

42. Zusman, J., and Lamb, J.R.: In defense of community mental health, Am. J. Psychiatry **134**:887, 1977.

■ ANNOTATED SUGGESTED READINGS ■

Bachrach, L.L.: Young adult chronic patients: an analytical review of the literature, Hosp. Community Psychiatry **33**:189, Mar. 1982.

This article analyzes the impact of an emerging new psychiatric service group, young adult chronic patients. This population presents a highly variable clinical picture constituting neither a uniform diagnostic category nor a population with fixed or predictable symptom pictures. They typically use psychiatric facilities in a "revolving door" fashion requiring considerable linkage among facilities if care is to be beneficial.

Bassuk, E., and Gerson, S.: Deinstitutionalization and mental health services, Sci. Am. **238**:46, Feb. 1978.

This article discusses the many problems related to deinstitutionalization and the care of discharged psychiatric patients in the community. Major issues addressed include deficiencies in follow-up care, lack of community facilities, inadequacy of insurance coverage for mental health treatment, and role conflicts among the psychiatric disciplines.

---

*Asterisk indicates nursing reference.

*Boondas, J.: The despair of the homeless aged, J. Gerontological Nurs. 11(4):9, 1984.

The homeless elderly, suffering from the effects of poor health, poverty, and social isolation, are in desperate circumstances. At least 1% of the nation's population (approximately 2.2 million people) lacks shelter. The increased homeless population is attributed to a variety of factors including deinstitutionalization and urban redevelopment.

Forstenzer, H.M.: Planning and evaluation of community mental health programs, Psychiatric Q. 52(1):38, 1980.

In recent years, an abundance of federal reports and legislation have emphasized and in some cases mandated the need for more effective planning for community mental health services. In the past, programs have been revamped without the benefit of research to support the direction being taken. Those who undertake planning efforts need to know about the regulations under which they operate, the nature of the community, the number and type of clients needing care, and what priorities exist.

Kurtz, L.F., Bagarozzi, D.A., and Pollane, L.P.: Case management in mental health, Health and Social Work 9(3):201–211, 1984.

This article reports on a survey of 403 case managers in community mental health centers in Georgia to identify their educational level, professional identification, and demographic characteristics influencing their performance. Findings indicated that workers with higher educational levels performed a greater number of case management activities and required less supervision.

Lowery, B.J., and Janulis, D.: Community mental health and the unanswered questions, Perspect. Psychiatr. Care 21(4):156, 1983.

This article examines the nature of conflicts inherent in the community mental health movement. The authors contend that complex issues exist and revolve around a series of fundamental questions including: Who is the patient? Who is the therapist? What is the process? What is the goal? What is the theory? And what is the role? The authors offer alternative responses to these questions, acknowledging that there is no one right or wrong answer to each one.

Lamb, H.R.: What did we really expect from deinstitutionalization? Hosp. Community Psychiatry 32(2):105, 1981.

The author asks "what went wrong with deinstitutionalization?" He posits the belief that severely disabled psychiatric patients have remained a marginal population with few continuity of care programs actually helping them to effectively assimilate back into the community. He contends that the goal of making it possible for these patients to live with dignity in a comfortable low-energy but satisfying life-style is a great step toward achieving the initial goals of deinstitutionalization.

*Lyon, G., and Hitchens, E.: Ways of intervening with the psychotic individual in the community. Am. J. Nurs. 79:490, 1979.

This article addresses an important problem—how to help the psychotic individual in a community setting. It is practical, realistic, and uses clinical examples to reinforce major points.

*Mackenzie, J.A.: Order out of chaos: changes in community health and home care, Nursing and Health Care 6:37, Jan. 1985.

The nature of community health, especially home health care, is changing dramatically. The community health nurse is ideally suited to serve as a case manager. In order to maintain the viability of agencies, administrators must look to new models of practice. One successful model is a corporate organizational structure in which the corporation is a tool for achieving tighter networks, for creating partnerships and mergers, and for achieving surpluses.

Pardes, M.D., and Stockdill, M.A.: Survival strategies for community mental health services in the 1980s, Hosp. Community Psychiatry 35(2):127, 1984.

According to these authors, widespread reduction of financial resources has created a growing concern about the survival of community mental health services and their inherent values and ideals. A variety of survival strategies have become essential including: incorporation, alternative services, innovative funding, and political activities. The authors urge the use of business techniques to make mental health services more efficient and cost-effective.

President's Commission on Mental Health: Report to the president, vol. 1, Washington, D.C., 1978.

This is a government report of a 1-year study commissioned by President Carter to review the mental health needs in the United States. It is strongly recommended that psychiatric nurses be familiar with the content of this report, although its actual impact on legislation and funding has been diminished with the Reagan administration.

Prindaville, G.M., Sidwell, L.H., and Milner, D.E.: Integrating primary health care and mental health services— a successful rural linkage, Public Health Reports 98 (1):67, 1983.

This article describes one successful linkage between a small primary health care center and a nonfederally funded, multicounty, mental health center. The services of the linkage project included direct clinical mental health services delivered at the primary health care site, consultation and education activities, and coordination of interagency services. The authors analyzed the key elements in the successful linkage and the subsequent attainment of goals.

Register, D.: Community mental health for whose community, Am. J. Public Health 64:866, 1974.

Eight conceptual models of community are presented with brief outlines of the implications of each model. Characteristics of community mental health centers that are described include target populations, staff, awareness of community needs, and the effect of center programs on the community.

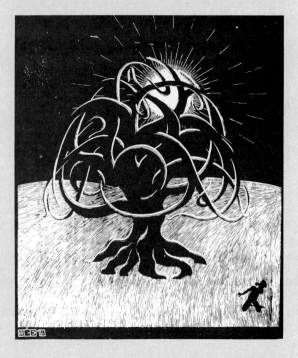

The greatest good we can do for others is not just share our riches with them but to reveal their riches to themselves.

Anonymous

C H A P T E R   2 6

LIAISON NURSING: A MODEL FOR NURSING PRACTICE

FRANCES G. LEHMANN

LEARNING OBJECTIVES

After studying this chapter, the student should be able to:

- relate the historical development of the liaison nursing role.

- identify the role characteristics and practice settings of the liaison nurse.

- state three categories of problems encountered by the liaison nurse.

- analyze the implications of the present economic environment for liaison nurses.

- describe a conceptual model and theoretical framework for liaison nursing practice.

- discuss the three phases of the liaison process, including the four steps that comprise the working phase.

- compare and contrast direct and indirect care functions of the liaison nursing role.

- discuss future trends and challenges for liaison nursing practice.

- identify directions for future nursing research.

- select appropriate readings for further study.

Historically there are many major and minor forces that have helped shape the role, need, and use of liaison nursing. Liaison nursing is a model for nursing practice that has developed from the consultative process, and within psychiatric nursing it is considered a subspecialty.[15] It was generated out of need: the psychosocial needs of the client in a general hospital setting and the ethical needs of nursing to deliver professional health care to the holistic client in the most practical and economical method available. The liaison nurse has a high degree of expertise in psychiatric nursing and a special ability to integrate these skills with knowledge in medical-surgical nursing to provide comprehensive nursing service.

The psychiatric liaison nursing role

There are various models of liaison nursing. Blake[2] perceives the nurse consultant providing indirect client services as a collaborative agent of change through an education process. Robinson's model[19] has the liaison nurse serving two basic functions: giving direct patient care and assisting the nursing staff in making their own care more therapeutic. The model used in this chapter is an adaptation of Caplan's model of consultation. Caplan's definition is "a process of interaction between two professional persons—the consultant who is a specialist, and the consultee."[4] In his model the focus of interaction is the consultee's difficulty with a work-related problem in which the consultant has specialized competency.

In this chapter the term "liaison nursing" is used to describe a particular professional process between two systems in which one of the systems (the user) has a current work-related problem and voluntarily requests help from an outside system (the provider), who is perceived to have a specialized competency in a defined area. Stated more simply, somone has a problem and believes an outside expert can help solve that problem. In addition, liaison nursing practice is viewed as a learned process that promotes planned change by use of interpersonal skills and specialized knowledge.[21]

■ Historical development

The present status of liaison nursing becomes more meaningful when viewed from the broader historical perspective of psychiatric nursing. A major influence on the evolution of psychiatric nursing was federal legislation (Public Law 88-164, the Community Mental Health Centers Act) passed in 1963, which created the authority for establishment of a comprehensive mental health delivery system in the United States to meet the psychiatric needs of all socioeconomic classes of Americans. This major mental health movement created a lack of qualified people to staff the centers. To help alleviate this deficit, several nonmedical professional disciplines, such as psychology, sociology, social service, and nursing, designed and implemented educational and training programs to prepare mental health workers. The significance of the legislation on nursing education can be measured by the number of schools of nursing that took advantage of federal training grant money and by the number of psychiatric/community mental health nurses prepared at the graduate level in the last two decades. Psychiatric nurse practitioners, using specialized education, have taken their place alongside other mental health specialists in the health care delivery system.

Along with the increased demand for professionally and competently prepared psychiatric nurses to serve as established program staff members, another force within the comprehensive mental health center movement created a visibility factor affecting this same human resources pool. Mental health consultation is provided by all mental health centers as well as many other health facilities. This basic service has resulted in mental health nurse specialists having regular contact with other human service agencies and institutions. Through this broad base of contact, many disciplines have had access to and have recognized the unique viewpoint of nursing in treating individuals in relation to one another and to their environment.

The thrust toward holistic health care is relatively new, becoming popular within the last 25 years. In nursing, however, total patient care is documented as far back as Florence Nightingale's time. In contemporary times, nurses continue to minister to human beings in a holistic manner. Nursing activities are concerned with those factors that influence both the client and his environment. Traditionally, interventions have focused on the client's mental, psychosocial, and spiritual needs as well as physical needs, regardless of the setting in which the nursing service is used.

The title liaison nurse came into popular use in the 1970s when primary care nursing demonstrated nursing's commitment to the delivery of comprehensive, individualized care. In general hospitals, the liaison nurse became a part of the nursing services department and consulted with staff and clients in all nursing units throughout the hospital.[1]

Not limited to hospitals, however, nursing has long been a proponent of its members being skilled in providing service to a client in his own environment, as evidenced by community health nurses going into the home, occupational nurses being available in work places, and school nurses being regular staff members of educational institutions.

By the 1980s, the title mental health nurse consultant had come into use. This umbrella title usually indicates that the person is professionally prepared to deal not only with the effects of disease on human beings but also with health promotion, human relations, and process consultation involved in organizational management and development. The mental health nurse consultant, as a facilitator of effective interpersonal and group relationships and communication, can be key to the successful growth of any organization in which human beings interact to produce services or products.[24]

A large number of psychiatric clinical nurse specialists are now available for both direct and indirect mental health services. Their visibility, accessibility, and proved value give credence to their viability. The evolving role of the psychiatric nurse from the traditional position of physical caretaker of patients in mental institutions to a leadership position as consulting nurse seems appropriate. The ability to provide on-the-scene direct and indirect consultation service in various settings is a natural unfolding of another chapter in the history of nursing.

■ Role characteristics

The psychiatric clinical nurse specialist can function in many professional roles, applying the knowledge and theory of mental health concepts. These roles may resemble each other but have different goals, outcomes, strategies, and methods. The role of liaison nurse offers an exciting method of working closely with other members of a health team in promoting effective problem management. The model of liaison nursing used here is that of an expert providing problem-centered consultation service in a coordinate relationship, with problem resolution being the mutually shared goal of both partners.[5]

Problem solving is a function of any nurse, regardless of educational preparation or defined roles. There are several essential qualities of the liaison relationship, however, that contribute to the specialized problem-solving activity of liaison nursing. It is also important to differentiate commonly blurred activities, such as supervision and education, from liaison nursing. The liaison nurse should have a way of distinguishing these various activities to define his or her own role, responsibilities, performance, and outcome.[10,20]

Essential differences between the liaison role and supervisor role are the authority base and administrative responsibility for outcome.[22] The liaison nurse should have a coordinate professional relationship with the user. This means she should have no administrative authority or coercive power over the user. Implicit in this aspect is the factor that the liaison nurse is not responsible for implementing recommended changes, just as the user is free to accept or reject any or all parts of the recommendation.

The organizational aspect of a liaison nurse position should be that of a staff rather than a line position. This differs from a supervisory role, in which authority is explicit to hierarchy rank. By definition, the liaison nurse is outside the user system. This means she is outside the regular chain of command within the user organization. This aspect also provides the liaison nurse with the necessary freedom to work with people at any level within any needed time frame rather than in a full-time line position that fills a slot within the organizational structure.

The power of the liaison nurse rests in her own authority of ideas based on an acknowledged specialized area of expertise. The user explicitly and voluntarily asks for help. The liaison nurse respects the user as a professional partner in problem-solving activities. While dealing with the current problem, the liaison nurse works in such a manner as to add to the user's knowledge base and thereby enables the user to deal more effectively with similar situations in the future. In this way the liaison nurse facilitates the user's potential and relates in a coordinate way by asking for and using his input.

The liaison process emphasizes that the provider and user deal with aspects of the problem that are unclear and confusing to the user rather than with the issue of people who are inadequate or incompetent. The liaison nurse should project the attitude that the user is an active, interdependent partner and ultimately responsible for implementing the proposed interventions.

Although the liaison nurse may provide new information and knowledge to the user, this aspect of the liaison process differs from an educational activity in that the stated goal is not to impart a specific body of knowledge to the user. The liaison process is an activity in which the liaison nurse provides support and guidance while helping the user to enlarge and deepen his own understanding of the issues. He can then, hopefully, develop more effective ways of handling the current problem and future similar situations. How the liaison nurse guides the consultee to creatively challenge and resolve the identified problem within his own resources can be the exciting synergistic application of her own talents to produce change and growth for all concerned.

Liaison nursing practice

■ Settings and functions

There are several ways of practicing liaison nursing. Some nurses are independent private practitioners who are employed for a specific assignment by the consultee organization on a fee-for-services basis. Other clinicians are staff members of an identified department within an organization that supplies human services.

The liaison nurse can provide either direct or indirect service. In both categories, the liaison nurse acts as an outside consultant, on a time-limited basis, and facilitates a person's, family's, group's, or organization's ability to develop and enhance personal knowledge and skills. In direct service, the liaison nurse is a direct care provider and intervenes in such a way that her activity has a measurable effect on the health status of a person,

group, or family. In indirect service, the liaison nurse functions as a human resource, supporting key people directly responsible for the operation of the consultee system.

Nurse practice acts in each state dictate a registered nurse's scope of practice and the educational preparation required to function in a specialty role. The accepted qualifications to function as a psychiatric liaison nurse are a master's degree in psychiatric–mental health nursing with identified and measureable knowledge, and clinical skills in specific areas of psychosocial nursing.[11] The setting in which a liaison nurse may function is limited only by imagination and demand. Her services may be utilized in acute or rehabilitative inpatient units of general hospitals, ambulatory health services, home health care organizations, community agencies, educational institutions, employee health components of industry or business, and special population settings such as extended care facilities, retirement communities, summer camp programs, and church-sponsored social support programs.[6,16]

■ Types of problems

The liaison nurse intervenes in various types of problems. The identified problem can focus on one client (**case problem**), a series of related problems (**program problem**), or a particular administrative problem (**organization problem**). In practice, there is generally an overlapping of these artificial categories. If, however, the liaison nurse has an awareness of the general nature of the identified problem and the level of the target system with which she is interacting, it helps in working through the entire liaison process from contract setting to outcome evaluation.

The **case** category relates to assisting the user to become more effective as a human being. The liaison nurse's primary focus is on ways to increase the user's skill and knowledge. The spotlight is on the client and alternative ways of problem resolution. The **program** category relates to helping the user define or meet particular professional goals. The liaison's primary focus is on ways to improve the user's professional functioning in an identified area of practice in dealing with more than one client. The **organization** category relates to developing new programs or improving existing ones that affect the basic structure or function of the organization. The liaison's primary focus is on the administrative system and an effective course of action that involves organizational change to produce a desired outcome.

Clinical example 26-1 illustrates each category of problems encountered by the liaison nurse.

CLINICAL EXAMPLE 26-1

CASE PROBLEM

Mr. C, a 68-year-old widower who had been living in a retirement home for about 6 months, began withdrawing from all social activities. Formerly he had been active and an initiator of planned outings for other members of the home community and generally appeared to be adjusting to the move after the death of his wife some 9 months previously. The staff of the home had vast experience in helping other clients work through similar life situations, but they believed that all the interventions implemented on Mr. C's behalf had minimum effect. The director of activities therapy and the director of nursing services requested a case consultation with Mrs. L, a clinical nurse specialist working as an independent practitioner. Mrs. L entered the user system at middle-management level and was asked to focus on Mr. C by working with the nursing staff to help it develop a more effective nursing care plan.

PROGRAM PROBLEM

The teaching staff in a private preschool facility went to the director of the program and requested more help. Mrs. B, the director of the program and a capable administrator, believed the present staffing pattern was adequate but also recognized that the faculty as a whole was experiencing more and more frustration in providing high-quality care for the children enrolled in the program. She requested Mr. G, a clinical nurse specialist working in a community mental health center, to consult with the faculty regarding the problem.

ORGANIZATION PROBLEM

A small manufacturing plant was in the process of expanding its product line and corporate structure. The organization had legally been a partnership with two principals of equal salary and stature. With the expansion, the organization became a legal corporation with a board of directors, major officers, and department managers. The growth and development of the organization had created a tremendous strain on the newly appointed officers, and their interpersonal relationships were dysfunctional.

The president recently had successfully completed family therapy with a clinical nurse specialist and decided that the company officers might profit from mental health counseling. He contacted the nurse therapist who agreed to serve as liaison nurse and consult with the company officers regarding their transition problems.

Economic considerations

As the largest health care provider, nursing is becoming more complex, specialized, and technical. Its latest challenge in the wave of cost containment is to provide nursing services to (1) sicker hospitalized clients who stay a shorter time, (2) clients with complex health problems in ambulatory settings, (3) clients in home settings with limited resources, and (4) increasing numbers of chronically ill, poor, and older Americans.[18]

The increasing demand for skilled and professional nursing services is a response to the ever greater requirement for cost-effective and efficient quality care. Decreased inpatient days and increased complex outpatient procedures demand accurate nursing assessments, diagnoses, and interventions. Quality, comprehensive nursing care is a key element affecting the clients' welfare and the fiscal foundation of the health care delivery system. Nursing leaders across the country are mandated to allocate resources to improve health care efficiency and reduce costs.[9] Nursing managers, wherever the setting, are results-oriented and business-minded.

In the backlash of cost containment, all specialized nursing positions have to be justified on a cost-benefit ratio basis. Logic suggests that liaison nursing has important economic as well as clinical benefits. As an advanced practitioner, the liaison nurse integrates a biopsychosocial perspective to client care, provides a holistic rather than dualistic approach to care, and serves in both direct and indirect ways to produce desired outcomes. Economy is the documented result when experts are used on a time-limited, consultative basis.[17] On an economies-of-scale principle, the liaison nurse as a member of the health care team can provide reduced labor-intensive indirect service. Resource sharing is an acceptable fiscal strategy that can be applied to offer psychosocial nursing expertise to a wider range of participants. The bottom line is cost-effective use of nursing hours to produce holistic quality care and individualization of services.

Liaison nurse positions, previously carried as line items in organizational budgets, are losing their institutional support. The paradox is that holistic interventions produce less relative costs. Not many health providers deny that too much anxiety interferes with the healing process. What better way to justify in the nursing department budget the actual cost savings of the liaison nurse who provides expert direct service to decrease the client's stress, diminish the degree of anxiety, and promote the healing process. This outcome would be cost-effective on a relative basis by shortening the client's recovery period.

Two other developments have created a ripple effect. The proliferating government and private prospective payment systems are emphasizing prevention. So too, industry and business are becoming aware that health promotion for the employee is cost-effective, and results in higher productivity and decreased costs for insurance and illness care. The aggressive approach to health promotion and wellness provides an opportunity for using liaison nurses' skills and knowledge. The liaison nurse, in whatever setting, can provide interventions to reduce stress and increase personal functioning. Employing liaison nurses in non–health care provider settings is on the cutting edge as employers begin to measure improved employee efficiency in terms of greater profit margins.

Community programming also should be considered in light of current economic attitudes. Use of the liaison nurse in this nontraditional setting can make mental health services available as community needs arise. It can provide greater accessibility to the expertise of a wellness-oriented health care provider with minimal threat or stigma to the service recipients. For example, in church-sponsored social programs for retired people, liaison nursing could play an active part in maximizing the wellness of the participating citizens.[23]

Given the present fiscal environment, it is essential that the liaison nursing role demonstrate its economic value. There is a need for documentation through nursing research of the outcomes associated with the role of the psychiatric clinical nurse specialist. In addition to quality of care measures, nurses need to justify the cost-effectiveness of their care as it impacts on the client, health care organizations, and governmental and private reimbursers. Such documentation is needed not only for the growth of this nursing role, but for its very survival.

The liaison process

■ Conceptual model

The liaison nurse should have a conceptual model and a theoretical framework for practice. It is this combination of style and method (structure and function) that will help the liaison nurse provide maximum return for her efforts and time and make the work exciting and rewarding. The conceptual model used in this chapter is a role model of a coordinate, nonhierarchical relationship between an outside expert and a participating human services system. This model sets the tone of the interactive relationship. Within this model, both provider and user bring distinct contributions to the problem-solving tasks, as depicted in Fig. 26-1.

■ Theoretical framework

It is the liaison nurse's professional responsibility to use sound principles, apply concepts to the information available, and provide practical and easy-to-understand interventions founded on carefully thought

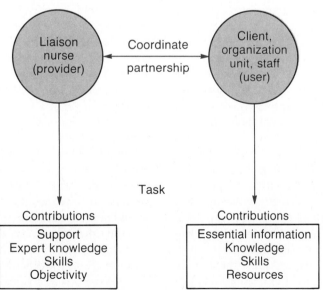

Fig. 26-1. Conceptual role model used by the liaison nurse.

out theory.[5] The practitioner therefore needs to develop a framework under which she functions in her role. The liaison nurse demonstrates a firm foundation of knowledge, organizes theory from a variety of disciplines, and uses this unique combination to formulate her own model for nursing. The theory base should include knowledge of systems theory, change theory, staff management, organizational behavior, problem-solving theory, growth and development, cultural and ethnic norms, stress and stress reduction theory, and crisis theory, as well as environmental, interpersonal, and intrapersonal psychiatric dynamics. In one situation organizational theory may become the primary focus, another time interpersonal relationships may be the frame of reference, and yet another situation will deal directly with an intrapersonal problem.

The theoretical framework serves as a flexible reference for the nurse as she adapts to the various expected and unexpected components of any liaison situation. The particular method and approaches chosen come about through her own sense of purpose and professional identity. Within a defined framework she can shift the focus and scope of the problem to meet the needs of the users on the basis of their organizational structure, institutional policies, and perceptions of the liaison nurse's role. This framework becomes a road map and a practical frame of reference for the liaison process. It is the liaison nurse's way of organizing a wide range of skills and in-depth knowledge. It is a way of visualizing her thinking. It reflects her beliefs about the nursing profession and influences her own practice.

■ Phases of the process

Although liaison nursing is a specialized type of nursing, the steps of the process can be compared to the traditional nursing process. Both are orderly, mutual, problem-solving activities; both relate to at least two people interacting in such a manner as to effect change; both processes hold the partners responsible for participation. The nursing process involves four steps: assessment, planning, implementation, and evaluation. These four steps comprise the working phase of the actual liaison process, with an orientation and termination phase marking the beginning and conclusion of the formal liaison activity. As with any "process," liaison nursing is an ongoing activity with any component step interrelated with all other steps.

■ **ORIENTATION PHASE.** As defined earlier, liaison nursing is a specialized professional activity in which the provider, as an outside expert, joins the user in problem solving in a nonhierarchical relationship. The nature of the relationship requires that certain issues in addition to the task at hand be attended to so that both

systems will find it mutually satisfying and beneficial.

It is important for the liaison nurse to make face-to-face contact with key members of the staff and the appropriate authority personnel in the system as soon as possible to make her purpose and presence known. This contact also serves as a way to gather data about the organizational structure and the communication network operating there. It is also important for the liaison nurse to have an idea of the nature and scope of services provided by the organization, the philosophy, and any operating policies relevant to the target unit within the organization.

Any role is defined in relation to the social system of which it is a functioning part. The entire liaison process is affected by the type of setting and the individual and collective professional background of the personnel involved in the relationship. Settings could include health care settings, such as acute care general hospitals, ambulatory care facilities, and nursing homes; non–health care settings would be industries, schools, churches, self-help groups, and human services agencies, such as welfare departments, judicial systems, penal systems, and child care services. Each type of setting will have its own unique philosophy, organizational structure, established protocol, and vague and specific expectations of how the liaison nurse will function in that particular setting. The liaison nurse's knowledge of and experience with organizational theory will benefit her intrapersonally and interpersonally as she functions within any setting.

The effectiveness of the liaison process is influenced by the user's concept of the liaison nurse's role. It is important for both sides to clarify the nature and scope of the liaison's role. This avoids two common causes of failure of a liaison process: the staff has unrealistic expectations or they distort the purpose for which the consultation was requested. The liaison nurse should also evaluate the accuracy of the user's perception of the present liaison nurse on the basis of past experience with other personnel in a similar role.

The liaison nurse will have the opportunity to work with intraprofessional (fellow nurses), interprofessional (other disciplines), and nonprofessional (technical) personnel. Needless to say, the liaison nurse will have to maintain the strength of her own identity as well as an awareness of the identities of others. The liaison nurse should interact with other people under the assumption that the other person has a sense of accountability, responsibility, and competency in his own area of work. This respect for the other person transcends educational background or professional experiences.

Effective communication. The liaison nurse's ability to communicate effectively with many levels of personnel is a skill that makes the process much smoother. The communication process depends on the liaison nurse, setting, and user of services. Developing communication channels involves identifying key formal and informal networks. It is important for the success of the liaison process that both sides have a working arrangement for obtaining and disseminating messages.

Basic conceptual differences will become apparent as people work together in the task of problem solving. Establishing a common language in which both partners are comfortable and feel productive will minimize differences. It is helpful for the liaison nurse to use words that are familiar to other people. Using words that others use will help prevent the nurse from talking on an inappropriate level or skirting the subject. Using abstract approaches or focusing on what seem to the user to be impractical or irrelevant issues will not promote their self-confidence. The liaison nurse's method of communicating with staff should not be by advice giving or using declarative sentences. It is preferable to use questions that guide the user to alternative ways of viewing the problem. Helping the consultee to reduce the complexities to relevant facts promotes clarity and mutual understanding of the situation.

It is important for the user to recognize that liaison discussions are confidential. This means that the liaison nurse guards against being a "switchboard" or carrier for messages that should be delivered directly within the organization. A liaison nurse should also make sure she does not take sides in differences of opinion among staff members. Promoting the attitude that any information gathered will not be used to purposely harm any person or the reputation of the organization is important. The focus of any interaction should be work difficulties and not the private personal needs of staff members. If personal issues are hindering a staff member's performance and interventions are indicated, this recommendation is not transmitted within the official liaison process. The liaison nurse restrains from gathering personal information that could turn the liaison session into a therapy session. Instead, she can tactfully encourage the troubled staff member to seek out an impartial skilled listener.

Contract. The need to delineate expectations on both sides is obvious. The informal liaison process is the ongoing way in which both user and provider continually work out, modify, and change ground rules of the relationship. The formal liaison process is guided and evaluated by a written agreement between the liaison nurse and the user. This agreement is simply called a contract. The contract represents an exchange between the partners of the terms of specific services to be rendered and the parameters of the complementary activ-

ity.[8] If the request for services comes through informal channels (via telephone or face-to-face contact), the liaison nurse needs to verify that permission at the appropriate level of authority is given for the liaison activity. The purpose behind requesting a letter of contract therefore is to prevent misunderstandings between the parties.

To avoid possible misrepresentation or ambiguity, a letter or memorandum from an authority person in the user organization should be directed to the liaison nurse. This document can describe the various aspects of the user's expectations. It eventually serves as a tool for outcome evaluation.

The contract is not so much a legal document as an agreement between professionals of two systems. It can be kept simple. It should be dated and signed by both user and provider. The main points to cover include the following:

1. A brief description of the problem situation
2. Expected goals
3. Estimated time to be used on the project
4. Means of compensation for the time
5. The key department and personnel involved, including the contact person

The liaison nurse can also use the contract to understand more fully the informal relationship. By expanding and examining the statement of problem in point 1, she can decide if it is a case, problem, or program consultation process. She can gather more background information as to what action has been taken so far to resolve the problem and what personnel have been involved in the activity to date. The stated goals in point 2 may end up as part of the original problem. Viewing both the expected goals and stated problem in context will show how the user perceives the entire situation.

Through points 3 and 4 the liaison nurse can learn about the organization's perception of both quality and quantity regarding time. It should also be established which possible dates or times are available for optimal productivity. Point 4 includes such considerations as whether the organization sees the compensation in terms of an hourly rate versus a job rate. If the consultant is in-house, it should be clear to which department the time is to be charged. Point 5 includes the communication network to be used, the names of staff and their jobs, a list of people who are available for discussion, the scope of confidentiality expected, the kinds of information appropriate for discussion with whom, and who the authority source is for permission.

■ **WORK PHASE.** After the orientation phase in which the initial contact and contract are completed,

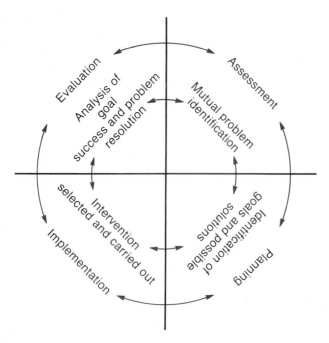

Fig. 26-2. Stages of the liaison process.

the actual liaison process begins. Fig. 26-2 is a representation of the process model, which depicts the four steps of assessment, planning, implementation, and evaluation. This same model is used on case, program, and organization problems. A more detailed discussion of the various steps follows. The model can be applied to both the direct and indirect care functions.

Assessment. This step actually begins when the contract is formulated. It continues with the two participating systems accumulating and classifying all data, clarifying the information available, and assessing it in a conceptual manner. The liaison nurse can ask questions in such a way as to stimulate the staff's thinking and communicate the message that they are capable. One technique that can guide the discussion to a deeper level is the liaison nurse asking herself aloud, questions about the complexities of the situation. By speculating aloud, she promotes new understanding among the staff. She also demonstrates a willingness to risk and act as a role model for the problem-solving process. Beginning sentences with "I wonder if . . ." facilitates a feeling of joint endeavor. During this stage the liaison nurse should assess the strengths and weaknesses of the user, identify the real and potential barriers to action, determine what impediments have kept the user from resolving the problem, and assess the general problem-solving ability of the partners.

This step ends when an identified problem is agreed on by the two systems. The activity in this stage is most critical to the rest of the liaison process and may be repeated a number of times until the focus of the identified problem is narrow enough to manage and realistic enough to be resolved by the user organization. A concise conclusion derived from the assessment stage makes the rest of the process easier.

Planning. This step starts with the liaison nurse reframing the problem in such a way that the user can view the situation objectively and, it is hoped, without feeling threatened. The liaison nurse does this by using theoretical concepts that promote learning and can be generalized to similar situations. She listens to and values the staff's ideas. She may modify them by adding depth and breadth to the proposed intervention or by suggesting unusual but theoretically sound ways to implement them. Any suggested intervention should be both feasible and practical within the setting and in line with the functioning skills and capabilities of those who are responsible for their implementation. This avoids upsetting the existing lines of communication and authority. The suggestions should also be sensitive to the rights and well-being of all those affected by the potential change. The planning should reflect what presently exists and not what ought to be. It is ethically improper for the proposed interventions to be based on an idealist level of problem management.

This step ends when possible solutions to the problem are arrived at through the coordinated efforts of the liaison nurse and the user. Goals should be stated based on the outcome desired. These goals provide a framework for interpreting, planning, and evaluating ongoing activities.

Implementation. This step begins with selection of the interventions to be tried. This decision rests with the users. In fact, this stage may actually take place after the liaison nurse has left the physical environment and the actual liaison process is terminated. This stage includes testing out any alternative suggestions that came out of the planning step. The step ends when the implemented interventions have been in effect long enough to assess observable change.

Evaluation. This step begins with ascertaining to what extent the interventions met their stated goals. If the liaison nurse does not plan to be involved with the actual evaluation stage of the process, it is important that she help the user devise specific ways to measure the expected outcome or the interventions; therefore, in a psychological sense, the liaison nurse is involved in the complete process. The evidence used to evaluate should include obvious data, although implied data are used on occasion. The evaluation focuses on the effects of the planned interventions and not on the staff who implemented the plan. This is an important difference in that the total situation is examined, not how individual people are functioning. Another aspect of evaluation is that information may be generated that indicates gaps of knowledge or lack of skill on the part of the staff. These needs may be met through an educational approach to the problem.

This step ends when the user determines whether the defined problem has been resolved, to what degree of success the solution worked, and what additional problems, if any, were uncovered during the process.

■ **TERMINATION PHASE.** Termination involves both physical and psychological closure. Wrapping up the work phase of the liaison process is important. Certain tasks such as report writing and leave taking are necessary. Much of the actual work involved in this phase depends on the liaison nurse's basic personality, the setting, and the formal contract. If the liaison nurse is a staff member of the user organization, her visibility will continue. If she has a one-time relationship, leave taking will be more formal.

Liaison report. Communication is not only a theoretical framework used in liaison nursing but a practical aspect of the experience. Throughout the interaction, progress may have been discussed, but, at the completion of the consultation activity, a formal written report is indicated. In this way all members of the organization who have been engaged in the process will have access to information relevant to the planned or implemented interventions.

The format of the report will vary with the type of consultation, the setting, the level of organization involved, and the issues under focus. The following areas should be included:

1. The purpose, dates, and activities during the process
2. A statement of the identified problem
3. An assessment of the situation
4. Alternative plans for problem resolution
5. Specific interventions
6. Suggestions on how to evaluate the interventions

This formal report can be brief but explicit as to what the liaison nurse believed happened in the total process. The report should be consistent with the theoretical framework on which she bases her practice.

Professional development. The contract and summary report serve as tools for the liaison nurse to use in evaluating her own performance in the process and for making revisions in using the process on the next occasion. The liaison nurse is constantly changing and growing in her own professional development as a consultant. Self-evaluation is a necessary part of the nursing

process. Areas that need evaluation are goal setting, problem solving, and communication skills (interpersonal and written), as well as theory application.

Performance evaluation is easier if criterion-referenced measurements are used. This is preferable over norm-referenced evaluation, since comparing oneself to others in the field is almost impossible. As with any profession, liaison nursing skills need constant nourishment. Attendance at professional meetings and conferences allows the liaison nurse to keep in contact with other professionals and helps her assess her own growth and development. Reading professional literature and theoretical and clinical textbooks is a way of increasing one's theory base and scope of knowledge.

Direct care provider

■ Role characteristics

The liaison nurse as a direct service provider acts autonomously as a psychosocial therapist to provide mental status assessment, nursing diagnosis, treatment, and evaluation services. The therapy modalities that might be used are individual, family or group therapy, crisis intervention, and stress reduction counseling. The liaison nurse expands the health services available to individual clients in nonpsychiatric settings by professionally intervening on an interpersonal level. Her direct services may be requested by the attending physician, the client, or a member of the nursing staff.

The types of problems that may be encountered in direct service are considered case problems and are client-centered. Most of the liaison nurse's time is spent with the client, and the interaction is primarily client-supportive and goal-directed. The identified case problem may be to

1. Establish the client's mental status
2. Assist the client through a crisis
3. Counsel and support the client who has impaired body functions; has experienced loss of self-esteem; is grieving; has suffered family abuse, violence, or rape; demonstrates impaired mental or emotional functioning; or needs guidance in coping with a personal life situation that presently or in the future could interfere with optimal functioning

The liaison process in the direct service function has the client and liaison nurse as the primary participants. The nurse uses advanced nursing skills and knowledge to provide direct care that effects predictable and measurable changes in the client's psychosocial welfare. The liaison nurse is directly responsible for implementing any strategies for change that will meet the defined ther-

CLINICAL EXAMPLE 26-2

Mrs. W, a 68-year-old widow, was admitted to a surgical unit of a general hospital for a colostomy after x-ray examination and biopsy revealed colorectal cancer. She had a history of three previous admissions for various somatic complaints over the last year since the death of her husband. During the presurgery workup, the attending physician requested a liaison nurse consultation to establish a therapeutic relationship with Mrs. W in anticipation of the colostomy, and to obtain an evaluation of Mrs. W's coping abilities.

ASSESSMENT

Mrs. H, the liaison nurse, reviewed the client's charts from the present and previous hospitalizations and talked with the family physician and the surgeon. She also talked with the ostomy service nurse and with Mrs. W's primary nurse. Mrs. H then met with Mrs. W in her private room for almost an hour.

After a thorough assessment of Mrs. W's physical, social, mental, emotional, and spiritual health, the nurse explored with her the meaning Mrs. W gave to the situation she was experiencing. The nurse also talked with her about her family and social support network and received permission to talk with her adult daughter. Rapport was established between Mrs. W and Mrs. H, and they mutually decided subsequent visits would be in order.

The nurse made the following nursing diagnoses:

1. Severe level of anxiety related to medical diagnosis of cancer
2. Disturbed body image related to the impending colostomy
3. Anticipatory grieving related to the loss of body functioning

PLANNING

The nurse conferred with the family physician and together they decided that Mrs. W, because of her high-risk stress factors, would benefit from six to eight psychosocial therapy sessions to be provided by the nurse, Mrs. H. The sessions were to be held in Mrs. W's hospital room at a mutually agreed-upon time. The scheduled surgery and Mrs. W's recuperation would be primary factors in the immediate treatment plan. The nurse charted her assessment, diagnoses, treatment recommendations, and therapeutic goals in Mrs. W's chart. She also talked with Mrs. W's primary nurse, and then stopped by Mrs. W's room to arrange another visit with her the next afternoon, the day before surgery.

IMPLEMENTATION

In this phase of the liaison nursing process, strategies would be based on a continuous evaluation of Mrs. W's changing health status and surgical intervention. Theoretical considerations shaping the therapeutic relationship would be life developmental stage, stress management, and the process of grieving for body changes. The strategies would include: (1) decreasing Mrs. W's level of anxiety; (2) providing therapeutic support for the grief and mourning process; and (3) reducing present and potential problems in the areas of self-esteem, body image, and personal control. The rationale for liaison nursing participation is preventive intervention to reduce the negative effects of stress, while improving Mrs. W's coping abilities at a time when she is dealing with a major health problem.

EVALUATION

Evaluation of the client's changing health status and how she is functioning is a shared responsibility of all health care team members. Specifically, the liaison nurse, functioning as a therapist, monitors the effectiveness of the psychosocial interventions and Mrs. W's mental, emotional, and social health status.

The following are a few of the liaison techniques used in this clinical example:

1. Focus on time-limited interventions and well-defined goals.
2. In promoting stress management, recognize the reality of the health-threatening situation and Mrs. W's compromised health status.
3. Build on the strengths of the client, her support network, and the team so that synergism enhances the healing process.
4. Use the liaison process as one component of the team's commitment to comprehensive care by participating in team conferences and communicating with the team members in an ongoing manner.

apeutic client-centered goals. The nurse is accountable for evaluating the service she provides. She is also responsible for making appropriate documentation of her liaison services. As a member of the health team providing comprehensive care, the liaison nurse is also responsible for providing other team members with client-focused information, conclusions, and evaluations that contribute to the client's total welfare.

Clinical example 26-2 illustrates the role of the liaison nurse as a direct care provider.

Indirect care provider

■ Role characteristics

When the liaison nurse functions in an indirect manner, the major responsibility for resolution of the identified problem remains with the consultee. The liaison nurse focuses her expertise on assisting the consultees to improve their problem-solving skills in the specific presenting situation and to handle similar work problems that might arise in the future. The liaison nurse is not expected to be an expert in the consultee-organization's specific operations. She is acknowledged as an expert in the process of maximizing human resources in order to resolve the current presenting problem and to enhance the consultee's own abilities and efforts.

Her indirect services may be used by a wide variety of consultees from nurses to other health professionals, schools, industries, business corporations, civic and community organizations, or church-sponsored social groups. The types of problems can range from employee-assistance brokerage service programs to interpersonal relationship enhancement among members of a corporate board of directors. The content of the identified problem is secondary to the human relationship dynamics surrounding the problem.

The indirect care functions can be applied in whatever setting the liaison nurse feels comfortable in using her specialized abilities to bring about desired change. The consultee maintains full coordinate partnership. Whatever the setting, the liaison process as previously described is the organizing framework for implementing the liaison role. Clinical example 26-3 illustrates the role of the liaison nurse as an indirect care provider.

A forward look

Psychiatric liaison nursing will continue to evolve and be influenced by movements within the general practice of nursing as well as forces within psychiatry and the comprehensive health care delivery system. As nurses improve their professional image and self-concept through education and quality performance, a

separate and equal identity with other health disciplines is achieved.

Cost control is the byword of the 1980s. Cost considerations in health care dictate allocation of resources.[13] Incentives from the federal government's pricing system and the private sector's initiatives to reduce hospital use have shifted the locale of health care services including nursing. In fiscally constrained eras, psychosocial aspects of health care are most vulnerable and yet greatly needed. Psychiatric liaison nursing, as an identified subspecialty, must continue to make itself visible,

---

CLINICAL EXAMPLE 26-3

ASSESSMENT

Mrs. L responds to a telephone call from Mrs. K, director of nursing of the retirement home.[3] Mrs. L, Mrs. K, and Mrs. P, director of activities, meet. After informal conversation regarding the case problem, a contract letter is drawn up by Mrs. K: "Whereas our home has a resident whose lack of participation in planned activities keeps him isolated from other residents, we would appreciate your help in developing a treatment plan that provides opportunity for Mr. C to increase his involvement in group activity. As mutually agreed, this project should entail approximately 3 hours of joint effort. Our standard pay rate for nurse consultants is $20 per hour with no employee fringe benefits. Please feel free to talk with any staff or residents at their discretion. Mrs. P or I will arrange our time to meet your schedule." Both Mrs. K and Mrs. L sign the contract and an appointment is set for the next day with Mrs. K and Mrs. P.

The next day Mrs. L meets with Mrs. K and Mrs. P in the latter's office. A report is given regarding Mr. C's current status. Mr. C's physician administered a tricyclic antidepressant the previous week. No therapeutic effects had been noted. Mrs. L encourages both Mrs. K and Mrs. P to recount past interventions that were tried. Mrs. L uses nonthreatening questions to ascertain how both staff members see Mr. C in relation to his environment, life stage, grief phase, and physical and mental capacities. By speculating aloud to herself, she brings out different aspects of the same information in such a way as to increase the complexities and broaden the focus of the stated problem. By elaborating on certain points, she increases the staff's knowledge base. She is able to assess the collaborative relationship between nursing and activity therapy. She re-

Continued.

flects her thoughts to the other two professionals in such a way that all three professionals engage in data gathering, investigating, and organizing the various information.

Mrs. K arranges for Mrs. L to talk with Mr. C during one of the structured activities held in the recreation room. During this time Mrs. L also talks informally with other residents and staff members in the same social setting. On returning to Mrs. K's office, Mrs. L encourages the staff to ask meaningful questions to increase their own knowledge regarding the total situation. After about 45 minutes of dialogue the three participants arrive at a concise conclusion. Mr. C is experiencing an anniversary grief reaction to his wife's death. They mutually agree upon the nursing diagnoses of: (1) delayed grief reaction related to his wife's death and (2) social isolation related to the grieving process. These diagnoses describe the response of the client and reflect the hypothesis on which the treatment plan will be based. This identification of the problem makes it easier for the staff to focus objectively on the client and not be threatened by feelings of guilt or inefficiency in not meeting his social needs.

PLANNING

The grief process is the theoretical concept Mrs. L uses to help the staff reframe Mr. C's situation. The emphasis is shifted from engaging Mr. C in more activity to evaluating his behavior in terms of the stages of grief as outlined by Kübler-Ross. The goal of problem resolution is to facilitate Mr. C's grief work. Although the aim is to provide individualized care for Mr. C, the staff benefits from learning about theoretical aspects of grief that can be generalized to other clients. The liaison nurse uses leading questions such as "Do you suppose Mr. C was in a state of denial when he first came here? That might explain how he got so busily involved in so many activities." Mrs. L provides information for discussing the various stages of grief and draws out examples of behaviors or attitudes that help assess which stages Mr. C has worked through. By increasing the staff's understanding of a specific need or reason for a particular behavior, approaches can be planned to help Mr. C relate to the emotional reactions manifested by his behavior.

At one point the discussion focuses on alternative housing for Mr. C. It is suggested he might live temporarily with his daughter. On closer eval-

uation it is ascertained that the daughter is unable to provide for her father at this time, since she recently changed jobs, moved to another city, and is living in an efficiency apartment until she decides if she likes the job and location. This alternative is discarded, since any recommendation should be sensitive to the rights of others. The treatment plan is written specific to actions of the patient with the underlying assumption that present behaviors are meaningful in helping him work through the loss of his wife, his home, his daughter, and his life-style. The liaison nurse uses the conference to have the staff look at Mr. C's behaviors as goal directed and to generate interventions that facilitate his emotional release. Mrs. K and Mrs. P mutually agree to reduce Mr. C's expected involvement in activities and to provide a psychologically appropriate environment for the various stages of grief.

Several strategies were discussed and it was agreed that Mr. C should be included in the planning stage of his treatment program. Mr. C's participation in the planning and implementing stages recognizes his strengths and allows him to remain self-reliant.

IMPLEMENTATION

Without describing specific interventions used in this case, a few guidelines are offered regarding this phase of liaison nursing. Short-term objectives can be used as selected steps toward reaching a long-range goal. In Mr. C's case "facilitating client's grief work" is one step toward helping him adjust to his life stage and life-style. The interventions should focus on specific, expected actions of the client and not nursing care provided by staff. The interventions should be written in short concise statements (e.g., "introduce Mr. C to Mr. O, who has successfully completed grieving for his wife"). Expected measurable outcomes are established and a time frame is placed on each suggested intervention. Mrs. L negotiates with the directors to be available as a resource for 2 months as the planned interventions are tried and the results are measured.

EVALUATION

Mrs. K receives a report from staff members in an ongoing manner regarding Mr. C's progress. A few minor revisions were made in the original plan. According to the evaluation of both Mrs. K and Mrs. P, the client profited, the interdepartment staff became more cohesive because of the cooperative effort

Continued.

at problem solving, and the staff's increased knowledge would benefit all residents of the home.

Mrs. L spent a total of 2 hours at the actual consultation site. The liaison project ended when she sent a summary letter to the retirement home at the end of the 2 months. The established relationship continued from time to time with other projects.

The following are a few of the liaison techniques used in this clinical example:

1. Keep the focus on the client's situation and away from the staff's handling of the situation so that the users recognize their work performance is not under investigation.
2. Avoid personal issues. If a staff member talks about personal or private material, gently and purposefully direct the discussion back on focus by asking a client-related question.
3. As information is reviewed, raise questions to discover additional details and enrich the staff's awareness.
4. Use inquiry in such a way as to show the staff's wealth of valuable information.
5. Avoid asking for information that the staff would perceive as testing its knowledge base.
6. Allow the staff to know when you are confused. Being open to your own confusion allows the staff to recognize that clarifying is one of the steps in problem solving and when the pieces are put together, the patterns and meanings become clear.
7. Whenever possible, interview the referred client and the staff members who provide direct service to that client.

accessible, and cost-effective in both health care and community systems. Special emphasis should be placed on developing practice opportunities focused on health promotion, wellness, and human resource enhancement.

Fundamental changes are taking place in how nursing services are allocated and reimbursed. Direct reimbursement through third-party and self-pay measures is increasing through state and federal legislation, expanded nurse practice acts, and demonstrated cost savings. Continued political activity at the policy-making level is needed to influence changing the shortcomings

of government, commercial, and prospective payor systems. Liaison nursing must continue to be responsible for strengthening its position as a necessary component of client care, especially in the general hospital and intermediate care facility. Cost-offset studies are imperative to specifically show the reduction of overall cost of health care by inclusion of a liaison nurse on the health team and the cost-benefit ratio of liaison intervention with medically sick clients.

Marketing is an absolutely needed skill of every liaison nurse. The scarcity of the health care dollar and the multitude of providers competing for the same clients make it mandatory for all of nursing to become proactive in guarding its service area. It is of even greater importance for psychiatric nursing to promote and document its contribution toward quality, cost-effective care. Finally, acceptance and use of mental health nurse consultants in traditional health care settings and nontraditional community and commercial settings depends on active political endeavors, especially on the part of independent practitioners. It also takes recognition and acknowledgment by nurse colleagues through client referral to provide support to the role and validation of its contribution to health care.[12,14]

There are three major dimensions in which liaison nurses can influence their own professional future. These and the tasks involved in each follow.

■ Accountability

1. Attain professional certification as advanced clinicians.
2. Develop instruments for self-evaluation, since most clinicians work independently and can learn from retrospective audit.
3. Document liaison services in an official manner to validate and justify needs as well as to promote referrals.

■ Accessibility

1. Participate in as many interprofessional and community activities as possible to provide role identity, visibility, and leadership.
2. Initiate liaison services to outreach agencies and rural and smaller consultees, even at the sacrifice of time or money, to promote improved and newly developed client care practices.
3. Utilize effective and creative marketing strategies to promote the consultation services. Competition for the declining health care dollar is a realistic component to consider in a cost-effective health care delivery system.

■ Application

1. Identify and practice within a sound theoretical framework.
2. Devise and implement research projects that test clinical theory and cost-effectiveness.
3. Use creative and flexible ways to effect change.
4. Be well prepared by keeping up with new developments through formal or continuing education.

■ SUGGESTED CROSS-REFERENCES ■

Roles of psychiatric nurses are discussed in Chapter 1. Therapeutic relationship skills are discussed in Chapter 4. The phases of the nursing process are discussed in Chapter 5. Elements of the psychiatric evaluation are discussed in Chapter 6. Strategies for promoting health are discussed in Chapter 8.

■ SUMMARY ■

1. Liaison nursing is a model for nursing practice that has developed from the consultative process. The liaison nurse has a master's degree, a high degree of expertise in psychiatric nursing, and an ability to integrate these skills with knowledge in medical-surgical nursing to provide expanded services. Liaison nursing is an interpersonal, coordinate, problem-solving consultation process that promotes planned change by the use of interpersonal skills and specialized knowledge.

2. Liaison nurses practice in a variety of settings, and they may be either private practitioners, employees on a fee-for-service basis, or employed staff of an organization.

3. Three categories of problems are encountered by the liaison nurse:
   a. Case problems that focus on the problems of one particular client.
   b. Program problems that focus on a series of problems related to the user's professional functioning.
   c. Organization problems that focus on developing new programs or improving existing ones within the organization.

4. Changing client populations and economic constraints strengthen the need for liaison nursing. Both direct and indirect services can be economically justified through application of sound business management principles.

5. The liaison nurse has no administrative authority within the problem-centered organization. She is not necessarily responsible for implementing recommended changes, and the user is free to accept or reject any or all parts of the recommendation. The provider-user relationship is voluntary and time-limited. The goal of the liaison nurse is to assist the user to advance in efficiency and increase one's ability to handle similar problems in the future. The liaison nurse should have a conceptual model and theoretical framework for practice.

6. The liaison process is based on the nursing process and consists of three phases: orientation, work, and termination.

DIRECTIONS FOR FUTURE RESEARCH

The following are some of the nursing research problems raised in Chapter 26 that merit further study by psychiatric nurses:

1. Cost analysis studies, especially in the area of the cost-effectiveness of liaison nursing services.
2. Whether liaison nursing direct care interventions promote shorter hospital stays or fewer nursing care hours for certain diagnostic-related groups in the general hospital.
3. The use of the liaison nurse role in health promotion in a nontraditional setting, such as a retirement center, particularly one in which nursing care is part of the self-contained health maintenance package.
4. Whether employee access to a liaison nurse within an organization has any effect on employee absenteeism or illness.
5. Ways in which liaison nurses are marketing their skills and knowledge.
6. Business strategies used by liaison nurses in clinical practice, in the documentation of direct and indirect service productivity.
7. The degree of interdependence present in the liaison nurse-consultee relationship at various stages of the nursing process.
8. The extent to which psychosocial dimensions are incorporated in the plan of care for medical and surgical clients in general hospitals.
9. Organizational aspects of the liaison nursing role within a health care setting.
10. The effectiveness of liaison nursing interventions in decreasing a hospitalized client's anxiety level.

   a. A written agreement or contract should be obtained during the orientation phase.
   b. The work phase consists of the four steps of assessment, planning, implementation, and evaluation.
   c. Termination involves both physical and psychological closure. Self-evaluation is another important activity at this time to further the nurse's professional growth.

7. The liaison nurse can be either a direct or indirect care provider. Either function can be carried out in case problems. Indirect service is generally involved in program or organization problems. Each type of function follows the entire liaison process in a coordinate partnership format.

8. Research is necessary in the liaison nursing role. Cost analysis studies involving both cost-offset and cost-benefit of liaison nursing practice are needed to demonstrate the relative

cost-effectiveness of this role.

9. Liaison nursing, as a subspecialty of psychiatric nursing, is evolving parallel to nursing in general. Three dimensions in which liaison nurses can influence their own professional future include accountability, accessibility, and application.

■ **REFERENCES** ■

1. Beraducci, M., Blandfor, K., and Garant, C.A.: The psychiatric liaison nurse in the general hospital, Gen. Hosp. Psychiatr. **1**:66, 1979.
2. Blake, P.: The clinical specialist as nurse consultant, J. Nurs. Admin. **10**:33, 1977.
3. Campion, E.W.: An interdisciplinary geriatric consultation service: a controlled trial, J. Am. Geriatr. Soc. **31**(12):792, 1983.
4. Caplan, G.: The theory and practice of mental health consultation, New York, 1970, Basic Books, Inc., Publishers.
5. Deloughery, G.W., Gebbie, K.M., and Neuman, B.M.: Consultation and community organization in community mental health nursing, Baltimore, 1971, Williams & Wilkins Co.
6. Fay, M.F.: Consult a nurse expert:, Nurs. Success Today **2**(3):34, 1985.
7. Forti, T.: A documented evaluation of primary prevention through consultation, Community Ment. Health J. **19**(4):290, 1983.
8. Gebbie, K.M.: Consultation contracts: their development and evaluation, Am. J. Psych. Health **12**:60, 1970.
9. Hoffman, F.M.: A finger on the pulse of change, J. Nurs. Adm. **15**(4):24, 1985.
10. Kolson, G.: Mental health nursing consultation: a study of expectations, J. Psychiatr. Nurs. **14**(9):24, 1976.
11. Lewis, A., and Levy, J.S.: Psychiatric liaison nursing: the theory and clinical practice, Reston, Va., 1982, Reston Publishing.
12. Mallison, M.B.: Editorial: preferring our own providers . . . be sure our referrals include as many nurses in private practice as possible, Am. J. Nurs. **85**(4):355, 1985.
13. McKibbin, R.C., Brimmer, P.F., Galliher, J.M., Hartley, S.S., and Clinton, J.: Nursing costs and DRG payments, Am. J. Nurs. **85**(12):1353, 1985.
14. Miller, L.E.: Resistance to the consultation process, Nurs. Leadership, **6**(1):10, 1983.
15. Nelson, J.K., and Schilke, D.A.: The evolution of psychiatric liaison nursing, Perspect. Psychiatr. Care **14**(2):60, 1976.
16. Pearson, G.S.: The development of mental health consultation to a foster care placement agency, Public Health Nurs. **1**(1):45, 1984.
17. Pincus, H.A.: Making the case for consultation-liaison psychiatry, Gen. Hosp. Psychiatry **6**:173, 1984.
18. Pyles, J.C.: Referral arrangements between hospitals and home health agencies, Caring **3**(2):54, 1984.
19. Robinson, L.: Liaison nursing: psychological approach to patient care, Philadelphia, 1976, F.A. Davis Co.
20. Smith, M.C.: Perceptions of head nurses, clinical nurse specialists, nursing educators, and nursing office personnel regarding performance of selected nursing activities, Nurs. Res. **23**:505, 1974.
21. Soda, D.: Consultation: an expectation of leadership, Nurs. Leadership, **5**(1):7, 1982.
22. Stetler, C., and Downs, C.: The supervisor/consultant: a difficult role, J. Nurs. Admin. **4**(4):50, 1974.
23. Tobin, S.S.: Embracing community mental health center and church collaboration for the elderly, Community Ment. Health J. **21**(1):58, 1985.
24. Well, P.: The nurse consultant, Imprint **31**(4):23, 1984.

■ **ANNOTATED SUGGESTED READINGS** ■

*Burch, J.W., and Meredith, J.L.: Help with problem patients: nurses as the core of a psychiatric team, Am. J. Nurs. **74**:2037, 1974.

   This article deals with the importance of a liaison nurse helping the nursing staff ventilate their feelings about their work and their relationships with medical staff, nursing staff, and family. The psychiatric nurse consultation role developed in this article focuses on both direct and indirect services.

Caplan, G.: The theory and practice of mental health consultation, New York, 1970, Basic Books, Inc., Publishers.

   This book is the acknowledged prototype for both consultation theory and practice. Many of the principles Caplan discusses are applicable to liaison nursing as a consultation process. It is an excellent resource book for a practitioner or student of liaison nursing.

*Critchley, D., and Maurin, J.: The clinical specialist in psychiatric–mental health nursing, New York, 1985, John Wiley & Sons.

   This book explores the various ways in which psychiatric–mental health clinical nurse specialists use their education, experience, knowledge, and skills. The liaison nurse role is discussed, as well as many other advanced practitioner roles. The authors have put together a wealth of information from which masters' prepared nurses can learn.

*Goldberg, R.J., Tull, R., Sullivan, N., Wallace, S., and Wool, M.: Defining discipline roles in consultation psychiatry: the multidisciplinary team approach to psychosocial oncology, Gen. Hosp. Psychiatry **6**(1):17, 1984.

   This article delineates the contributions of nursing, psychiatry, psychology, and social work professionals in the management of cancer patients through a consultation program in a general hospital setting. The authors propose a model of collaborative interaction. The multidiscipline team approach in the program can be generalized to other hospital units.

Haug, M.R., Ford, A.B., Sheafor, M., editors: Physical and mental health of aged women, New York, 1985, Springer Publishing Co.

   An excellent resource for all nurses. This book provides a

---

*Asterisk indicates nursing reference.

comprehensive view of older American women, presenting the biological, psychological, nutritional, and sociological factors that influence the aging process. Every professional nurse, whatever one's area of practice, can benefit from this practical guide.

Hess, R., and Hermalin, J.: Innovation in prevention, New York, 1983, Haworth Press.

With the thrust toward health promotion and wellness, this book provides basic reading for the creative liaison nurse who wants to market her abilities in today's competitive environment. They provide different approaches for applying advanced education to the current consumers of health care. As consultation struggles for fiscal survival, nurses should look to employers in industry and business as buyers of their skills.

*Lancaster, I.W., and Lancaster, J.: Models and model building in nursing, Adv. Nurs. Sci. **3**(3):31, 1981.

This article focuses on the concept of models and the model-building process. The article serves as an introduction to the relationship between model building and the role that models play in marketing the nurse practitioner's services as a consultant.

*Lewis, A., and Levy, J.: Psychiatric liaison nursing: the theory and clinical practice, Reston, Va., 1982, Reston Publishing.

This entire text is devoted to the liaison nursing role. It is a classic and excellent resource for developments in the field.

Mason, D., and Talbott, S.W.: Political action handbook for nurses, Menlo Park, Calif., 1985, Addison-Wesley Publishing Co.

In this era of competition, it is imperative that all nurses become skillful in the political arena, whether it be in the workplace or the state capitol building. This book is practical and useful to the nurse who wants to be an effective agent of change through political activities.

*Price, J.L., and Cordell, B.: So you want to try consulting, J. Cont. Ed. Nurs. **15**(3):103, 1984.

This article provides basic information for the nurse who is contemplating the consultation role. It gives encouragement to the emerging nurse consultant and proposes a model of service which can be used as a framework for structuring and planning appropriate interventions.

*Weinstein, L.J., Chapman, M.M., and Stallings, M.A.: Organizing approaches to psychiatric nurse consultation, Perspect. Psychiatr. Care **17**(2):66, 1979.

The article discusses the authors' experience as consultants involved in nursing rounds in a general hospital. The goal was to teach nurses how to better handle clients' emotional problems and to decrease the staff's anxiety under specific circumstances. The authors-consultants focused on areas of change and current concern during the consultation sessions which were both walking and kardex rounds. The article describes the joint effort of liaison nursing and staff nursing to produce improved quality of care.

SPECIALIZED TREATMENT APPROACHES

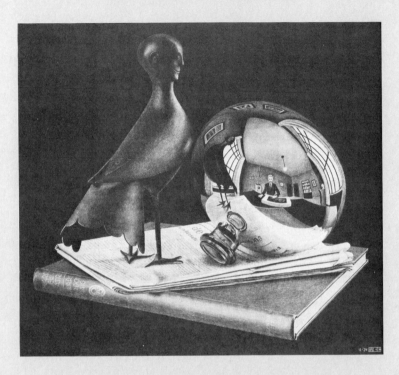

But humanism stands for the whole person, the whole individual striving to become as conscious and responsible as possible about everything in the universe. But now you sit there quite calmly and as a humanist you say that due to the complexity of scientific achievement the human being must never expect to be whole, he must always be frightened.

Doris Lessing, The Golden Notebook*

CHAPTER 27

BEHAVIOR MODIFICATION

HELEN R. PEDDICORD

*New York, 1973, Bantam Books. Copyright © 1962 by Doris Lessing.

LEARNING OBJECTIVES

After studying this chapter, the student should be able to:

- define behavior in specific terms.

- define behavior modification.

- analyze the application of operant conditioning principles to behavior modification.

- describe behavior modification techniques, including positive and negative reinforcement and positive and negative punishment.

- compare and contrast fixed interval, variable interval, fixed rate, and variable rate reinforcement schedules.

- discuss the ethical issues relative to the practice of behavior modification.

- identify directions for future nursing research.

- select appropriate readings for further study.

The principles described in this chapter are primarily the product of the field of psychology, particularly of B.F. Skinner's work. In 1953, *Science and Human Behavior*[13] by B.F. Skinner was published. This work presented the findings of animal behavior experiments and discussed their application to human behavior in an attempt to move toward a science of human behavior. Subsequent studies during the 1950s that applied the principles to profoundly retarded and psychotic institutionalized persons indicated their effectiveness. By 1958 the *Journal of the Experimental Analysis of Behavior* was published. This journal, although largely concerned with laboratory experiments with animals, printed some articles of applied behavior therapy with humans. In 1965 this journal published the results of the first experiment with the token economy.[1] The authors, Ayllon and Azrin, had developed and evaluated an environment that consistently and systematically reinforced patients diagnosed as psychotic for adaptive behavior. The motivating environment and operant conditioning principles they described were effectively applied later to populations such as the mentally ill, mentally retarded, juvenile delinquents, preschoolers, and slow learners.[2]

The late 1960s saw applied research in operant conditioning expand into the areas of education, classroom management, parenting, community work, and self-control. During the 1970s operant conditioning principles have been used by most of the helping professionals, including nurses, physicians, social workers, teachers, and psychologists. The impact of this work can be viewed from the perspective of published bibliographies. The 1967 bibliography by Barnard listed 866 references in behavior modification.[4] Britt's bibliography,[5] covering 1924 through 1975, lists 6780 publications. Assuming that Barnard's bibliography was correct, there have been well over 5000 publications in

behavior modification since 1967. These numbers give some indication of the many studies done in the area. During the 1970s textbooks on behavior modification appeared in the professions of medicine, social work, nursing, education, psychiatry, and rehabilitative medicine.

The last decade has brought an emphasis on cognitive behavior modification. This recognizes the value of both self-regulation and thought processes, as well as the fact that human behavior and experience are strongly influenced by internal phenomena. Much current research explores the internal (cognitive) antecedents and reinforcers which debilitate or habilitate.

Definition

Behavior modification involves the application of the findings of operant conditioning principles and procedures to human affairs. Operant conditioning, according to Reynolds, "refers to a process in which the frequency of occurrence of a bit of behavior is modified by consequences of the behavior."[12:1] Careful reading of this definition may lead one to assume it is an overly simplistic approach to the obvious complexities of human behavior; however, its empirical application breaks the complexities down to a manageable level and clarifies the multiple events that affect behavior.

The terms "behavior modification" and "behavior therapy" have some distinct meanings but are often used interchangeably. Martin and Pear[9] compare where and by whom each term tends to be used. "Behavior therapy" is the term favored by psychologists and psychiatrists who treat clients in traditional clinical settings. It is also associated with an experimental foundation that is based primarily on human studies in clinical settings. "Behavior modificaton" is the term favored for treatment carried out in schools, homes, and other natural settings outside the traditional psychiatric setting.

The subjects of its experimental research are animals and humans.

Within this chapter the term "behavior modification" will be used. It is an effective treatment modality for alleviating many human problems, among which are psychiatric disorders. Although behavior modification has not yet been proved to be the treatment of choice for strictly intrapsychic conflict, it can help to alter those behaviors which result from and exacerbate such conflict. A strictly behaviorally oriented therapist, for example, is not likely to treat a client who is experiencing a significant loss. These clients would benefit more from evocative or insight psychotherapy. A primary role of behavior modification within current treatment modalities is its emphasis on the effect of the environment on human behavior. As such, it provides an alternate way of diagnosing and treating problems.

The role of behavior modification in psychiatric nursing has been inadequately explored in nursing publications. In 1959 Ayllon and Michael[3] published an article entitled "The Psychiatric Nurse as a Behavioral Engineer" in a psychology journal. Perhaps if this had been published in a nursing journal, more inroads into this area would have been made by psychiatric nurses. A search of the nursing literature of 1984 and 1985 found behaviorally oriented articles almost exclusively in the somatic nursing journals. The April 1985 issue of *Journal of Psychosocial Nursing and Mental Health Services* focused on the borderline personality disorder and included two articles on behavioral contracting.[10]

An additional focus of psychiatric nurses using behavior modification techniques is evident in the application of various relaxation techniques as treatment strategies to reduce anxiety and foster more healthful physiological reactions. Progressive relaxation, which is the sequential tensing and releasing of large muscle groups, is employed to decrease anxiety; and biofeedback, which is the procedure of learned control of involuntary body reactions using electronic devices, is taught to alter physiology. Dossey[7] explains relaxation simply and concisely. The practicing psychiatric nurse should be alert to a paradoxical relaxation-induced anxiety in some clients.[8] Biofeedback techniques are best learned and practiced experientially. Connelly[6] presents an explanatory overview of this area. Chapter 12 discusses these interventions in detail.

This chapter merely introduces behavior modification principles, and it is not written with the expectation that the reader will be able to design, implement, and evaluate a behavioral treatment program without supervision. Appropriate application of behavioral techniques can be made in any setting in which psychiatric nurses work. The frequency with which psychiatric nurses do so depends on their experiences of success or failure when they use behavioral techniques, their exposure to a skilled and helpful behavior modifier, and their familiarity with behavioral literature.

Describing behavior

Behavior is any observable, recordable, and measurable act, movement, or response of the individual. It refers to everything a person does. It is observable, if only to the person performing the behavior. Although affect, cognition, and sensation, as well as imagery, are subject to behavioral treatment, the treatment is dependent on self-observation. This chapter focuses only on behaviors that are observed by others and subject to quantitative measurement.

Before a behavior can be measured, it must be defined or accurately described. One can, in defining behavior, break it into microscopic or macroscopic elements. For example, the fire setting done by a child can be defined microscopically as gathering flammable objects, striking the match, lighting the objects, fanning the lit objects, and watching the resultant blaze or macroscopically as lighting a fire that blazes. This shows that there are several different and accurate definitions of what at first glance appears to be a simply defined behavior. Behavior definition can be a difficult task. One starts by describing what is seen and/or heard and then clarifies this until pertinent observers can agree as to whether the behavior occurs.

Consider defining the behavior of fighting. It can be described as disagreement, accompanied by raised voices, exchanging epithets, and a physical struggle of reciprocal blows and kicks. In the process of clarifying this description, questions such as the following arise: Is it fighting if there is no yelling? Is it fighting if each person hits the other only once? Is it fighting if there is a physical struggle (similar to wrestling) with no hitting or kicking? As these questions are answered, definition that is both clear and pertinent to the purpose of the definition unfolds. If one is establishing rules and consequences for aggressive adolescents, it may be decided that there is a consequence imposed simply for one student hitting and/or kicking another student, since this is likely to prevent a fight such as that which was first described. If one is developing a treatment plan for a child who is said to "fight all the time" in a classroom, the clinician, teacher, and child together may arrive at a different definition. They may decide that the significant behavior is pulling classmates' hair or pushing them out of their seats.

These definitions exemplify that a behavior is what is observed—not conclusions, inferences, or interpretations drawn from observation. Hyperactivity is not a behavior but a conclusion about a multiplicity of behaviors. One cannot measure hyperactivity; one can measure the number of times a child looks away from an assignment within a specified amount of time, how many times he interrupts a conversation in a given time period, the number of toys he displaces, the pages of classwork completed, and the length of time he remains in one body posture. The behavioral treatment would not be directed toward hyperactivity but toward those specified behaviors which interfere with the child's success in the school, home, or community.

Other examples of conclusions instead of behaviors are psychiatric diagnoses and descriptions, such as uncooperative, aggressive, compliant, depressed, hostile, and withdrawn. When one thinks of a person to whom any of these adjectives or labels are attributed, one can readily describe behaviors associated with the adjective, but from person to person the behavioral components of the adjectives will vary. There is little chance that the conjured behavioral composite will be the same for more than one person. A clear definition of a behavior decreases the interpretative variability from person to person. A clear behavior definition is a statement of what

the person does, is accessible to measurement, and is not subject to interpretation.

Once a behavior is reliably described, one concludes that in the person's future that behavior will increase, decrease, or remain the same. Those procedures which increase, maintain, or decrease behaviors are given in Table 27-1. Each of these operant conditioning procedures will now be briefly described.

Increasing or maintaining behavior

A behavior may increase in frequency, complexity, or duration. In the acquisition of walking skills, for example, a step occurs more often; the complexity of the step increases (forward, backward, sideways, turning, becoming longer); and the amount of time walking increases. One can observe an increase in at least these three ways in the acquisition of most skills.

Operant behavior is that behavior which is maintained, increased, or decreased according to the environmental events that follow it. For clarity, the word "operant" instead of "behavior" will be used throughout the remainder of this chapter. **When the environment events following an operant increase the probability**

TABLE 27-1

OPERANT CONDITIONING PROCEDURES

Maintain or increase behavior	Decrease behavior
Positive reinforcement: Addition of an environmental event as a consequence of operant, increasing probability of operant's recurrence Operant → Consequence → Operant ↑	**Positive punishment:** Presentation of aversive stimulus following operant, decreasing probability of operant's recurrence Operant → Aversive event → Operant ↓
Negative reinforcement: Removal of part of an aversive stimulus as a consequence of operant, increasing probability of operant's recurrence Aversive stimulus → Operant → Removal of aversive stimulus → Operant ↑	**Negative punishment:** Removal of something following operant, decreasing probability of operant's recurrence **Response cost:** Negative punishment in which a reinforcer is lost or withdrawn following an operant Operant → Reinforcer withdrawn → Operant ↓ **Time-out from reinforcement:** Negative punishment in which no reinforcement is available following an operant Operant → No reinforcement available → Operant ↓
	Extinction: Withholding reinforcement following an operant that was previously reinforced Operant → No reinforcement → Operant ↓

that the operant will recur, the process is reinforcement. Reinforcement increases the probability that the operant will occur again. Positive and negative reinforcement both increase the chances of an operant occurring again.

The addition of an environmental event (consequence) contingent on the operant is **positive reinforcement.** An example of positive reinforcement is the response of a smile to a greeting. The operant, greeting, is followed by a smile from the person addressed. The chances that the greeting will happen in the future are increased by the smile given in response. The smile is an addition (positive in the mathematical sense) of an environmental event.

$$\text{Operant} \to \begin{array}{c} \text{Positive} \\ \text{reinforcer} \end{array} \to \begin{array}{c} \text{Probability of} \\ \text{operant recurring} \uparrow \end{array}$$
$$\text{Greeting} \to \text{Smile} \to \text{Greeting in future} \uparrow$$

There are occasions when the intent of the person responding to an operant is to **decrease** the frequency of the operant, but the operant actually increases in frequency or remains the same. A parent may yell at a young child whenever he climbs on the table; the process in operation is positive reinforcement if he continues to climb on the table or does so more often in the future.

$$\begin{array}{c} \text{Child} \\ \text{on table} \end{array} \to \begin{array}{c} \text{Parent} \\ \text{yells} \end{array} \to \begin{array}{c} \text{Child} \\ \text{on table} \uparrow \end{array} = \begin{array}{c} \text{Positive} \\ \text{reinforcement} \end{array}$$

It is important to understand in this example that the process is defined as positive reinforcement because the child climbs on the table more often. If the child decreased his climbing on the table as a result of his mother's yelling, the process would not be positive reinforcement. Any of a number of factors may possibly explain why the mother's correction did not result in a decrease in table climbing. The relevant point is that the intent of the person providing a consequence does not determine what process is in operation. The effect of the consequence on the future occurrence of the behavior determines the process.

When the reinforcer is the removal of an aversive stimulus contingent on the operant, the procedure is **negative reinforcement.** An example of negative reinforcement is putting on sunglasses in glaring sunlight. The sunlight is an aversive stimulus; the placing of the sunglasses over the eyes is the operant; the removal of, or escape from, the sunlight's glare is the negative reinforcer. It is a reinforcer because the glare's removal **increases** the probability that the person will, in future exposure to the glaring sunlight, make use of sunglasses. A reinforcer increases the probability that an operant will recur. It is negative when what was reinforcing was

the removal, or **subtraction,** of something from the environment. Negative, here, is to be understood in the mathematical sense.

$$\begin{array}{c} \text{Aversive stimulus} \to \\ \text{Glare of sun} \end{array} \quad \begin{array}{c} \textbf{Operant} \\ \to \text{Use of sunglasses in bright sun} \to \end{array}$$
$$\begin{array}{c} \text{Escape from} \\ \text{aversive stimulus} \end{array} \to \begin{array}{c} \text{Probability of} \\ \text{operant recurring} \uparrow \end{array}$$
$$\begin{array}{c} \text{Escape from} \\ \text{sun's glare} \end{array} \to \begin{array}{c} \text{Probable use of} \\ \text{sunglasses in future} \uparrow \end{array}$$

The example just given is one of **escaping** the glare of the sun. Putting on the sunglasses prior to going out into the sun would be an example of **avoiding** the sun.

Negative reinforcement is the procedure by which one learns to escape or avoid unpleasant situations. This is evident in the following examples.

EXAMPLE 1

A mother is reprimanding a young child; the child goes to his mother and kisses her, and her reprimand stops.

$$\text{Reprimand} \to \text{Kiss} \to \begin{array}{c} \text{Reprimand} \\ \text{stops} \end{array} \to \begin{array}{c} \text{Chance of child} \\ \text{kissing mother} \\ \text{when again} \\ \text{reprimanded} \uparrow \end{array}$$

EXAMPLE 2

Nurse A tells Nurse B she wants to discuss the conflicts in their work relationship. Nurse B becomes too busy to talk, thus avoiding the discussion. As a result, Nurse B is likely in the future to be busy whenever she sees Nurse A.

$$\begin{array}{c} \text{Sees} \\ \text{Nurse A} \end{array} \to \text{Busyness} \to \begin{array}{c} \text{Discussion} \\ \text{avoided} \end{array} \to \begin{array}{c} \text{Busyness} \\ \text{whenever} \\ \text{sees Nurse A} \uparrow \end{array}$$

EXAMPLE 3

An adolescent's parents are displeased with their son's misbehavior in school. The adolescent runs away, thereby escaping the direct experience of his parents' displeasure. In the future he may well run away again.

$$\begin{array}{c} \text{Parental} \\ \text{displeasure} \end{array} \to \begin{array}{c} \text{Run} \\ \text{away} \end{array} \to \begin{array}{c} \text{Escape from} \\ \text{displeasure} \end{array} \to \begin{array}{c} \text{Running away} \\ \text{when parents} \\ \text{displeased} \uparrow \end{array}$$

Negative reinforcement may also maintain some work habits. Employees in a work situation arrive on time for work to avoid a supervisor's reprimand or loss of wages.

Decreasing behavior

Negative reinforcement is not to be confused with punishment. **Punishment decreases the probability that the operant will recur.** Negative and positive, in the mathematical sense, describe punishing procedures. **Positive punishment** as Reynolds describes it, is "the presentation of an aversive stimulus following and dependent upon the occurrence of an operant."[12:111] In other words, an operant occurs and is immediately followed by an environmental event that is aversive to the person, and this results in a decrease in occurrence of the operant. A person wearing sunglasses on a bright sunny day removes them. Removing the glasses is the operant. Immediately the glaring light hurts the person's eyes; this is the aversive event. Subsequently the person removes the sunglasses less often in glaring sunlight. This is an example of positive punishment.

Operant →Aversive stimulus→ Operant ↓
Sunglasses off→ Glare in eyes →Sunglasses off ↓

The procedure is also occurring when the parent yells at a child immediately after he climbs on a table. If the child climbs on the table less often, then the procedure in operation serves as punishment, the operant being climbing on the table and the aversive stimulus being the yelling.

Child on table →Parent yells→Child on table ↓

As pointed out in the explanation of positive reinforcement, the process at work is not necessarily the one intended by the person who is responding to another's operant. One might praise a noncompliant adolescent for a particular operant whenever it occurs, but the operant may occur less and less often. The process then is not positive reinforcement but positive punishment.

Negative punishment, according to Mikulas, is "a contingent event whose offset or decrease results in a decrease in the behavior it is contingent upon. This generally consists of taking away something that is reinforcing from a person when he misbehaves."[11:97] The major forms of negative punishment are response cost and time-out.

Response cost is the loss of a previously available reinforcer following an operant. After hitting her young brother, the child is deprived of her allowance. An adolescent may lose the opportunity to use the family car after coming home beyond her curfew. A consumer pays the bank a fee after overdrawing his checking account.

Operant → Reinforcer →Operant ↓
                withdrawn
Child hits   →Loses allowance→Hitting ↓
Late coming in→Loss of car   →Late coming in ↓
                privileges
Overdraw   →Loss of money →Overdrawing ↓
account

Time-out (or time-out from reinforcement), according to Mikulas, is "the punishment procedure in which the punishment is a period of time during which reinforcement is not available."[11:99]

A young child throws toys at the wall. His mother places him on a chair in the corner. When he plays again, he is less likely to throw toys at the wall.

                    Loss of all
Operant   → environmental → Operant ↓
                    reinforcement
Throwing toys→No reinforcement →Throwing toys ↓
                    while in chair

Extinction is the final behavior-decreasing procedure to be discussed. Extinction is the withholding or removal of a reinforcer that was previously maintaining or increasing an operant. A fairly typical example of extinction involves temper tantrums.

A child has a temper tantrum. The mother tells the child to stop, and, because she is concerned that he will injure himself, hovers about the child. She then decides to no longer pay attention to future tantrums. When the next tantrum occurs, she completely ignores it. The previous reinforcer, mother's attention, is no longer presented. It is predictable that the tantrum will become louder and more intense, then gradually taper off. As the mother continues to ignore all tantrum behaviors, they will gradually decrease. The mother is employing the extinction process.

Operant→Previous reinforcer withheld→ Operant ↓
Tantrum→Mother's attention withheld   →Tantrum ↓

Extinction does not usually result in an immediate decrease in the operant. After an initial increase in rate, intensity, or duration, the operant gradually decreases.

An example, taken from group therapy, of several procedures in action follows. In human interactions there is an opulent interplay of operants, reinforcers, punishers, and aversive stimuli. When one observes a given behavior, it may be an operant of the person observed, a reinforcer to an operant of a second person, and an aversive stimulus to a third person. This example, for simplicity's sake, does not relate the content of the group's interaction. It deals only with a narrow aspect of the process to exemplify four operant procedures: positive reinforcement, negative reinforcement, positive punishment, and extinction.

Abraham, usually silent in the group, speaks. Zelda laughs while Abraham is speaking. Abraham is then silent, and Zelda speaks. While she does so, all group members look at her. Zelda verbalizes more frequently than the other group members. Each time she speaks, at least the majority of group members look at her. Later, Abraham speaks again; again Zelda laughs, and again Abraham stops speaking. He does not speak again in this session.

At least three operant procedures are in action. Zelda's laughter when Abraham speaks and Zelda's speaking are both reinforced; the former is negatively reinforced, the latter positively reinforced. The operant, laughter, is followed by Abraham's cessation of speech. Abraham's speaking is an aversive stimulus to Zelda, who removes it by the operant laughter. Zelda's laughter removes the aversive stimulus of Abraham's speaking, and her laughing when he speaks will increase. This is **negative reinforcement.** Zelda's operant of speaking is **positively reinforced.** The reinforcer is the eye contact of the other members. The frequency of her speaking increases. Abraham's operant of speaking decreases in frequency. Zelda's laughter is an aversive stimulus or punisher to his verbalizing. His speaking is punished by her laughter. This is **positive punishment.**

It is imperative to note that these processes are defined by what happens. The processes are not defined before they occur. The eye contact of others (added event—positive) is defined as a **positive reinforcer** to Zelda's speaking because this is what happens when she speaks and her speaking is maintained or increased in frequency. Zelda's laughter (added event—positive) when Abraham speaks is defined as a **punisher** to Abraham's operant of speaking because this happens when he speaks and his speaking decreases in frequency (punishment). Abraham's silence (removed or terminated event—negative) after Zelda's operant laughter is a **negative reinforcer** to the laughter because what happens is an increase in the probability that Zelda will laugh when the aversive stimulus (Abraham's speaking) recurs, and the laughter will remove the aversive stimulus.

In the next group session Zelda monopolizes the group during the first 10 minutes. All group members are looking at her at least occasionally during these 10 minutes. Gradually, one person stares out the window, another gazes at a picture, two others look at one another, and the last looks from one member to another but not at Zelda. As this starts to happen, Zelda's speech rate initially increases, then gradually decreases; finally, she pauses, then is silent.

This is **extinction.** The eye contact that had been reinforcing Zelda's verbalization is withheld, and her talking eventually ceases.

As mentioned earlier, this example indicates a narrow aspect of the behaviors in question for the sake of simplicity. There are, obviously, multiple reinforcers and punishers relative to any operant. In an analysis of an operant, one begins with what is most obviously presumed to be a reinforcer. If the operant is maladaptive and is to be altered, one starts treatment with what is seen as the reinforcer that is maintaining the maladaptive operant, removes the reinforcer for that operant, and provides reinforcement for an operant that is incompatible with the maladaptive one. Schedules of reinforcements have not yet been discussed, but will be considered in the following discussion of applications of behavior modification.

Applications of behavior modification

■ Increasing behavior

The simplest form of behavioral treatment is rearranging the environmental reinforcers. Sometimes this is not simple. A pediatric nurse consults with the psychiatric liaison nurse about an 8-year-old girl, Carole, whose treatment requires bed rest. The child is constantly out of bed playing despite the following interventions: the need for bed rest has been explained to the child and parents, parents have been cooperative, the child life worker has provided abundant activities for the child in bed, and there are other children in the room requiring bed rest who provide companionship. Carole's noncompliance with the bed rest requirement is now imitated by the other children, and they too are frequently out of bed. All involved adults are now scolding Carole.

Initially, one must define bed rest. Does it mean simply remaining on the bed? If so, is jumping on the bed within limits? In this situation bed rest means remaining in the bed and includes only those activities which can be done in a sitting or supine position. The second step is obtaining information about what happens when Carole is found out of bed (the undesirable operant) and when she is found in bed (the desirable operant). Staff will be able to describe these events, although it may be difficult to remember a time when Carole was found in bed. The third step is designing a data collection system and obtaining a baseline, that is, the frequency at which a behavior occurs prior to intervention. During waking hours Carole will be checked every 30 minutes and it will be noted whether she is or is not in bed.

After a half day of baseline data collection, it is observed that Carole was in bed only twice and that this was at mealtime. The staff reports that this is worse than usual. Each time Carole was observed out of bed, staff scolded her. This suggests that the scolding may be reinforcing the behavior, since the staff reports that she now seems to be out of bed more often, is being checked more often, and is therefore scolded more often. A current baseline is established.

The fourth step is to establish the desirable goal of intervention. Although it might be assumed that the goal is that she remain in bed 100% of the time, it is always desirable to state the intervention goal or terminal behavior clearly. The intervention goal should also include the time period during which it is to be accomplished. The intervention goal in this situation might well be "Carole will remain in bed 100% of the time within a week of treatment."

Now intervention can begin. Staff is instructed to continue checking every 30 minutes but to say nothing, maintain a blank expression, and simply place Carole in bed if she is not already there. A second staff person is to enter the room before Carole can get out of bed, to congratulate her about being in bed, and present the designated reinforcer. If two staff persons cannot be involved, then both roles can be accomplished by one person, who reenters the room immediately after placing the child in bed.

Data collection and constant evaluation should continue throughout the week, although once Carole is remaining in bed more often, she may be checked less often. All staff and family must be informed of the treatment to increase cooperation and prevent the inadvertent positive reinforcement that scolding provided to this child's being out of bed. In this situation the environmental reinforcer, staff attention, was rearranged. Staff no longer gave Carole attention for being out of bed. The attention is given for being in bed.

Let us take the same initial situation. Perhaps the initial data indicate that it is not staff attention but the gleeful laughter of her roommates that is reinforcing Carole's getting out of bed. This may be noted by Carole's increase in remaining in bed when a particularly lively roommate is not present or Carole's looking at her giggling roommates even when being corrected. One cannot suppress the children's spontaneous laughter, but one could devise a way for Carole to engage their laughter even while in bed, for example by providing a drawing pad large enough for the others to see on which she draws funny faces. One could also solicit the aid of the children by explaining the situation, but this is not likely to help unless one provides a group reinforcement contingent on Carole being in bed a certain number of times a day. The group reinforcement could be a staff person playing a game with all of them, an extra snack, parents staying some time past the end of visiting hours, or being the last group to be awakened in the morning.

The group in the room, including Carole, could easily be told that they will receive a specific reinforcer, such as one mentioned, if Carole is in bed at least half the times that she is checked. They can also be told that it is difficult for Carole to stay in bed when they laugh each time she gets up. In this way the group is involved in rearranging the reinforcement they provide Carole. The only way in which it will be known whether the reinforcer has been correctly identified or effectively altered is by the results: does Carole stay in bed more often?

Social attention is probably the most pervasive and readily available reinforcer for human beings. There are times, however, when primary reinforcers, such as food or activity, will be the reinforcers of choice. It may be that a client is not observant of or responsive to social attention. It may also be that the history for the client and the potentially reinforcing person may be so fraught with mutual anger and rejection that the quality of the attention that would be given could not be reinforcing. In these situations a primary reinforcer, such as food, or a material reinforcer, such as money, would be more immediately effective. At other times social reinforcers may be so multiply endowed that a primary reinforcer may be necessary to gain an immediate response from the client.

The first situation, that of nonobservance or nonresponse to social attention, is seen in a client who has been institutionalized for a number of years and gives no indication that he is aware of others. A piece of sugarless chewing gum contingently delivered for eye contact will be more effective than social attention. A goal of treatment for such a client is the development of social attention as a reinforcer. This is done by pairing the primary reinforcer, chewing gum, with social attention, then occasionally reinforcing with only social attention, and finally reinforcing with social attention and infrequently with a primary reinforcer.

The second situation, mutual anger and rejection, can be seen between an adolescent with a long history of behavior problems and his parents, whose many interventions have failed. In other words, the parents have received little reinforcement for parenting from the child, and the child has received little reinforcement for being their child. Reinforcers of choice may be money, privileges, or activities.

Multiply endowed reinforcers are constantly occurring, as, for example, in a young child who has many persons laughing at his misdeeds. The child will probably not be aware of a change in the quality of attention of one person if many are laughing, but he will notice if he receives a favorite treat when he behaves in a different way.

In each of the situations just described, primary reinforcers should be accompanied by social reinforcers so that the social reinforcers alone will, eventually, effectively maintain appropriate behaviors as the primary reinforcers are gradually attenuated.

■ **REINFORCEMENT SCHEDULES.** Another consideration is the timing of the data collection and the schedule of reinforcement. In the example of the child prescribed bed rest, the data were collected and the reinforcement was delivered (if Carole was in bed) every 30 minutes. Reinforcement can be delivered according to a time schedule, as in this example, or according to a performance schedule. The time schedule is called **in-**

terval schedule reinforcement; the performance schedule is called **ratio schedule reinforcement** (see accompanying box, which describes simple reinforcement schedules). Each type can be delivered on a fixed or variable schedule. An interval schedule refers to reinforcement being presented for the first designated behavior after a given period of time. If it is a fixed interval (FI) schedule, the time period is stable (e.g., every 5 minutes or, as in the example of Carole, 30 minutes). If a variable interval (VI) schedule is used, an average time lapse is designated (e.g., 30 minutes), as well as a minimum and maximum interval.

Behavior performance varies according to the reinforcement schedule (see accompanying box). On an FI schedule the operant increases just prior to the end of the interval and then, after reinforcement, decreases. One could predict that if Carole is checked and reinforced every 30 minutes, she will get out of bed soon

after being checked and given staff attention, then get into bed shortly before she thinks she will be checked again. If a VI schedule is employed, behavior is more consistent. If Carole cannot predict when she will be reinforced, she is more likely to remain in bed.

A fixed ratio (FR) schedule refers to reinforcement being provided after an operant is performed a designated number of times. A variable ratio (VR) schedule refers to reinforcement being provided for the performance of an operant a predetermined average number of times, with the minimum and maximum number of times also established.

FR and VR schedules result in higher rates of responding and greater resistance to extinction than either FI or VI schedules. If this fact is overlooked in clinical practice, one can expect treatment effectiveness to be short lived. Consider a child in residential treatment whose major problem is hitting peers in response to

---

Simple Reinforcement Schedules

TYPE OF SCHEDULE

Time or interval: Time lapse between behaviors before reinforcement
   Fixed interval: Specific lapse of time required for reinforcement (e.g., every 5 minutes, every month, every hour, paychecks)
   Variable interval: Various amounts of time elapse between possible reinforcement (e.g., 1 minute, 32 minutes, 3 hours, 5 minutes)

Performance or ratio: Number of times an operant is performed between reinforcement
   Fixed ratio: Same number of responses required for each·reinforcement (e.g., for every fifth performance of operant, piecework in factory)
   Variable ratio: Various numbers of responses required for each reinforcement (e.g., after 3, 10, 11, 19, 29, 33, 35 performances of operant; slot machines)

CHARACTERISTICS OF SCHEDULE

Fixed interval (FI)
High rate of performance before interval ends; low rate after reinforcement, the rate gradually accelerating until interval ends
Response to extinction: Responding ceases abruptly, recurs at a high rate, ceases, and recurs, with pauses increasing until rate is zero; relatively susceptible to extinction

Variable interval (VI)
Stable high rate of performance, rate lower than VR schedule
Response to extinction: Steadily decreasing rate until response is zero; of all simple schedules, most susceptible to extinction

Fixed ratio (FR)
Quickly developed high rate of performance; rate stable; especially if ratio is small
Response to extinction: Alternating pauses and high performance rate, the pause increasing until ratio is zero; relatively resistant to extinction

Variable ratio (VR)
High rate of performance, developing less quickly than FR; high rate stable even if average ratio is relatively high, except when average ratio is increased too quickly
Response to extinction: Responses continue at high sustained rate with alternating pauses until pauses lengthen and rate gradually reaches zero; of the simple schedules, most resistant to extinction

being teased. The child is taught an alternative response to being teased and is heavily praised every hour if he has engaged in the alternative response. This treatment is effective and the child is discharged. Suddenly the child is receiving no praise for his relatively new skill, and he quickly resorts to his old immediate feedback system of hitting.

The reinforcement schedule, while the child was in treatment, could easily have been altered to a variable ratio with the average ratio gradually increased until the reinforcement was being received at a rate closely approximating that in the natural environment. The child would thereafter have a greater chance at permanently incorporating his new skill.

■ **SELECTING A REINFORCEMENT SCHEDULE.** The choice of reinforcement schedules during clinical intervention depends on the severity of the presenting problem, the intended duration of the operant to be learned, the age of the client, the number of available persons, and many other factors. If the presenting problem behavior is life-threatening, one preferably designs an FR schedule with a very small ratio, graduates slowly to a VR schedule with a small average ratio, and then slowly increases the average of VR reinforcement. For example, a child with poor judgment runs away from a residential treatment center several times a day. While away, he engages in such behaviors as fire setting, theft, and running into heavy traffic. The initial FR schedule might reinforce him every time he walked by, instead of running out of, an exit door. The schedule is altered to every second time he walks by an exit door, then every third, then gradually a VR schedule is introduced.

The intended duration of the operant influences the choice of schedule. In Carole's case there is a time limit on her bed rest requirement; a small-interval FI schedule is likely to result in Carole rapidly learning to be in bed as the interval end approaches, although after reinforcement she is likely to get out of bed. The advantage is that Carole is receiving reinforcement for appropriate behavior. As the reinforcement becomes more important to her, a VI schedule is introduced, assuring her remaining in bed more constantly. The VI schedule is appropriate, since one need not be concerned with the operant of staying in bed as necessary for an extensive time period. Operants reinforced on a VI schedule cease quickly when reinforcement is withheld (extinction). Also, busy staff in a hospital setting seem more likely to provide reinforcement on the VI schedules.

On the other hand, if the treatment goal is a child's acquisition of appropriate classroom behavior, the ratio schedules seem more desirable. These are operants that will prove helpful to the child for many years. The re-inforcement schedule should be one that will result in the operant's resistance to extinction, as well as its maintenance by the reinforcers that will occur in the natural environment.

The age of the child seems to affect the rapidity with which the fixed schedules can be increased in ratio and interval length and with which they can be changed to variable schedules. A 2-year-old learns operants so rapidly that the new behavior may be maintained simply by reinforcers as they occur in the natural environment in a few days. By the time a child is 4 years old, it seems to take longer. By adolescence, the reinforcement history is so long and complex that months of intervention may be necessary before reinforcers in the natural environment can maintain newly learned operants.

The number of persons available to implement reinforcement schedules and the number of persons in treatment affect the schedule chosen. In general, ratio schedules require more persons because behaviors must be counted. Token economies in psychiatric hospitals and residential treatment centers usually are designed on FI and VI schedules. The number of staff needed to provide reinforcers on an FR or VR schedule to 20 to 50 clients would be exorbitant. Although the general reinforcement design of token economies is interval schedules, some provision is usually made for ratio schedules.

■ **Decreasing behavior**

Punishment and extinction are the operant procedures used to decrease behaviors. Most behaviorists do not recommend punishment except in situations in which the behavior is physically dangerous. There is no question about the effectiveness of punishment, there is question about the concomitant effects of punishment, and there are ethical considerations that do not make punishment a desirable treatment. A behaviorist is not likely to recommend hitting a child, except in situations in which his behavior must be immediately altered for his safety. If a young child, for example, runs into a busy street or picks up a sharp knife, the parent wants the child to immediately alter this behavior.

Extinction, withholding what was previously reinforcing an operant, is recommended while positive reinforcement is provided for an incompatible behavior. For example, a patient may, in verbal interactions, express a great number of nonsequential and nonsense remarks that make conversation impossible. The psychiatric nurse may note that typically when this happens the staff person comments on this to the patient and talks to him about the irrelevant material. She observes that this may well be reinforcing the nonsense talk and instructs all staff to ignore such statements, bring the conversation back to the topic at hand, and give the patient attention for attending to the topic. Extinction is being used for the irrelevant material, and positive reinforcement for relevant conversation. Whenever extinction is used, one should be careful to assure that reinforcement is given for a behavior that is incompatible with the one being treated by extinction.

Clinical case analysis

Clinical example 27-1 describes behavioral treatment initiated and carried out by a nurse.

The procedures used in this treatment were behavioral and included punishment, satiation behavior rehearsal, overt differential reinforcement, and covert positive reinforcement. The punishment was the "no" yelled at Joe as he opened the book of matches when the behavior rehearsal started. This punishment was almost immediately effective, having to be used only twice.

Satiation is what we experience when overdoing a good thing. We may frequent a favorite restaurant so often that we are tired of it or overindulge in a food until we do not want to see it again. This is satiation. There are theorists who assert that the effects of satiation are temporary. Satiation was certain to inhibit Joe's current interests in matches. The possibility that satiation's effects are temporary necessitated the development of the behavior rehearsal. In the behavior rehearsal Joe practiced an alternative response to matches, which could be reinforced. The practice response was incompatible with lighting a match; the reinforcement of this response was gradually altered from overt to covert so that it would not be dependent on others. The covert reinforcement was important also because Joe had played with matches and set the fires when he was alone. Future interest in match play and fire lighting would probably occur when Joe was alone. Having covert reinforcement in his repertoire would probably help him resist the enticement of returning to his former play with matches.

Ethical issues

Behavior modification intervention has raised many ethical issues. They are indeed issues that any therapeutic endeavor should raise, but the straight-forward assertion of behavior modifiers that they can change behavior has made them and their techniques the focal point of ethical considerations. In addition, behavior modification techniques can be applied to the environment and result in behavior change. Even as antithetical a treatment as psychoanalysis is described as successful or not by behavior change or the lack thereof. All psychiatric treatments that come to mind have at least a component of behavior change as their goal. Therefore

CLINICAL EXAMPLE 27-1

Joe, a 7-year-old child, was in serious jeopardy of being removed from his home because of his playing with matches and setting fires. It was agreed that treatment would be limited to 5 days from 9:30 AM to 12 PM and from 1 to 3 PM while the child continued to live at home. The boy had within the 2 years preceding treatment set three fires that caused damage, the last fire precipitating the referral. The mother and family were frightened but were not rejecting of the child.

Prior consultation and experience with a satiation procedure treatment suggested that intensive use of the procedure might be more effective than daily 1-hour sessions. The satiation procedure for fire setting involved the client lighting and blowing out matches one by one in a well-ventilated room in the presence of the therapist. The therapist supervised the activity, maintaining a minimum of verbal interaction, neither reinforcing nor punishing the child as he lit the matches. Records were kept of the endeavor.

On the first treatment day Joe lit matches during two sessions for a total of 4 hours. Over a thousand matches were lit and blown out during this time. The child's initial response to being allowed to light matches was surprise and some confusion. It was explained that it was all right for him to light the matches only in this particular room. His rate of lighting matches remained relatively constant. The mean number lit during intervals of 5 minutes was 34, the range from 22 to 45, the mode 34, and the median 33.

Observation of Joe outside the satiation sessions revealed how much he enjoyed being praised and hugged, as well as his affinity for all social contact. Joe initiated interpersonal interactions frequently, laughed and talked while playing with peers, and often sought physical affection from staff. These observations supplied data useful in Joe's subsequent treatment sessions.

On the second day Joe lit matches for only 55 minutes; the mean rate for a 5-minute interval dropped to 21, the range being 15 to 27, the mode 20, and the median 22. During this session Joe tried avoidance maneuvers, wanting to practice throwing matches away, and stating at least five times, "I don't want to strike more." Each time he made the statement he was told quietly, "Keep doing it." Finally, he stated firmly, "I ain't gonna strike no more" and walked away from the matches.

This was greeted with a hug and praise from the nurse and a discussion with him about alternative

Continued.

CLINICAL EXAMPLE 27-1—cont'd

treatment. Joe then identified, in response to questions, several areas in his home where he found matches. A book of matches was placed on the window, and Joe then rehearsed, both physically and verbally, finding the matches in a specific place at home. Initially he was not instructed what to do with the book of matches. After picking it up, he opened the book and the therapist immediately yelled, "No!" Joe replaced the matches, went through the rehearsal a second time, and the same sequence occurred. At the third rehearsal he was instructed to say aloud, "I'm not going to open up the matches" when he approached them. When he did so, he did not pick up the matches and was given a hug. Joe looked elated. His pleasure with himself increased as the rehearsals went on for over an hour and covered in his own imagery every place in his house where he could find matches.

Throughout the rehearsals several changes relating to his self-cueing and the reinforcers were gradually and progressively introduced. By the session's close, the self-cueing was inaudible and the reinforcing hug was being imagined each time he picked up and replaced a book of matches. Joe's facial expressions were so spontaneous and revealing that they left no doubt about his repeating the cue to himself and fantasizing the hugs.

These alterations were developed to increase the likelihood of Joe's continuing the behavior when not in the therapist's presence. The change from not picking up the book of matches to picking it up and replacing it was introduced to break the behavior chain of picking up matches, pulling out a match, and lighting it. It seemed important for Joe to realize that he could see and pick up matches without lighting them. Although not of major concern in comparison to fire setting, consideration was given to the possibility of the child developing a phobia of matches. A phobic response seemed more likely if he learned not to touch a book of matches. Being able to hold the matches and replace them made matches simply another object in his environment over which he had control.

On the following day, when Joe entered the room, the equipment for the satiation procedure was still in the room. Since Joe spent a few minutes looking at it, it was suggested to him that he again light the matches. Because the environmental conditions were vastly different from the previous day's rehearsal and because Joe's expression indicated a curiosity about lighting the matches, it was appropriate to continue the satiation.

The satiation session was 55 minutes long, 158 matches were lit. The 5-minute mean was 15, the range 0 to 25, the mode 20, and the median 15. During the last 10 minutes no matches were lit. There was also a qualitative difference in this session. After the first 5 minutes, during which Joe lit 25 matches, he was increasingly bored and disinterested.

The rehearsals were then started and Joe was again lively, spontaneous, and happy in his endeavor. The rehearsals were broadened to include areas outside his home where he might find matches. Joe and the therapist then went throughout the building, where he found and replaced many books of matches after the activity was explained to the occupant of each office. The social contacts, needless to say, were reinforcing to Joe, and he was lavished with encouragement and praise (perhaps too much) for his efforts.

During these rehearsals Joe was instructed to imagine his mother giving him a hug when he replaced the matches. Since it was his mother who would be giving him real hugs in the future, it would be easier over time for him to fantasize a hug from her. His image of the therapist would dim as the actual contact became a progressively distant memory.

On the final treatment day Joe showed no interest in the satiation equipment. Some time was spent on the rehearsals, but the major portion of the day Joe devoted to good-byes and playing with peers. The mother, who could not attend any of the sessions, was informed of the treatment and instructed to give Joe affection and praise periodically for not playing with matches. Phone contact with her was continued for 3 weeks. Follow-up contacts over a period of 2 years indicate that Joe has neither played with matches nor set fires since treatment.

it is not behavior change per se that has resulted in behavior modification being questioned on ethical grounds. It is that the behavior change can be effected by alterations of environmental responses to the behavior. The evocative psychotherapies seem to do so by working directly with the client, not the environment. Therefore it seems that the evocative psychotherapies alter nothing for a client without his direct cooperation and knowledge. The possibility of using behavioral techniques without such involvement necessitates special consideration.

The techniques that have been presented in this chapter are indeed effective, not always, not everywhere, but they are effective. The most basic issues related to them at present are the following: Does one human being have the right to control another? Who decides what the goals of treatment are? There are other issues also, such as obtaining client consent, guaranteeing basic human rights, weighing potential risks and benefits of treatment, evaluating treatment, and accountability for treatment.

The two major issues of control and goals of treatment will be explored. Control is a strong word—one that arouses fear in most people when they think they are being controlled by others. It arouses anger when people in power are seen to be abusing their power by controlling others. There is in this word a connotation of totality—a totality that allows no escape. It is this totality which worries people when they think there may be a behavioral technology that can control everyone. The strong public reaction to behavior modification indicates that most people do not believe that one human being has the right to control another. Whether the behavioral technology available at present can indeed allow control, even benign control, is not as central an issue as what individuals and society as a whole can do to protect themselves from being subjected to control and to what degree control should be allowed. In a society it seems to be expected that certain human behaviors be controlled. Some of these behaviors are murder, theft, assault, and property destruction. Laws are established to ensure compliance, and a judicial system is responsible for punishing the violators of the laws. Basically these laws state that a person may not abuse others or their property.

When one gets beyond these behaviors, the issues become less clear. What about emotional abuse: the way in which one slowly or quickly pecks away at another through ridicule, sarcasm, disapproval, or bitterness. Should this be controlled? Would a society in which people are encouraged, supported, openly disagreed with, and congratulated be preferred? Many people would prefer such a society, but few would want such

behaviors legislated or designed into the judicial system and controlled by a behavioral engineer. This is not desired even if it were possible because that would involve adding to the power of the government and behavioral engineer, and history documents how easily power is abused.

The fact that most behavior therapists have as their goal of treatment specific and limited behavioral change does not alter the fear that behavioral technology could, in the wrong hands, be abused. Such is the case in every scientific advance. Does this mean that it should not be used at all? Hardly. It means that one must use knowledge carefully and disseminate information about the technology as widely as possible so that use and abuse of the knowledge can be readily recognized. This is particularly helpful, since all people are affected by the reinforcers and punishments in the environment. As behavioral technology becomes more widely understood, this fear of control by others should decrease, because familiarity with it and its ensuing application increases each person's control of himself. It also becomes more evident that behavioral techniques indicate how one is influenced, not controlled, by the environment, and that influence allows for a wide range of choices.

The issue related to the specification of goals can be a complex one. Ideally the goals of treatment are the client's goals. In reality a client's goals may be at odds with those of the therapist and the first test of the therapist may then be to establish goals with which both the client and therapist can agree. An extreme example of conflicting goals could be seen in a parent asking that a behavioral therapist help design a program, the goal of which is silent sitting in a chair 4 hours a day by a 4-year-old child. No competent therapist could agree to such a goal. The therapist in such a situation may spend a great deal of time helping the parent establish more reasonable goals. The goal of the therapist during this time is the development of such reasonable parental goals. However, is this use of time unethical because it is clearly not the parent's goal? An immediate response is that this question is nonsensical; however, it points out that glibly recommending client input into goals is not as simple as it may appear. The client who is actively hallucinating or contentedly masturbating for hours on end may want nothing more than to remain in such a state. It is most unlikely that a therapist could share this same goal.

With these and other issues in mind it is possible to offer general guidelines for the ethical use of behavioral modification:

1. Treatment is to be preceded by informed con-

DIRECTIONS FOR FUTURE RESEARCH

1. Validate composites of behavior amenable to behavior treatment
2. Identify long-term outcomes of behaviorally oriented milieus versus psychodynamically oriented milieus
3. Describe various levels of behavioral treatment on inpatient units
4. Compare outcomes of patient-determined reinforcers versus staff-determined reinforcers
5. Identify results of behavioral treatment by diagnostic categories
6. Describe outcomes associated with teaching patients behavioral principles
7. Correlate noncontingent nursing behaviors with improved treatment effectiveness
8. Specify treatment goals that can be reached within specified inpatient length of stay (e.g., 30 days, 45 days, 60 days)
9. Describe reinforcers that staff inadvertently provide for maladaptive behaviors
10. Explore effective change mechanisms used by staff for eliminating inadvertent reinforcement of maladaptive patient behaviors
11. Report effects of nurse-monitored, but patient-initiated and patient-implemented behavioral self-treatment
12. Examine mother/child relationships in which prenatal teaching includes behavioral principles

sent; specification of procedure, goals, and measures to be taken; and client input.

2. Once begun, treatment should include an ongoing assessment of progress.
3. Before and during treatment the therapist should recognize that the treatment should be relevant to the client's adjustment to his natural environment.

Although these guidelines are not complete answers, they may help to prevent potential abuses of therapy and contribute to client growth, and these are worthwhile pursuits for all therapy modalities used by psychiatric nurses.

■ SUGGESTED CROSS-REFERENCES ■

Ethical decision making is discussed in Chapter 7. Child psychiatric nursing is discussed in Chapter 30.

■ SUMMARY ■

1. Behavior modification is the application of operant conditioning principles and procedures to human affairs. Operant conditioning is modification of the frequency of occurrence of a bit of behavior by the consequences of that behavior. Behavior modification is an effective treatment modality for alleviating many human problems, and it can be used by psychiatric nurses in many areas of their practice.

2. Behavior refers to everything a person does and is observable. Behavior may be defined in specific or general terms. Specific measurable definition facilitates behavior modification.

3. Behavior modification techniques may be applied to increase or decrease the occurrence of behavior. Positive reinforcement and negative reinforcement both maintain and increase behavior. Positive punishment, negative punishment, and extinction decrease behavior. Negative punishment includes response costs and time-out from reinforcement.

4. Reinforcement schedules may be based on fixed or variable intervals or fixed or variable ratios of reinforcement. Advantages and disadvantages of each were discussed. FR and VR schedules result in higher rates of responding and greater resistance to extinction than either FI or VI schedules.

5. An example was given of the use of behavior modification techniques by a nurse in therapy with a fire-setting child.

6. The techniques of behavior modification have raised many ethical issues. The two major issues of control and goals of treatment were explored. General guidelines for the ethical use of behavior modification were presented.

■ REFERENCES ■

1. Ayllon, T., and Azrin, N.: The measurement and reinforcement of behavior of psychotics, J. Exp. Anal. Behav. **8:**35, 1965.
2. Ayllon, T., and Azrin, N.: The token economy, New York, 1968, Appleton-Century-Crofts.
3. Ayllon, T., and Michael, J.: The psychiatric nurse as a behavioral engineer, J. Exp. Anal. Behav. **2:**323, 1959.
4. Barnard J., and Orlando, R.: Behavior modification: a bibliography, Nashville, Tenn., 1967, J.F.K. Center for Research on Education and Human Development.
5. Britt, M.: Bibliography of behavior modification, 1924–1975, 1975, privately printed by Dr. Britt, 3000 Erwen Rd., Durham, N.C. 27705.
6. Connelly, G.: New medicine or old tricks, Nursing Times **81:**41, Sept. 11, 1985.
7. Dossey, B.: A wonderful prerequisite, Nursing **14:**42, Jan. 1984.
8. Heide, F., and Borhovec, T.D.: Relaxation-induced anxiety: mechanisms and theoretical implications, Behav. Res. Ther. **22:**1, 1984.
9. Martin G., and Pear, J.: Behavior modification: what it is and how to do it, Englewood Cliffs, N.J., 1978, Prentice-Hall, Inc.

10. McEnany, G., and Tescher, B.: Contracting for care, J. Psychosoc. Nurs. Ment. Health Serv. **23**:11, Apr. 1985.
11. Mikulas, W.L.: Behavior modification, New York, 1978, Harper and Row, Publishers.
12. Reynolds, G.S.: A primer of operant condition, Glenview, Ill., 1968, Scott, Foresman and Co.
13. Skinner, B.F.: Science and human behavior, New York, 1953, The Free Press.

■ ANNOTATED SUGGESTED READINGS ■

Arkin, A.M., et al.: Behavior modification: present status in psychiatry, N.Y. State J. Med. **76**:190, Feb. 1976.

This article provides a comprehensive overview of the many issues related to behavior modification. The reader is introduced to the types of behavior modification approaches. Of particular significance is the discussion of ethical issues related to this therapeutic modality, particularly when aversive techniques are used.

Becker, W.C.: Parents are teachers: a child management program, Champaign, Ill., 1971, Research Press Co.

This book contains clear programmed instruction of behavioral techniques for use by parents.

Behavioral Disorders, Lancaster, Pa. Quarterly journal of the Council for Children with Behavioral Disorders.

Oriented toward special education teachers. Articles helpful for psychiatric nurses working with children and adolescents.

Behavior Modification, Beverly Hills, Calif., Sage Publication.

This interdisciplinary journal is published four times a year and prints research and clinical papers on applied behavior modification in a broad scope of settings.

Behavior Research and Therapy, Great Britain, Pergamon Press, Ltd.

This bimonthly, international, interdisciplinary journal publishes articles relating to the application of Behavior Theory to maladaptive behaviors.

*Berni, R., and Fordyce, W.E.: Behavior modification and the nursing process, ed. 2, St. Louis, 1977, The C.V. Mosby Co.

Particularly recommended is the chapter on ethical issues. The book is appropriate for all levels of nursing students.

Focus on Exceptional Children, Denver, Co.

Monthly publication addressed to those concerned with special education.

*Hauser, M.J.: Cognition commands change, J. Psychiatr. Nurs. **19**:19, Feb. 1981.

The author discusses cognitive models of behavioral change as they relate to work with disturbed children. The models presented include cognitive restructuring as exemplified by rational-emotive therapy, self-instruction, and problem solving. She also advocates teaching the treatment approach to parents. Cognitive restructuring and self-instruction are rather sophisticated methodologies that should only be implemented by nurses with advanced training in child psychiatric nursing.

Journal of Applied Behavior Analysis, Lawrence, Kan., Society for the Experimental Analysis of Behavior, Inc.

This quarterly journal reports primarily experimental research.

Journal of Behavior Therapy and Experimental Psychiatry, Great Britain, Pergamon Press, Ltd.

This quarterly journal publishes papers on behavior therapy and experimental psychiatry as well as some that are intended to assist nonbehaviorally educated clinicians.

Lazarus, A.A.: Multimodel behavior therapy: treating the "basic id." In Franks, M., and Wilson, G.T., editors: Annual review of behavior therapy theory and practice, New York, 1974, Brunner/Mazel, Inc.

This work is appropriate for graduate students. It assumes basic knowledge of behavioral principles and their application.

Mikulas, W.L.: Behavior modification, New York, 1976, Harper and Row, Publishers.

An overview of the whole field of behavior treatment is provided. This book is recommended to both undergraduate and graduate students.

*Peterson, K.A., and Erickson, E.A.: Use of reinforcement principles to reinstate self-care activities in a deaf and blind psychiatric patient, J. Psychiatr. Nurs. **15**:15, June 1977.

This is a good illustration of the application of behavior modification principles to the care of one patient who presented a particularly challenging constellation of nursing care problems. There is a detailed discussion of nursing intervention and patient response.

Reynolds, G.S.: A primer of operant condition, Glenview, Ill., 1968, Scott, Foresman and Co.

This excellent, basic, and brief text presents findings of behavioral laboratory experiments.

Skinner, B.F.: Science and human behavior, New York, 1953, The Free Press.

This is a basic reading in the area of behavior therapy. It is a "classic" in the field.

*Steckel, S.B.: Contracting with patient-selected reinforcers, Am. J. of Nurs. **80**:1597, 1980.

This article has value for nurses who are working in a variety of settings. The author describes her extensive experience with the use of performance contracts with patients who select their own reinforcements. A sample of a recommended contract is included.

---

*Asterisk indicates nursing reference.

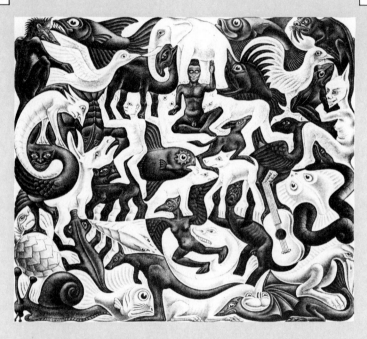

Self and world are correlated, and so are
individualization and participation . . .
Participation means: being a part of something from
which one is, at the same time, separated.

Paul Tillich, The Courage To Be

C H A P T E R   2 8

SMALL GROUPS AND THEIR THERAPEUTIC FORCES

KATHRYN G. GARDNER
PAULA C. LaSALLE

LEARNING OBJECTIVES

After studying this chapter, the student should be able to:

- define the group as a type of social system.

- compare and contrast the various types of groups, including identification of the nurse's role with each.

- identify and describe the two basic functions of groups.

- analyze group process in terms of the dynamic dimensions of communication, roles, norms, cohesion, and power.

- identify the four stages of group development.

- discuss the therapeutic aspects of group experiences.

- compare and contrast informal, therapeutic, and psychotherapeutic groups, describing indications for each and differentiating leadership roles.

- describe a variety of group psychotherapy models and theoretical frameworks.

- discuss the phases of development of a psychotherapy group, including therapist responsibilities and commonly encountered group behaviors.

- identify the need for nursing research relative to the therapeutic use of groups.

- identify directions for future nursing research.

- select appropriate readings for further study.

Groups play a powerful role in forming society's organizational structure, influencing social behaviors of individuals, and shaping individual identities. In the last few decades the potential and actual therapeutic force of groups has been increasingly recognized. At least since 1947 when Lewin[20] observed that individuals under certain conditions are influenced more easily in group rather than individual settings, groups have been more formally studied by many disciplines. From studies on groups some phenomena of groups have become clear. These phenomena have to do with the processes that occur in groups, the structure and common dimensions of small groups, and the therapeutic aspects of groups.

Historically, nursing has been relatively slow in realizing the implications of working with groups and studying groups. This slowness is partially because of the traditional model of acute care nursing, the emphasis on the one-to-one nurse-patient relationship, insufficient knowledge about groups, and, until recently, the lack of sufficient numbers of nurses educated and experienced in group work. However, in the last two decades several things have occurred that have fostered nurses' interest in group work. The concept of the therapeutic community, the community mental health movement, the emergence of self-help groups and ther-

apeutic groups, and the growing acceptance of group psychotherapy as a desirable treatment modality have kindled nurses' interest in groups. Additional factors that have enhanced group work in nursing have been the changing health care delivery patterns, the emphasis on preventive psychiatry, the increased amount of research in training and therapy groups, and health professionals' increased accountability to consumers and their representatives.

Diagnostically related groups (DRGs), a system of determination of insurance payment based on the diagnosis given to a patient, have influenced current nursing practice and have put great pressure on inpatient, transitional, and outpatient treatment facilities as well as private practitioners to provide cost-effective care.

The attendance in group therapies is one requirement for insurance reimbursement for psychiatric service. This requirement increases the need for accurate diagnosis and specific treatment objectives for patients in group therapy. Evaluation of outcomes and decisions regarding the diagnostic classification of patients increases the importance of nurses understanding and participating as an active member of the interdisciplinary team in the diagnosis, treatment, and evaluation of each patient. The specificity required to accomplish the above also is necessary for effective discharge planning. The type of treatment needed, who is to provide and evaluate it, and preparation for discharge itself are all within the nurses' range of responsibility.

The continued advances in the refinement and development of psychotropic medications make group treatment available to more people. The nurse-leader of group therapy has an essential responsibility to be aware of side effects of these medications as they might affect the behavior of individual group members.

Because of the increased numbers of elderly persons and the possibility that many patients will live longer, increased emphasis on psycho-gerontology programs is needed. Since the number of elderly patients can be expected to rise, the number of chronic patients needing treatment will also rise. More group treatments that involve long-term patients and that can be provided in community homes and day-treatment programs and by mobile group treatment teams that move from site to site will become necessary. The rise in elderly patients suggests the need for more teaching for family members who are trying to cope with aging loved ones.

All the above clearly indicate that psychiatric nurses need to be effective group leaders. From both the cost-effective and treatment points of view, group therapy skills must be an ongoing emphasis in nursing education, continuing education, and clinical supervision.

From 1960 to the present time nursing literature has increasingly described nursing interventions within small groups. By the 1970s, groups and therapeutic intervention in groups began to be a part of both the undergraduate and graduate curricula in nursing. In the 1980s nurses have begun to study the groups they lead.

In addition to the importance of groups in clinical work, the knowledge of the group process is critical in team practice, community work, supervision, and management. The nurse often uses knowledge of groups in working with colleagues and as a team member, team leader, and administrator. With the increased complexity of the health care system, it has become a necessity for nurses to be able to effectively participate in groups as a guest, member, and leader.

Groups as a potential therapeutic tool

To be consistently effective in therapeutic group work, one must have an understanding of some of the frequent and complex processes that occur in small groups and a knowledge of various approaches that use these processes to increase the therapeutic potential of the group for its members. This chapter will focus on these processes and approaches only as they relate to small groups. The study of processes and therapeutic techniques of large groups, such as ward or community meetings, is beyond the scope of this chapter.

■ Definition of group

The average size of a small group is six to twelve members. A basic definition of a group is that it is a collection of individuals who have a relationship with one another, are interdependent, and may share some common norms.[8] Thus the term "group" often refers to the interaction or relationship between three or more people. A group may be perceived as a separate entity or social system. As a separate system, it has its own structure and dimensions or properties. In other words, a group is not just a gathering together of three or more persons, but rather it is a separate entity that emerges only after the persons involved start interrelating with each other. As such, it is distinguishable from other groups within the environment and it has characteristics that differ from the sum total of all its parts.

Common dimensions in a group

■ Group functions

All groups have two basic needs or functions: the need to work on or complete a task or goal (there may be more than one), and the need to satisfy some psychosocial or emotional need or needs of its members. The latter function is sometimes called the group maintenance function.[28] If these two basic needs are not met, the group's effectiveness will decrease and the group may dissolve. The task or goal is usually one that connects the group to its external environment. The task of the group may or may not be well defined. The task of a group can be further divided into a primary task, which is necessary for the group's survival or existence, and secondary, or ancillary, tasks, consisting of those tasks which may enhance the group but are not basic to its survival.[25] An example of a primary task for a group of mothers might be to gain further mothering skills; a secondary task might be to improve the mother's social network. The psychosocial aspect of the group may either impede or enhance the group's accomplishment of its task.

■ Group structure

Group structure refers to the underlying order of the group. It describes the boundaries, communication and decision-making processes, and authority relationships in the group. The structure of the group offers it stability and helps to regulate behavioral and interactional patterns in the group. Structure describes the arrangement of the group similar to the arrangement of steps to a dance. Some of the major aspects of group structure, which will now be discussed, are communication, roles, and power. Attention will also be given to pragmatic considerations such as qualification for membership, where, when, and how long meetings are held, and handling of absenteeism.

■ Communication

The examination of communication patterns within the group is a common method used to study how a group approaches its task and psychosocial functions. Among the verbal and nonverbal aspects of the group's communication which can be observed are: (1) individual member communications, (2) spatial and seating arrangements, (3) common themes expressed by the group, (4) how frequently and to whom members communicate, (5) how members are listened to in the group, and (6) what problem-solving processes occur in the group. Through studying these aspects, an observer can note interpersonal conflict in the group, the roles assumed by some of the members, the level of competition in the group, and the degree to which the members understand and are working on the task.

One of the primary tasks of the group leader is to observe and analyze the communication patterns within the group. Utilizing feedback, the leader helps members become aware of the group dynamics and communication patterns so that they may realize the significance of these for the group and for them individually. The group or individual members may then experiment and may change these patterns if they choose to do so.

■ Role

In studying groups, it is important to observe what roles members assume in the group. Role is the position members assume in the group. Each role has certain expected behaviors and responsibilities.

The role a member of a group assumes can be determined by observing the communication and behavioral patterns of that member while in the group. The following factors influence role selection: personality structure of the individual, the group size, the group's tasks and their significance to a member, the interaction in the group, and the individual's position in the group. Benne and Sheats[4] catalogued three major kinds of roles individuals can play in groups: (1) group building or maintenance roles—concerned with the group processes and functions, (2) group task roles—concerned with completing the group's task, and (3) individual roles—not related to the group's tasks or maintenance and may be self-centered and distracting for the group. These roles are summarized in Table 28-1. A person in a maintenance role would, for example, be an individual who acts as a harmonizer and peace maker. An example of

TABLE 28-1

GROUP ROLES AND FUNCTIONS

Maintenance Roles	Function in Group
Encourager	To be positive influence on the group
Harmonizer	To make/keep peace
Compromiser	To minimize conflict by seeking alternatives
Gatekeeper	To determine level of group acceptance of individual members
Follower	To serve as interested audience
Rulemaker	To set standards for group behaviors (e.g., time, dress)
Problem-solver	To solve problems to allow group to continue its work

Task Roles	Function in Group
Leader	To set direction
Questioner	To clarify issues and information
Facilitator	To keep group focused
Summarizer	To state current position of the group
Evaluator	To assess performance of the group
Initiator	To begin group discussion

Individual Roles	Function for Individual
Victim	To deflect responsibility from self
Monopolizer	To actively seek control by incessant talking
Seductor	To maintain distance and gain personal attention
Mute	To passively seek control through silence
Complainer	To discourage positive work and ventilate anger
Truant/late comer	To invalidate significance of the group
Moralist	To serve as judge of right and wrong

Chart is extrapolated from structure provided by Benne, K.D., and Sheats, P.: J. Soc. Issues 4(2):41, 1948.

a person in a task role would be an individual who clarifies and seeks new information. The importance of group maintenance and task roles has been observed by Bales and Slater,[3] whose studies demonstrate that there is some evidence that groups encourage members to specialize in one of these two role functions.

Persons may experience a conflict when there is a discrepancy between the role they seek or assume and the role ascribed to them by the group. In addition to roles that members bring to the group, such as nurse or parent, there are group roles. For example, a member may assume and be given the role of the group historian. In this role the member may be encouraged by other members to reminisce important events in the group.

Lewin's analysis[20] of groups describes a role pertinent to all groups, the gatekeeper. The function of this role is to provide entry into the group. Health professionals often need to determine who occupies this role when they are trying to influence families and informal groups or other social support systems in the community. One way to determine the person who occupies this role is to ask the group with whom they prefer the outsider to talk. The person who occupies this role tries to maintain and strengthen the group in its interactions with the external world.

■ Power

All groups have a power structure or hierarchy. Power is the member's ability to influence the group and its other members. The power structure in the group is usually resolved in its initial stages. Power implies a reciprocal relationship. To be successful all members in a power structure must have their needs met. To determine the power various members have, it is helpful to assess which member(s) receive the most attention, which members are listened to most, and which members make decisions.

Resolution of the power struggle does not mean necessarily, however, that everyone will be satisfied with the arrangement. It is not uncommon for continual struggle for power to occur within the group. Such a struggle may be functional if the members are trying to attain new leadership which is more conducive to their therapeutic goals. It can also be dysfunctional in that it takes the energy and attention of the group away from other tasks.

■ Norms

Norms are standards of behavior that are adhered to by the group. They are statements (verbal or nonverbal) of the perceived expectations of how the group will react in the future based on the past and present experiences of the group. It is important to understand the norms of a group because they influence the quality of communication and interaction within the group. The observance of norms results in conforming. If a member does not follow the norms, he may be considered a deviant by the other group members. Groups differ in how much deviancy they will allow.

Norms may be expressed or communicated overtly or covertly. Overt expression of norms may be written or clearly stated. For example, members may clearly state to a new member that smoking is not allowed in the group. Covert expression of norms may be implied through the behaviors of members in the group, for example, a member who uses foul language may be ignored by the other members.

Norms are created to facilitate accomplishment of the group's goal(s) or tasks, control interpersonal conflict, interpret social reality, and foster group interdependence. An example of the importance of group norms is the influence of norms on health practices. For example, a family group may not eat meat and may bathe once a week.

■ Cohesion

Cohesiveness is the strength of the desire of the members to work together toward common goals and to support one another—the esprit de corps. It is related to the attraction to and the satisfaction derived from the group by each member. Cohesiveness is a basic fiber of any group because it is directly related to the life span and success of the group. It is the force that acts on members to remain in the group.[8] Since cohesion is such an important dimension, some group leader interventions are aimed toward promoting cohesiveness. The method to foster cohesion is application of communication theory, such as encouraging members to talk directly with each other, discussing the group in "we" terms, and encouraging all members to be in similar spatial arrangements, for example, not permitting some members to move their chairs away from the group. A leader can also foster cohesion by pointing out similarities among group members, assisting members in listening to each other, and encouraging cooperation among the members.

It must be noted that a highly cohesive group may have appropriate or inappropriate norms. For example, a group of patients may unite to help a patient sneak a cigarette when such behavior is contraindicated because of that patient's health problems. The group may also unite to do what it can to prevent that patient from smoking.

The group leader is continually concerned with the level of cohesiveness in the group. There are various ways to measure cohesiveness in a group. Group leaders might observe to what degree members express interest in each other and to what degree members recognize each other for their individuality. Another way to measure cohesion is to determine the degree of member identity with the group as a whole and the expression of members' desire to remain in the group.[8]

Many factors contribute to the level of cohesiveness in a group. Some of these are the agreement of members on group goals, interpersonal attractiveness between the members, degree to which the group satisfies individual needs, similarities among members, and satisfaction of members with the style of leadership. For a more detailed discussion on cohesiveness the reader is referred to *Group Dynamics: Research and Theory* by Cartwright and Zander.[8]

■ Group development

Another important factor that will influence a leader's behavior and determine the evaluation of the group's effectiveness is the developmental stage of the group. Groups, like individuals, have an innate capacity for growth and development. Likewise, they have an ability to regress and to resist working effectively. Many authors and researchers have studied phases or developments in groups. Small groups are recognized as having various definable stages of group development. Bennis and Sheppard[5] studied phases of group development in sensitivity groups and theorized that central concepts of group development are dependent and interdependent issues. They relied heavily on Freudian theory and viewed the issues of power, authority, and intimacy to be important to the group's life. Martin and Hill[24] studied the various phases of psychotherapy groups. The described six phases of group development, ranging from the individual's unshared behaviors in a derived structure to the individual's use of a group as an effective and creative problem-solving agent. Schutz[32] stated that every group developed according to three sequential interpersonal states: inclusion, or being "in or out"; control, or being "top or bottom"; and affection, or being "near or far." Each stage is characterized by members expressing various aspects of the same interpersonal issue or conflict. Tuckman[36] in discussing the development of the group, believed that any group is concerned with the completion of the task. He referred to the group structure as being the interpersonal relationships among the members and task activity as being the interactions directly related to the task. Tuckman summarized the various phases of group development as forming, storming, norming, and performing. These phases have been confirmed as occurring in at least one research study that observed groups in a classroom setting.[30] Table 28-2 summarizes Tuckman's categories and model.

Tuckman does not mention the termination phase. In a reclassification of Tuckman's theory of development, Lacoursiere (as cited by Dolgoff[13]) proposed that a mourning phase be added and combined in the norm-

TABLE 28-2

DEVELOPMENTAL PHASES IN SMALL GROUPS

Phases	Definition	Task activity	Interpersonal activity
Forming	Group members concerned with orientation	To identify task and boundaries regarding it	Relationships tested; interpersonal boundaries identified; dependent relationship with leaders, other group members, or preexisting standards established
Storming	Group members resistive to task and group influence	To respond emotionally to task	Intragroup conflict
Norming	Resistance to group overcome by members	To express intimate personal opinions around task	New roles adopted; new standards evolved in group feelings; cohesiveness developed
Performing	Creative problem solving done; solutions emerge	To direct group energy toward completion of task	Interpersonal structure of group becomes tool to achieve its task; roles become flexible and functional

Modified from Tuckman, B.: Psychol. Bull. **68:**384, 1967.

ing stage with the performing and storming phases. Termination occurs when the group dissolves because the task is accomplished. It may also occur when interpersonal issues prevent the group from accomplishing its task.

Group development does not occur in distinct phases. Phases may overlap each other, and a group may regress to a previous phase. For example, group regression can occur with the addition of a new member. Phases of group development can be thought of as a path that a group takes to form and accomplish its objectives. The leader's task is to understand and assist the group as it goes along its growth path. Examples of specific leadership behaviors will be noted later in the discussion of the leader's responsibility in therapy groups.

Therapeutic aspects of groups

Groups have the potential of being positive (constructive) or negative (destructive) forces. The history of civilization abounds with examples of both types of groups. Persons interested in behavioral sciences have begun to isolate some of the factors that occur in groups which influence their members. Nurses and other health providers need to understand how a group can exert influences on its members so that they may consciously use these forces to enhance or modify the effects on individuals in the group.

Dr. Irvin Yalom,[39] a group therapist, has clearly described some of the positive forces that occur in group therapy. Yalom listed eleven curative factors that may occur in every type of therapy group (Table 28-3). Yalom's curative factors do not occur in isolation from each other. Although these factors may be more pertinent to therapy groups, they are important factors to consider in all groups, especially those that have health-related goals for their members. In the last several years researchers have begun to study various groups for their curative factors. Because of the limited number of studies, no conclusions can be made at this point. However, several studies indicate that cohesiveness, catharsis, and interpersonal learning are rated by group therapy practitioners as the most important curative factors in their groups.[22]

In a study by Lieberman, Yalom, and Miles[21] on encounter groups, cognitive learning appeared to be the most important factor in differentiating those who learned from those who did not learn from the encounter group experience. Cognitive learning is the derivation of information or insight that is useful to oneself. Cognitive learning is a frequent activity that is used by many nurses working with groups. Examples of this are groups that have the learning about a condition or disease as a primary task. In this same study on encounter groups, four major leadership dimensions were identified: caring, emotional stimulation, meaning at-

---

TABLE 28-3

YALOM'S CURATIVE FACTORS

Factor	Definition
Imparting information	Receiving didactic information and advice
Instillation of hope	Increasing hopefulness of group members
Universality	Realization that others experience same thoughts, feelings, and problems
Altruism	Experience of sharing part of oneself to help another
Corrective reenactment of primary family group	Ability of members to alter learning experience previously obtained in their families
Development of social interaction techniques	Opportunity to increase one's awareness of social interactions and develop social skills
Imitative behaviors	Opportunities to increase skills by imitating behaviors of others in group
Interpersonal learning	Ability to engage in wider range of interpersonal exchanges, thereby increasing each member's understanding of responsibility and complexity of interpersonal relationships and decreasing member's interpersonal distortions
Existential factors	Ability of group to help members deal with meaning of their own existence
Catharsis	Opportunity to express feelings previously unexpressed
Group cohesion	Attraction of member for group and other members

Modified from Yalom, I.: The theory and practice of group psychotherapy, ed. 3, New York, 1985, Basic Books, Inc.

tribution, and executive functioning. Caring included warmth, affection, acceptance, encouragement, and communication of positive regard. Emotional stimulation was when the leader challenged and encouraged the revelation of feelings and personal values. Meaning attribution involved increasing cognitive dimensions, and executive functioning included limit setting and managing activities. In this study, the leaders who were rated most effective were high on caring and meaning attribution and moderate in emotional stimulation and executive functioning. Although, as of yet, these leadership dimensions have not been adequately studied in further encounter groups or other types of groups to be conclusive, they do offer a group leader a different way to think about leadership skills.

Groups commonly encountered in nursing practice

Many groups have therapeutic value for their members. Through belonging to a group, an individual's needs may be gratified and growth may be facilitated. Except for psychotherapy groups, most groups have not identified their primary task as the alleviation of emotional stress. However, the prevention and alleviation of emotional stress often becomes a secondary task of groups that have as one of their goals, or concerns, the promotion of health and adaptation of their members. The therapeutic impact of groups may occur spontaneously from an already formed group or when individuals form a special group because of their vulnerability, stress, and reactions to illness. These groups are in various phases of group development, have different primary tasks, and may or may not have designated leaders. Five common types of groups that either potentially or actually have therapeutic value for their members are the family group, informal group, sensitivity training group, therapeutic group, and psychotherapy group. An understanding of these five types of groups is essential to the practice of psychiatric nursing. Knowledge of individual behaviors in these groups can be used in any of the five components of the nursing process: data collection, nursing diagnosis, planning, implementation, and evaluation.

■ Family

The family is a specific kind of group, often called the primary group. A primary group fosters warm, intimate and personal relationships among its members.[28] Members of a primary group can exert great influence on each other. Often stress in one member of a primary group will cause stress in other members. Thus illness in one member of a family group is felt in some way by all members.[31] When a member of a family is ill,

nurses' use of the nursing process can assist families to optimize their therapeutic impact. Nurses can assess the amount of stress the individuals are experiencing, and, through a constructive use of themselves, they can intervene to decrease the stress. A common method of intervention employed by nurses is to use the curative factor of imparting information. A nurse will give information to a family regarding a patient's condition or treatment. Nurses have begun to research the relationship between family-oriented nursing interventions and the patient's rate of improvement and adaptation. For example, Eisenberg[15] studied the effects of nursing interventions with husbands of women undergoing mastectomies. This study compared the wives' perceptions of their adaptation to two different nursing approaches used with their husbands.

In another study[9] nurses were able to increase the recovery rate of patients after heart surgery by training their families how to do reality orientation and be reassuring to the family member immediately after surgery. This nursing intervention increased the families' therapeutic potential by decreasing the patients' post-surgical complications.

■ Informal groups

Informal groups are perhaps the most frequent type of group the nurse encounters. Although significant to nursing practice as a whole, they are especially significant to the practice of psychiatric nursing in a therapeutic environment or community. In a psychiatric ward setting the nurse's participation in informal groups can influence the therapeutic effectiveness of the environment. Likewise, observations of patient's participation in informal groups enhance the nursing assessment and nursing evaluation of the patient and the progress he has made.[17] An example of this is for the nurse to observe which patients tend to play cards with each other, or share snacks, or who join together to exclude a third person.

Another setting in which informal groups play an important role is the waiting room.[18] Depending on the nature of these groups, they may be more or less helpful and may align themselves with or oppose the health care staff. These groups usually form because the members share a common problem, need to communicate and share information, and need to be helped as well as to help. For example, families waiting for reports from the operating room may support one another and form an informal group. Each informal group will develop its own properties and culture and each has the potential of becoming a supportive group for its members.

Informal groups are groups that do not have a formalized structure and task and are often more spontaneous in nature than formal groups. Examples of these groups are various patient and staff groups that spontaneously form on a unit. Informal groups often consist of persons who are in some way interdependent and interrelated to each other. In organizations the presence of informal groups often supplements or counteracts the deficiencies of the formal group. Informal groups often improve and expedite information and communication processes. These groups may exert considerable influence among their memberships as well as on groups who interface with the informal group. For example, an informal group of patients may supplement or decrease the effectiveness of therapeutic interventions with a patient.

Because of the importance of the informal group, psychiatric nurses should consider nursing interventions with informal groups as essential. These groups provide a setting in which assessment of the patient's interpersonal communication and social skills can be done. The nurse, by participating in these groups, can use them to make effective and powerful therapeutic interventions. As participants, nurses should be aware of the group process, aware of their role as well as that of others in the group, and ready to capitalize on some of Yalom's curative factors.

Nurses can deliver many nursing services in an informal group setting, such as patient teaching and emotional support. Nurses may enter initially or join an already formed group, and in each case their behavior will partially determine the groups's therapeutic outcome. In joining informal groups, nurses must be prepared to be rejected at times by the members. The goals, roles, and norms of a group may not be enhanced by permitting a new member to join. When rejection occurs, the nurse would do well to consider the group's primary task and how she might facilitate or perhaps inhibit accomplishment of this task.

As time progresses, it has become more apparent that nursing intervention in informal groups is a skill necessary for the practice of psychiatric nursing and is increasingly useful in other areas of nursing practice. It is an area that warrants more critical study by the nursing profession. In the acute and community health care setting, informal groups of patients and families may influence the patient's compliance, self-esteem, satisfaction, and health outcome. Working with informal groups is a daily challenge. It requires that the nurse be astute in determining the tasks and roles of the various members, make quick assessments, and communicate clearly and honestly. In some respects all informal groups represent unharnessed energy of human beings who want to care for each other.

■ Sensitivity training groups

Although nurses without specialized preparation should not lead sensitivity training groups, nurses often participate in these groups to increase their understanding and effectiveness in group work. These groups are usually small, comprise eight to twelve members, and vary considerably in duration. The purposes of these groups are to increase self-awareness, increase an understanding of group processes, and/or increase an awareness of the effects of one's behavior in groups. These groups usually focus on present individual and group behaviors. Most sensitivity training groups will advocate a specific theoretical framework. These theoretical frameworks may range from being individual to being group oriented, and the interventions and techniques used by the leader may vary greatly. Some of these theoretical frameworks are that of the National Training Laboratory (NTL), which has the widest range of goals and leadership flexibility; the Tavistock model, which is mainly concerned with understanding the process of a group as a whole and the member's relationship to the leader; gestalt, which emphasizes awareness of the total person; and Esalen, which emphasizes the individual and interpersonal relations in the group. It is important before participating in a training group to know the leader's qualifications and the theoretical model that will be used. Participation in training groups is viewed by most group therapists as a valuable learning experience.

■ Therapeutic groups

Therapeutic groups are groups that have a broad goal of preventing emotional turmoil or disturbances. They are theme-centered and educational in nature. Their primary aim is to teach members to cope with emotional distress and to eliminate the sources of stress if possible.

Research on day treatment transition groups[14] emphasized the importance of "socialization and communication skills in a non-threatening peer group atmosphere." The frequent evaluation of patient's emotional functioning made timely intervention possible to prevent decompensation and rehospitalization. This supportive psychotherapy approach was used to attain the following goals: (1) decrease sense of isolation; (2) promote readjustment to outside including relationships with significant others, work, and community participation; and (3) enhance the skills of problem solving, socialization, and communication.

Two other current clinical research studies on the use of therapeutic groups evaluate the effectiveness of relaxation training for psychiatric outpatients[19] and the use of administering Prolixin conjointly with group therapy as compared to administering Prolixin by itself.[33] The use of a "Prolixin Group" in comparison to patients receiving neuroleptics in a variety of settings examined the rate of recidivism of group members. This study concluded that a Prolixin Group not only can reduce return to the hospital but is a cost-effective way to administer and monitor medication as well as offer therapy.

In the last decade nurses have become more involved in therapeutic group work and have begun to write about their effectiveness in these groups. Nurses have led therapeutic groups for parents whose children have a disease,[7,16] for patients who are coping with a disease or stress,[2,6,10] and for patients' spouses.[11] Because of the emphasis on prevention, these groups seem especially relevant to nurses in all health care settings, especially the community. For example, these groups are useful with schoolchildren who are coping with a problem such as obesity, parents who want to improve their parenting skills, the elderly to decrease social isolation, and families of the elderly in discussing coping with an aged parent.

Therapeutic groups, when possible, focus on the preparation of the individual for the next life stage. Preparation includes knowledge, such as daily living skills and discussion and improvement of coping mechanisms. When preparation is not possible (e.g., myocardial infarction patients), the focus is on adjustment, accurate information, and modification of daily behaviors and thinking patterns.

Patient and family education groups that focus on education, mutual support, problem identification, and problem solving may be conducted by the nurse therapist for the patient or the patient's family. Some examples of these groups include: significant others group for families of chronic psychiatric patients; medication group for people on psychotropic medications; grieving or losses groups; adult children of alcoholics; eating disorders group; stress management group; assertion training and conflict management groups. These groups have didactic as well as experiential segments. Participants are helped to develop skills and to apply the material learned to their lives. Role playing, audiovisual materials, homework assignments, bibliotherapy, and experiential exercises may be utilized to enhance the learning process.

The nurse needs to be an active member as well as a leader/facilitator for staff groups in organizations. Nurses are frequently involved in intense personal interactions with people in crisis and therefore require continued support, education, and supervision to maintain themselves personally and professionally. Staff groups may be effective in dealing with conflict on a nursing team, enhancing communication, seeking new options for behavior, consensus, and resolution. An interdisciplinary team which has experienced a mutual loss or success may benefit from a timely group experience as an opportunity to share their personal reaction to this event and enhance individual and group learning. For example, a staff group may discuss and work through their feelings about the death of a popular patient.

More recently nurses have written about groups in medical settings. According to the group's goals, they may be preparatory or adaptive groups. The preparatory group provides information in anticipation of the event, such as a preoperative surgical group. The adaptive group helps its members face an event, such as diagnosis. DeMocker[12] describes the following major helpful factors in nurse group care:

1. Providing information
2. Providing emotional catharsis
3. Sharing members' perceptions
4. Sharing feelings of fear, loneliness, and frustration
5. Improving interpersonal communication
6. Being in a helper role
7. Learning and rehearsing new skills
8. Providing role models
9. Helping to confront reality

All of these factors can be readily incorporated into Yalom's curative factors, but some of Yalom's factors are deleted in this list.

Most of the writing about these groups has been descriptive. There needs to be more systematic investigation of selection of members, leadership strategies, therapeutic interventions, and adequate measurement of therapeutic outcomes in these groups. Most of the nurse authors write enthusiastically about their perceptions of the therapeutic benefit of these groups, and there is little, if any, mention of negative aspects. The involvement of nurses in therapeutic groups seems to parallel or reflect the consumers' and nurses' increased attention to psychosocial factors in healing and health. Nurses, as demonstrated in the literature, have increasingly viewed leading or co-leading therapeutic groups as a part of their nursing practice, responsibility, and right.

The self-help group is another type of group that is often viewed as therapeutic to its members. The responsibilities of these groups lie within the membership. Professional persons, in their professional practice, are not directly involved with these groups. The extent of professional involvement is usually to refer members to a specific group or to act as a resource to the groups. Examples of self-help groups are Recovery Incorporated, Make Today Count, Alcoholics Anonymous, Weight Watchers, and colostomy groups. Self-help groups are usually formed around a specific problem or stress. Goals of these groups may include education about specific coping or adaptive techniques, suppression of harmful impulses that are related to a specific problem, and socialization. Some of these groups may be highly structured and have overt rules and norms. These groups often help and support their members with other social systems in their environment. They also instill hope in their members by giving new members successful role models.

In addition to these groups nurses have often led small groups for patients on inpatient psychiatric units. These groups often have the following goals: (1) resolving interpersonal issues that arise from living on inpatient units, (2) helping patients increase their problem-solving ability, (3) providing information, (4) helping patients gain or regain social interaction skills, (5) preventing maladaptive regression from occurring, and (6) helping patients to integrate back into their natural communities. These groups can often be a reflection of the larger treatment milieu. The group leader(s) must be aware of individual patient goals and approaches and significant events in the milieu. Because of the complexity of leading these groups, group leaders should always have adequate preparation for group leadership and have supervision or consultation available to them. Usually these groups will require the leaders to be more flexible in their activity structure and involvement than in other types of groups.

Psychotherapy groups

Group psychotherapy is the treatment of emotional stress and disorder through the means of a group method and group process. As treatment, the group psychotherapeutic processes are systematic, planned, goal oriented, and based on theoretical formulations. The therapist, on the basis of a theoretical framework, uses knowledge of group process to enhance the therapeutic effectiveness of the group.

Group therapy differs from individual therapy in several major ways. The most obvious difference is that the group itself is used as a treatment tool. Group therapy is effective in treating disturbances in interpersonal relations. A disadvantage of group therapy is that individuals may feel more frightened. In contrast to individual therapy, group members may feel more vulnerable and a higher sense of risk. Self-disclosure is usually viewed as being more difficult in a group setting. Compared to individual therapy, group therapy may not deal as effectively with in-depth material. Group therapy often allows for a corrective emotional experience that will facilitate a change in behavior. The therapist in group therapy is not as powerful as in individual therapy. Transference—the displacement of thoughts, wishes, and feelings from a significant person to another person—is more diluted in group therapy than in individual therapy. Group therapy allows for more reality testing than individual therapy. Some advantages of group therapy are that it allows for consensual validation, increases experiences in risk taking, and gives experiences of feeling mutually supported. An important element in all group therapy is that members feel a sense of belonging and thus feelings of isolation are decreased. Individuals learn that they may act as therapeutic agents for each other.

At this point there is no clear evidence establishing either the individual or group treatment modality as being more effective or superior. Both treatment modalities can be viewed as complementing each other. Recently there has been work on outcome studies involving specific patient populations, problems, and/or target complaints. In Parloff and Dies'[29] review of group therapy research literature, they reported that studies on schizophrenics, addicts, and offenders do not clearly endorse group therapy as the most effective independent treatment modality. However, many studies on group therapy have methodological problems and do not adequately describe the specific approaches and techniques used in treatment groups.[29] Thus before one draws conclusions about the effectiveness of group therapy, more specific research studies with better descriptions of the independent variables and designs are needed.

Group therapists are from the four disciplines that practice psychotherapy—psychiatry, psychology, social work, and nursing. Within these four disciplines, nursing has been the last to practice group therapy. Within the last decade there has been wide acceptance that nurses prepared with a master's degree in psychiatric—mental health nursing are able to practice effective group psychotherapy. The American Nurses' Association's *Statement on Psychiatric and Mental Health Nursing Practice* emphasizes that nurse therapists can use groups as a "primary treatment modality."[1] The development of group therapist skills requires specific and extensive preparation, usually including graduate study and several supervised clinical groups by qualified and experienced group therapists. A trained group therapist usually has a knowledge of dynamics of human behavior and psychopathology, has taken courses in group process and group therapy, participated in a sensitivity or encounter group, observed therapy groups, and conducted several supervised psychotherapy groups.

From the mid-1960s until the present time, some nurse authors have stated that nurses, regardless of formal education, who have the appropriate experience, knowledge, and personality are capable of doing group psychotherapy.[34] This position of the importance of experience, maturity, and knowledge over arbitrary educational criteria finds some support from authors in other health disciplines. Most nurse authors, however, suggest that nurses with less than a master's degree preparation should not do insight-oriented psychotherapy. As evidenced by the literature from 1965 until the present, nurses who are not clinically prepared at the master's degree level have functioned as group therapists for supportive therapy groups. At present there is no agreement as to what are the qualifications necessary to lead these supportive therapy groups. Nevertheless, this confusion should not be understood to mean that supportive groups are less complex or easier to lead than other therapy groups, but may indicate that these groups require a different kind of leadership skill.

■ Types of group psychotherapy

As already implied, a wide range of treatment techniques are used in group psychotherapy. Yalom[38] presents a clear concise description of a lower level psychotherapy group in his book, *Inpatient Group Psychotherapy*. This working model is useful to nurses because it includes specific recommendations for group size (4–7 members), patient selection criteria, and structural framework for this 45-minute group. The group, called a "focus group," has as one of its major goals to provide the lower functioning, frequently a psychotic, person with a successful low-anxiety group experience. Yalom specifically considers the role of the leader in focus groups.

He encourages overt positive reinforcement for minimal function, attention to maintenance of low levels of anxiety, and selective use of self-disclosure to enhance contributions of group members. He states that the goals of the leader of these groups must be sufficiently low to be attainable by members. Flexibility of the group leader is emphasized with consistency of leadership strongly recommended.

With the current emphasis on community psychiatry, models and techniques of group psychotherapy have expanded to accommodate more diverse populations. Group psychotherapy has become more acceptable and, in some situations, the preferred treatment. The various models of group psychotherapy can be best studied by considering them to be on a continuum, ranging from supportive to psychoanalytical group psychotherapy.

Marram[23] described the various groups on this continuum to be support, reeducation and remotivation, problem solving, insight without reconstruction, and personality reconstruction.

The first four groups described by Marram rely heavily on theoretical frameworks of ego psychology, learning theory, social psychology, and communication therapy. All these groups are concerned with increasing the members' adaptation, self-esteem, and state of emotional well-being. The goals of **support groups** are aimed at reinforcing the group members' healthier defensive operations. The focus of these groups is on what the members are experiencing presently in their lives and in the group. The interactions in the group are mainly at the conscious level. The therapist is usually active and keeps anxiety engendered by the group at a minimum level.

The **remotivation and reeducation groups** also may use behavior theory. Usually goals of these groups are to increase communication and interaction among members and to learn more socially appropriate and adaptive behaviors. These groups are frequently used for withdrawn, socially isolated, and institutionalized patients. Remotivation, or social skills, groups commonly use activities such as having coffee, going on a shopping trip, or doing an art project as a vehicle to motivate members' interaction with each other. In reeducation groups the therapist may act as a teacher. In these groups the therapist assists the patients to learn more adaptive and socially desirable behaviors. An example of a reeducation group is a group in which members learn social behaviors such as dining out.

Problem-solving groups focus on resolving specific problems that a patient may be experiencing. These groups assist the patient in better understanding the problem, suggest possible solutions, and evaluate the results of implementing a solution. These groups may be designed to focus either on one specific problem, such as admission or discharge, or on broader problems, such as those encountered while living in the hospital. The problem-solving technique is the main technique used by the therapist in these groups.

Insight-without-reconstruction groups emphasize interpersonal communication and psychodynamic theoretical frameworks. Group interventions are mainly focused at the conscious and preconscious levels. The group goals are aimed at alleviating emotional stress and effecting change by increasing an individual's cognitive and emotional understanding of his problems. Alternative ways of solving problems and behaving are explored. The interpersonal behaviors that occur among group members are studied and used to enhance their knowledge about themselves.[23]

Personality reconstruction groups actively use psychoanalytical theory and emphasize understanding unconscious materials. When appropriate, interpersonal concerns among members are worked through. These groups emphasize understanding the impact of former relationships on the present interpersonal concerns and conflicts. Dream analysis and free association may be used. Whereas some analysts emphasize the individual in the group, other therapists and analysts also work with the group process. The goals of these groups are for individuals to understand their personality and defensive structure and to modify behavioral patterns and defensive mechanisms.[23]

■ Theoretical frameworks of group psychotherapy

In leading a psychotherapy group, the therapist should act from a theoretical framework. The theoretical framework that is chosen serves as a guide to assess the group, determine the therapist's behaviors and interventions in the group, and evaluate the effectiveness of the therapeutic techniques employed. The theoretical frameworks of group therapy are mainly derived from various theories in psychiatry, such as psychoanalytical, interpersonal, and behavioral theory, and from social psychology. Differences in theoretical frameworks may range from emphasizing the individual in the group to emphasizing the group as a whole.

To enable the reader to grasp the various types of group psychotherapy theories that can be used, a few theories will be discussed briefly. However, to obtain a working knowledge of group psychotherapy theory, the reader must do further reading.

■ **FOCAL CONFLICT MODEL.** One theoretical framework that nurse therapists have found useful is Whitaker and Lieberman's Focal Conflict Model.[37] This model is based on the assumption that the therapist's primary interventions are at the group, rather than the individual level. This theory is based on the principle that therapy groups will develop unconscious conflicts that have meaning to all members. The conflict arises from the group experiencing simultaneously a wish (a disturbing motive) and a fear (a reactive motive). When confronted with such a conflict, the group seeks resolution that may alleviate the fear and/or, at the same time, gratify the wish. The therapist's task is to help the group to understand the conflict and to arrive at a successful solution. Successful solutions will be shared by all members of the group, will reduce reactive fears, and may also partially satisfy the wish.

An example of how this model may be used can be shown through the issue of a therapist's vacation. The disturbing motive or wish is to express anger at the therapist for taking a vacation; the fear or reactive motive is fear of retaliation if anger is expressed. For example, the group may fear the therapist will not return to the group after the vacation. A possible partially successful group solution to the conflict would be for all members to be silent about the therapist's vacation and instead discuss their own past vacations. A successful solution would be for the group to openly discuss their fears and anger regarding the therapist's vacation. The therapist could facilitate the group in arriving at this solution by giving the members permission to express their anger and fears and by demonstrating acceptance when the members discuss these fears.

■ **COMMUNICATION MODEL.** A communication model is another theoretical framework commonly used by nurses working in groups.[23] This model uses principles of communication theory and therapeutic communication. This model assumes that dysfunctional or ineffective communication in groups may lead to members' dissatisfaction, inadequate feedback, decrease in group cohesion, and further pathological problems. In using this model, the leader's interventions are aimed at facilitating efficient communication of group members. Through successful communication, individual members' problems and the group problems can be identified and solved, and successful feedback channels can be established.

Through the use of communication theory the leader can illustrate that (1) it is impossible for members not to communicate, (2) members must take responsibility for what they communicate, (3) communication is a phenomenon with many levels, such as verbal and nonverbal and overt and covert informational levels, (4) to be effective, a message must be understood by other members of the group, and (5) members can use communication theory to help each other communicate more effectively. An example of the application of communication theory is a therapy group that has the primary goal of helping members improve their social interactional and interpersonal skills. Communication theory is used in helping members to realize how they nonverbally communicate and in assisting them to practice different ways to communicate. One member of the group may learn that because she is always looking down, other members think she is disinterested in them. The group also learns to acknowledge a member's nonverbal communication (shaking); their concern can motivate her to describe what her shaking means (she feels anxious about being with new people). The leader in this group, when appropriate, briefly explains some principles of communication and illustrates how these principles can be used in the group. The leader uses interventions to model effective communication and utilizes Yalom's curative factor of imparting information. She also assists in the group in deciding when it is advantageous to analyze a specific message or communication sequence.

■ **INTERPERSONAL MODEL.** The interpersonal theory of interactional group theory is derived from Sullivan and the interpersonal school of psychiatry. In this theory therapists work on both the individual and group level. Group members learn by examining their transactions and feelings among themselves and between themselves and the therapist. Through this process members' disturbed perceptions are corrected and socially effective behaviors are learned. Feelings of anxiety and loneliness are focused on especially. The therapist presents herself as a humanist who is an expert in human relations.[35]

An example of the use of this theory is a women's therapy group in which the primary goal was for the members to improve their interpersonal relationships. When an interpersonal conflict occurred in the group, the leader used this situation to encourage members to discuss their feelings that were aroused by the conflict, to learn what in the conflict made the member or members involved feel anxious or emotionally distressed, and to determine the behaviors the members used to avoid or decrease the anxiety during the expression of the conflict. Through this learning, it was expected that members would be able to correct their previous maladaptive ways of relating and learn more adaptive behaviors.

■ **PSYCHODRAMA.** Psychodrama, which was introduced by Moreno,[26] is another form of group therapy that also requires specialized training. In this model, members are encouraged to act out immediate pressing or past life situations. Members in the group are structured and given temporary assigned roles, such as the audience, stage, protagonist (the patient selected to be the major subject for the specific enactment), auxiliary egos (the therapeutic actors to whom the protagonist is responding or reacting), director, and producer. Psychodrama is a therapeutic intervention based on spontaneity, reality testing, catharsis, and role reversal. Psychodrama allows members to act out specific situations, conflicts, or problems. One example of a situation enacted is a disagreement between a group member and his landlord regarding dissatisfaction with repairs that were made. The patient (protagonist) could play himself, and another member (auxiliary ego) would play the landlord. The group leader would direct the scene. As the script is acted out, the patient would gain further understanding of himself and his behavior during the disagreement. This understanding would also increase when other members (the audience) give feedback to the patient. At another time the roles of the patient and the landlord might be reversed. The role reversal would facilitate the patient's understanding the landlord's predicament and how the patient might communicate more effectively. Additional information about psychodrama is presented in Chapter 24.

In addition to these group theories, there are many other theories that can be employed in group therapy. Specific theories, such as transactional analysis, behavior therapy, and gestalt therapy have gained acceptance in group work. These theories use specific techniques, games, and rules. References about these theories can be found in this chapter's annotated suggested readings.

As stated before, many other theories can be used by the group therapist. Some group therapists use an eclectic theoretical approach and technique with groups. What is most important is that the therapist be well versed in the theories and techniques that she uses in group work and that they are chosen appropriately.

Responsibilities of leaders in group psychotherapy

Nurse therapists or leaders in therapy groups must be concerned about many factors regarding the group. Some of these factors are the manner in which the group is working toward achieving its goal or goals; the relationship of the individual members to the group; the anxiety level of individual members; the anxiety level in the group as a whole; the amount of cohesiveness in the group; the process, including communication and behaviors that occur in the group; and the leader's reaction to the group. Thus the group leader must be able to study the group and interact in the group at the same time. The leader is constantly monitoring the group and is, whenever necessary, ready to help the group toward achieving its goals.

To aid in understanding some of the many responsibilities of group therapists, the task of a group therapist will be described fully in the following discussion of the developmental sequence of a therapy group. From this discussion, the reader should not conclude that all therapy groups and all therapists function in the same way. Some groups, by decision or default, do not progress through these developmental stages, and the leaders' techniques and styles vary according to their personalities, beliefs, and their goals for their group. The principles outlined for leadership behavior will be generalized and may usually be used for therapeutic and psychotherapy groups.

■ Pregroup phase

The first task is to determine if the group will have one therapist or co-therapists or co-leaders. Co-leadership exists when there are two or more designated leaders for the same group. Co-leadership provides an opportunity for peer feedback and growth. Co-leadership facilitates members' work by increasing the possible assessments and areas to be covered in their analysis of the group, and, in some cases, allows for the reenactment of the primary or family group. If co-therapy is chosen, the nature of the co-therapy relationship must be identified. For example, co-therapists may choose to be equal partners, focus on different areas, or have a junior-senior relationship. Throughout the working relationship, conflicts between the co-therapists must be quickly resolved or usually they will be mirrored or reflected in the group. Co-leaders need to be aware of why they want to work with each other, allow for flexibility, be able to give and receive both positive and negative feedback, and plan sufficient time to become comfortable with each other and their respective leadership styles.

The most important factor to consider in starting a group is its goal or goals. The purpose of the group will greatly influence many of the leadership behaviors in the life of the group. There may be more than one group goal, and, if so, the primary goal should be clearly identified. To guarantee the success of the group, the goals of the group must be clearly understood by all persons involved, including the members and the agencies that sponsor the group. An essential task of the leader in the life of the group is to clarify and assist the group in achieving its purpose.

Once the purpose is established, the leader must be certain that administrative permission is given to have the group. A written group proposal is one effective way to discuss the group with the administration. A guide of what to include in a group proposal is shown in the accompanying box. To avoid possible future problems, the therapist should determine if there are any administrative limitations imposed on her in leading the group. For example, an agency may not want a group to meet beyond its physical facilities or may prefer that the therapist not use certain techniques in the group. Also, any financial cost factors to the agency should be clearly identified.

The leader is also responsible for obtaining the physical space for the group. In choosing a room, the leader should identify the room requirements in relationship to the purpose of the group. For example, in a therapeutic group that has didactic teaching, educational resources such as a blackboard or movie projector or screen may be needed. Likewise, in a psychotherapy group, space may be needed for comfortable chairs to

---

Group Proposal Guideline

1. List the group goal(s).
   a. Primary goal
   b. Secondary goal
2. List group leader(s) and their related expertise.
3. List theoretical framework(s) utilized by the leader(s) to meet the group goals.
4. List criteria for membership.
5. Describe the referral and screening process.
6. Describe the structure of the group.
   a. Meeting place _____
   b. Meeting time _____
   c. Length of each meeting _____
   d. Number of members _____
   e. Length of group _____
   f. Expected member behaviors _____
   g. Expected leader(s) behaviors _____
7. Describe the evaluation process for members and the group.
8. Describe resources needed for the group, such as coffee, a movie projector, or audiovisual equipment.
9. If pertinent, describe the expected cost and financial benefits incurred by the group.

be placed in a circle without a table. In a group that plans to use human relations exercises, a more spacious room will probably be needed. In all cases the room in which the group meets should be comfortable, private, and free from intrusive noises and interruptions. The room selected should remain consistent throughout the duration of the group. Leaders often have to adapt inadequate space to fit the needs of the group. It is more important that the group be conducted than where it is conducted.

The next step usually undertaken by the group therapist is to select patients or members for the group. The therapist develops selection criteria based on purposes of the group, solicits referrals to the group, and, ordinarily, interviews members to determine their appropriateness for the group. In obtaining individuals to be screened for the group, the therapist and/or the agencies must provide information to selected persons or groups about the group. All information given should clearly identify the purpose of the group, some broad criteria of membership eligibility, and the time, place, and duration of the group. The therapists' names and the appropriate professional credentials should be stated also.

The selection of patients or members of the group is one of the most important tasks of the therapist, because the composition of the group will greatly influence its outcome. In selecting members of the group, the leader should determine which variables will foster group cohesion and therapeutic problem solving. Generally, selection criteria should be based on both heterogeneous and homogeneous patient or member variables. Homogeneous variables will increase attractiveness to the group. Examples of possible homogeneous variables are individual adaptation styles, age, and education levels. Yalom[39] advocates that the therapist use cohesiveness as a primary guide for selection of patients for therapy groups and that heterogeneous factors be chosen from demographic variation. Selection criteria to be considered by the therapist include problem areas, motivation, age, sex, cultural factors, educational level, socioeconomic level, ability to communicate, intelligence, and coping and defensive styles.

If possible, the therapist should choose whether the membership of the group will be closed or open before she screens members for the group. A group is closed if no new members are added once the group is started. In an open group, members leave and new members are added throughout the duration of the group. Open-ended groups may maintain the same purpose, with both members and leaders changing. They usually continue indefinitely and have no termination date for the group as as whole. The closed group offers the advantage of consistency of leadership, norms, and expecta-

tions. The open group, on the other hand, continually brings fresh ideas and opportunities for learning to its members.

The screening interview's primary purpose is for the therapist and patient to determine the appropriateness of the potential member to the group. Many secondary purposes are simultaneously accomplished during the screening interview:

1. To begin to develop a relationship between the therapist and the member
2. To determine the motivation of the possible member
3. To determine if the candidate's goal or goals are in agreement with the group goals
4. To educate the candidate about the nature of the group
5. To determine the kind of group experience the individual has had
6. If appropriate, to begin to review the group contract

In addition to or replacing the screening interview, some clinicians use a group intake. A group intake is when several new members meet in a group for one to three sessions to learn about the group psychotherapy process and identify some possible treatment goals. This approach is less costly and has the same objectives as the screening interview.

As soon as possible a decision should be made about group membership. If a person is not selected for a group, other possible treatment should be made available to him, and he should be told the reasons for not being selected. If it is appropriate, the referring person should also be given these reasons.

■ Initial phase

The initial phase is comprised of those meetings in a new group in which the group's members begin to "settle down" to work. This phase is characterized by anxiety regarding inclusion (being accepted by the group), the setting of norms, and the casting of various roles. Curative factors such as catharsis and universality begin to operate in this phase but become more influential in other phases. This phase has been subdivided into three stages by Yalom[39]: the orientation, conflict, and cohesive stages. The stages correspond to Tuckman's first three stages of group development.

■ **ORIENTATION STAGE.** During the first stage of this phase the therapist is more directive and active than in other stages. Two tasks of the therapist in this stage are to orient the group to its primary task and to assist the group in arriving at a group contract. Some common factors that therapists may include in the group contract are goals of the group, confidentiality, meeting times, honesty, structure of the group, and communication rules (e.g., only one person may talk at a time). Since an important part of this phase is norm setting, the therapist should actively see that the norms set by the group will facilitate the group's achieving its primary and secondary tasks. Another task of the therapist in this stage is to foster attractiveness or cohesion among the members. In fulfilling this task, the therapist encourages interaction among members and maintains the group at a working level of anxiety. For example, the therapist could state that the group is "our" group and can suggest how group members help each other. One method would encourage members to state what they hope to learn from the group. The therapist would then reinforce the expectations that are realistic for the group to accomplish and give examples of how the group might meet these expectations.

During the first stage the members are evaluating each other, the group, and the therapist. In this evaluation process they are deciding if they are going to be in or out of the group and are determining what their level of participation in the group will be. Some common conscious or unconscious fears or concerns of members during this stage are the fear of being rejected, fear of self-disclosure, and fear of not being seen as an individual. Social amenities are important, and the members are searching and attempting to develop their social roles. The roles members assume during this stage are often renegotiated during other stages. The group, at this time, is a dependent one and frequently members will test out their dependency needs and wishes on the leader. Members look to the leader for stucture, approval, and acceptance, and they may try to please the leader with reward-seeking behaviors. The leader, in not gratifying all the dependency wishes of the members and by encouraging members to interact more with one another, supports group members in becoming more interdependent on each other and less dependent on the leader. The dependency issue between the leader and the members may lead the group into conflict and thus into the second stage.

■ **CONFLICT STAGE.** This stage of the group corresponds to Tuckman's storming stage of group development. Issues related to control, power, and authority become of prime importance. Members are concerned about the "pecking order" or determination of who is "top or bottom" in regard to issues related to control and decision making.[32] The dependency conflict may be openly or covertly expressed, with members being polarized between independent and dependent issues. Bennis and Sheppard[5] describe this stage as being a struggle between the counterdependent and dependent mem-

bers, with the counterdependent members waiting to assume the leader's role. An example of this phase would be a group that was divided over the issue of whether they could telephone each other. Some members wanted the leader to give them the correct answer, whereas others thought that the leader's statements were irrelevant and not helpful. During this phase the counterdependent members might sit in the leader's chair and let the leader know her directions have been unsuccessful or unheard. The dependent members could ask the leader for more directions. Other members who are neutral (neither dependent nor counterdependent) eventually may assist the group in resolving this conflict.

Subgroups usually form within the group and hostility is expressed. Often the hostility is directed toward the leader, but it may also be expressed toward other members. The therapist's tasks are to allow for the expression of both negative and positive feelings, to help the group to understand the underlying conflict, and to prevent and/or examine nonproductive behaviors such as scapegoating. This phase is usually the most difficult for the new therapist, because some members in the group may lead the therapist to believe she has failed the group by not living up to its unrealistic expectations. Yalom[39] described some reasons that commonly lead certain members to express resentment toward the leader: the member's awareness of the therapist's limitations, the therapist not fulfilling a "traditional leader" role, and awareness that the therapist will not give each member a favorite standing.

The therapist must be careful not to avoid or suppress the group members' anxiety and, at times, should encourage the group to express its hostility. If hostility toward the therapist is expressed indirectly, such as anger toward other authority figures (staff members, teachers, parents), the therapist should assist the group in expressing its anger more directly. A useful technique is for the therapist to give the group permission to discuss its anger, which she may do by expressing the possibility to the group that it may be disappointed or angry at the leader.

By the end of this stage the therapist may be dethroned and her omnipotent role with its magical solutions may be discarded. Slowly the therapist becomes humanized. Members learn that responsibilities for the group are shared and are not only invested in the leader. Members may also learn that expressions of anger and disappointment do not destroy the leader and may assist the group to more accurately assess its resources and limitations. The resources of the group can then be used to facilitate the group in achieving its primary and secondary tasks. Members of the group may realize that conflicts need not be avoided and, instead, through discussion, may serve to increase the group's maturity and usefulness.

■ **COHESIVE STAGE.** Tuckman's norming phase is closely related to this stage. Group members, after resolving the conflicts in the second stage, feel a strong attractiveness toward one another and a high attachment to the group. Expressions of positive feelings toward one another and toward the group are frequently verbalized and expressions of negative feelings are usually suppressed.

Members of the group feel free to give self-disclosing information and share more intimate concerns with one another. However, the group's problem-solving ability is restricted in that negative feedback and communication is usually avoided in order not to decrease the high group morale. The therapist's task is to facilitate the group in further exploring the members' disclosures in relationship to the primary task of the group. The therapist while not hindering the basic cohesiveness of the group, should encourage the group to eventually use its problem-solving ability. Through this behavior, the therapist role models how a group member can have individual concerns and values and still be a productive member of the group. In other words, the therapist demonstrates that differing and opposite opinions may not destroy the group identity.

At the resolution of this stage, members may learn that self-discoveries and differences should not be feared. They also learn that similarities and differences between the group members may help the group to achieve its tasks. At the end of this stage, task achievement is begun to be seen by the group as a reality. The group gains a more realistic and honest view of its ability to work together and accomplish its primary and secondary tasks.

■ **Working phase of the group**

The working phase of a group can be compared with Tuckman's performing stage of group development. During this stage the group becomes a team. It directs its energy mainly toward completion of its tasks. Although they are hard at work, this phase is an enjoyable one for both the leader and members. Responsibility for the group is more equally shared, anxiety is usually decreased and is tolerated better than in the previous phases, and the group is more stable and realistic.

In a psychotherapy group, members begin seriously to work through their concerns related to their therapeutic goals, which were identified during the pregroup and initial phases. They begin to do a more in-depth exploration of the various goals related to the tasks of their group. For example, in a psychotherapeutic group

for mothers with chronically ill children, the members may discuss their various reactions to the children, their ambivalent feelings, some of their thoughts regarding the reason for their feelings, and various alternative ways to cope with their present daily realities.

The major role of the leader is to facilitate the group's completing its task or tasks. This is accomplished by maximizing the group's effective use of its curative properties. Because the group members are fully participating in the work of the group, the therapist's activity level decreases in this phase. The leader now acts more like a consultant to the group. The leader helps to keep the group on its proper course and, if possible, tries to decrease the impact of any factors that may regress or retard the group.

Because this phase is mainly characterized as the group's creative problem-solving and resolution phase, there are few, if any, specific guidelines for the leader. The leader's interventions are mainly based on her theoretical frameworks, experiences, personality, intuition, and needs of the group and its members. In addition to monitoring the group's maintenance function through fostering group cohesion, maintaining its boundaries, and encouraging the group to work on the group tasks, the leader's interventions may be directed toward helping the group solve specific problems. Because these problems are unique to the group, many of them are not universally predictable. Some of the more common problems identified by Yalom are[39]: the formation of subgroups, the management of conflict, and determination of the optimal level of self-disclosure.

Subgroups that conflict with the goals of the group and are not acknowledged by the group are restrictive to its work. Other members of the group may feel excluded, and loyalties will be divided between the subgroup and the group as a whole. For example, in a women's group, two of the members become close friends. They keep secrets from the group and engage in many private conversations during the group session. Other members feel excluded from this dyad and are ineffective in working with them. To decrease the negative impact of a subgroup, the consequences and reactions of the subgroup should be openly discussed by the group.

Conflict is unavoidable and can be used to foster group and individual growth. However, at some time the expressions of conflict need to be controlled so that their intensity does not exceed the group's tolerance. Examples of conflict are competition among members for the leader's attention and a disagreement between two members of a group. Some ways a leader may manage conflicts are acknowledgment that the conflict does exist, expression of the value that conflicts are natural occurrences and can be growth producing, encouragement of members to discuss the reasons behind the conflict, and thorough discussion by members giving feedback to each other. The tolerance for successful conflict resolution is related to the amount of group cohesiveness, trust, and acceptance felt by the members.

The amount of self-disclosure is usually related to the amount of acceptance and trust the discloser feels. Self-disclosure is always risky. If a person gives pertinent or private information too quickly, he will feel vulnerable and perhaps untrusted. Likewise, during the working phase if a person discloses too little, he may be ineffective in forming interpersonal relationships; thus his growth potential in the group may be decreased.

Resistance, or the forestalling of the therapeutic process, is one form of behavior that can be expected in therapy groups. Resistance to working on the therapeutic goal can occur at both an individual and group level. For both the individual and group, it is one matter to agree on the therapeutic goals and another to work on obtaining the actual therapeutic outcomes. Resistance by individual members may take many forms, such as avoiding discussion of a conflict area, frequent or prolonged silences, attempting to become an assistant therapist, absence of members, pairing between two members, and prolonged expression of hostility. Resistance by the group or a majority of group members also takes on many forms, some of which are similar to the previously mentioned ones. Other examples of group resistance include shared silence among the members, unusual amounts of dependency toward the leader, an unusual amount of hostility in the group, scapegoating, subgroup formations, and the wish for magical solutions to resolve the group conflict. Resistance can be perceived as occurring because of individuals' or group's increased anxiety, which is experienced around conflict or change. The managment of resistance depends on the type of psychotherapy group, the group contract, and the therapist's theoretical framework. Some ways resistance can be decreased by the therapist are to make observations regarding the group process or individual behaviors, offer interpretations, counteract the resistant behavior, and demonstrate more adaptive behavioral patterns.

By the end of the second phase, members have learned that they, at least partially, have achieved their goals and hopefully have a sense of their own productiveness and accomplishments. The need for the group or their involvement in the group has become less apparent. The group or members of the group must begin to deal more actively with its final task—separation.

■ Termination phase

The work of termination begins during the first phase of every group. However, as the group or members of the group approach termination, certain processes are more likely to occur. The termination phase is not always discussed as a definite phase in the literature on groups. However, it is discussed as a separate phase here because of the significance that termination may have for the members.

There are two types of termination: termination of the group as a whole and termination of individual members of a group. A closed group usually terminates as an entire group; in an open group, members (and perhaps the therapist) terminate separately. Members and groups may terminate prematurely, unsuccessfully, or successfully.

Termination is a highly individualized process. Individuals and groups will terminate in ways that are unique to themselves. If the group has been successful, termination is a painful process. Termination may often cause the group to experience increased anxiety, regression, or a feeling of accomplishment. To permit members to avoid this subject would be the same as preventing individuals from having a possible successful growth experience. Useful or common behaviors used by therapists are to encourage an evaluation of the group or its terminating members, reminisce about important events that occurred in the history of the group, and encourage members to give feedback to each other. An evaluation usually is restricted to the achievement or lack of achievement of the group's or the individual's goals. The therapist must be careful not to collude with members in denying termination; rather, the leader must encourage termination to be fully discussed. Termination should be talked about several sessions prior to the actual "last" session to allow members time to work with issues that surface during the discussion. Termination may lead to the discussion of many related topics such as other separations, death, aging, and the use and passage of time. Members, if terminated successfully, may eventually feel a sense of resolution about the group experience and may use their experiences obtained in the group in many of their other encounters in life.

■ Evaluation of the group

Evaluation of the group and the progress of individual members in the group is an ongoing process that begins in the selection interview of possible group members. Most clinicians use record-keeping mechanisms as a way to remember the critical events in the group. These records can later be used to evaluate the group from a descriptive point of view. To make record keeping easy it is usually helpful to have a "group notebook." In this notebook leaders can write pertinent data on individual members, such as their group goals, their telephone numbers(s), their addresses, the screening note, any individual comments, and a termination summary note. In another section of the group notebook, the leaders can describe each group meeting. One suggested format on how to quickly record each group meeting is given in the accompanying box.

In addition to these measures, it is sometimes helpful to determine each individual member's goal attainment. This can be done using subjective ratings by the group leaders, or obtaining an individual member's perceptions on how they are meeting their goals. A slightly more objective evaluation is to write the members' goals down and ask them to rate their goal achievement on a Likert scale. The evaluation of members' goal achievement should always be done at termination, and, depending on the nature and length of the group, it may be done on a regular interview basis.

In addition to the descriptive evaluation, the clinician may decide to administer a before and after group paper and pencil test(s). The test(s) selected should be congruent with the expected changes in the group. For example, an anxiety scale could be administered to members attending a group whose major goal is to reduce anxiety. If this type of evaluation is used, it is critical that the clinician use the most appropriate scale available and that the agency and the patients' permissions are obtained. It is paramount that all parties involved know the intent of using such test(s) and the disposition of test results.

Future role of nurses in group work

In the last decade nurses have increasingly become aware of the therapeutic potential of groups and have begun to incorporate group work in their practice. Yet, if literature is an accurate reflection of the past, nurses have not yet fully incorporated group work in their practice. As observed by Nakagawa,[27] in the early 1970s nurses began to agree that nurses with advanced preparation did group therapy. Nurses mainly focused on the neglected or chronically mentally ill patient in the early 1970s. Examples of patient populations in which nurses practice as group therapists are geriatric patients, chronically schizophrenic patients, and chronically hospitalized patients. However, by the late 1970s nurses began to write about their group work with different populations, including crisis groups, groups for the acutely ill patient, and family groups. As reflected in the

---

Group Session Note Outline

Date _____ Group Meeting No. _____
1. Membership:
   a. List members attending (state if new member).
   b. List members who were late.
   c. List absent members.
2. List individual members' pertinent issues or behaviors discussed in the group.
3. List group themes.
4. Identify important group process issues (such as developmental stage, roles, norms).
5. Identify any critical leadership strategy used.
6. List proposed future leadership strategies.
7. Predict member and group responses for the next session.

---

literature, nurses, like other health professionals, have recently placed more expectations on themselves in describing and evaluating their clinical work in groups.

Psychiatric nurses have been slow to view themselves as group psychotherapists. As compared to their role as individual and family therapists, their ability to work in insight-oriented group psychotherapy has only begun to be adequately illustrated in the literature. As nurses and other professionals increase their understanding of the usefulness and effectiveness of group work, they become more accurate in documenting their skills and techniques and in evaluating the treatment outcome. Only then can concepts that are systematically applicable to nursing practice in groups be taught and studied.

It is expected that pressures for nurses to work with more groups will come from within and without the nursing profession. The increasing cost of health care, the amount of stress in our society, the awareness of the benefits of primary prevention, and the increased awareness of the effectiveness of groups are all bound to increase nurses' incentives to work with groups. As nurses gain more experience in group work, they are also bound to influence the profession internally. Within the next decade it is hoped and expected that nurses will describe their work with groups in a wider population and will scientifically document these skills and the resulting patient outcome behaviors.

Exclusive of psychotherapy, there are several exciting areas of group work for nurses. The first is work with informal groups. Nurses in acute health care settings have first-hand knowledge of patients' daily experiences and can easily interact with those patients in informal settings. Nurses have not yet fully realized the possibilities for nursing assessments and interventions in informal groups. Once nursing intervention in informal groups is understood, these interventions will need to be studied in relationship to outcome. The second area in which nurses should expand their group practice is with therapeutic groups. Nurses may make a special contribution in therapeutic groups that focus on coping with illness and on situational or developmental crises. A third area in which nurses can utilize their group skills is within their work group. Working with other nurses, as well as other professionals, often requires that the nurses be comfortable in group situations and can utilize the group process to assist the group in accomplishing its task. Without knowledge of group process issues, the nurse may be more likely to avoid identifying some helpful or destructive group behaviors. How nurses behave in groups of health team members warrants further study.

In the 1970s nurses had just begun to use group skills in their practice. It is expected that work with groups will expand nurses' effectiveness in at least the cognitive, psychological, and sociological aspects of their practice. Working with groups, similar to working in a one-to-one nurse-patient relationship, will become as essential part of the science and art of nursing practice.

The emphasis in the 1980s and 1990s needs to be on not only therapeutic effectiveness but also cost effectiveness—on efficiency and evaluation of group as a treatment modality. These directions necessitate greater knowledge of training methods and of clearly defined treatment objectives within short-term modalities. Transition, long-term, and educational groups need to be examined for their effectiveness. Delivery systems (who, where, how, when) for these groups need to be compared and evaluated.

◼ SUGGESTED CROSS-REFERENCES ◼

Working with groups in promoting mental health is discussed in Chapter 9.

◼ SUMMARY ◼

1. Groups are a specific social system that can be defined and studied. A group consists of individuals who are interrelated and interdependent and who may share common purposes and norms.

2. All groups have two functions: a task and a maintenance function.

3. Some common dimensions that are often used to eval-

DIRECTIONS FOR FUTURE RESEARCH

The following are some of the nursing research problems raised in Chapter 28 that merit further study by psychiatric nurses:

1. The role of nurses as group co-leaders with professionals of other disciplines (e.g., social work, psychiatry, psychology)
2. The efficacy of self-disclosures by the nurse/leader; nurse as therapist, educator, or both
3. Short-term modalities within DRG constraints
4. Evaluation of short-term modalities
5. Effectiveness of transition groups on adjustment to post-hospitalization
6. Role of psychiatric nurse as in-house consultant to general hospital staff and patients
7. Examination of effect of including family members in group treatments
8. Comparison of behavioral, analytical, and cognitive-behavioral treatment methods
9. Cost-effectiveness of group as a therapeutic technique
10. Comparison of heterogeneous versus homogeneous groupings according to DSM-III-R
11. Effect of community meetings on small group cohesiveness
12. Effectiveness of groups for medical patients (e.g., post-myocardial infarct patients) in coping with disease process and its implications
13. Training modalities of nurse therapists
14. Utilization of groups for staff team building, skill acquisition, and support
15. Effectiveness of patient/family peer support groups
16. Use of videotape as a feedback device

---

uate a group's progress are communication processes, membership roles, norms, power structure, cohesion, and stages of group development.

4. There are identifiable curative or therapeutic factors that may occur in groups.

5. Nurses can use informal groups to enhance their assessments and to provide a therapeutic experience for the group's members.

6. The leading of therapeutic groups, which prevents or decreases emotional disturbances or stress, should be viewed as being in the realm of nursing practice.

7. Group psychotherapy is a useful and beneficial treatment modality for alleviating emotional disturbances.

8. There is a wide range of models of group psychotherapy from supportive therapy to personality reconstruction.

9. Specific theoretical frameworks should be used by group therapists. Theoretical models can be used to assist therapists to assess the group, intervene in the group, and evaluate the effectiveness of their interventions.

10. A group psychotherapist has specific responsibilities in leading the group. Some of these responsibilities may be studied in relationship to the phases of group development.

    a. During the pregroup phase, therapists determine the purpose of the group, arrange for a place for the group to meet, determine criteria for membership, and select group members.

    b. In the orientation stage, therapists facilitate the group's arriving at a group contract, orient the group to its task, and promote group cohesion.

    c. In the conflict stage, therapists may encourage members to express their disillusionment and hostility and maintain the group's activity within a working level.

    d. During the cohesive stage, therapists assist the group to improve its problem-solving ability by helping the group to use negative feedback and disagreement.

    e. In the working stage, therapists facilitate the group's accomplishing its tasks by acting as a resource person to the group, assisting the group in handling problems such as subgroup formation, and managing conflict and resistance.

    f. In the termination stage, therapists assist the members in evaluating what they have learned and in separating from each other.

11. Nurses need to do more clinical research in their work with groups; specifically, their intervention techniques need to be documented more scientifically and related to outcome.

■   REFERENCES   ■

1. American Nurses' Association: Statement on psychiatric and mental health nursing practice, Kansas City, Mo., 1976, The Association.
2. Armacost, et al.: A group of "problem" patients and a staff of nurses at the other end of their tether, Am. J. Nurs. **74**:289, 1974.
3. Bales, R., and Slater, P.: Role differentiation in small decision-making groups. In Parsons, T., and Bales, R.F.: Family socialization and interactional process, Glencoe, Ill., 1955, Free Press.
4. Benne, K.D., and Sheats, P.: Functional roles and group members, J. Soc. Issues **4**(2):41, 1948.
5. Bennis, W., and Sheppard, H.: A theory of group development, Hum. Rel. **9**:415, 1956.
6. Bilodeau, C.B., and Kackett, R.P.: Issues raised in a group setting by patients recovering from myocardial infarction, Am. J. Psychiatry **128**:73, July 1971.
7. Burke, C.: Working with parents of children with hemophilia, Nurs. Clin. North Am. **7**:787, 1972.
8. Cartwright, D., and Zander, A., editors: Group dynamic research and theory, ed. 3, New York, 1968, Harper & Row, Publishers, Inc.
9. Chatham, M.A.: The effect of family involvement on pa-

10. Cohen, R.: ECT + group therapy = improved care, Am. J. Nurs. **7**:1195, 1971.
11. D'Afflitti, J.G., and Swanson, D.: Group sessions for the wives of home hemodialysis patients, Am. J. Nurs. **75**:633, 1975.
12. DeMocker, J., and Zimpfer, D.G.: Group approaches to psychosocial intervention in medical care: a synthesis, Int. J. Group Psychother. **31**:247, 1981.
13. Dolgoff, T.: Small groups and organizations: time, task and sentient boundaries, Gen. Systems **10**:135, 1975.
14. Echternacht, M.R.: Day treatment transition groups—helping outpatients stay out, J. Psychosoc, Nurs. **22**:10, 1984.
15. Eisenberg, A.: The effects of working with husbands on adjustment of mastectomy patients, master's thesis, Rochester, N.Y., 1976, University of Rochester School of Nursing.
16. Ferguson, B.: A parents group, J. Psychiatr. Nurs. **17**:24, 1979.
17. Gardner, K.: Patient groups in a therapeutic community, Am. J. Nurs. **71**:528, 1971.
18. Gardner, M.E.: Notes from a waiting room, Am. J. Nurs. **80**:86, Jan. 1980.
19. Griffin, W., Ling, I., and Staley, D.: Stress management groups, J. Psychosoc, Nurs. **23**:1, 1985.
20. Lewin, K.: Group decision and social change. In Newcomb, T.M., and Hartley, B.L., editors: Readings in social psychology, New York, 1947, Holt, Rinehart & Winston, Inc.
21. Lieberman, M.A., Yalom, I., and Miles, M.: Encounter groups: first facts, New York, 1972, Basic Books, Inc.
22. Long, L.D., and Cope, C.S.: Curative factors in a male felony offender group, Small Group Behavior **2**:889, 1980.
23. Marram, G.: The group approach in nursing practice, ed. 2, St. Louis, 1978, The C.V. Mosby Co.
24. Martin, E., and Hill W.: Towards a theory of group development: six phases of therapy group development, Int. J. Group Psychother. **7**:20, 1957.
25. Miller, E.J., and Rice, A.K.: Selections from systems of organization. In Colman, A., and Bexton, W.: Group relations reader, Sausalito, Calif., 1975, GREX Publishing.
26. Moreno, J.L.: Psychodrama and group psychotherapy, Sociometry **9**:249, 1941.
27. Nakagawa, H.: The state of the art of psychiatric nursing: the theory and practice of group work, presented at the State of the Art in Psychiatric Nursing Conference, Rutgers—The State University, New Brunswick, N.J., Apr. 8–9, 1974.
28. Olmsted, M.: The small group, New York, 1959, Random House, Inc.
29. Parloff, M., and Dies, R.: Group therapy outcome research, 1966–1975, Int. J. Group Psychother. **23**:281, 1977.

tients' manifestations of postcardiotomy psychosis, Heart Lung **71**:995, 1978.

30. Runkel, P., et al.: Stages of group development: an empirical test of Tuckman's hypothesis, J. Appl. Behav. Sci. 7:180, 1971.
31. Satir, V.: Conjoint family therapy, rev. ed., Palo Alto, Calif., 1967, Science & Behavior Books.
32. Schutz, W.: Interpersonal underworld, Harvard Bus. Rev. **36**:123, July–Aug. 1958.
33. Selander, J.M., and Miller, W.C.: Prolixin group, J. Psychosoc. Nurs. **23**:11, 1985.
34. Smith, A.: A manual for the training of psychiatric nursing personnel in group psychotherapy, Perspect., Psychiatr. Care **8**(3):106, 1970.
35. Spotnitz, H.: Comparisons of different types of group psychotherapy. In Kaplan, H., and Sadock, B., editors: Comprehensive group psychotherapy, Baltimore, 1971, The Williams & Wilkins Co.
36. Tuckman, B.: Developmental sequence in small groups, Psychol. Bull. **63**:384, 1965.
37. Whitaker, D., and Lieberman, M.: Psychotherapy through the group process, Chicago, 1964, Aldine Publishing Co.
38. Yalom, I.D.: Inpatient group psychotherapy, New York, 1983, Basic Books, Inc.
39. Yalom, I.: The theory and practice of group psychotherapy, ed. 3, New York, 1985, Basic Books, Inc.

■ ANNOTATED SUGGESTED READINGS ■

Group dynamics

*Beeber, L.S., Schmitt, M.H.: Cohesiveness in groups: a concept in search of a definition, Adv. Nurs. Sci. **8**:2, 1986.

This well-documented article strongly suggests need for nursing research in the conceptualization and measurement of group cohesion.

Bennis, W., and Shepherd, H.: A theory of group development, Hum. Rel. **9**:415, 1956.

This article reveals an often quoted and useful theory of group development. The theory, derived from the authors' observations of sensitivity groups, is based on psychoanalytical theory. Some readers may find this article a little difficult to read.

Bion, W.R.: Experiences in groups, New York, 1959, Basic Books, Inc.

This book describes the basic premises in the Tavistock theory of groups. It is a somewhat difficult but very rewarding book to read.

Cartwright, D., and Zander, A., editors: Group dynamic research and theory, ed. 3, New York, 1968, Harper & Row, Publishers, Inc.

This book is an excellent summary and classic collection of research studies on group dynamics. The theoretical presentation and its clinical implications are especially useful to the clinician.

Conyne, R.K.: The group workers' handbook: varieties of group experience, Springfield, Ill., 1985, Charles C Thomas.

This book considers group counseling and psychotherapy in traditional form but also examines groups as used to impart specific skills, for organization development, and for community change. There is also an interesting "Group Work Grid" created by the author to conceptualize the handbook.

Luft, J.: Group processes: an introduction to group dynamics, ed. 2, Palo Alto, Calif., 1970, National Press Books.

This quick-reading introductory book to the study of groups is especially useful in applying communication theories to the group or small group.

Olmsted, M.: The small group, New York, 1959, Random House, Inc.

This is a good classic introductory book for the study of small groups. It summarizes many theories of small groups that were derived from sociology and psychology.

Tuckman, B.: Developmental sequence in small groups, Psychol. Bull. **63**:384, 1965.

This excellent article summarizes many theories of group development. It may be necessary to read the article several times to obtain the full benefit of the author's work.

Vander Kolk, C.J.: Introduction to group counseling and psychotherapy, Columbus, Ohio, 1985, Charles E. Merrill Publishing Company.

This book is a good, clearly written basic group counseling text. The chapter on group dynamics is especially useful in its consideration of facilitative and anti-group roles assumed or ascribed to group members. Marital groups, skill acquisition groups, peer self-help groups, and other uses of groups not usually found in group texts are covered.

Whitaker, D.S.: Using groups to help people, Boston, 1985, Routledge and Kegan Paul.

This book includes in-depth consideration of preparation, "life cycle" of the group, and post-group aspects of group therapists.

Group therapies

*Adrian, S.: A systematic approach to selecting group participants, J. Psychiatr. Nurs. **18**(2):37, 1980.

This article explores how to assess candidates for group participation by utilizing inclusion and exclusion criteria offered by the literature. An assessment format is presented and illustrated by clinical examples.

*Affonso, D.D.: Therapeutic support during inpatient group therapy, J. Psychosoc. Nurs. Ment. Health Serv. **23**:11, 1985.

This article focuses on the nurse-patient interactions and their impact on patient progress. Milieu analysis, patient values and responsibility, and empathy are examined as they relate to therapeutic interactions.

Anzieu, D.: The group and the unconscious, Boston, 1984, Melbourne and Henley.

Psychoanalytic examination of group is presented, including examination of the oral fantasies in the group, group as a fantasy machine, and analytic psychodrama.

*Armstrong, S.W., and Rouslin, S.: Group psychotherapy in nursing practice, New York, 1963, The Macmillan Co., Publishers.

This is one of the first books written to introduce group therapy to nurses. The authors forcibly state the importance of group work to psychiatric nursing practice. It was designed to be an introductory textbook on group psychotherapy. A person who is

---

*Asterisk indicates nursing reference.

interested in the historical development of group work in psychiatric nursing would find this book to be a rich resource.

*Baier, M.: Group therapy with parolees in a community mental health center, J. Psychosoc. Nurs. Ment. Health Serv. **20**:26, Feb. 1982.

This is a good example of a creative use of group intervention by a nurse. The author describes a short-term group that she established for recently paroled offenders. She characterizes the group as a modified self-help group.

Berger, M., et al.: Practicing family therapy in diverse settings, San Francisco, 1984, Jossey-Bass Inc.

This book considers the family group in mental health settings including community mental health centers, psychiatric inpatient units, and private practice, as well as educational settings and community settings.

Berne, E.: Group treatment, New York, 1966, Grove Press, Inc.

This book is divided into two sections. The first gives a broad and practical guide for group treatment and the second describes transactional analysis and its application.

*Birckhead, L.M.: The nurse as leader: group psychotherapy with psychotic patients, J. Psychosoc. Nurs. Ment. Health Serv. **22**:6, 1984.

This article examines the unique opportunity for psychiatric–mental health nurses to assume leadership roles in group psychotherapy. It focuses on nurses as advocates of the most regressed members of an inpatient population and indicates the qualifications of nurses to lead these groups.

Bloch, S., and Crouch E.: Therapeutic factors in group psychotherapy, New York, 1985, Oxford University Press.

By use of a concept of a "therapeutic factor" the authors proceed to examine such factors as cohesiveness, self-disclosure, and catharsis. They define and examine theoretical aspects and empirical research.

Brabender, V., et al.: A study of curative factors in short-term group psychotherapy, Hosp. Community Psychiatry **34**:7, 1983.

This study examined the effect of context on patients' perceptions of curative factors in a short-term group and the variability in the factors identified as useful by the group over time.

*Collison, C.R.: Grappling with resistance in group psychotherapy, J. Psychosoc. Nurs. Ment. Health Serv. **22**:8, 1984.

This article examines resistance as it is commonly seen in groups. Types of patient resistance and therapist resistance are explored, and interventions are suggested.

Dies, R.R., and MacKenzie, editors: Advances in group psychotherapy: integrating research and practice, New York, 1983, International University Press, Inc.

This book is an attempt at collaborative review of the "unique curative processes inherent in group interaction from a clinical and research perspective." It includes a series of articles uniting empirical with applied work in groups.

*Dinnauer, L., Miller, M., and Frankforter, M.: Implementation strategies for an inpatient women's support group, J. Psychosoc. Nurs. **19**(8):13, 1981.

This article describes how three nurses implemented an inpatient women's group, including group objectives, supervision,

organizational endorsement, educational materials, and evaluation.

*Echternacht, M.R.: Day treatment transition groups—helping outpatients stay out, J. Psychosoc. Nurs. Ment. Health Serv. **22**:10, 1984.

This article describes the use of combined group therapy and major tranquilizer therapy to treat chronic schizophrenic outpatients. The goals for patients in these transition groups include decreased isolation, enhanced readjustment to life outside the hospital, and enhanced social and problem-solving skills.

Eklof, M.: The termination phase in group therapy: implications for geriatric groups, Small Group Behav. **15**:4, 1984.

This concise article focuses on the dynamics frequently seen at termination. It cites the particular difficulties of geriatric patients in the ending of a group.

Erickson, R.C.: Inpatient small group psychotherapy: a pragmatic approach, Springfield, Ill., 1984, Charles C Thomas.

This is a more advanced text about the group in-patient setting. Practical considerations are included.

Erickson, R.C.: Inpatient small group psychotherapy, Springfield, Ill., 1983, Charles C Thomas.

An especially interesting segment of this book is "Problem Patients and Problematic Populations." It is clearly written and focuses on clear interventions to be utilized by the group therapist in short-term psychotherapy groups.

Fidler, J.: The relationship of group psychotherapy to therapeutic group approaches, Int. J. Group Psychother. **20**:473, 1970.

This is a thoughtful description and discussion of the differences between psychotherapeutic and therapeutic groups for patients. Group psychotherapy is differentiated from other therapeutics in the psychotherapist's diagnosis, plan, and treatments.

*Fochtman, G.: Therapeutic factors of the informal group, Am. J. Nurs. **76**:238, 1976.

This short article illustrates, with clinical examples, how nurses can therapeutically intervene in informal patient groups.

*Gardner, K.: Patient groups in a therapeutic community, Am. J. Nurs. **71**:528, 1971.

This article describes various types of informal groups in the therapeutic milieu of an inpatient setting.

*Goldberg, C., and Stanitis, M.A.: The enhancement of self-esteem through the communication process in group therapy, J. Psychiatr. Nurs. **16**(12):5, 1977.

The authors describe their interventions used in a therapy group. Communication theory is used to explain the formation of self-esteem and the leader's therapeutic techniques. This article is easy to read and is a good example of how a group therapist can apply specific theory to assess, lead, and evaluate a group.

*Griffin, W., Ling, I., and Staley, D.: Stress management groups, J. Psychosoc. Nurs. Ment. Health Serv. **23**:1, 1985.

This is an excellent practical article on the teaching and the benefits of group relaxation training in a psychiatric outpatient setting.

*Hager, R.: Evaluation of group psychotherapy—a question of values, J. Psychiatr. Nurs. **16**(12):26, 1978.

The focus of this paper is on the evaluation that takes place during the course of group psychotherapy rather than afterwards.

The role of evaluator and criteria for evaluation are discussed.

Harman, R.L.: Recent developments in gestalt group therapy, Int. J. Group Psychother. **34**:3, 1984.

This article examines gestalt therapy as applied to groups.

Kanas, N.: Inpatient and outpatient group therapy for schizophrenic patients. Am. J. Psychother. **39**:3, 1985.

This article presents a clear discussion of theoretical constructs of group therapy for schizophrenic patients.

Kanas, N., and Barr, M.D.: Homogeneous group therapy for acutely psychotic schizophrenic inpatients, Hosp. Community Psychiatry **34**:3, 1983.

A group of acutely psychotic schizophrenic patients were grouped and treated with the concomitant use of neuroleptics. Group behaviors and leader approaches were researched and the researchers concluded that such homogeneous grouping was clinically indicated.

Kaplan, H.I., and Sadock, B.J.: Comprehensive group psychotherapy, ed. 2, Baltimore, 1983, Williams & Wilkins.

This book covers a broad range of subject areas concerned with group psychotherapy. It is divided into basic principles, specialized group psychotherapy techniques, groups for special categories of patients, training and research and international group psychotherapy.

Krumboltz, J., and Potter, B.: Behavioral techniques for developing trust, cohesion and goal accomplishment, Ed. Technol. **13**:26, 1973.

This article describes leadership behaviors that facilitate group members' developing trust and cohesion and accomplishing their goals. An excellent article for any beginner in group work.

Lonergan, E.C.: Group intervention: how to begin and maintain groups in medical and psychiatric settings, New York, 1982, Jason Aronson.

This interesting group resource covers such topics as practical ways to work within a system, cost-effectiveness, humanizing the hospital experience, and patient education.

*Loomis, M.: Group process for nurses, St. Louis, 1979, The C.V. Mosby Co.

A basic book on small group dynamics that is written to assist a nurse leading or participating in a group.

Maves, P.A., and Schulz, J.W.: Inpatient group treatment on short-term acute care units, Hosp. Community Psychiatry **36**:1, 1985.

Recent literature on short-term acute care groups is reviewed. The authors present an approach to therapy based on containment, support, structure, involvement, and validation. Application issues are also discussed.

Power, M.J.: The selection of patients for group therapy, Int. J. Soc. Psychiatry **31**:4, 1985.

Selection criteria for inclusion of patients in a group are discussed. Prevention of premature termination based on clinical judgment, self-report questionnaires, and observation of patients in preparatory groups is also examined.

*Rew, L.: Intuition: concept analysis of a group phenomenon, Adv. Nurs. Sci. **8**:2, 1986.

Intuition as a group phenomenon is clarified through the process of concept analysis. Applications to nursing education, nursing administration, and professional organizations are discussed.

Rogers, C.: On encounter groups, New York, 1970, Harper & Row, Publishers, Inc.

Carl Rogers' perceptions, beliefs, and techniques in encounter groups are discussed in this book.

Rosenbaum, M., editor: Handbook of short-term therapy groups, New York, 1983, McGraw-Hill Book Co.

This is a collection of articles on short-term group therapy with different focal audiences.

Sampson, M., and Marthas, M.: Group process for the health professional, New York, 1977, John Wiley & Sons, Inc.

This introductory textbook is aimed at acquainting the reader with major theories of group process. An excellent book for undergraduates who are beginning to use study groups and want to learn how to work effectively in them.

*Selander, J.M., and Miller, W.C.: Prolixin group, J. Psychosoc. Nurs. Ment. Health Serv. **23**:11, 1985.

The treatment and cost effectiveness of prolixin groups are examined in terms of reducing recidivism rates.

*Slimner, L.: Use of the nursing process to facilitate group therapy, J. Psychiatr. Nurs. **16**(2):42, 1978.

The author describes and illustrates three group theoretical models: the focal conflict model, the communication model, and the group dynamics model. Examples of these models are given to demonstrate how they can be used as group assessment guides.

Spitz, H.I.: Contemporary trends in group psychotherapy, Hosp. Community Psychiatry **35**:2, 1984.

This article provides a brief history of group therapy and a survey of current literature in the field linking past trends with recent developments. It looks at group therapy for specific populations, for example, borderline patients and geriatric patients. Recent innovations in group entry, retention and enhancement of the group experience are also discussed.

*Van Servellen, G.M.: Group and family therapy: a model for psychotherapeutic nursing practice, St. Louis, 1984, The C.V. Mosby Co.

This book is for advanced students in psychiatric–mental health nursing but may also be useful to beginning therapists. It is divided into four segments: (1) Conceptual perspective for nursing practice in group and family work, (2) the scope of nursing practice in group and family work, (3) the basic interventions utilized, (4) special considerations including special techniques, and evaluation and research issues.

Weiner, M.F.: Techniques of group psychotherapy, Washington, D.C., 1984, American Psychiatric Press, Inc.

In addition to being a clearly organized basic group psychotherapy text on technique, this resource offers extras including an extensive bibliography and a listing of teaching and training aids of films and videotapes on group psychotherapy.

*White, E.M., and Kahn, E.M.: Use and modifications in group psychotherapy with chronic schizophrenic outpatients, J. Psychosoc. Nurs. **20**:14, Feb. 1982.

The authors have analyzed their experiences as leaders of psychotherapy groups with chronic schizophrenic patients. They are advocates for the helpfulness of group approaches to these patients. Specific suggestions are made for the modification of group intervention techniques to meet the needs of chronic schizophrenic patients. This article should be very helpful to nurses who work in outpatient settings serving deinstitutionalized populations.

*Williams, R.: A contract for co-therapists in group psychotherapy, J. Psychiatr. Nurs. **14**:11, June 1976.

This article discusses ten basic points that should be a part of a contract for co-therapists who are working with groups.

Wilson, W.H., Diamond, R.J., and Factor, R.M.: A psychotherapeutic approach to task oriented groups of severely ill patients, Yale J. Biol. Med. **58**, 1985.

This article examines the therapeutic potential of many types of groups through use of direct, noninterpretative actions. Discusses use of structure, overt agendas, and dynamic group processes.

*Witt, J.: Transference and countertransference in group therapy settings, J. Psychosoc. Nurs. **20**:31, Feb. 1982.

This article provides a good overview of the application of psychoanalytical concepts of transference and countertransference to group interaction. The illustrative clinical example should be of particular interest to beginning group leaders.

Yalom, I.D.: Inpatient group psychotherapy, New York, 1983, Basic Books, Inc.

This excellent reference for beginning and experienced group therapists includes practical suggestions for formation, structure, and leadership of inpatient groups.

Yalom, I.: The theory and practice of group psychotherapy, ed. 3, New York, 1985, Basic Books, Inc.

This excellent book on group therapy is extremely useful for both the new and experienced therapist. The author cites relevant research and uses many clinical examples to illustrate his ideas.

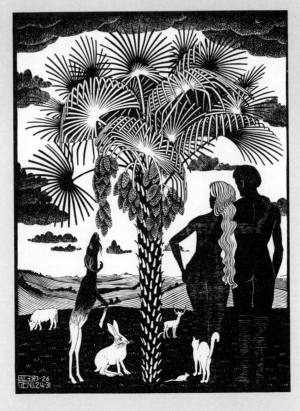

We are truly heirs of all the ages; but as honest men it behooves us to learn the extent of our inheritance. . . .

John Tyndall, "Matter and Force" in vol. 2, Prayer as a Form of Physical Energy

CHAPTER 29

FAMILY THERAPY

PATRICIA E. HELM

After studying this chapter, the student should be able to:

- state the focus of family therapy and the indications for it.

- identify the role of both the generalist and specialist in relation to family therapy.

- analyze the family systems model, structural model, and strategic, or brief, model of family therapy with regard to the following elements: theoretical basis, goal of therapy, and dynamics of treatment.

- within the context of a family systems model of therapy describe the relevance of differentiation of self, triangles, nuclear family emotional system, multigenerational transmission process, family projection process, sibling position, and emotional cutoff.

- within the context of a structural model of therapy describe the relevance of subsystems, subsystem boundaries, and restructuring operations.

- assess the importance of communication theory to the development of strategic, or brief, family therapy.

- identify directions for future nursing research.

- select appropriate readings for further study.

In the 1950s, if a nurse therapist acknowledged that she was seeing anyone in the family other than the patient, she risked censure by the entire psychoanalytical community. She could be accused of breach of confidence and of failure to protect the boundaries of the therapeutic alliance between the nurse and patient from contamination. Today, 30 years later, the "growing edge" of family therapy encompasses many well-known persons in the field, numerous conferences and workshops, a panoply of books and videotapes, and a number of training programs in family therapy.[1]

Family therapy seeks to view the gestalt, the context in which an emotional problem is generated and played out between family members. Rather than viewing one member as sick or one relationship as pathological (such as the much-researched "schizophrenogenic mother" and symbiosed child), the family therapist focuses on the symmetrical process between family members that perpetuates and enables the "sick" behavior of one identified member. All family members are equally involved. For example, the school-phobic boy's overclose relationship to his mother can be seen as her solution to the problem of her husband's emotional withdrawal from her into his business for 16 hours of the day. The boy's attention-demanding behavior saves both spouses from confronting their conflicts with each other and the problem of their intimacy within the marriage. Seen in this context, there is no one member of the family who is to blame, no one victim to bolster with supportive therapy, but rather a skewed family process that has become fixed and requires rebalancing.

Viewing symptoms within this context requires a theoretical reorientation. To view family therapy as a modality of treatment is obsolescent; rather, it is a different way to conceptualize human relationship problems. It broadens the isolating, individual point of view to include the context in which relationship events take place.

This chapter will provide a summary of three of the major, current theoretical approaches to family therapy and delineate some of the main techniques that have evolved from these theories. The best guides to the history of family therapy, highlighting the work of the "first generation" personalities, are works of Chris Beels and Andy Ferber[5] and Phil Guerin.[25] The goal of the chapter is to develop an informed interest in the field and facilitate the pursuit of further reading and perhaps training in family therapy. For those nurses who do not work in psychiatry but who work with patients' families in some capacity, this chapter will provide some theories to help organize the wealth of information and stimuli that impinge on any observer of a family in stress.

Role of the nurse in family therapy

Nurse therapists have evolved with psychiatry. "Insanity" moved out of the hands of priests who would exorcise it, out of prisons that would contain it, and into the hands of physicians who would cure it. When "insanity" was conceived of as "mental illness," it was brought under the rubric of medicine. As medicine became more psychologically sophisticated, the intimate connection between the soma and the psyche was established. Psychiatry has struggled to gain a position of legitimacy in the medical field. The development of psychosomatic medicine and psychiatric liaison services in medical hospitals attests to the increasing recognition that the emotional and psychological needs of patients must be met to maximize physical healing.

As medicine became more complex, the number of available physicians proved inadequate to perform multiple treatment procedures. Under these circumstances nurses were asked to assume more and more responsibility for total patient care. Observing emotional stress in patients and patients' families has always been an integral part of this care. Nurses responded intuitively to stress in their patients long before intrapsychic and interpersonal theories of psychiatry were conceived. Public health nurses observed the emotional stress of illness and social deprivation in patients and families in community settings. Inasmuch as one goal of psychotherapy is to reduce acute stress in a patient, family therapy is a natural evolution of the traditional role of the nurse.

■ Functional families

Contact with patients' families is an inevitable part of patient care. For many years nurses have been making intuitive observations about functional and dysfunctional families and intervening with families without formal training in family therapy. A well-functioning family is a flexible one that can shift roles, levels of responsibility, and patterns of interaction as it passes through periods of varying stressful life changes. A well-functioning family may, under acute or prolonged stress, produce a symptomatic member, but this family rebalances in such a way that function of all members is restored and symptoms fade. A functional family has the following characteristics.[2,22,34]

1. It maintains a homeostatic balance and flexibility and adapts to change as it passes through transitional stages of family life and periods of stress.
2. Emotional problems are viewed as partially a function of each person, rather than residing entirely in one family member.
3. Emotional contact is maintained across generations and between family members without blurring necessary levels of authority.
4. Overcloseness or fusion is avoided, and distance is not used to solve problems.
5. Each twosome is expected to resolve the prob-

lems between them. Bringing a third person in to settle disputes or to take sides is discouraged.
6. Differences between family members are encouraged to promote personal growth and creativity.
7. Children are expected to assume age-appropriate responsibility and to enjoy age-appropriate privileges negotiated with their parents.
8. The preservation of a positive emotional climate is more highly valued than doing what "should" be done or what is "right."
9. Within each spouse there is a balance of affective expression, careful rational thought, relationship focus, care taking, and object orientation, and each spouse can selectively function in the respective models and roles.

■ Dysfunctional families

Dysfunctional families lack one or more of these characteristics. All nurses, regardless of their area of expertise or practice setting, encounter dysfunctional families in which problems may be overt or covert and member satisfaction is low. Some of the more common dysfunctional family patterns nurses may observe include the following: the overprotective mother and the distant father (distant at work, in alcohol, or absent from the home) with a timid, whiny child or a destructive acting-out teenager; the overfunctioning "superwife" or "superhusband" and the underfunctioning passive, dependent, and compliant spouse; the spouse who maintains "peace at any price" and who whitewashes difficulties in the marriage but who suddenly feels wronged and self-righteous when the mate is discovered to be in legal difficulty or to be having an affair; the child who evidences poor peer relationships at school while attempting to parent younger siblings to compensate for ineffective and emotionally overwhelmed parents; and the overclose three generations of grandparent, parent, and grandchild in which lines of authority and generational identity are ill-defined and the child is acting out because of a lack of effective limit setting by an agreed-on parental figure.

The decision as to when family therapy is appropriate or especially indicated over individual or group therapy is a controversial issue. Partially this decision is dictated by resources; many settings do not have anyone trained in family therapy. Even if the resources are available, the therapist's bias will have an influence. Some family therapists believe family therapy is the treatment of choice for any presenting problem or symptom. They make no distinction because they conceptualize all emotional problems within the family framework. Other family therapists recommend certain guidelines in determining which problems should be treated in family therapy. They may suggest that family therapy is indicated in the following situations*:

1. The presenting problem appears in system terms, such as marital conflicts, severe sibling conflicts, or cross-generational conflicts (parents vs. offspring; parents vs. grandparents).
2. Various types of difficulty and conflict arise between the identified patient and other family members.
3. The family is experiencing a transitional stage of the family life cycle, such as beginning a family, marriage, birth of the first child, entrance of children into adolescence, the first child leaving home, retirement, or the death of one spouse.
4. Individual therapy with one family member results in symptoms developing in another family member.
5. There is no improvement with adequate individual therapy. Enlarging the conceptual field to include the family in therapy may produce therapeutic movement.
6. The individual in treatment seems unable to use an intrapsychic or interpretive mode of individual therapy but primarily uses therapy sessions to talk about or complain about another member.

In the majority of cases clinical training programs in family therapy are open to nurse specialists with graduate degrees. Workshops in family therapy are offered across the United States. They vary in duration, theoretical model used, and in the level of clinical sophistication required of participants. The nurse therapist doing family therapy should have some formal graduate training or on-the-job education through didactic and clinical seminars. She should seek out and obtain individual or group supervision for her clinical work in treating families to refine her clinical skills and deepen her theoretical understanding of family systems.

■ Practice settings

Family therapy is being done in inpatient and outpatient settings. In the home it is used by crisis intervention teams, and it is being used with groups of families of chronically ill patients in aftercare clinics at state psychiatric hospitals. It is also being done by mental health professionals who volunteer their time to private or nonprofit associations, such as the Cancer Foundation, to work with families stricken with a specific dis-

ease. Some intensive care units, such as kidney dialysis and coronary care units, are using therapists to do family therapy when a severe psychological disturbance is recognized in the patient or family as a result of the acute medical illness.

Because family therapy is practiced in a wide variety of settings and involves families at all levels of functioning, the generalist nurse, without a graduate degree, will be exposed to it in many areas of her practice. Understanding theoretical models of family therapy will benefit this nurse in many ways. She may apply certain principles of these models in her work with families of medically hospitalized patients to promote their functioning and support their methods of coping with stress and illness. Just as the functioning of the family as a whole is affected by the illness of one of its members, so too the family's method of coping with a member's illness can affect the outcome of the illness, either positively or negatively. Knowledge of family therapy theories will help her make more acute observations, more readily identify problems within family systems and assist her in selecting effective nursing interventions and evaluating the accuracy of her assessment by the interactional or functional change evident in the family. It may also assist her in initiating appropriate referrals.

The theoretical views of family therapy presented in this chapter—family systems therapy, structural family therapy, and problem-solving, strategic, or brief therapy—are three distinct and, at times, conflicting views. They represent three major approaches in family therapy that have clearly articulated theoretical frameworks developed from clinical research with families. The opinion about which treatment approach is most effective with a family is primarily a function of the nurse therapist's theoretical orientation. There are no well-defined criteria or conclusive research in this area.

Family systems therapy

Family systems therapy was developed by Bowen[9] in the 1950s. The therapy has continued to evolve and refine as more people trained in systems theory have studied increasingly larger numbers of families and developed more training and research programs. A premise of this therapy is that a family is a homeostatic system, and a change in fuctioning of one family member results in a compensatory change in the functioning of other family members.[9] It could be likened to a centerless web in which, when one strand moves, the tensions in the entire web readjust.

Systems therapy explains emotional dysfunction in human relationships, specifically in the family system. Symptoms in any member of the family, whether social (e.g., child abuse, delinquency), physical (e.g., alco-

---

*I am indebted to Behnaz Jalali, M.D., for her ideas on this subject.

holism, chronic illness), emotional (e.g., depression, schizophrenia), or conflictual (e.g., marital conflict), are viewed as evidence of dysfunction in the family relationship process. Although the family is only one of the multitude of emotional systems in which an individual is involved, it is probably the most intense and influential one. Extra-familial relationships rarely carry the voltage or toxicity of the family emotional system. This is not to say that one's family system totally determines one's behavior and function but rather that family systems foster or inhibit function. The individual's responsibility for his actions is never lost.

The purpose of any theory is to understand, predict, and thereby gain some control of the phenomena being studied. Understanding, as applied to family systems therapy, does not entail uncovering intrapsychic motivations but rather identifying the functional facts of a relationship—what happened, when, where, how, and who was involved. These observable facts are more important than the reasons why the problematical behavior occurred. A systems therapist gathers from family members descriptions of behavior rather than feeling states. The absence of conventional psychodynamic jargon in family systems writing reflects a conscious attempt by Bowen and early systems researchers to remove the cause-and-effect medical model or "why thinking." Systems therapy coined a new working language using simple descriptive words.

Bowen[7-12] has described in detail the team research he conducted in the early 1950s on schizophrenic families in a live-in hospital setting. From this live-in research evolved a new theory of family psychotherapy. This theory, which is based on clinical observations of the research families' behavior, proved applicable to relationship patterns in more functional family systems also. Bowen proposed the following:

. . . Schizophrenia and all other forms of mental illness belong to a continuum, the difference being one of *degree* of impairment rather than a qualitative difference between schizophrenia and the neuroses.[9:391]

He believed that "patterns originally thought to be typical of schizophrenia are present in all families some of the time and in some families most of the time."[12:61]

A cornerstone of systems therapy developed from a central pattern observed in research families, which was their failure to distinguish between the intellectual process of thinking and the more subjective process of feeling. It was as if the thinking processes were so flooded with feeling that they were unable to separate intellectual opinion and belief from affective content. Routinely a person would say, "I feel that . . ." when "I think/believe that . . ." would have been more ac-

curate. The families' efforts were toward fostering feelings of togetherness and agreement in relation to others, avoiding statements of opinion or belief that would establish one member as different or separate from the family "party line."

A key goal of systems therapy therefore is to clarify and distinguish thinking and feeling processes in family members. Bowen's belief in the importance of distinguishing between feeling and thought is reflected in his use of the term "emotional illness or dysfunction" rather than "mental illness." He views emotional illness as a phenomenon deeper than a disorder of the mind and the thinking process; it is rather a disturbance in the basic life processes of a person.[9] The observation of this fusion between thinking and feeling led to the concept of the "undifferentiated family ego mass" (what Virginia Satir refers to as "people salad") and the conclusion that people with the greatest fusion between feeling and thinking function the most poorly and inherit a high percentage of life's social, psychiatric, and medical problems.[12]

Family systems theory consists of seven interlocking concepts. There are three concepts that apply to overall characteristics of family systems: differentiation to self, triangles, and the nuclear family emotional system. The remaining four concepts, the multigenerational transmission process, the family projection process, sibling position, and the emotional cutoff, are elaborations of the central family characteristics.

All these concepts refer to family processes that inhibit or promote individual family members' rising out of the emotional "we-ness," or fusion, that binds us all to our families. Bowen believes forces toward fusion are as instinctual in a person as opposing forces toward differentiation, and a member's movement toward either increased emotional closeness or distance is reflexive and predictable. The higher the level of differentiation in a person, the higher the level of functioning. Differentiating the self from the "we-ness" is therefore the goal of treatment. Guerin, on the other hand, sees the goal of family systems therapy as attainment of emotional freedom in the context of the family system. He is less militantly opposed to "we-ness" in the system than Bowen. In restating the goal of treatment in this way, he "leaves room for the ability either to be fused into a period of relationship refuge or to clearly draw one's boundaries and hold a functional position against the weight of the system."[25:19]

■ Differentiation of self

The concept of differentiation of self is Bowen's attempt to measure all human functioning on a continuum from the greatest emotional fusion of self boundaries, such as the folie à deux phenomenon, to the highest degree of differentiation or autonomy. A concise description of the differentiated person is the person who is less anxious than the family system and who is able to bring up toxic issues in a nonassaulting way without anxiety. In Bowen's earlier work he refers to the "undifferentiated family ego mass" or the "conglomerate emotional oneness" that exists in varying degrees of intensity in families. The intensity of emotional closeness in a family can be such that members know each other's thoughts, feelings, and fantasies.

There is a cyclical quality to this closeness. As the emotional intensity or fusion between two individuals increases and the self of one is incorporated into the other self, the relationship is perceived to be uncomfortably close. This is usually followed by distance-creating behavior in which there is hostile rejection of the overcloseness and the two individuals actively repel each other.[10] Relationships can cycle through these phases, since anxiety in the relationship ebbs and flows at frequent intervals. Relationships can also become fixed at an angry, repelling standoff. In people who operate at this lower reactive end of the continuum, their intellect and emotions are so fused that they are dominated by the automatic emotional system. These people are less adaptable, less flexible, more emotionally dependent on those about them, and easily stressed into dysfunction. People at the upper end of the continuum maintain a degree of separation between thought and emotion. In periods of stress they can retain a relative amount of intellectual functioning and are more flexible, adaptable, and more independent of the reactive emotionality around them.[12]

The concept of differentiation eliminates the notion of normalcy, even in its poorly defined state. It has no direct connection to presence or absence of symptoms, although Bowen believes people at the lower end of the scale tend to inherit more of life's problems. People at the upper end of the continuum, if they are stressed into dysfunction, tend to recoup rapidly.

■ Triangles

The concept of triangles is the key to understanding the systems approach to emotional function, and many techniques evolve from this concept. The idea of triangles is certainly not a new one. Freud's theory of the oedipal complex describes a sexual triangle. Bowen has called the triangle the basic "building block of an emotional system." A triangle is a predictable emotional process that takes place in any significant relationship when there is difficulty in the relationship. The three corners of the triangle can be composed of three people; two people and a group, such as a religious affiliation or Al-Anon; two people and an issue, such as drinking or success; or two people and an object, such as the house or drugs.[21] Obviously the possible list of groups, issues, or objects is endless; it requires only that they have an emotional significance equal to that of a person.

All people seek closeness in emotional systems. Emotional closeness but separateness is difficult for two people to maintain; the tendency is to fuse, to lose self, or parts of self, in the other. There is a natural urge to seek completeness of self by accumulating parts of other. The old adage "opposites attract" reflects this assumption. The balance is precarious between two people trying to maintain a comfortable distance so that there is sufficient emotional closeness without fusion. The inevitable result is emotional distancing, and the system is then ripe for the formation of a triangle. For example, the husband wants more expression of affection and closeness from an emotionally constricted wife. The more he pursues her, the more she withdraws, most commonly into preoccupation with her child. The husband starts working longer hours. Husband and wife then start arguing circularly: "You care more about making a new account than you do about your wife and children!" "You expect to have nice things and then blame me for working extra hours!" The key to the function of triangles is stabilizing and maintaining the status quo while at the same time avoiding tension, conflict, or talking about sensitive emotional areas. The two people can then focus on the new issue (or person or object) and avoid discussing the painful issues between them. Feelings are thus drained off, focus is taken off self and one's own part in the problem, and change in self is avoided.

The reciprocal function of a triangle and the idea of equal responsibility can be a difficult concept to convey to a couple when the distancing mechanism used by one spouse is as emotionally charged as an extramarital affair. If the wife distances from the painful issues in the relationship, by "triangling" an affair, it is difficult for the husband to relinquish his self-righteous position of the "wronged husband" and to see his behavior of working 14 to 16 hours a day as serving the same distancing function in the relationship. The specific nature of the distancing mechanism has meaningful content (whether it is overwork, extramarital affairs, homosexuality, psychotic symptoms, religious preoccupation, suicide gesture, depression, or psychoanalysis), but all serve the same function as a triangular relationship within the family.[19]

The concept of a family scapegoat originally served to broaden the individual pathological view to include the part the family played in the symptomatic behavior. The tendency, however, is to view the scapegoat as the

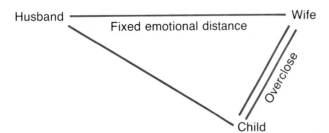

Fig. 29-1. A commonly occurring family triangle.

helpless victim of a persecuting family. With this bias a nurse therapist would see two patients who are unable to settle their differences and wish to avoid their marital discord by focusing on the "victim child." This leads to blaming the parents. From a systems view, with the concept of triangles, this process operates with all three twosomes that make up the triangle. A diagram of this triangle is presented in Fig. 29-1. Father and mother avoid conflict by focusing on the son, mother and son avoid dealing with their overcloseness by having a common enemy in the father. Father and son avoid awareness of their emotional distance by relating through the mother as go-between. Recognizing how this emotional dysfunction process is promoted by each family member invalidates the label of victim and victimizer. Fogarty stresses, "All members of a triangle participate equally in perpetuating the triangle and no triangle can persist without the active cooperation of all its members.[21]

It is not a problem to be in a triangle; in fact, it is impossible to stay out of all triangles. Triangles form and re-form rapidly and are the daily reflexive way most people handle conflict or tension. Problems will arise if a triangle becomes fixed when it involves significant relationships of deep friendship, blood ties, or marriage. Triangles are not static but form and re-form around toxic, emotion-laden issues, such as money, sex, child rearing, religion, alcohol, and education. A person's position in a triangle alters depending on the issue. A mother and father may be distant on the highly charged issue of how to spend their money but may be close and in accord about the loaded issue of their adolescent daughter's sexual activity. Judgments about these issues are most often based on emotion rather than careful thought.

■ **OPERATING PRINCIPLES.** To determine what a person's operating principles are, that is, the governing laws of his conduct, they must be inferred from what the person does in regard to an emotion-laden issue rather than what he says. Operating principles may thus vary from intrinsically valuable ones based on conscious conviction to more immature, reactive, impulsive prin-

ciples. Immature principles are other-focused rather than self-focused and lead to a loss of freedom of self-determination. Any behavior that is predictable (as in behavior operated by a triangle) is not free. The loss of freedom impairs self-functioning, perpetuates problems, causes a deterioration in family functioning and promotes symptom development.[19]

Other-focused, triangle-promoting operating principles are reflected in such ways as declaring feelings "right" or "wrong"; using plural pronouns "we" or "us" rather than "I"; accusing the other person of "you made me mad/do it"; stepping in to settle, side taking, or blaming in two other people's conflict; telling or holding secrets; telling the other person what to do; and assuming responsibility for the other person's feelings, for example, "I want to make her happy" or "I couldn't tell him because it would hurt him." These statements may commonly be interpreted as thoughtful or being very responsible. In fact, avoiding one's own feelings by focusing on the other person is fundamentally irresponsible. From taking responsibility for another's feelings it is a small leap to taking charge of the other person's behavior. Everyone tends to fall into this pattern, especially in a marriage or parent-child relationship. When a person becomes anxious, it is more comfortable to project the problem outside the self onto the other person and then work to change the other. The implicit assumption here is "I can't help my behavior, but he is behaving that way deliberately."[26]

In more dysfunctional, closed family systems, interaction between family members becomes determined by fixed interactional patterns, as observed in schizophrenic families, for example. These fixed triangles are an effort to maintain a homeostatic balance and to avoid stress. When an additional stress occurs outside or within the family, such as a job change or the birth of a new member, symptoms may arise in a dysfunctional attempt to reduce stress and restore balance. This is evident in Clinical example 29-1.

■ **INTERVENTIONS.** A major focus of treatment is to get key figures in key triangles to identify their emotional "triggers." This involves having the person identify the verbal or behavioral cues of the other person to which he reflexively reacts with a predictable behavior, maintaining his position in and perpetuating the dysfunctional triangle. When the person pinpoints what cues activate his triggers, he can take control of his part in the process. Once one person takes control and changes his part in a triangle, the whole system changes.

An example of this was a mother who was overclose to her 16-year-old daughter, who had become school phobic and stayed home from school for a year before the family sought treatment. The father would come home from work, see the daughter had missed school another day, and angrily attack her with "shape-up speeches." The mother, who bitterly complained about the daughter being home all day doing nothing, would then become protective of the daughter and launch an attack on the father: "How can you say those things to her; you know how upset she gets." Once the mother was able to get a "handle" on her emotional trigger and stop feeling sorry for her daughter (the mother had always been terrified of her "drill sergeant" father), she was able to control her protective reflex, step back, and permit the father to become more effective with his daughter.

The nurse must not only identify key triangles in a family and identify operating principles of family members pertaining to specific issues, but also she must be tuned into her own vulnerability to her emotional triggers. She must assume that the family will attempt to triangle her into the family's emotional system to reestablish equilibrium. The nurse's job is to maintain sufficient emotional distance to watch the process unfolding between family members while at the same time maintaining emotional contact with each family member.[14] Bowen[46] has enumerated many of the reactions a therapist might have which would indicate that the therapist is part of a triangle: feeling sorry for or pitying the other, feeling angry at the system or member, being overly positive about the system, or seeing someone doing something horrendous and feeling one has to

correct it. The nurse knows she is part of a triangle in the family process when she finds herself without questions or responses in the session. The idea is to avoid becoming part of a triangle, thus diffusing the emotional process, and to limit the action to the two family members. Once the therapist steps in to take sides, progress stops and status quo is reestablished.[47] If side taking is used by the therapist, it should be a planned strategy in which she maintains the freedom to realign with specific family members.

Systems therapists do not believe they can change family members; change is possible only when it is generated within the self. Just as family members are coached on taking responsibility for and control of self within the family system rather than trying to change the other, the family therapist's responsibility is to stay relevant to the emotional flow of the family without becoming part of a triangle in the system. One way for the nurse to get out of an emotional process she reacts to in the session is to elicit the member's responses. For example, if she finds herself getting irritated at a critical intrusive husband, she can turn to the wife and ask, "What happens to your insides when your husband interrupts with criticism?" This feeds the process back into the system, keeping it between the spouses.

One of the areas of controversy in the field of family therapy is the importance of the therapist's working on her own family of origin (referred to as TOF, therapist's own family).[42] Systems therapists contend that it is a major aspect of training as a family therapist. "Working on" means the nurse differentiates herself in her own family of origin. She identifies the issues in her family that she is reactive to and with whom she is part of a triangle around these issues. She then works to get out of the triangle by gaining control of her reflexive distancing and fusing in her family in order to have the freedom of emotional closeness and of some emotional distance with each family member (without using geographical distance to create emotional space). Unless a therapist is conscious of the triangles she is a part of in her own family, she will be vulnerable to the same roles and behaviors in the families she is treating.

■ Nuclear family emotional system

The nuclear family emotional system refers to patterns of interaction between family members and the degree to which these patterns promote emotional fusion.[20] These patterns of interaction, called operating principles, are the ways the person behaves in most significant relationships. All marriage relationships reflect a balance, or complementarity, of operating principles and reciprocal function.[26] There is the spouse who is reasonable, object oriented, and emotionally distant married to the affectively expressive, relationship oriented, emotional pursuer. These differences in operating principles provide the attraction and the balancing stability to the marriage relationship. One spouse is the subject overfunctioner, the other the emotional overfunctioner. Difficulty arises with time when dependence on attributes of the spouse reduces functional attributes in the self. Self borrows on the functioning of the spouse, and self boundaries are blurred. This is referred to as **ego fusion.** When these reciprocal functions become fixed positions of overfunction-underfunction, emotional dysfunction and symptoms occur, such as chronic depression or physical illness. In such a relationship, to view one spouse as strong and independent and the other as weak and dependent fails to recognize the overfunctioner's dependence on the underfunctioning of the other spouse. The underfunctioner must be one-down for the other to appear one-up.

Emotional fusion operates in all marriages to a lesser or greater extent. When the relationship is unstressed, the reciprocal function works smoothly. When stress occurs, each spouse becomes more like oneself. The distancer seeks space and objects (the job, art, alcohol); the pursuer seeks togetherness and expression of personal feelings. Both are efforts to avoid personal anxiety. The pursuer takes the distancer's withdrawal as personal rejection and reactively withdraws. No longer feeling crowded, the distancer then moves in emotionally, only to be met with "Where were you when I needed you; get lost." The distancer then pulls back, baffled and angry at the rejection, and, in time, a fixed emotional distance sets in.[26] These are the bitter standoff relationships nurses see in their practice just before the couple decides on a divorce. These relationships are ripe for triangulation with an affair or with an unsuspecting therapist.

People pick spouses who have equivalent levels of differentiation of self.[9] The greater the undifferentiation, the greater the tendency toward fusion and potential problems. If there is a high degree of ego fusion and intensity in the nuclear family, this intensity can be diffused and attenuated through active contact with the family of origin. In periods of stress, contact with the extended family or family of origin can stabilize the nuclear family. Promoting such contact can be an effective therapeutic strategy.

Bowen[10] has identified two patterns in the nuclear family emotional system, which he labels the explosive family and the cohesive family. Family units of a cohesive family are geographically close, in frequent contact and communication. The person who geographically separates from his family of origin because of the fusion or intensity of attachment there may marry a spouse from a cohesive family. The person's unresolved attachments to his own family of origin lie dormant until ritualized contact (at a wedding or funeral) stirs them up. In a nuclear family in which both spouses are detached from their families of origin the spouses tend to be more dependent on each other, and the process between them is more intense. These are the explosive families.

Bowen[9] postulates three mechanisms by which spouses maintain sufficient emotional distance from each other to handle the anxiety associated with fusion. All three mechanisms may be used by the couple, or tension may be focused in one area. If tension is great enough, it will spill over into other social systems such as mental health centers or school counselors. The three mechanisms used are (1) marital conflict, (2) dysfunction in one spouse, and (3) projection of the problem onto one or more children.

■ **MARITAL CONFLICT.** Conflictual marriages are built on a perpetual struggle between spouses to get "their fair share" (of needs met, of freedom, of love, of attention, or of control) and neither spouse is willing to compromise. A high percentage of the self is wrapped up in the "happiness" of the other, and functioning of the self is enmeshed in the function of the other. Because of the amount of investment in the other, whether positive ("Anything to make her happy") or negative ("I sacrificed the best years of my life helping him be a success; I'll never let him go now"), these relationships tend to be stable, predictably cycling through periods of intense closeness, distance-creating conflict, making up, then renewed closeness. Although it is commonly believed that this amount of conflict would harm the children of such marriages, Bowen[9] postulates that the children are, in fact, protected from overinvolvement because tension is focused between parents.

Intervention in conflictual marriages usually involves working with the most motivated spouse at first. If both spouses are seen together, frequently the uproar between them is too great to tolerate in the session. They are so reactive to each other that limit setting such as laying ground rules of no interruptions and one person talking at a time or strategies such as a "listening chair" or turning one spouse's chair to the wall to listen are ineffective. In such situations spouses must be seen separately initially. The approach is to get the focus on the self and to decrease the amount of blaming and attack and efforts to change the other. The nurse strives to focus on what part the spouse plays in the situation and gain some control of one's own reactive triggers. Once blaming is reduced, the spouse can then reevaluate his or her own set of beliefs and values without the need to attack the other. Such reevaluation entails going back to one's family of origin in phone or letter contacts or planned visits, gaining a broader view of the source of the nuclear family conflict, and working to establish more personal relationships with one's family of origin. Bowen calls this process coaching. Usually before this point is reached in the treatment, the absent, less-motivated spouse has sought to join the sessions because of the changes that have occurred.

Significant changes in the marriage system occur when one spouse withdraws emotional overinvestment in the other and focuses on self. The spouse making changes must be warned of predictable efforts by the other to reestablish status quo by an escalation of anger-provoking behavior, threats to leave, etc. If the spouse making changes can maintain a self-focused position through the resistance, both partners may become actve in the treatment. While temporarily working with one spouse, the nurse must guard against becoming part of a triangle in the system by emotionally siding with the spouse initially in treatment or by becoming the only support for the spouse in treatment. This can be especially difficult for the nurse when the unexpressed plan of the unmotivated spouse is to deposit the husband or wife in treatment and then obtain a divorce, expecting the nurse to "take care of" the spouse. Whitaker and Miller[54] explore this issue in depth.

■ **SPOUSE DYSFUNCTION.** The second mechanism used by spouses to maintain emotional distance is the dysfunction of one spouse. As mentioned earlier, one spouse may be emotionally, socially, or physically disabled to varying degrees. The degree to which the one underfunctions is the degree to which the other overfunctions. This ensures that emotional equilibrium is maintained, since both partners are locked into a mutually dependent relationship. Interventions with such a relationship are similar to those used with the conflictual marriage. Bowen suggests working with the overfunctioning spouse first, getting this spouse to tone down and pull back. Since nature abhors a vacuum, the underfunctioning spouse then moves in to take up the slack.

A striking example of pulling the overfunctioning spouse back with a resulting shift in the emotional and functional balance is evident in Clinical example 29-2.

■ **PROJECTION ON CHILD.** The third distancing mechanism used by spouses to control the intensity of fusion between them is the projection of the problem to one or more of the children. Prior to development of a theory of family pathology, the parents of a symptomatic child would be excluded from therapy, further reinforcing the dysfunction in the family by focusing on the child as "the problem." Child-focused families tend to be particularly entrenched in viewing the prob-

---

CLINICAL EXAMPLE 29-2

Mr. and Mrs. S are a couple who sought treatment because the husband was missing so many days at work. The couple would get into huge battles about the husband not feeling like working and the wife feeling outraged at the financial stress he was creating. It became apparent that Mrs. S. treated Mr. S like one of their adolescent boys. She overfunctioned to the point of cleaning up after her husband's destructive temper tantrums. Over a period of time, with considerable coaching, she was able to pull back in several areas, refusing to wake the husband or clean up after him, leaving it up to him to pay the bills, and generally holding back her critical nagging. The first sign of progress was at the husband's next temper tantrum (he did delicate electrical work and had a low frustration tolerance). He carefully selected which objects he would throw or smash in his workroom, not throwing a box of small nuts and bolts, for example. He cleaned up his own workroom and began going to work regularly. As the husband's functioning improved, the wife became significantly depressed and began addressing unresolved issues in her family of origin. This couple demonstrated the reciprocity in the mechanism of underfunctioning and overfunctioning in a marriage.

---

lem as exclusive to the symptomatic child, or else they deny the existence of a problem entirely. When the school or probation officer recommends treatment, they passively comply but participate reluctantly. When a couple centers on their children, it is easier to avoid marital confrontations because there is always something to worry, criticize, or complain about with the children. These families exhibit strong dependency on the children's symptoms, and they tenaciously resist exploring larger issues in therapy.[3]

How one child gets singled out as the focus of parental concern is a complex process that may have its roots in several previous generations. Key triangles tend to repeat themselves over generations; so the parent's natural tendency is to put one child in the parent's old position in the triangle. Nodal events are the normative events that occur in every family life but which generate anxiety because change ensues. These include such events as birth, death, sickness, marriage, job changes, school changes, divorce, and family relocation. Carter[15] suggests that the amount of stress generated around a nodal event is contingent on the amount of change resultant. If a significant developmental stage of the

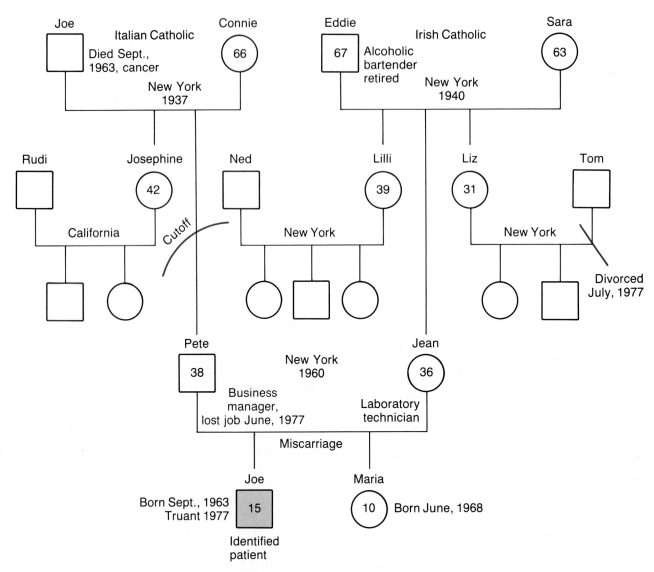

Fig. 29-2. A hypothetical family genogram.

child (e.g., in utero, birth, entering school for the first time, adolescence) coincides approximately with the occurrence of a nodal event, this child is vulnerable to the focus of family stress and impairment. The first born and the last born are also particularly vulnerable to the position of family focus.

Intervention with such families cannot be a frontal assault with logic or the family will be lost to treatment. The primary goal is to remove the focus from the child and place the conflict between the parents where it belongs. This is accomplished by placing the dysfunctions of the child within the context of the family system by taking a family history and drawing a family genogram. Drawing a three-generation family genogram is a structured method of gathering information and graphically

symbolizing a large amount of factual and emotional relationship data in the initial interview.[27,37,42] A sample genogram is presented in Fig 29-2. Drawing a family genogram in full view of the family on large easel paper or a blackboard broadens the family's focus and stimulates their thinking of the extended family system. The therapist's questions and comments are geared toward change of self rather than changing the child.

Strategies used to defocus the identified child as the problem include identifying or defining the behavior of other family members as problematical to spread the problem and anxiety around. Another strategy is to move the problem up one generation by asking how grandparents might handle the problem or opening discussion on conflict about disciplining the children between grandparents. With some families the nurse can coach the overinvolved parent, for example, the mother, to pull back from the focused child and send a note to her own mother telling her one thing about herself that she does not want her to know. This reveals the three-generational aspect of the presenting problem. Guerin recommends working with the sibling subset at times, separately from the parents, to promote a more positive support system among sibs. Frequently sibs mimic their parents' negative behavior toward the focused child or resent the excessive attention he gets from parents and are aggressive toward him.

Families with an acting-out child and two parents in the ineffective helpless position (or one parent set up as the "heavy" and the other as "the nice guy" saboteur) need a direct approach initially. An effective way to point out how the adults are relinquishing their authority to a young child is to use an extreme example: "If your child had third-degree burns, could you get her to take the horribly painful treatments?" or "If your child had heart disease, could you limit her activities?" Following are four guidelines for parents locked in a triangle with the acting-out "problem child":

1. The person who sets the rule must be present to enforce it.
2. With two parents in the home, divide the areas of responsibility (e.g., allowance, bedtime, nights out) so that when a dispute comes up, it is clear with whom the child must negotiate.
3. Yelling is ineffective and preempts thinking. Parents need to control their reactive buttons.
4. Calmly decide the consequences of repeated disobedient behavior and inform the child of them. When the behavior occurs, without yelling, carry out the consequence even if the parent's personal plans must be changed to do so.*

As soon as the child focus is sufficiently reduced, the child is removed from the sessions. The therapist then forms the third corner of the triangle, actively relating to both spouses without taking sides and thereby keeping conflict between the spouses.

■ Multigenerational transmission process

The roots of the family emotional system extend back through generations. When there is emotional dysfunction, it can be scattered throughout the family tree.[24] Drawing a three generation family genogram frequently reveals certain relationship patterns that might otherwise seem to be isolated phenomena peculiar to

one nuclear family. For example, suicide of younger brothers, divorce among female siblings, or alcoholism might appear to be a pattern across a family system when four or five generations are mapped out on a genogram. A difference between family systems therapy and other forms of family therapy is the underlying assumption that a symptom in one family member in one generation has its origin several generations before, although families seeking treatment usually present symptoms as a nuclear family problem.

■ Family projection process

The concept of the family projection process refers to the way anxiety about specific issues is transmitted through the generations. These are the issues that are emotionally powerful, such as money, sex, child rearing, religion, work or school achievement, alcohol, politics, illness and death, and around which a rigid "party line" develops. Family members polarize around these issues, taking the family position or the direct opposite. Neither position allows freedom or flexibility of thought. Positions are reactive and fixed. Coaching a person to work on the family of origin involves helping him identify his predictable position in family triangles around specific loaded issues. By thinking about the issues he normally reacts to emotionally, he can plan strategies that will get him unhooked from his triangled position.

The family projection process also refers to the process that labels and assigns characteristics to certain members of the family. Whether the labels are over-positive ("Mary Sunshine," "The Genius") or overnegative ("the crazy one," "dummy,"), they are equally unrealistic and confining. After years of family labeling or pronouncements, the labeled person will come to volunteer for the label and deserve it.

■ Sibling position

The concept of personality profiles based on sibling position is borrowed by family systems theorists from Walter Toman, a Viennese psychiatrist. Toman's basic thesis[49] is that important personality characteristics are determined by the sex of one's siblings and one's birth order. For example, the younger brother of two older sisters will present a profile quite different from the older brother of a brother. Using the 10 personality profiles Toman developed, one can fairly accurately predict marital discord or harmony on issues of rank or sex. A younger brother of brothers would have more difficulty relating to his spouse than a younger brother of sisters would have. If this younger brother of brothers married a younger sister of sisters, they would both have discomfort with the opposite sex. In addition, they would be struggling for juniority rights (who's going to take

---

*I am indebted to Betty Carter for her ideas on this issue.

care of whom). Recognizing a possible source of conflict to be sibling rank and sex can help a couple live with their differences.

■ Emotional cutoff

The emotional cutoff is a way some families deal with intense unresolved attachment between children and parents. The cutoff can be in the form of emotional isolation, although members still live geographically close, or in the form of physical distance from the family of origin.[12] The cutoff creates the illusion of having achieved separation from one's parents. The more intense the emotional cutoff, the more likely it is the person will recreate the same problem in his own marriage. The strongest argument for a person to reconnect emotionally with his cutoff family is to prevent the same process from occuring with his own children. Such patterns tend to repeat over the generations.

■ Modes of therapy

Several modes of therapy have been mentioned thus far, including therapy with both spouses or both parents present and therapy with one spouse or parent in preparation for the other spouse joining. Another mode of family therapy is therapy with one family member. This is most frequently used with the young adult who is single and self-supporting. This method involves learning about the functioning of family systems and triangles, keeping an active emotional relationship with important members of the family by planned phone calls, letters, and visits, and developing an ability to control emotional reactiveness to avoid becoming part of an emotional triangle during visits with the family.[9] The goal here, as with other modes of family therapy, is to achieve more self-differentiation from the family of origin, as well as to develop a person-to-person relationship with important family members. This therapy is referred to as coaching. Once the person is knowledgeable about triangles and methods of detriangling within his own family, coaching sessions can be held monthly or as needed to supervise ongoing self-differentiation efforts.

The last mode of therapy is multiple family therapy (MFT) developed in its present form in the late 1960s. MFT is to be distinguished from multiple family group therapy. The latter uses role playing and psychodrama and promotes interfamily group process to achieve the goal of changing family interaction and increasing its sensitivity to the family environment.[45] MFT, from a family systems framework, is different. Sessions are structured so as to ensure against emotional exchange between families, which, Bowen believes, encourages a fusion of other families into a large undifferentiated ego

mass.[45] The idea behind MFT was to conserve teaching time of families, provide contact with a greater volume of families, and allow the opportunity for families to learn from the efforts and experiences of other families. While other families observe, the nurse therapist works with each family the same as she would if she were working alone with that family. She asks numerous detailed questions about the family's problem, defocuses feelings, and addresses one spouse while the other spouse listens. Then she turns to the silent spouse, asking for thoughts or reactions to what the other spouse has said. The family members observing can talk to the therapist about another family but cannot directly talk to the other family. For an updated review of the research and clinical literature dealing with multiple family therapy as an identifiable treatment approach, see O'Shea and Phelps.[37]

Structural family therapy

Structural family therapy is a body of theory and techniques based on a view of the individual within his social context. The assumption is that behavior is a consequence of the organization of the family and the interactional patterns between family members. With this view, changing the family organization and the feedback processes between members changes the context in which a person functions, which thereby changes the person's inner processes and behavior. The therapist temporarily becomes part of the context. This approach is most clearly conceptualized by Minuchin[34,36] and those associated with the Philadelphia Child Guidance Clinic.

The implicit question of a structural family therapist is "In what way is this family structure maintaining this dysfunctional symptom?" Family structure is the invisible set of functional demand that organizes the way in which family members interact. A family is a system that operates through transactional patterns. Repeated transactions establish patterns of how, when, and to whom to relate, and these patterns determine whether the system is functional or dysfunctional.

■ Components of structural family therapy

■ **FAMILY IN TRANSITION.** The first component of this family model is the family as a social system in transformation. The family system must maintain its continuity so family members can grow while at the same time it must adapt to stresses both internal and external to the system. With this view, what traditional therapists would label pathological might be seen as the normal anxiety that characterizes a transitional stage in accommodation to new circumstances. This is described in Clinical example 29-3 by Minuchin.[34]

The interventions of a structural family therapist are toward changing the relationship between a person and the familiar context in which he functions, thereby changing his subjective experience and enabling new, more functional behavior to emerge. In this case the therapist's interventions protected the woman from the unfamiliar and frightening environment until she could "grow a new shell." He blocked the environmental feedback that was serving to confirm her paranoid fears as friends and family withdrew to secretly discuss her frightening behavior. As her experience of her environment changed, her symptoms disappeared.

■ **STAGES OF FAMILY DEVELOPMENT.** The second component of Minuchin's model[34,36] of a viable functional family is that the family undergoes predictable stages of development over time that require adaptive restructuring. Each stage has appropriate developmental tasks that must be accomplished for the family to pass on to the next stage. One stage is the courtship period when the young person is shifting from juvenile to membership in the adult community, establishing status in relation to others, and selecting a mate. This is one of the major times when professional help is sought.[28] The stage at which a new family unit is formed by marriage is preceded by negotiation of the spouses' relationship with respective families of origin. In addition, the families of origin must adjust to partial separation of one member, inclusion of a new member, and accommodation to a new spouse subsystem in the family system functioning. Unless families of origin undergo this transformation, the new family unit may never succeed. Equally unsuccesful are couples who cut themselves off from extended families.

During the marriage stage, multiple and complex rules and transactional patterns must be established between partners. Some ways of relating are reinforced and others are shed in the process of mutual accommodation as a new family system is formed. When a child is born, the functioning of the spouse unit must be modified to include parenting functions. It must shift from an intimate unit of two to a system of three. Frequently the new child becomes the repository of or the excuse for new and unresolved old conflicts between spouses. Many old battles are fought in the arena of child rearing because the couple cannot separate parenting functions from spouse functions.

In the middle years of marriage a major task is the weaning of parents from children. For families in which spouses established communication through the children and the children are leaving (or struggling to leave) home, this is a particularly stressful time. This can be a

---

CLINICAL EXAMPLE 29-3

An elderly widow decided to move from her apartment where she had lived for 25 years because she came home one day and found it had been robbed. Soon after a moving company moved her, she sought treatment from a psychiatrist. She complained that the people who moved her were trying to control her and had purposely lost and misplaced precious possessions. They were leaving sinister messages for each other on her furniture, and when she went outside, people followed her and signaled to each other. The psychiatrist diagnosed her as psychotic with paranoid delusions and prescribed tranquilizers. When this did not help, she sought a second psychiatrist who recommended hospitalization. The third therapist she sought out was a context-related therapist. He understood her symptoms as an ecological crisis precipitated by feeling forced to move into an unfamiliar environment. He explained to her that she had lost her shell—the familiarity of objects in her apartment, the neighborhood, the neighbors. As any crustacean who has lost its shell, she felt vulnerable and was experiencing reality differently than before. He instructed her to go home, unpack, and place her familiar objects, books, and pictures in the new apartment. He told her to do her daily chores in a routinized way, go to the same shops and checkout counters, and for 2 weeks make no effort to meet neighbors. She was to visit old friends and family but not discuss her recent experiences. If anyone asked, she was to explain that those had just been the problems of an illogical fearful old woman.

---

period of enrichment for spouses if (typically) the husband is enjoying a degree of career success and the wife is freer now to pursue career plans or interests she set aside earlier to rear children. Finally, a family member enters the stage of retirement and old age. This can be a period of relative harmony or it can be problematical as spouses are thrown together 24 hours a day. In time, one of the partners dies, and adult children then face the crisis of caring for an aging parent. The family cycle continues to unfold, and as the family is transformed over time, it must adapt and restructure itself to continue functioning. It is when a family adheres inappropriately to previous structural schemas that stress builds and symptoms develop. For an amplified discussion of the family life cycle, therapeutic considerations relevant to each stage, and normative interruptions of the family life cycle (divorce, remarriage, illness, and death), the reader is referred to Carter and McGoldrick.[16]

■ **FAMILY STRUCTURE** A third component of Minuchin's model of a viable functioning family relates to the structure of the family. The major elements of structure are power and influence, sets of relationships, and boundaries (individual, sexual, generational). Structure can become dysfunctional in any or each of these areas.[43] As in any organization, the family system must have a power hierarchy with different levels of authority to function efficiently. There must also be a complementarity of functions, a team effort among family members. Over the years mutual expectations of particular family members evolve. These expectations may be openly negotiated but more often are implicit, with patterns of behavior developing around small daily events.

The family system differentiates and carries out its functions through subsystems. Subsystems can be made up of individuals or dyads and can be formed by generation, sex, interest, or function.[34] Each person belongs to a multiplicity of subsystems with different levels of power and in which differentiated skills are learned. The boundaries of a subsystem are the rules defining who participates in subsystem functions and how. Each subsystem has specific functions and interpersonal developmental tasks to be accomplished. Subsystem boundaries must be free of intrusion if functions are to be performed and interpersonal skills developed. For example, patterns of mutual accommodation as well as healthy competition cannot develop among siblings if parents or grandparents perpetually interfere. A central principle of structural family therapy is that subsystem boundaries must be clear for proper family functioning. They must be defined well enough to prevent intrusion or interference but must also permit emotional contact among members.

Minuchin[34,36] describes families with extreme boundary problems as either enmeshed or disengaged. Enmeshed boundaries are weak and fluid; personal space and subsystem boundaries rapidly change and impact on all subsystems. This diffuseness of boundaries inhibits the development of autonomy and competence. Perceptions of self and others are poorly differentiated.[35] A child in such a family might be so sensitized to conflict between parents that he is unable to perform in school. The parents in such a family can become upset because the child refuses his vegetables at dinnertime. Such families flood with anxiety at times of stress and have poor adaptive capacities to change.

Disengaged families have rigid boundaries. Communication between subsystems is poor; supportive or protective contact is minimal. Members of such systems may function autonomously but have a skewed sense of independence and lack feelings of loyalty and belonging and the capacity for interdependence. Stierlin[44] hypothesizes that the product of a disengaged family is the sociopath. Because of the rigidity of subsystem boundaries, members may fail to respond adequately or entirely when one member is stressed. In such a family a child's reading disorder might go unnoticed or a husband's suicidal behavior be disregarded.

The nurse often functions as a boundary maker. She may clarify diffuse boundaries by blocking interruptions or encouraging the shutting of bedroom doors. She may open overly rigid boundaries by recommending that a distant parent and child spend time together or calling attention to the expression of a nuance of feeling by a family member that would otherwise go unnoticed by other members. The nurse's assessment of family subsystems and boundary functioning provides a rapid diagnostic picture of the family and indicates the direction and goals of therapeutic interventions.

As mentioned earlier, each subsystem has specific functions and interpersonal developmental tasks to be accomplished. The spouse subsystem must develop patterns of mutual support for each person's functioning in many areas. Couples must develop a complementary routine that enables decisions to be made and arguments to be settled without domination or relinquishing of self by either spouse. Ideally, they will bring out the best in each other, with each promoting personal growth and creativity in their spouse.

What commonly occurs in most marriages, to a greater or lesser degree, is that spouses engage in an "other-improvement program." They bring into the marriage certain expectations of their spouse and work very hard to get the spouse to meet them. Interpretations in this area should be balanced and directed to both spouses and the part each plays in perpetuating the destructive process should be pointed out. A mutual interpretation would be to say to the wife, "In your efforts to make contact with your husband, you are driving him away" and to the husband, "Your strong silent style is alluring and elicits nagging." Balanced interpretations such as this emphasize the complementarity of the system, join the positive and negative in each spouse, and eliminate judgmental implications of motivation.

The parental subsystem must perform the tasks of socializing the children without sacrificing the function of mutual support and accommodation between the spouses. Children must have access to each parent but be excluded from spouse functions. Minuchin speaks with a clear voice to parents regarding the importance of parental authority in an era that tends to promote "pure democracy" between parents and children. He validates the difficulty parenting entails, noting that few do it to their own satisfaction. Parenting processes are different depending on the age of the child. Part of promoting differentiation in the family is making the differentiation in ages clear. Adolescents have certain responsibilities and certain privileges that 12-year-old siblings do not. Children must learn to negotiate with their parents to learn to navigate in a world of unequal power relationships.

The sibling subsystem is where children first learn about peer relationships. They learn how to make friends, compete, negotiate, cooperate, and gain recognition of their skills. Knowledge of growth and development of children is valuable for the nurse who must, at times, translate age-appropriate skills, needs, and values to baffled parents. The nurse should support the child's right to autonomy while at the same time supporting the parents' authority.

■ Goals of the initial interview

A vital component to structural family therapy is the process of joining the family.[31,34,36] The nurse temporarily becomes part of the family system by adapting her behavior to the rules and manner of the particular family. She can do this either purposefully or unconsciously. The aim is to accommodate herself to the family to gain experiential entrance into the family system. Unless she does this at the outset, restructuring and change is impossible. Following are methods of joining:

1. Mirroring or mimicking—matching the family's mood, pace, communication patterns, or kinesthetic cues (e.g., becoming jovial or somber, communication becoming terse or punctuated with long pauses, becoming fidgety)
2. Respecting families' values and hierarchies (e.g., if one spouse is the central switchboard, addressing all communication through that spouse first)
3. Keying in culturally when possible or finding elements of kinship (e.g., "I have an adolescent boy too")
4. Searching for strength—observing for the minutest positive detail about individual family members that the nurse can highlight and thereby confirm the individual's sense of self and make contact with him (e.g., appreciating a clever phrase or a preteen's poised manner)
5. Supporting family subsystems (e.g., giving smaller children toys to play with while talking to older ones or having parents sit together as they discuss their difficulty with the children)
6. Tracking—asking for elaboration with concrete details and examples of specific content in the family's discussion, which serves to confirm individuals who are speaking as well as to explore family structure (e.g., tracking a mother's mentioning that she and her son are close by asking what time of the day and in which part of the home they are closest, thus learning that the mother and son sleep together while father sleeps in another room)

Another task of the nurse during the initial formation of the therapeutic system is the struggle to assume leadership in the session. The nurse therapist must accommodate sufficiently to the family to enter the system while at the same time maintaining the leadership position. She must join while still retaining the freedom to confront and challenge. She can assume leadership by presenting herself as an expert, gaining the family's confidence and instilling hope. She establishes the rules of the system, such as who attends the session, that no one talks for another, and that no one interrupts. She controls the flow of communication and directs who is to speak to whom.

At the beginning of the session she must contact each member. At that point, she will be presented with the public mask. She must not spend more than 15 to 20 minutes with an individual before moving to contact the next member or she will get sucked into the system. Very soon she must ask two people to interact directly to enact a problem they have been describing. The public mask then falls away and the nurse can make direct observation of dysfunctional interactions. Rather than going from content issue to content issue or participating in a litany of the past, the nurse therapist can introduce the conflict inherent in small events. She can be immediately involved in a conflictual situation by highlighting a nonevent and creating an affective event.

Minuchin is a master of this technique of transforming minute simple nonevents and ballooning them for therapeutic intervention. For example, in a demonstration videotape, within the first 5 minutes of the session Minuchin transformed the nonevent of a father "helping" the identified patient, the adolescent son, adjust his video microphone wire into a therapeutic intervention around the family's infantalization of the son. Minuchin maintains that the amount of knowledge needed about the family to diagnose and begin restructuring dysfunctional interactions is available quickly.[41] Structural family therapy does not explore or interpret the past. It is active and immediate.

Diagnosis in family therapy is based on the nurse's accommodation and joining the family and observing and experiencing the pulls of the family on her behavior as well as observing her impact on the family. The interactional diagnosis is not fixed in time but alters as the family accommodates to or resists the therapist's restructuring interventions. It also varies depending on which family subsystem is active in the therapeutic situation at any one time. In this way diagnosis and therapy are inseparable.

■ Restructuring interventions

The aim of restructuring interventions is to transform the dysfunctional transactional patterns that maintain symptomatic behavior. The nurse is concerned not only about symptom removal but also about changing the organization of the family so the symptom does not get passed on. However, if an area of organization such as the parents' relationship does not contribute to the symptom Minuchin does not enter there. He believes that therapy should be constrained by the family's presenting symptom.

Minuchin identifies seven categories of restructuring operations: enacting family transactional patterns, marking boundaries, escalating stress, assigning tasks, using symptoms, manipulating mood, and supporting, educating, or guiding.

■ **ENACTING TRANSACTIONAL PATTERNS.** Enacting transactional patterns, as described earlier, involves family members actively discussing an event that they might otherwise be describing to the nurse.[34] Instead, the nurse instructs specific members to discuss the matter between themselves. In this way she disengages from the interaction to observe and watch for nonverbal confirmation or contradiction of the content, patterned sequences, interruptions, distractions, alliances, and coalitions. Thus the nurse can see the family in action and make direct observations of how they naturally resolve conflicts, support each other, or diffuse stress.

The nurse may find it difficult to stay outside these transactions, permitting the family to drag her back into direct discussion. Going behind a one-way mirror after giving the family clear directions is a way to avoid this temptation. Manipulating space by rearranging seating or position can be an effective way of encouraging or intensifying dialogue. The seating pattern a family assumes when it first walks into a session provides clues to alliances, coalitions, centrality, and isolation. The nurse's manipulation of seating and space can be a diagnostic probe to see how flexible the family is to such change, as well as a graphic indication to the family of a therapeutic goal. For instance, seating the spatially isolated father next to his son where the mother was seated and placing her next to the nurse suggests the

goal of more direct involvement between father and son, with the mother outside that relationship.

■ **MARKING BOUNDARIES.** The marking of both individual and subsystem boundaries in a family promotes clarity in the enmeshed families and reduces rigidity in disengaged families. Simple rules such as that family members speak *to* each other and not *about* each other, no one speaks for another, no one may interrupt, and no one acts as another's memory bank promote individual autonomy. Subsystem boundaries are encouraged by the nurse's inclusion or exclusion of various subsystems attending a session. She would ask children to leave or not attend a session in discussing spouses' sex life. The assignment of tasks such as instructing the father and daughter to go out for a pizza once a week without the mother or younger siblings also promotes subsystem boundaries. Having the sibling subsystem interact in a session, with the mother behind a one-way mirror, gives the children the opportunity to find alternate ways to resolve conflicts normally interrupted by mother's interventions. At the same time, this gives mother the opportunity to identify more positive interaction among the children when before she could only reflexively react to their anger, rebelliousness, and selfishness by intruding on their boundaries. Rigid triads involving cross-generational interactions can be especially resistant to boundary marking.

■ **ESCALATING STRESS.** Escalating stress in a family forces members to develop alternative, more functional, ways of resolving stress. In families seeking treatment, dysfunctional patterns have developed around the symptomatic member. Operations that escalate stress can include blocking the usual transactional patterns and emphasizing differences the family was glossing over. Asking for the customarily silent spouse's opinion following the dominant spouse's statements or asking a member to describe a disqualifying facial expression serves to highlight unspoken family disagreements. Developing implicit conflict involves making covert conflict overt.

Families develop methods for diffusing conflict rapidly, such as the noisy teasing or shoving between two young brothers that occurred before the parent's conflict could surface openly. Blocking the sibling conflict forced the parents to contact directly. Polarizing extant conflict in a family provides the nurse with an opening into the system. A husband and wife were presenting to the nurse a picture of equal helplessness in the face of their adolescent son's delinquent activities. Asking the husband if he had ever tried telling his wife she was "messing up" with the son polarized the positions of the overprotective mother and the "reasonable" distant father.

The nurse can also produce stress by temporarily joining one member or subsystem in alliance or coalition. This operation must be carefully planned and requires the nurse's ability to disengage or else she will be sucked into the system. She can do this serially to help members take differentiated positions or can form a coalition, usually with a spouse, when the system rigidly resists open conflict. Joining a husband's attack on the wife makes the conflict too intense for the wife to diffuse stress onto the son. She is forced to address the conflict between herself and the husband.

■ **ASSIGNING TASKS.** The assigning of tasks, either in or outside the session, structures the setting for alternative interactions and behavior to occur between family members. In designing tasks the nurse must have a clear idea of the family's structure and dysfunctional patterns and have specific interactional goals to be accomplished through the task. Tasks can be such simple directions in a session as asking a husband and wife to sit next to each other as they discuss an issue. In a family in which the wife carries all discipline functions with the children, excluding the father, the father is assigned the job. The mother is instructed to handle only emergencies; otherwise, the father is to be informed of infractions he does not directly observe himself. The wife may not interfere with her husband's disciplinary tactics. She is to take note of the results of the discipline on the children's behavior. This can shift the skewed balance of parental authority so both parents become active and effective.

In assigning tasks it is good to give all critically involved members a portion of the task to complete. It reduces the likelihood of one member sabotaging the new behavior of another if each has a focus on himself. It also makes it easier to relinquish a fixed behavior if another behavior is assigned to replace it. Whether the task is completed or not, the family and nurse have new information about family patterns and progress.

■ **USING SYMPTOMS.** Symptoms can be used in restructuring operations in various ways.[34] Symptoms may be focused on, as in a family Minuchin describes in which the daughter was a fire setter. The focus remained on the daughter, but the mother was instructed to spend time daily teaching the daughter how to light matches safely. This promoted a closer mother-daughter relationship, which was previously obstructed, while retaining a helpful focus on the symptom. Symptoms can be exaggerated to increase their intensity and mobilize family resources, such as by telling a severely depressed middle-aged husband to sit Shiva (Jewish tradition of 7 days' mourning) for the part of himself that is dead. A symptom can be relabeled, as in the case of a mother who continually nagged critically at the son. Redefining her nagging as concern opened the way for more positive caring interactions. Moving to a new symptom entails shifting the family's focus and intensity onto another family member temporarily. In the family in which the husband was failing to go to work and the wife alternately protected him and threatened to leave him, identifying her behavior as seriously depressed reduces her intense focus on the husband. A symptom's effect can also be changed, thereby altering interactions around it. An example would be in the family with the fire setter when the mother was encouraged to interact with the daughter in a competent, educating fashion.

■ **MANIPULATING MOOD.** Manipulating the family's mood is another restructuring operation. An exaggerated initiation of the predominant family affect might mobilize counteraffect in the family, thereby initiating a wider range of expression. The nurse can also model a more appropriate affect for the family, for example, reacting with strong indignation to a young boy's criticism of his mother. This promotes respect and clarifies the boundaries of a passive enmeshed parental subsystem.[34,36]

■ **SUPPORTING, EDUCATING, GUIDING.** Support, education, and guidance can be a restructuring operation. They can take the form of modeling, assigning tasks, or sharing of concrete information. Minuchin repeatedly points out to families how they program each other in the circular process of a family system.

The goal of structural family therapy is not a change in behavior but a change in the organization of the whole family, allowing individual members a new experience in the family.[34,36] Using a model of an effectively functioning family, the therapist joins the family in a therapeutic system with the intent of restructuring it in a defined way. The restructuring either facilitates the maintenance of functional subsystems or helps to form new subsystems that will promote healing and growth.

Strategic, problem-solving, or brief family therapy

Communication theory has undergone evolutionary changes since the well-known double-bind theory was first proposed by a group of researchers in Palo Alto, California, in 1956.[4] These changes have revolutionary implications for the practice of psychotherapy. Out of communication theory has developed strategic short-term, or problem-solving, family therapy.

The original communication theorists included Gregory Bateson, John Weakland, and Jay Haley, with Don Jackson and William Fry consulting. The focus of their early study was the nature of observable face-to-face communication, verbal and nonverbal, among members of a family or other ongoing social group, and its significance for the shaping of actual behavior.[53] The clearest explication of early communications theory is in *Pragmatics of Human Communication* by Watzlawick, Beaven, and Jackson.[51]

■ Assumptions of communication theory

Communication theorists contend that *all* behavior, not only verbal productions, is communication, and since there is no such thing as nonbehavior, it is impossible not to communicate.[50] The theorists recognized that most communication does not consist of simple declarative messages but rather a multiplicity of levels of communication between sender and receiver. The verbal and nonverbal levels of a message necessarily modify and qualify each other. That is, the significance of any message depends on how it is reinforced, confirmed, contradicted, or specially framed by other simultaneous, preceding, or following messages. These (along with the setting and the relationship between sender and receiver) constitute the context that must be considered in interpreting any message.[53]

Another basic tenet of communication theory is that communication is an ongoing process. Originally, for purposes of analysis, communication was broken down into discrete units of "stimulus" and "response" in a linear structure reflecting cause-and-effect thinking. It later became apparent that this was both inaccurate and inappropriate. There is no beginning point or end point in the stimulus-response-reinforcement pattern of human interaction (referred to later as a positive feedback loop). Obviously, in most relationships, the behavior of each participant is predicated on the behavior of the other. In families, complex, highly patterned, repetitive interactions become established.

With the communications model, when a two-person (or more) system is dysfunctional in its communication, there is potential for a pathological condition. Studying communication patterns in schizophrenic families, the researchers identified several forms of "pathological communication." Disqualification in communication includes self-contradictions, inconsistencies, subject switches, tangentializations, incomplete sentences, misunderstandings, obscure mannerisms of speech, and literal interpretations of metaphor and vice versa.[51] An example of disqualification is a question an older brother used to baffle his younger sister: "Do you walk to school or carry your lunch?" Disconfirmation in communication involves ignoring or invalidating essential elements of a significant other's view of himself, telling the person you do not feel the way you feel, need what you need, or experience what you experience.[43]

Incongruent communication is delivering two conflicting messages simultaneously, whereby if the receiver responds to either message, he will be charged with badness or madness. This is the basis of the double-bind or paradoxical injunction. An example is the command "Be spontaneous!" or, from Greenberg's collection of maternal communications, "Give your son Marvin two sport shirts as a present. The first time he wears one of them, look at him sadly and say in your Basic Tone of Voice: 'The other one you didn't like?' "[50:111] Finally, symptoms are means of communication; the symptomatic person is convinced the symptoms are out of his control, while the symptoms can serve as a controlling mechanism in the family. Psychosomatic symptoms come under this description.

The treatment goals of family therapy, based on the early communicational view of behavior, were to correct pathological patterns of communication and to promote functional communication between family members in which members express themselves clearly and directly and ask for and receive feedback. Thus behavioral change would occur in the family as a result of direct, clear, unambiguous communication.[43] From their research of schizophrenic families, the Palo Alto group expanded their research and practice to other kinds of clinical problems, recognizing that the manifestations of schizophrenia included much that was characteristic of other clinical problems. From their observations of here-and-now communication in families, it was a short conceptual leap to the formulation of strategic family therapy.

■ Components of strategic family therapy

In 1966 Fisch proposed the establishment of the Brief Therapy Center of the Mental Research Institute in Palo Alto, California. He was joined by Watzlawick and Weakland, all previously involved in the communication research under Jackson at the Mental Research Institute. They shared an attitude toward treatment concerning the function (the "what") rather than the meaning (the "why"), of behavior and they were looking for tools to shorten treatment and facilitate change. Initially, the therapeutic interventions that seemed to do this appeared gimmicky, but they gradually evolved a conceptual framework to explain these successful interventions. Their focus was on how symptoms or human problems arise and how they are resolved, especially through paradoxical intervention.[50] Simultaneously with their work on the West Coast, Haley[29] developed the problem-focused family therapy approach through his association with Minuchin, Erikson, and Montalvo on the East Coast. What sets strategic family therapy apart from structural and systems therapy is its primary goal: the removal of the presenting symptom through directives or tasks in conjunction with the use of paradox.

Whether one speaks of problems or symptoms, they are not an entity in their own right. A problem is only a problem when it is labeled as such by those involved. A problem is behavior between two or more people that one or more persons do not like and which persists despite efforts to change.[24] Strategic therapists make a distinction between difficulties and problems. Difficulties are either undesirable states of affairs that can be removed by a logical solution or undesirable, common life problems that must simply be lived with.[52] Problems commonly stem from small difficulties that escalate and are maintained by mishandling of attempts to solve them. Mishandling most frequently occurs around adaptation to ordinary life events and ranges from (1) ignoring or denying difficulties on which action should be taken to (2) attempting to resolve an ordinary life difficulty that is unnecessary (e.g., a husband who would not talk to his wife before breakfast) or impossible to resolve (e.g., the generation gap) to (3) a wide area of difficulties where action is needed but the wrong kind is taken.[53]

Strategic family therapists are not concerned with the history of the problem or the motivation behind it. They are not interested in characteristics of people (passive, hostile, hysterical) and they place no importance on insight. Little distinction is made between acute and chronic problems. Chronic problems are simply ones that have been mishandled longer. The presenting problem behavior and the problem-maintaining behavior is the primary focus of treatment.

Communication theorists borrowed from cybernetics when they identified a positive feedback loop in human interaction. This is the vicious cycle that develops from efforts by family members or the identified patient himself to stop or "help" undesirable behavior. For example, the rebellious teenager, when faced with parental discipline, will become increasingly rebellious. As the discipline becomes harsher, the boy's behavior escalates further. Thus "the action which is meant to alleviate the behavior of the other party, in actual fact, aggravates it."[18:610] From this view, the cause and the nature of a problem are essentially the same process. People try to change behavior in the most logical way possible. Common sense suggests prevention or avoidance of undesirable behavior by means of the reciprocal or opposite behavior. If this does not work, they try harder with the same behavior. The resolution of problems therefore requires a change of the problem-maintaining behaviors so as to interrupt the vicious positive feedback cycles.[53]

■ Problem-solving interventions

Interdiction in the system can be either at the point of the identified patient, the nonidentified patient, or both, depending on who is the "customer," that is, the person most uncomfortable or most concerned with the problem and thus most willing to change. Effective intervention can be made through any member of the system to break the positive feedback loop. This is illustrated in Clinical example 29-4.

These examples demonstrate the use of reversal or symptom prescription, which carry the message "do not change" or "more of it," both of which stop the family or patient from trying to stop. The task of persuading people to change the very behavior that common sense tells them should help often requires treatment strategies which appear "weird," illogical, or paradoxical.

Since the focus of treatment is symptomatic, the nurse's first task is to obtain a clear statement from the patient of the presenting complaint in specific concrete terms. As Haley states, "Problems . . . should be something one can count, observe, measure, or in some way know one is influencing."[29:40] After the nurse obtains a detailed description of the problem and determines what about the behavior makes it a problem, she then gathers

---

CLINICAL EXAMPLE 29-4

A colonel is being militarily strict with his son, and the boy is becoming increasingly defiant. The therapist tells the father his son is "going to the dogs." The therapist then suggests that the father hold back on his discipline to get a baseline measurement of just how bad the boy's behavior will get. As pressure on the boy is reduced, his behavior improves.

Another example is a woman who suffered from urinary frequency. She was isolated both at home, feeling unable to leave the house to socialize, and at work because she had her machine set by the bathroom door where there were no co-workers. She worked from 12 to 8 P.M. The therapist instructed her to urinate as many times as she felt she had to each morning before going to work but to use the toilet only three times; after that she was to urinate sitting in the tub. She was to make no effort to change her pattern at work. The next week the woman reported she had been in agony the first morning but was unable to urinate sitting in the tub. She then figured that if she could limit herself at home, she could do so at work, and had no further urinary frequency.[6]

an account of what solutions the family has tried. This tells her which remedies to avoid and indicates the problem-maintaining behavior.

Next the nurse asks what the family's or patient's minimal goal of treatment would be—what smallest identifiable change would signify progress or some success. General goals such as "improved communication" are not acceptable, nor are feeling changes such as "to feel happier" or negative goals such as "to stop certain behavior." Rather, the nurse seeks positive statement-of-action goals that delineate what people would be doing to reflect an attitude or feeling change. According to the cybernetic view, if a small but significant change can be made in what appeared to be a hopeless situation, a so-called ripple effect may occur. That is, "once a patient is mobilized and regains confidence in his ability to solve problems, he sometimes finds that he can tackle other difficulties."[40:47]

As soon as possible, the therapist attempts to grasp the patient's "language" and the ideas and values that appear central to him. "Tuning into" the family's view and then extending that view is the critical step that precedes the therapist's concisely formulated strategic intervention. This step is known as reframing. To reframe means to change the conceptual or emotional setting or viewpoint in relation to which a situation is experienced and, by using language that is congenial to the family's world view, place it in another frame that fits the "facts" of the same concrete situation equally well and thereby changes its entire meaning.[24,50] An example of reframing includes using the component of hostility when it is present in a woman's frigidity and reframing the problem as one produced by her over-protecting the male. Since, assuming there is a hostile component and protecting the husband is the last thing she would want to do, the new frame to the problem uses the hostility as an incentive to release her inhibited sexual feelings. When Tom Sawyer reframed white-washing the picket fence as an artistic entertaining enterprise rather than a dreary chore, he utilized his derisive friends' competitiveness to vie for the opportunity to whitewash. Reframing brings about an attitudinal change and a change in emphasis of the facts of a situation. This thereby changes the meaning of the situation to permit new behavior while the concrete facts remain unchanged.

A team of Italian family therapists, led by the psychoanalyst Mara Selvini Palazoli, has gained increasing recognition in the United States for its successful short-term therapy with anorectic families[38] and more recently with schizophrenic families.[39] The team functions with two co-therapists working directly with the family while their two colleagues observe and support them behind a one-way mirror. Interventions, designed by the whole team, address each family member's cyclical behavior that perpetuates the problem. At the heart of their therapy is the use of paradoxical injunctions. Interventions are designed to produce resistance in the family, which in turn brings about the desired change in behavior.

Strategic therapists place no importance on the therapist having therapy. This is seen more as residue from earlier psychoanalytical thought. The nurse can be trained in this theoretical framework and learn the skills consistent with this approach without understanding her own involvement with her family. Structural therapists share this view.[29]

Strategic therapists are attacked for the "manipulative, insincere" nature of their approach. They emphatically acknowledge that this is the case. Communication research made clear that it is not possible not to communicate. An extension of that is that it is not possible not to influence. A nondirective, dynamically oriented therapist influences the patient's communication in hundreds of subtle ways, including body movement, intonation, and leading responses. If the therapist does this out of conscious awareness, she is said to be not manipulating. The "insight" school and the non-directive school of therapy influence patients outside of the patient's awareness throughout the process of therapy. Strategic therapists do so openly. The patient's "awareness" of the manipulation itself is irrelevant as long as the directive or strategy is given and followed. The difference between the two schools of psychotherapy is a conceptual one rather than an ethical one. The "insight" school believes that change in people comes about through the therapeutic relationship with a change in their understanding of themselves. The strategic school persuades a person to change "spontaneously" by arranging a situation so that the person initiates the change in behavior.[29]

The strategic therapy model views the therapist as an active and deliberate change agent who is expected to formulate a strategy that will bring about the change the patient is paying money to achieve. The responsibility for success or failure therefore rests on the nurse, although the nurse never takes the credit for change in the patient's eyes. In this therapy the point at which termination takes place is clear. According to Fisch and co-workers:

If a therapist accepts the patient's complaint as a reason for starting therapy with him, he should, by the same logic, accept his statement of satisfactory improvement as a reason (and time) for terminating treatment.[18:599]

Recent developments in family therapy

The family self-help movement is an important development in the mental health field. Families of schizophrenics have long been blamed by professionals for the family member's illness. Two of the family therapy theories discussed in this chapter, Bowenian and strategic, originated from the study of families of schizophrenics. These families feel guilty, bewildered, angry, frustrated, and, ultimately, exhausted and hopeless about the catastrophic and chronic illness of their family member. For the most part, these families live in isolation from their extended families and communities which fear and misunderstand the behavior of the ill member.

In the 1970's some families began forming local self-help and consumer-advocacy groups for families of the mentally ill. In 1979, about 100 such groups together formed the National Alliance for the Mentally Ill, organized with the goal of improving treatment and services for the chronic mentally ill. As a national organization the Alliance advocates increased funding for research, training, and public education, and more progressive attitudes in public policy affecting services for the mentally ill. As enlightened consumers, its members pressure mental health professionals for access to information about services needed for their ill member and themselves during the various phases of the illness. For participant families, local self-help groups offer mutual aid, intimacy with others, and involvement beyond the immediate family needs.[30,32,33]

Renewed interest in family treatments of schizophrenia has resulted in the development of psychoeducational programs for families of schizophrenics. The impetus for these programs came from Brown and Birley's compelling British studies. Although there is wide variation in these programs, there are certain common features. The family intervention programs begin during or just after hospitalization of the schizophrenic member. The approach of the programs is mainly educational and pragmatic, in a multiple family group setting. The aim of these programs is to ameliorate the course of the illness, reduce relapse rate, and improve psychosocial functioning of the patient by educating the family about the illness, treatment approaches, and helping the family reduce stress on the patient. Families are taught techniques to cope with symptomatic behavior of the ill member, and effective communication skills. Not all programs include the ill member, but all programs promote regular contact with other affected families. The effectiveness of these treatment programs has been tested and favorable outcome results have been published.[17,23,48]

Conclusion

The theoretical models of family therapy presented in this chapter are diverse and at times conflicting. There are, however, threads of similarity in the characteristics of a well-functioning family identified by the various theoretical views. These common characteristics suggest directions any nurse might take when intervening with families to promote health or prevent illness. Reducing the intensity of anxiety and stress in a family reduces the likelihood of secondary stress symptoms, such as divorce, exacerbation of disease, death or accidental injury of a family member, or conflictual interpersonal relationships. In the high-stress setting of the general hospital, anxiety in a family escalates when their questions, feelings, and fears are not openly expressed to medical staff or when medical staff fail to listen attentively or answer directly. Family and staff mutually attempt not to "upset" the other person by bringing up emotion-laden subjects, such as terminal illness, death, or disfigurement. In an atmosphere of mutual avoidance of taboo subjects a closed communication system develops between medical staff and family. The nurse who can handle her own anxiety about the issues of acute and chronic illness and death can listen and respond empathically but nonreactively to patients and families, share factual information clearly, and thus promote open communication systems. Opening a closed communication system reduces the intensity of a family's emotional reaction to illness and death.

Nurses working in obstetrics and pediatrics are in contact with families at the outset of a normative crisis in family life, that is, at the addition of another member into a homeostatic family system. The expectation of families at this time (except when the pregnancy is an unwanted one) is that the event will be joyful and satisfying. Mothers especially, when confronted with feelings of helplessness or inadequacy, severe anxiety or panic, and, perhaps, occasional almost homicidal rage at the spouse or infant, are frightened and believe something is wrong with them. They fail to perceive their reactions as predictable reactions in a crisis situation. As nurses educate families to the concept of normative life crises, the family's anxiety diminishes. They are less likely to view their emotional reactions as problems and more likely to see them as normal responses to transitional family stress.

For the nurse therapist working with couples or families in treatment, the sense of bewilderment and information overload, which is characteristic of the therapist in a family treatment situation, is what makes this work the most exciting as well as the most difficult. To stay afloat in this sea of data, it is important for the nurse to develop a thorough understanding of one conceptual framework for herself. She can then use treatment strategies and techniques from various models that are congruent with the theoretical framework she has developed. Her choice of strategy would depend on her assessment of the specific family and the level at which she decided to intervene.

The essence of family therapy is conceptualizing the nature of human relationship problems or behavioral disorders within the natural context in which they arise within the family. The family, as a system, seeks to maintain a dynamic equilibrium. Change in any one part of the system shifts the balance, resulting in alterations throughout the system. By recognizing this and using it as leverage for therapeutic change, family therapy aims to be effective.

■ SUGGESTED CROSS-REFERENCES ■

Assessment of families is discussed in Chapter 5. Vulnerable families are discussed in Chapter 9. Working with families of psychiatric patients is discussed in Chapters 10 and 11. Intervening in family abuse and violence is discussed in Chapter 32.

■ SUMMARY ■

1. Family therapy is not a modality of treatment but rather a way of conceptualizing human relationship problems. It focuses on the context in which an emotional problem is generated. The process between family members that supports and perpetuates symptoms is considered to be the focus of treatment rather than the individual family member who manifests the family's problems.

2. Characteristics of the well-functioning family, common dysfunctional family patterns, and indications for family therapy were described. The role of both the generalist and specialist nurse in family therapy was identified.

3. Bowen's family systems therapy was the first theoretical model discussed. It moved away from the medical model and a psychopathological point of view to conceptualize all family systems on a continuum ranging from total dysfunction to high levels of functioning. A cornerstone in systems theory is separating the thinking and feeling processes of family members. The goal of systems therapy is for individual family members to differentiate themselves from the family emotional "we-ness" system.

Seven central interlocking concepts of systems theory were discussed:

    a. *Differentiation* reflects sufficient separation between intellect and emotions so that one is not dominated by the reactive anxiety of the family's emotional system.

    b. A *triangle* is a predictable emotional process that takes place in any significant relationship when there is difficulty in the relationship.

    c. The *nuclear family emotional system* refers to patterns of

---

DIRECTIONS FOR FUTURE RESEARCH

The following are some of the nursing research problems raised in Chapter 29 that merit further study by psychiatric nurses:

1. Empirical validation of Bowen's self-differentiation scale
2. The relationship between the therapist's level of self-differentiation and the highest level of self-differentiation achieved by the treatment family after completing family therapy
3. Comparison of the effectiveness of one model of family therapy vs. another model with specified presenting problems
4. Personal exploration by the therapist of the issues into which he or she is most vulnerable to being triangled
5. Comparison of the effectiveness of individual family therapy vs. multiple family therapy with a specified presenting problem
6. Outcomes of types of family therapy utilized at different phases of schizophrenic illness
7. Comparison of nurse-run multiple family therapy groups to non–nurse-run groups measuring comparable effectiveness and cost
8. The effectiveness of doing therapy with the single generation sibling group when the parental dyad or single parent refuses to participate in the target child's treatment
9. Outcomes associated with creating a ritual with a family suffering unresolved grief due to loss through death, miscarriage, or abortion, to promote freer affect or grieving
10. The effect of nurse-run multiple family support groups for families suffering from chronic medical illness on measures of quality of life and family coping
11. Outcomes of a group composed of nursing staff and family caregivers (of the chronically medically ill family member) on the quality of care and utilization of services of respite care in a hospital or nursing home setting
12. The adjustment of new parents when content on the normative crisis aspects of birth of the first child is included in prenatal classes

---

interaction between family members and the degree to which these patterns promote emotional fusion.

    d. The *multigenerational transmission process* is the assumption that relationship patterns and symptoms in a family have their origin several generations before. A four- or five-generation genogram reveals such patterns.

e. The *family projection process* is the projection of spouses' problems onto one or more children to avoid the intense emotional fusion between the spouses.

f. One's *sibling position,* that is, birth order and sex, is a determining factor in a person's personality profile.

g. The *emotional cutoff* is a dysfunctional way in which some family members deal with intense family conflict by using either emotional isolation or geographical distance.

Various modes of therapy from a family system framework were described.

4. Structural family therapy, as conceptualized by Minuchin, assumes that behavior and the family's level of function are a consequence of the organization of the family and the interactional patterns between family members.

a. According to the structural view, a family is a social system in transformation.

b. The family goes through predictable developmental stages over time, requiring adaptive restructuring of the family.

c. The major elements of a family structure that enable the viable functioning of the family were identified as: **(1)** a power hierarchy with different levels of authority, **(2)** differentiated subsystems that have different functions and levels of power, and **(3)** subsystem boundaries that are sufficiently well defined to prevent intrusion but sufficiently permeable to permit emotional contact between members.

Tasks of the nurse according to this structural model include defining boundaries and supporting the functions of family subsystems. Restructuring interventions serve to transform dysfunctional transactional patterns that maintain symptomatic behavior and include: enacting transactional patterns, marking boundaries, escalating stress, assigning tasks, using symptoms, manipulating the family mood, and support, education, and guidance of the family.

5. Strategic, or brief, family therapy evolved on the West Coast from the earlier work of the communication theorists. Important principles of communication theory include the following:

a. All behavior is communication; therefore it is impossible not to communicate.

b. The meaning of a message includes the content and the context in which it was sent.

c. Communication is an ongoing process of stimulus-response-reinforcement. Communication theorists studied the interactional patterns in schizophrenic families and identified pathological communication patterns. Correcting these patterns became the goal of treatment.

Strategic therapists are concerned with the removal of problematical behavioral patterns or symptoms. Effective therapeutic intervention frequently involves the use of paradox and reverse psychology. The goals of strategic therapy include obtaining a clear statement from the client of the presenting complaint in specific concrete terms and reframing the problem, which thereby changes the meaning of the situation and thus permits new behavior to occur.

6. Knowledge of theoretical models of family therapy can assist the nurse when intervening in health promotion and illness prevention with families in a variety of settings. The nurse therapist should use a conceptual framework in work with families and integrate various treatment strategies and techniques as appropriate.

■   **REFERENCES**   ■

1. Ackerman, N.: The growing edge of family therapy. In Sager, C., and Kaplan, H., editors: Progress in group and family therapy, New York, 1972, Brunner/Mazel, Inc.

2. Barnhill, L.: Healthy family systems. The Family Coordinator **94,** Jan. 1979.

3. Barragan, M.: The child-centered family. In Guerin, P., editor: Family therapy theory and practice, New York, 1976, Gardner Press, Inc.

4. Bateson, G., et al.: Toward a theory of schizophrenia, Behav. Sci. **1**:251, 1956.

5. Beels, C., and Ferber, A.: Family therapy: a view, Fam. Process **8**:280, 1969.

6. Berensen, D.: An interview with Richard Fisch, The Family **3**(1):24, 1976.

7. Bowen, M.: Intrafamily dynamics in emotional illness. In D'Agostino, A., editor: Family, church, and community, New York, 1961, P.J. Kennedy & Sons.

8. Bowen, M.: Family psychotherapy with schizophrenia in the hospital and in private practice. In Bosormenyi-Nagy, I., and Framo, J., editors: Intensive family therapy, New York, 1965, Harper & Row, Publishers, Inc.

9. Bowen, M.: Family therapy and family group therapy. In Kaplan, H., and Sadock, B., editors: Comprehensive group psychotherapy, Baltimore, 1971, The Williams & Wilkins Co.

10. Bowen, M.: Multigenerational transmission process. In Haley, J., editor: Changing families, New York, 1971, Grune & Stratton, Inc.

11. Bowen, M.: The use of family therapy in clinical practice. In Haley, J., editor: Changing families. New York, 1971, Grune & Stratton, Inc.

12. Bowen, M.: Theory in the practice of psychotherapy. In Guerin, P., editor: Family therapy theory and practice, New York, 1976, Gardner Press, Inc.

13. Brown, G., and Birley, J.: Crises and life changes and the onset of schizophrenia. J. Health Soc. Behav. **9**:203, 1968.

14. Cain, A.: The role of the therapist in family systems therapy, The Family **3**(2):65, 1976.

15. Carter, B.: In a family therapy workshop, Bridgeport, Conn., 1976.

16. Carter, E., and McGoldrick, M.: The family life cycle, a framework for family therapy, New York, 1980, Gardner Press, Inc.

17. Faloon, I., Boyd, J., and McGill, C.: Family care of schizophrenia. New York, 1984, Guilford Press.

18. Fisch, R., et al.: On unbecoming family therapists. In Ferber, A., Mendelson, M., and Napier, A., editors:

The book of family therapy, New York, 1972, Science House, Inc.

19. Fogarty, T.: Family structure in terms of triangles. In Bradt, J., and Moynihan, C., editors: Systems therapy, Washington, D.C., 1971, The Groome Child Guidance Center.

20. Fogarty, T.: The family emotional self system. A day with a family workshop, New Rochelle, N.Y., CFL sampler, Jan. 4, 1975.

21. Fogarty, T.: Triangles. The Family 2:165, Spring-Summer 1975.

22. Fogarty, T.: System concepts and dimensions of self. In Guerin, P., editor: Family therapy theory and practice, New York, 1976, Gardner Press, Inc.

23. Glick, I., and Spencer, J.: Commentary on D. Hunter, On the boundary: family therapy in a long-term patient setting. Family process **24**:349, 1985.

24. Goolishian, H.: Problem focused family therapy, Orthopsychiatry Workshop, New York, Apr. 1977.

25. Guerin, P.: System, system, who's got the system, The Family 3(1):13, 1976.

26. Guerin, P.: Theoretical aspects and clinical relevance of the multigenerational model of family therapy. In Guerin, P., editor: Family theory and practice, New York, 1976, Gardner Press, Inc.

27. Guerin, P., and Pendagast, E.: Evaluation of family system and genogram. In Guerin, P., editor: Family therapy theory and practice, New York, 1976, Gardner Press, Inc.

28. Haley, J.: Uncommon therapy, the psychiatric techniques of Milton H. Erickson, M.D., New York, 1973, W.W. Norton & Co.

29. Haley, J.: Problem solving therapy, San Francisco, 1976, Jossey-Bass, Inc.

30. Hatfield, A.: What families want of family therapists. In McFarlane, W., editor: Family therapy in schizophrenia, New York, 1983, Guilford Press.

31. Klugman, J.: Owning and disowning: the structural dimension, Fam. Process **16**:353, 1977.

32. Lamb, R., et al.: Families of schizophrenics: a movement in jeopardy. Hosp. Community Psychiatry **37**(4):353, 1986.

33. McFarlane, W., editor: Family therapy in schizophrenia, New York, 1983, Guilford Press.

34. Minuchin, S.: Families and family therapy, Cambridge, Mass., 1974, Harvard University Press.

35. Minuchin, S., et al.: A conceptual model of psychosomatic illness in children, Arch. Gen. Psychiatry **32**:1031, 1975.

36. Minuchin, S., and Fishman, H.: Family therapy techniques. Cambridge, Mass., 1981, Harvard University Press.

37. O'Shea, M., and Phelps, R.: Multiple family therapy: current status and critical appraisal. Fam. Process **24**:255, 1985.

38. Palazoli, M.: Self-starvation, New York, 1978, Jason Aronson, Inc.

39. Palazoli, M., et al.: Paradox and counterparadox, New York, 1979, Jason Aronson, Inc.

40. Rabkin, R.: Strategic psychotherapy, New York, 1977, Basic Books, Inc.

41. Ritterman, M.: Paradigmatic classification of family therapy theories, Fam. Process **16**:29, March 1977.

42. Starkey, P.: Genograms. A guide to understanding one's own family system. Perspect. Psychiatr. Care **19**(5 & 6):164, 1981.

43. Steidl, J., and Wexler, J.: What's a clinician to do with so many approaches to family therapy? The Family **4**(2):59, 1977.

44. Stierlin, H.: The dynamics of owning and disowning: psychoanalytic and family perspectives, Fam. Process **15**:277, 1976.

45. Strelnick, A.H.: Multiple family group therapy: a review of the literature, Fam. Process **16**: 307, 1977.

46. Terkelsen, K.: Bowen on triangles—March, 1974, workshop. I, The Family **1**(2):45, 1974.

47. Terkelsen, K.: Bowen on triangles—March, 1974, workshop, II. The Family **2**:1, 1974.

48. Terkelsen, K.: Schizophrenia and the family: II. Adverse effects of family therapy. Fam. Process **191**:204, 1983.

49. Toman, W.: Family constellation, New York, 1961, Springer Publishing Co.

50. Watzlawick, P.: Some basic issues in interaction research. In Framo, J., editor: Family interaction, New York, 1972, Springer Publishing Co.

51. Watzlawick, P., Beaven, J., and Jackson, D.: Pragmatics of human communication, New York, 1967, W.W. Norton & Co.

52. Watzlawick, P., Weakland, J., and Fisch, R.: Change, principles of problem formation and problem resolution, New York, 1974, W.W. Norton & Co.

53. Weakland, J.: Communication theory and clinical change. In Guerin, P., editor: Family therapy theory and practice, New York, 1976, Gardner Press, Inc.

54. Whitaker, C., and Miller, M.: A re-evaluation of psychiatric help when divorce impends. In. Sager, C.J., and Kaplan, H.S.: editors: Progress in group and family therapy, New York, 1972, Brunner/Mazel, Inc.

■ ANNOTATED SUGGESTED READINGS ■

Anderson, C., and Stewart, S.: Mastering resistance: A practice guide to family therapy, New York, 1983, The Guilford Press.

As the title suggests, this useful book offers beginners and advanced students from any of the various "schools" of family therapy, accessible strategies for confronting the commonly encountered forms of family resistance to treatment. The book's orderly structure of problem heading, followed by suggested interventions is enriched by prolific clinical examples.

Anonymous: Toward the differentiation of a self in one's own family. In Framo, J., editor: Family interaction: a dialogue between family therapists and family researchers, New York, 1972, Springer Publishing Co.

Originally published anonymously, this work by Bowen describes his efforts to differentiate himself from his family of origin. He effectively demonstrates the application of family systems theory with his own family. It is a classic in systems theory.

Bowen, M.: Family therapy in clinical practice, New York, 1978, Jason Aronson, Inc.

The development of Bowen's thinking is collected in one volume containing all his previously published articles plus several original ones. Most of the earlier articles in this volume have become "classics." This is an important text for any student who wishes to understand systems theory in depth.

Bradt, J., and Moynihan, C.: Systems therapy, Washington, D.C., 1971, Groome Child Guidance Center.

This is a collection of outstanding papers presented at the Georgetown Family Symposia from 1966 to 1971. It includes theoretical papers, research, and descriptions of clinical application and technique from a family systems framework. It is a good text for the beginning family therapist.

*Cain, A.: The role of the therapist in family systems therapy, The Family **3**(2):65, 1976.

A nurse therapist describes the process of systems therapy, and the pitfalls involved in working with a family in treatment.

Carter, E., and McGoldrick, M.: The family life cycle, a framework for family therapy, New York, 1980, Gardner Press, Inc.

This volume contains a series of original contributions from well-known practitioners in the family therapy field. The chapters systematically cover the developmental stages of the family life cycle and commonly encountered family problems that disrupt the life cycle, including chronic illness and death, divorce and remarriage, and poverty. This is a valuable text for beginning and advanced students alike.

*Clements, I., and Buchanan, D.: Family therapy: A nursing perspective, New York, 1982, John Wiley & Sons.

This text offers beginning students of family therapy a historical view of family therapy. It reviews five family therapy models, operationalizes them, then compares and contrasts central concepts within these models. Finally the authors provide the means by which the nurse can effectively utilize specific interventions or tools within one's clinical practice with maladaptive families.

Ferber, A., Mendelsohn, M., and Napier, A.: The book of family therapy, New York, 1972, Science House, Inc.

In conversational style many well-known persons in the family therapy field discuss personal and theoretical views of their own work. This is a recommended book for a beginner in the field.

Fogarty, T.: Triangles, The Family **2**:11, Spring-Summer 1975.

This article thoroughly examines the family systems concept of triangles. It is an important article for the advanced student.

Guerin, P., editor: Family therapy and practice, New York, 1976, Gardner Press, Inc.

This book contains a series of original contributions from the most distinguished leaders in the family therapy field. It is an excellent reference text for the beginning and advanced student. Theory and technique from several frameworks are presented in a clear organized fashion.

Gurman, A., and Kniskern, D., editors: Handbook of family therapy, New York, 1981, Brunner/Mazel.

A comprehensive reference book covering an array of major current clinical concepts in family therapy. While chapters represent divergent approaches, certain editorial features facilitate readers' task of critical assessment, comparison, and integration of the divergent approaches. Recommended for beginning or advanced students.

Haley, J., editor: Changing families, New York, 1971, Grune & Stratton, Inc.

This is a well-selected collection of articles by well-known authors in the field covering a spectrum of theoretical approaches to family therapy. Many of the articles contained in this volume have become "classics."

Haley, J.: Uncommon therapy, the psychiatric techniques of Milton H. Erickson, M.D., New York, 1973, W.W. Norton & Co.

Milton Erickson is a highly regarded pioneer and leader in the family therapy field. In this volume Haley has carefully edited and explicated hours of recorded cases Dr. Erickson has treated. The use of paradoxical intention is demonstrated in multiple examples.

Haley, J.: Problem solving therapy, San Francisco, 1976, Jossey-Bass, Inc.

In this book the author presents the problem-focused, strategic approach to family therapy in a clear, organized manner. Theory and technique are richly supported with case examples. This is an important text for beginners and advanced students alike.

Haley, J.: Leaving home: the therapy of disturbed young people, New York, 1980, McGraw-Hill, Inc.

This practical, down-to-earth book focuses on the problems and solutions surrounding the transition of leaving home, when young people become self-supporting and independent of their families. It suggests and explicates a model of therapy to be used with families who are stuck in this crucial transition point. Case histories and interview excerpts illustrate the methods of therapy.

Jones, S.: Family therapy, a comparison of approaches, Englewood Cliffs, N.J., 1980, Prentice-Hall, Inc.

As the title implies, this book comprehensively reviews and compares different theoretical models of family therapy currently in practice, including Bowenian, structural, strategic, behavioral, psychoanalytical theories. It is a valuable resource for beginning students in the field.

Klugman, J.: "Enmeshment and fusion," Fam. Process **15**:321, 1976.

This concise article examines and contrasts the differences between two seemingly synonymous concepts from the structural and systems framework respectively.

Lederer, W., and Jackson, D.: The mirages of marriage, New York, 1968, W.W. Norton & Co.

This book is intended for families and therapists alike. It explodes false myths and assumptions about the marriage relationship and offers some no-nonsense suggestions for solving readily recognized marital problems from a communication theory framework.

Madanes, C.: Strategic family therapy, San Francisco, 1981, Jossey-Bass, Inc., Publishers.

This book, by a leader in strategic family therapy, focuses on destructive unequal power structures in symptomatic families. She describes both straightforward interventions and paradoxical interventions with commonly encountered family, marital, and parent-child problems.

McFarlane, W. editor: Family therapy in schizophrenia, New York, 1983, Guilford Press.

As increasing emphasis has been placed on biochemical and genetic factors contributing to the etiology of schizophrenia, the family therapies of schizophrenia have undergone revolutionary changes. Where in the past families were held culpable for schizophrenia in a member, in the treatment approaches presented here, the families are recognized as the principal caregiver of the schizophrenic patient, and working allies of the therapeutic team. In this volume, the most recently developed practical, tested treatment approaches are presented, some including outcome studies. The reader is confronted with the controversy which surrounds the two basic approaches: the medical model approach, which includes a "psychoeducational" component, and the communications theory approach. The final chapter by Beels and McFarlane, attempts to synthesize the various treatment approaches by offering a "decision-tree model." This book is recommended for any level practitioner interested in family therapy of schizophrenia.

McGoldrick, M., and Gerson, R.: Genograms and family assessment, New York, 1986, W.W. Norton & Co.

The authors present a standard format for constructing genograms and clearly outline the principals underlying their interpretation and application. Using genograms of famous people, such as Alexander Graham Bell, Virginia Woolf, and John F. Kennedy, to name but a few, the beginner is introduced to this essential tool in systems therapy.

McGoldrick, M., Pearce, J., and Giordano, J., editors: Ethnicity and family therapy, New York, 1982, Guilford Press.

The editors have compiled a long needed volume in the field. Each chapter describes ethnic and cultural characteristics of a specified group. Attendant values, social and religious beliefs, which influence individual and family behavior are identified and examined.

Minuchin, S.: Family kaleidoscope, Cambridge, Mass., 1984, Harvard University Press.

With this book, Minuchin wishes to challenge our society's predilection to explain human nature with the individual-oriented framework (epistomology). When families confront institutions with problems, as they do during divorce, remarriage, in therapy, with the judiciary and medical systems, and when there is violence, too often the result is dismemberment of the family. Using a potpourri of avenues by which to examine family problems, Minuchin makes a passionate bid for more accurate perceptions of the human reality as seen within the complete family system.

Minuchin, S.: Families and family therapy, Cambridge, Mass., 1974, Harvard University Press.

This volume contains a clear exposition of structural family therapy. Numerous case examples are well integrated into theoretical discussion. This book is an important text for beginning and advanced students.

Minuchin, S. et al.: A conceptual model of psychosomatic illness in children, Arch. Gen. Psychiatry **32**:1, Aug. 1975.

This article compares the medical model of psychosomatic illness to a systems, multiple feedback model within the family structure. In describes the necessary conditions in a family for the development of severe psychosomatic illness in children and the family therapy strategies used to treat it.

Minuchin, S., and Fishman, H.C.: Family therapy techniques, Cambridge, Mass., 1981, Harvard University Press.

This highly practical book provides clear definitive coverage of the techniques and skills utilized in structural family therapy. Techniques are described, and then excerpts of parts of sessions are included to illustrate and amplify theoretical descriptions. This is the logical theoretical sequel to Families and Family Therapy.

Minuchin, S., Rosman, B., and Baker, L.: Psychosomatic families, anorexia nervosa in context, Cambridge, Mass., 1978, Harvard University Press.

In this book by Minuchin and his associates he describes his successful treatment and research with the families of anorexics. Over half the book consists of clinical interviews and case examples.

Palazoli, M. et al.: Paradox and counterparadox, New York, 1978, Jason Aronson, Inc.

This book reports the early results of clinical research of the Milan Center for Family Studies with acute schizophrenic families. The unique short-term therapy approach of Palazoli and her team is described. Their use of paradoxical interventions to change the paralyzing circular patterns of disturbed communication in schizophrenic families is explained and elucidated by clinical examples. This book is recommended for the advanced student.

Rabkin, R.: Strategic psychotherapy, New York, 1977, Basic Books, Inc.

This book offers a thorough discussion of strategic therapy. It discusses in depth the use of reverse psychology, which employs the patient's resistance and paradox.

*Smoyak, S.: Family therapy. In Psychiatric nursing 1946 to 1974: a report on the state of the art, New York, 1975, American Journal of Nursing Co.

Through an extensive review of the literature, the author identifies the evolving role of the nurse in family therapy. Because of its thoroughness and historical review, it is an excellent resource for nursing's involvement with families.

Toman, W.: Family constellation, New York, 1961, Springer Publishing Co., Inc.

This book describes personality profiles based on a person's sibling position, considering birth order and sex. This book is a classic and should be read by all students of family therapy.

Watzlawick, P., Beaven, J., and Jackson, D.: Pragmatics of human communication, New York, 1967, W.W. Norton & Co.

This book describes the effects of human communication, with special attention to behavior disorders. The authors define general communication theory, present basic characteristics of human communication, and offer examples of pathological communication. This is a basic text for understanding the origins of strategic, or brief, family therapy.

Watzlawick, P., Weakland, J., and Fisch, R.: Change, principles of problem formation and problem resolution, New York, 1974, W.W. Norton & Co.

The authors' efforts to understand their effective but seemingly irrational treatment strategies stimulated the development of a theory of change, which evolved into strategic family therapy.

This book offers a clear explication of the use of paradox in treatment. It is the logical theoretical sequel to Haley's Uncommon Therapy *for the advanced student.*

Weitzman, J.: Engaging the severely dysfunctional family in treatment: Basic considerations. Family Process **24**:473, 1985.

The beginning clinician who has felt overwhelmed by the problems of the severely dysfunctional family, and has felt confused by the theoretical controversy surrounding the process of engaging these families in treatment, would do well to read this article. The author recommends a generic approach toward these most difficult to engage severely dysfunctional families. He proposes an attitude of acceptance of and sensitivity to the family "as is" before initiating more traditional interventions.

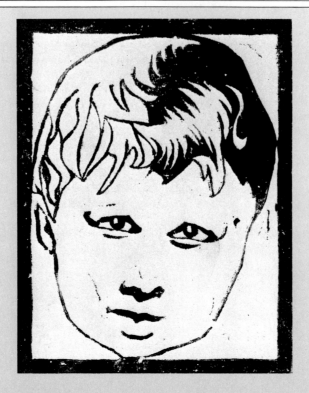

Youth's love
Embracingly integrates
Successfully frustrates
And holds together,
Often unwittingly
All that hate, fear, and selfishness
Attempt to disintegrate.

R. Buckminster Fuller, And It Came to Pass—Not To Stay

C H A P T E R   3 0

CHILD PSYCHIATRIC NURSING

RITA L. RUBIN

LEARNING OBJECTIVES

After studying this chapter, the student should be able to:

- describe the major influences on the development of child psychiatry.

- state the levels, scope, and settings of child psychiatric nursing practice.

- assess the purpose and importance of the *Standards of Child and Adolescent Psychiatric and Mental Health Nursing Practice.*

- discuss the elements of the latency period of child development, including Piaget's cognitive processes, the functions of the ego, and the role of Mahler's individuation theory.

- identify the major categories of data that should be collected by the nurse with regard to the child's health status.

- describe common medical diagnoses used with children with ego deficits.

- compare and contrast the characteristics of the following diagnostic groups: autistic-presymbiotic, symbiotic-psychotic, and borderline.

- discuss common areas of conflict for children with ego deficits and the nursing diagnoses appropriate to them.

- analyze the indications for and implications of the various therapeutic modalities that can be included in the plan of care.

- describe the phases, techniques, and components of nursing intervention with disturbed children.

- assess the importance of evaluation of the nursing process when working with children.

- identify directions for future nursing research.

- select appropriate readings for further study.

Historical antecedents

The field of child psychiatry had its beginnings in the early 1900s. It developed from four major bodies of knowledge: psychoanalysis, education, psychology, and an outgrowth of information from work with delinquent youth. Sigmund Freud's major influence on child mental health was his recognition of the role of early childhood experiences in the mental health of the adult. He also treated a phobic child, Little Hans, by coaching his father in the technique of analysis.[17] Child psychoanalysis owes it development and practice to two analysts, Melanie Klein, who initially worked in Berlin in the 1920s and 1930s, and Anna Freud, who worked simultaneously in Vienna. Klein is considered to have utilized play in the same way an analyst would use adult free association. Thus the term *play therapy* became the key to treating mentally disturbed children.[20] Anna Freud utilized the medium of play as well, but differed from Klein somewhat in her approach. Anna Freud's major emphasis was the development of a positive transference with her child patient. Play with toys was a technique of communicating and relating to the child in a way he could understand.[13] Both child analysts were uprooted by World War II and resumed their work later in the United States and England.

The field of education promoted the idea that children needed a combination of nurturing and learning experiences to become responsible adults. As early as the mid-1800s, students of educational science recognized that children progressed through developmental stages and learned spontaneously by doing. Contributors at the turn of the twentieth century included Sully,[35] who recognized the importance of play in children's communication, and the normative studies of Binet,[5] Catell,[8] and Gisell,[18] who developed the concept of intelligence and set the groundwork for the developmental theory of Erikson.[15]

The educational psychologists, Dewey and James, furthered the study of the range of normal and also asked questions about how the child learns. Their work was instrumental in bridging knowledge from education to psychology for application in the teaching and testing of children. Influential in the field of psychology were Pavlov, Watson, and Skinner, who established the behaviorist school.[40] Their descriptions of stimulus–response (S–R) learning have been applied not only to the education of children, but also to modifying troublesome behaviors of children. In addition, Jean Piaget, a Swiss psychologist, has provided child psychiatry with a developmental theory of cognitive growth.[14]

The contribution stemming from concern about juvenile delinquents and orphans came in response to the great influx of immigrants and the Industrial Revolution, both of which occurred in the early 1900s. During this time, almshouses and foster homes were established to keep children off the streets. In 1909, Healy[21] studied the problem of delinquency in Chicago and concluded that aberrant behavior was produced by multicausal factors, not the least of which was the role of the family. Another important name associated with the treatment of delinquency is Aichhorn, who treated delinquent youths in Vienna in the 1920s, using psychoanalytical principles.[20]

A final major influence on the field of child psychiatry was the child guidance movement that began around 1930. The psychiatric treatment of children was initiated through the court system, later becoming community based. This classic team approach is still utilized widely, in which a therapist sees the child, a psychologist does the testing, and a social worker works with the family, in addition to coordinating community resources.

The multidisciplinary team approach in the practice of child psychiatry has its parallel in theory. Theory remains a "mixed bag," pulling from a wide variety of frameworks, yet having no theory unique unto itself. Despite the criticism imbued by so-called purists, there remains the fact that no one method of treatment has been of help to all children in need of psychiatric intervention. Consequently, the field of child psychiatry continues to be the product of psychology, education, psychiatry, nursing, and social work.

Child psychiatric nursing practice

Nurses entered the field of psychiatry initially as custodial caretakers. Then with the advent of the somatic therapies between 1930 and 1940, some effort was placed on educating nurses in psychiatry to improve the care of psychiatric patients. The second half of the twentieth century has seen nurses functioning in ever-expanding roles, their advanced training mandated by federal legislation. The National Mental Health Act of 1946 provided funding for advanced training of psychiatric nurses (among other professionals) in undergraduate and graduate nursing programs. This became the stepping stone to recognizing that psychiatric nurses needed specialized training. Within the next decade Boston University had a graduate program for child psychiatric nurses. In 1955, Mental Health Law 182 charged the Joint Commission on Mental Health and Illness to conduct a study of mental illness and ways to prevent it. Significant among the findings was the recommendation that nurses be utilized more efficiently to provide mental health care in the face of a shortage of personnel.[27]

One could argue that since that time little progress has been made in meeting the mental health needs of children. It is estimated that the prevalence of mental disorder in children and youth is about 12%, which represents over 7 million children.[19,23] The American Academy of Child Psychiatry expects the incidence of psychiatric disorder in children and youth to remain the same or increase in the next decade.[11] It has also been estimated that only 7% of the children and youth who need mental health services receive them because of the lack of both professional personnel and clinical services.[22] Child psychiatric nurses are prepared to diagnose and treat mental disorders in children, but a recent survey demonstrated that there is a gap between the need for services and the utilization of prepared specialists in child and adolescent psychiatric nursing.[28] Thus, gaining access to populations in need of services remains one of the major challenges facing this area of nursing at the present time.

■ Scope of practice

Presently there are two levels at which child psychiatric nurses practice: generalist and specialist. Educational preparation differentiates the two levels. The registered nurse is considered to be a **generalist** and may intervene independently to provide care for nursing problems or dependently, through physicians' orders, for medically diagnosed problems. A generalist may assume the role of therapist with qualified supervision.[1] The **child psychiatric nurse specialist** has earned a master's degree and has a clinical background in child psychiatric nursing. At present nine schools offer graduate programs in this field (see accompanying box). With successful completion of certification by the American Nurses' Association, the specialist may choose to engage in private practice. When employed by a health care facility she may assume indirect and direct care duties specified by the current state nurse practice act.

Another professional organization, Advocates for Child Psychiatric Nursing, Inc., has provided a position statement on the education of a child psychiatric clinical nurse specialist, which concurs with the American Nurses' Association definitions of the specialist.[10] In addition, they specify the need for a nursing framework and a theory of human behavior to apply to practice. They see the specialist as a therapist who demonstrates her competence through the certification procedure and maintains her competency by continued formal and informal educational experiences.

Graduate Programs in Child and Adolescent Psychiatric and Mental Health Nursing

Boston University
School of Nursing
Boston, Mass. 02215

Columbia University
School of Nursing
New York, N.Y. 10027

Lehman College
City University of New York
New York, N.Y.

University of Alabama
School of Nursing
Birmingham, Al. 35294

University of California at Los Angeles
School of Nursing
Los Angeles, Calif. 90024

University of California, San Francisco
School of Nursing
San Francisco, Calif. 94143

University of Cincinnati
College of Nursing
Cincinnati, Ohio 45221

University of Illinois, Chicago
School of Nursing
Chicago, Ill. 60680

University of Maryland
School of Nursing
Baltimore, Md. 21201

Wayne State University
School of Nursing
Detroit, Mich. 48202

Yale University
School of Nursing
New Haven, Ct. 06520

■ Practice settings

The nurse in child psychiatry may assume positions in primary, secondary, or tertiary prevention settings. In **primary prevention settings,** the aim is to prevent emotional problems. Nurses with knowledge in child psychiatry may provide services to prenatal clinics, day care centers, nursery schools, and other child care programs. Preventive care includes health education in the areas of infant and child development, child rearing and parenting, and counseling for life stresses such as divorce, death, or chronic illnesses. The child psychiatric nurse specialist may provide consultation to day care centers, nursery schools, and pediatric floors in hospitals.

Secondary prevention settings are geared toward early intervention in mental illness to minimize its disabling effects. Examples of such settings in child psychiatry include outpatient clinics and partial hospitalization programs. The nurse-therapist in this setting may use a variety of therapeutic modalities to help chil-

dren and their families cope with high levels of stress. During crises the nurse may be called on to consult with schools to provide coordination of services and disseminate information relative to the child experiencing emotional difficulties.

Tertiary prevention settings provide rehabilitation to reduce the severity of mental illness. Common settings include child psychiatric inpatient units of general hospitals, residential treatment in psychiatric hospitals, transitional care settings, such as day care and group homes, and outpatient clinics. The child psychiatric nurse in such settings serves predominately as a milieu therapist. She provides therapeutic experiences by helping the child deal with daily life occurrences and providing a healthy adult-to-child relationship and role model.

STANDARDS OF CHILD AND ADOLESCENT PSYCHIATRIC AND MENTAL HEALTH NURSING PRACTICE

The American Nurses' Association, in cooperation with Advocates for Child Psychiatric Nursing, Inc. published standards for child and adolescent psychiatric nursing in 1985. These standards may be applied to inpatient, outpatient, and community practice settings. They are divided into professional and performance practice standards, and parallel the generic standards of practice presented in Chapters 1 and 5.

PROFESSIONAL PRACTICE STANDARDS

STANDARD I. THEORY
The nurse applies appropriate, scientifically sound theory as a basis for nursing practice decisions.
Rationale

Child and adolescent psychiatric and mental health nursing is characterized by the application of relevant theories to explain developmental and behavioral phenomena of concern to nursing, and to provide a basis for intervention and subsequent evaluation of that intervention. Primary sources of knowledge for practice are the scholarly conceptualizations of child and adolescent psychiatric and mental health nursing practice and research findings generated from intradisciplinary and cross-disciplinary studies of child and adolescent development, cultural differences, human behavior, and treatment issues. The nurse's use of appropriate theories provides comprehensive, balanced perceptions of client characteristics or presenting conditions and ensures accurate diagnoses. The nurse focusing on children, adolescents, and their families needs to use a broad range of theories, including developmental theory, systems theory, theories of prevention, and nursing theory.

STANDARD II. ASSESSMENT
The nurse systematically collects, records, and analyzes data that are comprehensive and accurate.
Rationale

Effective interviewing, behavioral observation, and developmental and systems assessments enable the nurse to reach objective conclusions and plan appropriate interventions with and for children and adolescents.

STANDARD III. DIAGNOSIS
The nurse, in expressing conclusions supported by recorded assessment data and current scientific premises, uses nursing diagnoses and/or standard classifications of mental disorders for childhood and adolescence.
Rationale

Nursing's logical basis for providing care rests in the recognition and identification of those actual or potential health problems that are within the scope of child and adolescent psychiatric and mental health nursing practice.

STANDARD IV. PLANNING
The nurse develops a nursing care plan with specific goals and interventions delineating nursing actions unique to the needs of each child or adolescent, as well as those of the family and other relevant interactive social systems.
Rationale

The nursing care plan is used to guide therapeutic intervention and move effectively toward the desired outcomes.

STANDARD V. INTERVENTION
The nurse intervenes as guided by the nursing care plan to implement nursing actions that promote, maintain, or restore physical and mental health, prevent illness, effect rehabilitation in childhood and adolescence, and restore developmental progression.
Rationale

Mental health is one aspect of general health and well-being. Nursing actions reflect an appreciation for the hierarchy of human needs and include interventions for all aspects of physical and mental health and illness not only for the child or adolescent but also for the family.

STANDARD V-A. INTERVENTION: THERAPEUTIC ENVIRONMENT
The nurse provides, structures, and maintains a therapeutic environment in collaboration with the child or adolescent, the family, and other health care providers.

Rationale

The nurse works with children, adolescents, and families in a variety of environmental settings that can themselves contribute to the movement toward mental health. The nurse can structure the environment in a goal-directed manner to assure that the environment is therapeutic.

STANDARD V-B. INTERVENTION: ACTIVITIES OF DAILY LIVING

The nurse uses the activities of daily living in a goal-directed way to foster the physical and mental well-being of the child or adolescent and family.

Rationale

The nurse is the primary professional health care provider who interacts with young clients on a day-to-day basis around the tasks of daily living. Therefore, the nurse has a unique opportunity to assess and intervene in these activities to encourage constructive changes in behavior so the children or adolescents can realize their potential for growth and health or maintain the level previously achieved.

STANDARD V-C. INTERVENTION: PSYCHOTHERAPEUTIC INTERVENTIONS

The nurse uses psychotherapeutic interventions to assist children or adolescents and families to develop, improve, or regain their adaptive functioning, to promote health, prevent illness, and facilitate rehabilitation.

Rationale

The nurse diagnoses actual and potential health problems in the child or adolescent which impede or impair the client's normal, healthy development. The nurse assists the child or adolescent and family to become aware of dysfunctional behavior, to modify or eliminate the behavior, and to develop functional behaviors.

STANDARD V-D. INTERVENTION: PSYCHOTHERAPY

The child and adolescent psychiatric and mental health specialist uses advanced clinical expertise to function as a psychotherapist for the child or adolescent and family and accepts professional accountability for nursing practice.

Rationale

Acceptance of the role of psychotherapist entails primary responsibility for the treatment of a child or adolescent and family and entrance into a contractual agreement. A contract includes a commitment to see a child or adolescent and family through the problem presented or to assist them in finding other appropriate assistance. It also includes an explicit definition of the relationship, the respective role of each person in the relationship, and what realistically can be expected of each person.

Treatment modalities are selected based on the developmental and system needs of the child or adolescent and family.

STANDARD V-E. INTERVENTION: HEALTH TEACHING AND ANTICIPATORY GUIDANCE

The nurse assists the child or adolescent and family to achieve more satisfying and productive patterns of living through health teaching and anticipatory guidance.

Rationale

Health teaching and anticipatory guidance are an essential part of the nurse's role with the child or adolescent and family who have actual or potential health problems. Many nursing interactions can be teaching-learning situations. Formal and informal teaching methods can be used in working with children, adolescents, families, and groups. The emphasis of the teaching and guidance is on the principles of mental health, normal development, and developmental needs, and on developing appropriate coping and adaptation patterns.

STANDARD V-F. INTERVENTION: SOMATIC THERAPIES

The nurse uses knowledge of somatic therapies with the child or adolescent and family to enhance therapeutic interventions.

Rationale

Various somatic treatment modalities may be needed by the child or adolescent and family during the course of treatment. Pertinent clinical observations and judgments are made concerning the effect of drugs and other somatic treatments used in the therapeutic program.

Continued.

STANDARD VI. EVALUATION

The nurse evaluates the response of the child or adolescent and family to nursing actions in order to revise the data base, nursing diagnoses, and nursing care plan.

Rationale

Nursing care is a dynamic process that incorporates ongoing alterations in data, diagnoses, or care plans.

PROFESSIONAL PERFORMANCE STANDARDS

STANDARD VII. QUALITY ASSURANCE

The nurse participates in peer review and other means of evaluation to assure quality of nursing care provided for children and adolescents and their families.

Rationale

Evaluation of the quality of nursing care through examination of the clinical practice of nurses is one way to fulfill the profession's obligation to ensure that consumers are provided excellence in care. Peer review, clinical supervision, consultation, and other quality assurance procedures are used in this endeavor.

STANDARD VIII. CONTINUING EDUCATION

The nurse assumes responsibility for continuing education and professional development and contributes to the professional growth of others studying children's and adolescents' mental health.

Rationale

The scientific, cultural, social, and political changes characterizing contemporary society require the child and adolescent psychiatric and mental health nurse to be committed to the pursuit of knowledge that will enhance professional growth.

STANDARD IX. INTERDISCIPLINARY COLLABORATION

The nurse collaborates with other health care providers in assessing, planning, implementing, and evaluating programs and other activities related to child and adolescent psychiatric and mental health nursing.

Rationale

Child and adolescent psychiatric and mental health nursing practice requires planning and sharing with others to deliver optimal psychiatric and mental health services to children and adolescents and their families. Through the collaborative process, different abilities of health care providers are used to communicate, plan, solve problems, and offer a variety of treatment modalities.

STANDARD X. USE OF COMMUNITY HEALTH SYSTEMS

The nurse participates with other members of the community in assessing, planning, implementing, and evaluating mental health services and community systems that attend to primary, secondary, and tertiary prevention of mental disorders in children and adolescents.

Rationale

The high incidence of mental illness in contemporary society and the increasing incidence of emotional disorders in children and adolescents requires greater effort to provide effective prevention and treatment programs. Child and adolescent psychiatric and mental health nurses must participate in programs that strengthen the existing health potential of children and adolescents in society. Concepts such as primary, secondary, and tertiary prevention and continuity of care can guide nurses in providing services to address a wide range of health needs of children and adolescents in the community. The nurse uses organizational, advisory, and consultative skills, as well as advocacy, to facilitate the development and implementation of such mental health services for children and adolescents.

STANDARD XI. RESEARCH

The nurse contributes to nursing and the child and adolescent psychiatric and mental health field through innovations in theory and practice and participation in research, and communicates these contributions.

Rationale

Each professional has responsibility for the continuing development and refinement of knowledge in the child and adolescent psychiatric and mental health field through research and through testing new and creative approaches to practice.

Development of the school-age child

■ The latency period

The school-age child from ages 6 to 12 years has become quite an independent human being. When compared to earlier stages, he is competent in many areas. He is able to leave his parents for the 6-hour school period and consequently comes under the influence of a complex world of teachers, peers, and other adults. He has established gender identity and is increasingly concerned with measuring up to his peers' accomplishments. Cognitively, he is able to reason, based on the perception of his senses. Emotionally, he has the potential of reaching "latency," which is, according to Sarnoff, ". . . the ability to achieve a state of calm, educability and pliability, using an age-appropriate organization of defenses."[33] The child achieving latency has an ego developed sufficiently to exercise control over his impulses; therefore he is able to behave appropriately to the situation. In the classroom, he may sit in a seat for several hours and attend to intellectual tasks, provided that he is able to release pent-up energy at intervals on the playground.

Erikson describes the task of latency to be that of the achievement of a sense of competency.[15] The 6-year-old is aware of his "inferiority" to adults and sets about with "industry" to learn the many skills and attain the necessary knowledge to achieve a feeling of competency. Originally the latency period was conceptualized by Freud, who believed that during this phase of psychosexual development the sexual impulses of the id were quiescent or repressed. The ego psychologists concentrated their efforts on explaining the developing ego and less on the role of the id. Consequently, theorists such as Erikson, Mahler, Chess, and others have posed explanations for psychopathological conditions based on deficits in ego strength. Disturbances of the ego are believed to be caused either by organic defects, as in the case of autism, or by some distortion of the experiential history within the family during the child's development, as in borderline states.[9] It is less clear which is causative in childhood schizophrenia, and both organicity and family environment are believed to play a role.

■ Functions of the ego

The cognitive domain of the ego is the seat of thought, sensory perception, memory, and language. Piaget, in his cognitive developmental theory, calls the school-age years the **concrete operations stage** and notes that here begins the "age of reason." A concrete operation is a thought process based on a concrete (as opposed to abstract) point of reference. The ability to perform concrete operations moves the school-age child beyond the magical thinking of preschool years. Learning is enhanced by the cognitive developments in this age range as is the skill of relating to others. Cognitive growth and its affective correlates that occur during the concrete operations stage as described by Piaget are presented in Table 30-1.

Another function of the ego is that of defending against instinctual drives using defense mechanisms. Sarnoff believes a major defense during latency is reaction formation. The anxiety of the oedipal period is harnessed during latency by converting one's drive to disorder into a desire for order and neatness. An example of this is the enthusiasm with which many children engage in collections of baseball cards, stones, small model cars, and the like.

Fantasy plays an important role in reducing anxiety for the child achieving latency. When able to engage in fantasy, much of the impulsiveness may be eliminated without it actually being acted out. Reading fairy tales performs this function, as does the fantasy material that occurs in spontaneous play.

The ego also functions to provide an individual with a sense of identity. Mahler has developed a theory whereby the child must separate from the mother and "individuate" in order to develop a sense of self.[24] Between birth and 6 months of age, the mother and infant are partners in a symbiotic relationship. Mahler postulates that the infant's awareness of self is limited to physical sensations from his body. He has no external reality and therefore mother and infant are fused into one amorphous unit.

In the latter half of the first year of life the infant begins the transition into Mahler's **separation-individuation phase**. His ability to locomote allows the external world to broaden under his control. His improved visual apparatus and memory help him realize he has one mother. During the following months the infant will continue to apply his physiological and cognitive growth to experimenting with leaving his mother. The crisis occurs between 18 and 24 months when the walking toddler realizes that he is separate from his mother, and, more important, has no control over her.

The reality of separating provides a benefit to the child in the form of increased ego strength. Mother's former help in the areas of impulse control, frustration tolerance, and reality testing are now part of the child's own repertoire of ego functions.[25] Mother encourages and supports the child's attempts to achieve autonomy and so cushions him from being overwhelmed by a sense of abandonment. Successful resolution of the rapprochement, or crisis, subphase in the separation-indi-

---

TABLE 30-1

COGNITIVE PROCESSES OF THE EGO IN PIAGET'S CONCRETE OPERATIONS STAGE

Ego function	Cognitive process	Affective correlate
Sensory perception	Takes in information more rapidly Organizes perceptions	Perceives reality in organized way
Thought	Demonstrates cause and effect thinking Problem solves and reasons Can follow rules	Learns and profits from formal education Behaves appropriately to given situation
Language	Knows basic rules of grammar Vocabulary increases Comprehension increases	Engages in meaningful communication and becomes more social
Memory	Mental representations are symbolic of objects, thus has increased ability to store and retrieve information	Establishes interpersonal relationships based on past events that give relations value

---

viduation process results in mother and child forming a reciprocal partnership, known as object relations, trading gradual maturity of the child for ego support from the mother.

Implementing the nursing process

In the specialty of child psychiatry the nurse may be called on to intervene with children who have insufficient ego strength to function outside of the inpatient setting. Many theorists contend that this is because of a lack of differentiation among family members and especially a failure of the separation-individuation phase to progress according to Mahler's formulation. Consequently, the child is unable to function when he reaches school age and must leave the comfortable hub of his family. The anxiety of separating, coupled with a fear of abandonment, inhibit the calm period of latency that should allow the child to take his place in the school environment. Manifestations of this poor sense of identity, or lack of ego strength, are diverse and many have biological and organic overlays. Examples of psychiatric conditions from the Draft of the DSM-III-R in Development[2] that may be seen among some children are attention deficit–hyperactivity disorder, conduct disorder, autistic disorder and disorders of elimination.

In the remainder of this chapter a nursing process orientation is presented to the treatment of the child with deficits in ego strength. The practice setting to be explored is an inpatient setting, such as in a psychiatric or general hospital, residential treatment center, or group home. The nurse is an integral part of a multidisciplinary team, comprised of professional and paraprofessional staff members, all of whom are involved in the treatment of the child with severe ego deficits.

■ Assessment

A child may be found in an inpatient child psychiatric setting for several reasons. At times the primary consideration in the decision to admit the child is that an accurate and thorough diagnostic evaluation has not been possible with the child as an outpatient. Other times, outpatient therapy has not been helpful to the child, and his behavior threatens to deteriorate further. In this case it is hoped that hospitalization will minimize regression, as well as rehabilitation time. Moreover, the child's behavior may have become bizarre and irrational, making the child difficult to manage in the home setting or at school.

Yet another criteria for inpatient admission is to protect the child from a severely pathological or abusive family. When this is the case, it might be helpful to admit the child to an inpatient facility to serve as a transition to foster home placement. Finally, "any child lacking the ego strength to control drives and instincts sufficiently enough to engage in the tasks of mastery and growth, and being unable to establish interpersonal relationships in the home, school or community for psychosocial development is a candidate for inpatient admission."[32]

The assessment phase of nursing care begins as the child is admitted to the unit. It is often useful to bring the child in to visit and become orientated before admission to alleviate a traumatic separation whenever possible.

The nurse will begin to collect data to formulate a picture of the whole child, including his strengths and weaknesses. The first data obtainable are his response to the admission procedure and presenting symptoms. Does he separate easily from his parent or significant other? If his separation is difficult, does he react by demonstrating feelings of abandonment or by masking his feelings with a violent and aggressive explosion? Lack of affect or a disinterested attitude will also give the nurse data relative to the child's relationship with his parents.

■ **MENTAL STATUS.** The psychiatric hospitalization of the child enables the nurse to gather information relative to several areas. The first area is the mental status of the child. A mental status examination produces a picture of the ego functioning of the child and may be used to document the functioning of the child during a single contact or over a longer period of time. When focusing on a narrow time frame, however, one must bear in mind that generalizations and conclusions about the child are limited only to that time being considered. Its greatest value is in comparing the child's behavior and level of functioning from one time to another.

The mental status of a child should ideally be assessed over a period of time, and there should be a relaxed atmosphere with minimal stressors. The use of play materials is valuable in displacing focus from the child (which is anxiety provoking) to an imaginary doll or character. Data should be recorded as observable behaviors to maximize the objectivity of the assessment, and impressions, feelings, and opinions should be labeled as such. A list of areas that are commonly covered by the mental status examination with a brief explanation of each part follows:

appearance Description of the physical size, manner of dress, hygiene, posture, and any obvious handicaps

defense mechanisms Description of major defenses the child uses to cope with anxiety

neuromusculature Description of the child's ability to locomote in a coordinated fashion and execute gross and fine motor movements

thought processes Description of the child's thoughts (verbalized). Are they logical, cohesive, and secondary process, or are flight of ideas, loose associations, and primary process thoughts present? Is the child preoccupied or having hallucinations or delusions?

fantasy Description of the child's ability to fantasize and know the limits of fantasy. This gives data relative to wish fulfillment, dreams, etc.

concept of self Description of the child's level of self-esteem, self-image, and self-ideal

orientation Description of the child's concept of time and ability to perceive who and where he is

super ego Description of the child's value system, ability to discern right and wrong, and ability to respond to limit setting

estimated IQ Description of the child's general fund of information for his age and other age-appropriate tasks.

A more detailed explanation of mental status and children can be found in Simmons's book.[34]

■ **INTERPERSONAL RELATIONSHIPS.** Observations relative to how the child relates to peers are important in assessing the child. Knowledge of age-appropriate behaviors for peer relations will help the nurse know what she is looking for. The following are a few of the many questions one should bear in mind:

■ Are the relationships formed with those of the nearest age to the child? With the same or opposite sex?
■ What is the child's position in the power structure of the group?
■ How good are the child's social skills in approaching other children and getting along with them?
■ Does the child have a "best friend"?

The child's ability to relate to adults is also of great importance. The child's comfort and skill in forming these relationships is of interest. Also the age and sex of the adults sought out will reflect his needs for role models and nurturance. Does the child use adults for support or see them as hostile enemies? Is he able to sublimate sexual interest? Is he able to accept limits from adults?

■ **ACTIVITIES.** Another information source is found by observing the child's response to activities. Observations relative to the type of activities the child enjoys and in which he or she does well, the energy level and response (bored, excited), and the ability to engage in solitary, as well as group pastimes, should be noted.

■ **PERSONAL AND FAMILY HISTORY.** In addition to observing the child's behavior in the inpatient setting, the nurse should be familiar with the child's background. A thorough history, including the precipitating problem, history of symptoms, growth and development, family life, school adjustment, and medical status, is usually compiled by one or more members of the multidisciplinary team. This information serves as a backdrop against which the child's current functioning appears. It provides the nurse with an understanding of the child's behavior and helps in setting goals for treatment that are realistic and achievable. For example, the treatment goals of a child who has had several foster home placements would differ with reference to adult relationships from goals for a child growing up in a traditional home environment.

As the picture of the child approaches completion, the data must be analyzed to make a diagnostic formulation. The diagnostic formulation serves as a basis for planning further treatment for the child. In some instances inpatient treatment ceases at this point. For the child with severe ego deficits, however, a comprehensive long-term treatment program usually is recommended.

▪ Nursing diagnosis

Children with severe ego deficits fall into a variety of diagnostic categories and comprise the majority of child psychiatric inpatient admissions. There are various ways of conceptualizing the diagnostic categories based upon the underlying psychodynamics, etiology of the disorders, and background of the mental health professional.

▪ **MEDICAL DIAGNOSES.** The nurse should be familiar with the major medical classes of disorders in order to identify related nursing diagnoses. The Draft of the DSM-III-R in Development[2] classifies disorders usually first evident in infancy, childhood, or adolescence by separating them into eight major groups. These Draft of the DSM-III-R in Development[2] diagnostic categories are listed in Table 30-2. In addition, the Draft of the DSM-III-R in Development[2] notes that a variety of other diagnostic categories will often be appropriate for children and adolescents, such as schizophrenic disorders, substance abuse disorders, mood disorders, and adjustment disorders. Some of the major classes will now be described.[29]

Mental retardation is defined as significantly subaverage general intellectual functioning, resulting in impaired adaptive behavior with the onset before the age of 18. Children in this category are likely to have associated impairment in the areas of emotional, behavioral, neurologic, and developmental functioning.

Pervasive developmental disorder and autistic disorder are Draft of DSM-III-R in Development[2] correlates of childhood psychosis. School-age children with pervasive developmental disorder are grossly dysfunctional in social relationships, anxiety levels, affect, and response to environmental change and stimulation, and tend to engage in self-mutilation. The disorder tends to be chronic with a high degree of impairment and poor prognostic outcome.

Attention deficit–hyperactivity disorder (ADHD) is characterized by inattentiveness and impulsity. Children typically are diagnosed around the age of entry into school when they are unable to maintain concentration and complete tasks. Hyperactivity further disrupts participation in classroom activity, and the child may be labeled as a discipline problem. ADHD is attributed to a neurological deficit, and children frequently improve with stimulant medication. The disorder is prevalent in 3% of prepubertal children and is

---

TABLE 30-2

DRAFT OF DSM-III-R IN DEVELOPMENT* DISORDERS USUALLY FIRST EVIDENT IN INFANCY, CHILDHOOD OR ADOLESCENCE

Mental retardation
  Mild (50–70 IQ)
  Moderate (35–49 IQ)
  Severe (20–34 IQ)
  Profound (below 20 IQ)

Pervasive developmental disorders
  Autistic disorder

Specific developmental disorders
  Language and speech disorders
  Academic skills disorders
  Motor skills disorders

Disruptive behavior disorders
  Attention deficit–hyperactivity disorder
  Oppositional disorder
  Conduct disorder

Eating disorders
  Anorexia nervosa
  Bulimic disorder
  Pica
  Rumination disorder of infancy

TIC disorders
  Tourette's disorder
  Chronic motor or vocal TIC disorder
  Transient TIC disorder

Disorders of elimination
  Functional enuresis
  Functional encopresis

Other disorders of infancy, childhood or adolescence
  Reactive attachment disorder of infancy and early
    childhood
  Stereotypy—habit disorder
  Elective mutism
  Separation anxiety disorder

---

*American Psychiatric Association: Draft of the DSM-III-R in Development (subject to change), as proposed by the Work Group to Revise DSM-III. American Psychiatric Association, October 1985.

ten times more prevalent in boys than in girls. Adolescents may have some residual impairment or show little of the behaviors.

Oppositional disorder is characterized by defiance of adult rules, anger, loss of temper, vindictive behavior, obscene language, and blaming others for one's own mistakes.

Conduct disorder is demonstrated by a repetitive and persistent pattern of conduct in which the basic rights of others are disregarded and societal norms are violated. Behaviors may include running away from home, fighting, cruelty to people or animals, firesetting, lying, and stealing.

Eating disorders with onset in childhood include pica, or eating nonnutritive substances, and rumination, or repeated regurgitation without nausea or associated gastrointestinal illness.

Disorders of elimination include functional enuresis, or the repeated voiding of urine during the day or night into bed or clothes, whether voluntary or involuntary by a child at least 5 years old. Functional encopresis is the repeated passage of feces into places not appropriate, whether voluntary or involuntary, by a child at least 4 years old.

Reactive attachment disorder results from the psychological or physical abuse or neglect of the child or repeated changes in the primary caregiver, as characterized by the inadequate or disturbed social relatedness of the child.

Separation anxiety disorder is characterized by the child's excessive anxiety about separating from those to whom the child is attached, as evidenced by persistent worry, refusal to go to school, nightmares about separations, social withdrawal, avoidance of being alone, and complaints of physical symptoms or excessive distress when anticipating or experiencing separation from attachment figures.

■ **EGO DEFICITS.** Another way of categorizing the disorders of childhood has been offered by Rinsley.[32] This classification is based on the ego deficits of the child and divides children into the autistic-presymbiotic group, the symbiotic-psychotic group, and the borderline group.

The **autistic-presymbiotic group** constitutes the following medical diagnostic labels: nonremitting schizophrenia, infantile psychosis, pseudoaffective schizophrenia, nuclear or process schizophrenia, and early infantile autism. The onset of symptoms is 3 to 5 months of age, and symptoms are pervasive. The child is considered fixated in the presymbiotic phase of development according to Mahler's theory. The child does not achieve a symbiotic relationship with the mother and does not differentiate self from mother. The symptoms include failure to learn, communicate, and form relationships. Consequently, these children are often mistaken as mentally retarded. It must be mentioned that there is approximately an equal split among those attributing the cause to emotional or organic causes.

The **symbiotic-psychotic group** is differentiated from the autistic-presymbiotic group by age of onset of symptoms, which usually appear between 3 and 4 years of age. These children are fixated in the symbiotic phase and are poorly individuated from their mothers. This group of disorders is characterized by disrupted and distorted body image and boundaries, pananxiety, fluctuating hyperactivity and withdrawal, delusions, distorted perception, and cognitive, adaptive, and coping failure.[31] In adolescence this group takes on the classic picture of adult-onset schizophrenic thought disorder.

The **borderline group,** like the autistic-presymbiotic group, consists of several medical diagnostic labels: character disorder, adjustment reactions of childhood or adolescence, delinquency, and conduct or behavior disorder. Onset of symptoms usually occurs at about 10 to 12 years. In this disorder, the child is believed to be fixated in the separation-individuation phase of development according to Mahler. The mother of the borderline child is also fixated in this phase and therefore is unable to provide the child the support he needs to separate from her. Consequently, he has the biological drive and emotional need to separate from the mother but cannot do so without an overwhelming fear of abandonment and ensuing depression. The depression is characterized by feelings of rage, fear, passivity, helplessness, and emptiness.[24] Clinically, the borderline child or adolescent uses acting out as a defense against the abandonment depression.

■ **PSYCHODYNAMICS AND MALADAPTIVE RESPONSES.** The children in all three groups may be commonly characterized as having deficits in ego strength. These deficits are because of organic causes or developmental arrests during critical periods of early childhood. The period in which the child becomes fixated will determine the extent to which his ego functioning will be impaired; the earlier the fixation, the more likely the child will appear psychotic.

Pioneers in the topic of the ego functioning of emotionally disturbed children were Fritz Redl and David Wineman.[30] Their description of the "ego that cannot perform" was derived from work in a Detroit group home for boys and for the next 20 years was virtually unchallenged as far as literature dealing with understanding and treating the aggressive child.

The first problem a child has with a poorly functioning ego is controlling his impulses. The child cannot stand even minimal frustration and insists on immediate gratification. Furthermore, when faced with a frustrating situation, panic overwhelms the child, and he becomes aggressive and destructive. The child is extremely susceptible to temptation; mere accessibility lures the child into the forbidden. The excitement of the forbidden then quickly spreads to the whole group of children. This "group intoxication" presents problems in many areas as ego boundaries blur and the atmosphere thickens with the excitation of aggressive impulses. The children show limited ability to use play materials for their intended use and destroy them, unable to see that this prevents the pleasure of future use.

New situations are frightening and overstimulating to the child with a poorly functioning ego. They may be the stimulus for a paranoid distortion, or the newness may be denied to squelch the anxiety of confronting the new experience honestly. Buffoonery and ridicule, as well as overly rough manipulation of materials, are used to master new situations, however maladaptive the results may be.

The child's social savvy is virtually nonexistent, and his presence in public places is painfully obvious. He is insensitive to feelings of others and cannot read the code of the informal social structure or abide by its mores. In fact, rules are often perceived as persecuting and, without external control, are all but forgotten by the child.

The child's ability to see his role in problems and bad experiences is severely limited. The few times when guilt feelings are predominant, the anxiety-panic-aggression cycle is triggered once again. The child does not have the capacity to learn from his mistakes or the mistakes of others, something that is taken for granted in the normal child. Normal doses of challenge, success, or failure totally disintegrate the fragile hold of the ego's control.

Perhaps the most devastating problem posed by the child with deficits in ego functioning is his resistance to forming relationships with mature and emotionally healthy adults. The very need they have for a nurturant role model sets off feelings of mistrust and fears of rejection. Communication is hampered by the child's secretive, guarded, and aloof nature. The usual social reinforcers an adult uses to show he is willing to form a relationship with a child, such as smiles, praise, or attention, are met with indifference.[35] Consequently, many therapists believe that the classic one-to-one relationship is ineffective and even contraindicated when working with such children initially.

Table 30-3 summarizes some of the psychodynamics and maladaptive responses occurring in children with severe ego deficits. From an understanding of the child, his stressors, and environment the nurse can arrive at an appropriate nursing diagnosis.

■ **FAMILY PSYCHODYNAMICS.** The child experiencing severe emotional problems is usually considered to be a "symptom bearer" for the larger family unit. Over the past 30 years attention has been increasingly placed on a systems theory view of psychopathology. In other words, the "problem" does not necessarily lie entirely within the identified patient, rather, the patient is one part of the problem. Certain children seem to be set up to have emotional problems, particularly those having special meaning to their parents at birth, such

---

TABLE 30-3

SOME PSYCHODYNAMICS AND MALADAPTIVE RESPONSES APPLICABLE TO CHILDREN WITH SEVERE EGO DEFICITS

Psychodynamics	Maladaptive responses
Failure of normal repression	Sexual acting out
Persistence of primitive defense mechanisms	Extreme use of denial and projection
Pervading anxiety	Severe level of anxiety
Failure of ego to synthesize perceptual, cognitive, and motor functions, thus disrupting child's relationship to environment	Impaired reality testing
Lack of basic trust	Withdrawn and self-isolating behavior
Impaired object relations	Inability to establish intimate relationships
Persistence of narcissism	Lack of insight into own problems
Persistence of primary process thinking	Hallucinations
Failure of sublimation of impulses	Aggressive and destructive behavior
Various degrees of impairment of self-mother differentiation	Negative self-concept

as the first born, the only child, or the child with a chronic illness or handicap. Parenting begins under anxious conditions and the child responds anxiously, eventually manifesting symptoms.

Along these same lines, parents who have been inadequately parented themselves are impaired in their abilities to parent. Winnicot's concept of the "good enough mother" requires that she be able to respond to the child's cues to separate and individuate with support and encouragement.[25] If she experiences the growth process of her child as abandonment, she will be unable to facilitate the process without becoming depressed herself.

Another phenomena of the pathological family is the double-bind communication pattern described by Bateson and co-workers.[3] The double bind is a pattern of communicating between two people in which there are two conflicting messages, from which there is no escape, and when repeated over time are not even recognized as conflictual by the victim. It is believed that the anxiety caused by this distorting experience can lead to schizophrenia.

A final family phenomenon is the blurring of ego boundaries. This is manifested in several ways. Roles may overlap or be reversed, such as a child being expected to parent his parent. Feeling states may be blurred, such as when a mother projects her feelings onto the child. Yet another example is the way in which the family handles anxiety. High levels of anxiety in one family member may be easily picked up by other members, causing confusion and disorganization.

Perhaps the most interesting family discovery was made in the research of Bowen.[6] He found that all of these faulty mechanisms occur to some extent in most every family. The ability to improve family adaptation rests on learning to separate and differentiate from other family members in a nonreactive and emotionally mature way. He believes that the symptomatic child in a family is representative of a family having a poor capacity to tolerate differentiation of family members.

■ Planning

Once a thorough assessment is completed and the child's major problems have been identified, a comprehensive treatment plan must be formulated. The nursing responsibility is generally for milieu therapy, but involvement is not confined to that area entirely. The nurse may take an active role in other therapeutic modalities, such as group therapy or family therapy, depending on level of practice and specialized training.

The inpatient setting provides various functions for the child psychiatric patient. First, the inpatient admission may be merely intended for diagnostic and evaluative purposes, and treatment will be carried out elsewhere. A second function is the case finding of children who could most benefit from a residential treatment center. The inpatient setting makes possible a comprehensive treatment plan in which individual, milieu, group, family, drug, occupational, and recreational therapies are all readily available. Finally, it provides a setting and stimulus for family treatment of pathogenic relationships.[32]

■ **GOALS.** Based on the identified problems, goals should be set that are individualized to the child's needs. Treatment goals usually include intervening in one or more of the following areas: modification of intrapsychic processes, altering peer group interactions, altering interfamily functioning, modifying the child's adjustment to school, and changing the child's environment. Wilson and Kneisl[39] have formulated the following broad goals for child psychiatric inpatients:

1. To meet the child's needs so tension will be reduced and the need for defensive behavior will be decreased
2. To help the child form a relationship with another person
3. To help the child develop a sense of self-identity
4. To offer the child an opportunity to regress and relive previous developmental stages that were unsuccessfully resolved
5. To help the child learn to communicate effectively
6. To prevent the child from hurting self or others
7. To help the child maintain physical health
8. To help the child form relationships with others
9. To promote reality testing by the child

In addition, most hospitalized children will need to develop internal impulse control to some degree.

Specific objectives for nursing care further specify the treatment approach. For instance, a child with a Draft of the DSM-III-R in Development[2] diagnosis of conduct disorder may have a nursing diagnosis of noncompliance to therapeutic milieu. Initially, the objective might be to have the patient admit to breaking rules. At a later time, the objective would be modified to have the patient comply to rules and finally to comply to limit setting without arguing or becoming combative. In this way, the treatment plan is individualized and based on the nursing diagnosis. When progress is made, the plan is revised to build upon the changes in behavior.

Once goals are set, the appropriate therapeutic modalities must be chosen to help the child reach the goal. One must be reminded again of the "mixed bag" nature of child psychiatric treatment and the useful combination of various therapies. The practice of the following psychotherapies are fully explained in other chapters in this text. A few highlights specific to child psychiatry are appropriate to mention here.

■ **FAMILY THERAPY.** Ideally, each child's family should be involved in family therapy (Chapter 29). From a systems perspective, expecting a young child to assume responsibility for changing when the family system opposes those forces toward change (in hopes of maintaining homeostasis) is absurd. Consequently, parents should be involved from the outset and slowly be educated as to their role in the problem and responsibility for change. The family must be dealt with carefully, since they are being asked to give up their symptom bearer (the hospitalized child) and are often overwhelmed by the task of changing their viewpoints. On the other hand, parents who are allowed to view their child as the only problem will be ill prepared to deal with him as the hospitalization reaches termination and, often, they become willing to abandon their problem (the child) after a significant time lapse has occurred. Some families will resist adopting a systems perspective, a phenomenon discussed by Bradt and Moynihan.[7] In such cases, special techniques are offered to avoid alienating families from involvement in treatment.

■ **GROUP THERAPY.** Group therapy (Chapter 28) is often a useful adjunct to inpatient milieu therapy. It may take the form of an activity group or a talking group. It is helpful in promoting reality testing, impulse control, self-esteem, growth, maturity, and social skills. The group therapeutic environment allows members to form relationships and experience a positive social situation in a controlled environment, which hopefully will be transferred to the outer world environment over time.

■ **PSYCHOPHARMACOLOGY.** Drug therapy (Chapter 23) is a controversial issue in the field of child psychiatry. However, when used under a physician's supervision and the appropriate guidelines are followed, they often are helpful in decreasing symptoms sufficiently for other therapies to be of increased value.[37] Drugs should be chosen based on a target symptom, rather than a diagnosis.[4] Dosages are prescribed on the basis of an effective *range,* rather than by body weight, because of the variability of response. Symptoms that have been most successfully treated with drugs to date are hyperactivity, depression, impulsivity, and anxiety.[38] Tables 30-4 and 30-5 include common child psychiatric disorders with the drug of choice and dosage most widely used.

■ **INDIVIDUAL THERAPY.** Individual psychotherapy in latency usually makes use of play equipment appropriate to the child's age. A variety of individual therapies exist, including psychoanalytical play therapy, psy-

choanalytically based psychotherapy, experiential play therapy, and various eclectic approaches. Play therapy provides a controlled stable environment for the child to work through conflicts and master phase-specific developmental tasks with the aid of an adult therapist. Play serves as a tool for communication with the inner self and with the therapist and as a way to master past experiences that have been problematic to normal adjustment and development. In the older latency age child, play often serves as a diversion that is employed to help the child express anxiety-provoking thoughts and feelings, such as in artwork or board games. The relationship between the child and the therapist provides the opportunity for experiencing a positive adult relationship tempered with judicious amounts of nurturance and reality testing.

■ **MILIEU THERAPY.** This occurs in an inpatient setting (Chapter 24). The milieu is the actual background of daily events and interactions occurring in the unit or ward. A therapeutic milieu is present when the daily life events are exploited to provide learning experiences to the patients. Just how this is managed will be the major topic explored in the discussion that follows.

■ **PARENT EDUCATION.** Parent education is a vital ingredient to preventive mental health as well as the promotion and maintenance of long-term gains from hospitalization. Parent education programs should cover a variety of subjects. Growth and development milestones are taught so parents have age-appropriate expectations of their children's behavior. Values clarification is helpful to parents in identifying what type of person they want their children to be when they get older.

Communication skills promote understanding and empathy between parent and child. Appropriate child-rearing techniques are necessary to help children develop self-discipline. Other helpful topics for an effective educational program would be family psychodynamics, concepts of mental health, and use of medications.

■ **Implementation**

Inpatient treatment in child psychiatry usually comprises three major components. The first is the life space interview, a group of techniques used to manage the behavior of children with weak ego strength. The second is some form of token economy that serves as a sanction for positive behavior. The third component is the establishment of therapeutic one-to-one relationships.

Treatment is best provided by professionals who have a genuine interest and concern for children. They need to have the capacity to withstand the multiplicity

TABLE 30-4

CHILD PSYCHIATRIC DISORDERS AND DRUG TREATMENTS

Disorder	Drug class	Comments/nursing considerations
Attention deficit–hyperactivity disorder	Stimulants	Used when primary symptoms are manifest in school
		Less reliable in pre-school and adolescence
	Antidepressants	Once a day dosing and improved monitoring of compliance and toxicity using plasma levels
		Monitor cardiac status and signs of overdose
	Antipsychotics	Sometimes used in combination with stimulants
Conduct disorders	Antipsychotics	May improve a child's capacity to benefit from social and educational interventions
Functional enuresis	Antidepressants (imipramine)	Used when an immediate therapeutic effect is necessary
Eating disorders	Antihistamines (cyproheptadine)	Anorexia nervosa
	Antidepressants (imipramine)	Bulimia
Affective disorders: depression	Antidepressants	Careful diagnosis is necessary to differentiate depression from normal feeling states
TIC disorders: Tourette's disorder	Antipsychotics (haloperidol)	Stimulants are avoided because they worsen symptoms
	Alpha-adrenergic agonist (clonidine)	
Pervasive developmental disorders	Antipsychotics	Used to treat agitation, insomnia, stereotypic movements
Mental retardation with psychiatric symptoms and behavioral problems	Antipsychotics	Used to control behavioral and psychiatric complications
	Antidepressants	Treat affective symptoms
	Stimulants	Treat attention deficit–hyperactivity disorder
	Lithium	Helps control aggression
Separation anxiety disorder	Antidepressants (imipramine)	Effective at high doses
		Speculative: panic disorder symptoms
Schizophrenic disorder	Antipsychotics	Lower dose instead on concomitant antiparkinsonian drug therapy

of moods and emotional outbursts that occur in these children. In other words, the nurse and co-workers must have sufficient ego strength to cope with a fairly high level of anxiety in the emotional atmosphere. The nurse's role as a good parent demands that she be able to provide an environment with open honest communication and clearly delineated adult-child boundaries that is free from pseudointimacy.[32] The therapeutic milieu should provide the child with sanctuary from the pathological family dynamics that were detrimental to growth prior to hospitalization.

■ **PHASES OF TREATMENT.** A comprehensive treatment plan for the child with weak ego strength can be expected to be of considerable length, as long as 3 or 4 years. Treatment usually proceeds in three phases.[32] The first phase is the testing, or resistance, phase. In this phase the child is orienting himself to the setting and "casing it" for the purpose of finding out who is in charge and with whom he may align. After this brief "honeymoon," the pseudocompliant front falls away and the child begins to test limits and demonstrate his problem with ego functioning. This entails negativism, reluctance to follow the program or form relationships, and destructiveness. The message is, "There is nothing wrong with me. I don't need to be in this place." The phase may last as long as 1 year.

The second phase is termed the definitive, or working-through, phase. During this time the child drops

TABLE 30-5

DRUGS COMMONLY USED IN CHILDHOOD PSYCHIATRIC DISORDERS

Drug	Description	Daily dose (mg/kg of body weight)	Side effects
Stimulants			
Dextroamphetamine	short acting (2–4 hr)	0.3–1.5*; 1–3 doses daily	*Short term:* Decreased appetite; sleep disturbances
Methylphenidate	short-acting (2–4 hr)	0.3–1.5*; 1–3 doses daily	*Long term:* Possible minor effects on growth; associated with onset of Tourette's syndrome in children with family history of tics
Pemoline	long-acting (2–4 week delay in therapeutic effect)	0.5–3*; 1 daily dose	*Abrupt discontinuation:* Behavioral deterioration
Antidepressants			
Imipramine	10–17 hr. half-life; immediate response with enuresis or ADD; 2–4 week delay in response with depression	Usual daily dose should not exceed 5 mg/kg/day	*Short term:* Dry mouth, blurred vision, constipation; EKG changes
MAOI and newer drugs: inadequate information on efficacy and toxicity			*Abrupt discontinuation:* Gastrointestinal symptoms
Mood stabilizers			
Lithium	12 hr half-life	Maintain plasma level between 0.6 and 1.2 mm/l	*Short term:* GI symptoms; polyuria, polydipsia, tremors, sleepiness, impaired memory
			Long term: Decreased calcium metabolism and thyroid function; possible kidney changes
Antipsychotics			
Chlorpromazine	low potency	3–6	*Short term:* Drowsiness, weight gain; dry mouth; blurred vision; nasal congestion; acute dystonia; parkinsonism
Thioridazine	low potency		
Trifluoperazine	high potency	0.1–0.5	
Perphenazine	high potency		*Abrupt discontinuation:* Withdrawal dyskinesias
Haloperidol	high potency		

*Doses are lower for younger children.

his resistance and begins to face his problems. There may be a significant regression during this time that often scares the child's family enough to withdraw him from treatment. However, the stormy phase gives way to therapeutic work toward separation-individuation, and the child begins to show improved ego functioning. This phase usually lasts 1 or 2 years.

The final phase, resolution or separation, hallmarks the child's successful achievement of object relations. The rapprochement crisis is resolved, and the child is able to move toward age-appropriate relationships with significant others. The child is able to handle extra privileges, visits home, and works through termination with the staff and other patients. This can also last up to a year.

■ **THERAPEUTIC MILIEU.** The concept of a therapeutic milieu is built on daily events in the child's life. In the inpatient setting this comprises a daily routine of meals, school, sports, group and individual activities and pastimes, outings, and bedtime. Trieschman[36] delineates the various ways in which deficient egos are supported by the milieu. One way is through *shared ego,* in which the child behaves appropriately to please those persons with whom he has positive relationships. The group of children and adult workers in an inpatient setting makes up a *group ego* to which conformity is exchanged for acceptance and a feeling of belongingness. The culture of the institution is made up of rules and routine, as well as tradition, which serves as an *external ego* that guides the children's behavior. Finally, the milieu therapist, through careful assessment, is able to pick out the *ego pieces* or functions the child has in the here and now and find ways for the child to use them in managing his own behavior.

■ **TYPES OF INTERVENTIONS.** With the daily routine, experiences arise that prove problematical to the child with inadequate ego strength. The nurse, as milieu therapist, extracts these problematical events as they take place and chooses one of two basic types of interventions to manage them: ego supportive or ego interpretive. A *supportive ego intervention* serves as a method of easing the child who is about to lose control, out of his panic-aggressive cycle and back into control, so that he may continue with the daily activity. These interventions serve to maintain the child at his current level of ego function through external control and over time set the stage for improving ego function. When conditions are ripe, the nurse is able to use *interpretive ego interventions,* which help the child to gain insight into his problematic behavior and use this insight as a basis for change, thus internalizing ego control. These two types of interventions were first described by Fritz Redl and are collectively known as **life space interview techniques.**[30] The

life space interview is an interaction that takes place outside the context of individual therapy. It occurs between the child and the adult involved in the situation. The focus is on improving the child's sense of self-identity and ego functioning within the developmental process.

Ego supportive techniques. This group of techniques can also be called "emotional first aid on the spot."[29] When the child inpatient confronts a developmental challenge or a demanding life situation, the milieu therapist may need to assist the child in coping with it. One technique for this is draining off the overwhelming frustration, caused by an interruption in the child's fun or routine, by communicating sympathy for the child's frustration and inconvenience. During periods when the child loses control and slips into his panic-aggressive cycle, it is important that the adult show support by staying with the child. This provides a sense of security and also affords the adult the opportunity to talk the child back into the daily routine after the stormy period wanes.

Often the child withdraws from relationships in times of emotional turmoil. To prevent this, Redl advocates dropping the issue that is being confronted in an endeavor to keep the child engaged, however trivial the subject may be. This prevents the phenomenon of "winning the battle, but losing the war" from occurring.

The milieu therapist also functions as a police officer in regulating and enforcing the social behavior of the children. This entails the act of benign and neutral reminding of rules and routines. "Enforcing the law" serves as an external booster to the children's ego at times when behavior is on the verge of slipping from the established norm. Along this same line the presence of an umpire is often necessary in settling arguments. A neutral outsider prevents breakdown in fair play or "petty swindling" in the children's transactions.

Ego interpretive techniques. The real therapeutic gains the child makes in ego strength occur as a result of self-examination and learning alternate behaviors to those which pose difficulty. In working with children who are prone to distorting and misinterpreting their experiences, insight may never be reached without a "reality rub in." This technique involves repeated confrontation with the reality that the child plays a part in his own self-defeating transactions.

Another intervention strategy is symptom estrangement. This interview situation focuses on enlisting the child to see his symptom as problematical, rather than as a tool that is used to manipulate and control. Symptom estrangement is accomplished by piling up evidence from past life events which provides proof that the symptom costs more than it pays to keep it.

Appealing to a sense of fairness and equality is helpful in awakening a value system in the children. The importance of developing an internalized standard for behavior may begin by this initial adherence to a code of fair play.

The technique Redl calls new-tool salesmanship has been enlarged on by Trieschman who calls it learning alternative or new behaviors.[36] This new behavior improves the child's coping ability, adaptation, and social acceptability as well. Selling a new way to handle frustration or guilt takes time and is often a by-product of a one-to-one relationship the child has with an adult. Substituting a mature behavior, from the adult model, for the old self-defeating behavior provides a step toward increased ego functioning.

The inclination to group contagion that many child psychiatric inpatients possess must eventually be countered. The life space interview in this situation focuses on increasing the child's boundaries so that he may withstand the group's atmosphere of excitement. In this way the child is educated as to how the process works and helped to remain outside the lure of misbehavior.

In summary, the clinical exploration of life events offers the opportunity to learn new behaviors and gain insight into the futility of old ones. The process of change takes time and often the stage must be set first through the use of ego supportive techniques.

Use of natural and logical consequences. Natural and logical consequences are an effective tool for teaching children responsibility for their own behavior.[11] Natural consequences occur in the natural course of events (i.e., one becomes hungry if one does not eat). Logical consequences are formulated by the caretaker and facilitate learning from the reality of social order (i.e., not completing homework will result in falling behind in school work). Nurses can utilize those concepts in managing a child's behavior and also teach them to parents. The consistent exposure to natural and logical consequences of behavior over time enables the child to eventually see his behavior as self-defeating and avoids many power struggles.

Behavior modification. Many inpatient settings utilize some behavioristic principles (Chapter 27) to manage the aggressive and limit-testing child. This is usually in the format of a token economy, in which socially acceptable behavior is rewarded or reinforced with points or tokens. The tokens are redeemable for extra privileges, such as an extended bedtime, a favorite food, or a special outing.

Maladaptive behavior is either ignored or punished by the use of time out. A time out requires that the child spend a brief period away from the group following acting out behavior. This serves as a time for the child to gain self-control and talk to an adult about the difficulty and also inhibits the spread of the child's acting out to other group members.

Yet another behavioristic program is contingency management. In this system, the milieu schedule promotes the use of positive or "on task" behavior with naturally occurring reinforcers, such as meals, free time, and outings. This is simply a variation of "grandma's law," which states, "If you want to eat dessert, you first must eat your peas."

All of these intervention strategies may be used together or singly with excellent results. One principle, however, should be kept in mind. The focus is on the positive, self-esteem enhancing aspects of the program. The nurse and co-workers should avoid slipping into a negative or threatening attitude by emphasizing that points are earned by the child, rather than taken away by the adult. Target behaviors should be clearly understood by the children and, whenever possible, positive reinforcement used instead of punishment.

A problem encountered in some behavior programs is that the child, after many acting out episodes in one day, has so few tokens that he gives up and completely decompensates. A way to provide further incentive to regain control is to build into each program a way in which the child can make up a portion of the points he has not earned. In doing so, he may not be able to reach the highest privilege status, but he will be able to rise above the lowest with some additional effort.

Also important to bear in mind is that the end point of behavior management is to internalize or learn self-control. Therefore it is hoped that social reinforcers such as praise will be paired with the token or extrinsic reinforcers so that the child eventually will reward himself for good behavior by feeling good about himself.

One-to-one relationships. Children with deficits in ego strength have great difficulty forming relationships with adults. They are often distrustful because of their past experiences and, unable to discriminate a trustworthy adult, they withdraw from everyone. Therefore some special effort is usually required on the nurse's behalf to seek out and work toward the establishment of contact with the child.[26]

In the early stages of a relationship small talk is usually all that can be tolerated. Topics such as the child's reason for admission and other psychotherapeutic issues will actually hinder the child's ability to view the nurse positively in the milieu setting. Instead, the child should be approached casually, for the purpose of becoming acquainted with his interests and reactions to various situations or activities in the milieu. Exchanges should be short to avoid provoking the child's suspicious nature.

The adult working in this setting walks a precarious tightrope between appearing unapproachably square and disrespectfully "hip." It is important for the child to view the nurse as an adult to promote his sense of security. Therefore gossip and off-color humor should be avoided, since they are tests of the adult's ability to abide by the rules of socially correct behavior. On the other hand, current fads in music, television, or movies may provide openings for conversations that demonstrate the adult's genuine interest in the child's world.

The adult will maximize his attractiveness to a child if he is able to find a common interest or skill to share with the child. This allows for many hours of diversional activity that serves as a backdrop for conversation in later stages of the relationship. It is important for the adult to demonstrate his inability to be manipulated. Since these children need external control, they will be unable to trust someone they are able to con.

Another important consideration in establishing and maintaining relationships is minimizing adult aversiveness.[36] One way in which this is accomplished is by staying out of power struggles. Sometimes potential altercations may be avoided merely by the adult failing to pick up a challenge. For instance, the child is asked to take a seat and responds by saying, "Make me!" The adult immediately picks up the child's cue and counters with "All right, I will." Avoiding a power struggle might be the answer here and the response could be, "For those who are seated, let's begin to clean up for a snack." The child is left to stand if he pleases while the rest of the group moves on with their activity. It is not always possible to avoid power struggles, but a concerted effort should be made at least in the case of minor or petty squabbles.

The nurse must actually prove her own trustworthiness to the child. One way she does this is by being as open and honest as possible with the child at all times. Being able to admit mistakes to a child communicates one's humanness and should be a firm operating principle. One can demonstrate increasing trust of the child by offering him small amounts of responsibility.

Once a positive relationship has been formed with the child it becomes more natural and the adult does not need to pursue the child quite so intensely. Topics will be centered around daily activities. The techniques outlined in the life space interview should then be incorporated into the adult-child interaction.

▪ Evaluation

Most treatment facilities for child psychiatric patients have programs designed for specific periods of time. The brief hospitalization is usually 2 or 4 weeks in length and is planned for diagnosis and evaluation, crisis intervention, and comprehensive case planning. Therefore when the presenting symptoms have receded sufficiently, the clinical picture of the child is completed, and a long-term plan has been formulated, the child will be discharged.

The success of brief hospitalizations in terms of patient outcome is determined mostly by the patient's follow-up care. Consequently, the ability of the multidisciplinary team to formulate a plan that is mutually agreeable to the child and his family will be vital. Emphasis on the parent's responsibility to comply with the treatment plan for any persistent long-term gain should be made to the parents in the earliest contacts.

Long-term hospitalizations are more complicated in terms of determining readiness for discharge. Generally, the nurse's observations focus on basic changes in the child's behavior. The child should hopefully demonstrate some insight and understanding of himself through self-reflection and increase his ability to make rational decisions. Behavior should become less impulsive and drive ridden. Instead, the child should begin to live adaptively in his surroundings.

When the child's behavior has become more socially acceptable to the inpatient setting, it is important to begin expanding his or her environment to the community. The use of the public school system provides an excellent opportunity for the hospitalized child to stay "tuned in" to the outside world and also to demonstrate his ability to handle his environment prior to discharge. The child should be given home visits or visits to wherever it is that he will be placed after discharge. This also broadens the child's environment and tests his ability to internalize ego control. Social outings into the community should be ongoing in the course of treatment and should be handled age appropriately prior to discharge. In this way institutionalization is avoided.

When evaluating the child's overall therapeutic gains, it is important to examine the problems or symptoms, goals, and interventions on a regular basis. The treatment plan is kept up to date, and, as problems resolve, the lower priorities may be integrated into the plan. Sometimes the original goals must be reconsidered or interventions may not work so alternatives must be found. The use of team planning conferences is often helpful in the ongoing process of evaluation. Aspects of the treatment plan that need special scrutiny include the following:

1. Effectiveness of interventions in managing behavior
2. Ability to relate to peers, adults, and parents appropriately

3. Ability to carry out self-care and care of possessions
4. Ability to utilize program activities in recreation and learning (including school)
5. Response to limits, rules, and routines
6. Development of insight into problems and willingness to change
7. Overall mental status as outlined earlier
8. Discharge coordination and planning

■ **TERMINATION.** Terminating a therapeutic relationship is difficult for many nurses. This is in part because of the universally experienced feeling of emptiness described by Fogarty.[16] Many people "use" relationships, albeit unconsciously, as a mechanism to avoid the empty feelings of loneliness, abandonment, and incompleteness. Termination stirs up these feelings within oneself and causes discomfort. Unfortunately, one must acknowledge these feelings to allow the termination to proceed therapeutically with the child.

The child also has problems in leaving. Behavior often regresses as the hospitalization draws to an end and a discharge date has been set. It is as if the child wants to prove that he still needs the hospital and its staff.

Some guidelines are helpful in terminating with children. Introducing the idea that there is an end point should be done early in treatment and stressed again when discharge nears. This allows ample time for the child and staff to experience the concomitant feelings and talk about them. Positive aspects of the termination process can be pointed out, such as the fact that discharge into family and community means the child is moving into a new phase of life where new relationships will be established in place of the old. Enumeration of the child's gains from hospitalization increase the child's confidence in facing a new environment. Finally, it is a valuable experience for the child to learn that one does not have to be mad or hurt to end a relationship, and a successful positive termination will be achieved when the child is able to grasp this.[9]

The use of ritual is a helpful method of handling "last days." Parties or special activities may be planned in the departing child's honor. Children sometimes enjoy autographs with special messages written to them from staff and other patients. All of these suggestions are merely aids to soften the finality of terminating, a painful fact of life for all people.

■ **FOLLOW-UP AND DISCHARGE.** The discharge of a patient should occur only when the health teaching plan has been completed. The child and his family should have information relative to the nature of the child's illness and his status at discharge, including the

family's role in the pathological condition. They should also know how stress relates to emotional illness and ways to cope more effectively with it. In addition, anticipatory guidance is often helpful in forewarning parents and children about future developmental or situational stressors that might have deleterious effects on the child's or family's functioning.

If the child is discharged and will be receiving drug therapy, it is extremely important that the child and family know the reason for the drug's prescription, the dosage, times of day it is to be given, and side effects that should receive medical attention. This cannot be overemphasized because of the common experience of many nurses with well meaning parents who do not understand the way in which many psychoactive drugs build up in the body. The layman's perception that the drug works much in the same way as an "aspirin stops a headache" may lead to the drug being ineffective or abused.

Follow-up care usually consists of some type of ongoing psychotherapy, whether it be individual, group, or family. Medication monitoring is carried out according to the specific indications of the prescribed drug. Sometimes vocational and school placements are part of the posthospitalization plan. Dispositions are made to the family of origin whenever possible. If this cannot be accomplished, placements with extended family members, boarding schools, and foster homes or group homes are considered.

Clinical case analysis

■ **Assessment**

The following case study involves psychiatric nursing care provided to a 6-year-old male child, Ted, and his family. He was admitted to an inpatient unit for assessment due to temper tantrums and inability to accept limits set by the parents. The mother was also concerned about his dislike of school. The father's perception of his son's problem consisted primarily of his belief that he and his wife had been unable to provide effective discipline.

The temper tantrums would erupt in a variety of situations, but most typically when limits were set on Ted's behavior. He would be verbally abusive toward either parent involved, calling them names and swearing, and at times, he would hit his sister and threaten to destroy his toys or surroundings. Cruelty to animals was not reported by either parent.

Both parents had tried to avoid spanking and relied on other forms of discipline such as sending Ted to his room or denying him a privilege, such as TV. These techniques of managing Ted's temper outbursts were not helpful, and Ted was successfully making everyone in the family miserable when he was punished. Ted's parents were getting into arguments over his behavior.

■ **PSYCHOSOCIAL HISTORY.** Ted was the first child born to his parents. They had been married 7 years prior to his birth, having met in high school and dated through college. Ted's mother had required surgery for endometriosis in order to be able to bear children. Ted was born by cesarean section 2 weeks prior to his mother's EDC, without complications. He was bottle-fed and was an easy baby to care for according to both parents. No feeding problems, colic, or the like were reported. He was weaned at 10 months with no problems. All development milestones were within normal limits (sat—5 months, crawled—6 months, walked—13 months, 1 word—8½ months, sentences—15 months, toilet trained—3 years).

Ted was reported to have a special interest in natural sciences and particularly animals from his toddler years. He demonstrated the capability of memorizing names of animals from a picture book and by 6 years of age was attached to a pet hamster and had a wealth of knowledge about animal behavior.

Ted's mother returned to work as a school teacher for a brief period prior to the birth of her second child. This was due to their financial situation. Ted was taken to a babysitter in the morning by his father and retrieved in the afternoon by his mother. He cried when he was left, but his caretaker was considered to be very capable and he was left with her consistently. Ted's mother did not return to work after the birth of her daughter.

Ted was 18 months of age when his sister E. was born. He was somewhat jealous of her and balked at giving up his crib. Consequently, he was allowed to use a porta-crib until he was convinced that he was ready to sleep in a twin bed. He also shook his sister's crib when he was unaware that his parents were watching and reported that she was "bubnoxious." Ted's mother had prepared him for his sister's birth in the later stages of her pregnancy. It seemed that Ted's strong will and intense anger became noticeable around this time and persisted *after* he had accepted his sister's existence.

Ted attended nursery school without problems. Kindergarten presented no problems academically, but his teacher reported that he and another male child were distracting to the class with their talking.

Ted's sexual behavior presented no problems, and he asked questions and received age-appropriate answers.

Ted's mother sought help with her son's behavior 1 month after he entered first grade. He had resisted going to school the first 2 weeks and his behavior at home had deteriorated.

■ **FAMILY HISTORY.** The father of the patient was born in 1941 in a small midwestern town. He was the third of six children and was raised in the Catholic faith. His father worked in a feed plant in a managerial capacity, and his mother was a housewife. They were described as strict, and they used authoritarian parenting styles. Anger was dealt with openly, and conflict was part of the family atmosphere along with other warm and loving feelings expressed equally.

Of the six children, the eldest brother had problems with alcohol abuse and had numerous marital separations over his drinking. A younger brother had recently had an extramarital affair and had divorced his wife. The other children were considered to have successful marriages and careers and had achieved varying levels of higher education.

Ted's father identified himself as being the most troublesome child in the family, requiring frequent discipline including physical punishment. He graduated from a state university in 1963. After 2 years in the army he entered a field of business requiring considerable time and effort.

The mother of the patient was born in 1942 in the same small town that her husband was. She was the second of three daughters and was raised in the Protestant faith. Her father worked for a utilities company, and her mother was a housewife. The family was described as closely knit, and angry feelings were seldom expressed. The parents did not use physical punishment, relying mainly on "talking things out."

Ted's mother described herself as making the most waves in her family. She was closest to her older sister who was nearest in age to her.

The parents met in high school and dated throughout college. They were married after a courtship of over 7 years, and moved to the east coast shortly thereafter. Ted's father pursued his business career, and his mother worked as a schoolteacher.

Ted's birth followed a long period of infertility, and his parents were ecstatic following the birth of Ted.

■ **MENTAL STATUS.** Ted appeared as a well nourished, white, male child who was neatly groomed and dressed casually. He was very cooperative with the admission procedure and required minimal reassurance to separate from his mother. He was willing to play with toys and talk about nonthreatening topics, but resisted any attempt to discuss problems. Mental status was assessed over a week's time.

Ted was oriented to person, place, and time and was alert and attentive. His general fund of knowledge was above average as he shared his indepth knowledge of natural science with the interviewer. He also had some idea of current events and knew his address, phone number, etc. His judgment was considered to be appropriate to his age. He utilized a right versus wrong set of values to distinguish moral dilemmas.

Ted was able to express himself verbally. His speech was clear, organized, and grammatically correct. His vocabulary was well developed and he liked to use "big words." His ability to spell was poor, although he knew the first letters of most words.

Ted shied away from fantasy in play except in terms of stereotyped games of cowboys and Indians. His concrete thought processes seemed to block attempts to become more intimate with the nurse. Attempts to ask questions about play themes were firmly resisted by Ted. His response to what his three wishes would be were: a seagull so he could fly; "to have a hood in the back of me like a cobra, so I can scare people when I'm angry"; and to live in "Bubble Gum Land." Ted spontaneously shared his knowledge of different kinds of fish, butterflies, and the like.

Ted's concept of self was considered to be well developed. His manner of relating was self-assured, and he portrayed a bravado of the tough guy who was able to take care of himself. He confronted the nurse about various injustices, such as not offering him chewing gum while she had some. He asked a few personal questions as well. The self-ideal was expressed in the form of superheroes with supernatural powers, such as Batman and Popeye.

The common theme in play was the bad guys against the good guys. Ted had issues such as freedom in mind to explain the conflict, and the good guys did win. He refused to utilize the doll house figures which were more real and stuck to monsters, cowboys, and Indians. This could indicate resistance to exposing threatening materials or sex role behavior that would inhibit doll play.

Ted's dominant mood seemed to be bright and cheerful, although he was somewhat concerned about why he was in the hospital. He had considerable self-control in a one-to-one situation. However, he quickly disregarded hospital rules in a less structured setting. No self-destructive behaviors were noted or reported.

■ Nursing diagnosis

The Draft of the DSM-III-R in Development[2] diagnosis for Ted was oppositional disorder. The mental status exam revealed no evidence of thought disorder, depression, hyperkinetic behavior, or separation problems. His difficulty seemed to lie in the area of accepting limits and following instructions. Personality features such as his bravado and unwillingness to try things he could not do well were considered to be part of his willful behavior. His perception of self seemed to border on feeling omnipotent in view of the control his temper tantrums held over the family.

The parental histories suggested a moderate degree of family psychopathology. In both families, one or two children functioned at a lower level than the others, and Ted's sister was seen as having no problems. Both parents recognized similar willfulness in themselves as children. In addition, there was a high degree of conflict over the childrearing practices. Consequently, one nursing diagnosis was identified as alteration in parenting, related to conflict between parents over parenting styles, with the child responding in an omnipotent and controlling manner. Alteration in family process and social isolation were also identified as nursing diagnoses.

■ Planning

The nurse proposed that treatment should be focused on learning about effective parenting behavior and discussing their ideas and philosophy of parenting. Treatment goals were as follows:

After completing a parent education program the parents will:

1. Describe three parenting styles—authoritarian, democratic, or inconsistent/laissez-faire and identify the type they utilize.
2. Describe democratic parenting techniques.
3. Set consistent limits on Ted's behavior.
4. Learn to apply logical consequences of Ted's behavior when he does not accept parental limits.
5. Praise Ted for positive behavior.
6. Allow appropriate ventilation of anger from Ted in the form of verbalization of complaints and sublimation of aggression in play and sports.
7. Conceptualize Ted's problem with temper tantrums in a family context.
8. Examine their own relationship and describe the effects of focusing their emotional energy on Ted and his problems.

A related treatment goal for Ted was that he would:

Accept and respond to limits set by his parents or experience logical consequences of his behavior.

■ Implementation

The first priority in working with the parents was to have positive or negative attention. Specific guidelines for handling temper outbursts were given. The parents were able to follow these guidelines while Ted was visiting home, and they achieved initial success in that Ted's outbursts were of shorter duration, less frequent and intense, and the parents were less angry at him for throwing tantrums. However, they had to be reminded to keep using the techniques consistently. They had the expectation that their son would learn to control himself in a short time period and not slide back into old habits from time to time.

The success in handling the temper tantrums was encouraging and made them more able to hear and practice effective limit setting. Again, specific guidelines were given. The parents were encouraged to record their efforts at setting limits so that they could be examined and discussed with the nurse. In this way, application of the specific guidelines could be evaluated. They required additional coaching in applying logical consequences.

After achieving some success in handling temper tantrums and setting limits, the parents could turn to more positive aspects of parenting. They were instructed to get a copy of *Parent Effectiveness Training* by Thomas Gordon to learn about communicating more effectively. They were reminded of the importance of praising good behavior and also for allowing appropriate ventilation of anger and frustration by talking to him and throughout his play.

Later, parent education meetings were utilized to teach the importance of keeping up interpersonal contacts with one's family of origin to avoid emotional overinvestment in one's own children. In addition, the nurse recommended that the parents continue to carve out time for relating as a marital pair, spending time together as a twosome, and talking about issues that concerned their marriage other than the children. These interventions were geared towards defocusing Ted as the problem child and helping to prevent further development of dysfunctional behavior in the future.

■ Evaluation

Ted returned home after 3 weeks of hospitalization. He and his parents had achieved the treatment goals and had obtained symptom relief. Upon discharge, Ted's behavior had improved, and the parents had more realistic expectations of their son's behavior. They had some conception of the family dynamics and had learned a variety of democratic parenting techniques.

■ SUGGESTED CROSS-REFERENCES ■

Behavior modification is discussed in Chapter 27. Group therapy is discussed in Chapter 28. Family therapy is discussed in Chapter 29. Adolescent psychiatric nursing is presented in Chapter 31. Intervening in family abuse and violence is discussed in Chapter 32.

DIRECTIONS FOR FUTURE RESEARCH

The following are some of the nursing research problems raised in Chapter 30 that merit further study by psychiatric nurses:
1. The number, settings, and scope of practice of child psychiatric nurses throughout the country
2. The amount and nature of primary, secondary, and tertiary activities engaged in by child psychiatric nurses
3. The effectiveness of primary prevention activities in avoiding maladaptive responses in children
4. Outcomes associated with long-term hospitalization of children
5. Curative factors of the milieu of child psychiatric inpatients
6. Motivating factors that help parents alter child-rearing practices
7. Attitude change of parents toward their child following psychiatric nursing intervention
8. Methods for establishing relationships with children who have difficulty trusting adults
9. Identification of children at risk for specific psychiatric disorders and maladaptive health responses
10. Prospective studies of child patients to identify factors associated with the development of adult psychiatric disorders
11. Retrospective studies of the childhood environment of adults with psychiatric disorders
12. The use of p.r.n. medication for the behavioral management of children
13. Child psychiatric nurses' knowledge of effective childrearing practices
14. Frequency and type of family interventions provided by child psychiatric nurses
15. The effect of locked-door seclusion on child psychiatric patients
16. Types of nursing diagnoses utilized when working with child psychiatric patients

■ SUMMARY ■

1. Child psychiatry evolved from the fields of psychoanalysis, education, psychology, and social welfare.
2. The child psychiatric nurse functions in a therapeutic role as a milieu therapist. Her expanded role as an independent practitioner requires advanced study on the master's level. Care settings in child psychiatry are diverse and vary from primary to tertiary prevention.

3. Standards of Child and Adolescent Psychiatric and Mental Health Nursing Practice were enumerated with rationale.

4. Latency has a potential for growth that is reached by the school-age child by sublimating basic instinctual drives to reach a calm and educable phase. Cognitive ego functions facilitate the child's emphasis on learning so that he develops a sense of competency about self. Children with ego deficits are believed to have developmental delays in differentiating from their mothers and developing object relations. Theorists differ in their views of the etiology of weak ego states.

5. The data collection phase involves the development of a profile of the child that includes presenting symptoms, mental status, interpersonal relationships, activities and behaviors, and personal and family history. Brief hospitalizations are often used for diagnostic purposes.

6. Nursing diagnoses are devised from the psychodynamics specific to each child's problems. Common problem areas include faulty impulse control, negative self-concept, impaired reality testing, poor interpersonal relationships, and lack of insight. Major medical diagnoses were described.

7. Children hospitalized in child psychiatric inpatient settings fall into three main categories of diagnostic labels: autistic-presymbiotic, symbiotic-psychotic, and borderline. Families of such children are often found to have faulty communication patterns, poorly defined ego boundaries, and difficulty identifying their role in the child's problem.

8. Helping children with deficits in ego strength requires a comprehensive treatment plan and specific nursing care goals. Residential treatment programs serve as therapeutic milieus in which daily living experiences are used to help children learn more adaptive behaviors and gain a stronger sense of self-identity.

9. Interventions such as the life space interview, behavior modification programs, and one-to-one relationships are helpful in facilitating the child's growth and development, and therapeutic modalities have an impact on the child in residential treatment. Individual, group, family, drug, special education, and recreational therapies are a few.

10. The child who has been hospitalized on a long-term basis should achieve some measure of insight into his problems, impulse control, and reality testing prior to discharge. Termination may bring about temporary symptom recurrences, but can be handled through adequate communication and cultural ritual. Health teaching and follow-up care have important prognostic value on the child's outcome after discharge.

11. A clinical case analysis was presented and analyzed using the framework of the nursing process.

■ **REFERENCES** ■

1. American Nurses' Association, Division on Psychiatric and Mental Health Nursing Practice: Standards of psychiatric-mental health nursing practice, Kansas City, Mo., 1976, The Association.

2. American Psychiatric Association: Draft of the DSM-III-R in Development (subject to change), as proposed by the Work Group to Revise DSM-III. American Psychiatric Association, October 1985.

3. Bateson, G. et al.: Towards a theory of schizophrenia, Behav. Sci. **1**:1, 1956.

4. Biederman, J., and Jelliner, M.: Psychopharmacology in children, N. Engl. J. Med. **310**(15):968, 1984.

5. Binet, A., and Binet, S.: The development of intelligence in children, Baltimore, 1916, The Williams & Wilkins Co.

6. Bowen, M.: Theory in the practice of psychotherapy. In Guerin, P., editor: Family therapy, New York, 1976, Gardner Press, Inc.

7. Bradt, J.O., and Moynihan, C.J.: Opening the safe: a study of child-focused families. In Bradt, J.O., and Moynihan, C.F., editors: Systems therapy, Washington, D.C., 1972, Groome Child Guidance Center.

8. Catell, J.M.: Mental tests and measurements, Mind **15**:373, 1890.

9. Chess, S., and Hassibi, M.: Principles and practice of child psychiatry, New York, 1978, Plenum Publishing Corp.

10. Child psychiatric–mental health nurse clinician, position statement, Chicago, 1980, Advocates for Child Psychiatric Nursing, Inc.

11. Child psychiatry: a plan for the coming decade, Washington, D.C., 1983, American Academy of Child Psychiatry.

12. Dinkmeyer, D., and McKay, G.: The parents' handbook: systematic training for effective parenting, Minnesota, 1982, American Guidance Service.

13. Ekstein, R.: Psychoanalysis. In Noshpitz, J., editor: Basic handbook of child psychiatry, vol. 3, New York, 1979, Basic Books, Inc.

14. Elkind, D.: Children and adolescents: interpretive essays on Jean Piaget, London, 1974, Oxford University Press.

15. Erikson, E.H.: Childhood and society, New York, 1950, W.W. Norton & Co., Inc.

16. Fogarty, T.F.: On emptiness and closeness. I. The Family **2**(1):22, 1975.

17. Freud, S.: Sexual enlightenment of children, New York, 1963, Macmillan, Inc.

18. Gisell, A.L.: Infancy and human growth, New York, 1928, Macmillan, Inc.

19. Gould, M., Wunsch-Hitzig, R., and Dohrenwend, B.: Estimating the prevalence of childhood psychopathology, J. Am. Acad. Child Psychiatry **20**:462, 1981.

20. Halpern, W.I., and Kissel, S.: Human resources for troubled children, New York, 1976, John Wiley & Sons, Inc.

21. Healy, W.: Twenty-five years of child guidance, Chicago, 1934, Institute for Juvenile Research.

22. Joint Commission on the Mental Health of Children: Crisis in child mental health: challenge for the 1970s. New York, 1969, Harper & Row Publishers.

23. Long, K.: Are children too young for mental disorders? Am. J. Nurs. **1985**:1254, Nov. 1984.

24. Mahler, M.: The psychological birth of the human infant, New York, 1975, Basic Books, Inc.

25. Masterson, J.F.: Intensive psychotherapy of the adolescent with a borderline syndrome. In Caplan, J., editor:

American handbook of psychiatry, ed. 2, New York, 1974, Basic Books, Inc.

26. Meeks, J.E.: The fragile alliance, Baltimore, 1971, The Williams & Wilkins Co.

27. Middleton, A.B., and Pothier, P.C.: The nurse in child psychiatry—an overview. In Fagin, C., editor: Readings in child and adolescent psychiatric nursing, St. Louis, 1974, The C.V. Mosby Co.

28. Pothier, P., Norbeck, J., and Laliberte, M.: Child psychiatric nursing: the gap between need and utilization, J. Psychosoc. Nurs. Ment. Health Serv. **23**(7):18, 1985.

29. Rappaport, J.: DSM-III training guide for diagnosis of childhood disorders, New York, 1984, Brunner/Mazel, Inc.

30. Redl, F.: Life space interview, Am. J. Orthopsychiatry **1**:1, 1957.

31. Redl, F., and Wineman, D.: The aggressive child, Glencoe, Ill., 1957, Free Press.

32. Rinsley, D.B.: Principles of therapeutic milieu with children. In Sholevar, G.P., editor: Emotional disorders in children and adolescents, New York, 1980, Spectrum Books.

33. Sarnoff, C.A.: Latency-age children. In Sholevar, P. et al., editors: Emotional disorders in children and adolescents, New York, 1980, Spectrum Books.

34. Simmons, J.E.: Psychiatric examination of children, ed. 2, Philadelphia, 1974, Lea & Febiger.

35. Sully, J.: Studies of childhood, London, 1903, Longman Group.

36. Trieschman, A.E., Whittaker, J.K., and Brendtro, L.K.: The other 23 hours, New York, 1969, Aldine Publishing Co.

37. Weiner, J.: Diagnosis and pharmacology of childhood and adolescent disorders, New York, 1985, John Wiley & Sons.

38. White, J.H.: Psychopharmacology in childhood, Psychiatr. Clin. North Am. **3**:443, 1980.

39. Wilson, H.S., and Kneisl, C.R.: Psychiatric nursing, Reading, Maine, 1979, Addison-Wesley Publishing Co., Inc.

40. Wingfield, A.: Human learning and memory: an introduction, New York, 1979, Harper & Row, Publishers, Inc.

■ ANNOTATED SUGGESTED READINGS ■

Arnold, E.L., editor: Helping parents help their children, New York, 1977, Brunner/Mazel, Inc.

This book discusses general principles of parent guidance and offers advice for helping parents of children with specific problems. It is an excellent reference for people working with children and families.

Axline, U.M.: Play therapy, Boston, 1947, Houghton Mifflin Co.

This classic work describes the author's unique art and style of play therapy.

Bradt, J.O., and Moynihan, C.J.: Opening the safe: a study of child-focused families. In Bradt, J.O., and Moynihan, C.J., editors: Systems therapy, Washington, D.C., 1972, Groome Child Guidance Center.

This is highly recommended to the student interested in viewing the child psychiatric patient from a systems theory perspective.

Chess, S., and Hassibi, M.: Principles and practice of child psychiatry, New York, 1978, Plenum Publishing Corp.

This is a comprehensive text with its main emphasis on etiology and description of syndromes.

Dinkmeyer, D., and McKay, G.D.: The parents' handbook: systematic training for effective parenting. Minnesota, 1982, American Guidance Services.

This is an essential teaching aid for parents. It also provides basic skills for the nurse beginning to work with children. Content includes parenting styles, the meaning of a child's misbehavior, communication skills, natural and logical consequences and more.

Elkind, D.: Children and adolescents: interpretive essays on Jean Piaget, New York, 1974, Oxford University Press, Inc.

For the student interested in cognitive developmental theory, this book is a readable interpretation of the extremely technical writing of Jean Piaget.

*Fagin, C.M., editor: Readings in child and adolescent psychiatric nursing, St. Louis, 1974, The C.V. Mosby Co.

This book provides the child psychiatric nurse with an interesting look at her beginnings and also provides a variety of intervention techniques for use in specific situations.

Freud, A.: The psychoanalytic treatment of children, New York, 1965, International Universities Press, Inc.

This classic in the field of child psychoanalysis is highly recommended to the nurse interested in advanced study.

Gordon, T.: P.E.T.: parent effectiveness training, New York, 1970, Wyden Books.

The author presents an alternative approach to child-rearing based on Rogerian communication techniques. It is helpful for parents as well as professionals.

Guerin, P.J., editor: Family therapy theory and practice, New York, 1976, Gardner Press, Inc.

This book is the bible of the family systems therapist, offering many valuable chapters on theory and technique. It provides in-depth knowledge about the child as a symptom bearer of family problems.

Noshpitz, J.D., editor: Basic handbook of child psychiatry, vols. 1-4, New York, 1979, Basic Books, Inc.

These volumes represent a wealth of information for the advanced student. Subjects included are child development, assessment, deviations and syndromes, therapeutic interventions, and community mental health. An excellent, if somewhat costly, addition to the child psychotherapist's library.

*Pothier, P., Norbeck, J., and Laliberte, M.: Child psychiatric nursing: the gap between need and utilization, J. Psychosoc. Nurs. Ment. Health Serv. **23**(7):18, 1985.

This is the report of a survey by the authors of child psychiatric specialists including their preparation, practice settings, and utilization.

---

*Asterisk indicates nursing reference.

Rappaport, J.L.: DSM-III training guide for diagnosis of childhood disorders, New York, 1984, Brunner/Mazel, Inc.

Provides specific instructions for diagnosing childhood disorders using the DSM-III manual. Provides information on the adult disorders that appear in childhood and those specific to infancy, childhood, and adolescence.

Redl, F.: The life space interview, Am. J. Orthopsychiatry **1**:1, 1959.

The author presents his classic work in concise form.

Redl, F., and Wineman, D.: The aggressive child, Glencoe, Ill., 1957, Free Press.

This book is required reading for milieu therapists because it describes the ego pathology of the aggressive child and delineates the life space interview techniques. It is replete with clinical examples.

Schaeffer, C., editor: The therapeutic use of child's play, New York, 1976, Jason Aronson, Inc.

This is a compilation of individual and group approaches to treating the child. Psychoanalytic and humanistic theory and clinical applications predominate.

Schulman, J.L., and Irwin, M.: Psychiatric hospitalization of children, Springfield, Ill., 1982, Charles C Thomas.

A comprehensive description of treatment for children requiring acute and chronic levels of care.

Simmons, J.E.: Psychiatric examination of children, ed. 2, Philadelphia, 1974, Lea & Febiger.

Simmons offers a compact and concise paperback manual explaining mental status and psychiatric examination of children. A case study and suggested format are included.

*Special issue: Focus on the child, J. Psychosoc. Nurs. Ment. Health Serv. **22**(3):11, 1984.

This entire issue is devoted to exploring various aspects of child psychiatric nursing. Recommended to all nurses interested in this area.

Trieschman, A.E., Whittaker, J.K., and Brendtro, L.K.: The other 23 hours: child care work with emotionally disturbed children in a therapeutic milieu, New York, 1969, Aldine Publishing Co.

Many aspects of milieu therapy are included in this book which is available in paperback. The concept of milieu therapy, therapeutic relationships, program development, and recording are covered to make a basic text for beginning practitioners.

Weiner, J.M.: Diagnosis and psychopharmacology of childhood and adolescent disorders, New York, 1985, John Wiley & Sons.

An up-to-date compilation of research information on the use and effectiveness of drug therapy for psychiatric disorders in children and adolescents.

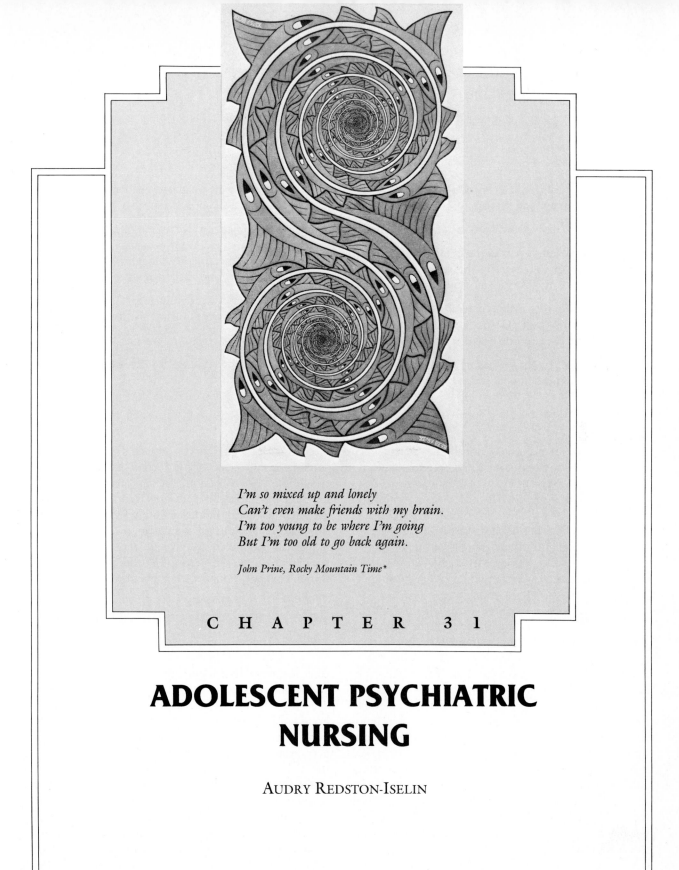

I'm so mixed up and lonely
Can't even make friends with my brain.
I'm too young to be where I'm going
But I'm too old to go back again.

John Prine, Rocky Mountain Time*

ADOLESCENT PSYCHIATRIC NURSING

AUDRY REDSTON-ISELIN

*Song from album "Diamonds in the Rough," 1972.

LEARNING OBJECTIVES

After studying this chapter, the student should be able to:

- state the scope and function of adolescent psychiatric nursing practice.

- list the developmental tasks of adolescence.

- compare and contrast the following theoretical views of adolescence—biological, psychoanalytical, intellectual, and cultural.

- identify the major categories of data that should be collected by the nurse with regard to the adolescent's health status.

- discuss common areas of conflict for adolescents and the implications of them.

- describe the nursing diagnosis relative to specified problematical adolescent behaviors.

- analyze the indications for and implications of the use of patient education, family, group, and individual therapies by the nurse working with adolescents, and their parents.

- assess the importance of evaluation of the nursing process when working with adolescents.

- identify directions for future nursing research.

- select appropriate readings for further study.

Adolescence is a time of transition—an age when one is not an adult and not a child. Yet the issues reflected in the adolescent experience are central to one's development as a person. Of profound proportion in adolescence, they are often recapitulated later in life. The intense feelings during the teenage years are perhaps the most meaningful of any experienced in a lifetime. Assisting adolescents during this conflictual period of development can be an enlightening and rewarding experience.

In this chapter an attempt is made to understand adolescent behavior and the nurse's role in facilitating growth during this developmental phase. An overview of various theoretical models is presented to illustrate a number of diverse perspectives of the adolescent experience. In addition, areas of conflict such as identity, social role, sexual behavior, independence, and body image are examined. The "normal" behaviors of adolescents result from these conflicts and are experienced by virtue of the biological and subsequent psychological growth that occurs.[8] An exploration of these conflicts and resulting behaviors is presented to help the nurse in assessing the adolescent and his functioning. When these conflicts are intensified, certain maladaptive coping patterns may be seen, and a nursing diagnosis of the adolescent's problem can be made. These maladaptive behaviors and nursing diagnoses, such as delinquency, hypochondriasis, weight problems, sexual promiscuity, and drug abuse, are discussed here as well. These lead to the formulation of a plan of action that aids the nurse in assisting the adolescent in productive movement on the developmental continuum.

This chapter attempts to provide the nurse with the assessment skills necessary to formulate therapeutic interventions. The collection of data in an organized fashion is reviewed to facilitate diagnosis and action. Finally, various therapeutic modalities are reviewed. Concrete suggestions for the implementation of these techniques are presented to provide the nurse clinician with some of the skills required to initiate and follow through on a productive therapeutic experience with adolescents.

Role of the adolescent psychiatric nurse

Adolescent psychiatric nurses are prepared in psychiatric–mental health nursing and are characterized by specific interests in meeting the needs of this age group. They focus on adolescents as they develop toward adulthood—considering social, emotional, and physical aspects of their adjustment in their family, school, and peer groups. These nurses concentrate on facilitating the adolescent's successful movement in the growth process toward adulthood. Adolescent psychiatric nurses become experts in identifying deviations or stalls in the developmental process and work closely with the adolescent's support systems to further enhance the growth process. This is in contrast with adult psychiatric nurses, who work with people who have attained some level of maturity and often need a reeducative experience to correct deficiencies in developmental areas.[4]

The scope of adolescent psychiatric nursing practice encompasses direct and indirect care in the areas of prevention, intervention, and rehabilitation. Direct nursing functions focus on actions toward the particular adolescent and include the following:

1. Psychotherapy (individual, family, and group therapy)
2. Intake screening and evaluation
3. Home visits (or substitute dwellings)
4. Provision of therapeutic milieu
5. Counseling (time limited on a specific problem)
6. Health teaching (role model and didactic teaching, usually on sex and health)
7. Support and medication surveillance
8. Community action (resource person to others dealing with adolescents; help formulate programs needed)
9. Crisis intervention

These functions attempt to alleviate emotional difficulty and discourage maladaptive relating patterns.

Indirect nursing functions focus on actions taken to assist another person who actually carries out the care given to the adolescent. These functions are usually done by an adolescent psychiatric nurse specialist in the following roles[4]:

1. Educator
2. Administrator
3. Clinical supervisor
4. Consultant
5. Nurse researcher

Developmental stage of adolescence

Adolescence is a unique and distinct stage of development that, although often seen in the context of contemporary social change, has great significance in the understanding of human behavior. A look at human development reveals a progression of movement from one stage of life to the next, from infancy through old age. The common age range for adolescence (11 to 20) indicates that during that time period a shift in the developmental and learning process occurs. It is more accurate to view this progression as continuous in which each stage overlaps the next. Goals and tasks within the specific stage of adolescence, and the way each stage of life moves into the succeeding ones, have been studied by various theorists.

The new developmental tasks that emerge during adolescence stress the individual's defenses and can either stimulate growth in the form of new ways of coping or lead to regression and disorganization from failure to cope. Long-standing difficulties from the past may contribute to disorganization, and the current environment may help or hinder the adolescent's attempt to deal with these issues. Beginning at infancy, development is often marked with episodes of disintegration at the onset of learning a new skill, with movement toward integration as the new skill is acquired. The pattern of dealing with developmental stress contributes to how the adolescent will cope with current anxieties. Skills established during latency do little to ward off anxieties associated with changing body image and new instinctive feelings. Past coping skills, if integrated with success, can assist toward healthy integration of adult functions.

During adolescence major events are encountered and attempts to resolve these events are made. These result in behavior uniquely "adolescent."[25] Havighurst delineated tasks that should be accomplished during adolescence[15]:

1. Achieving new and more mature relations with age mates of both sexes
2. Achieving masculine or feminine social roles
3. Accepting one's physique and using the body effectively
4. Achieving emotional independence from parents and other adults
5. Preparing for marriage and family life
6. Preparing for an economic career
7. Acquiring a set of values and an ethical system as a guide to behavior and developing an ideology

Different theoretical concepts of adolescent development have evolved in conjunction with how these developmental tasks are encountered and resolved to produce an adolescent moving toward adulthood.

Theoretical views of adolescence

■ Biological theory

Gesell, Ilg, and Ames[13] believed that biological influences are the major determinants of adolescent development. They studied humans from birth to age 16, placing great emphasis on observable behaviors of the child and adolescent and the role of environmental influences on adolescent development. They believed that growth patterns followed certain principles of maturation. Through maturation and environmental influences a person learns how to adjust. Behavior is therefore a conscious growth experience. Gesell and associates described adolescent development as consisting of intense physical growth changes which are so dramatic that they affect all aspects of the human being. He presented a normative theory, categorizing through his observation certain behaviors that occur at particular points in the maturational development of most adolescents. Gesell's specific normative data consist of feelings, thoughts, and behaviors seen at each age. He indicated differences in equilibrium ranging from stormy disequilibrium to calm equilibrium and maintained that these changes are caused by maturational states which cause the adolescent to grow.

■ Psychoanalytical theory

Freud also believed that human development was biological and was marked by stages. He put more emphasis on the first year of life, concluding that adolescence and adulthood have their roots in the resolution of childhood developmental stages. These stages originated in the sexual instinct he called the id, which he viewed as a primary factor in determining an individual's successful personality development. The rational, reality-based part of humans he called the ego, which helped control and modify the id and created coping mechanisms to deal with the environment. The superego was described as the conscience, which assisted the ego in establishing socially acceptable behaviors and attitudes. Freud constructed five stages of development from birth to adolescence: oral, anal, phallic, latency, and genital.

During puberty (ages 13 to 18), which is Freud's genital stage, there is a reawakening of sexual interest. The adolescent with new sexual urges looks for gratification outside the home. This renewal comes from physiological maturing. The genitalia mature, and there is an increase in the release of sex hormones. Sexual exploration and maturation often occur. Freud stressed that the first years of life were important in establishing traits that become permanent in adolescence.[11]

The more modern psychoanalytical theories of today are the most descriptive in defining adolescence. Classically, they, as did Freud, define it as the stage between childhood and adulthood correlated with the biological changes of puberty. Adolescence is described by Josselyn[17] as the psychological development that attempts to deal with pubescent changes and is therefore initiated by them. The biological changes of puberty upset a balance that previously existed between the ego and id during latency. Increased drives or impulses initiated by the greater hormonal secretion cause a personality reorganization in adolescents as they attempt to adjust to their new physical status. These increased impulses confront a relatively weak ego. Most evident at this time is a resurgence of the oedipal complex, which brings along with it derivatives of pregenital drives, oral and anal impulses, and aggressive drives. Adolescents therefore return to earlier modes of adaptation in an effort to reevaluate and reestablish mastery over the environment. Many solutions to problems caused by instinctual pressures are tried.

Psychoanalysts believe that sexual development does not begin with puberty but that new avenues for dealing with drives and the growth spurt come to the forefront in adolescence. The simple solutions of drive satisfaction that a child used no longer work, and efforts toward new solutions are made. The ability to make these adjustments comes about by the ego's capacity to renegotiate between the id, the superego, and the environment. The groundwork for this is laid earlier in development. If there has been inadequate accommodation in earlier stages, this is often reflected by difficulties in adolescence. Adolescence is a developmental maturational process in which the individual attempts to work through his life experiences to achieve maturity. Related to the oedipal conflict is the adolescent's task of freeing himself from dependency on parents. This detachment from incestuous objects can be evident in rejection, resentment, and hostility toward parents and authority. For this reason Blos[9] calls adolescence a "second stage of individuation," the first occurring during the oedipal period.

The classical psychoanalytical description of adolescence has been modified by Erikson, Fromm, Horney, Sullivan, and others who emphasize the effect of social factors on these developmental processes. Erikson[12] speaks about ego identity, or the relationship between what a person seems like to others and what the person himself thinks he is. To Erikson, adolescence represents an attempt to establish an identity within the social environment. This search is described as "normal adolescent identity crisis." Erikson outlined this in the theoretical framework of his eight stages of human beings. He called the stage of adolescence "identity vs. identity diffusion," which is followed in young adulthood by the stage of "intimacy vs. isolation." He stressed that identity must be established before intimacy can occur.

■ Intellectual development theory

Cognition was most completely described by Piaget.[23] By gradually internalizing actions, one evolves a system of thought processes. A child learns to reason by a process he described as "concrete operations," based on concrete objects. Adolescence was defined as an advanced stage of cognitive functioning in which one is able to reason beyond concrete objects to symbols or abstractions, or what Piaget called "formal thought." Piaget believed the adolescent has the ability to deal with propositional logic, to grasp metaphors, and to reason about thought. This develops in a continuous fashion from the concrete thinking of childhood to (at about age 12) a rapid progression toward free reflection. This Piaget called the "formal operational period." The concern with realities and tangible objects manipulated toward real action is transferred to an ideational plan, permitting one to draw conclusions and reflect in the absence of the object. This ability he called "logic of operations."

■ Cultural theory

Anthropologists who studied adolescent behavior concluded from studies of adolescents in different cultures that primitive cultures had less stressful periods than those experienced by American teenagers. Mead[20] concluded that the experience of adolescent rebellion was culturally determined by the changes in generations and not biologically based. Anthropologists believe adolescence is a period when the person feels he deserves adult privileges that are not given to him, and it ends when the full power and social status of an adult are delegated to him by society. Anthropologists see growth as a continuous process and a cultural phenomenon, with individuals reacting to social expectations. The more clearly defined these expectations are, the less stressful and ambiguous the adolescent period. The more the culture has changed, the greater the generation gap.

Today's adolescents have the culture of the present times to cope with, which can exacerbate conflicts awakened by increased drives and changes in body image. Several issues in the complex and changing American society bear mentioning, since they directly influence the support an adolescent is able to obtain from the environment. Blurring sexual roles is one phenomenon affecting contemporary adolescents. Women today have less traditional attitudes, expectations, and behaviors. Men are increasingly aware of women in changing and evolving roles, and they are consequently more involved in functions that were previously believed to be predominantly in the woman's domain and vice versa. The anxiety associated with these role changes has begun to be identified and explored.

The current economic reorientation from abundance to conservation has brought a new focus on such issues as economic stability, restraint, and budgeting. There are fewer jobs, particularly for adolescents. The cost of higher education has increased dramatically, which has resulted in an extended adolescence beyond the previously described time frame because of prolonged economic dependency. In today's world, women are developing careers and entering the work force, which requires a new perspective on two-parent working families. There has also been an increase in divorce rates and single-parent families. The results of these changes can only be speculated on; however, it is obvious that these issues increase the complexity of society and add new pressures to adolescents who are becoming adults and attempting to define their role in today's cultural milieu.

There is evidence suggesting that historical and cultural factors often have a greater impact than developmental or age-related factors on adolescents. Even though adolescence is thought of by some as "an experience of the 20th century," today's adolescent experience is a very different experience from that of the past. There is a large amount of interaction between development, with its psychological tasks, and the world in which the developmental tasks take place.[22]

Assessment

Collection of data through clinical observations, which are based on theoretical knowledge, is an important aspect of the nursing process model. It involves observation and interpretation of behavior patterns in an organized way, which may indicate a need for growth-promoting relationships. The collection of data about the adolescent's health status is often referred to in other disciplines as the developmental history. It specifically includes the following information:

1. Growth and development (including developmental milestones)
2. Biophysical status (illnesses, accidents)
3. Emotional status (relatedness, affect, mental status—including evidence of thought disorder, and suicidal or homocidal ideation)
4. Cultural, religious, and socioeconomic background
5. Performance of activities of daily living (home, attending school)
6. Patterns of coping (ego defenses such as denial, acting out, withdrawal)
7. Interaction patterns (family, peers)
8. Adolescent's perception of and satisfaction with his health status
9. Adolescent's health goals
10. Environment (physical, emotional, ecological)
11. Available and accessible human and material resources (friends, school and community involvement)

These data are collected from adolescents, their families, and other significant persons, such as school personnel and the physician, by interviews, examinations, observations, and reports.

The importance of detailed information on the psychological development of adolescents has been challenged by many, since it places an emphasis on past occurrences. Data collection by the nurse is based on current, as well as past, functioning in all realms of adolescent life. It helps to give a view of the adolescent experience and aids the nurse in assessing the success of the adolescent's attempts to complete the prescribed tasks.

An examination of the common behaviors that adolescents display reveals that adolescence is a time of anxiety and conflict. Conflictual issues such as body image, identity, independence, sexuality, social role, and social behavior are the most common. These conflicts can produce adaptive or maladaptive behaviors in an attempt to master the tasks at hand. The extent of these conflicts, or the qualitative response of the adolescent's attempt to master and move toward adult functioning, is the key to the necessity of intervention with conflicted adolescents.

■ Body image

Chronological age is not a valid guide for physical maturation, since growth often occurs in spurts and there are individual differences. Since the grouping of adolescents is usually done chronologically, the adolescent must face being with others who vary greatly in physical development and interests. This explains the predominance of imitative behavior resorted to in adolescence as an effort to keep within the expected range of conduct and be compatible with peers. The greater the divergence from the rest of the group, the greater the adolescent's anxiety. The lack of uniformity of growth often puts great demands on physical and mental adaptability. Growth being uneven and sudden, rather than smooth and gradual, causes a change in body image.

Adolescents reevaluate themselves in light of these physical changes, particularly the onset of primary and secondary sex characteristics, which are so pronounced. They tend to compare themselves and their physical development to that of their peers. They are very concerned about the normality of their physical status. The absence of clear-cut norms only adds to this uncertainty. The physical changes of puberty cause adolescents to be self-conscious of their changing bodies. Often they are reluctant to have medical examinations because they fear abnormalities will be found. Examinations may intensify masturbatory conflicts, sexual fantasies, and guilt feelings. Extreme concern with body changes may lead to deviant behaviors such as hypochrondriasis, in which physical complications are the focus of underlying conflicts.[8]

Usually there is an increase in self-esteem over the period between early and middle adolescence. However, in recent studies, girls show a decrease in self-esteem at this time, which is associated with negative feelings about body image and their comparison of themselves to older adolescents. Offer and co-workers present evidence that this is a vulnerable time for girls and may be associated with the onset of differences that begin to appear at this age and coincide with an increase in the incidence of depression in girls.[22]

■ Identity

In an attempt to adjust to the physical changes of puberty, adolescents experience a surge of excitation and tension. Methods of gratification and defenses against these feelings that were used in infancy and childhood are renewed. This mixture of previous infantile solutions, plus new adult attempts at mastery, accounts for the often bizarre and regressive nature of adolescent behavior. As they attempt to cope, adolescents sometimes act as adults and other times as children.

They can be seen to be experiencing a second individuation process, similar to the first one noted at about age 2. Blos[9] equates the characteristic "no" predominating in the 2-year-old's effort to differentiate between self and nonself with the rebellious and oppositional behavior of the adolescent. Adolescents exhibit behavior marked with experimentation, testing the self by going to extremes. This has a usefulness in the establishment of self-identity. The rebelliousness or negativism shows a movement toward individuation and autonomy that has greater complexity but also elements similar to the 2-year-old's "no." Adolescents assert themselves in affirmation of their self-identity by being negative to parents and other authority figures whom they feel are not allowing them to be separate and unique, as illustrated by Clinical example 31-1.

The individuation process is accompanied by feelings of isolation, loneliness, and confusion, since it brings childhood dreams to an end and attributes them to fantasy. This realization of the end of childhood can create intense fears or panic. Many adolescents therefore attempt to remain in this transitional stage. The awakening of emotional ties with the family also occurs in

---

CLINICAL EXAMPLE 31-1

David, although an avid football fan for several years, suddenly switched his interest to basketball. He quit his local football team despite his father's urgings to continue. His father, also a football fan, could not understand David's sudden negative attitude toward football and newly found interest in basketball.

the establishment of new, more interdependent relationships. This fearful, yet exciting, entrance into adulthood is a profound personal experience that is not totally resolved in adolescence but is dealt with throughout the course of one's lifetime. Adolescents mourn the loss of childhood, and the feelings of loneliness and isolation that accompany this loss establish an intense need for closeness, love, and understanding. If they are unable to obtain support during this struggle, an intense nontransient depression may result.[8]

■ Independence

There is an unconscious longing by adolescents to give in to their dependency needs. It is also a time of profound movement toward independence. Adolescents reveal this ambivalence by responding to petty annoyances and irritations with outbursts more intense than seem warranted. They see the process toward independence as being free of parental control. They do not view attainment of independence as a gradual learning process but as an emancipation accomplished by acting "differently." If one acts adult, then one is adult. Therefore they expose themselves to situations beyond their capabilities and then become overwhelmed and frightened. They seek reassurance in an attempt to alleviate their anxiety by returning to childlike ways and being dependent on those with whom they feel most secure, usually their parents. This accounts for the inconsistency of adolescent behavior.

Well-adjusted adults usually use a problem-solving approach and do not feel as threatened when inexperience requires dependency on others. Adolescents, however, already tempted to give in to dependency needs, feel as if they are regressing to childhood, which deflates their self-esteem. They must deny their need for their parents. Sometimes they will criticize their parents for treating them as a child and not allowing them freedom and then remark that their parents are not helpful enough. When adolescents seem to be rebelling against their parents, they may be rebelling against their own childhood conscience or superego. They project their ambivalence onto their parents, since they were the original source of restrictions. This projection actually reveals a movement toward a more mature standard and also indicates their insecurity about relinquishing childhood standards. By blaming their parents for their childish actions, they can avoid blows to their fragile self-esteem and protest that their actions result from parental demands, not their own.

■ Sexuality

Most adolescents accept the sexual mores of our culture, which dictate that sexual feelings be directed toward persons of the opposite sex. This is not achieved without confusion, since the adolescent is capable of a greater depth of emotional experience than the child. The biologically induced sexual feelings that are intensified during adolescence go along with intensified emotional feelings. The fusion of sexual impulses with love means that sex is the usual mode of discharge of feelings of deep affection. The strongest emotional ties are felt toward the parents, but the channeling of these sexual impulses creates a conflict. The adolescent interprets love for the parent of the same sex as suggestive of homosexuality. At the same time, feelings of love toward the parent of the opposite sex are equally conflictual, since they are viewed as incestuous. Movement toward independence complicates this issue, necessitating defensive activities toward these new emotions.

Rejection of parents, so frequently expressed by adolescents, can also be seen as a defense to diminish ties to the parents and therefore avoid sexual arousal. Efforts to resolve this conflict can be seen in experimentation through heterosexual and sometimes homosexual relationships. Ambivalence is apparent, since adolescents are often flirtatious one moment and rejecting the next, and parents may find these flirtations enjoyable. Clinical example 31-2 is an example of this ambivalence.

■ Social role

Adolescents respond to persons and events with great intensity. They may be totally invested in one interest and then suddenly change to something different at a moment's notice. This intensity of feelings and lack of stable identity can account for their extreme sensitivity to the response of others. They are easily hurt, disappointed, and fearful of others. There is a tendency toward "hero worship" and "crushes," but with poor discrimination in evaluating the individuals to whom these feelings are directed. Adolescent relationships serve many functions. Frequently adolescents relate to a chum as if neither person were a separate individual. They often mimic each other's dress, speech, language, and thoughts. These relationships help in the development of self-identity and establishment of a social role.

CLINICAL EXAMPLE 31-2

Debbie, at age 13, would not let her father kiss her. She was often distant and aloof when he attempted closeness. In contrast, she was often teasing and flirtatious, often remarking about his muscular body structure.

The peer group is of extreme importance to adolescents, since within the security of the peer group, adolescents can attempt to resolve conflicts. They can relate to peers in a way in which they cannot relate to others, and with peers they can test out their thoughts and ideas. Their thoughts may be different from their peers, but through mutual sharing, they can attempt to find an answer. The peer group explores more autonomous ways of dealing with problems in life. A peer group that shares these explorations offers its members companionship, protection, and security, with acceptable elements of dependent gratification. In the peer group, adolescents can accept dependency, not as a child but as one of the gang, testing out ideas and trying new values. Within the safety of the peer group they can observe, comment on, and evaluate the activities of other peer groups. Adolescents usually are very loyal to their group of friends. Sometimes group security is so important that it is necessary at all costs. Then destructive experimentation may occur to preserve acceptance in the group.

Adolescents often test out ideas pertaining to values. They either eventually abandon them or incorporate them gradually into their adult personality. They react to many stimuli and drain off the tension created by new drives and impulses by investment in many interests. They do this with great intensity, and that is why adolescents are susceptible to many brief fads. This is often seen in their dress, love for music, or hobbies.

Close relationships with the opposite sex provide adolescents with security (often by "going steady") and a person with whom to discuss problems and evaluate solutions. Often the partner may take on similar characteristics. This reciprocal relationship enhances self-esteem by demonstrating sexual attractiveness to the self and to the world, and it indicates that one is lovable. It also allows for bisexual expression, since the girl expresses her partner's feminine parts and her boyfriend represents her masculine parts. It is frequently observed that people tend to marry someone resembling the parent of the opposite sex. However, adolescents may purposely choose someone different to free themselves of their ties to their parents, which are sexually tinged, or may choose someone who is an acceptable substitute for parents.

■ **Sexual behavior**

Fantasy is used by adolescents to discharge tension meant for sexual play. Secretly they can be participant and observer and try out means of direct sexual discharge. They may, however, feel guilt and shame about sexual feelings, or they may experience the incompatibility of their fantasies with their ideal of themselves. Fantasies usually are an attempt to find solutions and evaluate consequences. Most adolescent fantasies are of a problem-solving nature. They may indicate a disturbance if they continually occupy the adolescent's thoughts, are not converted into constructive actions, or are not modified by reality. Then they may disrupt other activities that are important to adolescent functioning and indicate a withdrawal from reality.

Masturbation is also a frequent mode of discharge of tension for adolescents, particularly when alone, unhappy, or frustrated, and it serves to fuse psychological and physical sexuality. It is not always associated with sexual fantasies. The value of masturbation may be lessened by the shame and guilt that accompany it. Male adolescents often fear discovery of evidences of ejaculation and females often fear changes in their genitalia as a result of masturbation. Fears are not limited to discovery by others but also are caused by the expansive experience of orgasm, with the resulting feelings of loss of ego boundaries. If masturbation is used as a continual source of comfort or with inappropriate exposure (exhibitionism), it is indicative of disturbance.

Mutual masturbation can also serve the purposes of tension release and fusing of identity. If mutual masturbation is the primary focus of the relationship, without the enrichment of other aspects of a relationship, then it may be maladaptive. Mutual masturbation is often acceptable to adolescents as long as it does not lead to intercourse. It can help to dispel anxieties about sexuality by assuring adolescents that they are sexually adequate.[17]

 Nursing diagnosis

Behaviors that cripple growth and development may warrant nursing intervention. The nurse should consider the degree of destructiveness and the nature of the defense and regression that the adolescent experiences. If the difficulty is predominant and not transient, it may mean intervention is needed. These destructive behaviors become the basis for the identification of specific problem areas.

■ **Sexually active adolescent**

The sexual behavior of adolescents is often not as much an outlet for sexual passion as a desire to achieve closeness with another individual. The sexual expression seems to fulfill needs of love and security. Adolescents tend to use their sexuality to sublimate other needs. Josselyn[17] mentions some of the common interpretations sexual relations may have:

1. Finding an alternative choice to replace incestuously laden parental object of the opposite sex
2. Identifying with the parent of the same sex and trying to do what they do
3. Attempting to camouflage homosexual feelings
4. Expressing anger or hostility toward the parent of the opposite sex

Personal anxiety about sexual adequacy and peer group pressure also seems to add to the possibility of using sexual relations inappropriately. Some adolescents use sexual relations in a self-destructive way as a means of punishing themselves. Their promiscuity elicits external control and condemnation from others. This is apparent when there is an exhibitionistic quality, and subtle efforts to "get caught" are seen. Periods of extreme prudery may alternate with periods of extreme sexual activity. Adolescents often attempt to have the nurse take a stand against their behavior and thereby avoid the underlying conflictual issues.

Meeks[21] suggests exploring the meaning of sexual behavior in adolescents by asking the following questions:

1. Does the adolescent desire sexual gratification for punishment?
2. Do the adolescent's goals match the situation or is he deceiving himself?
3. Is he demanding adult privileges while acting irresponsible and dependent?
4. To what extent is the behavior a defense for depression, anger toward others, or exploratory experimentation?
5. Is the behavior to avoid anxiety-producing fantasies?
6. How close is the relationship to a mature one?

Clinical example 31-3 illustrates inappropriate use of sexual activity.

Another example of inappropriate use of sexual activity is a new thrill-seeking experience, used by teenagers across the country, based on an old Japanese act of heightening the sexual experience by asphyxiating the adolescent male just at the point of ejaculation. This has unfortunately accidentally sent several adolescents to an early death.

■ Pseudohomosexuality

Adolescents who are uncertain of their sexual identity often misinterpret certain characteristics as being masculine or feminine. The anxiety that results can precipitate a fear of homosexuality. This triggers additional feelings of depression and anxiety that exaggerate the initial ones. This is common in males who see charac-

> ### CLINICAL EXAMPLE 31-3
>
> Janet, a 14-year-old adolescent, had apparently been sexually active since age 12. She was brought to the clinic by her parents when they had been told by a neighboring friend of Janet's exploits. Janet had bragged to the neighbor of her sexual ventures. Two years before referral her parents had placed Janet in a more controlled parochial school because they were concerned she was "acting wild." It became apparent that Janet had wanted her parents to know about and put limits on her behavior. She admitted to not enjoying sexual intercourse very much. She seemed to be trying desperately to get approval from her distant and punitive mother. Her father, who was a policeman, was what she described as "a hopeless case," secretly wishing that he would be a better policeman for her.

teristics such as passivity as castrating and diminishing their maleness. Their fear of homosexuality increases their anxiety, causing them to withdraw into a cycle of failure. They may then feel dependent, have trouble asserting themselves, and respond by "acting out." It is important to differentiate between deviant behavior and defects in socialization skills in this regard. Defects in socialization skills causing a pseudohomosexual response may result from the absence of an adequate male figure, the mother or father's expressed fearfulness of aggressiveness, physical disabilities, seduction by an older adult, or a personality temperament of passivity.[21]

■ Overt homosexual activity in adolescence

During adolescence, when identity is unclear and much experimentation occurs, the individual may have both homosexual and heterosexual experiences. This does not mean that the adolescent is homosexual or bisexual.[18] If he is not severely conflicted either in his experimentation or in his regular homosexual relationships, he probably will not reach the nurse therapist. If he does, it may be to appease a conflicted family. Sometimes, however, homosexual relationships may interfere with establishing an adequate sexual identity. In this case homosexual behavior may be indicative of anxiety about heterosexuality. Because it is usually complex, the meaning of continued homosexual behavior must be assessed individually. This is evident in Clinical example 31-4.

CLINICAL EXAMPLE 31-4

Joanne, age 15, was engaged in homosexual experiences with an 18-year-old girl. She claimed she enjoyed sexual experiences more with girls than boys. She had poor sexual experiences with boys because she believed boys wanted girls for their sexual exploits. This was understandable because her history revealed that she was sexually abused by her paternal grandfather several times and once by her father at about age 5. She had painful experiences and minor medical complications with her menstrual period. This, in addition to her early traumatic experiences, caused Joanne much confusion about her sexual identity. Her mother experienced sexual confusion of her own and related better to the boys in the family. Joanne always wanted to be close to her mother and gain her approval. Joanne, in her confusion, assumed that if she could be a boy (male counterpart of a homosexual relationship), she could do to women what had been done to her (express her anger about early sexual traumas by identifying with the aggressor), could get her mother's approval (being a boy and not having sex with Daddy or boys), could gain closeness (sex with a girl), and could avoid mother's anger (for sex with Daddy). In her attempt to gain a comfortable sexual identity, she was trying out a homosexual identity because it seemed the least threatening.

CLINICAL EXAMPLE 31-5

Susie, a 16-year-old adolescent, had run away for the second time, only to return home to the same chaos. She had tried to run away with her boyfriend. Her alcoholic mother and psychotic 19-year-old brother were making life unbearable. Her mother was surprised to learn about 3 months after her return that Susie was pregnant. Susie was delighted because she had hopes that now she could get out of the house, knowing her mother would now approve of her marriage to her boyfriend Jim.

An added dimension to homosexual activity in adolescence is the AIDS epidemic. Anxiety over sexual identity issues are heightened by fears of contracting this fatal illness. Although the full ramifications of this are not yet clear, it may be that the epidemic has heightened stigma about homosexual preference and experimentation.

■ Unwed motherhood

The meaning of pregnancy in adolescence is a complicated issue because there are social, as well as intrapsychic, factors involved. Some adolescent girls fear inadequacy of their femininity. These fears may stem from dependent attachment feelings toward the mother, which are frequently experienced during regressive periods and mistaken as signs of homosexuality.[8] To ease these fears, the adolescent girl may become pregnant. Sometimes pregnancy is an effort to escape a difficult family situation or to force the parents to agree to a marriage that may be inappropriate, as shown in Clinical example 31-5.

Occasionally, emotionally deprived adolescents hope to give their child what they feel they have never received (or, probably more accurately, get from the child what they have not gotten). Sometimes pregnancy appears to be a device to allow parents to relinquish parental responsibility for the adolescent. In some cases the adolescent has lived out a scapegoat role as the bad one in the family, thereby justifying parental neglect and hostility. The pregnancy can then improve family relationships because, with the adulthood the pregnancy implies, parents may be freed of guilt and may then not need to encourage the adolescent to do things that make her unlovable.

Pregnancy in adolescence may have other origins. It can occur accidentally after sexual exploration. The adolescent may not be aware of contraceptive methods. Pregnancy in an unmarried adolescent is often associated with sexual promiscuity, and, if it is, the girl may be ostracized. Sometimes pregnancy occurs from a close interpersonal relationship. Both the circumstances and the adolescent's level of maturity need to be assessed. Peer groups can be supportive to a girl who becomes pregnant as a result of a meaningful relationship yet intolerant of one whose pregnancy is the result of promiscuity. In some cultures out-of-wedlock pregnancies are an accepted part of adolescence.

The decisions involving abortion, placement of the baby, and marriage are difficult ones. Attitudes and laws influencing these decisions are diverse. Many believe that to force the adolescent to have the baby and then give it up is more traumatic for her than abortion. Others believe that abortion can be more disturbing. Marriage is another alternative. Forcing a marriage to avoid societal condemnation usually adds to the adolescent's problems, but a mature couple might do well in marriage. All the alternatives should be presented to the adolescent with the consequences clearly stated. The adolescent should come to her decision with the aid and support of her partner, her family, the nurse, and other involved health care professionals.

■ Adolescent suicide

Sleep

I want to sleep
But with no fears
I know if I do
There will be tears.

Tears of sorrow
Tears of pain
Make no difference
They're both the same.

Asleep where you never awake
The times just go past . . . nothing
Too slow and nothing too fast.
There is no one to cheat you or lie
To you. Nothing to make you sad or blue.

This is the sleep of peace
Of Eternal Rest . . . This is the
Sleep I feel is best. This is
The sleep I long to have . . .

Spice, age 14

The most common factor in adolescent suicide is lack or loss of a meaningful relationship.[16] Many researchers think suicide is an attempt for attention and does not necessarily represent a true desire to die. Regardless, it is a bid for help that must be recognized. Subtle references, as well as attempts, should always be taken seriously and explored. Suicidal gestures are more often seen in girls, with boys expressing their depression by bravado that results in accidents,[24] as in Clinical example 31-6.

The adolescent may be prevented from acting on suicidal feelings by parental concern and the establishment of new relationships. Adolescents may avoid the depression triggered by separating from their parents by expressing it through delinquent behavior. This behavior serves as a defense against self-destructive impulses that accompany feelings of self-loathing. The attempt to manipulate parents, which can motivate the runaway as well as the suicidal adolescent, often has secondary gains that are less important than the internal conflict causing this manipulation. Feelings of helplessness and worthlessness can be initiated by threatened abandonment, being asked to take the adult role, and lack of opportunities to be dependent. Sometimes these adolescents perceive themselves to be expendable because the family unconsciously wishes them dead.

The nurse must make it clear to the adolescent that

CLINICAL EXAMPLE 31-6

John, a 12-year-old depressed adolescent, had just gotten a small dirt bike. Six months earlier John's grandfather, his only friend, had died. John's father had died when he was 2 years old, and he had lived with his mother and grandparents ever since. John, feeling hopeless, had ridden his bike into a car. Luckily, after medical treatment for his broken arm and rib and multiple bruises, John was able to come to therapy. He described feeling helpless and lonely, especially without his grandfather.

---

suicidal behavior is something that is not confidential and that one's parents must be alerted. Involvement of the family is essential to circumvent angry, hostile, and hopeless feelings of abandonment, and create a reality of support and caring.

In working with suicidal adolescents, the nurse should explore the following areas:

1. The seriousness of the attempt (What are the chances of rescue?)
2. The mental status of the adolescent (Was he psychotic?)
3. The extent of environmental stress—especially family disintegration
4. The adolescent's wider social environment and the strength of his support systems (social isolation, school performance, parental loss, disruption of friendship or romantic alliance)
5. The likelihood of repeated suicidal attempts (especially if conditions remain the same)

Clinical examples 31-7 and 31-8 illustrate suicide attempts by adolescents.

■ Adolescent runaways

Adolescents attempting to free themselves from an unbearable living situation may run away. The exit can indicate unconscious conflicts, and the running away usually points out difficulties between the parents and the adolescent. Parental rejection is often experienced from birth, and the parent may alternate between extreme punitive measures and a "laissez-faire" attitude toward the adolescent. Adolescent runaways are often conflicted, especially regarding dependency-independency, and feel embarrassed, helpless, and defeated by their dependency wishes. This can result in a panic that motivates running away to prove autonomy and escape painful circumstances. They usually run away from dis-

CLINICAL EXAMPLE 31-7

Maria, a 15-year-old girl, was referred to her local community mental health center from the neighborhood emergency room after ingesting pills. Maria had taken five of her mother's "arthritis pills" after an argument with her father about her 17-year-old boyfriend, José. Her father, who came home only on weekends, told her to stay away from him. After he left, the other family members noticed Maria had become sleepy while playing cards in the living room. Maria admitted to taking the pills and was rushed by her mother to the emergency room. Maria claimed she would never do it again. She had clearly wanted to be rescued, not really wanting to die. She had had poor school performance for the last year since her father had left the family. She had many friends and had been dating José for the past year. Maria had always been her father's favorite. When she reached puberty at age 13, that relationship changed a great deal. Maria's position as her father's favorite was delegated to a younger female sibling, causing Maria to feel angry and rejected. Her father left the family a year later and returned for weekend visits, during which he mainly disciplined the children. Maria's attempt to get close to José as a replacement for her father was sabotaged by her father as well. Her only recourse was to elicit her father's caring and concern through a suicide attempt. Maria and her family are currently in outpatient treatment.

CLINICAL EXAMPLE 31-8

Donald, age 13, was brought to the emergency room after cutting his wrists one evening when he thought his family was asleep. His mother had awakened and found him bleeding. She rushed him to the local emergency room where he received medical treatment. It was then revealed that this was Donald's second suicidal attempt. The first attempt occurred a year ago when he had ingested pills. Donald had received therapy for about a month. It was then discontinued because of the family moving to a new location, despite recommendations to continue with a new therapist. Donald was always an isolated child. He was never very close with anyone but had two friends. Since the move he had become more withdrawn. He had done well in school in the past but now had given up and was failing almost every subject. The youngest of nine children, Donald had little relationship with his siblings, who were all older than he and not at home much. Donald's parents, both approaching old age, seemed not to notice that he had become increasingly upset. Donald was hospitalized, since the risk of his attempting suicide again was high. He was an isolated and depressed adolescent, seeking refuge from loneliness and defeat in death. He had not wanted to be rescued. The last year, especially, revealed many unsuccessful attempts to find meaningful relationships.

appointment toward something viewed as favorable and supportive. Parents often feel guilty and ashamed and have difficulty acting on practical issues, although some, relieved of their responsibility, are secretly pleased. Frequently the adolescent becomes involved in dangerous activities after running away. Most runaway adolescents want to return home if they believe their parents really want them.[21] Clinical example 31-9 illustrates home conditions that may lead to an adolescent's running away.

■ Conduct disordered adolescent

Conduct disordered adolescents often experience poor parent-child relationships. Antisocial acts enable the adolescent to express anger toward parents, who are punished for the adolescent's acts. Parents are often scapegoated because the child is seen as a helpless victim. It is important to keep in mind that some parents are not effective with some adolescents. Children are socialized mainly by the parents and, hopefully, learn from the parents acceptable behaviors that become part of the internalized self or conscience. A good relationship between parent and child facilitates this process.

However, adolescents learn not only from their parents but also from others in their environment. The school and peer groups are influencing factors, as are the social, economic, and cultural environments. The self-destructive behaviors seen in conduct disordered adolescents may be indicative of need for punishment, anger at the family, peer group pressure, depression, feelings of self-defeat, a search for opportunities to take what they feel emotionally deprived of, and testing omnipotence through exciting experiences. Alignment with delinquents gives a defeated adolescent a feeling of self-respect and companionship through a sense of belonging to a subculture.[17]

A classical work on juvenile delinquency, *Wayward Youth*,[3] was written by August Aichhorn in 1935 and revised several times, most recently in 1966. This is a classical Freudian look at juvenile delinquency and attempts to apply psychoanalysis to the treatment of de-

CLINICAL EXAMPLE 31-9

Karen, age 14, ran away from home to a friend's house. Her mother had often expressed a desire to leave; in fact, she had once left the family to the charge of Karen's father when Karen was 9 years old. Karen's mother had suddenly told her she could not see her boyfriend for a month because she had come in late the night before. This caused a tremendous scene because Karen had been out late every night the week before without her mother even noticing. Karen's friend's mother was different. She spent a lot of money on her children, talked to them, and never limited their activity; thus the friend's home appeared attractive to Karen.

CLINICAL EXAMPLE 31-10

John, 13 years of age, was referred by the juvenile court for psychotherapy because he had been picked up for the second time after breaking into a store with another boy. John's parents were separated for the past 2 years after John's father had served a sentence in jail for tax evasion. John, very attached to his father, was extremely upset when his parents separated and rarely saw his father. His antisocial acts caused his father to become more involved with him, since his father claimed he did not want John to go through what he had experienced in prison. John gained his father's attention during these times, even though his father was angry. His delinquent actions therefore enabled John to express his anger at his father's leaving, as well as to fantasize about having his father return.

linquents. Aichhorn continues and extends his classical understanding of delinquency in a more recent work entitled *Delinquency and Child Guidance,*[2] in which he applies these principles and explores how the court and other systems handle these problems.

Recent research by Offer and co-workers[22] supports the idea that when there is a mixed picture of depression and conduct disorder the central problem approximates depression. Their research found little support for the notion of masked depression, and mentions features that best differentiate depression from conduct disorder. Adolescents reporting helplessness where there is the expectation that someone should do something for them, and reporting fewer sad moods and lethargy are probably conduct disorders. They also found distinct patterns of characteristics of both depressed and conduct disordered adolescents. Although they both share problems with morals and superego, a difference between them is that conduct disordered adolescents had more family problems than depressed adolescents. A similarity is that depressed adolescents with eating disorders and conduct disordered adolescents all had problems with impulse control.[22]

Clinical example 31-10 of an adolescent who steals illustrates the many factors that may lead to adolescent delinquency.

John's actions illustrate that adolescents may not differentiate between their stealing and their parent's business dealings. Stealing may also be an effective way to rebel against parents. Adolescents may perpetuate childhood through stealing by indulging in immediate gratification rather than maturely working for things. Sometimes adolescents steal in hopes of getting caught and obtaining help. Parents may consciously or unconsciously condone stealing. Adolescents may act out their anger with the justification that they deserve the stolen items. The reasons for stealing must be established for the individual adolescent, since causation may be diverse.

The conflict of dependence vs. independence can be expressed in poor school adjustment. Some adolescents view teachers as parental surrogates who do not help or who merely apply rules of attendance and homework. Dependent feelings are sometimes elicited by these rules, and adolescents, in proving their independence, may become negative about learning. They may think that schoolwork is secondary to other more important things that they are attempting to master. Daydreaming may interfere with schoolwork as adolescents concentrate on and fantasize about achieving an independent identify.

Adolescent students may drop out of school for practical financial reasons, or they may be rebelling against education laws. The adolescent may be part of a peer group that denounces school attendance and involvement. Parents may overtly or covertly discourage education. This is conveyed through lack of support and approval for education or by their making it difficult for the adolescent to follow through with school expectations, as illustrated by Clinical example 31-11.

■ Violent adolescents

Most adolescents displaying aggression have experienced frustration and observed violent models during their childhood. It seems appropriate to speculate that

CLINICAL EXAMPLE 31-11

Debbie, a 15-year-old adolescent, dropped out of school after several years of poor school performance and truancy. She would occasionally go shopping with her mother on a school day. Her mother never knew the names of her teachers or guidance counselor, and no provisions for a place or time to study were made.

CLINICAL EXAMPLE 31-12

Ricky was a 15-year-old boy referred for treatment for violent outbursts at home. When frustrated, he would break and destroy objects in his path. Ricky was an only child, adopted shortly after birth by a couple in their forties who were unable to have children. Now Ricky's parents, who were about 55 years of age, were increasingly frightened by his aggressive outbursts. They had also felt powerless with his childhood temper tantrums and had consistently responded to outbursts by attempting to limit frustrating situations. They felt guilty and inadequate about his being an adopted child and continually made attempts to reassure Ricky of their love for him. They consequently reinforced his lack of control by assuming these outbursts were results of his fear of being unloved and would offer peace offerings of gifts and rewards. Ricky assumed he was omnipotent, successfully controlling his parents, but was fearful that he could not control his anger. Acknowledging Ricky's fear of loss of control, applying external controls, and pointing out areas of Ricky's ability for responsibility and control resulted in a gradual decrease in outbursts. First the outbursts became more limited as Ricky began breaking specific things that he did not value. Then he progressed to an elimination of violent outbursts.

aggression is a human impulse which must be channeled constructively by a learned process that occurs within a supportive loving relationship. Under favorable conditions a child learns the healthy expression of aggression by involvement in activities that result in pleasure and active problem-solving attempts. Under less ideal conditions the expression of aggression can occur in destructive activities that are harmful to self and others. In adolescence, when aggressive as well as sexual impulses are increased, the energy that strengthens these impulses also strengthens the adaptive and defensive aspects that go along with aggression.[5]

Much anxiety of adolescents is therefore related to the fear that they may be unable to control their destructive aggression. Adolescents often have violent dreams and fantasies that they express in threats, even though in some the potential for violence is minimal. Pointing out the harmlessness of these thoughts is helpful to adolescents, since it is instrumental in showing that these thoughts are not as powerful as they fear. Some adolescents, however, are genuinely fearful that they will be unable to stop their thoughts from becoming actions. They require the recognition of their fear and the reassurance of the existence of external limits. Pointing out to the adolescent the necessity of self-responsibility and control is paramount. Their defenses against aggressive outbursts should be reinforced and supported. Focus should be on the behavior and feared loss of control, not on the roots of the anger.[21] Clinical example 31-12 is an example of management of a violent adolescent.

Most adolescents fear violence; others pose a real risk. Adolescents who have committed extreme acts of violence, or homicide, are often from families in which violence is the norm. These adolescents may have experienced physical abuse, and, if not, they may have witnessed it between their parents. Behavior toward them has often alternated between seductiveness and physical brutality, adding to the adolescent's confusion and arousing intense frustration. Many times these ad-

olescents are encouraged to be violent, since their outbursts are not firmly limited. Sometimes parents can predict the adolescent's ability to injure or kill. Frequently there is a history of dangerous assaults on family members and pets. In severely violent adolescents, violent acts can be followed by a calmness and lack of sorrow or guilt, since they claim that outside forces provoked them. Many homicidal adolescents will freely discuss their violent plans or fears. These should be explored and homicidal intent evaluated. Does the adolescent have a victim, weapons, or plan? This information, along with the history, shows the level of success or failure in controlling feelings and delaying gratification. Poor rapport with the therapist and evasiveness may indicate disturbing paranoid tendencies, revealing a greater potential for violence.

■ Adolescents and drugs

Adolescents may turn to drugs for relief of tension when pressures are intense. Meeks[21] and other theorists have spoken of the following types of drug users:

1. **Casual users—"the experimenters."** These ad-

olescents use mostly marijuana in small quantities to substantiate their position in the peer group and to decrease the anxieties experienced because of their movement away from the family. Alcohol has often been used this way in the past, and there currently seems to be a return to alcohol for this purpose.

2. **Sociological users—"the seekers."** These adolescents are very aware of social realities, and they want to be active participants in the social process. They believe society's shortcomings to be their own inadequacies. They tend therefore to form separate communities in which they idealistically attempt to create a society of their own free of social conventions. Many seek relief from boredom through drugs and membership in this society. They lack the ability to express their inner feelings and tend to deal with their loneliness through mystical revelation and the group connection, with the hope of a conflict-free life with others.

3. **Sick-users—"the heads."** Adolescents using drugs for cultural or neurotic reasons must be differentiated from those who use drugs to mask or correct maturational difficulties. This distinction is difficult to make. Those with serious interpersonal difficulties often are in a group that is bonded together by a high frequency of drug usage. They turn to drugs in times of stress and prefer drug-induced pleasures to those arising from interpersonal relationships and competitive efforts. This group also includes those who are socially critical and use the drug group as a personal justification rather than with any real social concern.

There are social implications connected with drug usage that must be considered. Our "pill relief" society gives a backdrop for pharmacological abuse. Drug abuse can reflect a general discontent with society's shortcomings in values and organization. The awakened interest in magic and mysticism also adds the potential of drug-induced exploration of life.

The meaning of drug usage in adolescence is a difficult and complex question. The adolescent's individual motivation must be explored, the nurse keeping in mind that it may be an expression of rebelliousness with support of a peer group, as well as a way of obtaining gratification of instinctual needs at a regressed level. It may also indicate an effort to come to grips with feelings of vulnerability and inner emptiness.

Adolescents often report a wish for closeness that is satisfied by sharing a drug experience with friends.

CLINICAL EXAMPLE 31-13

Tommy was a 16-year-old adolescent boy who had been school phobic since age 10. He had been on home instruction since that age and was referred for a yearly assessment to get approval for a continuation of home instruction services. Tommy proudly spoke of his drug episodes. He and his small group of friends were close and had a repertoire of exciting experiences induced by various hallucinogens and amphetamines. Tommy had little support in the real world, since he had been isolated at home and experienced interpersonal relationships primarily in terms of obtaining and experiencing the effects of drugs.

Drug users can experience an illusion of closeness because drugs decrease anxiety and users can share anticipation of use of the drug. Some adolescents fill the void of isolated loneliness with drugs and would otherwise feel suicidally depressed. Drugs can be crippling and delay healthy maturity by promoting the avoidance of the development of an adult identity in a real world, as illustrated in Clinical example 31-13.

It is rare that adolescent drug usage precipitates difficulties when the adolescent was previously well adjusted. This is especially true with soft drugs such as marijuana. Adolescents have been known to become psychotic, panicked, and assaultive after drug ingestion, especially of harder drugs. PCP, or "angel dust," has been noted to produce violence and incoherence. Sometimes "angel dust" is mixed with marijuana and other drugs without the adolescent knowing it. Bad trips have been reported with hallucinogens, as well as belladonna and opiate drugs. Often friends help to deal with upsetting reactions, but occasionally medical care is sought. Amphetamines have been known to produce psychosis. Belladonna can produce acute maniclike psychotic states accompanied by hallucinations.

One of the more commonly abused drugs at present is cocaine. This drug is snorted, free-based, injected, or smoked, producing euphoria, grandiosity, and increased feelings of confidence and esteem. In addition to emotional euphoria, it produces a sense of physical well-being that exceeds the normal body capacity.

Another trend among teenagers across the country is to sniff typewriter correction fluid which produces effects similar to alcohol. Teenagers become lightheaded, euphoric, and confused. The danger is that it can also cause irregular heartbeats. Six teenagers died suddenly in New Mexico after sniffing typewriter correction fluid.

Alcoholism among teenagers is currently on the rise and seems to be similar to drug abuse dynamically. Addeo and Addeo[1] have suggested some possible origins for alcoholism in adolescents, including parental and social influence, peer pressure, and emotional disturbances. Many researchers believe teenagers are currently switching from drugs to alcohol and alcoholism is the greater social problem.[10]

■ Hypochondriasis

Adolescents are preoccupied with their bodies and body sensations. There are many reasons for this concern and preoccupation. Adolescents are uncomfortable with their bodies because of the rapid changes in size, contour, and functioning. In an attempt to establish their identity, adolescents try to become familiar with their changing bodies. They respond to sensations with increased intensity. When an adolescent appears overly concerned, it may indicate underlying difficulties in the formation of a self-image.

Hypochondriasis occurs when the adolescent has intense anxiety about his health. This anxiety may be diffuse or directed toward one specific area. Focus on the body may conceal vague fears of catastrophe. Adolescents' concerns that their bodies are inadequate, that they will be rejected by others, or that they are unable to reach adulthood may predominate. Hypochondriasis may be a way of avoiding activities that expose these and other stressful fears. Fears such as inadequacy at school, either socially or in schoolwork, may be a projection of general fears of inadequacy. Lack of knowledge of the normality of body changes may be a simple precipitating factor. This can be tackled by reassurance that these changes are normal. If reassurance does not alleviate anxiety, then it is possible that other more intense fears are involved.

Reassurance and support can frighten the adolescent who uses body concern to mask an intense conflict. This is important to consider—the adolescent may then have no means to discharge the pressures of the basic anxiety, since the defense is removed. Support may imply to adolescents that the nurse or parents do not care for them. It is important to communicate to adolescents that people are aware something is wrong and that their concerns will be taken seriously until the core difficulty is alleviated. Intense body concern is a signal that something is not right and help is needed. Physical status must be assessed first before a psychological basis for concern is assumed. Sometimes body preoccupation is an effort to recreate infantile dependency by eliciting care giving. This is particularly seen in adolescents who

---

CLINICAL EXAMPLE 31-14

John, age 12, was referred for treatment from the local hospital after having been seen for chest pains. The physician found no medical problems. John was embarrassed and angry about the episode, insisting that the physician was wrong. The chest pains had disappeared, but he now had injured his arm. He also was often plagued by genuinely uncomfortable attacks of tonsillitis and middle ear infections. John had experienced early emotional deprivation because he was often moved around in his living arrangements. He was born out of wedlock and lived occasionally with his mother, often with his maternal grandmother, and infrequently with his father. He generally had the feeling that no one really cared for him. Further exploration revealed that John's body concerns were to precipitate care giving by those around him, who he feared really were not there for him. He performed well in school and had friends, but none of these compensated for his feelings of inadequacy.

---

experienced early emotional deprivation.[17] John in Clinical example 31-14 is an interesting example of this.

■ Weight problems

Another disturbance often seen in adolescence is anorexia nervosa, or loss of appetite and refusal to eat, leading to emaciation. This life-threatening behavior often appears to be similar in psychodynamics to bulimia, obesity, or overeating. Many authors suggest that the underlying conflict in these disorders is sexual. A denial of a wish to be sexual is expressed by the unattractiveness of being extremely thin or the camouflage of feminine or masculine characteristics with childlike heaviness. Often heaviness is equated with pregnancy, which represents sexuality.

Another speculation is that anorexia nervosa is a reaction formation to the desire to be gluttonous, whereas excessive eating is the symbolical taking in of love. Extreme restraint of gluttonous wishes or giving in to these wishes represents a desire to return to infantile dependency, often precipitated by emotional deprivation. The possibility of a physical origin must always be considered and ruled out before the syndrome is attributed to psychological determinants. Obesity or loss of weight may be the result of abnormal glandular functioning. Clinical example 31-15 illustrates the development of anorexia nervosa in a young girl.

CLINICAL EXAMPLE 31-15

Janet, age 15, was admitted to the hospital because it was feared that her extreme loss of weight was endangering her life. Exploration revealed that Janet was petrified of her sexual feelings and the response of others to her budding sexuality. Her father, provocative and teasing toward Janet, was continually kidding her about her oncoming sexual attractiveness and implied that he really preferred her to her mother. This created panic and Janet refused to eat. She liked her thinness, which was protection from sexual desires. In the hospital, the area of concentration was not the behavior of not eating, but rather the underlying panic feelings about her sexuality and her relationship with her father. This provided freedom for normal sexual growth and development.

CLINICAL EXAMPLE 31-16

Donna, a 13-year-old girl, had always been shy with others. She was referred for therapy after the third week of classes in her new junior high school because she was not attending school on account of illness. Her mother claimed that despite her efforts to get Donna to school, she would return home with an upset stomach or headache. Her mother had taken her to school the 2 days she had attended, only to have her return home 3 hours later. A medical work-up provided no medical basis for her stomach and head pains. As the evaluation proceeded, it became clear that Donna had an extraordinarily close relationship with her mother. In the past her mother had worked as a teacher's helper at the elementary school Donna attended. Treatment dealing with the mother-daughter dyad was instituted.

■ School phobia

School phobia is an example of neurotic anxiety often seen in adolescence. Some school dropouts may be suffering from undiagnosed school phobia. This differs from other disturbed behaviors in that school represents the focus of their fears. The parents (most often the mother), although verbalizing the wish for the adolescent's maturity, often unconsciously want the adolescent to remain at home, limited in opportunities to move toward adult development.[17] Other possible causes may be fears experienced by the adolescent concerning maturing and leaving childhood protection, the meaning of new knowledge, exposure to feelings and wishes stimulated by close relationships with peers and adults, and failure to meet the adolescent's idealized self-image.[7]

Adolescents may use destructive means of obtaining attention, demonstrate their poor conception of themselves, or hide from dealing socially with the opposite sex by remaining at home. Clinical example 31-16 is an example of school phobia.

❦ Planning and implementation

When dealing with the adolescent, it is advisable whenever possible for the nurse to have an initial contact directly with the adolescent. Many adolescents are concerned that the nurse therapist is aligned with the parents. Other adolescents take a passive role, letting the adults straighten things out for them. By initiating contact with the adolescent, an alignment is made with the independent mature aspects of the adolescent. Parents asking for advice on how to present coming to a therapist to the adolescent should be advised to be honest, stating the true nature of the visit and their reasons for requesting it. Many agencies and institutions use a child guidance approach, seeing the parents first to get a full developmental history. Family sessions have also been used in the diagnostic evaluation, helping to reveal family interaction and later being helpful in establishing family support.

■ The nursing care plan

A solid knowledge of normative adolescent functioning is necessary to differentiate between age-expected behavior and maladaptive responses. The majority of adolescents are well adjusted, have good relationships with family and friends, and generally accept societal values. Studies by Offer and co-workers,[22] however, suggest that professionals view normal adolescents from an analytic perspective as more disturbed than they really are. Despite new data refuting this view, professionals still persist in describing normal adolescents as having a disturbed self-image based on the "analytic turmoil" theory.

Identifying maladaptive responses and defining the problem in behavioral terms is the first step in planning intervention. The nurse can then explore the underlying conflicts. All adolescents may have conflicts in some areas but many are able to respond to them in an adaptive manner. It is problematic when conflicts are expressed in a maladaptive or destructive way. Establishment of short-term goals based on the maladaptive responses is done after the adolescent's strengths are recognized. Long-term goals and rationale are also listed. Recommend treatment with rationale or recommended referral completes the plan.

Review of nursing care plans is necessary periodically to update situations, note progress, and consider new problem areas. Short- and long-term goals are reassessed at this time and, based on new developments, are revised if indicated. Most important, nursing process is assessed and re-evaluated.

■ Patient education

The psychiatric nurse is in an important position to educate the adolescent, his or her parents, and the community as a whole. Basic health information can be transmitted in such areas as drugs, sex and contraception, suicide prevention, and crime prevention to name a few. The nurse is also in an excellent position to educate parents, teenagers, and the community on healthy emotional functioning. In addition, by educating parents and the community on normal adolescent behavior and interpreting the underlying conflicts, parents, teachers, and other members of the community are better prepared to react supportively to adolescents and can encourage healthy independent functioning. Very often parents and community members become frustrated, angry, and confused by the independent strivings of adolescents. Encouraging independence and lessening power struggles can produce a marked difference in adolescents' relationships with adults as well as feelings about themselves. That is not to say that adults should not set limits. Limit setting and providing structure can be done in a way as to encourage the adolescent's independent functioning. Many parents are conflicted about their children becoming adults. That mixed with the adolescent's own ambivalence and fears about independence can create havoc.

One of the best ways to educate parents on adolescent development is through a parents' group. In this way, the nurse can enlighten parents on normal adolescent functioning, as well as provide them with much needed support from other parents in the same situation. The sharing of mutual experiences and searching for solutions in a supportive environment can be extremely helpful to parents. It is important to remember that parents have nurtured children to reach this juncture of adolescence, moving toward adulthood. Many feel that "showing them how" is their primary parental responsibility. It is a difficult change for them to suddenly switch from the "how to" of the child to the "try to" of the budding adult. The process of increased responsibilities based on a gradual progression of inde-

---

CLINICAL EXAMPLE 31-17

Mr. and Mrs. B came to the attention of the psychiatric nurse by their distressed calls to the community mental health center. Mrs. B tearfully explained that they had lost all control of their 14-year-old daughter. She had become arrogant and hostile, locking herself in her bedroom after an argument they had about her going to the movies with a 14-year-old boy she had met at school. Further exploration revealed that Emily was an honor student at school, maintaining a solid A average. She had many friends at school, was on the volleyball team, and babysat regularly on weekends for the neighbors' two children. She had always been pleasant, happy, and friendly. Suddenly this boy that the parents did not know called her at home. After many phone conversations he asked Emily to join him on a weekend evening at the movies. Mr. and Mrs. B felt Emily was much too young to date, that she could get involved with drugs, sexual promiscuity, and the like. They were sad and worried that they had lost their little girl who always did what she was told. Emily was hurt and furious. She thought her parents were being totally unreasonable. She felt her parents did not trust her. Further exploration revealed that Mrs. B had gotten into trouble sexually as a young girl. She didn't want Emily to make the same mistake. Her parents had been very lenient. She blamed their lack of guidelines for her error. Mrs. B became aware of her overreaction. She was able to understand that dating was a normal part of adolescent development after discussion with the psychiatric nurse. A compromise was arranged after she recognized Emily's competent and responsible functioning. After Mr. and Mrs. B met the boy at Emily's house, Emily was able to go to the movies with him and two other friends on a Saturday afternoon.

---

pendent functioning is a strategy that parents can learn. In spite of their fears of their teenagers "getting into trouble," or "goofing up," they can be educated to promote self-reliance in their adolescents. Clinical examples 31-17 and 31-18 show the need to educate parents and community members.

■ Family therapy

Family therapy is particularly useful to an adolescent when chronic disturbed family interaction is seriously interfering with the adolescent's development. Sometimes a series of family sessions may be enough, and the adolescent may benefit from either individual or group

Barbara, an adolescent girl starting high school, had always functioned adequately. Beginning high school was a totally different experience. She became overwhelmed by the large building, increased academic responsibilities, and complex peer relationships. She began school in September with much anxiety. By October she began having numerous illnesses that prevented her from attending school. It came to the attention of the school guidance counselor, who noticed her increased absences. The guidance counselor saw her and after no medical etiology was found, offered to have Barbara come to her office whenever she felt sick at school. When this didn't help, she suggested Barbara receive some home-bound instruction until she felt less anxious. This suggestion validated Barbara's fears that she could not handle high school and its increased pressures. Her solution of retreat was supported. Fortunately, her parents sought the help of a psychiatric nurse, who encouraged immediate return to school with entry into a peer support group with individual sessions initially as needed. This enabled her to talk out her fears and get support from her peers. This also strengthened her confidence and fostered healthy functioning. She found she could handle high school after all. The nurse educated the guidance counselor on ways to be supportive while encouraging independent functioning.

approaches to offer greater support to his effort to separate emotionally from his family. Occasionally, after a few family sessions, it may become clear that the adolescent may not need the intervention directly. Engaging the parents may free the adolescent to progress on the developmental continuum.

The techniques used in family therapy are reviewed in detail in Chapter 29. Whatever modality is selected in working with the adolescent, a family orientation and the adolescent's attempt to separate from his family and become an independent adult should be considered.

■ Group therapy

Group therapy uses adolescents' propensity to gain support from their peers. The conflict of dependence-independence with adults becomes somewhat diluted by the presence of other adolescents. Conflicts, especially about authority, can be detected by peers rather than adults, making the modality particularly desirable for adolescents. Many nurses use group therapy as a catalyst and combine it with individual therapy. It is a valued modality in reaching skills in relating and dealing with others. It helps fulfill the adolescent's need for a positive, meaningful peer group for ego identity formation.

Adolescent groups, in contrast to other groups, are difficult in that many adolescents turn to peers in a defensive and tenuous connection. Sibling rivalry often disrupts group cohesion. Many groups suffer from poor attendance, a high dropout rate, antisocial behavior, and a lack of group cohesion. However, group therapy with adolescents has proved to be successful in many community mental health centers, outpatient clinics, and hospital settings.

Berkovitz[6] believes that coed groups decrease homosexual anxiety and anxious disruptiveness. Often, beginning groups with some activity helps to provide a stabilizing factor for young adolescents. The number of members to include in the group depends on the type. For example, it may not be feasible to limit an outpatient "drop-in" group. Because of the age spread among adolescents, it is usually preferable to form at least two groups. A possibility is an early adolescence group consisting of 13 to 15 year olds who have conflicts of separation from parents as well as homosexual and incestuous anxieties. An older adolescent group, age 15 to 17, would probably consider issues such as the further establishment of identity, the beginning of dating or exploration of relations with the opposite sex, experimentation with drugs, handling money, responsibilities of driving, and vocational plans. Mixing the two age-groups with varying concerns may not be productive.

The most ideal situation is to have male and female co-therapists; however, this is not always feasible. If there is a single therapist for an unmixed group of the opposite sex, anxiety of group members may be shown by disruption or flight. Conflict between therapists, if there is an open and honest discussion, can provide a corrective experience because adolescents can see adults disagree without devastating consequences. If therapists are of the opposite sex, a parental similarity is often apparent and members often play on the therapist's feelings and try out tactics as they would with their own parents. Even if both therapists are of the same sex, one is usually more active, and a member may project a good or bad image onto each therapist that corresponds with his view of his parents.

Group process with adolescents is often similar to that with adults, and specific aspects of group therapy are reviewed in Chapter 28. Resistances such as silence, passivity, disruptiveness, and intellectualization are often seen with adolescents, since they tend to act out rather than verbalize anxiety. Differences among various types of groups, for examples, residential groups vs. outpatient groups, must be considered.

■ Individual therapy

Individual therapy done by the psychiatric nurse specialist can consist of brief goal-directed therapy, behavioral therapy, or insight therapy. A description of insight therapy is presented here, since the principles are helpful in other types of individual therapy as well. Once the decision to engage in individual therapy is made, a pact or contract between the therapist and adolescent is established, depending on the approach and type used.

■ **THERAPEUTIC ALLIANCE.** This contract in insight therapy is described by Meeks[21] as a "therapeutic alliance" in which the nurse aligns herself with the healthy, reality-oriented aspect of the adolescent's ego and moves toward an honest and critical understanding of the adolescent's inner experience. This alliance is created through the orderly interpretation of the adolescent's feeling states and defensive behavior, especially toward the nurse.

The alliance in dealing with adults differs from that with the adolescent in that with adults there is a promotion of a regulated and controlled regression. This is not useful for the adolescent. Adolescents' alliances are focused toward links between their feelings and behavior in the present. Brief regressions occur anyway, and focuses usually are aimed at efforts to recover from regressions and at reinforcing and supporting progressive development. The alliance is a central aspect of individual therapy, and, once it is established, a feeling of working together is apparent. Meeks[21] mentions helpful specific hints to establish and maintain this alliance:

1. Point out that behavior is motivated by feelings. Often, early in treatment, adolescents may express feelings of impatience, helplessness, and failure at having to see a therapist. Defenses are often seen in rebelliousness, passivity, shyness, negativism, and intellectualization. Adolescents generally have a propensity to act out and avoid feelings.
2. Limit acting out by pointing out how it interferes with the therapeutic process and that it must be controlled to proceed. Maintain a neutral but interested attitude toward all behavior.
3. Point out the adolescent's tendencies to be judgmental and self-critical. This is supportive and helps to encourage the adolescent to look for sources of behaviors, attitudes, and feeling states.
4. Establish that the adolescent's behavior is the end result of many inner feelings. Some of these unknown feelings sabotage freedom. This knowledge strengthens motivation for therapy and maintains an alignment with the adolescent's wishes for autonomy. Encourage therapeutic efforts as a means to alter rebellion into true self-direction and freedom.
5. Point out the adolescent's propensity to see things in extremes; the desire to be complete master opposes the feelings of total helplessness. Reveal areas of strength and competence that are often unrecognized. Avoid focusing exclusively on problems and weaknesses. This shows neutrality and is supportive. Giving the adolescent as much information as possible to be prepared to make his own decision helps the adolescent work toward self-direction.
6. Distinguish between thought and action, discouraging impulsiveness. Encourage open expression of strong feeling but not strong action. For example, anger does not mean killing; sexual feeling does not mean intercourse. Adolescents sometimes confuse discussion with permission to experiment with action, especially with sexual issues.
7. Encourage real emotion in sessions by expressing interest in and acceptance of feeling states appearing in relation to the nurse and feelings expressed in description of events outside the session. Point out the importance of feelings.
8. Watch out for the defenses of denial and reaction formation. Maintain neutrality and encourage objectivity without directly assaulting essential defenses. Adolescents will resort to pathological defenses when threatened by emergencies.
9. Adolescents often act provocatively to get important adults to delegate punishment. This puts the nurse in alignment with the self-hatred aspect of the adolescent's conscience and should be avoided. The nurse is supportive by continuing therapy even during these difficult periods.

The work of the nurse therapist is to recognize the adolescent's anxiety and try to assist him in finding ways to deal with emerging impulses. Defenses suggested by the nurse are rarely useful, but pointing out, supporting, and accepting any healthy defense of the adolescent strengthens his sense of ego mastery. Adolescents often have wishes that they regard as crazy and frightening. Open discussion of fears of homosexuality, incest, or homicide helps adolescents realize these feelings do not lead to psychosis and are uncomfortable but harmless thoughts.

■ **TRANSFERENCE.** Transference, as with the adult patient, is an important aspect of adolescent treatment. Pointing out that these irrational projections originate in the adolescent's mind and not in reality and that they usually represent a meaningful person such as a parent is necessary. It is often good to point out the commonality of this response. Transference is interpreted to diminish its impact on the therapeutic situation. Several common transference patterns have been identified[21]:

1. **Erotic-sexual**—especially if the nurse is young and of the opposite sex. Usually, this transference is shown by awkward blushing and agitated confusion by the adolescent. It is usually best to emphasize value in the mutual work of emotional growth while establishing, tactfully, the nurse's unavailability as a sexual object. Focusing on origins or encouraging elaboration of these feelings is not helpful and is anxiety provoking.
2. **Omnipotent**—expecting the nurse will have the answers to all questions. It is easy for the nurse to drift into this pattern, since often the adolescent appears to be a helpless cripple. The adolescent's secret desire for personal omnipotence is somewhat fulfilled by granting it to the nurse. The nurse then serves as a front, hiding the adolescent's fear of confronting reality without magical powers.
3. **Negative transference**—usually intense and pervasive. Negative feelings toward the nurse usually represent a negative attitude toward all adult authority figures. This transference is often defensive to cover feelings of shame, inadequacy, and anxiety, and it disappears as the adolescent respects the nurse's feelings. The adolescent tries to force the therapist to reject him. Open discussion to explore these feelings objectively and establish their origin is beneficial. Sometimes interpretations arouse anger toward the nurse because of the anxiety they create. These are reactions to the realities of therapy and are not to be confused with negative transference.

A true negative transference occurs when situations reactivate early experiences in which negative feelings toward important others predominate. The nurse is seen as a frustrator whenever she, representing reality, opposes gratification of impulses and ego drives. Negative transference tends to appear whenever the nurse refuses to gratify needs that the adolescent feels are important and legitimate. The nurse unavoidably will frustrate the adolescent, who often has trouble delaying gratification to reach long-range goals. The nurse should point out the true motive behind activities that express anger. Clarifying hidden hostile feelings frees them for expression towards the nurse, and irrational expectations may then be revealed. Negative transference is dealt with as any other resistant behavior through objective exploration, which includes seeking causes of anger and pointing out irrationality. This is often followed by an expected period of regression and depression. Empathic understanding that the adolescent is mourning a loss is helpful, but it should be emphasized that what was lost was an illusion.

Another negative transference occurs when the adolescent sees the nurse as his superego. Projecting his superego onto the nurse may cause all interventions to be seen as superego sanctions. Adolescents have trouble understanding the rationale for foregoing gratification of an impulse. It is important to point out that these are the adolescent's own taboos and to encourage open confrontation with these taboos rather than avoidance. A common occurance is for an adolescent to rebel against his conscience and then respond to guilt through self-destructive behaviors. Pointing out this pattern helps the adolescent to eventually become aware of this.

■ **TERMINATION.** Termination of therapy is an integral part of the therapeutic process. Often, leaving therapy symbolizes the process of loosening bonds to parental images, relinquishing accompanying desires to be passive and expectations of the omnipotence of these figures. One therefore expects defensive and regressive behaviors as the adolescent attempts to deal with the anxieties related to the termination process. This can mean the recurrence of emotional crises, symptoms, self-destructive fantasies, and even dependency behavior to provoke rescue.

Termination should be flexible and correctly timed. The decision should be made in line with adolescent norms, not adult ones. Often adolescents will verbalize appropriate interest in termination. When this occurs, it is often helpful to open it to discussion without commitment to a set time. This implies that further work needs to be done in a definite time span, and it maintains a focus on the adolescent's responsibility to finish. Gradually supporting and approving of the adolescent's independence and mature functioning prepares for a positive termination. Some adolescents leave therapy to return later. Some can never leave forever, seeing termination as a rejection rather than a vote of confidence. Gradual reduction of sessions without pressing for final termination may help as long as the overall situation is reviewed occasionally.[14]

Sometimes terminations occur prematurely because of either the lack of success in establishing an alliance or some external events. Occasionally terminations are forced because of a nurse's change of location, death, or illness. The adolescent will express anger at the new therapist until the feelings about the lost therapist are accepted and resolved. In working out this attachment, a new therapeutic alliance can be established.

■ Talking with adolescents

Adolescents are different from adults and children, and often interactions pose difficulties not as apparent with other age-groups. Following is a discussion of some important considerations in communicating with adolescents.

■ **SILENCE.** Silence is often effective with adults but frightening to the adolescent, especially in the beginning stages of treatment or evaluation. This anxiety often is reflecting the adolescent's feelings of emptiness and lack of identity. Brief silences can be creative and productive when the adolescent is engaged in treatment, and, when the adolescent is able to tolerate them without anxiety, it indicates growth in self-confidence and acceptance of inner feelings. More often, however, silence is used defensively by adolescents to avoid discovery of hostile feelings or fantasies that might appear. Older adolescents may tolerate interpretive remarks, but with younger adolescents it is usually helpful to suggest an activity to help facilitate discussion and establish a relationship. For some adolescents silence is a characterological defense of inhibition and withdrawal, since they have never learned to communicate in a positive way. In these cases the therapist must carry the burden of responsibility for dialogue.

■ **CONFIDENTIALITY.** Confidentiality is a concern to many, but especially to the adolescent who is fearful of the nurse reporting to his parents. A blanket promise to tell nothing to the parents is not advised, since the nurse may need to contact the parents if the adolescent reveals suicidal or homicidal behavior or the use of illegal drugs. It is usually best to tell the adolescent that the nurse will not divulge any information without informing the adolescent of the intention to do so in advance. It is also helpful to explain that feelings are confidential but that actions considered dangerous to the adolescent or others may need to be shared.

■ **NEGATIVISM.** Negative feelings are often expressed by adolescents, especially initially, because they are frightened of the implications of coming for treatment. The young adolescent's lack of objectivity and upsurge of instinctual impulses, as well as the tendency to confuse fantasy and action, make the discussion of feelings threatening. Usually, gently noting in a supportive way defensive techniques the adolescent uses during the session helps to gain cooperation.

■ **RESISTANCE.** Often adolescents begin by testing the nurse to see if she will be another authoritarian figure. The rebellious adolescent may claim he does not need therapy or help. If the adolescent appears anxious, it is best to be supportive and sympathetic, expressing interest in getting to know the adolescent and then discussing a neutral area. A more angry, rebellious adolescent may require a direct approach, with the nurse saying openly that she feels the adolescent is opposing the visit because he believes no help is needed. This can lead to a further discussion of feelings about the visit, for example, parental coercion to come to the session. A productive discussion of feelings about authority may then ensue. Some adolescents are just baiting and testing to see if the nurse is an anxious and defensive adult. If so, it is best to ignore their comments about not wanting treatment and move on. Often adolescents with an angry facade depend on their omnipotent control of the environment and are often successful in manipulating their families. They are angry at attempts to disturb this power, and the anger is expressed in their lack of cooperation in the session.[19]

■ **ARGUING.** Adolescents always argue and, although they do not admit it, learn from arguments. Often the adolescent goes against the viewpoint of the nurse and then in the next session states her opinion as his own. It is best not to comment on this and accept it as a harmless defense. If the nurse admits having areas of ignorance, it is productive to the adolescent, who may fear that he must be perfect.

■ **TESTING.** Adolescents often need and want limits. They are confused and cannot set their own limits. They experiment by trial and error to find a self-concept. Often an adolescent will test the nurse to see how firm and consistent she will be. Controls frequently are effective if there is a basic positive relationship with the nurse. Limits should be set only when they are essential for current and future well-being, and the adolescent will value the security they provide. The nurse represents a substitute parental figure allowing independence. Adolescents will dare to be independent if it is conveyed that the nurse will serve as a control against carrying independence too far.

■ **DREAMS AND ARTISTIC CREATIONS.** Adolescents are often creative, and a lot can be learned from studying their productions. As long as the discussion is relevant to achieving ego synthesis, it can be a productive source for exploring inner feelings that, along with dreams, can reveal valuable information about their real concerns, even when attempts are made by the adolescent to avoid them. The nurse must be careful not to engage in intellectual discussion irrelevant to the adolescent's inner life.

■ **BRINGING FRIENDS.** The adolescent who brings a friend to a session may be attempting to avoid the seriousness of therapy. There is some benefit in sharing the experiences with the peer group, since this lowers anxiety. Telling the adolescent that bringing friends is not allowed may not be successful because the nurse cannot always enforce such a rule. The reason for bringing friends may vary, but the action should be seen as communication to be explored and understood. Sometimes adolescents want to refer friends. This may be positive but may also focus attention away from the original adolescent. The nurse should insist on exploring motives behind the referral before accepting the new patient, since the adolescent may feel that the nurse's acceptance of another is a betrayal of loyalty. If the friend clearly wants and needs therapy, referral to a competent colleague is usually best. If a friend is brought late in therapy, it may mean the adolescent is getting ready to terminate.

■ **EMBARRASSMENT ABOUT BEING IN THERAPY.** Embarrassment may occur in any age group, but it is prominent in adolescents, especially during the early stages of treatment. It also can become an issue as therapy progresses because it often reveals the adolescent's embarrassment about his wishes for dependency. Therefore adolescents may become uncomfortable in the therapeutic relationship. This is usually dealt with effectively by indicating the normalcy of these types of feelings. Behind the fear of accepting help is the wish for care, and this can be dealt with by pointing out the adolescent's strengths and areas of independence. The nurse can then reveal that any wish or thought of care or dependency is thought by the adolescent to represent total dependency. This helps the adolescent to be more tolerant of his wishes, seeing them realistically as wishes that all people have.

Some adolescents, by expressing embarrassment about being in therapy, are actually revealing a fear or social stigma that they have heard from their parents. The adolescent who has feelings of inferiority often focuses these on the therapeutic process, blaming therapy for discomfort. It is best to encourage and be supportive to the adolescent, gently refusing to accept blame for this discomfort. The issue of whether to tell friends should be explored dynamically.

■ **REQUESTS FOR SPECIAL ATTENTION.** Some adolescents can develop intense dependency ties to the therapist. They reflect this in requests for additional appointments, extra time in appointments, frequent telephone calls, or social contact outside the therapeutic sessions. Late in therapy there is little advantage to meeting these primitive needs. The regressed adolescent needs an undemanding nurse who allows him to experience inner feelings of emptiness. The therapist cannot fill this emptiness and should avoid false promises.

Focus should be on the exploration of feelings of inner emptiness, deprivation, and incompleteness.

■ **Parents of the adolescent**

If group or individual treatment is selected for the adolescent, the nurse must still consider the family. Many parents overtly claim desire for their adolescent's maturity and independence but unconsciously need to maintain him as a child and covertly undermine growth. Parents may sabotage the adolescent's treatment if they are not helped to understand and accept it. It is possible to work with the parents without revealing confidential material.

Adolescents frequently try to avoid limits by playing parents against the nurse. If parents are angry with the restriction of their involvement in their child's therapy, there is a greater potential for this. The nurse can encourage healthier aspects of the parent-adolescent relationship and sympathetically accept parental anxieties and needs.

Not all parents of adolescents need treatment. Many adolescents do well despite parental difficulties. It is helpful for parents to have treatment if the adolescent is asked to assume an inappropriate destructive role at home, since this interferes with the therapeutic role. If the parents are resistant, the nurse must usually begin with the adolescent until the parents are more receptive.

Telephone contact is a helpful way to ensure cooperation and support by having the parent call when necessary. Parents should tell the adolescent when they call. Parents should be told of normal adolescent behavior they should expect. The nurse should avoid advising the parents about specific actions and focus on attitudes and feelings, especially concerning discipline. Parents can be helped with understanding the purpose of limit setting. Some parents exclude themselves entirely from their adolescent's life. They have brought the adolescent to treatment to assuage their guilt by doing all that is possible. They may often want the nurse to take over parenting functions. This should not be permitted, especially during crises. If the adolescent is suicidal or homicidal, the parents are informed and must take the responsibility for action with the nurse's help.

Adolescents often need help in dealing with their parents. At times, late in therapy, it is helpful to verify parental pathological behavior. If done too early in treatment, it can cause the adolescent to see himself as the victim. Later, well into the therapeutic alliance, it permits the adolescent to see his parents realistically, to forgive them, and to work on his own strengths and limitations. Parents should be discussed in an open exploratory manner, with emphasis on the fact that they have their own feelings on which their actions are based.

Adolescents can be helped to realize that if their parents are being controlling, adolescents must be free to reject or accept parents' goals according to their own needs and abilities, rather than merely rebelling. Even if the parents treat the adolescent as a child, that does not make him a child. The danger is the adolescent's own childlike wishes.

Sometimes adolescents want to leave home because they hope they will feel more adult away from their parents. It is usually best to support the wish to leave, emphasizing that it must be done in an adult way. If leaving is an impulsive thought with no feasible plan, it will ensure failure, parental rescue, and continued dependency. This is often recapitulated in termination from therapy if the adolescent quits early to avoid the pain of separation that a planned termination would bring.

Evaluation

Problems presented by adolescents, more frequently than those of any other group, activate the nurse's own unresolved conflicts. This countertransference reaction decreases the nurse's usefulness because of anxiety and confusion. Alignment with either the parents against the adolescent or the adolescent against the parents should be watched for. Most adults are resistant to reexperiencing the feelings of adolescence and have repressed these experiences. As a result of anxiety, the nurse occasionally may have trouble listening or may encourage the adolescent (for his or her own unrecognized wishes) to do what the nurse never dared do. The adolescent may be acting as the nurse did during his or her own adolescence. The nurse, in an effort to deny this, may see this adolescent behavior as nondeviant. Identification of the nurse with the adolescent can contribute to delays in exploring areas important for psychological growth. The nurse may relate well to the adolescent but because of unresolved, unrecognized conflicts or resentment toward his or her own parents, may be locked into his or her own adolescent rebellion. The nurse may overtly or covertly encourage the adolescent to express rage toward his family. Both the adolescent and the nurse then avoid facing the reality of adult burdens. It is easier for the nurse to do this if the adolescent's parents are indeed hostile, rejecting, and irresponsible.

Adults often have motives for emphasizing the inadequacies of adolescents, which can lead to an underestimation of the adolescent's abilities. These motives are often seen in protective or competitive attitudes of varying degrees that make it difficult for the nurse to let the adolescent do things on his own. In terminating with an adolescent, as with any valued human relationship, the nurse often has feelings of being abandoned and unappreciated. Many adolescents therefore often seem guilty and apologetic about their wishes to terminate and deal with things on their own. Just as many nurses hold on to adolescents too long, many times, unconscious hostile feelings on the part of the nurse can cause him or her to claim exaggerated progress. This allows the nurse to disguise unconscious angry rejection and avoid waiting for appropriate termination. Often the nurse's need to achieve quick success causes a superficial handling of necessary therapeutic work. Pressures from the family with financial troubles can hurry an insecure nurse. Fears of erotic feelings stirred up by closeness with the adolescent can lead to a panicked withdrawal and termination motivated by self-preservation.

Nurses owe it to themselves and the adolescents they treat to be honest and rely on intellectual and emotional strengths, using the same exploratory attitude with themselves that is required and encouraged with the adolescents they treat. Errors are unavoidable. Doing therapy should provide a growth experience for the nurse as well as the adolescent. Critical self-evaluation and reassessment of the effectiveness of nursing actions, as well as assessment of the client's progress, are paramount in the treatment of any human being of any age group. Supervision provides an opportunity to objectively explore and evaluate the therapeutic process with an experienced colleague and is a necessary tool to encourage and facilitate this process. Supervision is a necessity for all therapists, no matter how much experience they have, because of the highly emotional nature of the work in treating adolescents.

■ SUGGESTED CROSS-REFERENCES ■

Issues of identity and self-concept are discussed in Chapter 13. Suicide and other forms of self-destructive behavior are discussed in Chapter 15. Problems with the expression of anger are discussed in Chapter 17. Substance abuse is discussed in Chapter 19. Group therapy is discussed in Chapter 28. Family therapy is discussed in Chapter 29.

■ SUMMARY ■

1. The adolescent psychiatric nurse was defined as a person who assists adolescents in their growth toward adulthood. Nurses take on roles as therapists, evaluators, educators, community consultants, and administrators in attempting to assist adolescents with their struggles.

2. Adolescence, as a developmental stage, was identified as movement on a life continuum between the ages of 11 and 20. During this time, shifts in past developmental and learning processes occur. Tasks accomplished during adolescence were presented.

3. Various theories explaining the adolescent's resolution of these tasks were presented. The biological theory consists of Gesell's beliefs that adolescence is biologically determined by physical growth changes. The intellectual development theory bases adolescence on cognitive development and was conceived by Piaget. Psychoanalytical theorists, whose beliefs are based on the theories of Freud, were reviewed. Josselyn sees adolescence as the psychological consequence initiated by the hormonal changes of puberty. The increase in sexual and aggressive impulses causes a psychic restructuring. Blos described adolescence as the second individuation process. These analytical theories were modified by Erikson, Sullivan, and others. Erikson speaks of adolescence as a normal crisis with a great growth potential in facilitating adjustment to the new environment. Cultural theorists consisting of sociologists and anthropologists view adolescence as a societal phenomenon induced by society's lack of formal structure for passage into adulthood.

4. Areas explored in data collection reflect an understanding of the adolescent's experience and health status and include factors such as growth and development, physical status, emotional status, socioeconomic background, environment, daily activities, and support systems.

5. An understanding of normal behaviors seen in adolescents reveals basic conflicts adolescents experience. Conflicts considered were those involving body image, identity, independence, sexuality, social role, and sexual behavior. Body-image conflicts reveal behaviors such as self-consciousness, imitativeness, and body concerns. Conflicts concerning identity reveal regressive characteristics, rebelliousness, negativism, confusion, isolation, and depression. Independence vs. dependence conflicts lead to behaviors such as independent strivings, inconsistency, intenseness, and defensiveness. Sexuality conflicts produce behaviors attempting to deal with sexual impulses, such as heterosexual relationships, homosexual relationships, and parental rejection. In establishing a social role, adolescents exhibit behaviors involving hero worship, chums, crushes, peer group importance, and acting out. Fantasies, relationships with the opposite sex, masturbation, and homosexual activity reveal sexual behavior conflicts.

6. Various problem areas were described, including the sexually active adolescent, unwed mother, pseudohomosexual, overt homosexual, suicidal adolescent, runaway, conduct disordered adolescent, violent homicidal adolescent, substance abuser, hypochondriac, the adolescent with weight problems, and the school phobic adolescent. The planning and implementation of various techniques of intervention were presented.

7. Patient education by the nurse of parents, adolescents, and the community was described. Family therapy and group therapy, with its particular advantage to adolescents who can supportively use the peer group, were briefly explored. Individual treatment, which focuses on establishing an alliance, dealing with transference, and reviewing termination aspects, was presented in an attempt to provide the framework for a productive, growth-producing, therapeutic relationship.

8. The special difficulties in dealing with adolescents, including silence, confidentiality, negativism, resistance, limit

DIRECTIONS FOR FUTURE RESEARCH

The following are some of the nursing research problems raised in Chapter 31 that merit further study by psychiatric nurses:

1. The validity of the developmental tasks of adolescence as described by Havighurst
2. The relationship between coping skills in early life and later adolescent adjustment
3. Nurses' awareness and identification of normal adolescent functioning
4. The implications of new and blurred sexual roles in increasing anxiety for the adolescent
5. Evidence of an extended adolescence as a result of prolonged economic dependence
6. Exploration of the differences between the adolescent experience today and in the past, and the reasons for those differences
7. Indicators of increased depression associated with body image in girls during middle adolescence as compared with older adolescents
8. The effect of the AIDS epidemic on sexual exploration in adolescence
9. Analysis of the role of depression in conduct disordered adolescents
10. Criteria for psychiatric nurses to use in differentiating between depressed and conduct disordered adolescents
11. Exploration of the relationships between depressed and conduct disordered adolescents and problems with moral and superego development
12. Knowledge by psychiatric nurses of indications, actions, and possible side effects of psychotropic drugs on the adolescent
13. Effective nursing actions for dealing with resistence and negative transference in treatment of the adolescent
14. The effectiveness of limit setting interventions by nurses in response to selected acting out behavior in adolescents
15. The relationship between a nurse's comfort with assertive behavior and her effectiveness in setting limits with adolescents
16. Knowledge by psychiatric nurses of the techniques used to promote an alliance with an adolescent
17. The effect of the nurse's own adolescent experiences in creating countertransference problems when working with adolescents.

setting, power struggles, requests for special attention, embarrassment about therapy, bringing friends, and artistic creations, were discussed.

9. Dealing with the adolescent's parents is often a difficult task for the nurse, and some suggestions to facilitate parental support without sabotaging the therapeutic relationship with the adolescent were presented.

10. Evaluation of the nurse's intervention is a necessity. Adolescents arouse feelings within the nurse that must be dealt with if a therapeutic relationship is to be established. Supervision of the nurse is important to promote the evaluation process.

■ REFERENCES ■

1. Addeo, E., and Addeo, J.: Why our children drink, Englewood Cliffs, N.J., 1975, Prentice-Hall, Inc.
2. Aichhorn, A.: Delinquency and child guidance, selected papers, New York, 1964, International Universities Press, Inc.
3. Aichhorn, A.: Wayward youth, New York, 1966, The Viking Press.
4. American Nurses' Association, Division of Psychiatric Mental Health Nursing Practice: Statement on psychiatric and mental health nursing practice, Kansas City, Mo., 1976, The Association.
5. Bandura, A., and Walters, R.: Adolescent aggression, New York, 1959, Ronald Press Co.
6. Berkovitz, I.: Adolescents grow in groups. On growing a group: some thoughts on structure, process and setting, New York, 1972, Brunner/Mazel, Inc.
7. Bhoyrub, J.P.: School phobia, in-patient involvement, Nurs. Times **73**:1388, 1977.
8. Blos, P.: On adolescence, New York, 1962, The Free Press.
9. Blos, P.: The second individuation process of adolescence, Psychoanal, Study Child **22**:162, 1967.
10. Bragg, T.: Teenage alcohol abuse, J. Psychiatr. Nurs. **14**(12):10, 1976.
11. Brenner, C.: An elementary textbook of psychoanalysis, New York, 1974, Anchor Press.
12. Erikson, E.: Childhood and society, ed. 2, New York, 1963, W.W. Norton & Co., Inc.
13. Gesell, A., Ilg, F., and Ames, L.: Youth: the years from ten to sixteen, New York, 1956, Harper & Row, Publishers, Inc.
14. Harley, M.: Analyst and adolescent at work, New York, 1974, Quadrangle/The New York Times Book Co., Inc.
15. Havighurst, R.L.: Developmental tasks and education, ed. 3, New York, 1972, David McKay Co., Inc.
16. Jacobs, J.: Adolescent suicide, New York, 1971, Wiley-Interscience.
17. Josselyn, I.: Adolescence, New York, 1971, Harper & Row, Publishers, Inc.
18. Kappelman, M.: When your teenager needs you the most, Fam. Health. **9**:44, Aug. 1977.
19. Marshall, R.: The treatment of resistances in psycho-

therapy of children and adolescents, Psychother. Theory Res. Prac. **9**(2):143, 1972.
20. Mead, M.: Culture and commitment: a study of the generation gap, New York, 1970, Basic Books, Inc., Publishers.
21. Meeks, J.: The fragile alliance, Baltimore, 1971, The Williams & Wilkins Co.
22. Offer, D., Ostrov, R., and Howark, K. editors: Patterns of the adolescent self-image, San Francisco, 1984, Jossey-Bass.
23. Piaget, J.: Six psychological studies, New York, 1968, Vintage Books.
24. Reuben, R. et al.: Adolescents who attempt suicide, J. Pediatr. **58**:636, 1977.
25. Thornburg, H.: Development in adolescence, Monterey, Calif., 1975, Brooks/Cole Publishing Co.

■ ANNOTATED SUGGESTED READINGS ■

Blos, P.: The adolescent passage, developmental issues, New York, 1979, International Universities Press Inc.

This is a comprehensive view of Blos' look at adolescence in a developmental perspective.

Brandes, N.: Group therapy for the adolescent, New York, 1973, Jason Aronson, Inc.

This is a good primer for beginning group therapists dealing with adolescents.

*Danziger, S.: Major treatment issues and techniques in family therapy with the borderline adolescent, J. Psychosoc. Nurs. Ment. Health Serv. **20**(1):27, 1982.

This excellent paper focuses on five major issues in the treatment of the borderline adolescent and his family: separation-anxiety, lack of control, poor ego boundaries, inability to express feelings, and borderline defense mechanisms. Treatment techniques are suggested for each.

*David, P.: International trends . . . pregnancy and the unmarried girl, J. Psychiatr. Nurs. **15**:40, Feb. 1977.

This article addresses itself to the unmarried pregnant teenager. Difficulties such as isolation caused by fear of communicating with parents and the various consequences of the possible alternatives are discussed. There is a call for more education for teenagers and their parents.

*Duffey, M.: Factors contributing to the development of a cohesive adolescent psychotherapy group, J. Psychiatr. Nurs. **17**:21, Jan. 1979.

A nurse describes her experiences in setting up an adolescent group. Goals, guidelines, and a group contract are presented in this informative article.

Esman, A. H.: The psychology of adolescence, New York, 1984, International Universities Press Inc.

Here is a new source of ideas on the developmental aspects of adolescence.

*Fagin, C., editor: Readings in child and adolescent psychiatric nursing, St. Louis, 1974, The C.V. Mosby Co.

This is an excellent view of the role of the nurse with adoles-

---

*Asterisk indicates nursing reference.

cents. *Case studies are given (e.g., a nurse organizing and running an adolescent girls group).*

Feinstein, S.C., and Giovacchini, P., editors: Adolescent psychiatry, vols. 1-3, New York, 1971, 1973, 1974, Basic Books, Inc., Publishers, vols. 4 and 5, New York, 1976, 1977, Jason Aronson, Inc.

This is a collection of works that acts as a guide to present-day adolescent psychiatry. Numerous outstanding contributors present past and current developments in the field. Basic theoretical notions plus clinical findings are included.

*Fox, K.: Adolescent ambivalence: a therapeutic issue, J. Psychiatr. Nurs. **18**(9):27, 1980.

Through clinical examples the dynamics of adolescent ambivalence are explored and related nursing interventions are suggested.

Gamage, J.R., editor: Management of adolescent drug misuse: clinical, psychological and legal perspectives, Beloit, Wis., 1973, Reash Press.

This book contains articles on various drug issues, such as college students' perspectives of their parents' attitudes and practices regarding drugs, toxic reactions to marijuana, management of emergencies, long-term treatment of adolescent drug abuse, and drugs and the law. It is a good overview of various aspects of adolescents and drugs.

Guest, J.: Ordinary people, New York, 1976, The Viking Press.

This novel relates the story of an adolescent boy after his discharge from the hospital after a suicide attempt. It is sensitively written, with realistic views of his family and therapy.

Haley, J.: Leaving home: the therapy of disturbed young people, New York, 1980, McGraw-Hill, Inc.

This famous family therapist discusses ideas that plague therapists in dealing with adolescents. Using a family focus, he describes in detail specific issues using actual dialogue that provides easy, informative, and enjoyable reading. He discusses the therapist's support system, co-therapy, supervision, and the stages of therapy.

Hodgman, C.: Current issues in adolescent psychiatry, Hosp. Community Psychiatry **34**(6):514, June 1982.

The author reviews recent findings on selected topics in adolescent psychopathology. He also outlines findings on normal adolescent development and discusses problems of diagnosis.

Jones, V.: Adolescents with behavior problems: strategies for teaching, counseling and parent involvement, Boston, 1980, Allyn & Bacon, Inc.

This is a good overview of dealing with problematic adolescents. Issues such as talking to adolescents, understanding their behavior, working with parents, understanding school difficulties, and developing strategies to promote productive behaviors are considered.

Kiell, N.: The universal experience of adolescence, New York, 1983, International Universities Press Inc.

This is a new piece of research illustrating that the turmoil and disorder of adolescence are universal and only superficially affected by cultural aspects. The information is gathered from many disciplines and over a wide time frame.

Lewis, D., and Balla, D.: Delinquency and psychopathology, New York, 1976, Grune & Stratton, Inc.

The authors give psychiatric and social viewpoints of delinquency. The focus is on diagnostic evaluation of abused children, sociopaths, and the delinquent child with CNS dysfunction. Social issues and their important influence on delinquents are examined psychodynamically.

Marohn, R.: Juvenile delinquents: psychodynamic assessment and hospital treatment, New York, 1980, Brunner/Mazel, Inc.

This is a discussion of adolescent behavior describing developmental and psychodynamic theory. A description of the philosophy of treatment with disturbed teenagers who stayed on the unit follows with specific exploration of dynamics, environment and modes of intervention with case examples.

Masterson, J.F.: Treatment of the borderline adolescent, New York, 1972, Wiley-Interscience.

This book describes treatment of adolescents diagnosed according to the medical model as borderline.

Masterson, J., and Costelle, J.: From borderline adolescent to functioning adult, New York, 1980, Brunner/Mazel, Inc.

This is a follow-up report of Masterson's Treatment of the Borderline Adolescent.

McKuen, R.: Finding my father: one man's search for identity, New York, 1977, Berkley Publishing Corp.

This famous poet writes of his lifelong search for the father he never knew. Like the adolescent, he searches not just for his father but for his identity. This is an account of a lonely boy approaching manhood and looking for a caring and loving father of each boy's dreams.

*Mellencamp, A.: Adolescent depression: a review of the literature with implications for nursing care, J. Psychosoc. Nurs. Ment. Health Serv. **19**(9):15, 1981.

This article is true to its title. It treats this important problem in a scholarly and thorough way with clinical application to nursing care. Highly recommended.

*Meyer, A.: School phobia: care in the community, Nurs. Times **73**:1393, Sept. 1977.

This is a description of a nurse's successful work in the community with a 15-year-old adolescent boy who was school phobic for more than 12 months.

Miller, D.: Adolescence: psychology, psychopathology and psychotherapy, New York, 1974, Jason Aronson, Inc.

This is a good overview of adolescence that discusses theory, psychodynamics, and treatment.

Miller, D.: Development of psychiatric services for adolescents. In Schoolar, J., editor: Current issues in adolescent psychiatry, New York, 1973, Brunner/Mazel, Inc.

This chapter contains a helpful description of psychiatric services needed to treat adolescents and a projection of ideal settings to meet their unique needs.

Murphy, L.B., and Hirshberg, J.C.: Comprehensive treatment of a vulnerable adolescent, New York, 1982, Basic Books, Inc., Publishers.

This book presents a case study of a 12-year-old girl who is neurologically damaged. It presents a detailed account of work with her in psychoanalytically oriented Menninger Foundation. A developmental approach is used describing the therapist's view of how she negotiated her developmental tasks at hand and dealt with them in her therapy. This study is helpful in viewing comprehensive treatment strategies in an inpatient setting.

*Nakashima, L.: Teenage pregnancy—its causes, costs and consequences, Nurs. Pract. **3**:10, Sept.-Oct. 1977.

The issues involved with teenage pregnancies are reviewed. Possible origins of teenage pregnancy and the consequences of alternative solutions are discussed.

Novello, J.: The short course in adolescent psychiatry, New York, 1979, Brunner/Mazel, Inc.

This is an overview of a 2-day symposium at the Psychiatric Institute Foundation in Washington, D.C. It is a good encapsulated discussion of adolescent development, evaluation, diagnosis, and treatment.

Offer, D.: The psychological world of the juvenile delinquent, New York, 1979, Basic Books, Inc., Publishers.

The findings of a 5-year research project are presented in which juvenile delinquents were treated in a hospital setting.

Offer, D., Ostrov, E., and Howard, K.I., editors: Patterns of adolescent self image, San Francisco, 1984, Jossey-Bass.

This book is the second in a series on adolescents, under the editorship of H. Richard Lamb of New Directions for Mental Health Services Series. The Offer Self Image Questionnaire developed in 1962 is used in 120 studies on 20,000 adolescents. His studies reveal that professionals describe adolescents as being in turmoil and disturbed when in fact the majority are well adjusted, have good relationships with parents and peers, and generally accept societal values.

Ottenberg, P.: Delivery of adolescent services, In Schoolar, J., editor: Current issues in adolescent psychiatry, New York, 1973, Brunner/Mazel, Inc.

This article reviews the various programs available to adolescents and discusses the specific needs of adolescents.

Robichow, H., and Sklansky, M.: Effective counseling of adolescents, Chicago, 1980, Association Press.

This is a complete overview of adolescent stresses, ego, defenses, and regressions. Treatment is described with discussion of assessing treatability, engagement and continuing treatment, and termination.

*Schlesinger, B.: From A to Z with adolescent sexuality, Can. Nurse **52**:34, Oct. 1977.

In this article an attempt is made to understand adolescent motherhood. Schlesinger uses an alphabetical listing to discuss such issues as the double standard for the sexual act (girls responsible, boys not); including fathers in programs; limit setting with adolescents; adults being models, not judges; women's rights; and possible origins for teenage pregnancies.

Sorenson, R.: Adolescent sexuality in contemporary America, New York, 1973, World Publishing.

A valuable overview of sexual behavior is presented in this text. Every aspect of adolescent sexual behavior is explored from homosexuality and unwed pregnancy to sexual attitudes and uses of sexual behavior.

Stone, J., and Church, J.: Childhood and adolescence, New York, 1973, Random House, Inc.

A good review of normal growth and development, this book has been revised several times and brings a concise and contemporary view of normal behavior and age-specific guidelines. The combination of theory and observable behaviors makes this reference a must for beginners.

Thornburg, H.: Adolescence: a re-interpretation. In Neubauer, P., editor: Process of child development, New York, 1976, The New American Library, Inc.

A good description of adolescence, this book also defines and interprets in detail Robert Havighurst's developmental tasks in adolescence.

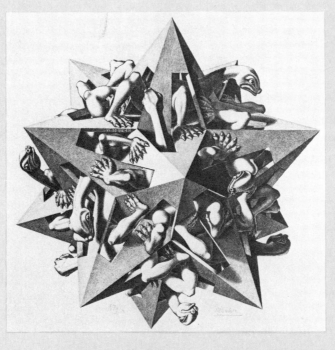

When I was a laddie
I lived with my granny
And many a hiding my granny di'ed me.
Now I am a man
And I live with my granny
and do to my granny
what she did to me.

Traditional rhyme, anonymous*

C H A P T E R   3 2

NURSING INTERVENTION IN FAMILY ABUSE AND VIOLENCE

THERESA S. FOLEY
BARBARA A. GRIMES

**From Davidson, J.L.: Elder abuse. In Block, M., and Sinnott, J., editors: The battered child syndrome: an exploratory study. College Park, Md., 1977, The University of Maryland Center on Aging.

LEARNING OBJECTIVES

After studying this chapter, the student should be able to:

- define and differentiate between the concepts of abuse and violence.

- report the incidence of family abuse and violence and factors that contribute to its occurrence.

- describe offenders and victims using reported demographic data.

- identify twelve characteristics of abusive and violent family systems.

- analyze the stress reaction process in abusive and violent families.

- relate types of violent behavior, motives of the offender, and targets of family violence.

- compare and contrast theories on the etiology of family violence.

- apply a systems theory model to assess and intervene in violent family processes.

- identify the data base needed for a nursing assessment of violent families.

- formulate individualized nursing diagnoses for abusive and violent families and their members.

- develop long-term and short-term individualized nursing goals for abusive and violent families and their members.

- describe nursing interventions in secondary prevention utilizing crisis, individual, group, and family approaches appropriate to the needs of the violent family.

- describe nursing interventions in tertiary prevention appropriate to the needs of the violent family.

- describe nursing interventions in primary prevention directed toward preventing family abuse and violence.

- assess the importance of the evaluation of the nursing process when working with abusive and violent families.

- identify directions for future nursing research.

- select appropriate readings for further study.

Family violence is an extremely unpleasant topic, one that most people do not bring up in public or social conversation. If the topic is introduced it often is met with complete silence or failure to pursue a discussion about violence and abuse. Nurses need to be aware of the problem of family violence because they work with children, their families, and society at all levels of prevention. Family violence is more than a family problem. It is a reflection of a sick society that fosters and sanctions violent behavior as a norm in response to the stressors of daily life. As a learned behavior, the cycle of violence is frequently passed from generation to generation—the child victims later resorting to violence with their own mates or children and perhaps again experiencing victimization as elderly persons by those whom they had previously abused. The statistics on the incidence of family violence are staggering, and projections of future trends indicate that it is likely to increase. Because of the many settings and roles nurses work in,

they are in an ideal position to contribute to the prevention, identification, treatment, and eradication of family violence.

Abuse and violence are two closely related concepts. Often the terms are used interchangeably in the literature; lack uniform definitions or parameters across research studies or social values, limiting generalization of the findings; and are subject to a wide variety of theoretical propositions to explain the phenomena. **Abuse** is generally defined as "an act of misuse, exploitation, deceit, wrong or improper use, or action so as to injure, damage, maltreat or corrupt,"[78] whereas **violence** is defined as "the exertion of extreme force or destructive action so as to injure or hurt; discordance, outrage, and sudden intense activity to the point of loss of control."[78]

Acts of physical injury and death are often contained within the definitions and use of the terms. For example, child physical abuse usually refers to overt, active, physical violence by an adult against a child, which causes injuries ranging from bruises and burns to fractures and death, or covert violence through neglect, which may have the same outcomes. Although child sexual abuse generally involves coercion to gain the victim's compliance, the phenomenon creates a condition of psychological violence that has long-term effects on the family system yet is not as easily detected or measured as physical signs of injury. This offense is primarily described in terms of abuse, yet it is not uncommon for a sexually abused child to also be subjected to physical violence by the parents or siblings.

Furthermore, a fine line exists between what one considers abuse as opposed to violence. There is, for example, a questionable distinction between corporal punishment and physical violence; the definition usually is determined by the parent or guardian. The situation is further complicated in that the abusive or violent family does not perceive their behavior as abusive or violent; the members tend to deny and discount the existence of the problem as do many professionals who have an awareness of or reason to suspect that a case exists.[40,43,71] For the purposes of this chapter the term **family violence** is used to refer to all forms of family abuse or violence and is defined as the physical, psychological, sexual, material, social violation, or exploitation of a person by a family member or their delegate.

Most of the literature discusses family violence according to the way in which the dysfunction is expressed: child physical abuse, child sexual abuse, sibling violence, spouse abuse, or elder abuse. This chapter attempts to examine what is common across categories of family violence, that is, what is common to violent family systems rather than to a specific form of family violence. The nature and scope of the problem, theories on the etiology of family violence, and treatment issues within a nursing process model will be analyzed in this chapter. Books and monographs have been written on each form of family violence, thus the following discussion is necessarily and intentionally limited in scope. It is assumed that the reader has a working knowledge of family theory and concepts and family therapy as discussed in other chapters of this textbook (Chapters 5 and 29), permitting fuller attention to the application of theory and concepts to intervention in family abuse and violence.

Defining the problem of family abuse and violence

The problem of family violence can be defined and described in a variety of ways. Questions frequently asked include the following: What is its incidence? Who is the abuser? What is this person like? Who is the victim and what is he or she like? Who could ever marry or live with such a person? How does family violence get started and perpetuated? What do the abusive or violent behaviors consist of?

■ Incidence

How serious is the problem of family violence? Statistics are, at best, only estimates of the incidence of family violence. Crime statistics should generally be doubled because it is estimated that 50% of violent crimes are unreported.[72] For a variety of reasons common to the problems of conducting any valid and reliable research study, as well as to the taboo and secret nature of the topic in our society, the statistics on family violence are limited. In the United States, it would seem that people would prefer to ignore both that it does exist and that it is as prevalent as it is. Attorney General Lois H. Harrington eloquently stated:

Every 23 minutes, someone is murdered. Every 6 minutes a woman is raped. While you read this statement, two people will be robbed in this country and 2 more will be shot, stabbed, or seriously beaten. . . . The criminal knows that his risk of punishment is minuscule. A study of 4 major states revealed that only 9% of violent crimes were resolved with the perpetrator being incarcerated . . . .

You cannot appreciate the victim's problem if you approach it solely with your intellect. The intellect rebels . . . . You must know what it is to have your life wrenched and broken, to realize that you will never really be the same. Then you must experience what it means to survive, only to be blamed and used and ignored by those you thought were there to help you. Only when you are willing to confront all these things will you understand what victimization means.[72]

Children who are molested suffer incalculable harm . . . . It is my firm belief that the values of society and the seriousness with which they're held can be measured by the penalty imposed when they're violated. What then does a 10 day sentence for the rape of a child say about the youngster's place in our society? We have not held our children in very high regard. And what can be said about a society that runs criminal history checks on those who handle its money in banks, but does virtually nothing to check the background of those who work with its children?[74]

Hundreds of thousands of Americans . . . are harmed, not by strangers but by those they trust and love. They are victimized, not on the street or in the workplace but in their own homes . . . . Anyone who lives in a violent home experiences an essential loss. The one place on earth where they should feel safe and secure has become instead a place of danger . . . . To tolerate family violence is to allow the seeds of violence to be sown into the next generation . . . . The problem of family violence is a very human one, and it is amenable to human solution. We as a society must undertake that solution. The time for standing idly by is past.[73]

Table 32-1 presents current data on the incidence of family violence.

■ Demographic data

It is known that family violence is evident at all socioeconomic levels, in all educational, racial, occupational, gender and religious groups, and regions in the United States. Table 32-2 presents a profile of the violent family, reporting data specific to each form of family violence. Data presented in Table 32-2 suffer from difficulties common to the field of victimology: the statistics are derived from a variety of sources (police files, hospital records); collection methods have not been uniform; definitions of terms differ; disadvantaged families are identified through care delivery systems, whereas middle and upper class families often escape detection and reporting; and unreported cases (estimates ranging from 10 to 20 unreported for every reported or founded case) ultimately skew a clear profile of the violent family.

These data do, however, offer a starting point in recognizing individuals who have most frequently come to the attention of authorities and professionals. Generally, the **offender** ranges in age from a toddler to about 60 years; is male, married, and living with a spouse or partner; is frequently not fully employed and has a semi-skilled job; has completed high school; is likely to have been a victim of childhood physical or sexual abuse; is of a minority religion or does not share the same religon as other family members; and can reside anywhere in the United States. The **victim** is generally a female; ranges in age from newborn to old age; is related to and living with the abuser; is not employed, has not developed an occupation, or has retired; does not have a high school diploma; can reside anywhere in the United States; and is usually in a captive position within the violent family as a result of emotional or economic issues in the system.

TABLE 32-1

INCIDENCE OF FAMILY ABUSE AND VIOLENCE

Category	Statistics
Child abuse	
Physical	3 in 5 families[64]; 1,712,614 cases reported in 1984[3] with reports increasing at a 9% annual rate[46] to 2.5 million per year[30]; every other household has abuse at least once a year[64]
Sexual	62% of random sample of 700 adult women retrospectively reported abuse occurred before age 18[81]; of 2008 adults surveyed, 40% of females and 26% of males retrospectively reported abuse before age 21[66]; 38% of 930 women reported unwanted sexual contact before age 18[66]; 123,000 cases reported in 1984 with reports increasing at a 9% annual rate[46]; 20 unreported for every reported case[37]
Sibling abuse	Most prevalent form of family violence[64]; 4 in 5 children (3 to 17 years old) experience sibling violence once a year[64]; 36.3 million children ages 3 to 17 years old[76]; 29 million children commit one act of violence per year[76]; affect 1 in 6 families[64]
Domestic violence	
Female	Over 2 million cases per year[64]; 50% are abused some time during their marriage[76]; 50% of female domestic violence victims report marital rape—this figure is estimated to be low as many women, due to socialization, do not identify that they have been raped or consider marital rape to be domestic violence[57,58]
Male	Over 2 million cases per year[64]
Marital rape	1 in 7 (14%) of women who have ever been married report forced vaginal intercourse; incidence of oral and/or anal rape (common to sexual assault) not investigated[57]
Elder abuse	Estimated incidence of between 1 and 2.5 million cases per year[28,35]; 9.6% of elderly clients are seen by an agency[40]; in 55% of 183 cases, there was one incident or more within 18 months[40]; 13.43% of 134 professionals surveyed reported a case[11]; 87% of service agencies, professionals, or elderly do not report suspected cases of abuse[11]; 4% of 73 elderly reported abuse[11]; 62.3% (151 of 228) service agency personnel report experience with elder abuse cases[21]

■ The violent family system

The question that continues to be explored by family therapists is: Why are some families violent and others not? Some families that come for therapy have the same characteristics as violent families but are not violent. What clinicians and researchers do agree on is that there are a number of characteristics that describe what a violent family is like, and yet these same characteristics can be found in nonviolent families with the dysfunction expressed in an alternative form (e.g., one member may be diagnosed as a schizophrenic).[20,75] **Family violence is, then, the mode by which a given family system expresses its dysfunction.** Why family violence is elected rather than an alternative form, such as schizophrenia, remains to be researched. Thus emphasis is placed on genetics and the context in which any given set of variables is present as important factors in determining violent behavior. Some researchers and clinicians believe that a healthy family system, if subjected to the right combination of stressors, could develop violent interactions. The concept of family violence therefore focuses on the system, not the individual members, as being "self-destructive." For example, in a violent family the individual members are usually at a low level of differentiation, but emphasis is placed on the fact that the entire system is undifferentiated. What is important is that these individuals formed a group but were unable to meet their own or others' needs, thereby setting up a context in which family violence is the outcome of dysfunctional relationships and emotional processes.

Because so much of the literature focuses on a specific type of family violence, a tremendous volume of data must be synthesized and ordered if one is to begin to understand the nature of a violent family system. This requires knowledge of both the characteristics of the violent family system and the stress reaction process involved in family violence. Both of these aspects are illustrated in Clinical example 32-1.

This situation could have had any number of different transactions and reactions. For example, Mr. F could have insisted that Mrs. F stay home (jealousy and possessiveness) and beat her up for even thinking about leaving him. Sue could have complied and been submissive with every verbal assault from her father but physically beat the younger siblings while putting them to bed. Mrs. F could have stayed home and gone on a spending spree the next day to lift her mood and get away from the hassle of the kids and use up money set aside for support of her elderly mother who now must do with little or no food until the next payday. This clinical example illustrates the interlocking nature of individual members' conflicts within the family system.

CLINICAL EXAMPLE 32-1

Mr. F came home from work after a "terrible day." The boss rejected a request for a salary increase yet hired a new employee, and arguments with co-workers had escalated. All Mr. F wants is a little love, attention, and nurturing. He feels lonely, depressed, and unappreciated. He handles his conflicts by pursuing companionship and shutting out the outside world.

Mrs. F had a hectic day with the three children, and the last thing she needs is to mother another person. She just wants to be left alone and feels depleted from giving to others. Mr. F's depression leaves her feeling angry and frustrated. She feels hopeless about things ever being any better in their relationship but ignores that feeling in trying to make it from day to day. Mrs. F handles her frustration by withdrawing from her husband and the family; she reads books for days at a time, goes on spending sprees to lift her mood, and plays bridge at least two evenings a week.

Mr. F started drinking after work to "get rid of his troubles" and followed his wife around until she exploded, telling him what a "no-good drunken provider" he is. An argument ensued, and Mrs. F left the house to play bridge with her friends. Mr. F retreated to the bedroom and drowned his misery by leafing through pornographic literature but continued to feel intolerably depressed and lonely. He was angry that he could not control his wife's activities so she would be exclusively with him.

The oldest daughter, Sue, entered the bedroom to inform him that the younger children needed to have dinner and be helped getting to bed. Mr. F picked a fight with her. He stormed out of the bedroom to take care of the children and dragged her by the arm downstairs to "teach her" how to be a "mother." Feeling intense irritation with his wife, he continued picking and nagging at Sue over little things—the way the table was set, which dishes were used, what food items were selected, and so forth—and eventually hit her. She cursed at him and ran to her bedroom.

The other children ran to the other room to escape the frightening situation. They played with toys but did mean things with them like hit them and pull their hair. The television was on and is their best friend most of the time. They watch more violence on television and learn that violence is a norm for solving tension in daily living, just like in their house.

Mr. F then tried to handle his frustration by pursuing closeness with his daughter. He'll "be damned" if he'll "let her get the best of me." He's

Continued.

TABLE 32-2

PROFILE OF THE VIOLENT FAMILY

Identifying data	Child physical abuse		Child sexual abuse	
	Abuser	Victim	Abuser	Victim
Age	Mother, average age = 26; father average age = 30; all ages	Most under 2 years; average age = 4 years; all ages	All ages; 21 to 30 years old most often; 11 to 20 years old next often	All ages; 6 to 9 years old at onset; 12 years old when disclosed; mean age = 7.9 years
Sex	Male and female; father more often than mother, but mother more violent	Not a factor	Male; accomplice sometimes female	Male and female; most reported cases are female (7 females to 1 male); in females, 63% are younger than 12 years old; in males, 64% are older than 12 years old
Relationship	Father or step-father; not a stranger most often, e.g., baby-sitter or guardian	Acquainted or known; oldest/youngest daughter or only child most often	Father more often than mother	Son/daughter or stepchild
Marital status	Married and living with spouse	Single	Married and living with spouse	Single
History of childhood physical/sexual abuse	60% of cases	Repeated multiple victimization or neglect	70% of cases	Repeated multiple victimization
Socioeconomic status (SES)	Evident at all SES levels; rate twice as high in reported cases of families under the poverty line ($5999) as in families of $20,000+ income		Evident in all SES levels; found cases most often lower SES	
Occupation	Reported cases most often skilled or semiskilled	Student	Found cases most often professional, skilled, or semiskilled	Student
Employment status	Unemployment not disproportionately prevalent; abuse twice as high if father is employed part time	Not employed	Employed; higher rate if part time or unemployed	Not employed
Race	Blacks and minorities inaccurately represented; all races	Same as abuser	Not a factor	

Data from references 11, 15, 19, 27, 30, 34, 36, 60, 64, 76.

TABLE 32-2—cont'd

PROFILE OF THE VIOLENT FAMILY

Spouse abuse		Sibling abuse		Elder abuse	
Male	Female	Abuser	Victim	Abuser	Victim
Often 17 to 30 years old at disclosure; all ages; seen in abuse of elders		All ages; most reported cases are 17 years old or less; rate decreases as age increases		40 to 60 years old	60 years old and older
Male and female; most reported cases have female victims		Male most often; higher incidence in all male—sibling families	Male most often; higher incidence in all male—sibling families	Female	Not a factor; more elder are female
Spouse or partner		Brother to brother as victim most often; brother to sister as victim next often		Son/daughter, relative, or caretaker	Parent of abuser most often
Married most often; living together next often		Single	Single	Married	Widowed
Most were subject to repeated victimization as children		Live in abusive/violent home; often victims of parent/guardian as well		Data not widely available; positive history in some cases	Positive history in some cases; repeated victimization
Evident at all SES levels; five times more common in families at or below poverty line than in families over $20,000 income in reported cases		Evident at all SES levels		Not a factor; evident at all SES levels; founded cases mostly lower to middle class and found through health care systems	
Reported cases skilled or semiskilled most often		Childhood (or history of delinquency)		Professional or semiskilled	Not employed
Violence two or three times higher if man is unemployed or has part-time employment		Not employed		Least violence in homes of retired men; victim often physically/mentally impaired	
All races; reported most by minorities; black more than whites (2:1)		Highest, racial minorities; lowest, blacks		Highest, American Indians, orientals, minorities; blacks = 12%, whites = 88%[11]; also reported as no difference[63]	

Data from references 11, 15, 19, 27, 30, 36, 60, 64, 76.

Continued.

TABLE 32-2—cont'd

PROFILE OF THE VIOLENT FAMILY

Identifying data	Child physical abuse		Child sexual abuse	
	Abuser	Victim	Abuser	Victim
Religion	Highest, one or more parents of minority religion; lowest, Jewish	Mixed religious background	Highest, highly religious family, rigid inflexible belief system; lowest, realistic balance of religion in family belief system	
Education	Most violent, high school diploma for both men and women; least violent, grammar school dropout or some college education	Mostly preschool; if in school, performance may be poor (stress symptom)	Inaccurately presented Often high school and some college	Grammar and high school student; performance may be poor (stress symptom)
Residence	Large city most often Evenly distributed in United States		Evenly distributed in United States	

CLINICAL EXAMPLE 32-1—cont'd

determined to prove that *he* is right; he can't stand feeling powerless. He already felt like a miserable creature and wouldn't allow her to have power over him. He felt kind of rotten for having hit her and was determined to see that she kept that a secret from mom. Mr. F entered the bedroom, apologized to Sue for having hit her, but told her it was for a good reason given her "mouthy disrespectful behavior and attitude." He insisted that she talk the conflict out with him and began to rub her back. Sue started to tell father how she felt; Mr. F listened and soothed her and gave her a back rub. Sue appreciated the attention because she was feeling worthless after her father's demeaning verbal assault earlier. Mr. F's back rub gradually progressed to her genitals, and he con-

vinced her that he should "teach her about sex." He taught her about oral sex and used his pornography to show her other sexual behavior he wants to teach her about. He told her about all the terrible things that would happen to her and the family if she ever tells anyone about tonight and that he wouldn't want that to happen because he truly loves her, sometimes more than mom. Mr. F felt relieved but left Sue's room because he was nervous about his wife returning to discover him.

Mrs. F returned from her evening out, her frustration temporarily relieved after having withdrawn from the family. Mr. F argued with her (wanted to know why she was home so early, why she didn't get the food at the all-night store as he had asked),

TABLE 32-2—cont'd

PROFILE OF THE VIOLENT FAMILY

Spouse abuse		Sibling abuse		Elder abuse	
Male	Female	Abuser	Victim	Abuser	Victim
Highest, minority religions and Jewish women; lowest, Protestants and Jewish men		Highest minority religions (excluding Jewish, Catholic, or Protestant)		Protestant	
Victim more often without high school diploma and less often with college education		Most violent if father/male highly educated and mother/female high school diploma or some college education		High school diploma or some college	
Most violent husbands, high school diploma; least violent, grammar school dropout or some college	Most violent, wives without high school diploma				
Evenly distributed in United States	Abused by male in large city or rural area; rate decreased by half in suburbs	Higher rates in rural area and large cities Not Southern phenomena		Limited data, evenly distributed with more reports in large cities Not Southern phenomena	

CLINICAL EXAMPLE 32-1

cont'd

and she gave him "the silent treatment," going to bed for the night with a book. Mr. F retreated to the living room to drink a few beers and watch the late show but found that he was, instead, obsessively preoccupied, recalling highlights of the tantalizing sexual intimacies with Sue.

■ **CHARACTERISTICS OF THE VIOLENT FAMILY AS A SYSTEM.** Although specific forms of family violence may differ somewhat on family system characteristics, the literature and clinical practice suggest some general patterns. First, violent families have **boundaries** that seem impermeable to outsiders. Until disclosure, no one is aware of what is going on in the family, often including other members of the family. In therapy the family is extremely resistant to being opened up for change to occur. When "in trouble" (for example, when charges are pressed and the family is facing separation by legal authority) the system will usually loosen its boundaries, if forced or pressured to do so, and become more permeable to the degree that people or agencies are believed to further the family system's direction and can be co-opted (for example, by obtaining home-care aids or professionals who will testify in their behalf). When outsiders attempt to permeate the system's boundaries, the action is felt to be an invasive assault, and the family becomes more firmly entrenched, cutting off contact with the outside world, which is a perceived threat. It is not surprising therefore for the abuser* to assert and believe that his own assaultive

---

*Since most reported abusers are men, the abuser is referred to by the male gender here, but we acknowledge that women also fall into this category as the identified patient, signaling the system's distress and dysfunction.

behavior within the system was justified, given his intent of preserving the family, and for him to ignore the reality of the destruction his violence creates. In Clinical example 32-1, the father ensured that boundary lines would be maintained by convincing the daughter to keep the violence a secret; the system was sealed off by a conspiracy of silence. In addition, the father crossed over generational boundaries by seeking companionship with the daughter and excluding the mother. Finally, in terms of boundaries, it is found that violent families are socially isolated; they have few friends and little contact with helping persons. The family is "roped off from the outside world, which only serves to create a pressure cooker within the system that eventually explodes in violence.

The **mood,** or **feeling tone,** in such families is one of pain and desperation. The members compete for affection, caring, attention, and nurturance as if the supply were insufficient and limited and generally ignore the needs of the other members. When two adults with low self-esteem who are unable to meet their own needs merge, the relationship system can be potentially explosive. No one person can possibly meet all the needs of another person, yet that is often what violent couples expect of each other. The violent couple have frequently married or moved in together when quite young and have many unresolved separation-individuation issues that get transferred onto their new relationship. Cutoffs or fusion with the family of origin are also quite common. When marriage fails to resolve these residual developmental issues, the couple becomes disillusioned, and disappointment with the mate creates tension that explodes in family violence.

Add elderly persons or children to that system and the situation becomes even more volatile. The child or elderly person is expected to meet the adult's needs, and his or her needs for care and love place an intolerable burden on an adult already stressed by demands made by a mate. The elderly person or child then becomes at high risk as a target for physical or sexual violence by adults who focus only on gratifying their own needs while disregarding, denying, and discounting the needs of the developing child or elderly person. In the clinical example the mother was unable to meet the father's needs for empathic listening because of her own need, withdrew from his intense unhappiness, and the tension was subsequently released between the father and daughter through physical and sexual violence.

Another characteristic of violent families is their lack of **autonomy,** or **differentiation.** Unlike adequately functioning families, violent families tend to be characterized by low levels of differentiation and fusion with others to attain a sense of self. Family members operate on an emotional level and are threatened by the individuation of other members.

A characteristic related to lack of autonomy is the violent family's inability to **trust.** Usually violent adults have experienced a history of one or more premature separations, neglect, or episodes of childhood physical and sexual violence. The violence experienced in childhood is a predisposing factor to violent behavior in adulthood in response to high levels of stress. It emerges as difficulty with object loss or separation from those emotionally depended on. No matter how terrifying the family environment is, the members desperately work to keep the system intact rather than lose another member; hence the fusion of spouses with their families of origin, each other, or one of the children. Staying together is a painful rather than joyful process, with an absence of humor, flexibility, caring, genuine empathy, excitement in exploring an adventuresome world, recognized productivity, and clear communication. The result is that violent families have no real intimacy, only a pseudointimacy.

The violence can thus be viewed as a misguided and desperate attempt by the system to gain closeness and companionship and provide a release for accumulated frustration. It is also a way of coping with a world that is viewed as threatening, demanding, unrewarding, and problematical. Through repetitive episodes of family violence, the family ignores and denies a multitude of daily living problems, and members experience an absence of empathy, traumatic loneliness, and a high degree of both overt and covert conflict.

Conflict is expressed overtly through violent aggression and covertly through constant power struggles, depending on the motive of the abuser and the needs of other members in the system. In some families, conflict is the way in which closeness is expressed or communicated. It is as if the message communicated in the system is, "I only know that you care about me when you are really (violently) upset." The result is a confusion of closeness and caring with violence. Many professionals hypothesize that it is at this point that sexuality and aggression become confused and fused, resulting in rape within domestic violence and marriage. Although colleagues discuss that viewpoint in their clinical work, the question has yet to be researched. What is known about conflict in the family system is that the release of frustration and accompanying relief is only temporary. The emotional cycle rebuilds gradually, arguments are frequent, and relief is again sought through violent behavior. Violent behavior thus becomes a learned mode of response to reduce stress or tension, and the relief felt from the violent behavior acts as a positive reinforcer to the maladaptive coping style.

Conflict resolution in families is closely related to their **regulation of duties,** such as aggression and sexuality. Violent families are characterized by a lack of impulse control and self-discipline and a reduced capacity to delay gratification. With inadequate internal controls and limit setting, they tend to "act out" their needs without regard for others. Their very acts of abuse and violence speak to their lack of ability to tolerate frustration and regulate drives.

The violent family thus focuses on getting their needs met in the present—for example, decreasing an immediate state of loneliness or low self-esteem. The result is that an awareness of past, present, and future, known as **time binding,** is poor or minimal. However, an awareness of the passage of time surfaces acutely when the victim begins to physically separate from the system or becomes less available as a target of emotional release, such as in puberty and adolescence when peer relationships are built and separation from the family system is in process. Another instance of the awareness of the passage of time is when the system's direction is impeded, as when an elderly person is brought into the family home and home care responsibilities interfere with the wife's ability to achieve career goals. The members define time, then, in terms of the narcissistic self rather than the family system, and the nurse will note that the violent family is unable to tolerate interference with need gratification. Thus long-range goal-directed behaviors that often interfere with need gratification (for example, years of education prior to gainful employment and a successful career) are often absent or weak.

This leads to problems with **task performance,** which can affect all aspects of the family's life. Frequently, members have difficulty obtaining and retaining jobs. If employed, they may experience job dissatisfaction and interpersonal problems with co-workers. Financial problems are recurrent. Problems also spill over into parenting and social situations. There may be early or forced marriages, unplanned children, lack of parenting skills, and the generalized inability to problem solve effectively. The adults tend to have unrealistic and magical expectations of other members of the family system, and conflicts around discipline and child rearing or care for an elderly parent are quite high. The problem is further escalated in that the system is cut off from the outside world, which could provide inputs to reduce the tension. For example, they do not discuss their problem child with "outsiders" and therefore do not hear others say, "That's normal behavior for a 3-year-old. Yes it does drive you up a wall, but it will pass. . . . What I did when my kid was that age was. . . ." Violent families have a need to learn not only normal aspects of growth and development, but also how to meet their needs through their own resources and the resources available outside the family. This is a significant area for preventive interventions by nurses and other health professionals.

Communication in violent families is characterized by mixed or double messages, an emphasis on nonverbal messages, and an absence of direct communication that is believed to be intolerably threatening. Communication is frequently used to keep the family cut off from the outside world. For example, the victim is told not to tell anyone about the violence or she will be responsible for the family being dissolved and broken up or the father going to jail. The victim thus learns to subject her own needs to the violent system, feels like an object that is used and discarded or is valued by the violent system only as a target for discharge, and may have long-term conflicts because of the sense of worthlessness conveyed by the system. Communication can also be quite threatening and intimidating to gain the victim's compliance. For example, an elderly person may be threatened with being abandoned to a nursing home or losing control over his will and inheritance unless certain demands by the family system are met. Food, clothing, and other necessities may be denied or used in barter as a trade-off or pay-off. Meanwhile the terror and rage felt in response to the violence continue to be denied, ignored, or discounted.

This denial process contributes to a faulty **belief system** and perception of reality. The family system may believe that violence is what happens in all families, violence is a norm, the victim is responsible for the assault, or violence is the way to solve problems. The family system can teach its members faulty or impaired cognitive processes in coping with daily stressors. In Clinical example 32-1 Mr. F taught Sue that she was responsible for the violence because of her "mouthy disrespectful behavior" and thus taught her to discount the reality that his violent behavior was out of bounds.

Distorted perceptions and communications may also be used by the abuser to maintain an imbalanced **power ratio** in the system, giving the abusive person an advantage over the other members. For example, the abusive person may tell the members they are worthless for any number of reasons, which may or may not be rational; have them convinced of their worthlessness, powerlessness, helplessness, and hopelessness; and keep them from reaching out to others for help or taking any assertive action in their behalf. Or the abusive person may tell the victim that the violent behavior was justified given the victim's behavior and have the victim attribute the fault to himself, thereby excusing the violent member for the abuse. Essentially, the abusive person has learned to be a master "con" artist who can talk almost anyone into believing his point of view. The net effect is that the members in the system learn to abuse power; use people to achieve personal or narcissistic aims with a disregard for the individual being abused; use manipulation, lying, and deceit as coping mechanisms and use covert passive-aggressive power to control relationships that can ultimately result in the development of mental illness, psychophysiological stress reactions, and characterological behaviors, such as prostitution and drug and alcohol abuse. Thus the covert use of power is ultimately self-destructive, with the victim perpetuating the victim's role as a scapegoat for the family system's focus of attention (for example, an adolescent's drug habit is of more concern than the factors contributing to it).

Competition and the abuse of power was evident in Clinical example 32-1. The mother was powerful by withdrawing and refusing to give empathy to father; the father was powerful in hitting the daughter, insisting that the daughter talk with him and winning her closeness; the daughter was powerful in fleeing from her father, refusing to interact with him, and granting or denying him satisfaction of aggressive and sexual drives; the siblings wielded power by removing themselves as potential scapegoats and by making demands on the system for care and attention. The power ratio is also evident in the structure of relationships within the system so that the abusing person usually assumes a dominant role, the victim a passive and submissive role, and the other members silently collude in the abuse if only to escape the scapegoat position in the system. The members often have good reasons to be frightened of the one holding the power and do not challenge that person.

The clearest example of power inherent in a relationship structure is seen in the family's **role stereotyping** and belief system, which is quite rigid, absolute, and traditional: a woman's work is at home taking care of everyone else, children are to be seen and not heard, older siblings have the right to discipline younger ones with physical punishment, elders are seen as having nothing to contribute to the family or society and are best left alone, and so forth. Any departure from a prescribed role can precipitate violence (for example, if a woman decides to get a job, if a younger sibling challenges an older sibling's authority, if an elder refuses to turn over a savings account to the family and become dependent on them). Rigid roles control the members by keeping them from growing or developing and reduce the threat of system dissolution, since the members feel unable to leave or separate. Finally, in relation to this issue, it is common to observe that the parental coalition is absent or in shambles. In the clinical example the father and mother were not allied in their parenting responsibilities. They were, in fact, emotionally oppositional. The father fused with the daughter to meet emotional needs and excluded the mother, while the siblings fled the frightening situation.

Table 32-3 summarizes these 12 characteristics of violent family systems. They are common aspects of all violent families, regardless of the form in which the system dysfunction is expressed. However, as summary sketches, the nurse needs to realize that not all characteristics will apply to each family. Rather, they describe background dimensions that can be useful in working with these families.

■ **STRESS REACTION PROCESS.** Effective intervention in family violence requires that the nurse understand the interactional sequence of events leading up to the system's explosive dysfunction. In therapy the members demonstrate their individual reactivity to problems in the family that fuel the dysfunctional process. Ultimately a composite of the interlocking variables may be worked out, with the family actively contributing to developing cognitive awareness of the process. Fig. 32-1 depicts an overview of the stress reaction process in abusive and violent families.

■ **Forms of family violence**

Forms of family violence are described in three ways: (1) the types of violent behavior, (2) the predominant motive expressed by the violent behavior, and (3) the target of the violent release of tension. **Types of violent behavior** include psychological, physical, sexual, material, and social acts as follows:

1. **Physical abuse/violence:** Beating, withholding personal care, food, and medical care; lack of supervision; bruises, wounds, cuts, punctures, and bone and skull fractures; sprains and dislocations, abrasions, and lacerations; an environment of dirt and vermin in the house, an odor of urine, or inadequate heat[11,40]

2. **Psychological abuse/violence:** Verbal assault and threats, provoking fear, and isolation; disturbed communication patterns and cognitive processes[11,40,71-74]

3. **Material abuse/violence:** Theft of money or property; misuse of money or property[11,40,71-74]

4. **Social abuse/violence:** Violation of rights, such as forceful eviction from one's residence and relocation in another setting,[10] being locked out of the refrigerator or one's home,[10] being restrained from seeing one's friends or helping persons, being pressured or forced into isolative behaviors[71-74]

5. **Sexual abuse/violence:** Pressured or forced sexual activity or stimulation that "includes physical acts

TABLE 32-3

CHARACTERISTICS OF ABUSIVE AND VIOLENT FAMILY SYSTEMS

Criteria	Assessment data
Boundary	Impermeable to outsiders; generational boundaries are crossed over, blurred, nonexistent; others' boundaries are intruded; system is socially isolated; permeation felt as invasive assault
Mood/feeling tone	Pain; depression; competition for caring, affection, and nurturance; longing for closeness but allergic to it; intense tension and anger; fear; great intensity, force, and fusion; lack of empathy; constant crises; extreme deprivation and neediness; helplessness and hopelessness
Autonomy/differentiation	Nonexistent autonomy or pseudoautonomy; low level of differentiation; threatened by separation-individuation of members; own needs subjected to those of the family system; fused with others for a sense of self; members propelled by feelings; intergenerational transmission process (over one or more generations)
Trust	Absent or shattered sense of trust; history of premature separations/neglect; high-level denial and discounting of problem; pseudointimacy; fear of authority figures; inability to trust self or others in or outside system; no reaching out to others; staying together is a painful process
Conflict	High level of conflict that is overt and covert; conflict exacerbated by drug/alcohol abuse; may be either denied or condoned; intense triangulation; closeness and caring confused with abuse/violence; learned behavior to reduce stress
Regulation of drives (aggression/sexuality)	Little or no impulse control; low frustration tolerance; acts out drives without regard for others; abuse of alcohol/drugs; projection and acting out of self-hatred on scapegoat (victim); inadequate limit setting; reduced capacity to delay gratification
Time binding	Ignored or minimal awareness; focus on self and daily crises; awareness emerges as victim escapes field or is less available; panic sets in to locate replacement for gratification/discharge of tension; time defined in terms of narcissistic self vs. family system; long-range goal-directed behaviors are absent or weak; severe stress reaction to loss
Task performance	Inefficiency; high unemployment and conflict with co-workers/family system around tasks; child/adult role responsibilities reversed; discipline problems; dysfunctional may be expressed as "workaholic"; high-level job dissatisfaction; recurrent financial problems; ineffective problem-solving skills; unrealistic and magical expectations of others
Communication	Poor communication; double messages; mixed nonverbal messages; threatened by direct messages; discounts problems and people affected; threatening or fear inducing; incongruent; abusive; blaming; confusing; demeaning; failure to talk and share with others; unkept promises
Belief system	Faulty perception of reality; family's view not congruent with assessment by outsiders; members taught faulty or impaired cognitive processes
Power ratio	Imbalance in power ratio; usually male dominated; struggle for power and dominance acted out; self-esteem determined by power wielded in system; need for constant refueling through abuse/violence; abuse of power often maintained by distorted communication; master con artists; members are impersonal objects to achieve narcissistic aims; power often maintained through lying, deceit, manipulation, and passive-aggressive behaviors; members learn and perpetuate victim roles
Role stereotyping	Traditionalist; absolute; rigid rules; serves to control the system; departure from prescribed role can precipitate violence; members' growth and development restricted; members feel unable to leave or separate; parental coalition is nonexistent or in shambles; adult role model is of abuse/violence; role confusion and reversal

Data from references 7, 11, 15, 36, 42, 64, 68–74, 76.

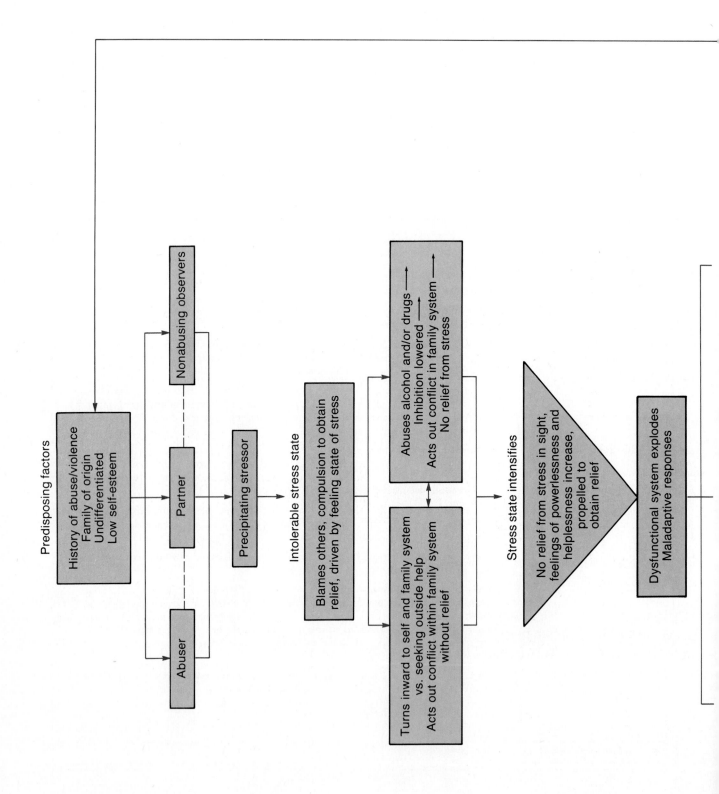

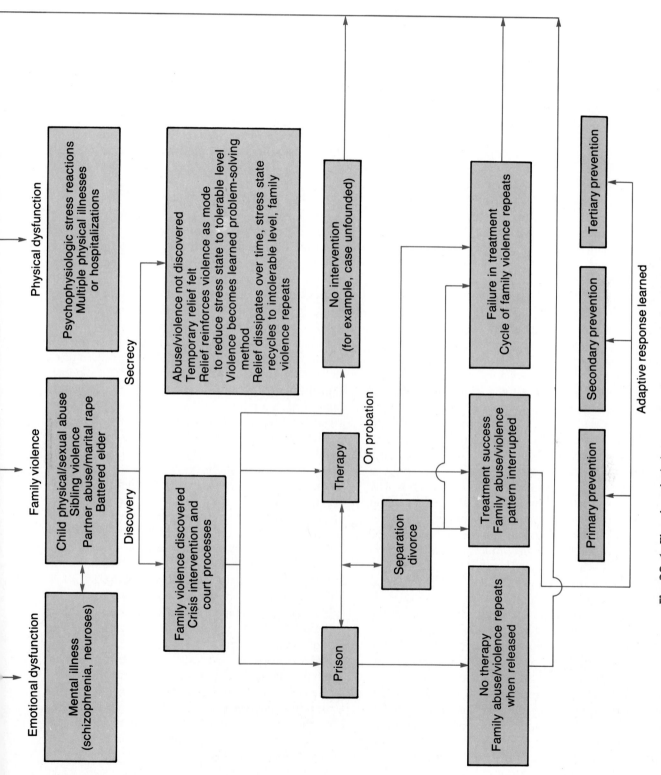

Fig. 32-1. Flowchart depicting stress reaction process in family abuse and violence.

of kissing, fondling of genital areas, mutual masturbation, fellatio or cunnilingus, sodomy, attempted or actual coitus, and nonphysical activity or stimulation which includes acts of exposure of the genitals, use of pornographic materials, voyeurism and verbalized sexual fantasies"[13,65,71–74]

The family system will respond differently to violence depending on the predominant **motive** of the abusive/violent person throughout the episode. For example, the system responds to extreme aggressive violence with high levels of anxiety and fear for physical safety and survival, whereas power violence tends to generate responses of guilt, repressed anger and hostility, reactive depression, and an impaired ability to trust.[30] Although family violence may contain elements of both aggressive and power motives, usually one of the two elements will be predominant.

If the violent behavior is **aggressive,** it is characterized by an extreme use of force, causing physical injury to the victim. It is episodical, unplanned, and often impulsive. The language tends to be abusive with the use of obscenities and swearing. The abusive person's mood is one of depression and rage over unmet needs and perceived wrongs, injustices, or "put downs," and the assault is usually of a short duration.[30] The most frequently identified forms of aggressive violent behavior are families of domestic and sibling violence and child physical abuse.

In contrast, if the violent behavior is a result of unresolved **power** issues, it is characterized by anxiety because of intolerable feelings of inadequacy, insecurity, loneliness, and low self-esteem. Force is used only to subdue, dominate, or gain the victim's compliance. The language is inquisitive or instructional and demanding to control the victim's and other family members' responses. The victim is usually not harmed but may be held captive for long hours while the abusive person attempts to relieve stress. The assault is usually premeditated and planned with "props" or fantasies that are acted out as part of "the act," and the behavior tends to be repetitive and increase in violence over time as the abuser's needs continue to be unmet and his sense of desperation intensifies to relieve pent-up stress.[30] The most frequently identified forms of power violence include child sexual abuse and elder abuse.

Last, the form of family violence is defined by the **scapegoat,** or **target,** of released aggression or unresolved power issues within the emotional and relationship subsystems. Forms of family violence defined by aggression and unresolved power issues include:

1. **Child physical abuse:** Any mistreatment, physical or mental, brought about through acts of commission or omission by parents or other care givers[43]

2. **Child sexual abuse:** The forced or pressured sexual acts on a child or adolescent by another person[27]

3. **Spouse partner/abuse:** The physical, social, psychological, material, or sexual violation or injury of one's mate/partner

4. **Sibling abuse:** Violence between and among siblings that includes physical, psychological, material, social, or sexual acts

5. **Elder abuse:** The physical, psychological, material, medical, social, or sexual abuse or injury of a person 60 years of age or older who resides in the home of a son, daughter, or other relative or with a caretaker[71]

Theories on the etiology of family violence

Theories on the causation of family violence are abundant, overlap with each other in explaining determinants of family violence, and are incomplete in explaining family violence when standing alone. The greatest focus of debates on the etiology of family violence centers around whether the behavior is the outcome of external pressures or internal intrapsychic conflicts. It is important for nurses to be aware of theories on the etiology of family violence because the nurse's theoretical framework will affect the treatment approach implemented. Several theoretical models explaining family violence will be discussed briefly.[36]

Psychodynamic theories assert that the abuser was deprived of the necessary nurturance and mothering in childhood to be able to give to and nurture his own family as an adult. The focus is at the individual level on the abusive person's potential for abuse, and history of physical or sexual abuse as a child is recognized as a contributing factor. Attention is given to impaired trust and unrealistic expectations of others, a nonsupportive relationship with a mate, and a tendency toward emotional and social isolation. Within the psychodynamic theories are contained theories about the characterological structure of the abusive person's personality. In particular, emphasis is placed on antisocial behaviors, drug and alcohol abuse, evidence of a criminal record, and lack of impulse control.

Many people are inclined to believe that the violent family and the abusive member in particular are mentally ill. Researchers and clinicians agree that family violence is the result of personality and system dysfunction; however, they disagree on whether that dysfunction constitutes mental illness. According to the DSM-III, a mental disorder is a "clinically significant behavioral or psychological syndrome or pattern that occurs in an individual typically associated with a painful symptom or impairment in one or more areas of functioning."[5]

According to the earlier discussion on the nature of the problem, family violence does fit the definition of mental disorders. Antagonists of the mental illness theory of family violence caution that the proponents of the theory tend to excuse the perpetrator's behavior as "sickness," rather than viewing it as irresponsibility and poor impulse control, for which the perpetrator is held responsible. Theories about mental illness focus on individual intrapsychic dynamics and thus fit under the category of psychodynamic theories of family violence.

Social learning theories emphasize the absence of healthy role models of parenting and problem-solving in childhood, which impairs a person's knowledge of and ability to provide parenting to others as an adult. Attention is given to behavior as a learned process that can be unlearned if the sequence of behaviors, precipitants, and preceding events are clearly identified.[8,54] Complementing social learning theories are psychosocial theories, which account for the influence of socialization processes, cultural scripting in society, social class, the community, and a variety of stressors such as unemployment, unwanted or too many children, or a "problem" child or elderly family member.

Environmental stress theories emphasize stress as the determinant of family violence. Proponents of environmental stress theories set up social programs to remove stress that results from poverty, poor education and occupational skills, and economic conditions that contribute to unemployment and poverty. Environmental theories also address factors in society that promote and maintain the expression of violence in relationships. Many of these factors were brought to public attention by the women's movement in the 1960s. The most predominate factor identified explains violence as the result of the inequity that exists between men and women, stronger and weaker persons, and older and younger people in our society. Proponents of this theory criticize western society for being patriarchial in that men and women are socialized to believe that males are inherently in positions of power because of their sex; women and children are socialized to be submissive and passive and taught to be subservient. This message of inferiority conveyed to females and children interferes with their development of self-esteem and identity, and contributes to their emotional and economic dependency on males or authority figures. Further, the dynamics of power and control are expressed through the societal belief of "property ownership" in which the acknowledged authority (e.g., caretaker of an elder or spouse) can do as one desires with one's "property." This socialization increases the vulnerability of a person to become a victim of violence, and interferes with his or her ability to terminate such relationships.

Family structure theories assert that violence is the result of problems around the system's enmeshment and disengagement, alliances, coalitions, boundaries, and role relationships.[50] It is believed that violence results from a faulty structure in the family system and that the behavior can be stopped by a reordering of structural properties among the members. Structural reorganization of the family system is believed to provide the members with a new emotional and relationship experience in a context different from that which caused the violence.

Family systems theories complement structural theories and incorporate many of the same formulations. It is believed that violent family members are at a low level of differentiation and are driven by feeling states (anxiety, low self-esteem, inadequacy, loneliness, depression, and so forth) to seek relief. Relief is sought by fleeing oneself and fusing with another person. This process creates intolerable tension, which is released through family violence in one or more dysfunctional processes: triangulation; marital conflict; dysfunction in a spouse, child, or elderly member; physical illness or psychophysiological distress; or emotional illness of a member. Treatment is directed toward helping individual members achieve higher levels of differentiation, ideally resulting in a family system that is more differentiated. The differentiation process requires changes in the members' emotional and relationship processes that result in higher and more adaptive functioning. It requires that family members gain an awareness of certain processes which operate in their family, for example, feeling states that drive individual members' behaviors and how other members in the system respond to them or fuel the process. Thus the system is taught to acquire impulse control; to stop, look, and observe instead of reacting to every stressor; and to "ride the wave" of stressors in a manner that puts self, and ultimately the family system, in command. Working on "self" in the system puts individual members in charge and in control of self, bringing the system into balance with a different form of equilibrium than that maintained by family violence. Feedback processes result in higher levels of self-esteem that reverberate throughout the family system, resulting in a wide range of positive outcomes, including higher levels of functioning, goal-directed behaviors, reaching out to others, and a realistic world view.

Epidemiological theories attempt to identify the incidence, distribution and control of family violence and incorporate all of the foregoing theories, taking into account the following: the agent (abuser, violent family system), environment (social and physical dimensions), host (child or adult victim, family scapegoat), and vector (socialization processes, cultural scripting in society).

TABLE 32-4

PRECONDITIONS FOR SEXUAL ABUSE

	Level of explanation	
	Individual	Social/cultural
Precondition I: Factors Related to Motivation to Sexually Abuse		
Emotional congruence	Arrested emotional development Need to feel powerful and controlling Re-enactment of childhood trauma to undo the hurt Narcissistic identification with self as a young child	Masculine requirement to be dominant and powerful in sexual relationships
Sexual arousal	Childhood sexual experience that was traumatic or strongly conditioning Modeling of sexual interest in children by someone else Misattribution of arousal cues Biologic abnormality	Child pornography Erotic portrayal of children in advertising Male tendency to sexualize all emotional needs
Blockage	Oedipal conflict Castration anxiety Fear of adult females Traumatic sexual experience with adult Inadequate social skills Marital problems	Repressive norms about masturbation and extramarital sex
Precondition II: Factors Predisposing to Overcoming Internal Inhibitors	Alcohol Psychosis Impulse disorder Senility Failure of incest inhibition mechanism in family dynamics	Social toleration of sexual interest in children Weak criminal sanctions against offenders Ideology of patriarchal prerogatives for fathers Social toleration for deviance committed while intoxicated Child pornography Male inability to identify with needs of children
Precondition III: Factors Predisposing to Overcoming External Inhibitors	Mother who is absent or ill Mother who is not close to or protective of child Mother who is dominated or abused by father Social isolation of family Unusual opportunities to be alone with child Lack of supervision of child Unusual sleeping or rooming conditions	Lack of social supports for mother Barriers to women's equality Erosion of social networks Ideology of family sanctity
Precondition IV: Factors Predisposing to Overcoming Child's Resistance	Child who is emotionally insecure or deprived Child who lacks knowledge about sexual abuse Situation of unusual trust between child and offender Coercion	Unavailability of sex education for children Social powerlessness of children

Reprinted with permission from Finkelhor, D.: Child sexual abuse: new theory and research, New York, 1984, The Free Press, pp. 56–57.

Epidemiological theories are comprehensive in attempting to explain family violence. Treatment is multifactorial, since no single factor is believed to exist in isolation from the others in causing family violence.

Finkelhor[23] applied epidemiological theories in another model that incorporates psychosocial characteristics of the offender, victim, and family specifying four preconditions to abuse: (1) motivation to abuse, (2) overcoming internal inhibitors to abuse, (3) overcoming external inhibitors to abuse, and (4) overcoming the resistance of the victim. Table 32-4 depicts the individual and social/cultural factors within these four preconditions that are necessary for child sexual abuse to occur. While the information is specific to child sexual abuse, many of the factors are common to more than one form or type of family abuse/violence. For example, in domestic violence the motivation to abuse would be the need to dominate, control, and feel powerful; overcoming internal inhibitors would be lack of impulse control; overcoming external inhibitors would be isolation of the family; and overcoming the victim's resistance would be the victim's low self-esteem.

Systems theories are a more contemporary perspective for understanding the etiology of family violence. In the systems theory model, four factors are identified as contributing to family violence: (1) individuals (offender, victim, observers), (2) family system, (3) environment, and (4) society. As in epidemiological models, the systems theory considers the etiology of family violence to be multifactorial. It occurs when the interaction of these four factors reaches a severely dysfunctional state such that the conflict in the system is acted out in an abusive or violent manner. Assessment is aimed at evaluating dimensions within each of these four factors for the extent to which any given factor contributes to the violent condition. Intervention is then specifically targeted to ameliorate the dimensions within these four factors that contributed to the violence. Assessment of and intervention in dimensions of one factor often overlap to include dimensions of other factors, for example, evaluating individual psychodynamics of the offender will often reveal characteristics about his family of origin which need to be considered when planning the intervention.

 # Assessment

■ Self-awareness

Self-awareness is the beginning of a nursing assessment. The moment the nurse comes into contact with a violent family, personal or subjective responses are elicited. It is particularly important for nurses to be aware of and in control of such responses. Violent families have a history of mistreatment that makes them extremely sensitive to any potential present mistreatment. They anticipate abuse and mistrust helping persons or authority figures. The nurse who unleashes a strong negative emotional reaction on the family is only continuing to fuel the maladaptive emotional climate and dysfunctional family processes. The family can then be expected to become more entrenched and impermeable, closing off the nurse, and thereby becoming resistant to therapy, since the nurse cannot impact on the system as a change agent.

Also, the nurse who is not aware of and in control of personal feelings is not in a position to provide objective and competent nursing interventions. In effect, the nurse will have fused with the violent family system. Negative feeling responses that violent families elicit in nurses include, but are not limited to, the following:

Anger	Intimidation
Betrayal	Mistrust
Disgust and revulsion	Powerlessness
Fear	Sadness
Frustration	Sympathy
Hopelessness	

Violent families can also elicit positive feeling states in nurses, such as humor, warmth, laughter, and pride in their achievements. These are responses that foster family healing rather than having destructive consequences.

Violent families also provoke a number of cognitive, attitudinal, and behavioral responses in nurses such as, but not limited to, the following:

Blaming the abuser, victim, or family members
Believing that change is hopeless
Commitment to prevention and eradication of family violence
Memories of personal experiences with abuse or violence
Research and publication of findings
Search for intervention methods that are effective
Social action

The nurse's thoughts and attitudes will affect what one does in response to family violence as a social problem and in therapy with violent families. Effective mental health therapists working with violent families believe that change is possible; the violence can and will stop. They refuse to give up on the family or feel hopeless and continue to search for, research, and report effective intervention methods. They also support social action that reduces or eliminates psychosocial environmental stressors which contribute to family violence.

■ Clinical assessment

Clinical assessment of the violent family incorporates all that is known about the nature of such a family discussed earlier in this chapter. The goal of clinical assessment is to identify which vulnerability factors present in the family made them particularly at risk for expressing violence, what precipitants were typically involved, what the family's strengths are, and where they are lacking in coping strategies. Based on this information a treatment plan is developed to reduce the family's vulnerability and reduce the use or occurrence of possible violent or abusive episodes. Treatment plans, then, are specific to the needs of an individual family and are developed to intervene in the dysfunctional state of both the family as a system and its members. A comprehensive assessment usually requires a minimum of four to six sessions and usually includes the use of individual, dyadic, family, and collateral (e.g., extended family, school personnel, clergy) sessions.[7,68,69]

Although the emphasis is on data collection for assessment purposes, these initial sessions also include elements of intervention. For example, the safety of the victim must be ensured, a contract is made to establish control over impulses such as suicidal attempts or further violent behavior, and rapport is established with the family. For the assessment phase of treatment, data are collected from the following sources[29,62]:

1. Face-to-face interviews with the complaintant, the victim, the mother or adult ally for the victim, the perpetrator, and collateral interviews
2. Physical evidence and medical examination
3. Behavioral observation
4. Field investigation
5. Documents
6. Referrals
7. Psychometric tests
8. Physiological measurements

Not all these data sources are utilized in every case. However, the more comprehensive the assessment is, the more able the clinician is to be "on target" with an effective intervention. Increasingly, clinicians and experts in the field of abuse and violence are using objective, reliable, and valid psychometric instruments in completing family assessments to complement and validate their subjective clinical assessments. If educated in the use and analysis of such instruments, nurses can complete this testing with families, otherwise another qualified member of the interdisciplinary team completes the testing. Since these instruments are completed by individual family members, the level or lack of congruence among family members in their perception of the family can be obtained, compared, and discussed in

treatment sessions. The data from these instruments also provide an objective measure of treatment progress and can be used, in addition, by the nurse or other health professional in testimony as an expert witness in legal proceedings. In addition to psychometric testing and data collection from the above cited sources, a variety of procedures are implemented to assess the family. These include the use of family sculpting, family drawings, eco-map completion, genograms, family role-playing, family story-telling, and observing the communication flow of who talks to whom, when, and how.[7,68,69]

In conjunction with the above measures, the nurse completes an assessment of a violent family system according to a given conceptual framework or model. Each of the concepts of the systems theory model will now be described.

■ **FAMILY SYSTEM.** The family system consists of those individuals who contribute to the functional state of the family as a system. Contemporary views about factors contributing to abusive or violent behavior use a vulnerability[30,82] or diathesis-stress[56] framework. Using these frameworks, Trepper and Barrett[68] assert that all families are endowed with a degree of vulnerability to be dysfunctional based on individual, family, and environmental factors which may be expressed in a particular form of violence if a precipitating event takes place and the family's coping skills are low. In their assessment model the individual, family, and dyadic interactions are evaluated based on the following vulnerability factors[44,46–49]:

1. **Family of origin.** The family of origin of the adult(s) in the household is viewed as a possible contributor to the violence in the nuclear family. Often current or presenting violence is the result of a multigenerational transmission process where these adults were themselves childhood victims or observers of violence in the nuclear family. Such a history increases the likelihood of violence being expressed in the family being evaluated.[52,55,80] Other factors that are assessed include the degree of childhood emotional deprivation or neglect including alternating periods of overinvolvement, conditional love, actual or emotional abandonment, and the style of discipline including physical abuse. It is recommended that this history be corroborated with information from extended family members.[7,68,69]

2. **Family style.** Family style is defined as those pervasive patterns characteristic of the family's interaction. A rigid family style of interaction is characterized by inflexible rules, traditional sex-role stereotyping, and a strict hierarchy. A cha-

otic/disorganized family style is characterized by being leaderless with inappropriate and fluctuating formal roles, and constantly changing family rules. For both rigid and chaotic/disorganized types of family styles, satisfaction of the emotional needs of individual members is sought primarily or entirely within the family, outsiders are perceived as threatening, and the family is socially isolated from the community.[7,68,69]

3. **Family structure.** Family structure refers to the way in which the family is organized according to roles, rules, power, and hierarchies. Building on the work of Minuchin,[44] Barrett and co-workers[7] identified five family structure classifications which are most common in maintaining and promoting family violence: (1) father executive; (2) mother executive; (3) third generation; (4) chaotic; and (5) estranged father (see Table 32-5).

4. **Family communication.** The style of communication among family members is the final dimension evaluated in assessing a family's vulnerability to violence. Typically, communication patterns between adult-adult and adult-child evidence conflict avoidance or high overt and covert conflict levels, hostility, and double-binding communication. These families usually lack the ability to communicate emotions or feelings effectively.

In addition to these vulnerability factors, the following family characteristics should also be assessed:

1. Boundaries
2. Mood/feeling tone
3. Autonomy/differentiation
4. Trust
5. Conflict
6. Regulation of drives
   a. Alcohol and/or substance abuse[53]

TABLE 32-5

FAMILY STRUCTURE CLASSIFICATIONS IN ABUSIVE AND VIOLENT FAMILIES

Father executive	The father or male adult is in charge, controls, and directs the family. The adult male tends to have a family style that is characterized by rigid, dominant-aggressive patterns, and stereotypic sex-role views. The executive male rules the family like a dictator expecting the family to be responsible for meeting his needs, and demands economic and emotional dependence. He will usually isolate the family physically and socially to ensure their dependence on him and his power. The victim is forced to be submissive and compliant, and is passive with little or no power.
Mother executive	The mother or adult female is the sole person in charge, controlling and directing the family. The adult male or father functions in many respects as "one of the children" with little or no parental responsibilities and may, in fact, be "parented" by the executive female. In an attempt to alleviate his sense of powerlessness, he may resort to aggression and violence against the children.
Third generation	The mother or adult female interacts and reacts in the same manner and style as a grandparent or third generation extended family member. She has a polar relationship with the children and "parents" the executive male. At times she acts like an observer of the family, very removed and distant emotionally; at other times she moves in with great executive force and emotional closeness.
Chaotic-disorganized	No person is in charge or available for the executive role to direct the family system. Rules, boundaries, and formal roles are not enforced by any one person as parents and children function on the same level as peers. Most of the family members have little tolerance to control impulses, seek immediate gratification, evidence immature judgment, and interact like siblings exploiting one another.
Estranged father	The adult female or mother functions similar to the executive mother style. The adult male is divorced, literally or emotionally, from the executive female and holds no power in directing the family system. The emotional or physical absence of a partner to satisfy basic needs typically results in one of the family members being victimized.

Modified and adapted from references 7, 68, and 69.

b. Aggression
c. Sexuality
7. Time binding
8. Task performance
9. Communication
10. Belief system
11. Power ratio
12. Role stereotyping
13. Relationship and social skills[53]
 a. Intrafamily interpersonal: Husband-wife, father-child, mother-child, child-child, adult-elder, child-elder
 b. Adult sexual: Relationships between adults, between adults and children
 c. Child sexual: Relationships with adults, peers, younger children
 d. Interpersonal/social: Outside of family, larger external systems
14. Health problems of any family member[53]
15. Form of family violence[30]
 a. Type of acts committed
 b. Motivation for the offense
 c. Style of attack
 d. Selection of the victim
 e. Response to attack by perpetrator and family members
 f. Safety or protection issues: Presence of functioning adult ally for the victim or history of threats, use of force or violence

A descriptive statement should be made for each factor as illustrated in the following example:

Criteria	Example
Boundaries	Mr. and Mrs. X are closed to outsiders and helping persons. The family is socially isolated, and they have few friends.
Mood/feeling tone	The family is engaged in intense competition for caring, attention, and nurturance. The mood is one of depression and pain, with members lacking empathy for each other.
Autonomy/differentiation	The children demonstrate precocious maturity and responsibility for the family. The elders depend on the family because of impairments from aging. The mother is fused with her family of origin, which creates marital conflict with her spouse.

Completing such an assessment gives the nurse data on the nature of the family as a system, and areas requiring intervention are specifically identified.

■ **ENVIRONMENT.** Environment refers to the circumstances, objects, or conditions that surround and have an immediate influence on the life of the family and its members.[77] Assessment of environmental factors takes into account physical and social variables. In making an assessment of the family the nurse evaluates the following stressors:[30,36,67,76]

1. Employment
 a. Present status part-time, full-time, unemployed
 b. Pattern of employment
 c. Job satisfaction
 d. Self-actualization
 e. Number of members employed combined with role stereotyping
 f. Marketable skills
2. Financial status
 a. Management techniques
 b. Recent increases or reductions in income
 c. Type of occupational preparation
 d. Resources
3. Housing
 a. Adequacy
 b. Crowded conditions
 c. Cleanliness, order, upkeep
4. Transportation
 a. Use of a car
 b. Use of public transportation
 c. Financial burden
 d. Refusal to use available means or social mobility
5. Support services
 a. Nature of the relationship with extended family including noncontact, high conflict, triangulation, projection processes, and scapegoating
 b. Nature and extent of relationships with neighbors and friends
 c. Degree of religious beliefs and use of church and religious affiliates
 d. Availability and use of a local support group
 e. Use of social service agencies
 f. Perception of coping resources and support systems
6. Precipitating stressors
 a. Nature
 b. Origin
 c. Timing
 d. Number
7. Criminal justice system
 a. History of criminal/delinquent offenses
 b. Current probation status
 c. Present and past status of criminal charges

An attempt is made to identify both predisposing and precipitating stressors that contribute to family violence. Frequently cited stressors include unemployment or part-time employment, limited education and support systems in achieving career goals, and financial difficulties. No single factor is believed to be causative of family violence, but rather it is the accumulation of multiple stressors that cannot be accommodated or dissipated within the family system that leads to violence.

■ **SOCIETY.** Society refers to a nation, community, or broad grouping of people who establish particular aims, beliefs, or standards of living and conduct.[77] Society is the mode by which cultural scripting and socialization processes are communicated to and within the family system. Cultural variables that the nurse assesses include, but are not limited to, the following:[30,36,76]

1. Attitudes
   a. Toward the family and individual members
   b. Toward outsiders, support services, and helping persons
   c. Toward the use of physical punishment
   d. Toward sex and sexual relationships
2. Value systems
3. Sex-role stereotyping
4. Way of life
5. Language
6. Ethical positions

Cultural scripting often includes positions that uphold the sanctity and privacy of the family and view outside help as interference in the private domain of the family. The family is likely to report a belief in traditional sex roles and sanction the use of physical punishment in "disciplining" its members.

Professionals and social activists focus on the means by which cultural scripting is communicated, such as the way in which mass media portrays and sanctions violence as a way of life or solving problems. Intervention then focuses on altering learned attitudes, value systems, and behaviors and is often combined with teaching the family members different or alternative attitudes and behaviors, such as more effective child-rearing practices. The final factor to consider is that of the victim and the impact of family violence on that person.

■ **INDIVIDUALS.** The final dimension to be evaluated is the personality characteristics of individual family members including: the offender, victim, and nonabusing observers such as other adults of children.

Offenders. Offenders are defined as persons who perpetrate violence on others. Their violent behavior usually follows a cyclical nature (see Figure 32-1) with a calm period, followed by a build-up of tension producing violence, and ending with a "honeymoon" or "make-up" phase. It is this "honeymoon" phase that is addictive in two respects: (1) the offender acts like such a "nice guy" through presents, courting behaviors, and apologies, that the victim often dismisses the seriousness of the abuse and attends only to the attractive qualities of the offender; and (2) the relief of tension experienced by the offender from the outburst of violence becomes addictive in itself, such that the cycle rebuilds and tension relief is sought through the same violent behavior.

Not all offenders follow a cyclical pattern. For some offenders, their violent behavior is episodic or considered a "regressed" behavior under high levels of stress, rather than what is sometimes referred to as a "fixated" life-style.

Offenders tend to be immature, insecure, dominant, aggressive, rigid, and moralistic within the family. They generally lack impulse control, need immediate gratification, and do not feel guilty for their violence. These persons usually have symbiotic personalities expressed by their undifferentiated state and behaviors, expect all of their needs to be met within the family, and are constantly searching for love and adoration. Their interpersonal relationships are poor or unsatisfying, and they have a diminished capacity for intimacy. Substance abuse is not uncommon and is frequently used as an "excuse" for their behavior. A sexual disorder may be present and, in some cases, leads to blaming the victim for the dysfunction or violent act. Although a diagnosis of psychosis is uncommon, its presence contributes to a vulnerability to express violence.

Victims. The victim is defined as the scapegoat, or target, of family violence and includes children, adults, and the elderly. Victims are generally selected by the offender based on a variety of or a set of circumstances such as old age and infirmity. Victims will present on assessment with evidence of low self-esteem, passivity, dependency, and submissiveness. These qualities are a direct result of being victimized as well as learned behaviors in the interest of survival. The victim often has a special status such as "daddy's little girl," "adoring wife," or "infirmed parent," and may have learned to use the status position as a means of gaining affection and preventing or postponing repeat victimization. Thus, "manipulative" behavior is a learned behavior in response to victimization. In addition, role-reversal such as a child assuming adult responsibilites, or an elderly adult relegated to a child's position, is also a frequent characteristic. The emphasis in assessing these personality characteristics of the victim is not to convey that this person caused or is responsible for their victimization. Rather these qualities are assessed so that the nurse can help this person change these qualities to ensure that future violence does not occur.[39]

Nonabusing observers. Observers consist of those adults and children in both nuclear and extended families who neither perpetrate the violence nor are the victim. Frequently they are aware, on some level, of the violent behavior, yet report feeling helpless to do anything about it. On assessment "observers" evidence low self-esteem, emotional or economic dependence on the abuser or family system, submissiveness or compliance, placating or peacemaking behaviors, little or no use of outside resources, social isolation or restriction, and self-blame.

In assessing individuals, data are collected in relation to: (1) the personality characteristics of individual family members that contribute to the violent behavior; and (2) the acute and long-term impact of the violent behavior on individual members' psychosocial function.[7,68,69] As with family system assessment, objective and projective psychometric testing such as the MMPI, TAT, and Purdue Sexuality Questionnaire are being used more often to complement subjective clinical assessments of individual family members' personality characteristics. Specifically, data on individual family members include the following:

1. Developmental life state
   a. Tasks accomplished
   b. Tasks not accomplished
2. Feelings about self
3. Power
4. Relationships
5. Intrapsychic conflicts
6. Regulation of drives
7. Boundaries
8. Psychosocial values/belief system
9. Coping style
10. Skills/task management
11. Family background
12. Crisis state

Assessment of individual members tends to be specific to the form of family violence and can be quite comprehensive. Most of the clinical assessments reported in the literature tend to focus on the violent member. This is in keeping with the fact that many health care settings and therapists focus on the individual rather than the entire family as a system. As more care providers take a family approach in treating family violence, more tools will be developed, reflecting the dysfunctional state of the other members in the system. The results of a careful assessment are utilized to formulate a nursing diagnosis of the problems requiring intervention.

 Nursing diagnosis

A comprehensive nursing diagnosis of family violence includes the family's maladaptive responses and related stressors, as well as the family's assets and resources. These assets or resources are then used in planning interventions related to the family's problem areas or stressors. For example, the nurse could emphasize that the family is able to "get done those things which need to be done," such as housework, or that they are a good team together. Such a family has the skill to solve the dilemma around who does what in the house. They may reverse roles to get the work done by having the son or daughter do the laundry, cooking, and cleaning instead of the parents. The nurse emphasizes that the family's asset is one of management skills whereas its liability is in functioning as a group related to the assumed or assigned responsibilities and tasks. Or the nurse might assess and emphasize that the family members have a sense of humor, which decreases tension in the family. The family has the ability therefore to respond with warmth and empathy to each other. However, its liability is in their use of humor to discount serious problems, such as financial difficulties. The nurse role models how to talk about stressful topics (financial difficulties), while using humor to balance working out the problem operationally. The asset identified by the nursing diagnosis is thus used to the family's advantage in making changes in the system's dysfunctional patterns and interactions.

After a list of maladaptive responses and stressors is compiled, the listings can be conceptualized as meeting the criteria of one or more nursing diagnoses approved by the North American Nursing Diagnosis Association (NANDA). Selected maladaptive responses and related factors that frequently arise in working with violent families are depicted in Table 32-6. A maladaptive family response can apply to one or more nursing diagnoses. The outcome of this process is to identify a pattern of responses, stressors, and related factors that can guide the nurse in planning interventions for the dysfunctional aspects of the family system, while capitalizing on family assets.[1]

The maladaptive family pattern that emerges from this conceptualization will then meet the criteria and defining characteristics of one or more of the following NANDA nursing diagnoses that are related to coping:

- Ineffective individual coping
- Ineffective family coping: compromised
- Ineffective family coping: disabling
- Family coping: potential for growth

Other nursing diagnoses that the nurse would consider based on a case specific family assessment include: anxiety, impaired communication, alterations in family processes, fear, potential for injury, knowledge deficit, noncompliance, alterations in parenting, posttrauma response, hopelessness, impaired social interaction, powerlessness, rape trauma syndrome, sensory-perceptual alterations, sexual dysfunction, social isolation, spiritual distress, alterations in thought processes, and potential for violence.[17]

TABLE 32-6

MALADAPTIVE RESPONSES AND RELATED FACTORS IN ABUSIVE AND VIOLENT FAMILIES*

Maladaptive family responses	Related factors			
	Personal factors of family members	Style of interaction on average daily basis	Historical or developmental factors	Social factors
Denial of violent behavior related to extreme emotional deprivation and low self-esteem	X	X	X	X
Compulsive acting out of violent behavior related to failure of family to disclose the act and of society to respond	X	X		X
Obsessive fantasies of violent acts and accompanying behaviors related to loneliness and low self-esteem	X			
Impaired ability to trust related to violation of rights and lack of physical safety	X	X	X	
Poor social skills related to social isolation of family	X	X		X
Inadequate ego strength and emotional deprivation related to childhood neglect and violence	X		X	
Inadequate controls and limit setting related to severe low esteem	X	X	X	
Magical expectations related to coping style of denial and discounting	X	X		
Fear of authority related to violence by authority figures	X	X	X	
Depression related to self-hate and lack of achievements	X	X		X
Blurred role boundaries and role confusion related to reversal and family coalitions		X		
Repressed anger and hostility related to abuse of power and poor communication patterns	X	X		
Lack of empathy related to competition for nurturance and attention	X	X		
Isolation related to feelings of inadequacy, low self-esteem, and fear	X	X		X
Repetitive violence related to denial, discounting, and low self-esteem	X	X	X	
Pseudomaturity coupled with failure to accomplish developmental tasks related to role reversal, family coalitions, and boundary violations	X	X		
Guilt related to participation in violence with failure to resist or disclose it	X	X		
Negative self-concept related to negative appraisals by family system and outsiders	X	X	X	X

*Family assets and resources should also be assessed for each family.

The nursing diagnosis is best completed with the family participating in the process. However, at this time, the majority of violent families do not acknowledge that a problem exists and often are in treatment only as a result of a court order. Developing a collaborative relationship with the family in involuntary treatment is often a major task of the nurse in the first phase of therapy. Despite these limitations, the nurse needs to make every effort to formulate a nursing diagnosis and treatment plan with the family.

🔸 Planning and implementation

▪ Goal setting and formulating a treatment plan

The general goal of the nurse working with a violent family is to help them achieve a higher and healthier level of functioning. Goal setting is specific to the individual and system functioning of a given family, and is directed by the following:

1. Vulnerability factors
2. Coping skills
3. Strengths and resources
4. Precipitating stressors
5. Environmental context
6. Societal influences
7. Nursing diagnosis, specifically the presenting maladaptive response
8. Intensity of the problem or level of illness (e.g., compulsive acting out of violent behavior in contrast to obsession with violent behavior)
9. Form of family violence
10. Role, setting, and point in time at which the nurse sees the family (e.g., general nursing care, family therapy, follow-up care, or prevention program)

Most violent families come to the attention of professionals when the violence is initially disclosed or reported. Short-term goal planning at this time requires that three key questions be answered[30]:

- ▪ How probable is it that this family will behave in a way that will jeopardize the safety of another person?
- ▪ Under what psychosocial conditions is such behavior most likely to occur?
- ▪ What is the likelihood that these psychosocial conditions will prevail?

The treatment plan will be different, depending on whether or not it is probable that the family violence will be repeated and whether the conditions that contribute to the violence are removed. Initial plans address the following management areas[30,61,76]:

1. Report to authorities
   a. Police
   b. Child welfare
   c. Center for victims
2. Safety
   a. Physical: Is behavior repetitive?
   b. Environment: What family environmental stressors are present?
   c. Society: What standards, values, and beliefs of the family's community promote and maintain abuse or violence?
   d. Psychological: What characteristics of the family and its members contribute to the family's vulnerability for expressing abuse or violence?
3. Medical examination and evidence collection
4. Decision regarding separation
   a. Abuser from victim and family
   b. Victim from abuser and family
   c. Family from victim and abuser
5. Treatment decisions
   a. Outpatient therapy: Individual, group, family, community
   b. Residential treatment
   c. Incarceration
6. Essential life-support, therapeutic, and social services
7. Anticipatory guidance
8. Preparation for court

Once initial management decisions are made, the family is usually in treatment. The planning phase then reflects the type of therapy being implemented to eradicate target behaviors and processes, as well as to learn new behaviors and processes in the family system. For example, the work done in crisis intervention (removal of the abuser from the home and placement of children in a shelter) is very different from the work done in family therapy (restructuring role and emotional relationships in the system) or group therapy (individual members working on their own ability to identify feeling states, triggers, tools, sequences of behaviors, outcomes, and reinforcers as interplayed with the family system dynamics). The problems identified by the nursing diagnosis become the target areas for formulating goals of treatment and areas for nursing intervention. Such intervention may include short-term and long-term treatment at the secondary and tertiary levels of prevention. Several treatment models currently being implemented in therapy with violent families will now be presented.

▪ Interventions in secondary prevention

The discussion of intervention in family violence will begin with secondary prevention, that is, the point in time at which the violence comes to the attention of authorities, and outside help is usually legally brought to bear on the family system. It is at this time that a nurse with a master's degree in psychiatric–mental health nursing might see the violent family as a primary therapist or co-therapist. Furthermore, given the staggering statistics on the incidence of violence, it is expected that nurses in all fields of practice will see members of violent families for their various health needs.

■ **CRISIS INTERVENTION APPROACH.** Crisis intervention is the first model of care that can be implemented with violent families. A crisis is defined as an upset in a steady state when, temporarily, a person's usual mode of coping is ineffective and results in dysfunction, decompensation, or disorganization.[2,16] Crisis intervention theory (Chapter 10) asserts that if a person's perceptions of an event, coping mechanisms, and support systems are kept in balance, a crisis state can be avoided or reversed.[2] Usually when violent families come to the attention of authorities, all three balancing factors are separately and together in imbalance; for example, the family is no longer allowed to perceive violent behavior as tolerable or acceptable because of society's sanctions. The coping mechanism (violence acted out) is no longer effective if only because the violence is disclosed and the family's boundaries (secrecy) are permeated. Support systems are usually absent or cut off because of the family's maladaptive social isolation prior to disclosure of the violence and to society's stigma and social rejection of families involved in such violence. The violent family is thus in a severe crisis state. Given the extreme imbalance in the family's steady state, the system is particularly open to therapeutic intervention at this time. Unfortunately, the family is not often in therapy at this point but rather is coping with separation and prosecution. It is more often the case that the family will be seen by a therapist 3 to 6 weeks after disclosure of the violence, when the family is already beginning to "seal off" outsiders and is more entrenched in protecting itself from invasion.

Crisis intervention in family violence is well documented and discussed in the literature.[2,61,76] The reader is referred to these writings because each form of family violence has procedures and protocols that are varied, yet comprehensive. Intervention that can be provided is also influenced by legislation in the nurse's state of residence and other factors, such as the decision of the judge and the testimony of professionals or other witnesses. This is illustrated in Clinical example 32-2.

Clinical example 32-2 reflects the importance of professionals and legal officials working together in making decisions that affect therapy with violent families. It is particularly important that professionals arrive at a level of agreement about such cases before testifying in court. If not, they may act out the family's dynamics around power plays, a game the family is quite good at playing. The person who ultimately suffers is the victim who lives on a daily basis with the constant terror of abuse and violence.

During crisis intervention the following steps are usually implemented[67,76]:

CLINICAL EXAMPLE 32-2

Hearing: A hearing was held before a judge to determine whether it was safe for two children to be returned to the home of a child sexual abuser.

Accused abuser: Charges had been dropped against the abuser by his wife 2 weeks after the petition for prosecution. She "could not live without him." The accused denied ever having committed the crime, the charges were dropped, and no legal record reflecting conviction was "on the books." The accused and his wife wanted the children returned home. The accused stayed in therapy with the two co-therapists and a family therapist.

Co-therapists: Both testified that the accused was not in control of himself, that he was not working in therapy on himself, and that the children were at risk for sexual abuse if returned home. They recommended that the wife could care for all the children and the accused should be removed from the home or that all the children remain out of the home at this time until the accused, through work in therapy, was safe in the home.

Wife: Testified that their relationship had changed since the disclosure. She had assumed mothering responsibilities and their sex life had improved. She wanted her family together and would kill herself if she had to choose between her children and her husband. She cried on the stand.

Family therapist: Testified that the family relationships had been restructured with parents in their appropriate roles (Minuchin model). The accused had become less domineering in the home and was respected by his peers at church. He believed the accused was safe in the home and the children should be returned home, but he admitted that he never had dealt with the accused's sexually abusive behavior or dynamics. (The family therapist was from a different agency than the co-therapists.)

Children and youth services: Testified that they could not safely recommend that the children be returned to the home.

Grandmother: Testified that the children were not safe in the home. (The accused and wife testified that they thought the grandmother, who was currently caring for the children, was trying to split them up.)

Judge's decision: Return the children to the home.

I. Police/legal intervention
   a. Receiving the complaint
   b. Arriving at the scene
   c. Gaining entry
   d. Establishing control
   e. Protecting the victim
   f. Interviewing the victim
   g. Interviewing witnesses
   h. Interviewing the assailant
   i. Gathering evidence
   j. Arrest
      1. Prosecution
      2. Charges dropped
      3. No petition to prosecute
      4. Separation of the perpetrator from the family
II. Hospital intervention
   a. Treatment of injuries
   b. Collection of evidence according to protocol
III. Children and youth services
   a. Complaint filed with police
   b. Investigation of complaint
   c. Interviews with the victim, accused, family members
   d. Collateral interviews
   e. Assessment of the home situation and environment
      1. Welfare assistance as needed
      2. Homemaker services
   f. Separation of the victim, accused, or family as necessary
   g. Shelter, group home, or residential treatment
IV. Psychological intervention
   a. Hotline crisis counseling
   b. Therapy
      1. Specific to form of violence (e.g., Parents United/Parents Anonymous; rape crisis center)
      2. Community mental health center
      3. Private therapist
   c. Referral for long-term therapy with the same or a different agency
V. Community linkages initiated
   a. Medical institutions
   b. Social service agencies
   c. Criminal justice agencies
   d. Legal aid
   e. Vocational rehabilitation
   f. Support or self-help groups

Crisis intervention with violent families usually merges with and extends into longer term therapy, counseling, and social service intervention. It is this phase of therapy that is the least described or discussed in the literature. The following discussion presents some models currently being implemented in therapy with violent families. The extent of their effectiveness remains to be researched.

■ **INDIVIDUAL PSYCHOTHERAPY APPROACH.** Generally, violent family members are not in individual psychotherapy as the primary mode of therapeutic intervention. Individual psychotherapy is more often used as an adjunct to group or family therapy.[59] It is believed by experts in victimology that the character structure and life-style of the family members is not conducive to traditional or classic psychoanalytical psychotherapy. The level of denial is so severe that family members are extremely resistant to therapeutic change by classic methods. Another reason violent families are not seen primarily in individual therapy is that they desperately need to experience the curative factors that group therapy has to offer. The family needs to decrease social isolation and make new friends, have "input" from a variety of sources to open up their closed system, develop social skills, feel wanted and a sense of belonging, and feel accepted and cared about.[36]

When individual therapy is used for violent offenders and their family members, two goals are addressed. First, since therapy cannot successfully progress as long as any or all family members are in active denial, clinicians in the field have found that individual sessions with these persons helps to "break through" this process enabling the person to be more amenable and to benefit from dyadic, group, and family therapy. Active denial does not mean that therapy must be terminated; it simply means that different strategies need to be implemented to accommodate the denial.[68,69] Barrett and co-workers[7] identified at least four types of denial in violent families (see Table 32-7). When the victim evidences any of these types of denial it may be necessary that individual sessions be conducted to ameliorate this condition. These sessions also offer support and validation of the victim and begin the process of reversing personality characteristics that make one vulnerable to victimization.

In intervening in a state of denial, the basic principles of working through or mastering resistance in psychotherapy described by Weiner[79] and Anderson and Stewart[6] apply. First, the nurse must understand both what is behind the denial and its importance and function for both individual family members and the family system as a whole. With violent individuals and their families, the emotional need to deny is based on actual or fantasized fears, such as fears of divorce, abandonment, and poverty; verbal and nonverbal pressure to remain loyal to the family; conflictual feelings over choosing between the needs of the abuser and those of the victim and other family members; and the desire to protect the family from outside threats, rejection, or further isolation.

In individual therapy, the nurse establishes a paradoxical balance in which the person's emotional need to deny is supported, while being simultaneously challenged to accept the factual evidence of their violent behavior, such as medical reports, bruises, or broken bones. Such intervention requires that the nurse elicit and be empathetic to these concerns or fears, yet challenge the parent, partner, sibling, or caretaker, and for other family members to function in ways that prevent further violence. Since it is difficult for these persons to admit their violent behavior or role in contributing to the event, an effective strategy is to ask a hypothetical question in a paradoxical and puzzled manner such as, "If it were true (and I am not saying that it is), what do you fear would happen to you and your family?"[7,68] If active denial persists on the part of an offender or other family members, then legal counsel rather than therapy is needed.[7]

Second, maladaptive personality characteristics and issues important to the offender, victim, or nonabusing observers are the focus of individual therapy. The goal is to help these persons achieve effective levels of functioning as individuals and within the family system. All individual therapy sessions are usually provided by the family therapist and are coordinated with family therapy.[7,68]

Offender sessions. A number of issues are worked on in the individual therapy that help the offender become aware of and alter the many complex factors that contributed to his or her violent behavior. Active denial of the offender and the need for this defense are continuously challenged and worked through. Contributing factors from one's family of origin and psychosocial development are also focused on. In addition, life concerns that facilitate personal growth are explored, and personal goals are established and implemented. Individual sessions reinforce that the offender is not "crazy" because of his behavior but is simply not in control of impulses, and that one can learn this behavior. These sessions also provide an opportunity for the offender to share, often for the first time, many of the details of the event. Barriers that inhibit effective functioning and triggers to violent behavior are identified, and alternative coping skills are explored and implemented.[7,68,69]

Victim sessions. Therapeutic issues focused on in individual sessions with the victim include low self-esteem, feelings about being victimized, differentiation, and peer group issues. The therapist is often the victim's major ally or support system throughout the treatment process. A careful balance needs to be found in which the therapist protects (without overprotecting) the victim in bringing issues to the family sessions and encourages the victim to take appropriate risks related to personal growth and improving family functioning. The type of intervention implemented depends on the age of this person. With young children under the age of 5, the most common strategy is the use of play-therapy and parent-child sessions. Through the use of play therapy, the victim is encouraged to freely express feelings and thoughts, learn ways of protecting oneself, and adopt appropriate behavior. Through these sessions the child relearns to trust, has an opportunity to ameliorate feelings of guilt, and experiences intimacy that is not destructive. It is often helpful to include an adult ally of the victim in these sessions.

With juvenile or adolescent children, individual sessions focus on helping them work through feelings of guilt, responsibility for the event, shame, depression, and anger. Post-traumatic stress disorder symptoms are explained to them in language they can understand so that symptoms (such as flashbacks and nightmares) are predicted, described as time-limited, and normalized as part of the healing process. This provides the children

---

TABLE 32-7

TYPES OF DENIAL IN ABUSIVE/VIOLENT FAMILIES

Type	Parent	Child
Denial of facts	"It never happened"	"It never happened"
Denial of awareness	"I was drunk"	"I was asleep"
Denial of impact	"It didn't harm her"	"It doesn't affect me"
Denial of responsibility	"She came on to me"	"It wasn't my fault"

Reprinted with permission of Barrett, M.J., Skyes, C., and Byrnes, W.: A systemic model for the treatment of intrafamily child sexual abuse. Chicago, 1985, Midwest Family Resource Center.

with a feeling of control over their world which is essential to their post-trauma adjustment. In addition, the therapist focuses on ways in which the victim can prevent future experiences of being victimized through behaviors such as assertiveness, use of resources, personal growth and differentiation, and trusting intuitive feelings and judgments about safety. These sessions also provide a forum in which the victim can define, without pressure from the family system, how they would like their role in the family to be different.

Adult victims face some of the same issues that young people do. For example, individual sessions focus on describing, time limiting, and normalizing posttraumatic stress disorder symptoms as part of their healing process. Feelings of guilt, responsibility for the event, shame, low self-esteem, depression, and anger stemming from the victimization need to be worked through. Often, victims need to learn assertiveness skills and behaviors to protect themselves from repeat victimization. This intervention concurrently raises their self-esteem, sense of worth, and right to be treated with respect. Intimacy and relationship problems with both men and women are common. The victim must learn alternative ways of meeting needs and achieving goals without destructively "using" others. Trust needs to be relearned with the therapist and other people in the victim's life. The victim's human sexuality and, in some cases, sexual dysfunction, may need specific treatment with a sex therapist or qualified professional. Some victims need to learn that affection without sex can exist in a relationship and that sex does not need to be bartered or traded to gain affection or intimacy. Some victims may separate from or divorce, literally or emotionally, the offender or family, requiring a grief resolution process. With many victims it is important to help them ameliorate emotional and physical cut-offs and reconnect with their family of origin from a differentiated position. In some cases, the victim may be unable to leave the family. The nurse must then help this person to define what would make the quality of life in this family and the community more satisfying and fulfilling, and establish and implement feasible options.[7,68,69]

Finally, individual therapy reinforces the work done in group or family therapy. Patients might work on other problem areas, such as getting themselves out of financial difficulties or pursuing career goals, in individual therapy. What seems consistent across problem areas is the "powerless to power" dynamic, regardless of the issue being worked through or the approach to treatment.

■ **GROUP THERAPY APPROACH.** A variety of treatment approaches are used in group therapy with violent families ranging in focus from intervening in repetitive violent patterns to supporting personal growth.

Cognitive-behavior model. The cognitive-behavior model is built upon Beck's cognitive therapy of depression[8] and behavioral treatment models such as those used with persons who stop smoking or enter diet reduction programs. The treatment approach can be used in individual psychotherapy sessions, but group treatment has the advantage of the members helping each other by identifying the sequence of feelings, thoughts, and behaviors; confronting each other on rationalizations; and suggesting alternative coping skills. As a group approach, the model is applied with family members meeting in separate group sessions for offenders, victims, and nonabusing observers. The procedure described below may be implemented in separate steps; or steps 1, 2, and 3 may be implemented concurrently.

Step 1: Feeling States. Each group member begins by describing his or her own feeling states before, during, and after the event that either (a) led up to the violent behavior, (b) occurred in response to being victimized, or (c) occurred as a "silent" observer of the family process "in motion." The feeling states are "triggers" that put them "in motion" toward the event. The group member can then be helped to identify alternative coping skills at this very early phase of the cycle to prevent the event.

Step 2: Thoughts. The next step is to have each person describe the thoughts they experience before, during, and after the violent event. It is important to elicit without criticism or judgment as many thoughts as possible. Although many thought patterns reflect active denial and rationalization, these are not addressed at this time. It is important for the nurse to remain empathic and continue building rapport at this time.

Step 3: Behaviors. Step 3 involves recounting all behaviors that occur before, during, and after the event. It is important to get a detailed description of all behaviors because violent families often ignore, deny, or minimize these behaviors. This step gives them the opportunity to talk about the details of what they do when they are "in motion" or out of control. Offenders must learn alternative behaviors to cope with stress states; victims must learn behaviors to protect themselves; observers must learn to not be silent about family processes that result in violence.

Step 4: Family Composite. Family members can meet

for family or dyadic sessions to share their information, see how their patterns interlock, interact, contribute to, and maintain the event, and how their alternative coping skills are affecting their current family functioning. The nurse may choose to provide these sessions concurrent with any of the above steps to help family members early in therapy begin talking about alternative ways of coping.

Step 5: Restructuring. For each of the categories of feelings, thoughts, and behaviors, alternative coping skills are elicited. Rational-emotive therapy developed by Ellis[22] is particularly useful in refuting thought patterns and feeling states that promote and maintain violent behavior. Developing alternative behavior patterns that increase constructive coping skills will be specific to the situation of each group member.

Transactional analysis model. The transactional analysis model of treatment has been well developed and discussed in the literature over the last 15 years.[9,10] Application of the model in the treatment of violent families has been most thoroughly described by Justice and Justice[36] in their work with physically abusive families. In the transactional analysis model all three spheres of a person's functioning—cognitive, behavioral, and affective—are engaged in the treatment process. Justice and Justice treat the physically violent family by seeing the couple in group therapy with other couples who have the same problem; children do not attend these group therapy meetings.

Group treatment of the physically violent family involves the implementation of goals that arise out of the nursing diagnosis. In transactional analysis models of therapy the patients make a contract with the therapist to work on specific behaviors or problems, and goal achievement is specified by behavioral outcome statements. For example, a behavioral goal might be, "At the end of 1 week Mrs. X will have made one new friend" for the nursing diagnosis of "Severe social isolation related to feelings of inadequacy and worthlessness." Measurement of goal achievement is a way of systematically quantifying and measuring the effectiveness of treatment. Beyond the goals worked on in therapy, Justice and Justice also work on the following family system processes with physically abusive families. Behavioral outcomes are specified for each[36]:

1. *Symbiosis.* Shifting symbiotic relationship processes will be dissolved.
2. *Isolation.* Social and emotional isolation will be reduced.
3. *Talking and sharing with mate.* The couple will be able to talk and share with one another, intimately and superficially.
4. *Impatience/temper.* The family will demonstrate alternative nonviolent coping styles for working through frustrations.
5. *Child management.* The family will be knowledgeable about child growth and development and nonviolent child-rearing practices in parenting.
6. *Employment.* At least one spouse will obtain gainful employment within 3 weeks of entrance into treatment.

The behavioral outcome goals are then further operationalized for measurement. For example, dissolving the shifting symbiotic processes might include the following behavioral outcomes:

- Makes all or most decisions on one's own
- Offers suggestions to others when asked
- Takes responsibility for children when asked

These specific behavioral outcomes are then measured on a goal attainment scale (Table 32-8) that predicts the level of attainment on a five-point Likert scale of (1) most unfavorable outcome thought likely, (2) less than expected success, (3) expected level of success, (4) more than expected success, and (5) most favorable outcome thought likely.[36] The specific behavioral goals filled in are unique and individualized to each family's needs. The scale can then be used to monitor the family's progress in therapy.

In implementing goals of treatment, the transactional model of intervention utilizes the following approaches: (1) structural analysis of personality, (2) teaching about siamese-twinning life scripts, (3) relaxation and hypnosis therapy, and (4) gestalt and confrontation techniques.[36]

Structural analysis. As part of the work in helping patients gain a cognitive understanding of their difficulties, couples are taught in group therapy sessions how to structurally analyze their personalities. The couples come to recognize their Parent, Adult, and Child ego states involved in particular transactions. The couple also learns about the interlocking nature of their ego states. For example, the husband typically acts as if he has no Child ego state (exemplified by feelings states such as sadness, gladness, or fear), and the wife interlocks with the husband's ego states, acting as if she has no Adult or Parent ego states (exemplified by an absence of care-taking behaviors, decision making, and judgment capacities).[36] The "shifting symbiotic" relationship structure of the physically violent family who relate in this way is depicted in Fig. 32-2.

TABLE 32-8

GOAL ATTAINMENT SCALE FOLLOW-UP GUIDE FOR A PHYSICAL CHILD ABUSER

Goal headings	Level of predicted attainment				
	Most unfavorable outcome thought likely (−2)	Less than expected success (−1)	Expected level of success (0)	More than expected success (+1)	Most favorable outcome thought likely (+2)
Symbiosis	Talk, think, act for spouse; turn to children to be cared for		Do no talking, thinking, acting for spouse; seek no nurturing from children		Meet own needs, give support when requested to spouse; support two children
Isolation	Stay in house all day; visit no one; call on no one for help		Get out of house each day; visit neighbors; call on them or friends in crisis		Get out of house each day; go somewhere with a friend; go out with husband; call people in crisis
Talking and sharing with mate	Criticize and nag spouse; give no positive strokes		Give positive strokes instead of nagging and criticism to mate while talking and sharing for at least 10 minutes		Give positive strokes to mate while talking and sharing for at least 15 minutes
Impatience/ temper	Outbursts of temper and impatience at husband, children, and persons outside the home		No outburst of temper or impatience at children or husband		No outbursts of temper or impatience in home or elsewhere
Child development and management	Continue present disciplining; learn no child development or managment techniques; children not allowed to be children		Learn developmental needs; use "I messages" and reinforcement techniques; let husband do any physical disciplining; children allowed to be children		Learn developmental needs; use "I messages" and reinforcement techniques; stop yelling at children
Employment	Continue to remain idle at home and demonstrate "job phobia"		Overcome "job phobia" by getting and keeping job at least 3 months		Overcome "job phobia" by getting and keeping job at least 6 months

Modified from Justice, B., and Justice, R.: The abusing family, New York, 1976, Human Sciences Press, Inc.

Siamese-twinning life scripts. The couple is taught about their interlocking symbiotic relationship structure as they learn about life scripts: how these were communicated to them; how they fit with their spouse's life scripts in a complementary and reciprocal manner, and how they communicate the same life scripts to their children. Siamese twinning is explained as a process in which one spouse cannot act without the other going along with the action or direction either by doing nothing or failing to change the course of action.[36] Life-script messages are usually communicated verbally from Parent to Parent ego states, nonverbally from Child to Child ego states, with strong influences on later feelings and behaviors in life, and behaviorally from Adult to Adult ego states when the implementation of a life script is demonstrated or role modeled. Fig. 32-3 depicts a siamese-twinning script matrix of a child abuser's partner. It shows the way in which the physically abusive family is fused around transactional processes.

Most of the literature focuses on the abuser,

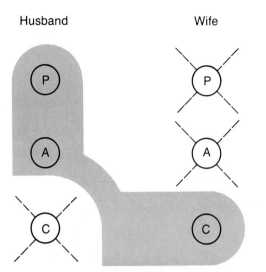

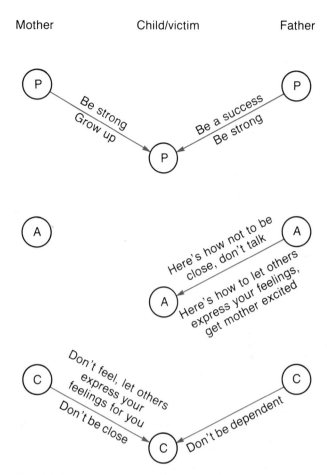

Fig. 32-2. Shifting symbiotic relationship structure that may characterize physically violent families. (From Justice, B., and Justice, R.: The abusing family, New York, 1976, Human Sciences Press, Inc.)

Fig. 32-3. Siamese-twinning script matrix of a child abuser's partner. (From Justice, B., and Justice, R.: The abusing family, New York, 1976, Human Sciences Press, Inc.)

whereas this model focuses on the family as an interlocking system. The dynamic processes are the same in the physically abusive family as in the sexually abusive family. Tension builds in one member until it can no longer be contained, and the feelings are relieved by the physically or sexually abusive act. Usually the nonabusive partner emerges from the violent episode "smelling like a rose," since the focus is typically on blaming the abusive or violent member for the system's dysfunctional processes. The nonabusive family member generally colludes in the violence by doing nothing to relieve or prevent high stress levels that build to a violent release, and, after the violence, takes care of the crisis calmly as if in command of the entire situation. Both adults have learned not to ask outsiders for help or show feelings, which "seals off" the family system from potential therapeutic intervention. This transactional interactional process is brought to the couple's awareness in therapy by visually diagramming the process on paper or a blackboard (Fig. 32-3). In this way, the transactional model implements the goal of helping patients gain control of themselves in transactions with others.

Relaxation and hypnosis therapy. Relaxation and hypnosis therapy use behavior modification strategies to teach patients to relax in tense situations and to prevent accumulation of tension to explosive levels. They are thus taught how to respond differently to stressful stimuli. The reader is referred to Chapter 12 and the literature for detailed discussion of these two approaches in treatment.[54]

Gestalt and confrontation strategies. Gestalt techniques are used to give members "permission" and

"protection" in disclosing painful feelings (sadness, depression, loneliness) and intense feelings (love, hate, jealousy, rage, fear) in a safe environment of people who care about each other.[36] Caring is communicated verbally through empathic remarks that reflect the therapist's and members' understanding and appreciation of a family's painful existence and struggle for healthier functioning.

The strongest confrontation strategy is to insist that the violence and abuse stop and may include close monitoring of the family.[36] In terms of a behavioral goal, the patient might be told, for example, that "under no circumstances is he or she to be left alone in the house with the child or elder." Confrontations are used throughout group therapy, such as when group members confront each other on denial, blocks, destructive communication, and responsibility for self.

■ **PERSONAL GROWTH GROUPS.** Personal growth groups include sessions where laypersons meet with each other to share a particular problem they have in common and help each other develop coping skills; a health professional may or may not lead or co-lead these groups. Attendance at these groups is part of the treatment plan, is coordinated with family sessions, and is based on the emotional readiness of the family members for these sessions.[7] Examples of therapeutic personal growth groups include: Alcoholics Anonymous, Al-Anon, Al-Teen; Parents United and Parents Anonymous; church groups; feminist groups; and groups that stress career development options and job interviewing skills, caring for elders or handicapped/impaired persons, and preparing for retirement.

■ **FAMILY THERAPY APPROACH.** Controversy characterizes the issue of using family therapy as the primary approach in treatment and whether it should precede or exclude other forms of intervention, such as individual counseling of victims. The family therapy approach most frequently reported in work with violent families is Minuchin's structural therapy.[44] Generally, it is agreed that all of the factors characterizing violent families, if present in a given family system, are in need of intervention. Thus one would see a family therapist work toward a variety of goals such as the following[18,51,62]:

1. Rebalance the power bases in the system
2. Build the relationship between the mother and daughter (through a shared activity) and break the closeness between father and daughter related to the sexual abuse
3. Open communication between the spouses (assign mom and dad to plan a picnic, talk about finances or the wife going to work)
4. Stimulate members' efforts toward independence and autonomy (family is assigned the task of dividing up household chores, teenage daughter is made responsible for mothering 2-year-old out-of-wedlock child, wife is instructed to learn to drive a car)

Midwest Family Resource model. Barret and co-workers[7] at the Midwest Family Resource Center in Chicago report a comprehensive treatment model which has been highly successful in ending family violence and allowing families to remain together. Preliminary empirical outcome results with over 250 individuals and families indicate that the program has a recidivism rate of about 2%. The treatment program implemented in this model usually requires 12 to 18 months for successful completion with these types of families; this is not considered a long period of time given the number of problems to be resolved by the family and its individual members. The model was developed with incestuous families, but it is presented here because the components are applicable to effective treatment with any abusive or violent family.

The Midwest Family Resource Model is a systems-oriented treatment approach that attends to the therapeutic needs of individual family members, the family as a system, and the needs of society. It is based on structural[45] and strategic[31,77] approaches of family therapy. There are three stages of treatment: (1) creating a context for change; (2) challenging patterns and expanding alternatives; and (3) consolidation. The model acknowledges the essential need for interdisciplinary, multi-system cooperation and coordination, and multiple treatment methods if treatment is to be effective with an abusive or violent family.[7]

Stage 1: Creating a context for change. Stage 1 consists of completing an assessment of the family and individual members and establishing the groundwork for ongoing treatment. Stage 1 is completed when the following two goals have been achieved: (1) a mechanism for coordination of services among protective services, state caseworkers, and the courts has been established to achieve ongoing effective network communication; and, (2) four family therapy goals have been achieved:

■ Therapists have joined with each family member and the family system
■ Assessment of individual family members and the family system has been completed
■ A therapeutic contract with the family has been established
■ "Workable realities" have been developed with the family that allow them dignity and flexibility to grow inter- and intra-personally[7]

For treatment to be effective it is mandatory that ongoing communication and mutual goals be established between the therapists, one's agency, and the legal and state systems. Ongoing clear communication serves as a role model to the family, avoids mirroring their symptoms such as chaos/disorganization or rigidity, and facilitates productive conflict resolution.

Stage 2: Challenging patterns and expanding alternatives. In this stage of therapy family members are helped to learn new sequences of emotional and behavioral expression and eliminate dysfunctional ones that are often reinforced by family of origin, society, personality, and peer group. Treatment approaches include the use of family, marital, sibling, individual, and group sessions.[7]

Stage 3: Consolidation. The consolidation phase of

therapy usually lasts about 3 months. Work completed in this phase of treatment solidifies the changes that have been made in therapy by the family, and explores concerns or potential problem areas in functioning they anticipate in the future. At this time, families evidence more skill and responsibility in conflict resolution, problem solving, and decision making. The family now has the ability to articulate a problem and describe how they effectively handled and coped with it as compared with past modes of functioning. The therapist complements them for their skill in these areas and points out family strengths.

The nurse will know that a family has reached this stage when they are able to be clear, direct, and constructive in their communication patterns. As with all therapy termination phases, emphasis is placed on the family's functioning independent of the therapist, and their newly acquired coping skills and strategies. It is important that the nurse explore and predict with the family any concerns they have about potential future problems such as developmental transitions. Although clinical evidence and post-assessment objective outcome measures suggest that they are ready to terminate therapy, the family is encouraged to return to therapy whenever they need or want help with a problem. At this time the family should be receptive to such a suggestion since they have experienced therapy as a helpful process and a resource ensuring their welfare rather than punishment. The consolidation phase gradually terminates the family from individual, dyadic, group, and family therapy. Its duration is based on the needs of a given family and the clinical judgment of the nurse.[7] Work begun as secondary prevention activities takes a long time to complete and is supported by tertiary prevention interventions.

■ Interventions in tertiary prevention

Tertiary prevention consists of interventions implemented after adaptation has occurred. Efforts are directed toward helping the family system stabilize, adapt, become educated, or be maintained at a desired level of healthy functioning. Furthermore, interventions are directed toward reducing the possibility of further episodes of violence in the family. A variety of tertiary prevention activities implemented with violent families are briefly described. Many of these activities, because of present governmental policies of budget cuts and financial constraints, will no longer be funded or available to many violent families as tertiary or primary prevention interventions.

■ **THERAPEUTIC EDUCATION.** Part of prevent-

ing repetition of family violence depends on the family becoming educated (1) with more information and teaching strategies that foster learning about the nature of their dynamic processes and (2) by achieving academic advancement through completing diplomas, certificates, and college. The family, staying in therapy at this time, learns how to restructure their lives so as to achieve positive and satisfying goals in their lifetime. Children also need to be educated about family violence because if they are made aware of the problem they will usually report it to a "grown-up." In this way children learn that they do not have to be victims of violence and become community monitors on the welfare of the family within its private inner sanctum.

The family needs to see how the abuser uses his attitudes and emotional states just prior to a violent episode. Tertiary prevention begins when the abuser is in control of his behavior and when the therapeutic focus can turn more deeply into the system's dynamic processes. For example, the wife of an abuser needs to see that she is not responsible for his feelings. However, then the wife needs to recognize the abuser's feeling states by which he calls attention to himself, indicating "where he is at." The message from the therapist to the abuser's wife is, "If you care at all about your husband you will see to it that he doesn't repeat the violence. And, to do that you need to deal with yourself. You need to deal with your dynamics because you contributed to this situation all these years. Therefore you need to get to know yourself better if you're going to help your husband. It doesn't have to happen again."

In the final phase of therapy the family continues to deal with the issue of powerlessness-to-power as a dynamic in their transactions and enmeshment.[33] The members need to learn to differentiate and discriminate affection from power because in the act of abuse or violence, affection and power are often fused and confused. Becoming aware of oneself and the family system, a learned behavior by this point, then generalizes to objectively assessing transactions outside the family. It becomes obvious to the violent family, depressingly so at times, how the powerlessness-to-power dynamic is "played out" in every aspect of their lives. It is often not confined or limited to the physically or sexually abusive or violent transactions. Awareness of the pervasiveness of the powerlessness-to-power dynamic, combined with awareness by patients of the tendency to fuse affection with power, is a sobering moment. It can be the turning point in therapy for making changes to replace faulty maladaptive processes. It can also be so painful that patients reactivate old coping patterns, such as denial and discounting, to flee acknowledging and accepting themselves. When families are able to be open and accepting of themselves, admit or acknowledge that changes are needed, and work continuously in therapy to achieve these changes, then the system is generally demonstrating a healthier level of self-esteem and reality testing.

Another area that is explored at this time is the relationship of the therapist with the family. Often the family's dynamic conflicts are worked through around the therapeutic relationship. One of the important relationship issues in this regard is the *power dynamic*.[20,33] For example, the therapist is caring, attentive, and committed to helping the violent family stop the violence. The family usually interprets this as, "That person genuinely cares about us," or "I have good feelings about that therapist because she cares enough to care about me. Even when I have temporary setbacks she sticks by me, expects me to change, and doesn't give up hope that I can and will change." At some point the family may test out the limits of their relationship with the therapist, who then needs to redefine that this is a therapy relationship. Exactly how families work through this power issue is quite varied and unpredictable. The only factor that is predictable is that the power dynamic in the relationship with the therapist does come to the fore and needs to be attended to. This can be seen in Clinial example 32-3.

The therapist had to do something about the situation presented in Clinical example 32-3. To not act would have meant she had been co-opted by the family system into permitting the violence to continue and ignoring it as a reality. The two daughters were placed in a shelter, and the father was returned to prison for parole violation. The mother was court ordered to not only attend, but to participate, in therapy as indicated by the therapist's progress report in 2 months. The mother was confronted with the dynamic way in which she contributed by default to the father's lack of control.

In this situation, the power dynamic was played out around the following questions: Would the therapist find out about the parole violation or rule-breaking behavior? Would the therapist do anything about it after the act was discovered? Did the therapist have any power to do anything about the violation? It is precisely at this point that the violent family translates and misconstrues the therapist's adult/responsible behavior of reporting and testifying in court as "not caring" about them, being "out to get us, to split up the family," and being "on a big ego trip." The issue then becomes, in some cases, the turning point at which reality is reevaluated, "I care about you because I won't let you continue to be violent and abusive." Caring and affection are gradually seen as mature adult behaviors, and gradually the therapist's intervention can be seen as caring rather than as a power trip. And so the family learns to separate caring and affection from power in the therapeutic relationship and is helped to generalize that learning experience to other relationships, particularly with authority figures, such as employers or supervisors.

It is clear at this point that therapeutic intervention with violent families continues for an extended period of time, and discussion is in terms of control rather than cure. Therapy must necessarily be supported by the use of programs in the community.

■ **COMMUNITY LINKAGES.** Since the beginning of the community mental health movement and federally funded social programs in the 1960s, many programs have been developed that offer both tertiary and preventive interventions to violent and highly stressed families. These programs are currently being reduced or eliminated because of cuts in the federal budget and the austere economic condition of the nation. This is a sad commentary because by eliminating such services one can predict that the level of family violence will increase in this nation, and agencies offering support after secondary intervention will no longer be as available to clients. In times of stress, healthy families usually become more permeable and activate extended family contacts. However, violent families do not act in this manner, and, when they do, usually at the encouragement of professionals, the family is exposed more intensely to family processes that are dysfunctional and intensify the family pathological conditions. Experts generally do not advise putting the victim with grandparents, since

---

CLINICAL EXAMPLE 32-3

Joe, a 30-year-old father of five, was convicted of sexually abusing his two stepdaughters. Joe claimed he did not commit the act because he does not remember doing it; he was drunk at the time. The judge ordered Joe out of the family home and to therapy. Since Joe has been living alone, the children have become physically and psychologically violent at home with each other, and their mother has not stopped the violent behavior. An uncle came from California to visit, and while he was there he sexually abused the daughters. The father moved back into the home, knowing he was breaking his parole regulation. The mother did nothing to stop the father from moving back into the family home. The two daughters, in group therapy with other adolescent victims, were very distressed and acted "strange," but it took a month before they found the situation intolerable and disclosed the events.

grandparents often violated their own children and may do the same with the victimized grandchild, or otherwise perpetuate the family's violent dynamic processes. Thus, for a variety of reasons, community programs have been an important mode of intervention in work with violent families. The following is a brief listing of some programs that have been available.

Foster grandparent programs or lay therapy. These programs are usually comprised of people willing to give of themselves to others. Foster grandparents can give to (and receive from) children a lot of love and attention; often the very kind of nurturing the child needs but the parents feel unable to provide. Lay therapists are usually viewed as adults who give to adults, one couple to a family, and provide the needed nurturing, attention, and caring that violent families so desperately seek.[36] As a peer experience it is particularly valuable for adults who have lacked the experience of intimacy with peers during adolescence, or the ability to give of self to another. As outsiders, the input into the violent family system of new experiences, perspectives, and feeling states, is particularly powerful. Professional therapists can strategically work with foster or lay therapists to create changes in a violent family system. However, the team must guard against arguing and fighting among themselves, playing out their own power dynamics, and, ultimately, diverting attention away from a concentrated multimodel approach in treating the violent family.

Support services. Support services consist of programs or services available in the community that, when used by the violence-prone family, will help prevent repetition of family violence. Thus support services are a tertiary intervention and also a primary intervention. Some of the support services available in the community include the following[36,76]:

1. Visiting or public health nurses
2. Homemaker services
3. Cooperative nurseries
4. Crisis nurseries
5. Day care centers/nurseries
6. Foster home care
7. Classes on child and elderly development and management
8. Telephone hotline services for violent families
9. Classes about personality and family dynamics
10. Transportation car pools or taxies
11. State and national hotlines for information and reporting
12. Self-help groups, such as Alcoholics Anonymous, Al-Anon, Al-Teen, Abusers Anonymous, Parents United/Parents Anonymous, and Daughters and Sons United
13. Financial assistance programs
14. Suicide hotlines and crisis intervention teams
15. Peer counseling (women's centers, rape crisis centers)
16. Assertiveness training
17. Divorce counseling
18. Meals-on-Wheels
19. Big Brother–Big Sister organizations
20. Foster grandparents

Many families need supportive follow-up care while establishing healthy network systems, and nurses are in a unique position to (1) provide the service, (2) monitor the family's adaptation, and (3) intervene to prevent future violence.

Social service intervention. An episode of family violence is frequently preceded by a precipitating event that stresses the family beyond its ability to cope. Precipitating events such as loss of employment, increased financial strain, loss of or inadequte housing, or loss of transportation may require the intervention of social service agencies. These agencies provide emergency services to (1) decrease the level of stress on families; (2) reduce the risk of families expressing abuse/violence under such stresses; and (3) free up the time and energy of abusive/violent families in treatment to work on treatment issues and prevent further abusive/violent events.

■ **Interventions in primary prevention**

The aim of primary prevention is to reduce the incidence of and, ideally, eradicate family violence. Primary prevention focuses on promoting optimum health and uses measures that will prevent maladaptation or disease. Research is directed toward identifying possible risk factors and associated stressors that place a family at high risk for violent transactions. Interventions are then directed at identifying those families at high risk and intervening to prevent the violence from happening. Primary prevention also strengthens current adaptive coping mechanisms of families, and interventions are directed toward preventing dysfunctional decompensation. The following discussion briefly outlines a variety of primary prevention programs that have been or could be implemented.

■ **VALUE EVALUATION.** By the time professionals become actively involved in primary prevention programs, the gravity of the problem of family violence has been fully realized. It is no longer sufficient to stop the violence; the professional becomes committed to preventing its occurrence based on an awareness of the destructiveness and devastation it creates. That process is a gradual experience over time, culminating in a full value clarification process with a commitment to action. This process is called a *value evaluation process*. It is very similar to a self-awareness, philosophical-meditative, self-exploratory process in which the professional comes to terms with what one thinks and feels about the problem of family violence and what action or inaction is taken as a result.

Value evaluation requires that the nurse take a value position about the problem of family violence. For example, if the nurse believes the problem of family violence is of epidemic proportions, there is greater likelihood that action will be taken to eliminate it. What one does about a problem is directly related to what one thinks about that problem or even if it is classified as a "problem."

At this point, it appears that not many professionals are involved in primary prevention activities.[36,76] Community and public health nurses could make an excellent contribution in primary and secondary prevention through case identification, referral, education, and agency collaboration. Nurses in every field of practice could contribute in similar fashion. At present most of the professionals working with violent families are providing secondary prevention services, and few people are qualified to do such work. It is only when the problem becomes epidemic in proportion that there is a massive, often federally funded, program to reduce or eradicate the epidemic, whereas prevention would have been less costly and destructive.

The people of this nation appear to value secondary prevention more than primary prevention.[36,76] Otherwise, more health professionals would be involved in clinical work to prevent family violence, and more social resources would be allocated to that end. Progress in that direction, however, is slowly occurring. For example, the American Nurses' Association Council of Specialists in Psychiatric–Mental Health Nursing passed a resolution on victimology. In passing that resolution, the council members made the following public commitment:

To include victimology in the curricula of basic nursing education programs, to encourage graduate programs in psychiatric—mental health nursing to assure adequate numbers of faculty to teach victimology and victimologist researchers to expand the scientific base for psychiatric and mental health nursing practice with victims, and to encourage clinicians who care for abused victims to write and report their information concerning clinical practice.[4]

A second nursing activity at the national level endorsing victimology as a legitimate field of practice has been the endorsement of a subspeciality interest group in victimology by the Council of Specialists in Psychiatric–Mental Health Nursing, and nursing research groups such as the Midwest Nursing Research Society. These activities reflect a beginning, but much remains

to be done. Specific strategies in primary prevention are clearly planned interventions aimed at a specific problem area. A number of different specific strategy programs will now be discussed.

■ **HIGH-RISK IDENTIFICATION.** Programs aimed at high-risk identification teach people how to identify cases that have a high risk or potential to become violent and then provide primary prevention to prevent an occurrence of violence.[12] For example, community health nurses might be alert to elders who are at high risk for family violence according to current, although rather limited, research findings, which suggest the following characteristics of families of abused elders:

1. A middle income family in which their dependency stresses a high-achieving, career-oriented family beyond its limits, with a son (daughter or relative) striking out in violence
2. Unemployment
3. Financial difficulties
4. No relief from the responsibility of care taking
5. A stressed economy

■ **TRAINING PROGRAMS IN VICTIMOLOGY.** The field of victimology is expanding at an exponential rate. It is difficult to keep up with all the literature that is being published on each form of family violence, as well as data on cases in which more than one form of family violence exists. Enough information exists at this time that it could legitimately be "institutionalized" by a training program.[14] Such a program would address issues such as the following:

1. Case identification for every form of violence
2. Crisis intervention in family violence
3. Therapy with violent families
4. Therapy with prisoners in prison systems who have been abusers, victims, or both of family and other violence
5. Programs to eradicate family violence that have been or could be developed
6. Workshops that teach self-defense
7. Therapy with the mentally ill who have episodes of violent behavior

This list is a small sampling of content that could be included in a training program. The programs that are currently being offered at a national level have been federally funded programs and generally have not been sponsored by nurses.

■ **PROFESSIONAL EDUCATION.** Curricula in schools of nursing need to include more content on all forms of family violence than is currently included in most existing curricula.[14,25,27] All professional schools need more content on family violence and intervention in their curricula. The 1982 President's Task Force on Victims of Crime,[72] as well as the 1984 Attorney General's Task Force on Family Violence[73] and 1984 national symposium Protecting Our Children: The Fight Against Molestation,[74] recommended that theoretical and clinical content on abuse and violence be included in the curricula of all health professionals, educators, and law enforcement officials. The educational process needs to be extended as well through continuing education to professionals who did not have this content in their curricula or who are in need of updated information, and to the community through public speaking engagements to meet the educational needs of both professionals and the public.

■ **LAY EDUCATION.**[43,76] Violent families are sorely lacking in knowledge in many fields of information. A prevention program could set up educational classes to provide people with information they need to achieve their developmental tasks with a minimum of stress. Examples of such programs include educational courses on relationships and marriage, child-rearing practices and development, and anticipatory guidance.

Relationships and marriage. Adolescents have demonstrated a need for courses on relationships and marriage.[41] What are relationships all about? How do you handle all the strange and stressful things that arise in a relationship? Are there some people who should not get married or have children? How does homosexuality fit into a relationship with someone? All kinds of other management and relationship questions should be examined: Who is in charge of the money or to what extent does that person have control over the funds? If there is a disagreement, who has the last word and is it the same person all the time? How do you get along with someone? Who is the family manager, plans the social life, meals, bedtimes, clothing, career schedule? These and many other questions are familiar to "elders" who have gone through more of life. They could be explored and discussed with the youth in this nation and hopefully help them achieve answers and emotional well-being.

Child-rearing practices and development. Violent families are often limited in their knowledge about child development and how to raise a child. Their paucity of information adds stress to an already stressed psyche. Nurses could preventively intervene by providing more families, particularly families at high risk for violence, courses on child development and child-rearing practices. Community health nurses entering family homes are in an excellent position to identify families who would benefit from such a nursing action.

Anticipatory guidance. In preventing a crisis from developing, one strategy that is often implemented is that of anticipatory guidance. The patients can be prepared for what is about to happen to them and their lives. The following are two important areas in which violent families could benefit from anticipatory guidance:[61]

1. *Therapeutic education.* The therapist talks with the patient about setbacks while in therapy and advises the patient to be on the lookout for clues or warning signals that indicate regression into a violent episode.

2. *The court process.* Patients undergo a painful process of having all the case data presented publicly, often in front of curiosity seekers who listen to court cases the way some people follow soap operas. The family needs to be prepared for what to expect, exactly what can happen, what some of the outcomes might be in the case, the consequences of any of those outcomes, and where to turn when they really need someone to talk to about what they are experiencing. It is important for the professional to be steadfast with the family at this time, and it is even more favorable if the nurse could begin therapy with the family during this critical period, which is usually perceived as a crisis by most families.

■ **COMMUNITY AWARENESS PROGRAMS.** Community awareness programs are prevention programs that are offered through public speaking engagements and are designed to inform the audience about the nature of a problem, how it is treated, its causes, and how to prevent it. Rape crisis centers have actively sponsored community awareness programs. Nurses could offer such programs to the public and become publicly identified as someone to turn to before, or in the event of, family violence. Such programs need to be more widely offered in relation to all forms of family violence. Groups who could be addressed include parent-teacher associations, church groups, children in school systems or after-school activities, Rotary Clubs, and a wide range of men's and women's groups.

■ **OTHER STRATEGIES.** Descriptions of prevention programs could be endless. They are only limited by the nurse's creativity and environmental influences, such as governmental policy, economic constraints, and personnel issues. The following list briefly identifies additional prevention programs nurses need to be aware of and can potentially offer as a service[36,76]:

1. Visiting or public health nurse programs provide support, aid, nurturance, and human contact to isolated individuals who are at high risk for violence.

2. Homemaker services provide teaching to parents who are poorly equipped or unable to perform functional tasks, such as doing the dishes or laundry, disciplining the children without corporal punishment, or cleaning house. These homemakers often become a friend of the family in the truest sense of a friend helping one out in a time of need.

3. Child care services offer care to children in crisis nurseries, emergency shelter care, cooperative nurseries, day-care centers, and foster care.

4. Transportation includes publicly organized car pool systems to help the disadvantaged, such as vans that chauffeur senior citizens around the city.

5. Telephone reassurance services consist of crisis hotlines available to people in times of crisis, such as Alcoholic Anonymous, Parents Anonymous/Parents United, and Suicide Crisis Intervention.

6. National networking is when persons concerned about victimology form a national group and stay in frequent contact with each other, such as members of the National Organization of Victims' Assistance and nurses belonging to the council's special interest group in victimology.

7. Family planning programs provide individuals with contraceptive options and education.

8. Political action includes activities directed toward public policy and getting legislators and politicians to support programs for preventing family violence. This is an area in which increased activity is needed by nurses and other health professionals.

Evaluation

In the 1960s physical abuse of children was brought to public attention, in the 1970s spouse abuse and sexual abuse of children became important social issues, and in the 1980s abuse of the elderly and sibling violence have come to greater public attention.[71] At this time, however, little is known about the effectiveness of treatment and even less is known from a strict empirical position. Professionals are only beginning to widely report treatment interventions (as opposed to assessment factors) with violent families. Most of these reports are descriptive and are clinical research studies that evaluate the effectiveness of a given treatment approach. The secondary interventions discussed in this chapter were presented as currently reported treatment strategies with violent families. However, much remains to be researched about these descriptive clinical impressions.

Research is even less available on primary and tertiary prevention programs. It is known that a certain cluster of variables (unemployment, limited education, and emotional deprivation) are high-risk factors for family violence; however, it is difficult to measure the effectiveness of any prevention program. That fact continues to present nurses in all fields of practice difficulty in designing primary prevention research studies. In terms of tertiary interventions, there are many influences, and it would require multivariate analysis to determine which variables were contributing to preventing further episodes of family violence. Research is also lacking in studies reporting longitudinal therapeutic work with violent families and follow-up assessment. Much remains to be done in the treatment and prevention of this mounting social problem.

■ SUGGESTED CROSS-REFERENCES ■

The transactional analysis model of communication and self-awareness of the nurse are discussed in Chapter 4. Primary prevention activities are discussed in Chapter 9. Crisis intervention is discussed in Chapter 10. Rehabilitation activities are discussed in Chapter 11. Relaxation techniques are discussed in Chapter 12. Group therapy is discussed in Chapter 28. Family therapy is discussed in Chapter 29. Interventions with victims of rape are discussed in Chapter 33.

■ SUMMARY ■

1. Family violence is the physical, psychological, sexual, material, or social violation of a person by a family member or their delegate. Family violence is the mode by which a given family system expresses its dysfunction.
   a. Abuse is an act of misuse, exploitation, deceit, wrong or improper use, or action so as to injure, damage, maltreat, or corrupt.
   b. Violence is the exertion of extreme force or destructive action so as to injure or hurt; discordance, outrage, and sudden intense activity to the point of loss of control.

2. The problem of family abuse and violence was defined in terms of its incidence, known demographic data, characteristics of the violent family as a system, and the stress reaction process. Types of violent behavior include physical, psychological, sexual, material, and social acts that violate another person. Motives of the assailant and colluding members include power and aggression. Both motives may be present throughout the event or act. Targets of released aggression and unresolved power issues in violent/abusive families were defined as child physical abuse, child sexual abuse, spouse/partner abuse, sibling abuse, and elder abuse.

3. Theories on the etiology of family violence are abundant, overlap with each other, and when considered alone are incomplete in explaining the phenomena. Theoretical models used to explain family violence include psychodynamic the-

DIRECTIONS FOR FUTURE RESEARCH

The following are some of the nursing research problems raised in Chapter 32 that merit further study by psychiatric nurses:

1. Identify the comparative effectiveness of specific types of individual, crisis, group, and family therapy treatment approaches with different types and forms of family violence.
2. Identify which combinations of treatment approaches (e.g., individual and crisis, group and family) and treatment methods (e.g., cognitive–behavioral vs. family of origin work) result in the most effective outcome specific to each type and form of family violence.
3. Develop a research method to support a given theory about the etiology of family violence.
4. Compare the differences in the nature, type and utilization of social support between nonviolent and violent families and their members.
5. Identify which vulnerability factors are most predictive of families at risk for expressing abuse and violence.
6. Compare the vulnerability factor differences between victims and observers of family violence.
7. Compare the differences in coping styles between victims and nonabusing observers in violent families.
8. Compare the differences in roles of men and women in communities with a high incidence of family violence and communities with a low incidence of family violence.
9. Compare the levels of self-esteem in nonvictim children or elders in violent families with that of children or elders in nonviolent families.
10. Identify which family processes (e.g., cohesion, adaptability, mutuality, conflict, communication, differentiation) are most characteristic of a specific form (e.g., elder) and type (e.g., psychological) of family violence.
11. Identify the type and amount of theoretical content and clinical experience students receive related to family abuse and violence in the curricula of schools of nursing.
12. Compare violent and nonviolent families on the extent to which they are exposed to specific types (e.g., television murders) and amounts (e.g., number of hours per day) of violence from public media.
13. Identify which type of family structure is most often associated with a specific form of family violence.
14. Compare the efficacy of specific treatment approaches for intervening in dysfunctional family structures associated with abuse and violence.
15. Identify the feelings and attitudes of nurses toward abusive and violent families.
16. Compare the knowledge level of nurses, other health professionals, and law enforcement officials related to assessing and intervening in violent families.
17. Investigate the relationship between cuts in federally funded programs for the prevention of family violence and changes in the incidence of specific forms and types of family violence.
18. Identify which nursing diagnoses and their defining characteristics are most common for specific types and forms of family abuse and violence.
19. Develop and test a model that is predictive of effective treatment outcomes with specific forms and types of family violence.
20. Compare the incidence of family violence in communities that provide educational programs addressing child development, parenting skills, and personal growth with communities that do not provide these programs.

ories, social learning theories, psychosocial theories, environmental stress theories, family structure theories, family system theories, epidemiological theories, and systems theories.

4. The nursing process model is used in assessing family violence and identifying ways in which to best intervene in the problem. Self-awareness by the nurse is essential. Clinical assessment of the violent family includes all that is known about the nature of such a family and can be completed by applying a systems theory model that assesses the individual, family system, environment, and society. Assessment of in-

dividuals and the family system is specific to the type of family violence and is comprehensive.

5. The formulation of a nursing diagnosis includes the precipitating stressor, the family's vulnerability, coping skills, maladaptive responses, strengths, and resources. It is completed with the family's participation.

6. The planning phase of the nursing process includes the general goal of helping the family achieve a higher and more effective level of functioning. Goal setting is directed by the nursing diagnosis; the intensity of the problem or level of illness; the form and type of family violence; and the role, setting, and point in time at which the nurse sees the family. Short-term goals require an assessment of potential repetition of the abuse or violence and victim safety, as well as initial management plans. Short-term goals merge with longer term goals in treatment and are directed by the type of therapy being implemented.

  a. Interventions in secondary prevention include crisis intervention, group therapy, individual therapy, and family therapy that applies both family structure and family systems theories.

  b. Interventions in tertiary prevention include therapeutic education and community linkages that offer support after secondary intervention.

  c. Interventions in primary prevention include value evaluation and programs directed at high-risk identification, training programs in victimology, professional education, lay education, and community awareness programs.

  7. Evaluating the long-term effectiveness of different treatment modalities has yet to be implemented as a strict empirical process. Nurses can make a significant contribution in this area. The problem of family violence is believed by experts to be the result of a dysfunctional family system in response to predisposing and precipitating stressors, including cultural and socialization processes, values, attitudes, and belief systems. The problem of family violence and its generational repetition/transmission will be eradicated only to the extent that such families are helped to achieve higher levels of differentiation and effective functioning.

■　　　　**REFERENCES**　　　　■

  1. Abraham, I.: Personal communication, Nov. 1981.
  2. Aguilera, D., and Messick, J.: Crisis intervention: theory and methodology, ed. 4, St. Louis, 1981, The C.V. Mosby Co.
  3. American Humane Association: Statistics collected for the National Center for Child Abuse and Neglect as of Nov. 1984, Aurora, Il., The Association.
  4. American Nurses' Association, Council of Specialists in Psychiatric and Mental Health Nursing: Resolution of victimology, Kansas City, Mo., June 9, 1980, The Association.
  5. American Psychiatric Association: Diagnostic and statistical manual of mental disorders (DSM-III), Washington, D.C., 1980, The Association.
  6. Anderson, C., and Stewart, S.: Mastering resistance: a practical guide to family therapy. New York, 1983, Guilford Press.
  7. Barrett, M.J., Skyes, C., and Byrnes, W.: A systemic model for the treatment of intrafamily child sexual abuse. Midwest Family Resource Center, Chicago, Ill. Paper presented at the Ann Arbor Center for the Family, Great Lakes Regional Conference on Families and Family Therapy, Nov. 2, 1985.
  8. Beck, A. et al.: Cognitive therapy of depression, New York, 1979, The Guilford Press.
  9. Berne, E.: Games people play: the psychology of human relationships, New York, 1964, Grove Press, Inc.
  10. Berne, E.: Principles of group treatment, New York, 1966, Oxford University Press, Inc.
  11. Block, M., and Sinnott, J., editors: The battered elder syndrome: an exploratory study, College Park, Md., 1979, The University of Maryland.
  12. Blumberg, M.: Treatment of the abused child and the child abuser, Am. J. Orthopsychiatry **31**(2):204, 1977.
  13. Brudnak, L.: Self-esteem levels, sexual knowledge, and sexual attitudes of male child sexual abuse offenders, master's thesis, Pittsburgh, 1981, The University of Pittsburgh School of Nursing.
  14. Burgess, A.W.: Personal communication, Oct. 1981.
  15. Burgess, A.W. et al.: Sexual assault of children and adolescents, Lexington, Mass., D.C. Heath & Co.
  16. Caplan, G.: Principles of preventative psychiatry, New York, 1964, Basic Books, Inc.
  17. Carpenito, L.J.: Nursing diagnosis: application to clinical practice. New York, 1983, J.B. Lippincott Co.
  18. Coleman, P.: Incest; family treatment model. In Holley, K.C.: Sexual misuses of children: tools for understanding, Tacoma, Wash., 1979, Pierce County Rape Relief.
  19. Davidson, J.L.: Elder abuse. In Block, M., and Sinnott, J., editors: The battered elder syndrome: an exploratory study, College Park, Md., 1977, The University of Maryland Center on Aging.
  20. Davis, B.: Personal communication, Oct.-Nov. 1981.
  21. Douglass, R., Hickey, T., and Noel, C.: A study of maltreatment of the elderly and other vulnerable adults, Ann Arbor, Mich., 1980. The University of Michigan School Public Health.
  22. Ellis, A., and Greiger, R. (editors): Handbook of rational-emotive therapy. New York, 1977, Springer.
  23. Finkelhor, D.: Child sexual abuse: new theory and research. New York, 1984, The Free Press.
  24. Finkelhor, D. et al.: The dark side of families: family violence research. Beverly Hills, Calif., 1983, Sage Publications.
  25. Foley, T.: The development and evaluation of an instructor's manual on nursing care of victims of rape, doctoral dissertation, Pittsburgh, 1979, The University of Pittsburgh School of Education.
  26. Foley, T.: Nursing intervention in family abuse and violence. In Stuart, S. and Sundeen, S. (editors): Principles and practice of psychiatric nursing. St. Louis, 1983, The C.V. Mosby Co.
  27. Foley, T., and Davies, M.: Rape: nursing care of victims, St. Louis, 1983, The C.V. Mosby Co.
  28. Geriatric Nursing **1**:153, Sept.-Oct. 1980.
  29. Gottschalk, L.A.: Vulnerability to stress. Am. J. Psychother. **37**:5–23, 1983.
  30. Groth, A.N., and Birnbaum, J.: Men who rape: psychology of the offender, New York, 1979, Plenum Press.
  31. Haley, J.: Problem-solving therapy. San Francisco, 1976, Jossey-Bass.
  32. Harbin, H.: Episodic dyscontrol and family dynamics, Am. J. Psychol. **134**:1113, 1979.

33. Hayes, P.: Personal communication, 1981.
34. Herman, J., and Hirschman, L.: Families at risk for father-daughter incest. Am. J. Psychol. **138**:967–970, 1981.
35. Journal of the American Medical Association **243**:1221, 1980.
36. Justice, B., and Justice, R.: The abusing family, New York, 1976, Human Sciences Press, Inc.
37. Justice, B., and Justice, R.: The broken taboo: sex in the family. New York, 1979, Human Sciences Press, Inc.
38. Kim, M., and Moritz, D.: Classification of nursing diagnoses: proceedings of the third & fourth national conferences. New York, 1982, McGraw-Hill Book Co.
39. Larson, N., and Maddox, J.: Incest management and treatment: family systems vs. victim advocacy approaches. Paper presented at the Annual Meeting of the American Association for Marriage and Family Therapy, San Francisco, Oct., 1984.
40. Lau, E., and Kosberg, J.: Abuse of the elderly by informal providers, Aging **12**:299, 1979.
41. Lidz, T.: The person, New York, 1968, Basic Books, Inc.
42. Martin, E.J.: Types of families continuum, Pittsburgh, 1981, The University of Pittsburgh School of Nursing.
43. McNairy, D. et al.: A community approach to child abuse and neglect, Popular Government **41**:10, Spring 1976.
44. Minuchin, S.: Families and family therapy, Cambridge, Mass., 1974, Harvard University Press.
45. Meiseleman, K.C.: Incest. San Francisco, 1978, Jossey-Bass.
46. National Committee for the Prevention of Child Abuse, Chicago. Survey data for 1984 (survey not necessarily conducted in same method every year).
47. Olson, D.H., Sprenkle, D.H., and Russell, C.S.: Circumplex model of marital and family systems. I: Cohesions and adaptability dimensions, family types, and clinical applications. Fam. Process **18**:3–28, 1979.
48. Olson, D.H., et al.: Family inventories. Family Social Science, St. Paul, 1982, University of Minnesota.
49. Olson, D.H., et al.: Families: what makes them work. Beverly Hills, 1983, Sage Publications.
50. Papp, P.: Symposium on strategic-structural family therapy, Ann Harbor, Mich., Oct. 16, 1981, Ann Arbor Center for the Family.
51. Porter, F.S., Blick, L.C., and Sgroi, S.M.: Treatment of the sexually abused child. In Sgroi, S.M.: A handbook of clinical intervention in child sexual abuse, New York, 1981, Garland Publishing, Inc.
52. Renshaw, D.: Incest: understanding and treatment. Boston, 1982, Little, Brown and Company.
53. Research Divison of Child and Family Services of Connecticut, Inc.: Child sexual abuse problem categories.
54. Rimm, D., and Masters, J.: Behavior therapy: techniques and empirical findings, New York, 1974, Academic Press, Inc.
55. Rosenfeld, A.: Endogamic incest and the victim-perpetrator model. Am. J. Dis. Child. **133**:406–410, 1979.
56. Rosenthal, D.: Genetics of psychopathology. New York, 1971, McGraw-Hill.
57. Russell, D.: Marital rape. New York, 1982, MacMillan Co.
58. Russell, D.: Sexual exploitation: rape, child sexual abuse, and sexual harrassment. Beverly Hills, 1984, Sage Publications.
59. Schwartz, R., Barrett, M.J., and Saba, G.: Psychotherapy for anorexia nervosa and bulimia. New York, 1984, Guilford Press.
60. Sexual abuse of children, San Francisco, 1976, Queen's Bench Foundation.
61. Sgroi, S.M.: An approach to case management. In Sgroi, S.M.: Handbook of clinical intervention in child sexual abuse, New York, 1981, Garland Publishing, Inc.
62. Sgroi, S.M.: Family treatment issues in parental incest families. In Sgroi, S.M.: Handbook of clinical intervention in child sexual abuse, New York, 1981, Garland Publishing, Inc.
63. Stevens, D.: Personal communication, July 7, 1981.
64. Straus, M., Gelles, R., and Steinmetz, S.: Behind closed doors: violence in the American family, New York, 1980, Anchor Books.
65. Summit, R., and Kryso, J.: Sexual abuse of children: a clinical spectrum. Am. J. Orthopsychiatry **48**:237–251, 1978.
66. The Minister of Justice and Attorney General of Canada, The Minister of National Health and Welfare. Sexual offences against children: report of the Commitee on sexual offences against children and youth. Aug. 1984, Ottawa, Canada.
67. Training Key No. 246: Investigating wife beating, Gaithersburg, Md., 1976, Police Management and Operations Divisions of the International Association of Chiefs of Police, Inc.
68. Trepper, T.S., and Barrett, M.J.: Vulnerability to incest: a framework for assessment. Midwest Family Resource Center, Chicago, Ill. Paper presented at the Ann Arbor Center for the Family, Great Lakes Regional Conference on Families and Family Therapy, Nov. 2, 1985.
69. Trepper, T.S., and Traicoff, M.E.: Treatment of intrafamily sexuality: conceptual rationale and model for family therapy. Family Studies Center, Purdue University Calumet and Southlake Center for Mental Health, Merriville, Ind. Paper presented at the Annual Regional Conference of the Michigan Association of Sex Educators, Counselors and Therapists, Dearborn Hyatt Regency, Nov. 1984.
70. U.S. Congress, House Subcommittee on Aging. Report for 1984 communicated to the National Organization of Victims, Washington, D.C., Jan. 1985.
71. U.S. Department of Health and Human Services: Elder abuse, Washington, D.C., 1980, Office of Human Development Services.
72. U.S. Department of Justice: President's task force on victims of crime: final report. Washington, D.C., 1982, U.S. Government Printing Office.
73. U.S. Department of Justice: Attorney General's task force on family violence: final report. Washington, D.C., 1984, U.S. Government Printing Office.

74. U.S. Department of Justice: Attorney General's protecting our children: the fight against molestation: A national symposium. Washington, D.C., 1984, U.S. Government Printing Office.

75. Vasquez, J.: Child-abuse neglect, substance-abuse family therapy project, Ann Arbor, Mich., The University of Michigan. (Unpublished.)

76. Warner, C.: Conflict intervention in social and domestic violence, Bowie, Md., 1981, Robert J. Brady Co.

77. Watzlawick, P., Weakland, J.H., and Fisch, R.: Change: principles of problem formation and problem resolution. New York, 1974, Norton.

78. Webster's New Collegiate Dictionary, Springfield, Mass., 1977, G. & C. Merriam Co.

79. Weiner, I.: Principles of psychotherapy. New York, 1975, John Wiley & Sons.

80. Will, D.: Approaching the incestuous and sexually abusive family. J. Adolesc. **6**:229–246, 1983.

81. Wyatt, G.: University of California, Los Angeles, Neuropsychiatric Institute. Research results reported at the N.I.M.H. Research Scientist Level I Awardee Meeting, N.I.M.H., Washington, D.C., June 1985.

82. Zubin, J., and Spring, B.: Vulnerability: a new view of schizophrenia. J. Abnorm. Psychol. **86**:103–126, 1977.

■ ANNOTATED SUGGESTED READINGS ■

Anderson, L., and Shafer, G.: The character-disordered family: a community treatment model for family sexual abuse, Am. J. Orthopsychiatry **49**(3):436, 1979.

An interagency model for treating sexually abusive families is presented. Inherent in the model is a view of the family as a set of character-disordered individuals who require a community approach for control of dysfunctional behavior, the use of many resources in cooperative concert, and more than one therapist.

Barrett, D., and Fine, H.: A child was being beaten: the therapy of battered children as adults, Psychotherapy: theory, research and practice **17**:285, 1980.

The authors discuss cultural and historical backgrounds of the battered child syndrome. Five case studies are used to demonstrate the way in which adults who were battered as children adapt, as well as various psychopathological disturbances that emerge as a result of traumatic childhood events.

Bavolke, S.: Primary prevention of child abuse and neglect: identification of high risk adolescents prior to parenthood, doctoral dissertation, Dissertation Abstracts Int. **39**:3511A, 1978.

The author developed an instrument to assess parenting and child-rearing attitudes of adolescents. The instrument could be used by nurses to identify those adolescents who may be at high risk for becoming abusive parents.

Beck, A., et al.: Cognitive therapy of depression, New York, 1979, The Guilford Press.

The authors describe the application of cognitive-behavioral therapy in the treatment of depression. The method has adaptability for nursing interventions in family violence.

*Burgess, A.W.: Child pornography and sex rings. Lexington, Mass., 1984, D.C. Heath & Co.

*Burgess, A.W. et al.: Sexual assault of children and adolescents, Lexington, Mass., 1978, D.C. Heath & Co.

Colao, F., and Hosansky, T.: Your children should know. New York, 1983, Berkeley Books.

This book is highly recommended by experts in the field of victimology for use with professionals and lay persons to teach children to recognize suspicious behavior, prevent assault, escape abduction, and stop sexual abuse.

Denicola, J., and Sandler, J.: Training abusive parents in child management and self-control skills, Behav. Ther. **11**:263, 1980.

The authors describe a research study in which parents were taught self-control techniques and given parent training with a two-variable withdrawal design. Parent training focused on inappropriate or punitive child management techniques. Cognitive-behavioral training focused on helping the parents cope with their aggressive impulses and feelings of anger and frustration.

*Elmer, E., Bennett, H., and Sankey, C.: A state-wide child abuse training program for public health nurses, Child Abuse Neglect **3**(1):131, 1979.

The authors describe a program for Pennsylvania public health nurses addressing their needs in relation to roles and responsibility in child abuse cases. Problems in nurses' dual role in the community and reactions that inhibit responsible reporting of cases are discussed.

Finkelhor, D. et al.: The dark side of families: current family violence research. Beverly Hills, 1983, Sage Publications.

This edited text presents research by experts in the field of family abuse/violence on domestic violence, child physical and sexual abuse, marital rape, and theories of intrafamily abuse/violence. It is highly recommended reading for professionals working in the field of victimology.

*Foster, P., Lanier, M., and Whitworth, J.: Expanding the role of nurses in child abuse prevention and treatment, J. Psychiatr. Nurs. **18**(21):24, 1980.

The authors describe a multidisciplinary program designed to meet family needs in times of crisis, help resolve problems that precipitate abuse, and coordinate with other agencies to plan longer term treatment as indicated. A case example is used to illustrate the multidisciplinary team's responsibility in assessment, planning, and treatment.

*Germain, C.: Sheltering abused women: a nursing perspective, J. Psychosoc. Nurs. Ment. Health Serv. **22**(9):24, 1984.

This article is a report of an ethnography-in-progress in which the authors indicate that participation by nurses in the health care of abused women and their children in community shelters offers an interdisciplinary opportunity for dealing with the victims of this major mental and physical health problem.

---

*Asterisk indicates nursing reference.

Harris, T.: I'm ok—you're ok: a practical guide to transactional analysis, New York, 1969, Harper & Row, Publishers, Inc.

The author's work is an excellent guide for nurses in learning how to apply transactional analysis concepts in therapy with patients. The book is easy to read and complements Eric Berne's original work in the field.

Herr, J., and Weakland, J.: Counseling elders and their families, New York, 1979, Springer Publishing Co.

The authors present practical approaches based on theory for working out some of the problems of the aging and their families. Problems such as physical and mental health, income, and loneliness are presented clearly and sensitively.

Hoopes, M. et al.: Structured family facilitation programs: enrichment, education, and treatment. Rockville, Md., 1984, Aspen Systems Corp.

This edited text provides an operationalized set of family facilitation programs that can easily be implemented in any service agency.

*Hunka, C., O'Toole, A., and O'Toole, R.: Self-help therapy in parents anonymous, J. Psychosoc. Nurs. Ment. Health Serv. 23(7):24, 1985.

This is a report of the results of nursing research to assess the effectiveness of Parents Anonymous. The authors conclude that participation of abusive parents in PA resulted in significant improvement. Additional nursing research similar to this is needed in the field.

Johnson, J., editor: Family violence, J. Fam. Issues, vol. 2, issue 4, 1981.

This special issue is devoted entirely to the many aspects of family violence. It reviews recent research and thinking on this problem area.

Meiselman, K.: Incest: a psychological study of causes and effects with treatment recommendations. San Francisco, 1981, Jossey-Bass.

The author presents information previously unreported on the causes and long-term effects of incest including adjustment difficulties—social, sexual, and psychological—in adolescence and adulthood. The author discusses multiple forms of incest with guidelines and recommendations for the evaluation and treatment of incest cases.

*Miller, V., and Mansfield, E.: Family therapy for the multiple incest family, J. Psychiatr. Nurs. 19(4):29, 1981.

The authors describe the incidence and types of family incest that are most prevalent. A case example is presented, discussed, and evaluated using Bowen's theoretical framework of family functioning.

*Murray, R., and Zentner, J.: Nursing assessment and health promotion through the life span, ed. 3, Englewood Cliffs, N.J., 1983, Prentice-Hall, Inc.

The authors introduce the reader to the person and his family throughout the life span. The text is an excellent resource for nurses in teaching families normal development, how to deal positively with behaviors, and what changes to expect in the future.

Nasjleti, M.: Suffering in silence: the male incest victim, Child Welfare 59:260, 1980.

The author explores why the male incest victim remains silent and the special meaning of victimization to males.

NiCarthy, G.: Getting free: a handbook for women in abusive relationships. Seattle, 1982, The Seal Press.

This is a self-help book directed to the abused woman which provides practical advice for: overcoming fears; finding shelter; dealing with the batterer and the children; evaluating lawyers, doctors and counselors; and finding new friends and relationships. Nurses would find it helpful reading to suggest to clients who are in abusive/violent relationships.

Pelton, L. (editor) The social context of child abuse and neglect. New York, 1985, Human Sciences Press.

This text presents empirical evidence supporting the assertion that social and economic factors, especially poverty, create stress in parents which can provoke maltreatment of children. The contributors describe innovative service, program, and policy recommendations that address the situational context of child abuse.

Rathbone-McCuan, E.: Elderly victims of family violence and neglect, Social Casework 61:296, 1980.

The author discusses noninstitutional aged persons as victims of nonaccidental violence. Intervention in this problem has been limited because of lack of community and professional awareness, absence of protective service legislation; personnel shortages among agencies; and restrictions on data availability.

Russianoff, P. (editor): Women in crisis. New York, 1981, Human Sciences Press.

This text contains the most important papers delivered at the first 'Women in Crisis' Conference held in 1979 in New York. The text is divided into three parts: (1) the issue of women in crisis, (2) problems and approaches in intervention, and (3) making change. The book is valuable for all health professionals, lawyers, legislators, judges, and public policy makers.

Sanford, L.: The silent children: a parent's guide to the prevention of child sexual abuse. New York, 1980, McGraw Hill Book Co.

This book offers a detailed and practical program designed for parents to make their children less vulnerable to the crimes of incest, child molestation or sexual abuse, and rape. Parents contributed a section to address the special needs of Blacks, Asians, Hispanics, Native Americans, single parents, and parents of handicapped or disabled children.

*Sharer, K.: Nursing therapy with abusive and neglectful families, J. Psychiatr. Nurs. 17(9):12, 1979.

The author presents a thorough review of the problem of child abuse and neglect, including explanatory theories surrounding the problem. A case study is presented, applying the theoretical framework of the six nursing subroles.

Steinmetz, S.: Women and violence: victims and perpetrators, Am. J. Psychother. 34:334, 1980.

The role of women as victims and perpetrators of violence is examined with a focus on violence within the family context. Violence against women is traced historically, and trends of increasing female criminal violence are briefly discussed.

Tsai, M., and Wagner, N.: Therapy groups for women sexually molested as children, Arch. Sex. Behav. 7:417, 1978.

The authors describe the results of group therapy with a total of 50 women. The primary curative component was identified as a sense of identification and emotional closeness in an environment that is warm and supportive of persons who shared a common bond.

U.S. Department of Justice: Attorney General's protecting our children against molestations: a national symposium. Washington, D.C., 1984, U.S. Government Printing Office.

This report presents the papers and addresses of 75 experts at a national symposium on the problem of child sexual victimization sponsored by the U.S. Dept. of Justice. The experts addressed the areas of prevention, education methods, counseling and care for the victim and family, the international scope of the problem as it affects our nation, recent research and future needs, and improving the response of the criminal justice system and all service agencies.

U.S. Department of Justice: Attorney General's task force on family violence: final report. Washington, D.C., 1984, U.S. Government Printing Office.

This report summarizes the findings of the attorney general's task force on family violence tht evolved as a result of findings from the earlier report on victims of crime. Of importance are specific recommendations for the type and scope of education for all professionals including national board exams, licensure, and certification.

U.S. Department of Justice: President's task force on victims of crime: final report. Washington, D.C., 1982, U.S. Government Printing Office.

This report summarizes the findings of the President's interdisciplinary task force on victims of crime in the U.S. The report is considered essential reading for all persons interested in preventing and intervening in abuse/violence as a societal problem in our nation.

Victimology.

An international journal.

Warner, C.: Conflict intervention in social and domestic violence, Bowie, Md., 1981, Robert J. Brady Co.

This is a collection of papers that includes theories about violence, its incidence, and suggestions for specific intervention techniques with victims and their families.

White, R., and Terrell, A.: Victim services bibliography: an annotation by subject. Washington, D.C., 1984, National Organization for Victim Assistance (1757 Park Road, N.W., Wash. D.C. 20010).

This annotated bibliography offers a comprehensive summary of current research and clinical reports in the field of victimology.

Wolkenstein, A.: The fear of committing child abuse: a discussion of eight families, Child Welfare 56(4):249, 1977.

The author describes a child abuse prevention program with eight families, five of whom were single-parent families and volunteered to participate in a program for potentially abusive parents. A life-line procedure was used so that staff were available to clients 24 hours a day, 7 days a week, for help as long as necessary.

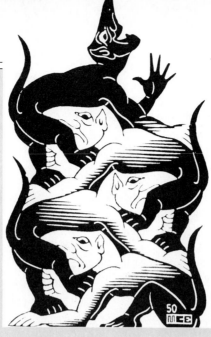

*One summer's night I was digging and tripping around
I found myself drinking with an old friend,
Then getting pinned to the ground
This was an occasion when I first found my true identity
with the cross,
As he pounded himself into me,
I lied motionless,
And to him it was a loss.
So yelling about God got me here.
But I trust Him so my day is near.
'Cause soon I'll be home and rid of this shit,
They will realize that I am a mere child of God
In the midst of a God-for-saken-fit.*

*A rape victim and mental hospital patient,
The Nut That Put Me Here[7]**

C H A P T E R   3 3

NURSING INTERVENTIONS WITH SEXUAL ASSAULT AND RAPE VICTIMS

Theresa S. Foley
Barbara A. Grimes

LEARNING OBJECTIVES

After studying this chapter, the student should be able to:

- define sexual assault and rape including the concept of nonconsent and its legal definition.

- discuss the incidence of sexual assault as a current problem in American society.

- compare and contrast thirteen common myths about sexual assault and rape, the results of believing the myths, and the facts.

- describe three phases of growth nurses experience as they work with sexual assault victims.

- relate common psychological responses of victims to a sexual assault.

- assess the influence of a sexual assault victim's coping style, social support, past psychiatric history, and nature of the assault on her subsequent adjustment.

- formulate individualized nursing diagnoses and a treatment plan for victims of a sexual assault and their significant others.

- identify assault-specific treatments for sexual assault victims.

- apply assault-specific treatments in the nursing care of sexual assault and rape victims and their significant others.

- identify criteria for referring sexual assault victims for long-term counseling and referral resources in the community.

- describe legal responsibilities in providing nursing care to sexual assault victims.

- evaluate the knowledge base and efficacy of treatment approaches for sexual assault and rape victims.

- identify directions for future nursing research.

- select appropriate readings for further study.

Nurses will see sexual assault victims of all age-groups and in every area of their practice, thus there is a need to focus on prevention, effective nursing interventions, and long-term counseling of victims. The term sexual assault is used in this chapter for two reasons: (1) experts in the field accept that "rape" includes a range of unwanted sexual acts beyond forced vaginal intercourse; and (2) legal definitions, which vary among the states, have changed to include a range of forced sexual acts as "rape" with degrees of charged offenses structured according to the type of offense committed. It is acknowledged that males are victims of sexual assault and that females are also sexual offenders, however for clarity in this chapter, the victim will be referred to as "she" and the sexual offender referred to as "he." Finally, the focus of this chapter will be limited to the adolescent and adult victim of sexual assault.

Sexual assault defined and described

The most widely accepted definition of **sexual assault** is that it is the forcible perpetration of an act of sexual contact on the body (female or male) of another person without their consent. The criminal sexual conduct statute in the nurse's state of residence will specify if:

1. The felony can be charged against one's spouse or partner
2. It includes completed or attempted sexual assault, whether homosexual or heterosexual
3. It includes the use of coercion, force, and bribery of children
4. It excludes victim resistance standards
5. It restricts use of the victim's sexual history as evidence in court
6. The sexual offense includes only vaginal intercourse (historically the requirement) or includes a range of other unwanted sexual acts such as oral intercourse, anal sodomy, touching of one's "private parts," or exploitation through photography

Many victims consider oral or anal sodomy to be more humiliating and traumatic than legal definitions limited to penile-vaginal assaults.

The concept of force includes verbal and physical force, threats, and intimidation in which the victim complies in the interest of survival or is unable to resist.

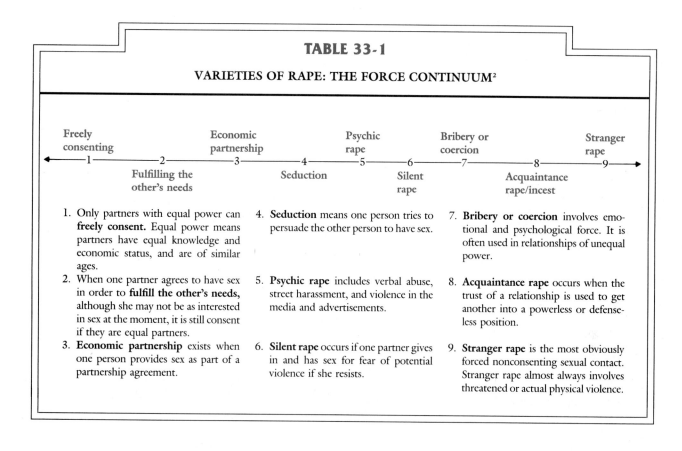

TABLE 33-1

VARIETIES OF RAPE: THE FORCE CONTINUUM[2]

Freely consenting — 1 — 2 — Economic partnership — 3 — 4 — Psychic rape — 5 — 6 — Bribery or coercion — 7 — 8 — Stranger rape — 9

Fulfilling the other's needs   Seduction   Silent rape   Acquaintance rape/incest

1. Only partners with equal power can **freely consent.** Equal power means partners have equal knowledge and economic status, and are of similar ages.

2. When one partner agrees to have sex in order to **fulfill the other's needs,** although she may not be as interested in sex at the moment, it is still consent if they are equal partners.

3. **Economic partnership** exists when one person provides sex as part of a partnership agreement.

4. **Seduction** means one person tries to persuade the other person to have sex.

5. **Psychic rape** includes verbal abuse, street harassment, and violence in the media and advertisements.

6. **Silent rape** occurs if one partner gives in and has sex for fear of potential violence if she resists.

7. **Bribery or coercion** involves emotional and psychological force. It is often used in relationships of unequal power.

8. **Acquaintance rape** occurs when the trust of a relationship is used to get another into a powerless or defenseless position.

9. **Stranger rape** is the most obviously forced nonconsenting sexual contact. Stranger rape almost always involves threatened or actual physical violence.

Nonconsent includes a range of dimensions such as: explicit refusal or resistance; substance intoxication that precludes consent; and cognitive, physical, or emotional impairment such as with mental retardation, developmental disabilities, mental illness, or old age. Evidence of force, therefore, demonstrates the presence of nonconsent by the victim to unwanted sexual acts. The concepts of force and nonconsent have recently been described on a continuum ranging from free consent in a sexually intimate relationship to stranger assault.[2] The continuum combines socialization processes that promote sexual assault and legal criteria for the felony in describing a variety of conditions based on the principle of inequality in a relationship (see Table 33-1).

The legal definition of sexual assault has its origin in the property rights of man. Historically, man has protected his property, progeny, and inheritance rights. With women as his property, he had complete, sole, and total access to a woman; she was barter in a trade. The rapist, when convicted, was punished for unlawful possession of property. The concept operating was that male rights of possession had been violated based on the bargain of marriage for the virginity, chastity, and sole consent to her person. Even today many criminal sexual assault statutes do not recognize the right of a woman to control her own body. They imply that one cannot steal what one already owns. They assume that once a woman signs the marriage license she cannot refuse sex, even if she is sick or unwilling. It is essential for the nurse to be informed of the criminal sexual conduct statute of one's state, and to support task forces working to update criminal statutes to meet contemporary criteria for this felony.

Another reason for failing to identify behavior as forced sexual assault is the socialization processes evident in our society that perpetuate belief systems historically contained in "rape" laws. Recent research reveals that most teenagers do not believe that forcible sexual acts on dates constitute a sexual assault, and that date/acquaintance rape is acceptable under some circumstances. Fisher[23] found in a random sample of 245 female and 194 male teenagers that only 24% of the total sample (19% of males and 5% of females) answered yes to the question, "Is forcible sex on dates definitely rape?" Goodchilds and co-workers[35,36,80] investigating responsibility and sexual behavior, found that of 432 teenagers surveyed in Los Angeles more than 50% of the males (n = 245) and 42% of the females (n = 194) agreed that it was all right if a male holds a female down and forces her to engage in sexual

> ### CLINICAL EXAMPLE 33-1
>
> Susan is a 20-year-old college student attending a university and living in an apartment. Susan awoke suddenly to find a man had entered her apartment through a window in her kitchen. She screamed and tried to escape but was unsuccessful and the man raped her.

> ### CLINICAL EXAMPLE 33-2
>
> Cheryl is a 16-year-old high school student who attended a jazz concert at the civic center. She lost her friends and became confused by the building when the concert was over. Two men offered to show her where to go. They escorted her down a hallway and shoved her into a closet used for cleaning equipment. They threw Cheryl on the floor and raped her. Cheryl felt betrayed. She was afraid to tell her parents about the rape because they did not want her to go to the concert and were concerned about her safety.

intercourse if she gets him sexually excited. In a survey of college students by Malamuth,[54] 51% of college males reported they would rape a woman if they knew they wouldn't be caught and punished, and they also indicated that they thought the victim would enjoy it. These responses reflect the persistence of societal socialization processes that exempt males from responsibility for inappropriate sexual conduct and condone their aggressive tendencies, blame females for sexual assaults, and are consistent with the statistics on date/acquaintance rape for college or adult women.

Because legal definitions of sexual assault vary, nursing research and other funded researchers continue to use the three main categorizations of sexual assault according to lack of consent specified by Burgess and Holmstrom in 1974[11]:

1. Rape—sex without consent
2. Accessory to sex—inability to consent or not consent because of the victim's stage of cognitive or personality development
3. Sex-stress situation—sex with initial consent in which something drastically went wrong; usually the male exploited the initial agreement

The authors also reported two main styles of attack. The first is the **blitz rape,** the least common form of sexual assault, in which the victim and assailant lack prior interaction, as described in Clinical example 33-1.

The second style of attack is a **confidence rape,** the most common form of sexual assault, in which interaction between the victim and assailant generally occurs prior to the assault, and the assailant obtains access to the victim through the use of deceit, betrayal, or violence, as in Clinical example 33-2.

In literature, myth, and culture, rape is sanctioned as an act of power intended to humiliate and degrade the person. Brownmiller defines the effect of rape as follows:

A sexual invasion of the body by force, an incursion into the private, personal inner space without consent . . . In short,

an internal assault from one of several avenues and by one of several methods . . . [It] constitutes a deliberate violation of emotional, physical and rational integrity and is a hostile, degrading act of violence.[6:376]

For the woman, rape implies total loss of self, in which she is reduced from a person to an object and a function. She experiences total isolation and emptiness from herself and society. The net effect is to simultaneously destroy the sense of person and the sense of community, to depersonalize the woman by separating her person from her humanity. A victim's ability to maintain coping defenses is challenged by a sexual assault because intense feelings of anxiety, guilt, and inadequacy are aroused. Rape is experienced as a loss, and thus the victim needs to be afforded all the rights and privileges of a period of mourning and grief.

■ **Incidence of sexual assault and rape**

In 1984 the FBI Uniform Crime Reports stated that 84,233 sexual assaults, or attempts to commit sexual assault by force or threat of force, were reported; this represents an increase of 11% from 1979 figures (75,789 cases) and a 127% increase from 1970 figures (over 37,000 cases).[73] It is estimated that the majority of all reported incidents are committed by someone the victim knows and believes she can trust. To understand the seriousness of this felony, these figures must be doubled because it is estimated that 50% of violent crimes are unreported,[73] and surveys of criminal victimization estimate that 40% to 50% of forcible sexual assaults are not reported.[48] The enormity of this felony is further evident from national statistics on date/acquaintance and marital sexual assault as research results are increasingly being reported (see accompanying box).

Sexual assault is the highest rising violent crime in

the nation and the most underreported of all Crime Index Offenses. Nonreporting is the result of victims' fears of nonbelief, fears of the assailant, feelings of embarrassment and guilt, and a socialized response of self-blame. It quickly becomes apparent that Western society reflects a culture of increasing violence and that the nurse can expect to see many victims of violence. For some victims, the nurse may well be the first person encountered subsequent to the sexual assault and may be the only advocate the victim will have throughout attempts to receive care. The treatment a sexual assault victim receives immediately after the event has been noted to be a critical variable in later resolution of the crisis. It is therefore imperative that nurses utilize in their practice what is known about sexual assault and interventions with victims to facilitate post-trauma adjustment.

Historical perspective

Abuse and violence against women and children as an inherent part of their lives has been recognized throughout recorded history.[6] As long ago as 1870 Susan B. Anthony wrote, "... I do pray ... for some terrific shock to startle the women of this nation into self-respect which will compel them to see the abject degradation of their present position."[10] The problem of sexual assault was brought to the attention of the United States by three important forces: (1) the "antirape movement" initiated by the women's movement in the 1960s; (2) federal funding that established the National Center for the Prevention and Control of Rape; and (3) the National Organization of Victim's Assistance.

Development of the women's movement was a gradual process that began with consciousness-raising

---

Incidence of Sexual Assault/Rape

- 44% of women have been a victim of an actual or attempted sexual assault at some time in their lives[65,66]
- 50% of women who have ever been a victim of an actual or attempted sexual assault reported more than one such experience[65,66]
- Only 12% of the time is the perpetrator a stranger to the victim[65,66]
- Only 2% of reported sexual assaults result in arrest[57,65,66]
- Only 2% to 5% of reported sexual assaults end in conviction of the perpetrator[57,65,66]

Date or Acquaintance Sexual Assault/Rape

- 52% of 7,000 women in college today surveyed among 35 college campuses have experienced some form of sexual victimization[46,71]:
    —Almost ¾ of sample who met the most conservative legal criteria for rape did not identify their experience as a rape
    —More than ⅓ did not discuss the experience with anyone
    —More than 90% did not report the incident to police
    —1 in 12 men admitted to sexual assault or attempts according to the most conservative prevailing legal definition yet virtually none of those men identified themselves as rapists
- 20% of college women in three separate surveys at three universities reported sexual assault by men they knew[71]

- 51% of college-age men reported they would rape a woman if they knew they wouldn't be caught and punished, and indicated they thought the victim would enjoy it[2,54]

Marital Rape/Sexual Assault

- 1 in 7 (14%) women in a random sample of 930 women who have ever been married have experienced as a result of force, threat of force, or inability to consent at least one completed or attempted rape by their husband or ex-husband; twice as many women have been raped by their husbands as by strangers. Results do not include experiences of forced oral/anal intercourse, women who submitted out of a sense of helplessness or duty, or women unable to identify or acknowledge that their husbands' behaviors were inappropriate. Thus, the statistics of marital rape are believed to be much higher.[55,57,65,66,78,79]
- It is a felony in 29 states and District of Columbia; a felony in 20 states pending exemption specification according to state law (e.g., legal separation filed, divorce filed); not a felony in 1 state[22,57,65]
- Of 210 cases filed, 48 dropped; of the remaining cases (75%) prosecuted the conviction rate is 80% to 90%[57]
- First Supreme Court decision occurred on November 1985 and ruled marital rape is definitely rape[57,77]

groups providing a supportive and intimate environment. In these groups women were able to share, often for the first time, experiences of childhood sexual or physical victimization and adult sexual assault. The women's movement confronted the political and social function of sexual assault in society as one of keeping women powerless. With the support of their peers and publication of the first newsletter on sexual assault by Laura X[79] women were given the impetus to speak out about the crimes that had been committed against them. In 1974 Germaine Greer was the first to interview a rape victim on national television. The New York Radical Feminists broke the silence of the crime by holding a "rape speakout," in which, for the first time in public forum, women began to tell of the horrors they sustained. The forum resulted in publication of a book, *Rape: the First Source Book for Women,*[18] exploring the reasons for rape, what a woman can do to protect herself, and how women can join forces toward resolution of rape as a problem. A movement against rape began throughout the United States with the joint efforts of dispersed grass roots groups that developed sexual assault crisis centers and combined the efforts of professionals and feminists toward further analysis and prevention of this problem.

Over the last 10 years these combined efforts have modified our understanding and conceptualization of this problem through three phases. *Phase 1* involved a proliferation of scientific and feminist literature that attacked society's prevailing view of sexual assault as a crime of passion versus a crime of violence. As stated by Brownmiller[6] in *Against Our Will: Men, Women, and Rape,* the intent of such random terrorizing is to keep all women "in their places." Brownmiller's book resulted in an explosion in national consciousness about the etiology of sexual assault. From a feminist perspective she argued that all men benefit, whether or not they consciously intend to, from the rape of women as a social-control exchange. Thus, like any class that is "kept in their place" women have fewer opportunities in all areas of life, and this reinforces and perpetuates a societal structure of male power and dominance over females. This first phase was a necessary historical development at the time.[79]

Phase 2 followed in which it was more readily accepted among professionals and in society that sexual assault and rape were "all violence" in which the dominant motivating factors are power and aggression rather than "all or only sex."[79] Public TV debates and literature in the field continued to refute myths such as, "You can't rape a moving target" or victim consent, and the victim's experience of violence and terror versus pleasure, passion, and romance was acknowledged.

Finally, research by feminists, sociologists, and psychiatric and mental health professionals moved us into *phase 3,* the current phase, with modified conceptualizations about this felony. In phase 3 current conceptualizations include[79]: (1) experts now recognize that the violence expressed through a sexual assault is inextricably connected to sexuality: (2) that taking control over, dominating, and humiliating a person through sexual assault is a "sexual turn-on" for offenders; (3) sexual assault is neither "all or only sex" nor "all violence" but a combination of the two in which violence is eroticized and sexualized; (4) sexual assault is therefore appropriately called a "sex crime" when forced sex and the expression of aggression, hostility, power, and dominance are motives; (5) that within a sexual assault the offender's aggression and sexuality have the potential to merge in sadism or murder[8,62]; and (6) marital and date/acquaintance rapes are paradigms of this phenomenon.

Thus, phase 3 not only acknowledges that sexual assault is eroticized, sexualized violence in which forced sex, power, and aggression are the motives but also combines historical perspectives on the "politics of rape." In addition, the clinical and scientific field has moved beyond describing victim responses to investigating which post-event treatments are most effective in facilitating adjustment to this life crisis. In the decade ahead, one can expect more research and feminist efforts to be directed toward: (1) understanding and preventing the sexualization of violence in society, particularly where juveniles are concerned; (2) changing existing sexual conduct statutes to reflect that "marital rape is rape" without restrictions; (3) educating the public about marital and date/acquaintance rape; and (4) finding effective assault-specific treatments to facilitate a victim's and her significant others' post-event adjustment.

■ Centers and organizations

Sexual assault crisis centers are structures developed "through which women can begin to take back control over our lives—control which is denied in part by the threat of rape."[72] Through the women's movement, victims recognized that they were more able to control what happened to them when they joined together to help each other. Women found that they could help each other after a sexual assault had occurred to obtain needed services, learn to protect themselves, and work to eradicate the crime in society. Included in the achievements of this era were the public attention brought to the poor way in which victims were treated by institutions which resulted in "secondary victimization" following a sexual assault, and changes in the quality of services provided.[71]

In 1972 there were only three centers whereas today

almost all cities and towns provide sexual assault crisis intervention and counseling services through an assault crisis or community mental health center, YWCA, or other specified local agencies listed in the phone book yellow pages. Sexual assault centers are located in a variety of settings ranging from the YWCA to rented office space and hospitals and function within varying organizational structures. Because of limited funding most centers are staffed by volunteers. Services provided generally include a crisis/telephone line for immediate support, information, and short-term counseling of victims. Most centers also provide advocates to go with victims to the hospital, the police, and court proceedings. When long-term counseling needs arise, victims are generally referred to other social service agencies. Rape prevention and treatment for victims is one of the 13 services mandated by the federal government to be provided by community mental health centers. Professionals in community mental health centers are now being challenged to demonstrate the effectiveness of treatment received by victims referred to them.

Most often professionals are welcomed in antirape projects. Feminists noted the need for professional involvement in rape crisis centers if victims were to receive better care and more sensitive treatment from professionals. However, the tendency to defer to professional leadership, as happened in the development of suicide crisis prevention centers, is a current trend feminists caution against. Working as peers within the system, professionals offer skills and knowledge that are valuable resources in a project. After two decades of work in this field, nurses have yet to demonstrate a significant impact on the opportunities available in this area of practice for using nursing expertise to open boundaries between themselves, victims of sexual assault, rape crisis centers, law enforcement and other disciplines, educators, and the community.

As a result of the women's movement, which brought public attention to the problem of sexual assault, legislation introduced by Senator Charles Mathias in 1973 established the National Center for the Prevention and Control of Rape (NCPCR) in 1975 within NIMH (Public Law 94-63, Section 231). The legal mandate of the NCPCR was for research, training, and public education related to: (1) the etiology of sexual assault; (2) the short- and long-term mental health consequences on children and adults from these crimes; (3) the design, implementation, and evaluation of treatment programs for victims, their families, and their communities; and (4) the effectiveness of programs designed to reduce and prevent sexual assault and acts of violence. As a result of projects funded under the above four categories, knowledge over the last decade has increased considerably, and the dissemination of this knowledge to professionals has gradually improved services victims and their families receive today.[52] After a decade of advancements in the field, the NCPCR was abolished in 1985 as a Division within NIMH due to changes in federal funding priorities and structural reorganization within NIMH under the Reagan administration.

The final force which brought attention to sexual assault as a societal problem was the establishment of the National Organization of Victim's Assistance (NOVA) in 1977. NOVA is a private, nonprofit organization of victim and witness assistance practitioners, criminal justice professionals, researchers, former victims, and others committed to the recognition of victim rights. NOVA's activities are guided by four purposes: (1) national advocacy, (2) helping victims, (3) service to local programs, and (4) membership support.

Myth dimension

The myths that exist about the crime of sexual assault are damaging to everyone involved. The victim will not be taken care of empathically when law enforcement and medical personnel subscribe to sexual assault myths. The victim will find her claims doubted by family and friends. If the victim believes sexual assault myths, as many do, she will have greater difficulty resolving shame and guilt. Finally, the crime of sexual assault is fostered as society plays out the myths in different health care settings that continue to excuse or condone the act.[53] All myths have a similar function: they result in the victim blaming herself.

Before the nurse can effectively assist the sexual assault victim, it is essential to be aware of biases held and the extent to which biases affect one's belief system about sexual assault and nursing care of victims. Brodsky and Hobart[5] note that on the basis of assumptions about the nature and causation of sexual assault, treaters and researchers develop differing treatment plans and decisions and act on these assumptions within the treatment plans, whether or not they are aware of doing so. The authors define blame as "attribution of responsibility and focus of attention," which is put into operation in one of four blame models[5]:

1. **Offender blame model.** In the offender blame model sexual assault takes place when a person with deficits in aggressive/sexual behavior makes forcible sexual contact. "He had to be crazy."

2. **Victim blame model.** Under this model sexual assault takes place when a woman has in some way, obviously or nonobviously, consciously or unconsciously, allowed herself to be in an interpersonal or physical position that antecedes forcible sexual contact. "She deserved what she got."

3. Situational blame model. Sexual assault takes place when environmental and structural circumstances, transient factors in mood or place, and assault-vulnerble parties merge to generate a forcible sexual contact by one person or another. "She should not have gone to the party, concert, bar."

4. Societal blame model. Sexual assault takes place when accumulated cultural and societal attitudes are manifested through the forcible sexual contact of one person on another. "Men dominate and abuse women."

Blame models suggest levels at which prevention, education, and intervention can occur. Table 33-2 is a composite presentation of existing sexual assault myths, the results of believing the myths, and the facts. There are many other myths not listed that need to be considered, for example, rape is not a serious problem for older women because they have experienced sex, or mental patients who claim rape cannot be believed and probably provoke rape. Nurses need to be aware of all rape myths.

 ## Assessment

■ Self-awareness

Self-awareness is the beginning of a nursing assessment. Counseling the victim of sexual assault can be emotionally fatiguing and raise many feelings within the nurse, particularly if the nurse is a woman. Effective nursing care emerges from working conditions that offer an arena in which feelings, experiences, problems, and cases can be freely discussed and provide the nurse with greater self-awareness. Nurses and others who begin to become informed about sexual assault and work with victims experience a variety of cognitive, affective, and behavioral responses. It is important that nurses be aware of these processes because, in the beginning, they can be frightening and the nurse needs a support network available to work them through. Later responses that are generated are more exhilarating as the nurse feels she is actively doing something about the problem.

Based on a value clarification framework, Foley and Davies[27] describe a three-phase process nurses experience as they work with sexual assault victims (see Fig. 33-1).

> Phase one: **choosing values,** nurses work through four affective or cognitive responses: (1) denial or belief in sexual assault myths; (2) resolving cognitive dissonance that results from becoming informed of empirical facts that refute myths; (3) anxiety that emerges from increased awareness about the prevalance of the phenomena; and (4)

anger about sexual assault and its long-term impact. Since these affective and cognitive states create intolerable tension over time, the nurse moves into the next phase.

> Phase two: **action,** the nurse engages in one of five activities: (1) seeking more information about the phenomena; (2) providing emergency nursing care to victims; (3) consultation to professionals and the public; (4) educating professionals and the public; and, (5) counseling victims of sexual assault. Nurses who are committed to reversing the incidence of sexual assault and identifying effective interventions for victims move into phase 3.

> Phase three: **prizing,** consists of four behaviors evidencing the nurse's level of commitment: (1) research on the nature of the problem and the efficacy of nursing interventions; (2) volunteering as a counselor in a crisis center to provide care to victims; (3) public education through speaking engagements; and (4) social action programs or activities that increase societal awareness of the problem and change conditions that promote, maintain, and sanction sexual assault.

In providing nursing care to a sexual assault victim, a number of specific factors need to be considered in the assessment process:[63]

1. **Philosophy.** The issue of "Who owns the rape?" or who makes the decisions is the most important issue in counseling to ensure that the victim regains control over her life as soon as possible.

2. **Confidentiality.** All that the victim tells the nurse should not be passed on to others without the victim's explicit permission. Consultation can be obtained while the victim's identity is protected.

3. **Neutrality.** By maintaining a neutral position, the nurse facilitates the victim's making her own decisions from information on alternatives and from the chance to review advantages, disadvantages, and options.

4. **Intense feelings.** The nurse needs to allow the victim to lead the conversation, help her explore her feelings, and meet her level of intensity through empathic responses. Encouraging verbalization and ventilation is one means of helping her regain control.

5. **Silences.** If the nurse can allow long pauses without becoming alarmed, she can use the time to think about what is going on with the victim, the situation, and possible actions.

TABLE 33-2

SEXUAL ASSAULT AND RAPE MYTHS, RESULTS OF THE MYTHS, AND FACTS

Myth	Result of myth	Fact
Rape is provoked by the victim; victims are responsible for their victimization either consciously or by default; all women really want to be raped	Blame is taken from rapist and responsibility for crime is shifted to victim; it fosters public statements incorrectly connecting sexual permissiveness with rape, such as that made by Judge Archie Simmons of Dane County, Wisconsin (since recalled from office)	About 80% of rapes are planned in advance by rapist, victim is usually threatened with death or body harm if she resists; rape is violent attack using sex as weapon; a woman does not ask for violence (rape) by accepting a date, acting polite, being friendly and cheerful, dressing and walking in socially defined attractive ways; no woman's behavior or dress gives a man the right to rape her; Federal Commission found only 4% of sexual assaults involved "precipitative behavior," which consisted of only a slight "gesture" in their definition
Only young beautiful women in miniskirts are raped; it can't happen to me; only other types of women get raped; only "bad girls" get raped; rape reflects demographic strain caused by sex–marital status imbalance in community; only promiscuous women get raped	Women deny rape could happen to them; belief in myth perpetuates unhealthy denial defense mechanism and lack of readiness for self-defense; rape is the only felonious, violent crime in which victim is held suspect and has burden of proof of innocence; women tend to blame themselves for crime, not report it or not seek support from others because of embarrassment, shame, and questions about where they can turn for empathy and help	Rapists choose victims without regard for age, race, or socioeconomic class; chances are 1 in 15 a woman will be raped in her lifetime; some cities report probability as high as 1 in 3; reported victims' age range is 6 months to 93 years; highest incidence is in women 15 to 24 years of age (target population)
Sexual assault occurs only among total strangers; if I avoid strangers, I will not be raped	Women who are acquainted with the rapist tend to blame themselves more and are less likely to report the crime or prosecute the assailant; fault is attributed to woman for "leading him on"; women deny that their spouse/lover could be rapist; one will not believe victim if one believes this myth; women do not report rape for fear of repercussions if they are raped by acquaintance/friend; they wonder if they will be believed, how others will react, and if offender will seek revenge (a common threat to keep rape secret); marital conflict and divorce are kindled by belief in this myth	Amir[1] found 66% of *reported* rapes took place between strangers, yet in 34% victim and offender were acquainted; in 14%, rapist was member of family, friend of family, or close personal friend. It is important to note that these statistics reflect only reported forcible rape and that woman is more likely to report rape by stranger than friend or relative, as is often the case with adolescents; victims report that spouses and lovers do not believe them, blame them, and separate or divorce in many cases

*Modified from Keller, E., and Remus, S.: Statistics on sexual assault, Minnesota Program for Victims of Sexual Assault, 430 Metro Square Building, St. Paul, Minn. 55101; Travis, M.: The most common myths concerning rape—and the facts, *Brainerd Daily Dispatch*, May 15, 1976; and the collected publications of A.W. Burgess and L.L. Holmstrom.

Continued.

TABLE 33-2—cont'd

SEXUAL ASSAULT AND RAPE MYTHS, RESULTS OF THE MYTHS, AND FACTS

Myth	Result of myth	Fact
Women are raped when they are out alone at night, primarily in dark alleys; if women stay at home, they will be safe	Belief is perpetuated that women are not raped by their husbands; it reflects a "just world" rationale, implying she would not have been raped had she been "in her place" or "undeserving"; it violates her right to freedom of movement by dictating self-defense strategies	Any woman can be victim of rape, regardless of social or economic class, appearance, age, or place of residence; woman's husband can rape her; half of all rapes occur in private residence and a third to a half of all sexual assaults are committed in victim's home; on October 5, 1977, Oregon was first state to amend its laws so that a woman could prosecute her husband for rape
Most rapes involve black men and white women; blacks are more likely to attack white women than black women; all rapes are interracial	A woman who was raped by someone of her own race would not be believed by one who believed this myth; myth perpetuates racial prejudices that exist in society	Amir[1] found that rape was intraracial, especially between black men and women; FBI statistics cite 3% of rapes involve black women and white men; most rapes involve victim-offender of same race and socioeconomic class
Rape is impulsive, uncontrollable act of sexual gratification (i.e., a sexually frustrated man sees attractive young woman and "just can't control himself")	One will expect victim to be accountable for actions of rapist; one will not hold rapist responsible for his behavior and will excuse and condone his "need" rather than challenge his violent lack of impulse control	Amir[1] found 71% of all rapes were planned, rapist had it in his mind to rape specific woman or any woman; in 11% of cases, rapist took advantage of woman in more "vulnerable" position—drunk, walking alone at night, hitchhiking, only 16% were rapes with no prior intent to commit crime; rapists describe their motivation as hatred, conquest, humiliation, and degradation, not in terms of sexual gratification and report a lack of sexual gratification afterward; Groth and Birnbaum found 58% of 170 convicted rapists experienced sexual dysfunction during rape and often dysfunction increased assailant's rage toward victim
Rapists are abnormal perverts or men with unsatisfied sex drive; only "sick" or "insane" men rape women; primary motive for rape is sexual; rapist is sexually starved psychopath	One would not believe that normal-appearing and acting man could have committed rape; one may expect rapist to stand out in crowd, to have special identifiable characteristics; attire worn at jury trials to convey respectable character reference plays on public's tendency to believe this myth	Rapists generally exhibit "normal" types of behavior, are generally sexually active with spouse or partner, and have normal sex drive; their major difference is lack of impulse control seen in greater than average tendency toward expressing violence, rapist is assessed as having abnormal tendency toward being aggressive and violent; otherwise his personality appears within "normal" limits.

Continued.

TABLE 33-2—cont'd

SEXUAL ASSAULT AND RAPE MYTHS, RESULTS OF THE MYTHS, AND FACTS

Myth	Result of myth	Fact
Any woman could prevent rape if she really wanted to; no woman can be raped against her will; victims generally do not resist their attackers; any woman who resists her attacker will be killed	One who believes this myth expects victim to be brutally beaten because of her resistance and does not believe her in absence of bruises and cuts, although only victim can assess what resistance is possible if she cannot escape assailant; myth fails to recognize that immobility or "freezing" is psychological response to extreme fear; carrying this myth to its "logical" extreme, it is better to be dead than alive	Amir[1] found in a majority of cases, victim was threatened with death if she resisted, rapist carried weapon or threatened death in 87% of cases, manhandled in 30%, verbally threatened in 20%, used no force in 15% (usually with child victims); almost all victims reacted with fear for their lives; in view of known humiliation, fear of injury or death, and loss of control over her life and body, it is amazing this myth still exists; suicide is a documented behavior of victim response to rape
Rape occurs only in large cities	One who believes this myth is less likely to believe victim who reports rape that occurred outside large city	Sexual assault happens everywhere—rural, suburban, and urban areas; majority of reported rapes occur in urban areas; rural rape crisis centers report high incidence of the community believing rape myths and thus difficulty in obtaining adequate care for victims; both factors affect underreporting of rape in smaller communities
It is easy to prosecute rapists; not to prosecute implies that woman is guilty of consent	One may believe that if woman was really raped, she will prosecute man; one fails to look at reasons she does not report or prosecute and work for change in those areas; one may have contempt for victim who does not win her case or who refuses to prosecute	Unless victim has "respectable character," filed prompt report with police, has eye witness to crime, is not acquainted with assailant, is assaulted by man of different race, is sexually inexperienced, and sustained physical injuries, case is unlikely to be taken to trial or receive conviction; Holmstrom and Burgess found that of 109 cases, 24 went to trial and 4 received convictions for rape; nationally approximately 3% of reported cases lead to conviction[40]; this means conviction rate as low as 0.3% if estimates of unreported rapes are taken into account; many cases are lost because of jurors' tendency to believe myths, failure to interview and exclude jurors holding myths beliefs, and improper collection of corroborative evidence

Continued.

TABLE 33-2—cont'd

SEXUAL ASSAULT AND RAPE MYTHS, RESULTS OF THE MYTHS, AND FACTS

Myth	Result of myth	Fact
Women frequently cry "rape"; there is a high rate of false reports	One will not develop or provide type of care victim desperately needs; one will be skeptical of anyone who reports rape or seeks care; victim who believes this myth will blame herself for attack; if she knows others believe myth, she may not report rape, fearing she will not be believed	False report rate for other kinds of felonies is 2%; rape has same rate
Rape is minor crime affecting only few women	One who believes this myth will act with disbelief when someone reports rape; one will not believe that sexual assault would occur in his area or to anyone he knows	Rape is the fastest rising violent crime in United States; in 1979 number of "founded" reported rape cases was 75,789; if this number is multiplied by factor of 10 to account for unreported cases, no less than 757,890 women were raped in 1979; these are epidemic proportions; it is estimated that chances are 1 in 15 that woman will be raped in her lifetime
Rape is predominantly hot weather crime; women provoke rape by their style of dress and behavior	One may believe that people who dress for warmer weather invite rape and are at fault for crime	Amir's[1] study found that thermic law of delinquency was not confirmed in his study; Denver Report found higher incidence of rape in summer months correlated to cold weather areas; person's dress style is not license for others to assault that person with impunity

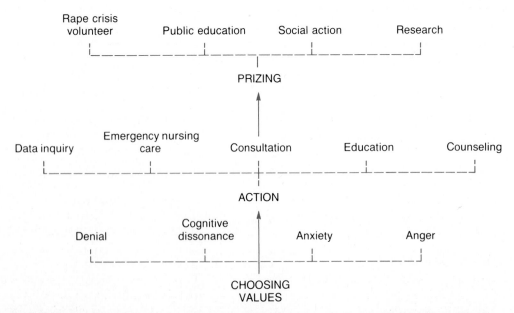

Fig. 33-1. Positive growth experiences of nurses in response to rape. (From Foley, T.S. and Davies, M.A.: Rape: nursing care of victims, St. Louis, 1983, The C.V. Mosby Company, p. 66. Reprinted with permission.)

6. **Keeping the nurse's problems in the background.** Focus needs to be maintained on the victim's concerns rather than the nurse's own "causes," such as abortion, politics, or reporting.

7. **Keeping the nurse's agenda out of the discussion.** The use of "should" or "ought" is to be avoided, since they cut short an exploring dialogue, may irritate or alienate a victim, and usurp her decision-making right. One way for the nurse to help the victim clarify values is to be in touch with her own feelings and values.

8. **Searching for alternatives.** Instead of giving overhelpful advice, the nurse can assist the victim to assess all possible alternatives, examining the advantages and disadvantages of each.

9. **Avoiding "why" questions.** The nurse needs to support the victim without putting her on the defensive or making her justify her plans or what she did. "Why" questions are for necessary information only, not curiosity.

10. **Recognizing the real issue.** The victim needs to be allowed to direct the conversation and decide what the real issue is, such as feelings vs. care system procedures.

11. **Message behind the statement.** The nurse can assist the victim in identifying a feeling position. The woman can then examine it, choose to keep it, reject it, or choose not to decide about it. Feelings that are identified and verbalized prevent long-term confusion.

12. **Hostility toward the nurse.** The nurse can avoid personalizing hostility when the care provided is competent. The nurse may be the first person the victim has come in contact with since the assault to whom she can safely express her rage. Finally, it is necessary for the nurse to be aware of the biases held, the myths believed, and their impact on nursing actions.

■ **Psychological responses of the victim**

Psychological responses to a sexual assault include: (1) the victim's emotional style; (2) psychological symptoms; (3) phases of response to an assault; and (4) the victim's coping style. Each of these factors will be influenced by the pre-event history of the victim and the response of her social support network post-event, including the response of mental health professionals.

1. **Emotional style.** Burgess and Holmstrom[10] identified two emotional styles: a predominantly expressed style and a controlled style. Some victims evidenced a mixed style of these two types.

Table 33-3 gives a description of these styles and defining characteristics.

2. **Psychological symptoms.** Early research in the field by Burgess and Holmstrom[10,38] described the psychological symptoms of the victim in response to a sexual assault in terms of a rape trauma syndrome. Rape trauma syndrome is now documented as fitting the criteria of an acute post-traumatic stress disorder that, without treatment, can become chronic.[6] Resolving issues of trust, betrayal, loss, and loyalty are central issues particularly traumatic for victims of marital rape or date/acquaintance sexual assault to work through.[57,71,78] As one victim stated, "I will never have blind trust in anyone again," and "I'm more afraid of having a relationship with someone than of being without one." Table 33-3 summarizes psychological reactions of a victim to a sexual assault.

3. **Phases of response.** Two reports are commonly referred to in the literature that describe a victim's phases of response in adjusting to a sexual assault: Burgess and Holmstrom[10] and Sutherland and Scherl.[70] Table 33-3 summarizes these findings. In addition, it is evident that there are many victims who experience a "silent rape syndrome" and seek treatment only years after the assault.[26] While most of these victims never reported their assault experience to anyone and carried the psychological trauma with them for 5 to 20 years or more, some victims received a medical or "rape" exam but refused crisis or follow-up counseling for a variety of reasons. These victims are called "delayed treatment seekers," and their responses comprise yet another phase of response to a sexual assault. On assessment these victims evidence a variety of clinical symptoms (see Table 33-4), which, when clustered together, meet the criteria of a post-traumatic disorder, chronic subtype. However, many nurses and other health professionals may not recognize that these symptoms represent a concealed history of sexual assault, and fail to inquire about such a history or to intervene in these symptoms as assault-specific outcomes. Thus, these victims experience "secondary victimization" when mental health professionals fail to intervene to ameliorate their chronic post-traumatic stress disorder symptoms.

4. **Coping style.** According to crisis theory (see Chapter 10) the coping mechanisms of a person are balancing factors in the resolution of a life crisis. Victims cope not only with assault-specific

TABLE 33-3

PSYCHOLOGICAL RESPONSES OF VICTIMS TO A SEXUAL ASSAULT/RAPE

Dimension	Defining characteristics
Emotional style	
1. Expressed style	Victim expresses feelings of anxiety, fear for her life, loss, concern about how to cope with men in future relationships, or anger by talking, shaking, crying, smiling, laughing to avoid crying, muscle tenseness, and restlessness
2. Controlled style	Victim masks feelings by a subdued, calm, or composed affect as if "in control" or only mildly distressed
3. Mixed style	Victim vacillates between an emotional and controlled style during the same interview
Psychological symptoms	
1. Acute reaction	Acute post-traumatic stress disorder symptoms; rape trauma syndrome
a. Emotional reaction	Fear of physical violence and death, anxiety, embarrassment, humiliation, self-blame, guilt, low self-esteem, depression, impaired social adjustment, anger and revenge, volatile or labile, incoherent, and agitated
b. Physical reaction	Gastrointestinal irritability, genitourinary irritability and discomfort, muscle tension, sleep disturbance
2. Long-term reactions	Working through repetitive nightmares, phobias, and issues of trust and betrayal in relationships with men; seeking family and social support; change of residence, work, or school
3. Silent rape syndrome	Does not disclose the assault to anyone; has not resolved feeling and reactions to the trauma; carries alone psychological trauma: often has a history of childhood sexual victimization and/or prior sexual assaults
4. Compounded reaction	Pre-event history of psychiatric, physical, or social difficulties. Characterized by psychotic behavior, depression, suicidal behavior, psychosomatic disorders, and acting-out behaviors (e.g., substance abuse, sexual promiscuity)
Phases of response	
1. Acute phase	Shock, dismay, disbelief, and disorganization expressed by victim's expressed and/or controlled style. Emotional and physical reactions described above
2. Outward adjustment	A few days or weeks post-event, victim resumes her usual pursuits at work, home, or school. Conceals a fragile adjustment based on denial and suppression of deeply felt anxieties and fears. Is not interested in talking about the event or seeking help at this time. Often will cancel, not show up for appointments, or drop out of treatment. May state she is "doing just fine"
3. Reorganization	Begins at different times for victim pending assessment of all factors under global traumatic reaction of victim, especially coping skills of victim and response of social support network. Integrates and adjusts to the traumatic event: new self-view accepting event as part of life-history; realistic appraisal of behaviors during the assault (survival); resolves feelings about offender; works through anger and resentment
4. Delayed treatment seekers	Silent rape syndrome. Chronic post-traumatic stress disorder symptoms. Rape trauma syndrome. Enters treatment following: precipitating event, an anniversary reaction, and/or unfulfilling or unsatisfying life. Perceived by others as competent and strong in instrumental roles, often associated with repeated exploitation of abuse. Impaired interpersonal relationships. Victimization history not explored on assessment or treated by "professionals"

Data from references 6, 10, 38, 57, 70, 71, 78.

TABLE 33-4

CLINICAL SYMPTOMS OF DELAYED TREATMENT-SEEKING VICTIMS OF SEXUAL ASSAULT/RAPE

Clinical symptom	Example	Post-traumatic stress disorder criteria
Depression	"I can't get out of bed in the morning." "I cry all the time when I'm by myself." "I'm not interested in doing anything anymore."	Markedly diminished interest in one or more significant activities
Nightmares and sleep disturbance	"I have trouble going to sleep at night and don't wake up rested. My boyfriend assaulted me in the dorm one night when I was going to sleep." "I woke up in a cold sweat dreaming he was after me again and no one responded to my screams for help."	Sleep disturbance Recurrent dreams of the event
Guilt and self-blame	"I feel people will blame me for being so naive as to 'let' it happen." "I wonder if I caused it because we were lovers at one time."	Guilt about behavior required for survival
Repression	"I can't remember what he did to me." "I don't want to remember what happened, it's too frightening/painful." "Only after I started therapy did I remember three other assaults when I was younger."	Avoidance of activities that arouse recollection of the traumatic event
Suppression	"All I remember is being attacked. I blanked out after that." "I saw his face and can describe him, but I don't think I can identify him." "Every man I see on the street looks like him (the assailant)."	Recurrent and intrusive recollections of the event
Lack of social support	"I was acting so weird trying to pretend that I was normal that my bridge group dropped me. I cried and cried for days." "Since the assault I've lost *all* my friends." "I avoid all parties now 'cause of the gang rape. So I don't have many friends."	Avoidance of activities that arouse recollection of the traumatic event
Extreme fears	"I'm afraid to go anywhere alone. I *run* from the car to my house." "I bought a car with automatic door locks." "When my husband started night shift I cried for days. If I needed him, I couldn't even scream for help."	Hyperalertness or exaggerated startle response
Emotional isolation	"I can't tell anyone what I'm feeling." "I couldn't stand one more rejection, so I won't give anyone a chance to know my *real* feelings."	Constricted affect
Impaired relationships and anger with men	History of multiple unsuccessful relationships with men, separations or divorces, or no intimate relationship with a male. Acknowledged use of men for sexual gratification without intimacy or commitment. Revolted by thoughts of a sexual or intimate relationship.	Avoidance of activities that arouse recollection of the traumatic event
Flashbacks	"When my husband touched me like (the assailant) I just started screaming. 'Get away from me.'" "I was so afraid during the physical exam. I felt like I was being assaulted again."	Sudden acting or feeling as if the traumatic event were reoccurring because of an association with an environmental or ideational stimulus
Triggers (symbolic)	"I won't take any 'crap' from my husband. Anytime he 'dumps' on me I just blow up and we have a terrible fight. I never used to be this way." "I can't get along with my boss now, his behavior reminds me of (the assailant) and he said if it doesn't stop I'll lose my job."	Intensification of symptoms by exposure to events that symbolize the traumatic event
Altered identity	"I am just *not* the same person anymore. I'm not who I was and I don't know who I am now, I'm different." "I don't think anyone understands how what happened has affected me, made me unhappy with myself and who I am, where I am, what my identity is."	Feeling of detachment or estrangement from others Constricted affect

symptoms such as anxiety and fear, but a genuine loss that many people fail to appreciate. Victims painfully discover an entirely different world view and loss in relation to: sense of control and ownership over their body, the ability to enjoy solitude and nature without having to plan for safety, the illusion that all people are basically trustworthy and that if you try hard enough you can cause or prevent anything, and disrupted relationships with significant others. Coping with both post-event symptoms, including loss and the grief work required, activates a variety of coping strategies that can be applied simultaneously or sequentially to a given problem.

Categories of coping strategies in response to stressful life events include: problem-solving behaviors, cognitive restructuring processes, seeking social support, avoidance behaviors, tension reduction behaviors, wishful thinking, detachment, affective or emotion-centered responses, and self-derogation or self-blame attributions.

Preliminary unpublished research results by Ergood,[20] a nurse researcher, indicate that the victim's coping style is the variable most closely associated with post-event adjustment, even when past psychiatric history and demographic data are also considered. Ergood found that cognitive restructuring responses ("I'm changing or growing as a person in a good way.") and, to a somewhat lesser extent, self-blame statements ("I criticize or lecture myself.") were most consistently associated with post-event levels of adjustment at 2 and 4 weeks. A cognitive restructuring coping style was most consistently associated with a reduction in post-event symptomatology, whereas a coping style of self-blame attributions was most likely to be associated with depression and impaired interpersonal or social adjustment. Treatment implications from these results are currently being explored.

■ Past psychiatric history

The influence of a victim's past psychiatric history on her post-event adjustment is assessed in relation to: the presence or absence of a compounded reaction; and a set of psychosocial variables associated with poorer post-event adjustment. In 1979 Burgess and Holmstrom[5] identified a set of past psychiatric variables among victims that were associated with greater difficulty in resolving a sexual assault and poorer adjustment post-event. The authors called this phenomena a compounded reaction. Table 33-3 lists the defining characteristics of a compounded reaction as psychotic be-

havior, depression, suicidal behavior, psychosomatic disorders, and acting-out behaviors.

Assessment of a victim's past psychiatric history as a predisposing variable associated with poorer adjustment post-event includes physical or sexual victimization; a diagnosed psychiatric disorder in the victim or first or second-degree relative; the use of mental health counseling or therapy; the use of prescribed psychotropic medications; suicide ideation; suicide attempts; and substance abuse. Empirical evidence[11,19,23,24,32,33,44,55,64] indicates that victims evidencing any of these variables in their history have higher global traumatic symptom levels and lower levels of social adjustment post-event.

■ Nature of the assault

Another one of the balancing factors that affects crisis resolution is a person's perception of the event. The crisis a sexual assault victim experiences differs from other crises because of nonsupportive societal attitudes. The nurse can make this crisis more, or less, like other crises depending on the way in which she works with the attitudes of others. When the victim has a distorted perception of the rape, perhaps from her belief in myths, there is diminished ability to recognize a relationship between the feelings of stress and the rape. It is important to consider what the rape means to the individual. How is it going to affect her future? Does she distort its meaning or can she look at it realistically?

Thus, the nature of the assault is important for the meaning of the event to the victim, particularly if it is perceived as a violation of one's most private inner space. This fact is supported by the research results of Ruch and Chandler[64] with 325 sexual assault victims. They found that "when the intensity of the victim's emotional response is examined, the nature of the attack is surprisingly unimportant . . . thus, prevailing stereotypes of rapes as being traumatic when they involve weapons, strangers, or multiple assailants—and as nontraumatic when they do not—are false." Frank[30] reports that the nature of the assault has only an indirect effect which is mediated by the response and supportiveness of the victim's social network. Specifically, when the victim was assaulted with a weapon or physically brutalized her social support network evidences less victim-blaming behavior and more support because she is more likely to be perceived as a "legitimate victim"; the victim evidences higher levels of adjustment in school or work, use of leisure time and social activities, and less conflict in interpersonal relationships with nuclear and extended family members.[28,30] The victim's adjustment post-event is thus also assessed in terms of the quality of her social support network pre- and post-event.

■ Social support network

Social support has been identified as a significant factor that affects a person's state of health and well-being. However, few clinical reports and research studies have investigated this variable for its influence on a sexual assault victim's adjustment. The few studies that are reported are consistent with other mental health research suggesting that social support may buffer or contribute to a victim's global traumatic reaction to a sexual assault.[13,14,15] Research on the social support of a victim varies in focus from partners or couples, to husbands or boyfriends, family members and in particular mothers, and to persons the victim identifies as important to them in their network, such as close friends.

Silverman[69] was one of the first to report observations from clinical assessments and interventions with the families and mates of victims. With family members Silverman found the response of fathers and brothers was primarily that of anger and thoughts of revenge, and victims perceived these responses as nonsupportive and increasing their stress level. Mothers frequently identified with the victim and experienced a post-event reaction comparable to that of the victim (e.g., anxiety, fear, rage, shock, physical revulsion, and a sense of helplessness) which impaired their ability to be supportive to the victim. Overall, the family responded by overprotecting the victim or attempting to distract her rather than supporting her grief work in response to the event. In assessing and intervening with the couples, Miller[55] found that the partners of victims focused on their own feelings of fear, self-blame, and rage. This response pattern contributed to problems in the couple's relationship and left the partner less able to be supportive of the victim.

Holstrom and Burgess[40] focused on the emotional difficulties experienced by mates and boyfriends of a victim. Factors that contributed to non-support of the victim and relationship difficulties included the mate/partner: (1) stigmatizing and blaming the victim for the assault; (2) wanting to injure the assailant which heightened the victim's level of fear; (3) focusing on their own distress rather than that of the victim; (4) experiencing difficulty in resuming sexual relations with the victim; and (5) insisting on prosecuting the assailant despite the victim's ambivalence, and being unable to support her throughout the legal process. Factors that contributed to support of the victim and effective relationships included the mate/partner: (1) focusing on the victim's psychosocial and physical injury from the assault; (2) giving the victim control over the decision of prosecuting the assailant and supporting her through the process; (3) being able to discuss the assault with their partner rather than avoiding the topic; (4) offering the victim their support with assault-related fears; and (5) giving the victim control over their sexual relationship and responding with gentleness during love-making.

Shore[68] found that while victims tended to contact family or friends within hours of the assault for their support, the response of these persons to the victim varied. Although victims more often initially informed their mother of the assault it was the father who was more supportive of the victim when he was informed. The mother's initial nonsupportive response during the acute reaction period abated and she tended to become more supportive of the victim as time progressed. Overall, the social network support lessened for the victim after the acute impact phase. The least supportive relationship to the victim over time was with husbands and boyfriends. Foley[24] found that families were frequently isolated from a social support network postevent, including emotional or physical "cut-offs" within nuclear and extended families, and the community. This pattern tended to increase their anxiety, fears, and concerns about the victim's adjustment and impaired their ability to support her; it also intensified their own global traumatic reaction to the assault and impaired their ability to be supportive of one another. When family members were nonsupportive of one another, the net effect was an increase in the overall level of family and marital conflict, often with one partner blaming the other for the assault or scapegoating or blaming the victim for the event. Adaptive and maladaptive family stress reactions to rape are presented in Table 33-5.

Appraisal by significant others tends to reinforce the victim's perception of herself. It is important to help the victim identify those persons who can be most supportive to her at this time. The nurse needs to recognize that those whom the nurse might automatically identify as supports, such as parents, may *not* be those whom the victim would have selected. Who are the members of her family and which ones will she talk to or avoid? Which family members are important to her? Which friends at work or school will she talk with about the rape? Does she have a therapist, counselor, or minister? Is she aware of the pathological risks involved in keeping the event secret or not using support systems? What groups is she a member of or participating in within her community—church groups, women's groups, single-parent groups, self-defense groups?

Discussion groups have proved an excellent support for victims. Often they are a first step in initiating long-term counseling with a professional. Victims cite a sense of universality, a decreased sense of isolation, a sharing of anger and pain, a catharsis in sharing their secret, an ability to do something constructive with feelings, a validation that intense feelings do not mean they are

---

TABLE 33-5

ADAPTIVE AND MALADAPTIVE FAMILY STRESS REACTIONS TO RAPE

Adaptive stress reactions	Maladaptive stress reactions
Care and concern for the victim	Concern primarily about how others will think of the family
Support of the victim	Contested feelings over who was raped, hurt most, or victimized
Feelings of shock, disbelief, dismay	Minimizing the victim's feelings or response
Feelings of helplessness and disequilibrium	Feeling guilty or responsible for not having protected the victim
Physical revulsion which may parallel the victim's affective responses	Rape trauma syndrome
Distraction tactics to keep the victim and themselves occupied	Patronizing or overprotecting the victim
Reacting to rape as a violent act	Viewing rape as a sexually motivated act and the victim as "damaged goods"
Anger and rage directed at the rapist or society	Direct or indirect anger and resentment as seen in communication difficulties
Blame directed at the rapist	Blame directed at the victim or family members
Thoughts about violent retribution or active retaliation	Act out violent retribution toward assailant or victim
Reaching out to extended family/significant others for support	Emotional cut-offs with extended family/significant others
Empathic with each other	Absence of empathic responses with each other; emotional isolation or withdrawal
Use of crisis counseling as needed	Failure to seek professional counseling when needed
Supportive of victim's medical or gynecological care needs and follow-up care	Failure to seek medical or gynecological care and follow-up care
Cooperation with criminal justice system to prosecute rapist	Inability to cooperate with criminal justice system
Participation in rape prevention programs	Belief in rape myths
Supporting the victim's decisions and wishes	Action pressured against victim's wishes, such as forced or pressured sexual relations with victim, informing others, dropping charges, or insisting that prosecution be carried out
Reevaluating previous relationship with the victim; unit stays intact	Divorce/separation

Foley, T.S., and Davies, M.A.: Rape: nursing care of victims. St. Louis, 1983, The C.V. Mosby Co. Reprinted with permission.

"crazy," and minimized feelings of guilt, depression, and suicide.

Finally, advocates from rape crisis centers, hospitals, or community mental health teams provide information, intervene, and support victims, particularly if the woman lacks assertiveness in meeting her needs within an authoritarian mystifying system. Advocates have specialized skills in helping victims, coordinate all systems with them, and are available for counseling long after the acute care is completed. They provide a needed support system and link in the continuity of care with victims. For this reason nurses are encouraged to welcome them when they accompany a victim.

■ Impact on sexual functioning

Sexual assault clearly has a negative impact on the sexual relationship of a couple, and raises a number of concerns for adolescent victims and their parents. Victims reported being adversely affected primarily by behaviors that were forced on them during the assault. These assaultive acts then acquire fear and pain-related associations that are generalized and result in decreasing their satisfaction level with their current sexual relationship.[75]

Follow-up studies with victims 1 to 2½ years post-event indicate that many victims continue to report worsened sexual relations with their partners; changes in sexual attitudes or difficulties with their partners; new suspiciousness of men; and husbands and boyfriends evidencing changed behavior including rape-related separations[5,19,40,43,56] Interventions with victims should therefore include sexual counseling designed to ameliorate post-event aversive sexual response patterns.

Adolescent victims and their parents have a different set of concerns to work through post-event. Parents are faced with confronting the fact of their child's sexuality, sometimes for the first time.[67] Parents and adolescents generally have divergent concerns. Parents report being concerned about the victim's future sexual disturbances and venereal disease, while victims report more concern about peer reactions and communication difficulties with their parents. Family members often blame adolescent victims for the assault, particularly if they are attractive or if the assailant was an acquaintance such as a family friend, boyfriend, or neighbor.[21] Thus sexual assault for an adolescent poses additional assessment challenges to the nurse.

■ Crisis and counseling requests

The last factor to be considered in a nursing assessment of a victim's response to sexual assault is the type of help or intervention requested. Identifying these factors will influence the individualized treatment plan for the victim. In a study of 146 adult and pediatric victims of sexual assault, Burgess and Holmstrom[9] found that victims identified what they wanted or needed if the nurse listened to their direct verbal statements. The victim's self-care requests became the clinical guidelines for nursing interventions. They identified five categories of crisis requests.

1. **Medical intervention,** or "I need a physician." In this category the hospital staff and emergency room services were viewed in a traditional medical role with the physician explicitly asked to do something to alleviate the victim's fears of disease and pregnancy.
2. **Police intervention,** or "I need a policeman." Here the police were viewed as the first official authority to turn to because of their traditional role of supporting, protecting, and defending the community against crime. The victim within the category had a strong desire to retaliate against the assailant and did not view psychological and medical care as first priorities.
3. **Psychological intervention,** or "I need to talk to someone." These victims wanted to talk with someone about the rape experience and viewed the hospital staff and emergency room services as providing both emotional support and medical care.

4. **Uncertain,** or "I'm not sure I want anything." These victims went to the hospital or police as a result of outside pressure or advice but did not necessarily view these persons as being able to help. In their ambivalence about what to do as a result of the rape/sexual assault they tended to seek out and be emotionally propelled along by the thoughts and feelings of others.
5. **Control,** or "I need control." These victims were incoherent because of the use of alcohol or drugs, a psychotic state, or mental retardation, which aggravated the current crisis and their general inability to verbalize their wants or needs.

Counseling requests made by rape victims included the following:

1. **Confirmation of concern,** or "It's nice to know you are available." These victims volunteered minimal information, were polite, and answered routine questions but tended to be guarded and controlled. They were satisfied that the counselor was available and concerned should they need assistance.
2. **Ventilation,** or "It helps to get this off my chest." These victims were relieved to share the burden with someone. They felt burdened psychologically by the crisis and had much to say about their experience in a spontaneous manner with a strong focus on feelings.
3. **Clarification,** or "I want to think this through." These victims explicitly wanted to think through and settle the crisis for themselves by sorting out conflicting thoughts and feelings to put the crisis in a realistic perspective.
4. **Advice,** or "What should I do?" These victims explicitly asked about alternatives or what to do about physical, social, legal, or psychological problems related to the rape and viewed the counselor as having the information to suggest possible alternatives.
5. **Nothing,** or "I don't need the counseling services." These victims did not indicate a wish for follow-up counseling, gave a false phone number and address or none, and tended to seek police intervention.

 Nursing diagnosis

There are many factors for the nurse to consider in completing an assessment of a sexual assault victim. At the end of the assessment process, the nurse will describe clinical impressions, formulate a nursing diagnosis, and identify the nursing services requested or needed by the victim. Formulating a nursing diagnosis of a victim's response to a sexual assault is based on a synthesis of all factors discussed above under assessment. Rape trauma syndrome was approved as a NANDA nursing diagnosis at the 1980 national conference on nursing diagnoses[45] and subsequently documented as meeting the Draft of DSM-III-R in Development* criteria of a post-traumatic stress disorder, acute or chronic subtype. Assessment may result in a variety of other nursing diagnoses such as: ineffective, compromised, disabling, or maladaptive individual and/or family coping patterns; spiritual distress or despair; disturbances in self-concept related to self-esteem, role performance, personal identity or body image; and dysfunctional grieving.[45]

⚜ Planning

A victim of sexual assault confronts two areas of need. One is inner-directed, concerning psychological adjustments and emotional well-being. The other is outer-directed in relation to the police, legal, and hospital systems. In both areas she enters seemingly hostile, foreign, and male-dominated systems. She faces medical examinations, possibly a long series of legal procedures that may be incomplete as much as a year later, and a long-term reorganization process. Figure 33-2 is a flowchart summarizing the self-care decisions a victim of rape makes after a sexual assault.[60] Often these systems present the victim with fragmented services, inadequate information, and little emotional support at a time when she most needs competent coordinated care and continuity of services. In any health care delivery system the victim of rape has the following rights†:

1. To transportaton to a hospital when incapacitated
2. To emergency room care with privacy and confidentiality
3. To be carefully listened to and treated as a human being with respect, courtesy, and dignity
4. To have an advocate of choice accompany her through the treatment process
5. To accurate collection and preservation of evidence in an objective record that includes signs and symptoms of physical and emotional trauma

---

*American Psychiatric Association: Draft of the DSM-III-R in Development (subject to change), as proposed by the Work Group to Revise DSM-III. American Psychiatric Association, October 1985.
†Modified from Pittsburgh Action Against Rape: Patient's rights handout, 1976-1977, 211 S. Oakland Ave., Pittsburgh, Pa. 15213, and Westmorland Alliance Against Rape: Patient's rights, 1978, 102 W. Otterman St., Greensburg, Pa. 15601.

6. To receive clear explanations of procedures and medication in language she can understand
7. To know what treatment is recommended, for what reasons, and who will administer the treatment
8. To know any possible risks, side effects, or alternatives to proposed treatment, including all drugs prescribed
9. To ask for another physician or nurse
10. To consent to or refuse any treatment even when her life is in serious danger
11. To refuse to be part of any research or experiment
12. To reasonable complaint and to leave a care facility against the physician's advice
13. To receive an explanation of and understand any papers she agrees to sign
14. To be informed of continuing health care needs after discharge from the emergency room, hospital, phyiscian's office, or care facility
15. To receive a clear explanation of the bill and review of charges and where to apply for compensation to cover costs

Professionals, volunteers, and rape crisis centers urge that the victim be actively involved in her own treatment program. The position if based on Orem's self-care model with the philosophy of maintaining and restoring the victim's self-respect, dignity, integrity, autonomy, and self-determination. The intent is to help the victim regain control of events and so renew mastery over her own life. The overall frame of reference is that each person needs to be listened to so that her current status and what she is experiencing within her environment can be determined. The victim should not be fitted into discrete response patterns. Response patterns overlap and are unique to each person.

If a victim is experiencing the **acute disorganization of phase 1,** the goal is to restore emotional control so that feelings do not reactively determine actions or dominate judgment. The first step is for the victim to get in touch with her own feelings. The nurse's task is to assist the victim's process of self-exploration through listening to and understanding her feelings and communicating to the victim that she has been heard and understood. The focus of the conversation, based on crisis theory, is what the nurse and the victim can do together to make the situation better. The goal is to develop a relationship with the victim that will help her sort out her thoughts and feelings prior to making a decision and acting on it.

Included in the planning is the working through of seven issues by the victim: legal matters and police con-

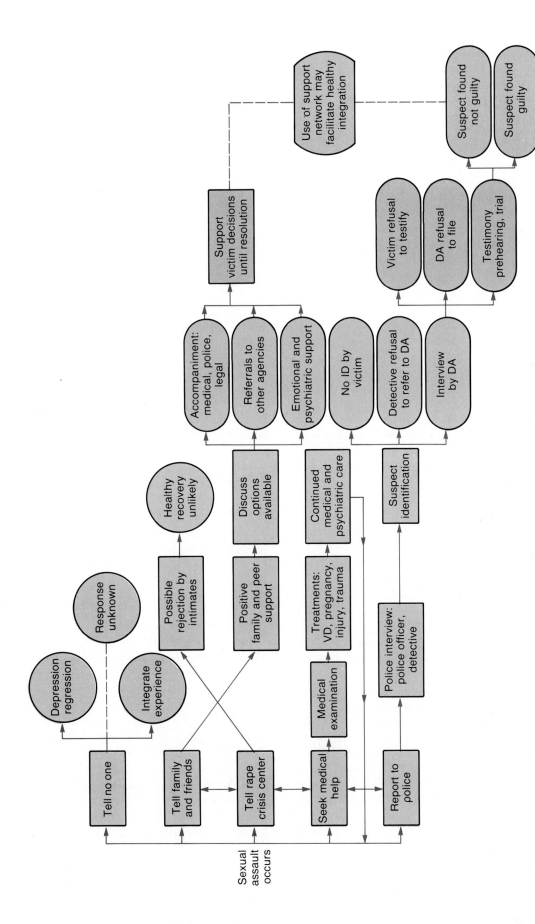

Fig. 33-2. Victim decisions following a sexual assault. (From Rape Crisis Services Division of the Greater Harrisburg YWCA, 215 Market Street, Harrisburg, Pa., 17101.)

tacts, clarification of factual information, medical attention, notification of family or friends, emotional responses, current practical concerns, and psychiatric–mental health consultation. Sutherland and Scherl[40] suggest the use of anticipatory guidance, or forewarning the victim of responses she might experience in later phases. Others disagree with that approach, claiming it gives the victim a preset that could become a self-fulfilling prophecy or precipitate self-doubt if later phases are not experienced.

In a **medical model** the nurse will attempt to ensure adequate medical care for all victims and watch for gynecological problems or somatic disturbances. In a **social network model** the nurse facilitates the victim's active involvement with her extended family and social network. In a **behavioral model** the nurse attempts to decrease the victim's stresses, anxieties, and fears while increasing her self-confidence and self-esteem. Assault-specific behavior modification programs are designed to help the victim with fears, phobias, sleep disturbance, and compulsive behaviors enabling her to achieve her pre-event level of functioning. In a **psychosocial model,** the painful parts of the experience are neutralized by talking about them. The nurse stresses three dynamic issues: (1) the need to be in control, which is approximated as the victim reorders her life, (2) the need to be cared about, which can be met by helping the victim with ways to tell people about her needs and by showing her ways to have more people concerned about her, and (3) the need to achieve, which can be channeled into such activities as enrolling in a self-defense course or working with the rape crisis center.

Intensive counseling at this time has three goals: further identification and acceptance of feelings; reorientation of perceptions, feelings, attributions, and self-statements; and resumption of a normal life-style. The nurse identifies the ways in which a victim processes and attributes causality to events connected to the sexual assault and how her daily behaviors are influenced by such processing.

If a victim of an assault is demonstrating the **outward adjustment or pseudoadjustment of phase 2,** the goal is to remain available and supportive to her. Concrete problems can be further explored now that intense feelings and cognitive disorganization characteristic of a crisis state have subsided. The nurse avoids challenging the victim's wish to forget the assault or get on with her life; she will resolve the event at her own readiness. The nurse can use energy to reflect back with greater clarity and in different words what it is the victim

seems to be feeling and thinking. At this point different alternatives for solving the presenting problem are explored. In addition, the nurse can help family and friends of the victim evaluate their responses to the victim and the assault. If their responses are negative, nonsupportive, or rejecting, the importance and need for counseling increases.

If a victim of rape has moved into the **integration and resolution of phase 3,** the nurse's goals are to assist the victim in (1) exploring feelings about the assailant, (2) exploring feelings about herself, and (3) making decisions for herself. Planning provides for the resolution of feelings of guilt, shame, and anger toward the assailant when these are experienced. Planning for an extended evaluation is indicated in the presence of one or more of the following: compulsive rituals such as cleaning or washing, sleeping or eating disturbances, fears that have generalized or a post-traumatic stress disorder, chronic subtype, which may be the result of assault symptoms persisting beyond an acute phase or may consist of symptoms presented on assessment by a delayed treatment seeker.

The overall goal is to help the victim acknowledge, face, and resolve the response she is feeling. Ultimately all planning will follow from the victim's crisis and counseling requests and the nursing assessment.

➡ Implementation

■ Telephone crisis counseling

Crisis theory and basic principles of counseling are applied in the process of counseling sexual assault victims on the telephone. Victims often call a crisis hotline or sexual assault center before they are seen in the emergency department, or the nurse may receive a crisis call in the emergency department directly from the victim. Wherever the call is received, the nurse assesses the victim for the absence of one or more balancing factors. The functional strengths the woman possesses are conserved as a useful resource. The nurse assists the victim to identify what services are needed. A set of recommended telephone interviewing guidelines for use with victims of rape is presented in the accompanying box. Not all of the questions are covered in any one interview; these guidelines represent categories of information and helpful questions to explore. The nurse uses clinical judgment in deciding which areas to explore. The guidelines are an instrument from which to obtain data useful in assessing the victim and suggest questions to consider in relation to services requested.

Telephone Interviewing Guidelines with Victims of Sexual Assault and Rape

Date _____ Time _____

General information

Introduction: Hello. This is _____ from _____
   How can I help you?
Name of victim/caller _____
Phone number calling from _____
Address or general area _____
   Location/neighborhood of assault _____
   Why in the area _____
When did assault occur (date, time)? _____
Are you in a safe place? _____
Are you hurt? _____
How are you feeling now? _____
Time between assault and call to crisis line _____

Demographic data

Age of victim _____
Race and sex of victim _____
Marital status _____
Description of assailant:
   Who did it? _____
   Age _____
   Race and sex _____
   Acquainted with victim _____
     Describe relationship:

Crisis status

Perception of the event _____
Response to the event _____
Situational supports _____
Coping mechanisms _____

Type of assault

_____ Rape
_____ Attempted rape
_____ Involuntary deviate sexual intercourse
_____ Indecent assault
_____ Sexual assault of a minor
_____ Other degrading acts
   Describe:
_____ Use of weapon
   Type:
_____ Struggle by victim
   Feelings now about that
_____ Threats (describe)
   Verbal _____
   Physical _____

Services requested and questions to consider

1. Medical intervention (hospital): Has the victim had a medical examination? Encourage going to the emergency room for treatment of injuries and collection of evidence pending decision to prosecute.
   a. **If not examined:** If she does not want to go to the hospital, does she know about the importance of testing for VD, gonorrhea, and pregnancy now and later? Is she injured other than the sexual assault? What supportive network is available to her? Does she want/need an advocate to accompany her to a shelter/care facility? Give her information about the local hospital procedure and what to expect, her rights.
   b. **If examined:** How did she get to the hospital? What did she expect would be done for her at the hospital? Were tests for VD, gonorrhea, and pregnancy done? Did she change clothes or get cleaned up before going to the hospital? Was medical evidence collected (what, where)? Was she treated for lacerations, abrasions, bruises? Is she taking any medications or DES? Specify these. Does she know their side effects and risks involved? Is she having any medical problems? Was follow-up care discussed/planned? How does she feel she was treated by the health professionals? What is her reaction to this experience? Did she decide to obtain help or did someone else pressure her to seek help?
   c. **Abuse:** Is there evidence of physical abuse to a child or elderly person or battered wife syndrome? Describe the data. Has the evidence been reported to the police, hospital, and/or child welfare office?

Telephone Interviewing Guidelines with Victims of Sexual Assault and Rape—cont'd

2. Shelter and transportation intervention: Does she need emergency transportation?
   From _____ to _____ Date _____
   Time _____ Does she need emergency shelter? _____
   Contributing factors _____
   Length of time requested _____
   Accompanied (children) or alone _____
   Economic/financial concerns (describe) _____

3. Police and legal intervention: Has she reported to the police?
   a. **If not reported:** Does she want to report? Does she want the report kept anonymous? Does she want to press charges? Does she want to talk about the pros and cons of not reporting/reporting? What feelings/ factors are contributing to a no-report decision? Does she know about victim compensation-restitution (that she can be compensated for unpaid medical expenses if she reports the crime within 72 hours)?
   b. **If reported:** Does she understand the legal procedure and what to expect at the preliminary hearing, pretrial, trial? Is she aware of the possibility of a trial postponement and of a not-guilty verdict? To whom did she report (which police station and name of officer taking the report)? Was a report taken? Was she encouraged or discouraged from prosecuting? What is happening with the police follow-up at this time? Is she aware of the procedures necessary to identify the assailant? Has the assailant been picked up by the police? Is the assailant in jail, out on bond? Is she being harrassed or threatened by him or others? Describe. Does she have any intent to retaliate against the assailant? Name of officer arresting the assailant and police station(s) he is assigned to? Who is the district attorney? How does she feel the police treated her? What is her reaction to the experience of reporting?

4. Psychological intervention:
   a. **The victim:** How did she feel at the time of the assault? And now? Does she feel the rape was her fault? Does she believe in the myths? Which ones and what impact are they having on her? Does she perceive anyone as able to assist her? Did she go or not go to the police/hospital as a result of outside pressure/ advice? Is she ambivalent regarding what to do? Describe. Is she seeking others' opinions? (Whose? What content? What action taken?) Was she or the assailant affected by the use of alcohol and/or drugs? (What ingested? When? Amount? By which party? Feelings about this?) Is she unable to verbalize her needs? Is she psychotic? Mentally retarded? History of social difficulties? History of physical difficulties? Hospitalized or under a physician's care now or previously? Mental status is (describe). What is the most painful part to recall/discuss? Has she been raped before? Is this her first sexual experience? What is her usual sexual style? What does this sexual assault mean to her? How did she react to acts demanded (feelings, behaviors [e.g., compliance, resistance])?
   b. **Family and friends:** Who are her friends, relatives? Where do they live? Quality and frequency of contacts? Persons most and least in touch with? Does she have a therapist, minister? Does she attend any women's groups, any rap sessions? Does she want to talk with other victims of rape? Can she rely on her support systems if she wants to talk about the rape? Will they listen? How will she feel if they do not listen or reject her? How is her church community a support system for her? Has she decided to talk about the incident? (Discuss pros/cons of doing so and with whom—she is the best judge of her situation.) Who knows about the assault? Describe their response. Do family/friends want to talk with a counselor, or does she want a counselor to talk with them? Is the family responding with (1) caring for the victim's welfare, empathy, support, anger directed at the assailant, ability to give to the victim or (2) blaming the victim, caring for their own welfare (e.g., what others will think), recriminations, anger directed at the victim, blaming themselves?

Telephone Interviewing Guidelines with Victims of Sexual Assault and Rape—cont'd

5. Narrative summary:

   Services requested _____ Medical
   _____ Police/legal
   _____ Shelter
   _____ Transportation
   _____ Advocate
   _____ Counseling (specify type)
   _____ Other

   Nursing diagnosis _____
   Plans _____
   Contacts made (e.g., police, hospital, name of person/agency) _____
   Referrals made or suggested _____
   Follow-up indicated and type _____
   Self-evaluation
   Describe feelings about the call, personal reactions, influence of biases/myths. List additional information/training that would help improve services. Delineate learning needs.

   Modified from Pittsburgh Action Against Rape: Crisis call form, 211 S. Oakland Ave., Pittsburgh, Pa. 15213, and Burgess, A.W., and Holmstrom, L.L.: Nurs. Res. **23**:198, May-June, 1974.

■ Hospital emergency department

Sexual assault victims arrive at the emergency room in varying degrees of emotional trauma. It is essential that careful and prompt treatment be provided. One recommended procedure for medical examination of victims of rape is given in the accompanying box. Preferably, a comfortable and private waiting room should be available. When a private room exceeds pragmatic possibilities and the victim must wait with others, it is advisable to refer to sexual assault patients by name or a code such as Code R. A code call system sometimes avoids insensitive comments such as "Where's the rape?" The examination should be done in a private area located near the emergency room. If the police later interview the victim, a similar facility should be made available to them. It is recommended that medical care be provided in advance of any interviews with the police. There is no valid reason to interrogate or interview a victim in a public area or waiting room. To protect the woman's rights, no information should be released without her consent.

In many communities there will not be an advocate to go with the victim through the medical and legal systems. The nurse may be her only advocate during a physical examination and may be able to assist her with the beginning phases of crisis resolution. Whenever possible two nurses need to be available, one to assist with the examination and evidence collection and the other to provide direct care to the victim, especially in the absence of an advocate. If the nurse has a clear idea of how the woman feels about herself, her level of self-esteem, and whether it is important for her to be in control, the nurse will have the necessary data to act as an effective advocate with the victim during a physical examination and interview.

The nurse begins by listening to the victim's account of the attack in a warm and empathic way. The nurse needs to convey acceptance of the victim's description of the use of threat or force, that the assault involved penetration, however slight, and that whatever her response to the assault was, it was appropriate. The nurse needs to strive to get as clear an idea as possible of what the woman would like the nurse to do for her. The nurse needs to let the victim know that, although she just survived a trauma she has some strengths to cope with and get over this event. Thus to help her begin the resolution process the nurse will not speak for her unless it is clear she wants help in conveying her needs.

Medical Examination of the Victim of Sexual Assault and Rape

History

A medical history should be obtained and a statement taken about the time and place of the event; relationship to the assailant, if any; nature of suspected physical and sexual acts; time lapse between assault and current examination; victim's physical state; and whether there have been any physical changes since the assault (e.g., if the victim bathed, douched, showered, urinated or defecated, changed clothes, used or removed a tampon, treated wound, etc., prior to examination)

Examination, treatment, and follow-up care

Equipment recommended for evidentiary material
1. Fresh-sealed package of microscopic slides with frosted ends
2. Eyedropper bottle with 0.9% saline
3. Six to twelve packages of sterile cotton swabs
4. Nine to twelve test tubes with stoppers
5. Urine container
6. Sterile new comb
7. Sterile scissors
8. Nail scraper—plastic or orangewood
9. Envelopes
10. Package of gummed labels
11. Glass-cutting pencil
12. Sterile gauze and envelope for saliva sample

Complete physical and gynecological examination
1. Evaluate vital signs, general appearance, and mental status.
2. Identify and measure cuts, and scratches; record and photograph (black and white only admissible in court).
3. Take fingernail scrapings, particularly if nails are broken or victim scratched the assailant.
4. Examine for extragenital sexual trauma to mouth, breasts, neck, and other body parts. Take swabs and smears from mouth, throat, or anus in the case of sodomy to check for semen presence.
5. Do a baseline check for venereal disease (VD) and gonorrhea, followed 6 weeks later with another set of tests. Sometimes massive doses of penicillin are given to help prevent VD infection. The victim should understand what is being given and may refuse any medication.
6. Discuss with the victim her birth control practices, use of oral contraceptives, and intrauterine devices, and belief system surrounding abortion. A discussion of possible types of postcoital contraception with a full explanation of possible effects is indicated (diethylstilbestrol [DES] has been shown to cause cancer in daughters born to women who have taken it during pregnancy).
7. Discuss with the victim the sexual functioning of the rapist (impotence, retarded ejaculation, premature ejaculation, masturbation)
8. Pregnancy testing and information on abortion, location of free clinics, women's health services, and crisis and counseling centers in the community should be provided.
9. Pelvic examination should include the following:
   a. Observation for matted or free hair
   b. Combings of pubic and head hair to find any traces of assailant's hair and collection of pubic and head hairs from victim for reference
   c. Description of vulvar trauma, redness, lacerations, and bruises and photography in black and white
   d. Examination of condition of hymen
   e. Determination of parity
   f. Determination of date of last menstrual period
   g. Determination of date and time of last voluntary coitus
   h. Determination of condition of anus and rectum
   i. Vaginal examination with lubricated, water-moistened speculum
   j. Specimen of victim's blood for matching if she is bleeding
   k. Examination of adnexa for hematoma
   l. Swabs and smears from vagina, vulva, rectum, and thighs to check for presence of semen

Medical Examination of the Victim of Sexual Assault and Rape—cont'd

10. Clothing should be checked for tears, blood, semen, and stains. Victim's clothing should be preserved, marked, photographed, and collected in a paper bag (never plastic).
11. Obtain 5 ml of blood for typing.

Evidentiary material

Evidentary material should be gathered and held for release to the police. It should not be released without consent of the patient or guardian, except by subpoena or court order. Specimens should be gathered and handled as follows:

1. Take swab from the vaginal pool and from any suspicious area about the vulva and protect in dry test tube. These can be examined by a hospital or police laboratory for the following:
   a. Acid phosphatase test
   b. Blood group antigen of semen test
   c. Precipitin test against sperm and blood
2. Examine wet sample from fornix immediately for motile sperm. This examination should be performed only by an experienced person who understands the limitations of examining sperm material.
3. Take separate smears from the vulva.
4. Culture for *Neisseria* organisms in appropriate medium such as Thayer-Martin.
5. Comb pubic and head hair for free hairs; pull (do not cut) a minimum of 25 of the victim's pubic and head hairs.
6. Take fingernail scrapings.
7. Chain of evidence: laboratory specimens should be gathered by a physician in the presence of a witness and personally handed to a technician or pathologist. Slides and containers should be clearly labeled with patient's name. The victim should be advised that turning bloody, torn, or stained clothing over to the police may help their investigation and prosecution of case (if she chooses to prosecute). It is critical that a chain of evidence be established identifying all persons responsible for handling or keeping evidentiary material.

Follow-up care

The patient should be examined for lacerations, contusions, and other wounds. Retesting and examining for pregnancy, VD, gonorrhea, herpes, and AIDS should be completed. Counseling to assess and prevent long-term psychological effects should be provided or made available.

Medical records

The medical record should contain complete documentation of the history, examination, and treatment provided. It should describe the physician's findings and what was done. It should state what evidentiary materials were given and to whom. Only the medical conclusions, opinions, and diagnosis should be in medical record. Above all, it must be legible, and preferably typed, to avert case dismissal in court proceedings. The medical personnel and record may be subpoenaed. Misinterpretations can be avoided if all data are exact and detailed. Negative findings are as important as positive ones and may assist in protection of all concerned parties.

Modified from The Hospital Association of Pennsylvania and the Pennsylvania Medical Society: Penn. Med. 79:73, June, 1976; Bragonier, R., and Nadelson, C.C.: In interact: new perspectives for the clinical management of sexual problems, Chicago, 1977, G.D. Searle & Co.; and the collected publications of A.W. Burgess and L.L. Holmstrom.

The nurse can provide the victim with adequate information about what her rights are and what she can expect from the hospital staff to reduce her sense of anxiety and helplessness. It is important to determine if the woman generally finds it easy or difficult to assert herself and whether she values that ability. Even a woman who is normally assertive may not ask what the physician is doing, given her emotional and physical pain. Later she may regret having been so passive in the examination and feel angry. Muscular tension is common during an examination for a victim of sexual assault. The nurse needs to encourage the victim to let the physician know her response as the examination proceeds. The nurse needs to try to get an idea of the woman's values and give her the opportunity to express her feelings. The nurse needs to let her know that whatever she is feeling is valid and acceptable and that victims respond in a wide variety of ways. The woman needs to be assured that current feelings may change with distance from the attack and that she can remove distorted perceptions by reviewing the incidence when she is in a period of greater calm. The woman will resolve the crisis better if she finds the nurse supports her beliefs and her own value system.

The sexual assault examination requires that the victim describe the kinds of sexual contact that took place. The nurse is often the person to conduct the interview and will find the process easier if the victim is given a rationale for the questions asked combined with empathy and good interviewing skills. Explaining the nature of and rationale for any tests done is a nursing action that can alleviate the victim's anxiety and fears. Since recall under high anxiety is minimal, it is recommended that these facts be given to the woman *in writing*, as well as in a packet of follow-up information. The nurse needs to also ask the woman how she feels about the morning-after pill (diethylstilbestrol [DES]), menstrual extraction, and abortion. The nurse can provide a full explanation of the use, side effects, and risks of DES. For more details *Our Bodies, Ourselves* and *Contraceptive Technology* are excellent resources.

Another area of nursing intervention is asking the woman if she is willing to answer questions that are nonmedical but which may be pertinent if she prosecutes the assailant. Valuable evidentiary material can be lost if she does not report the sexual assault during the first 24 hours or few days, and she may also lose an opportunity for compensation or restitution. She can decide later about signing a release form and concentrate for now on acquiring medical attention; thus the victim is not pressed for a decision she may not feel ready to make. The nurse can inquire if she is willing to sign a medical release form and find out if there is any information to appear on it that she might not want released. Only information obtained through the physical examination and interview should be released, not her entire medical history. The victim may later want to share the whole, detailed event at least once with someone with whom she feels secure. The nurse can offer to be that person. The nurse can ask to provide follow-up care by calling the victim in a couple of days to see how she is doing or referring her to a specified follow-up team (rape crisis centers, community mental health cen-

Assisting the victim during the medical examination is very important. The nurse needs to ask the woman if she wants to know what is going on during the physician's examination. Without medical information some women feel powerless; with it they may feel more in control of what happens to them and more able to knowledgeably participate in the decision-making process. It will be helpful to explain in detail all medical procedures in advance of their implementation and assist the woman in coping with any discomfort caused by the physical examination. The woman needs to be reminded of the body's excellent healing capacity, its tissue elasticity, and its rich blood supply. Any bleeding or discomfort needs to be discussed, as well as measures she can take to facilitate healing. The victim may fear infection, verification of damage to her body, pain, and even being repugnant. Before the victim leaves, she needs to be given a card or packet with follow-up information, appointments, and telephone numbers of local crisis and counseling centers. The nurse emphasizes the importance of a follow-up check for venereal disease, pregnancy, herpes, and acquired immune deficiency syndrome (AIDS) and asks permission to call in a day or two to see how she is doing.

■ **Principles of counseling**

Professional literature on intervention in working with victims of sexual assault recommends that nurses have a substantial working knowledge of theories of anxiety as they counsel victims. Anxiety is a response to a critical life transition, requiring that the nurse be familiar with means of working toward changes that are creative and positive. Since many victims experience a loss of self-respect, loss of virginity, threat of loss of one's life, and temporary loss of power, control, and autonomy, some experts in the field find it useful to perceive the victim's trauma in the context of a grief framework. The victim's response to rape closely approximates four interrelated feeling responses to loss or trauma in a grieving process: denial, depression, anger, and resolution or reconstruction.

One recommended counseling model for helping victims of sexual assault is called **active listening.** It is a method by which the counselor empathically responds to the feelings of another while being aware of the counselor's own thoughts and behavior. The model suggests that most people have difficulty understanding and responding to another's feelings at high levels of intensity that contrast with their thoughts or behavior. Growth of a person in counseling has been found to be related to certain dimensions present at high levels in the counselor. These core qualities are accurate empathy, respect for the other, objectivity, warmth, genuineness (self-disclosure), concreteness, and immediacy (see Chapter 4). While implementing these core qualities through active listening, the nurse assists the woman through three phases of a change process: self-exploration, self-understanding, and action (see Chapter 14). Recognizing that something is "wrong" and coming for counseling must be joined with a commitment on the part of the woman to change and to do something about the situation or herself. If this essential motivation is lacking, the whole counseling process will have limited value. No one phase of counseling is discrete. The victim may revisit each phase of the counseling process based on what she is working through and may experience more than one phase within a given session.

The first phase of the change process is **self-exploration,** which "leads to a better understanding of concerns and a commitment to change which, in turn, makes possible a more successful course of action."[37] Here the problem is explored in depth by identifying feelings, thoughts, and behaviors. The approach is usually nondirective (Rogerian framework), and the primary focus of the nurse is on responding empathically to the feelings of the other. The nurse's role is to help the woman begin to understand what she can do to change the situation. Sometimes this phase is full of confusion. For example, the sexual assault itself may be of minor significance for the woman, and something else (sexuality beliefs, her support system, society's response to her) may be more important. Clinical example 33-3 illustrates this self-exploration phase.

In the process of **self-understanding,** phase 2, identified feelings, thoughts, and behaviors are clarified, and causes and reasons are assigned by the victim to each as she explores her problems. The nurse assists her to make some sense out of the "pieces of the puzzle" when many nonspecific feelings arise by making these more concrete. The woman is then able to decide on what action she believes will resolve the difficulty and commits herself to a specific plan of action that is both reasonable and attainable. The nurse is more active at this time, sharing information such as how to contact the local crisis center. As a professional the nurse knows how to help the victim with the services requested, such as learning how to be more assertive or referring her to where the service can be obtained. The approach tends to be more psychosocial in nature. It employs analytical and conceptual thought processes as evident in the continuation of Clinical example 33-3.

In the process of **action,** phase 3, the woman decides precisely what she will do to accomplish life goals. Specific plans are devised from concrete and relevant information. In a facilitative position, the nurse acts on a philosophy that the victim's decision is her choice and

---

CLINICAL EXAMPLE 33-3

Gwen is a 17-year-old high school student who works part time at a shopping mall. She accepted a ride home from a teenager who frequented the mall and she casually knew. He talked her into a ride in his new jeep. Instead of taking Gwen home, he took her to a park where he raped her in the car.

During the self-exploration phase Gwen decided that she had been raped and betrayed and wanted to prosecute the assailant stating, "He's a real creep! He violated my body, even *I* don't do that. He deserves to be punished and has to be stopped from doing that to other women." A year later Gwen revisited self-exploration to gain understanding of homicidal feelings in response to a not-guilty verdict at the trial.

Gwen used counseling to understand many of her confused feelings and responses after the rape. She was able to see that she was not to blame for the rape and become more discriminating in trusting casual acquaintances. She shared the rape event with her parents when she felt she was able to cope with their response. She separated her own sexually active life-style from societal appraisals judging her as promiscuous and deserving of abuse. She understood her nightmares as an attempt to regain mastery over her life and make her life secure.

After the trial she saw the nurse counselor several times weekly because of unresolved anger. The nurse encouraged Gwen to fantasize and ventilate feelings of rage. The nurse directed Gwen's rage in multiple areas to help diffuse overfocusing on the rapist; all the errors made by the police and medical staff in evidence collection were highlighted, and the insinuations of the defense attorney were recalled ("So after you *sobered* up. . . ."). Gwen gradually realized her anger was in more than one area.

Gwen realized that she did not have to kill the rapist as she had thought to dissipate her rage or prove to others that she was truly raped. Gwen went about making the rapist lose power over her life by living a constructive life: she finished high school, worked on making her relationship with her boyfriend satisfying, and was accepted for training in the police academy where she felt she could fight crime.

---

includes a decision not to act. The nurse demonstrates objectivity and self-control by keeping her own agenda out of the counseling process. The action phase is identified by the woman's behavior, such as pressing charges, in contrast to her solely discussing what to do, which is characteristic of previous phases. This phase is emphasized within the counseling model. When a sexual assault victim remains depressed, she does not gain mastery over the rest of her life. Although she was unable to control the external event of the sexual assault the nurse emphasizes that the victim does have control over internal intrapsychic events and her own behavior. Although unable to avert her own rape, a sexually assaulted woman sometimes acts to help herself and other victims of assault by working on a crisis hotline, by joining consciousness-raising women's groups, or by taking self-defense courses. For women who like to help others, this has been noted to be useful in helping a victim regain a sense of control over her life.

■ Other assault-specific interventions

■ **BEHAVIORAL TECHNIQUES.** It may also be helpful to use behavior modification approaches at this time.[36] For example, cognitive restructuring techniques can be employed to stop the anxiety-producing chain of destructive self-statements. These include thought stopping, self-reinforcement, thought substitution, and the development of concrete plans. The nurse helps the woman consider her basic human rights and thus evaluate the legitimacy of self-blame attributions. In counseling, the nurse might ask, "Do you need to feel shame if you really did not have a choice of behaving in the matter?" Healthy anger directed toward the assailant replaces the victim's previous guilt-inducing statements, and negative self-evaluations tend to dissipate. Role playing and behavior rehearsal of such events as court proceedings or talking with one's family can help the victim develop the skills necessary to successfully implement a decision. When the woman experiences daily reinforcing events, the rape experience is more quickly put into proper perspective.

Relaxation training (Chapter 12) may also be helpful. A cognitive-behavioral procedure described in detail by Jacobson[41] has been modified to meet the needs of victims post-event. Due to a victim's hyperalert and anxious state it is often difficult for her to relax, fall asleep at night, or be without tension and fatigue from depressive symptoms or expectations to continue functioning in a variety of situations. Thus she is taught by these procedures: (1) a guided dialogue that induces relaxation; (2) deep breathing; (3) progressive, total body deep muscle relaxation; and (4) how to generalize her learned conditioned relaxation procedure to relax at will under a variety of stressful, anxiety- or tension-evoking circumstances.

■ **SOCIAL SYSTEM SUPPORT.** An additional form of help is available for the assault victim through groups in rape crisis centers. Rape crisis centers are modeled after the Washington, D.C., center, which was an outgrowth of a feminist group that was attempting to open a women's center. Several members of the group had been raped and were dissatisfied with the treatment received. They formed a group to meet the needs of rape victims that they perceived were being unmet by the community. Their interventions on the behalf of victims are felt throughout the health care delivery system today. The justice system is also changing, as are the laws surrounding rape. Some judges fine the assailant to pay for damages suffered by the victim, and programs such as victim compensation-restitution are being implemented.

In rape crisis centers victims can request to meet with other victims or counselors. The structure of the group varies from a nondirective approach, which gives the victim space to focus on her concerns, to having members write down specific problems they would like to work on, such as sexuality, fears, or assertiveness. The leaders vary from professionals to volunteers who use active listening skills and facilitate the verbalization of feelings. Most groups evolve and dissolve spontaneously, usually at a time somewhat distant from the assault, when the victim has had time for reflection. Many of the crisis centers' programs extend into the realm of prevention and education within established groups, such as school systems, parent and church groups, and police and health care systems. Intervention in these programs is directed at changing societal attitudes and behaviors.

■ **GOAL-ATTAINMENT SCALING.** Goal-attainment scaling (GTS) places the responsibility for change with the victim, not the nurse. The strategy, based on traditional short-term goal-oriented and cognitive-behavioral therapy methods, was developed by Ledray, a nurse, and involves the following procedures: (1) the victim identifying problem areas and changes she wants to make (e.g., developing a social support network, expanding social activities, decreasing fears of being alone); (2) weighting each area according to its comparative importance (e.g., from 1 = most important to 5 = least important); (3) selecting a follow-up time interval (e.g., 3 weeks or months); and (4) filling in a scale of potential operationalized outcomes for each area (e.g., none to 2–3 or 7–10 friends and social activities) using a five-point Likert scale (1 = much less than expected, 3 = expected or mostly likely results to 5 = much more than expected level of results); (5) identifying feasible strategies to achieve a desired goal and listing this by the goal (e.g., go out to safe places daily with friends); and (6) developing a summary goal attainment score by aggregating scores on individual scaled goals. The nurse then uses the GTS form as a structured, goal-oriented guide for counseling sessions. This method has been most successful when combined with supportive counseling.[49,51]

■ **SUPPORTIVE COUNSELING.** This approach, used in counseling victims the last two decades, has been formalized by Ledray as a "low treatment" condition for clinical practice and research. Ledray[50] identified seven components to this intervention in her nursing research: (1) being an empathic, accepting, and respectful listener to whom the victim can express her feelings at her own readiness; (2) responding to the victim as a normal, healthy person who is currently experiencing a serious life crisis and emotional disequilibrium; (3) being nonjudgmental of the victim by focusing on the victim's subjective experience of the assault rather than determining if she was "really" assaulted; (4) assisting the victim in regaining and maintaining control over her life, and ensuring her right and ability to make choices by providing her with information to make informed choices; (5) responding to the victim as a person separate from the assault; (6) assisting the victim in coping with responses from her social support network; and (7) ensuring the victim's personal safety.[4,50,51]

■ **ASSERTIVENESS TRAINING.** Many victims need help in learning assertiveness skills. This is important for two reasons. First, some victims lacked assertiveness skills pre-event which may have contributed to their victimization vulnerability. Second, one effect of the assault experience is that many victims fear any situation that even suggests aggressiveness which is too closely aligned to their assault experience. Thus, in their efforts to protect themselves from further trauma they cope by avoiding such situations, or respond by compliance and submission in these circumstances which sets them up for being further victimized or abused. Often they express difficulty discriminating assertiveness from aggressiveness, and when they are assertive report low self-esteem, feelings of anxiety and fear, and misguided self-blaming attributions. Thus, one or more sessions may be devoted specifically to assertiveness training (see Chapter 18).

■ **VICTIM GROUP SESSIONS.** This strategy is based on the curative factors of group therapy. Any of the strategies discussed above are structured into a treatment protocol for these sessions. The sessions vary from time-limited 8 to 12 sessions to open-ended formats depending on the program implementing the treatment. The group sessions achieve a number of goals such as: decreasing victims' sense of isolation and lack of support; concrete problem solving; normalizing responses to a sexual assault and validating members' feelings; encouraging and suggesting coping strategies in responding to others about assault-related issues such as

assault mythology; learning, from an infusion of group members' ideas, new coping skills in areas of daily life not related to but affected by the assault; and providing an array of information essential to adjustment post-event (see Chapter 28).[4]

■ **FAMILY SESSIONS.** This strategy is based on crisis theory and principles of intervention (Chapter 10) and family systems theory and therapy (Chapter 29). It is now recognized that a sexual assault represents a crisis not only for the victim but also her significant others who, in turn, facilitate or impede her adjustment. Sessions with these persons range from nonstructured approaches in which the clinician helps these persons work through a presenting complaint to structured treatment protocols implementing specific strategies to meet the needs of these persons.

Appropriate nursing interventions when working with the family include emphasizing the importance of nonjudgmental support of the victim in making her own choices, which helps her regain control. It is important to emphasize to friends, relatives, and parents the understanding, compassion, protection, and warmth that a victim needs after such an intimately disturbing experience. Family members are encouraged to put aside the desire to thrash the assailant in retribution and to direct their energy toward caring for the victim. She will need to be reassured, supported, soothed, comforted, and have attention to her immediate medical problems. Someone quiet and supportive is helpful while she resolves the event at her own pace.

■ **SPIRITUAL COUNSELING.** The goal of spiritual counseling is to help a victim and her significant others resolve a state of spiritual distress or despair in response to the trauma of a sexual assault. It is integrated into the holistic practice of nursing and may be combined with or enhance the effect of other scientific or humanistic treatments. It is important that nurses talk with trauma victims about how the event has impacted their spirituality, the defining characteristics of their distress or despair, ways they are coping with this, and the help they feel they need to achieve adjustment in this area. Nurses may be surprised that once the topic is opened up for discussion how grateful victims are for an opportunity to explore these concerns. Nurses are encouraged to seek out and use a wide variety of readings in spiritual and humanistic fields to help them with this area of practice. At times it is important for the nurse to work as a co-therapist with the clergy or ministry of a victim's religious denomination; the clergy or minister understands the dimensions of spirituality in depth while the nurse or other mental health professional understands the phenomena of sexual assault and victim response—each professional can be helpful to the other and the victim. It is also important that the nurse be aware of qualified clergy or ministry in the community to refer the victim to because many of these persons, like most professionals, have had little or no content on sexual assault in their curricula and may compound a victim's post-trauma responses.

■ **LONGER-TERM COUNSELING.** Some victims require longer-term counseling or therapy to work through their post-assault symptoms and concerns. Longer-term therapy is necessary for symptoms of a post-traumatic stress disorder that have become chronic, and may be necessary for victims who are less able to work through the acute symptoms of the assault experience due to one or more past psychiatric history variables. In addition, victims who are delayed treatment seekers often require longer-term therapy to ameliorate symptoms that have become chronic and impair their functioning or quality of life. The conduct of longer-term therapy by nurses requires advanced preparation.

■ **LEGAL RESPONSIBILITIES.** Nurses need to be knowledgeable about the role they may play as witnesses in legal proceedings. Prosecution is difficult when medical data are not properly recorded, if the evidence is not gathered completely and quickly, and if the signs and symptoms of physical and emotional trauma are not cited. The victim holds the burden of proof beyond a reasonable doubt for all of the elements of the crime. The nurse therefore has a responsibility to carefully collect and preserve corroborative evidence. Victims have lost their case in court when evidence has not been properly collected, and the professional is then faced with counseling a person experiencing dual legitimate rage: (1) the rape experience, and (2) negligent medical and nursing care. As part of an official medical record a nursing assessment becomes an objective record corroborating evidence in court proceedings and has the potential to increase conviction rates.

Burgess and Laszloa[18] discuss four particular areas in their assessment instrument:

1. **Signs of physical trauma,** which describe specific physical findings.
2. **Symptoms of physical trauma,** which include the patient's verbatim statements about the nature of the attack. The types of sexual acts demanded are especially important to include here, as well as how they were carried out and in what order. Should the victim's accurate recall about this falter later, the objective account stands witness to a jury and clarifies misinterpretations of evidence submitted in a courtroom. The jury is likely to believe the written record. If the victim

is in crisis, the nurse may have to ask what sexual acts occurred. These questions need to be carefully worded to obtain accurate facts, since the victim is under stress. Victims will also appreciate respect for their sensitivity at this time, as shown by the way the nurse asks questions about the interactive components of the sexual assault. It is important to convey one's intent to obtain information, not to judge the victim. This is especially important with sexual behavior other than vaginal intercourse. Avoid phrases that ordinarily connote lovemaking, those which the woman may not know the meaning of, such as fellatio or cunnilingus, and those which suggest that she took initiative in or precipitated the assault. The nurse could ask, for example, "Did the rapist put his penis in your mouth, vagina, or rectum?" Although the questions are more graphic, they suggest less than a passive reconstruction of the victim's behavior in the assault. In addition, such phrasing helps to defuse the victim's emotions and depersonalize the attack, which can serve as a healthy coping mechanism.

3. **Signs of emotional trauma** consist of the victim's behavior during the interview. Any precise, concrete signs should be recorded, such as withdrawn or quiet behavior, hyperventilation, signs of extreme anxiety, sobbing, or tears.
4. **Symptoms of emotional trauma** include the victim's verbatim statements about the method of force used and the assailant's threats. If a weapon was used by the assailant, this should be noted. The nurse's subjective impressions and opinions should not be recorded in the account. To try to discredit the victim or establish "character fault" by claiming that consensual intercourse occurred, the defense counsel will often use such subjective data.

■ **CASE EXAMPLES.** To increase the effectiveness of one's nursing care, it may be helpful to role play some case situations.[58,59] One person can act out the role of the nurse applying the nursing process, and the other can play the role of the victim in the context of a person-to-person contact or a telephone call. Following are sample situations*:

■ You are 25 years old and live alone. You dated a man you work with twice, and on the third

---

*Modified from Rape Crisis Center of Madison, Wisconsin: Counselor's manual, 1976-1977, P.O. Box 1312, Madison, Wis. 53701, and Rape Crisis Center of Syracuse, Inc.: Training manual, Sept., 1976, 601 Allen St., Syracuse, N.Y. 13210.

date you invited him over for dinner. He forced intercourse on you. You did not tell anyone and have broken off all communication with the man. This happened 6 weeks ago. You now think you may be pregnant and do not know where to turn.

- You are a married woman, age 36. After a fight with your husband one night, you went alone to a bar. When you left, you were intoxicated. Your car would not start, and you accepted a ride from a man you knew only slightly. He drove to a deserted area and beat and raped you. You reported it, but no one really believes you, especially your husband.

- You are an 83-year-old widow. One night when you were sleeping you were raped by the 27-year-old man who rents a room from you. He cut the telephone cord, ripped your pajamas, and tried to smother you with a pillow. During the actual rape, you passed out. You are suffering from extensive internal bleeding. You want to prosecute.

- A woman was hitchhiking at midnight wearing a halter top and cutoffs. A man picked her up, drove to a dark side street, and raped her at gunpoint. She was so exhausted, she sarcastically asked if she could have her ride home now and he gave it to her. You find out through the conversation that she is on drugs and has been in and out of therapy. How do you handle this?

- A woman was raped by an old acquaintance while out walking her dogs. She calls, feeling guilty and upset because she was afraid to fight and is afraid to be independent anymore. This incident has shaken her confidence in herself and her trust in people. What do you say?

Evaluation

There are no absolute counseling rules, since every situation has exceptions. Counseling does require a comprehensive knowledge base from which to make assessments, respond with compassion, plan appropriate interventions, and implement care effectively. The nurse can provide comfort and support in a time of need, assist the victim in problem-solving processes, intervene with brief assault-specific treatments and, when indicated, provide or refer the victim to longer-term counseling. As victims approximate and achieve post-assault adjustment, clinicians use the term "survivor" with them affirming that, indeed, they are a survivor of a traumatic life-event. This reinforces a positive self-concept and the reality that they are a competent and strong person,

capable of coping with and adjusting to a traumatic life event, and that they have grown or become a "better" person as a result of this unfortunate experience.

The nurse is not responsible for the victim's choices or for her working or not working out problems. By maintaining a facilitative position, she can help the victim work through her problems.

Research studies indicate that rape victim populations range from heterogeneous to homogeneous. There are also a variety of research methods, which include immediate interview and follow-up care, as well as retrospective interviews and standardized psychological or psychosocial measures of adjustment. There is a consensus that a sexual assault causes acute disorganization immediately after the trauma marked by anxiety, fear, and depressive and acute post-traumatic stress disorder symptoms which, without intervention, can become chronic. Response to a sexual assault resembles most stress responses to other traumatic crisis, and the crisis event sets in motion long-term reorganization processes. (See Clinical example 33-4.)

■ Research findings

Several conclusions are evident from research results on treatment efficacy with victims over the last 10 years. *First,* recent research results indicate that a victim's symptoms are reduced at 3 months post-event and further reduced at 6- and 12-month follow-up periods, and that with assault-specific treatment these symptoms reduce more rapidly than without treatment. *Second,* current findings indicate that thus far no statistically significant difference has been found at 3 months between symptom clusters (e.g., anxiety, fear, depression) of victims who receive assault-specific treatment and non-victim control groups. *Third,* no statistically significant difference has been reported to date for treatment efficacy of one assault-specific treatment over another (e.g., desensitization vs. assertiveness training) in reducing victims' symptoms at 3 months. *Fourth,* clearly a considerable number of long-term longitudinal studies with large samples need to be conducted comparing the adjustment over time of (1) treatment-seeking victims, treatment refusers, delayed recovery victims, and delayed treatment seekers; and (2) singular assault treatments, protocols combining various treatment techniques, no treatment, and low treatment conditions. *Finally,* research over the past two decades has focused primarily on the victims' responses to a sexual assault and treatments that facilitate adjustment. These studies by comparison to current research in the field[25,31,34,76] have failed, however, to investigate the context or environment, including the social support network in which the victim resides and the influence of these variables on her adjustment. Thus, all victim-focused research has necessarily been limited by failing to account for systemic variables such as those that affect adjustment to sexual assault as a significant life crisis.

The majority of research findings lack objectively measurable and quantifiable data. There are thus no systematical data regarding the long-term consequences of being raped or the impact it has on a woman's life. The various ways in which women respond to rape within the assault and the relationship of cultural, social, and personality variables is essentially unknown. Neither is it known how victims of rape differ from victims of other types of acute and chronic stress, such as battered women. As yet, long-term follow-up investigation is not well organized or implemented in many care systems in the nation. The professional literature needs to explore the work currently being done with nuclear and extended families and significant others in counseling.

CLINICAL EXAMPLE 33-4

Clair is a 17-year-old high school student who called the rape crisis hot-line and talked with a nurse on call that day. She wanted to know if she had been raped and what to do next. Clair said she was out with her boyfriend, Dave, and he had been pressuring her for sexual relations. Clair said she reluctantly agreed after much pressure because she didn't want to lose him or continue to make him angry but then changed her mind before sexual intimacies "got underway" and told him this. Dave was enraged and forced sexual relations on Clair despite her screaming, crying, and pleading. Clair said she felt responsible for what had happened. She wanted to know if she could get pregnant from the rape. Clair said she couldn't tell her parents because they wouldn't understand; they would blame her, and she was calling the hot-line while they were out of the house. She did not want to be called back, since it would divulge her secret. Clair said her best friend and only person she could confide in was out of town for the week on vacation. Clair cried during the phone call and said "I can't believe what happened. I didn't think anyone would ever do anything like that. I can't see him again, it's all over and so awful."

ASSESSMENT

The nurse assessed this situation as a confidence rape (style of attack) and a sex-stress situation (type of nonconsent). It was also agreed that Clair believed some of the rape myths (self-blame), that she was in a crisis state (without a support network, loss of boyfriend, not able to use customary coping mechanisms) but was able to express her stress (style of response).

PLANNING

The nurse planned for crisis intervention and follow-up care for Clair. She agreed to come in for individualized assault-specific interventions after school under the guise of attending after-school extra-curricular activities to protect her secrecy of the event from her parents.

INTERVENTION

The nurse provided crisis intervention and basic counseling for Clair by confirming that she had been raped, the nature and type of rape, including the element of betrayal that was adding to her sense of stress and disbelief (phase 1 response). The nurse encouraged ventilation of feelings (crying, disbelief, anger, fears of falling apart, sadness over the loss of her boyfriend). The nurse refuted Clair's faulty perceptions (self-blame for the assailant's behavior) and encouraged Clair to talk with her parents, which she continued to refuse to do for fear of their response. The nurse provided her with information on where she could get free pregnancy and venereal disease testing and said the crisis center could send a taxi to pick her up. Since Clair was in the middle of her menstrual cycle, the nurse encouraged her to obtain follow-up care in 6 weeks. The nurse told her that the local women's health center was open Monday morning, and an advocate could go with her to get medical care. The nurse gave her the phone number of the health clinic and the crisis center and encouraged her to stay in touch during this difficult time.

EVALUATION

Within the initial 2 weeks post-event Clair thanked the nurse for her help with her pregnancy and medical concerns. She continued to be seen for an individualized nursing treatment plan that addressed her assault-specific intervention needs. At the end of a 3-month period Clair reported that she did not feel the need for further intervention, that her life was "back to normal." Clair agreed to follow-up appointments to assess her post-event adjustment at 6, 12, and 18 months; she was assessed by the nurse at these time periods as evidencing reduced levels of post-event assault-related symptoms. Clair thanked the nurse for her help and agreed to contact her in the future if the need should arise.

DIRECTIONS FOR FUTURE NURSING RESEARCH

The following are some of the nursing research problems raised in Chapter 33 that merit further study by psychiatric nurses:

1. The post-event adjustment of adult sexual assault victims who have a history of child sexual or physical victimization compared to adult sexual assault victims who do not have this history
2. The incidence and impact of sexual assault on adolescent and adult male victims among the general population; identifying the assault-specific treatment needs of this population
3. The impact over time of a sexual assault on the family and significant others of a victim, and intervening and post-event variables associated with adjustment over time to this trauma
4. The effectiveness of assault-specific interventions as related to selected variables in a victim's pre-event history
5. The extent to which nursing and professional curricula in this nation include theoretical content on sexual assault and clinical practice experience with victims
6. Replication of nursing research investigating the relationship between a sexual assault victim's coping behavior, coping responses, and post-event symptomatology
7. The treatment efficacy of goal-attainment scaling as compared to selected other assault-specific treatments
8. Differences in adjustment over time between victims who prosecute and those who do not prosecute a known assailant
9. The relationship between types and levels of reciprocity in a sexual assault victim's social support to post-event symptomatology and adjustment over time
10. The post-event symptomatology and adjustment over time of sexual assault victims compared to the post-event symptomatology and adjustment over time of victims of other types of violent crimes (e.g., assault and burglary)
11. The effectiveness of a sexual assault prevention program for adolescents in preventing attempted (or completed) date/acquaintance sexual assaults
12. Differential mental health sequelae from a sexual assault experience over time for specialized populations (e.g., severely impaired or chronically mentally ill, elderly, developmentally disabled)
13. The quality of care victims receive from multidisciplinary health professionals who have completed a specified training program on victim care as compared to the quality of care received by victims from professionals without this training
14. Variables associated with effective treatments for juvenile and adult sexual assault offenders

Although counseling procedures have been described and implemented in various programs, they often lack internal and external evaluation with comparable treatment programs. Of particular relevance in the counseling of women is Bergin's challenge "that the effects of therapy are not uniform but that research should take into account which treatment by what therapist is effective for what client with what problem under what conditions."[39] Unfortunately, most authors that discuss sexual assault counseling lack empirical evidence for the effectiveness of their treatment approaches. In the absence of such research, there is no scientific way to know if treatment programs are more effective than either no treatment at all or "traditional" treatments. Nurses are encouraged to develop a structure in their work setting to provide long-term follow-up care for victims, to scientifically investigate the effectiveness of treatment programs, and to open the dialogue about this area of practice on local, state, and national levels with colleagues and others in victim assistance programs.

■ SUGGESTED CROSS-REFERENCES ■

Therapeutic relationship skills and self-awareness of the nurse are discussed in Chapter 4. Crisis intervention is discussed in Chapter 10. Interventions with violent and abusive families are discussed in Chapter 32.

■ SUMMARY ■

1. Sexual assault crisis centers are an outgrowth of the feminist movement and exist in most cities across the United States. Professionals volunteer their services in these centers. Treatment of rape victims is a service that also must be provided by community mental health centers.

2. Sexual assault is defined as the forcible perpetration of an act of sexual contact on the body (male or female) of another person without their consent. Legal criteria for specific sexual acts included in this crime and for marital rape vary among the states.

3. Sexual assault is neither "all sex" nor "all violence" but a combination of the two where violence is eroticized and sexualized. Many myths surround the crime of rape and all of them serve to place blame on the victim. Since many people believe these myths, they hinder the ability of the victim to receive adequate treatment in medical, legal, and sociocultural systems. Some of the facts related to rape include the following:

   a. Rape is the fastest rising violent crime in the nation, and among these it has the lowest proportion of cases closed by arrest and conviction.
   b. Chances are 1 in 15 a woman will be raped in her lifetime.
   c. The target population of victims is young women ages 15 to 24.
   d. By all appearances the offender is no different from the

accepted norm of other men in our society except for an exaggerated tendency to express violence and aggression.

4. Victims of rape respond with feelings of fear, guilt, anger, self-blame, denial, disbelief, shock, depression, and isolation. They may also exhibit phobic reactions, sexual dysfunction, motor activity, nightmares, and disruption of task expectations. The severity and duration of a victim's post-trauma responses are a function of: (a) psychological responses to the assault including emotional style, psychological symptomatology, and phase of response; (b) coping style; (c) past psychiatric history of the victim; and (d) the nature of the assault.

5. Four phases of response to a sexual assault experience have been identified:
   a. An acute phase characterized by shock, disbelief, and dismay
   b. An outward adjustment phase characterized by denial of the event's impact and a desire to get on with one's life.
   c. An integration and resolution phase in which the victim confronts her anger with the assailant and puts the event into realistic perspective
   d. A delayed treatment-seeking phase by a subsample of victims characterized by a "silent rape syndrome" and post-traumatic stress disorder symptoms, chronic subtype. Assault-specific treatments and longer-term counseling are indicated to ameliorate post-event symptomatology.

6. Rape trauma syndrome is the nursing diagnosis of a victim's response to a sexual assault experience, and this syndrome has now been documented as meeting the criteria of a post-traumatic stress disorder, acute or chronic subtype.

7. The nursing process is used in assessing the victim's crisis and counseling requests and the ways in which to best facilitate meeting the victim's identified needs. Self-awareness by the nurse is an essential component of the assessment process. There are many factors for the nurse to consider in completing an assessment and it needs to be carried out with adequate knowledge of one's legal responsibility.

8. The planning phase of the nursing process requires the active involvement of the victim and reflects her individualized needs. Plans can be formulated on the basis of the victim's phase of response—acute disorganization, outward adjustment, or integration and resolution. Areas for intervention include medical care, emotional support, legal concerns, social support network and family/significant others' responses, assault-specific interventions, and, when indicated, longer-term counseling. The overall goal is to help the victim acknowledge, face, and resolve the response she is feeling.

9. The type of nursing intervention implemented will be partially determined by the setting in which the victim is seen. If the woman appears in a hospital setting, the nurse can support her during the medical examination. The nurse can initiate counseling in a hospital setting or in a telephone contact. Counseling is focused on three phases of the change process: self-exploration, self-understanding, and action. Additional assault-specific treatments were also described.

10. Evaluating the long-term effectiveness of different treatment interventions has yet to be universally implemented. Current research results have yet to prove that one assault-specific treatment is more effective than another in reducing a victim's post-event symptomatology, or more effective than no treatment.

REFERENCES

1. Amir, M.: Patterns in forcible rape. Chicago, 1971, University of Chicago Press.
2. Adams, C., Fay, J., and Loreen-Martin, J.: No is not enough: helping teenagers avoid sexual assault. San Luis Obispo, Calif., 1984, Impact Publishers.
3. Anthony, S.B.: From a letter to a friend, Summer, 1870. In Largen, M.A.: The anti-rape movement: past and present. In Burgess, A. W., editor: Rape and sexual assault: a research handbook. New York, 1985, Garland Publishing, Inc., p. 4.
4. Assault Crisis Center of the Washtenaw County Community Mental Health Center, Ann Arbor, Michigan, Rape Victim Treatment Program, 1985.
5. Brodsky, S.L., and Hobart, S.: Blame models and assailant research, Crim. Justice Behav. **5**:379, 1978.
6. Brownmiller, S.: Against our will: men, women and rape, New York, 1975, Simon & Schuster, Inc.
7. Burgess, A.W.: Sexual victimization of adolescents. In Burgess, A.W., editor: Rape and sexual assault: a research handbook. New York, 1985, Garland Publishing, Inc.
8. Burgess, A.W.: Personal communication and consultation, October 11, 1985 and February 9, 1986.
9. Burgess, A.W., and Holmstrom, L.L.: Crisis and counseling requests of rape victims, Nurs. Res. **23**:196, May-June, 1974.
10. Burgess, A.W., and Holmstrom, L.L.: Rape trauma syndrome, Am. J. Psychiatry **131**:981, 1974.
11. Burgess, A.W., and Holmstrom, L.L.: Rape: victims of crisis, Bowie, Md., 1974, Robert J. Brady Co.
12. Burgess, A.W., and Holmstrom, L.L.: Rape: its effect on task performance at varying stages in the life-cycle. In Walker, M.J., and Brodsky, S.L., editors: Sexual assault, Lexington, Mass., 1976, D.C. Heath & Co.
13. Burgess, A.W., and Holmstrom, L.L.: Adaptive strategies and recovery from rape. Am. J. Psychol. **136**(10):35–47, 1979.
14. Burgess, A.W., and Holmstrom, L.L.: Rape: disclosure to parental family members. Women Health **4**:255–268, 1979.
15. Burgess, A.W., and Holmstrom, L.L.: Rape: sexual disruption and recovery. Am. J. Orthopsychiatry **49**:648–657, 1979.
16. Burgess, A.W., and Holmstrom, L.L.: Rape trauma syndrome and post-traumatic stress response. In Burgess, A.W., editor: Rape and sexual assault: a research handbook. New York, 1985, Garland Publishing, Inc.
17. Burgess, A.W., and Laszloa, A.T.: Courtroom use of hospital records in sexual assault cases, Am. J. Nurs. **77**:64, Jan. 1977.

18. Connell, N., and Wilson, C., editors: Rape: the first source book for women, New York, 1974, Lume Books.

19. Ellis, E.M.: A review of empirical research: victim reactions and response to treatment. Clinical Psychology Review 3:473–490, 1983.

20. Ergood, J.: The relationship between coping behavior, coping responses and post-rape symptomatology. University of Pittsburgh, Dept. of Psychology. Unpublished doctoral dissertation. Personal communication, January 1986.

21. Felice, M.: Follow-up counseling of adolescent rape victims. Medical Aspects of Human Sexuality 14(3):67–68, 1980.

22. Finkelhor, D., and Kersti, Y.: License to rape: sexual abuse of wives. New York, 1985, Holt, Rinehart and Winston.

23. Fisher, G.: Is forcible sex on dates rape? Washington State University. Paper presented at the Annual Meeting for Scientific Study of Sex, Session on Coercive Sexuality, San Diego, Calif., September 1985.

24. Foley, T.S.: Family response to rape: a pilot study. In Proceedings of the 5th Pittsburgh Family Systems Symposium. The University of Pittsburgh, Western Psychiatric Institute and Clinic, Pittsburgh, Pa., June 1982.

25. Foley, T.S.: Family response to rape. NIMH Clinical Investigator Award Grant # 1K08 and 5K08MH00557, July 1984–1987. The University of Michigan School of Nursing, Ann Arbor, Mich.

26. Foley, T.S.: Expert witness testimony in cases of victims filing civil suits against sexual offenders. The University of Michigan, School of Nursing, 1985–1986, and private practice.

27. Foley, T.S., and Davies, M.A.: Rape: nursing care of victims. St. Louis, 1983, The C.V. Mosby Co.

28. Frank, E.: Psychological response to rape: an analysis of response patterns. University of Pittsburgh, Department of Psychology. Unpublished doctoral dissertation, 1979.

29. Frank, E.: Personal communication and consultation, November 13, 1985.

30. Frank, E.: Rape and sexual assault: new innovations in treatment. Paper presented at The University of Michigan School of Nursing, November 13, 1985.

31. Frank, E.: Theoretical model of rape reaction. NIMH Grant #MH 2969208 The rape victim: her response and treatment, pp. 41–43. Rape Victim Treatment Project, Western Psychiatric Institute and Clinic, University of Pittsburgh School of Medicine, Department of Psychiatry and Psychology, 1985.

32. Frank, E., Turner, S., and Duffy, B.: Depressive symptoms in rape victims. J. Affective Disord. 1:269–277, 1979.

33. Frank, E. et al.: Past psychiatric symptoms and the response to sexual assault. Compr. Psychiatry 22:479–487, 1981.

34. Frank, E. et al.: Psychoeducational intervention manual. NIMH Grant #MH 2969208, The rape victim: her response and treatment, pp. 1–43. Rape Victim Treatment Project, Western Psychiatric Institute and Clinic, University of Pittsburgh School of Medicine, 1985.

35. Goodchilds, J., and Zellman, G.: Becoming sexual in adolescence. In Algier, E.R. and McCormack, N., editors: Changing boundaries: tender roles in sexual behaviors. Palo Alto, Calif., 1983, Mayfield Publishers.

36. Goodchilds, J. et al.: Adolescent perceptions of responsibility for "dating" outcomes. Paper presented at the Eastern Psychological Association Meetings. Philadelphia, Pa., April 1979.

37. Gzada, M., et al.: Human relations development: a manual for educators, ed. 2, Boston, 1977, Allyn & Bacon, Inc.

38. Heppner, M., and Heppner, P.P.: Rape: counseling the traumatized victim, Personnel Guidance J. 8:78, Oct., 1977.

39. Hill, C.E.: A research perspective on counseling women, Counsel. Psychol. 6:53, 1976.

40. Holmstrom, L.L., and Burgess, A.W.: Rape: the husband's and boyfriend's initial reactions. The Family Coordinator 28(3):321–330, 1979.

41. Jacobson, E.: Modern treatment of tense patients. Springfield, Ill., Charles C Thomas Publishers, Chaps. 4, 5, and 6.

42. Kilpatrick, D.: Tretment efficacy of current early, brief assault specific protocols, including comparison of results from treatment protocols using the same standardized outcome measures. Personal communication, October 1985.

43. Kilpatrick, D. Resick, P., and Veronen, L.: Effects of a rape experience: a longitudinal study. J. Social Issues 37(4):105–122, 1981.

44. Kilpatrick, D., Veronen, L., and Best, C.: Factors predicting psychological distress among rape victims. In Figley, C.R., editor: Trauma and its wake. New York, 1985, Brunner/Mazel.

45. Kim, M.J., and Moritz, D.A.: Classification of nursing diagnoses: proceedings of the third and fourth national conferences. New York, 1982, McGraw-Hill Book Co.

46. Koss, M.P.: National survey of inter-gender relationships. Preliminary results of NIMH grant funding survey of date/acquaintance rape on college/university campuses. Kent State University, Department of Psychology, Kent, Ohio in collaboration with Ms. Foundation for Education and Communication, Inc. New York, 1985.

47. Largen, M.A.: The anti-rape movement: past and present. In Burgess, A.W., editor: Rape and sexual assault: a research handbook. New York, 1985, Garland Publishing Inc.

48. Law Enforcement Assistance Administration: Criminal victimization surveys in 13 American cities. Washington, D.C., 1975, U.S. Government Printing Office.

49. Ledray, L.: Treatment efficacy results of current early, brief assault-specific treatment protocols, including comparative results on goal-attainment scaling and supportive counseling. Personal communication, Nov. 1985.

50. Ledray, L.: The impact of rape and the relative efficacy

of guide to goals and supportive counseling as treatment models for rape victims. Sexual Assault Resource Service, Minneapolis, Minn. Manuscript submitted for publication, November 2, 1985.

51. Ledray, L., and Chaignot, M.J.: Services to sexual assault victims in Hennepin County. Evaluation and Change, Special Issue: 131–134, 1980.

52. Lystad, M.H.: The national center for the prevention and control of rape. In Burgess, A.W., editor: Rape and sexual assault: a research handbook. New York, 1985, Garland Publishing, Inc.

53. MacLean, J.: Rape: what's being done to stop it? In these times: a special report, Chicago, 1975, New Majority Publishing Co.

54. Malamuth, N.: Rape proclivity among males. J. Social Issues **37**(4):December 1981.

55. Miller, W.R. et al.: The effects of rape on marital and sexual adjustment. Paper presented at the meeting of the Eastern Assoc. for Sex Therapy, Philadelphia, March 1979.

56. Nadelson, C. et al.: A follow-up study of rape victims. Am. J. Psychiatry 139, **10**:1266–1270, Oct. 1982.

57. National Clearinghouse on Marital Rape and Women's History Research Center, Inc. 2325 Oak St., Berkeley, Calif. 94708, (415) 524-7770. Personal communication, January 1986.

58. Rape Crisis Center for Madison, Wisconsin: Counselor's manual, 1976-1977, P.O. Box 1312, Madison, Wis. 53701.

59. Rape Crisis Center of Syracuse, Inc.: Training manual, Sept. 1976, 601 Allen St., Syracuse, N.Y. 13210.

60. Rape Crisis Services Division of the Greater Harrisburg Area YWCA: First night: flow chart—victim decisions following a sexual assault, 1977. 215 Market St., Harrisburg, Pa. 17101.

61. Resick, P.: Treatment efficacy of current early, brief assault-specific treatment protocols, including comparative results on assertiveness training, crisis intervention, and supportive counseling and protocols using the same standardized outcome measures. Personal communication, Nov. 1985.

62. Resseler, R., Burgess, A.W., and Douglas, J.: Rape and rape murder: one offender and twelve victims. In Burgess, A.W., editor: Rape and sexual assault: a research handbook. New York, 1985, Garland Publishing Inc., pp. 209–221.

63. Rey, D.: Counseling tips, Marin Rape Crisis Center, May 1976, P.O. Box 823, Kentfield, Calif. 94904.

64. Ruch, L.K., and Chandler, S.M.: Sexual assault trauma during the acute phase: an exploratory model and multivariate analysis. J. Health Soc. Behav. **24**:174–185, 1983.

65. Russell, D.: Rape in marriage. New York, 1982, MacMillan Publishing Co.

66. Russell, D.: Sexual exploitation: rape, child sexual abuse, and sexual harrassment. Beverly Hills, 1984, Sage Publications.

67. Schmidt, A.: Adolescent female rape victims: special considerations. J. Psychosoc. Nurs. Ment. Health Serv. **19**:17–19, 1981.

68. Shore, B.: An examination of critical process and outcome factors in rape. NIMH grant # MH30315. Report to the public, 1979 and final report, 1980.

69. Silverman, D.: Sharing the crisis of rape: counseling the mates and families of victims. Am. J. Orthopsychiatry **48**:166–173, 1978.

70. Sutherland, S., and Scherl, D.J.: Patterns of response among victims of rape, Am. J. Orthopsychiatry **40**:503, 1970.

71. Sweet, E.: Date rape: the story of an epidemic and those who deny it. Ms. Magazine October:56–59, 84–85, 1985.

72. The Feminist Alliance Against Rape Newsletter: Professionalism, Fall 1975, P.O. Box 21003, Washington, D.C., 20009.

73. Uniform Crime Reports. Federal Bureau of Investigation, U.S. Dept. of Justice, 1970, 1979, 1984.

74. Veronen, L.: Treatment efficacy of current early, brief assault-specific protocols using the same standardized outcome measures. Personal communication, November 1985.

75. Veronen, L., and Kilpatrick, D.: Self-reported fears of rape victims: a preliminary investigation. Behavioral Modification **4**:383–396, 1980.

76. Veronen, L., and Saunders, B.: The impact of rape on dyadic involvement and functioning. NIMH grant application #MH40360-01, April 1985.

77. *Warren v The State.* #42545, State of Georgia, Supreme Court Decision on "marital rape is rape." November 6, 1985.

78. Weingourt, R.:Wife rape: barriers to identification and treatment. Am. J. Psychother. **33**(2):187–192, April 1985.

79. X, Laura: Sexualization of violence in society and current conceptualizations of sexual assault. Personal communication, February 9, 1986. Women's History Research Center, Inc. and National Clearinghouse on Marital Rape, Berkeley, Calif.

80. Zellman, G.L. et al.: Adolescent expectations for dating relationships: consensus and conflict between the sexes. Paper presented at the American Psychological Association meetings, New York, September 1979.

■ ANNOTATED SUGGESTED READINGS ■

Adams, C., Fay, J., Loreen-Martin, J.: No is not enough: helping teenagers avoid sexual assault. San Luis Obispo, Calif., 1984, Impact Publishers.
  This is a book for persons and professionals to use in talking with teenagers about the nature of sexual assault, how to prevent it, factors that contribute to the crime, and what to do if one is victimized.

*Asterisk indicates nursing reference.

Brownmiller, S.: Against our will: men, women and rape, New York, 1974, Simon & Schuster, Inc.

The author presents a well-documented, thorough scrutiny of the history of rape. From a historical perspective the author reveals rape as embedded in and supported by our culture. Occasional generalizations without the necessary qualifications are sometimes made, yet the work remains an important and valuable contribution for anyone attempting to understand and eradicate the problem.

Burgess, A.W., editor: Rape and sexual assault: a research handbook. New York, 1985, Garland Publishing Inc.

This book contains a synthesis of current research results and perspectives in the field of sexual assault/rape by experts with a wide range of disciplines and backgrounds including the behavioral sciences, communications, criminal justice, criminology, history, education, law enforcement, medicine, nursing, psychiatry, psychology, social sciences, social work, victimology, and women policy studies.

*Burgess, A.W., and Holmstrom, L.L.: Rape: victims of crisis, Bowie, Md., 1974, Robert J. Brady Publishing Co.

The text presents a comprehensive analysis of a rape victim's counseling needs. Crisis centers and their purpose are discussed. Methods in telephone and home counseling and crisis intervention are presented. Special needs of the victim who prosecutes, the prostitute victim, the child and adolescent victim, and the victim with prior psychosocial problems are presented. This is a highly recommended reading for all those serving or involved with rape victims.

*Burgess, A.W., and Holmstrom, L.L.: Rape: crisis and recovery, Bowie, Md., 1978, Robert J. Brady Co.

The text contains a number of articles of the author's works from journal publications. It cuts across disciplines, addressing the nature of and reactions to rape, community, and forensic issues; crisis intervention, and counseling of victims, including long-term recovery.

*Burgess, A.W. et al.: Sexual assault of children and adolescents, Lexington, Mass., 1978, D.C. Heath & Co.

This book is designed as a handbook for persons who come into contact with either the victim or offender in their work. It attempts to provide some of the treatment answers in a manner that is easily understood and adaptable to both lay and professional counselors and their individual programs.

Dobash, R.E., and Dobash, R.: Violence against wives. New York, 1979, The Free Press.

The authors document violence against wives based on history, biography, institutional processes, cultural beliefs and ideals, statistical data, and the social sciences. They discuss factors associated with its emergence and continuation, and the relationship between community reactions and the perpetuation of that violence.

Finkelhor, D., and Kersti, Y.: License to rape: sexual abuse of wives. New York, 1985, Holt, Rinehart and Winston.

The authors refute the myth that marital rape is a contradiction in terms and compassionately present the victims' account of their trauma. They examine why marital rape remains legal in most states and is largely unrecognized as a social problem.

*Foley, T., and Davies, M.: Rape: nursing care of victims. St. Louis, 1983, The C.V. Mosby Co.

The book is a comprehensive and practical guide for understanding sexual assault, and for providing nursing care to victims and their family/significant others. It is divided into three parts. Part 1 presents facts about rape including sexual assault myths and facts, and information about sexual offenders and their treatment. Part 2 describes responses to rape by nurses, victims, family and significant others, and suggests intervention strategies related to specific response patterns. Part 3 presents the nursing care of victims including emergency care in the hospital; advocacy; basic counseling and crisis intervention; counseling through the court process; and a final chapter on the nature of child sexual abuse, the response of offenders, victim and family response patterns, and interventions. The text offers learning activities, annotated readings, and appendices relevant to clinical practice.

Gager, N., and Schurr, C.: Sexual assault: confronting rape in America, New York, 1976, Grosset & Dunlap, Inc.

Multiple dimensions of the crime of rape are presented in an informative, insightful, and thought-provoking survey. Legal, medical, and psychological aspects are considered.

Greer, J., and Stuart, I.: The sexual aggressor: current perspective on treatment. New York, 1983, Van Nostrand Reinhold Co.

The authors comprehensively present virtually all treatment methods for sexual offenders including: issues in assessment including a detailed protocol for evaluation of criminal insanity and competency to stand trial, treatment, and evaluating treatment effectiveness; and behavioral, psychotherapeutic, socio-educational, and biomedical intervention procedures.

Griffin, S.: Rape: the all American crime, Ramparts **10**:26, Sept. 1977.

This article offers a feminist analysis for the political meaning of rape as an aggressive act. Culturally rooted myths such as (1) rapists are insane, (2) women want to be raped, and (3) rape is an impulsive act are examined and refuted.

Groth, A.N., and Birnbaum, J.: Men who rape: psychology of the offender, New York, 1979, Plenum Press.

The text presents 15 years of research with more than 500 sexual offenders. Examined are psychological and social factors that predispose one to react to situational and life events with sexual violence: development factors, life-style and motivations. Diagnostical assessment and treatment of the offender are discussed in detail. Easy to read and nontechnical in style of presentation.

Halpern, S., editor: Rape: helping the victim—a treatment manual, Oradell, N.J., 1978, Medical Economics Books.

This text is a manual for use in emergency room and follow-up care with rape victims. Practical procedures, such as the medical examination, evidence collection, chain of evidence, and counseling of the family, are succintly outlined for ease in use.

Holmstrom, L.L., and Burgess, A.W.: The victim of rape: institutional reactions, New York, 1978, John Wiley & Sons, Inc.

The text describes how major institutions respond to rape victims and the often devastating effects of care received from hospital emergency wards up though court trials. Research findings substantiating the victim's plight are presented along with policy recommendations for change in institutional settings.

Katz, S., and Mazur, M.A.: Understanding the rape victim: a synthesis of research findings, New York, 1979, John Wiley & Sons, Inc.

An excellent reference book reporting and analyzing research findings and critiquing methodology across studies. The authors examine the facts about the victim prior to rape (risk factors, family and social background, personality, and sexual history), during the rape (setting, situation, transaction, reactions) and after the rape (reporting, prosecuting, counseling, and child sexual abuse) concluding with rape prevention and a summary of findings.

Kunz, D., editor: Spiritual aspects of the healing arts. Wheaton, Ill., 1985, The Theosophical Publishing House.

This book combines the writings of distinguished professionals offering a unique, in-depth survey of holistic healing. The book is an overview of uncommon, at times transcendental techniques used in the treatment response to stressful life events and illness.

Lederer, L., editor: Take back the night: women on pornography. New York, 1980, William Morrow & Co., Inc.

This book contains a thought-provoking collection of articles, interviews, research, and calls to action by women committed to stopping violence against women.

Lewis, M.: Trying a trauma case: don't let the defense throw the book at you. Trial (April):52–58, 1985.

The author is an experienced trial lawyer who shares his experience in civil suits for damages related to a traumatic event. He describes how the expert witness can most effectively use the diagnosis of a post-traumatic disorder in testifying, how a discussion of the client's symptomatology may be preferred to use of the diagnostic label, and what cross-examination "pitfalls" the expert witness should anticipate and how to respond to these. It is recommended that nurses preparing to testify as an expert witness read this article.

McCombie, S., editor: The rape crisis intervention handbook, New York, 1980, Plenum Press.

The text is a contributed work from experts in the field of victim care. It offers a practical handbook of treatment-oriented information for professionals working directly with victims and their families. Addressed are psychological, medical, and legal aspects essential in counseling rape victims.

McEvoy, A., and Brookings, J.: If she is raped: a handbook for husbands, fathers and male friends. Homes Beach, Fla., 1984, Learning Publications, Inc.

The book is a practical guide for counselors to use in helping a victim's significant others understand and cope with a sexual assault. It helps them become aware of their supportive role in the victim's recovery process.

Russell, D.: The politics of rape. New York, 1974, Stein and Day Publishers.

This book contains 22 sensitively conducted interviews with victims who recount their experience and an analysis of the political issues involved in the problem of sexual assault/rape.

Russell, D.: Rape in marriage. New York, 1982, Macmillan, Inc.

This book contains an analysis and interpretation of excellent sociological research on marital rape based on interviews with a random sample of 930 women. The book begins with an introduction about the "crime in the closet" and is divided into nine parts. The victims' accounts enrage and haunt the reader, and clearly refute the myth that wife rape is less traumatic than stranger rape.

Russell, D.: Sexual exploitation: rape, child sexual abuse, and workplace harrassment. Beverly Hills, 1984, Sage Publications.

This book discusses a variety of sexualized violence against women and children. It is divided into 5 parts.

Schultz, L.G., editor: Rape victimology, Springfield, Ill., 1975, Charles C Thomas, Publisher.

This is a collection of lectures and essays drawn from law, social work, medicine, nursing, sociology, the feminist movement, and victims that speaks to various dimensions of the problem of rape. Special focus is given to the social aspects of rape.

Schwendinger, J., and Schwendinger, H.: Rape and inequality. Beverly Hills, 1983, Sage Publications.

The authors draw on extensive historical, cross-cultural, and anthropological data to show how male violence against women is not a universal or inborn trait, rather it is an exploitive mode resulting from socioeconomic inequalities which increase violence.

Selkin, J.: Rape, Psychol. Today **8**:71, 1975.

The author identifies a five-stage pattern in stranger-to-stranger rape: target selection, testing, threat, sexual transaction, and termination. Types of rapists are subdivided into two categories; however, no further diagnosis is included. The importance of immediate resistance at the onset of the attack is emphasized throughout the article.

Weingourt, R.: Wife rape: barriers to identification and treatment. Am. J. Psychotherapy **39**(2):187–192, April 1985.

The nursing author discusses background of the problem of sexual abuse by women's husbands or long-term lovers, including prevalence of the problem. Special attention is given to initial assessment and evaluation of the client, treatment issues, and interventions that break down barriers between the client and therapist facilitating the treatment process.

Weis, K., and Borges, S.S.: Victimology and rape: the case of the legitimate victim, Issues Criminol. **8**:71, Fall 1973.

This article discusses the relationship between victimology and rape and the origin of the legitimate victim. It describes ways in which socialization and sex-role learning exploit both males and females, producing both offenders and victims.

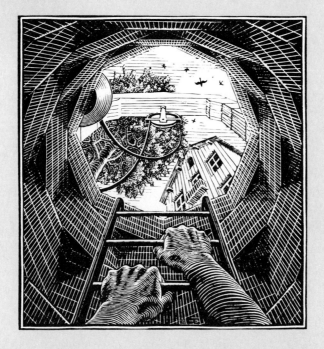

*What I ask for is absurd: that life shall have a meaning.
What I strive for is impossible: that my life shall acquire
 a meaning.
I dare not believe, I do not see how I shall ever be able to
 believe: that I am not alone.*

Dag Hammarskjöld, Markings*

C H A P T E R   3 4

CARE OF THE CHRONICALLY MENTALLY ILL PATIENT

RUTH WILDER BELL

*Hammarskjöld, D.: Markings, New York, 1966, Alfred A. Knopf, Inc. (Translated by L. Sjoberg and W.H. Auden.)
Reprinted by permission of Faber & Faber, Ltd., and Alfred A. Knopf, Inc.

LEARNING OBJECTIVES

After studying this chapter, the student should be able to:

- discuss the impact of deinstitutionalization on the care of the chronically mentally ill.

- identify legal issues that have had an influence on the treatment of the chronically mentally ill.

- describe the evolution of a chronic mental illness, including the development of primary and secondary symptoms.

- assess the nursing care needs of chronically mentally ill patients based on data concerning problem areas and strengths.

- compare and contrast the characteristics of chronically mentally ill young adults with those of older patients.

- describe the elements of psychosocial rehabilitation programs.

- describe the importance of psychoeducation for patients and their families.

- analyze the role of the nurse caring for seriously mentally disabled patients in community and acute care settings.

- discuss nursing interventions based on the assessed needs of chronically mentally ill people.

- identify directions for future nursing research.

- select appropriate readings for further study.

Before the advent of phenothiazines in the 1950s, persons with a chronic mental illness were relatively easy to locate. Primarily they were the residents of large public psychiatric hospitals which were located in rural areas, distant from the populations they served.

The identification and location of the chronically mentally ill and the nurses who care for them are more difficult in the 1980s. Since the CMHC movement of the mid-1960s, the resident population of state and county mental hospitals has decreased by two thirds.[5,10] It is estimated that of the three million Americans who are diagnosed as having a severe mental disorder, only 120,000 are residents of state mental hospitals.[7,26] The others live in the community in a variety of residential settings. Nurses now care for the chronically mentally ill in a multiplicity of health care settings: private and public psychiatric hospitals, psychiatric and medical-surgical units in general hospitals, emergency rooms, community-based treatment programs, and patients' homes.

As the "careers" of the discharged chronically mentally ill unfold, there are likely to be periods when they cannot be maintained in the community, and rehospitalization is necessary. As the patients alternate between community-based and hospital-based care, nurses in both community-based and inpatient facilities share responsibility for care of the same group of patients. Knowledge of the special needs and characteristics of the chronically mentally ill as a population is important

for all nurses who care for these patients, in whatever setting the care may be given.

Social perspective

■ Policy issues

Deinstitutionalization is the term used to describe the process of moving long-term mental hospital patients back into the community where they are to be supported by a "formal network of clinical, social, and vocational agencies, as well as by an informal network of family, neighbors, and local community resources."[31] Implicit in the concept, deinstitutionalization, is the assumption that a network of community resources exists and is available to meet the needs of the chronically ill.

The move to develop resources needed to return the long-term or chronic psychiatric patient to the community was initiated by a 1961 report of the Joint Commission on Mental Illness and Health. Actual construction of facilities to provide community-based treatment for these patients was made possible by the enactment of the 1963 Mental Retardation Facilities and Community Mental Health Centers Construction Act. Policy statements by Presidents Kennedy, Johnson, and Nixon further supported the goal of community-based treatment for the mentally ill. President Carter established a second commission on mental health in 1977, for the purpose of determining and making recommendations regarding the nation's mental health needs. Two of the many recommendations of the final report of the President's Commission on Mental Health were that a federal grant program be established for the purpose of developing "comprehensive integrated systems of care" and that the chronically mentally ill be one of the groups receiving funding priority.[32]

■ Legal issues

As health policy began to direct that there be alternatives to a lifetime in public mental hospitals, court decisions reflected increasing attention to protection of the rights of this patient population. The legal rights of psychiatric patients are discussed in detail in Chapter 7. Friedman and Yohalem,[24] however, specify five clusters of rights that most directly impact on the chronically mentally ill:

1. Civil commitment
2. The right to treatment and protection from harm in the least restrictive environment possible
3. The right to refuse treatment
4. Confidentiality
5. Employment

■ **CIVIL COMMITMENT. Paternalism** is the interference with the liberty of another or the controlling of another when such interference is justified in terms of what is ultimately good for the person being controlled. Paternalism reflects the attitude of a parent toward a child and in the concept underlying the state's right *(parens patriae)* to make decisions for those who are not able to make decisions in their own best interest. Involuntary commitment of the mentally ill is the paternalistic resolution of the conflict between the liberty of an individual and the consequences of his mental illness. Through the use of its **police power** to hospitalize mentally ill patients involuntarily, the state carries out its responsibility to protect its citizens from real or potential danger.[16,24] And, until the late 1960s evidence that a person was suffering and needed treatment for mental illness allowed for commitment of the mentally ill person.[4]

In 1975 Donaldson, a patient who had been hospitalized involuntarily (committed) for 15 years without receiving treatment, challenged the state's right to hold him against his will. The court *(O'Connor v Donaldson)* determined that the state cannot "confine a nondangerous patient who is capable of living safely by himself or with the assistance of caring others unless treatment is being provided."[8]

With increasing attention to protection of individuals' rights, "dangerousness" (to self or another) rather than "need for treatment" is likely to be the condition

necessary for commitment, or involuntary hospitalization. Although such a criterion provides for protection of the civil liberties of the chronically mentally ill, it makes it difficult for society to intervene paternalistically on their behalf.

With the implementation of dangerousness as a criterion for commitment, clinicians, of all disciplines expressed concern that the best interests of the mentally ill were not being served. In 1983, the American Psychiatric Association presented legislatures with a model commitment law hoping that provisions of the model law would be used to guide revision of commitment laws, and in so doing, achieve a better balance between the protection of civil liberties and the need for treatment. Under the provisions of the APA's model law, the criterion that an individual with a serious mental illness, suffers "substantial mental or physical deterioration, and lacks the capacity to make an informed decision regarding treatment," may be substituted for the criterion of dangerousness.[4]

■ **THE RIGHT TO TREATMENT IN THE LEAST RESTRICTIVE ENVIRONMENT.** In 1972 in a landmark decision *(Wyatt v Stickney)*, the United States Supreme Court ruled that "mentally handicapped persons involuntarily confined to a state institution had a constitutional right to treatment."[24] The court identified treatment as including a humane environment, an individualized treatment plan, and adequate numbers of qualified staff to implement the individual treatment plan. In 1975 in the Willowbrook case, the court further ruled that not only did involuntary patients have the right to treatment but they had the right to protection from harm, including protection from "seclusion, corporal punishment, degradation, medical experimentation, and the routine use of restraints."[24]

Although courts have consistently upheld the right of involuntary patients to treatment, they also have upheld the right to treatment in the least restrictive environment. In a class action suit *(Dixon v Weinberger, 1975)* patients at the federally run St. Elizabeth's Hospital in Washington, D.C., sued for their right to treatment in community-based facilities. The court ruled that an individual has the right to treatment in the least restrictive environment and, as a result, directed the federal government to develop community-based facilities for patients who could be therapeutically maintained in the community.[24,50]

Court decisions such as these provided energy for the deinstitutionalization movement. Although increasing numbers of community resources are available and greater numbers of mentally ill are being treated in the community, concern has been raised that the quality of care and life of the chronically mentally ill has not changed. Concerned about the isolation and lack of treatment available to many chronically ill living in board and care homes, Bachrach[6] voiced the possibility that the back wards of public mental hospitals have merely been transferred to the board and care homes in the community. The right to adequate psychiatric care *(Wyatt v Stickney)* is ironically a right belonging to involuntarily committed patients. At present, in the United States voluntary patients have no guaranteed right to adequate psychiatric care.

■ **THE RIGHT TO REFUSE TREATMENT.** To be valid, consent to treatment must be given by an individual who is knowledgeable about the nature and consequences of the choice being made, who is choosing voluntarily, and who is free to withdraw consent at any time without penalty. That is, the consent must be "competent, knowledgeable, and voluntary."[24] Nurses beginning to work with psychiatric patients often believe that the presence of mental illness negates the patient's competency to give informed consent. Given the intrusiveness of many psychiatric treatment interventions, particularly ECT and psychosurgery, it is imperative that patients are involved in deciding whether to participate in such treatments. Increasing evidence about the long-term side effects of psychotropic medications and the availability of long-acting intramuscular drugs, such as fluphenazine decanoate (Prolixin), has focused attention on the patient's right to refuse medication.[24] Voluntary patients have the right to informed consent as well as the right to refuse treatment. Although involuntary patients do not have the right to refuse treatment, they do have a right to information about their treatment.[3] When patients are not capable of making informed decisions about their care, they can be declared mentally incompetent by the court and a guardian is appointed. The court-appointed guardian then participates in the informed consent process and makes knowledgeable decisions about the patient's treatment.

■ **CONFIDENTIALITY.** As with civil commitment, the ethical and legal issues around confidentiality must strike a balance between the rights of the patient and society's right to protection from the consequences of the patient's illness. Additionally, insurance companies and health care professionals have legitimate needs for information from the patient's records. As the chronically mentally ill travel from agency to agency within the community, as well as between community agencies and psychiatric hospitals, the need for professional sharing of information about the patient increases. As a general principle, the patient's written consent must be obtained before health status information can be released or exchanged. At times agencies have patients sign a blanket permission for release of information on admission. This is not adequate protection of the patient's right to confidentiality. The patient has the right to know what information is being released, to whom it is being released, and for what purpose and under what circumstances it is being released. Such conditions require specific forms for each situation in which information is being released. As with other instances of informed consent, the patient has the right to withdraw consent, without penalty, at any time.[24]

At times, however, the right of society to information supersedes the patient's right to confidentiality. In *Tarasoff v Board of Regents of the University of California (1976)*, the California Supreme Court ruled that the therapist is required to violate the confidentiality of the therapeutic relationship in circumstances in which the therapist "knew or should have known that the patient posed a danger of imminent physical harm to others."[24]

■ **EMPLOYMENT.** Issues surrounding the employment and pay of the mentally ill are not limited to employment in the community. In the past, large public psychiatric hospitals were largely self-supporting, with the patients providing much of the labor to run the hospitals' farms, bakeries, sewing rooms, kitchens, laundries, and housekeeping departments. Although work assignments were therapeutic at times, there were many instances of abuse: long hours, working conditions, and lack of monetary compensation provided for labor. The conditions under which patients worked often contributed to their sense of exploitation and worthlessness and limited the therapeutic potential of such activities.

An important ruling protecting patients from providing labor without adequate compensation occurred as the result of *Souder v Brennan* (1973). A federal district court ruled that provisions of the 1966 amendments to the Fair Labor Standards Act applied to institutional residents who provided labor. Residents were to receive minimum wages and overtime pay. Since the Souder decision, a consortium of states successfully challenged the right of the federal government to regulate the minimum wages in state-run institutions. Thus the federal requirement that institutions pay their residents minimum wages applies to private, not public, institutions.[24]

Employment is an even more critical issue once the mentally ill return to the community. It is one variable used to evaluate treatment program effectiveness. Federal regulations protecting the handicapped from discrimination, apply to those with mental impairment, as well as those with physical impairment. Although the handicapped must be able to manage the essential features of a job to be hired, employers can be expected to make reasonable accommodation to special needs of handicapped persons. In job interviews the potential employer is prohibited from asking questions about the handicap and must limit questions to "specific abilities and talents." Furthermore, employers are prohibited from discriminating against the handicapped in terms of salary and benefits.[24]

The development of chronic mental illness

The chronically mentally ill are likely to have both primary and secondary symptoms of their illness. Primary symptoms are those associated with the intrinsic nature of the illness. For example, hallucinations, delusions, and inappropriate affect would be primary symptoms of schizophrenia, and elation and hyperactivity would be primary symptoms of manic-depressive illness. Secondary symptoms are a consequence of the illness process and are not only associated with the disability of chronic illness, but also perpetuate its existence. The progression from primary symptoms to secondary symptoms and ultimately the label "chronically mentally ill" is further understood by more specific examination of the interaction between an individual and his environment.

The behaviors of mentally ill individuals that are associated with the primary symptoms of psychiatric illness are likely to violate social norms and standards of proper conduct and may be considered deviant behavior. These deviant behaviors set in motion a social interactive process whereby society protects itself from the norm violation of the deviant. As this process unfolds individuals increasingly assume the self-identity "mentally ill" and relate to society more often in terms of this identity, rather than in terms of other available identities, such as wife, mother, husband, father, or worker. The ultimate acceptance of the deviant status mentally ill and adjustment to society in terms of this role are accompanied by the many secondary symptoms of chronic mental illness.

■ Social interaction model

The process by which society and the individual interact to the end of conferring/accepting the role of deviant (chronically mentally ill) has been outlined by Lemert[35] as the following eight-step process:

1. Individual instances of deviant behavior; role and status are not defined at this time in terms of a deviant identity
2. Social penalties
3. Further deviant behavior
4. Stronger penalties and rejection of the individual with the deviant behavior
5. Further deviant behavior, perhaps with hostilities and resentment beginning to focus on those doing the penalizing
6. Crisis reached in society's tolerance quotient, expressed in formal action by the community stigmatizing the deviant
7. Strengthening of the deviant conduct as a reaction to the stigmatizing and penalties
8. Ultimate acceptance of deviant social status and efforts at adjustment based on an associated role

■ Public health model

As Lemert's social interaction model demonstrates, the disability of chronic mental illness does not suddenly

---

TABLE 34-1

STAGES OF THE NATURAL HISTORY OF CHRONIC ILLNESS

Stage	Characteristics
Susceptibility	Presence of environmental, biological, behavioral, and emotional risk factors
Presymptomatic disease	No overt symptoms of disease; pathological changes begin; risk factors intensify; behaviors increasing susceptibility solidify and become patterns
Clinical disease	Anatomical and functional changes occur; presence of recognizable disease symptoms
Disability	Disease symptoms increase; anatomical and functional changes produce reduction in activity; impairment of instrumental or expressive function

Modified from Anderson, S., and Bauwens, E.: Chronic health problems: concepts and application, St. Louis, 1981, The C.V. Mosby Co.

appear, but develops over a period of time as an exchange between individuals with deviant behaviors and the world within which they live. Similarly, through their attention to the "natural history" of chronic illness, public health epidemiologists view chronic illness not as a state or end point but as a process of progressive deterioration. According to the public health model, individuals with a chronic illness show increasing symptoms of functional impairment and disability as they move sequentially through the four stages of the "natural history" of chronic illness. The first stage, **susceptibility,** is a period of exposure to risk factors; the second stage, **presymptomatic disease,** is the period within which pathological changes begin; the third stage **clinical disease,** is the period within which primary symptoms of the disease are recognizable; and the fourth stage, **disability,** is the period within which there are identifiable changes in both activity level and role performance.[1] See Table 34-1 for a description of the characteristics of these four stages. Psychiatric disability is the functional impairment occurring because the chronically mentally ill person does not have the skills necessary to meet the environmental role requirements.[32]

Description of the chronically mentally ill

Elaboration of the special characteristics of the chronically mentally ill portrays a population with difficulties with activities of daily living, maintaining interpersonal relations, lack of coping resources, and a need for long-term treatment.[16] Other characteristics influencing the course of their illness are their consistently low self-esteem and preoccupation with avoidance of failure rather than the achievement of success.[46] The chronically mentally ill, as a group, can be described not only in terms of the problems confronting the group but also in terms of the group's unique strengths and potentials. There is tentative evidence that the kinds of interpersonal strengths available to this population differ from those available to the general population.

■ Activities of daily living

When nurses refer to activities of daily living (ADL), they are usually referring to the complex of behaviors necessary to maintain independence in personal hygiene, dressing, and grooming. The use of the term when referring to the chronically mentally ill has an expanded meaning, referring to the skills necessary to live independently as an adult. At times professionals caring for the chronically mentally ill use the broader term **psychosocial rehabilitation** when referring to development of the many skills necessary for independent living.

If the premise that the chronically mentally ill relate to their world essentially in terms of the role "mentally ill" is accepted, it follows that these patients would have difficulty meeting the multiple functional requirements of an adult in the United States. Impairment in instrumental role performance is one of the characteristics of disability, the end stage of the progressive deterioration of individuals with chronic mental illness.[1] Individuals are considered legally disabled when they have impairment of instrumental role performance in at least three of the following areas: "self-care, receptive and expressive language, learning, mobility, self-direction, capacity for independent living, and self-sufficiency."[25]

■ Interpersonal relations

Over the years, patients in public mental hospitals have been described as apathetic, withdrawn, and isolated from other patients and their family. They have been described as possessing only the minimum of interpersonal skills. The process leading to impoverished interpersonal relations has been thought not to be a primary symptom of their mental illness, but rather a secondary symptom resulting from adaptation to life in a rigid and nonstimulating environment. The term **social breakdown syndrome** was coined to describe the progressive deterioration of the social and interpersonal skills of long-term psychiatric patients.[28] However, evidence is accumulating that chronically mentally ill patients who have spent most of their life in the community, with brief periods of hospitalization during acute crises, have the same deterioration of social and interpersonal skills as those who have had long-term hospitalizations. Studies of the social activities of the chronically mentally ill support the conclusion that these patients "lead an unusually barren and isolated existence."[37] Generalizing from a study of all nonhospitalized California residents who received Social Security because of a psychiatric disability, fewer than 50% were employed or had any structured activity around which to orient their lives.[33] The question must now be asked whether the social breakdown syndrome of the chronically mentally ill is in fact causally related to long-term hospitalization, or whether there might be another explanation for the syndrome's appearing in patients cared for in both the hospital and in the community. Minkoff[37] wrote, "Those who tend to be more active socially, tend to be less chronic, married and employed and characterize a group of high functioning mentally ill whose lives stand apart from the more dreary existence of the rest."

■ Lack of coping resources

The social isolation, lack of support systems, and functional impairment of the chronically mentally ill leave them with minimal coping skills to use in dealing with stress. Social margin, as defined by Segal, Baumohl, and Johnson,[48] is the sum total of "all the personal possessions, attributes, or relationships which can be traded on for help in time of need." It is, in effect, the sum total of resources available to the individual. With a nearly nonexistent social margin, the chronically mentally ill are likely to respond to stress and the necessity for adaptation as a crisis. (See Chapter 10.)

■ Need for long-term treatment

Implicit in the concept, "chronicity" is the notion of illness over time. Federal policy makers acknowledge the need for long-term treatment in labeling patients as having a "chronic mental disability" when they have had either one episode of at least 6 months of continuous hospitalization within the past 5 years or two or more hospitalizations in a 12-month period.[37] Given the marginal existence of the chronically mentally ill living in the community and their vulnerability to stress, it is not surprising that within a year of their discharge from the hospital, 40% are expected to be readmitted.[6] Treatment factors that facilitate patients' maintenance in the community are the patient's compliance with a medication regimen and the patient's involvement in aftercare programs.[37] Because of their need for long-term treatment, whether in residential institutions or from community-based facilities, the proper focus of treatment for the chronically mentally ill is care and rehabilitation rather than cure.

■ Low self-esteem

Self-esteem is the feeling or sense of regard that accompanies individuals' self-perceptions. It is "the personal judgment of worthiness that is expressed in the attitudes of an individual to himself . . . it indicates the extent to which an individual believes himself to be capable, significant, worthy."[17] As part of an extensive research project, Fitts[21,22] found the self-esteem of psychiatric patients to be lower, in all areas, especially in the areas of identity and behavior, than the self-esteem of the general population. The self-esteem of the chronically mentally ill parallels that of psychiatric patients,[12] and the chronically mentally ill suffer from the many perceptual and behavioral difficulties associated with low self-esteem. (See Chapter 14.) A description of the characteristics of an individual with low self-esteem is also a description of the chronically mentally ill individual.

Persons with low self-esteem . . . have come to believe they are powerless and without resource or recourse. They feel isolated, unlovable, incapable of expressing and defending themselves, and too weak to overcome their deficiencies. Too immobilized to take action, they tend to withdraw and become overly passive and compliant while suffering the pangs of anxiety and symptoms that accompany its chronic occurrence.[17:250]

■ Motivation

As described earlier, the chronically mentally ill have difficulty in achieving a level of psychosocial functioning that would allow them to live comfortably in the community. For many patients, success and greater competence are followed by increased anxiety and symptoms of regression, rather than by pride and the sense of improved well-being. Patients attribute their uneasiness with success to the fear that once they succeed, even more will be expected of them, and they may not be able to meet the new expectations.

Chronically mentally ill patients have experienced repeated failures. They have not met the expectations of family, friends, or society, but most important, they have not met their own expectations. New experiences, rather than being seen as opportunities for growth, are seen as opportunities for further failure. Studies of psychiatric patients, living both in institutions and in the community, support the observation that when compared with the general population, psychiatric patients are much more concerned with avoiding failure than they are with achieving success.[46] A pattern of motivation that is based on the avoidance of failure, rather than the achievement of success, not only produces resistance to involvement in new experiences, but also makes it difficult for the chronically mentally ill to acknowledge and assume responsibility for their personal achievements.

■ Strengths

Rehabilitation of the chronically mentally ill depends on the control of illness, as well as on the development of health potential by mobilizing patients' ego strengths. A strength is an "ability, skill, or interest" an individual has previously used.[38] Categories of individual strengths, as derived from work with assumed healthy nonpsychiatric patient groups are as follows:

Sports and outdoor activities
Hobbies and crafts
Expressive arts
Health
Education, training, and related areas
Work, vocation, job, or position
Special aptitudes or resources

Strengths through family and others
Intellectual strengths
Aesthetic strengths
Organizational strengths
Imaginative and creative strengths
Relationship strengths[39]

Although the assessment and description of patients' strengths are largely an individual matter and the profile of strengths will vary from patient to patient, there is initial evidence that the relationship strengths of the chronically mentally ill differ from those of a nonpatient population.

Concerned with the development of healthy interpersonal relationships, Porter[43] defined interpersonal strength as a "behavior trait . . . so employed as to enhance the production of mutual gratification between one's self and another person without violating the integrity of either person." According to Porter, interpersonal strengths cluster around three basic motivational patterns or orientations in interpersonal relationships. These are the "altruistic-nurturing" motivational pattern, the "assertive-directing" motivational pattern, and the "analytic-autonomizing" motivational pattern. Associated with each of the motivational patterns are positive goals in terms of interpersonal relationships. Individuals with strengths associated with the altruistic-nurturing motivational pattern report their goal in interpersonal relations to be that of being genuinely helpful, with little regard for what they consequently received from others. Individuals having strengths associated with the assertive-directive pattern report their desire to lead others in a way that does not interfere with others' rights. The goal or desire behind the strengths associated with the analytic-autonomizing motivational pattern is to create order, becoming self-reliant and independent. The interpersonal strengths of the nonpatient population are evenly divided among those of the three motivational patterns and represent nurturing strengths, leading strengths, and analyzing strengths (Table 34-2).

Initial evidence supports the premise that the relationship strengths of the chronically mentally ill are not evenly divided among the three motivational patterns as are those of nonpatients. When interpersonal relationships are going well, the chronically mentally ill preceive themselves as mobilizing the nurturing strengths of the altruistic-nurturing motivational pattern. They feel good about themselves when they are genuinely caring for someone else, with little regard for what they receive in return. In conflictual interpersonal situations their strengths are those of the peacemaker. Aware of the personal cost of their peacemaking efforts, they will insist, probably explosively, that their rights be respected if harmony and peace cannot be restored.[12]

TABLE 34-2

BEHIND THE WEAKNESSES ARE STRENGTHS

Altruistic-nurturing		Assertive-directing		Analytic-autonomizing	
Characteristic strengths	Risks	Characteristic strengths	Risks	Characteristic strengths	Risks
Trusting	Gullible	Self-confident	Arrogant	Cautious	Suspicious
Optimistic	Impractical	Enterprising	Opportunistic	Practical	Unimaginative
Loyal	Slavish	Ambitious	Ruthless	Economical	Stingy
Idealistic	Wishful	Organizing	Controlling	Reserved	Cold
Helpful	Self-denying	Persuasive	Pressuring	Methodical	Rigid
Modest	Self-effacing	Forceful	Dictatorial	Analytic	Nitpicking
Devoted	Self-sacrificing	Quick to act	Rash	Principled	Unbending
Caring	Smothering	Imaginative	Dreamer	Orderly	Compulsive
Supportive	Submissive	Competitive	Combative	Fair	Unfeeling
Accepting	Passive	Proud	Conceited	Persevering	Stubborn
Polite	Deferential	Bold	Brash	Conserving	Possessive
Adaptable	Without principle	Risk taking	Gambler	Thorough	Obsessive

From Porter, E., and Maloney, S.: Strength deployment inventory: manual of administration and interpretation, Pacific Palisades, Calif., Personal Strengths Assessment Service, Inc.

The young adult chronically mentally ill patient

■ Characteristics

The characteristics of the chronically mentally ill previously discussed describe the chronically mentally ill regardless of their age. However, researchers describe the "young" chronic patient, generally between the ages of 18 to 35, as differing in important ways from the chronically mentally ill who are over 35 years of age. Many of the differences in the two groups of patients can be traced to the deinstitutionalization movement and the development of community-based care as an alternative to hospital-based care.[40]

Generally, chronically mentally ill patients under 35 have not experienced lengthy psychiatric hospitalizations as have older psychiatric patients. For those under 35, recurrent short hospitalizations at times of crisis or during periods of acute exacerbation of symptoms have alternated with care in the community. The personal requirements for adaptation to long-term hospitalization are different from the requirements for adaptation to community life interspersed with short hospitalizations.

Patients who have spent years in psychiatric hospitals have been confronted over and over with their personal failure in terms of meeting their own, their family's, and society's expectations. In most instances older chronic patients have traded personal autonomy and adult functioning in roles such as father, mother, husband, wife, and employee for a life of personal dependence and the role of psychiatric patient. Through socialization into this role, chronic patients become compliant and nonassertive, and their social participation is likely to be limited to the social and geographical boundaries of the hospital or perhaps even the ward where they live. Although such adaptation may provide limited potential for growth, it does provide relief from the seemingly impossible demands of age-appropriate role expectations and continuing confrontation with failure.

Younger chronically ill patients do not have such protection from bombardment with messages as to their inadequacy and the resulting sense of failure. Alternating between hospital and community life, they compare themselves with others of their age and continue to expect of themselves behavior similar to that of their nonpatient peers. They expect that they should marry, have children and jobs, and perhaps even acquire advanced education. Given their failure in managing the role expectations of others their age and their limited ability to cope with the many tasks of community living, it is not surprising that the young chronically mentally ill are "acutely vulnerable to stress, and are characterized by a high incidence of alcohol and drug abuse, suicide and suicide attempts."[40,41] Generalizing from a study of nearly 300 patients, 42% of this population of young chronic psychiatric patients "present a risk of suicide for reasons that include the simple fact that they see no hope for the future."[40] They cannot see a future in which they will have the abilities to meet the ongoing demands of their daily lives.

Younger chronically mentally ill patients are not characterized by docile compliant behavior as are long-term hospital residents. They do not see themselves as mentally ill but as social casualties, unfortunate victims of social circumstances.[40] Not having been hospitalized for long periods of time, the younger chronically ill patient who is more likely to have a diagnosis of personality disorder than the older patient, has not been socialized into the compliant nonassertive behavior associated with the older chronically ill patient. Their self-concept, accompanied by their particular symptoms, especially disorders of impulse control and disturbances of affect,[47] have important consequences in terms of supporting their marginal life-style.

■ Involvement in treatment

Because they do not see themselves as patients, there is little motivation to become involved in aftercare or treatment programs or to comply with a medication regimen. For example, a study of more than 100 young chronically mentally ill patients living in New York City found that only 17% complied with their aftercare plan.[15] Involvement in aftercare programs and maintenance on a medication regimen have been previously identified as critical factors for maintenance of the chronically mentally ill in the community.

Further interfering with their involvement in a therapeutic relationship is the general affective response of anger, which manifests itself in the sarcastic and argumentive manner in which these patients relate to the caregivers from whom they seek help. Caregivers often report feelings of frustration and helplessness when confronted by the many problems of this group of patients, and the manner in which they seek help. This behavior has been labeled "help-seeking–help-rejecting behavior."

■ Drug and alcohol abuse

Many patients under 35 years of age have lived primarily in the community during the course of their mental illness and have been exposed to the same health risks as their contemporaries. It would be predicted then that young chronically mentally ill patients would have a higher incidence of drug and alcohol abuse than older patients. Evidence confirming this is accumulating.[13] A survey of clients in a suburban New York Community Mental Health Center found that 37% of those who were between 18 and 35 abused alcohol; another 37% abused drugs.[40] Schwartz and Goldfinger documented poly-drug abuse by this population.[47]

Drug and alcohol abuse compound the problems of the young chronically mentally ill in a variety of ways. Mentally ill clients with an additional diagnosis of alcohol or drug dependence have been less successful in rehabilitation outcomes.[11] In a study of the acting-out behavior of the young chronically mentally ill population, those who abused drugs and/or alcohol were more likely to be involved in acting-out behavior, both at home and in the community. As age itself was not directly related to acting-out behavior, the researchers concluded that drug and alcohol abuse "appear to be largely responsible for the increased acting out" of the younger clients in the study.[36] And since psychosis may be drug induced, the problem of identifying whether psychotic symptoms are the result of drug abuse or schizophrenia is a difficult one and may interfere with planning and implementing appropriate treatment.

■ Entry into the mental health system

Because their pathological condition interferes with voluntary involvement in treatment programs and ongoing participation in a therapeutic relationship, the younger chronically ill patient is likely to enter the mental health system through hospital emergency rooms or the legal system. Younger patients may seek help from emergency rooms either voluntarily or at the insistence of family or friends during times of personal or family crisis. Behavior resulting from their poor impulse control is often the precipitating event for the crisis. Schwartz and Goldfinger[47] reported that although suicidal threats and self-damaging acts are common, impulsive acts against others are less frequent. However, many of these patients enter the mental health system through involvement with the law for offenses such as "minor property damage" and "petty assault." Likewise, Caton[15] found the arrest rate of young chronically mentally ill patients to be eight times that of the general population in the areas in which the patients lived.

The symptoms and style of interpersonal relationships of the younger chronically mentally ill patients seem to interact nonproductively with present treatment resources.

■ Strengths

Initial descriptions of the special characteristics of this population essentially portrayed a troublesome group with particular deficits which interfered with both their adjustment to community life and their involvement in a rehabilitation program, but more recent research also identifies strengths which are more likely to be available to this population than to the older chronically mentally ill population. In a survey of 844 clients of New York State's Community Support Service program, 18% were under 35 years of age. When compared with the older client, the younger client was likely to be

better educated, more proficient and independent in performing community living skills, actively engaged in significantly more healthy adult leisure activities, more likely to be competitively employed, more capable of living on their own instead of in supervised housing, more likely to be utilizing sheltered workshops and other vocational services, and less dependent on the Community Support System . . . for medical care or transportation.[30:50]

Further description of this rapidly expanding subgroup must continue if programs suitable to their needs are to be developed.

Psychosocial rehabilitation: the Fountain House model

Ronald Peterson, a veteran of 10 years of residence in a state hospital, speaks poignantly of the loneliness and isolation he felt when he left the state hospital to live alone in a small hotel room. Since he had no job, knew no one, and lived on welfare, it never occurred to him that it could be any different. He said, "You take what you can get. There is no choice."[42] Now a staff member of Fountain House, a psychosocial rehabilitation program, Peterson speaks for many chronically mentally ill persons who are trying to adjust to community living when he describes their greatest need to be a place where they belong and are needed.

I think the greatest need is to have a place to go where you are expected each day, a place where you can be with people like yourself and do things that mean something to yourself and others . . . you have to remember that many of us did a lot of things in the hospital. If given a chance we can do lots of things in the community—if we have places to go and can be with people who need us to contribute, to take part, to help, and who notice when we're not present and do something about it.[42:41,42]

In making a judgment as to the effectiveness of any treatment program for the chronically mentally ill, the program's readmission and employment rates are compared with baseline readmission and employment data.[39] As a baseline it is expected that 6 months after leaving the hospital 30% to 40% of the patients will be rehospitalized. And, with regard to employment, 6 months after leaving the hospital it is expected that 30% to 50%

will be employed. The percentage decreases to 20% to 30% after 12 months and to 25% after 3 to 5 years. Despite a lack of adequate follow-up studies of the fate of chronically mentally ill individuals returned to the community, it is generally believed that community-based treatment programs, while increasing in both number and quality, are not adequate to meet the need.

Fountain House, in New York City, an early psychosocial program, has been described as an excellent program for assisting chronically ill psychiatric patients in making a place for themselves in the community, and has been used as a model in developing programs across the country.[2,14,49] Information regarding rehospitalization of Fountain House participants provides evidence of the program's effectiveness. For the first 5 years after returning to the community, Fountain House members have a 40% lower rehospitalization rate than the baseline percentage. After 9 years, Fountain House's rehospitalization rates are similar to the baseline rate. However, when hospitalization is needed, Fountain House members are hospitalized for only half the usual number of days.[18] Critical to Fountain House's success is attention to psychosocial rehabilitation, especially in terms of facilitating independence of living and employment.

Incorporating elements from the medical, rehabilitation, and social support models, psychosocial rehabilitation provides a variety of living and work opportunities to individually accommodate the needs and functional abilities of patients as they begin to live in the community. Staff not only help patients develop skills necessary to assume increasing independence in living and working, but they serve as buffers between the patient and the community, in a sense, by lending their own skills and competency to the patients until the patients can develop these skills for themselves. Compensating for patient's functional inadequacies while encouraging them to assume increasing responsibility, allows the patients to experience the pride of achievement rather than the pain and humiliation of failure. Basic to this rehabilitation process is focusing on the strengths of Fountain House members.

Fountain House attributes the state of isolation and alienation of its new members to the process of illness which initially brings the members to Fountain House—but it is the strengths and capabilities of each individual that validates his belonging and are the beginning of the discovery that he is worth something and may be able to achieve at least reasonably full participation in community life.[14:86]

Fountain House functions as a club in which patients are no longer patients, but members, and the usual hierarchical distinctions between staff (the healthy) and patients (the ill) do not exist. It is a place where members care about each other and pool their resources and abilities as they work toward increasing independence. Thus Fountain House combats loneliness and isolation while providing a variety of living and work situations that require differing levels of functional ability.

The first month at Fountain House is a residential phase, and residents are taught skills necessary for apartment living. Fountain House owns and leases apartments that have staff on call, although not in residence. These supervised apartments allow for a gradual transition to independent living situations in the community.

Fountain House runs several businesses itself and can provide work experiences in a protected environment in which patients can develop both self-confidence and transferable job skills. Progressing to a more complex work situation, Fountain House has creatively arranged for transitional employment placements, called TEPs. Recognizing that the job interview is a tremendously stressful experience for recently discharged psychiatric patients and is often seen as an obstacle that cannot be overcome, staff, rather than patients, seek out and contract with businesses for jobs. The jobs are assigned to Fountain House rather than to individual patients. Staff are then free to assign a patient to a transitional employment position for as long as needed. The employer is promised that if patients are unable to manage the job, or even portions of the job, or do not show up, Fountain House staff will cover for them. With such an arrangement, the dreaded employment interview is avoided. Fountain House members who share responsibility for a job with staff, can be delegated increasing responsibility as they are able to handle it, and a TEP can easily be transferred from one member who is ready for a more complex work experience to a member who needs a TEP. Furthermore, employers are satisfied because the quality of work is guaranteed by the staff. Again in the words of Peterson who tried a number of part-time TEPs:

If you have the chance to go to work without having to pass a lot of hurdles first, you discover things. All of us found we could do parts of the job real well, but we couldn't do so well on other things.[42:42,43]

Between 1977 and 1982, Fountain House, with funding from the National Institute of Mental Health, implemented a national training program in the principles of psychiatric rehabilitation upon which the Fountain House program is based. By 1982, as a result of this training program, the number of clubhouses based on the Fountain House model increased from 18 to 148; the number of transitional employment programs increased from 21 to 102; the number of participating employers increased from 122 to 507; and the number of job placements increased from 360 to 1154.[2] Spurred on by the mounting evidence from community-based programs, that the functional level and quality of life of the chronically mentally ill can be improved by the development of their physical, emotional, and intellectual skills, within a supportive environment, clinicians are beginning to use psychiatric rehabilitation principles in designing inpatient programs for the chronically mentally ill. There is initial evidence that recidivism decreases and employment and quality of life are positively affected, when an inpatient program is based on the principles underlying the Fountain House model.[11,19]

Psychoeducation

Psychoeducation is the use of educational methods, techniques, and principles to facilitate the rehabilitation and treatment of the mentally ill.[9] Psychoeducation is an important treatment component in psychosocial rehabilitation programs in which the primary concern is the development of skills rather than the development of insight. In addition to fostering skill development, psychoeducation is used to teach patients about their illness and its management. Providing patients with this information counteracts misconceptions about mental illness and invites patients to collaborate and actively participate in their treatment. For example, if patients are taught about psychotropic medication side effects, they will be better able to participate in finding the lowest dose that comfortably controls some of their symptoms; or, if patients are taught about symptoms of their illness, they can begin to recognize early warnings of relapse and be taught to appropriately ask for assistance in coping, perhaps averting rehospitalization. Psychoeducation is a powerful therapeutic tool in increasing patients' self-esteem and offering hope. By treating patients as though they are able to learn difficult information and expecting them to use that information in improving the quality of their life, patients are given some control over their life and a sense that improvement is possible.[2,9,32]

For families of patients experiencing a first admission, hospitalization provides the hope that "things will be different" in the future. However, at discharge, families express disappointment that the desired changes have not occurred, and they frequently view the patient as not ready for discharge.[34,45] After reviewing a number of studies, Goldman concluded that about 62% of hospitalized psychiatric patients are discharged to their families, and, of these about 25% were severely ill at the time of discharge.[25] Acknowledging that families are all too often asked to care for the chronically mentally ill without the necessary expertise, clinicians are beginning

to provide psychoeducation for family members with the hope that families' acceptance and ability to manage the illness will increase. Information about schizophrenia, its etiology and symptoms, treatment approaches, psychotropic medication, management of behavioral problems and how to deal with crisis is usually presented in the family sessions.[9] Families can be taught about the consequences of schizophrenia for an individual and how to assist patients in coping with their environment in a way which minimizes stress on the rest of the family.[29] The use of a family psychoeducational approach has been successful in decreasing symptomatology and the rehospitalization of chronically ill family members.[20]

Nursing care of the chronically mentally ill

Although there are many similarities in the needs of the chronically mentally ill, whether they are being cared for in inpatient units, community psychosocial rehabilitation progams, or emergency service, the health care setting in which the nurse cares for the chronically mentally ill influences the scope and priorities of nursing care.

■ Psychosocial rehabilitation programs

Nurses working in community-based psychosocial rehabilitation programs are ultimately concerned with assisting patients to achieve their fullest potential in terms of independent living and adequate interpersonal relations. In this situation nurses have the opportunity for long-term ongoing relationships with patients and the mutual setting of long-term goals. The nurses' functions will vary. For example, they may be on call for assistance to patients living in supervised apartments. Others may be active participants in a day treatment milieu, both creating situations for growth and serving as process observers to the patient so that he may benefit from analyzing his behavior as he functions in the therapeutic milieu. Nurses may also provide a formally structured educational experience, such as teaching patients about community resources, skills necessary for independent living, or self-care behaviors that facilitate health maintenance. They may participate in a variety of work programs with patients or may even be backing a patient up in a transitional work placement. If the nurse has had additional training and supervision, she may function in the expanded role of group leader or co-leader, conduct family meetings, or assume responsibility as the patient's primary therapist.

In most psychosocial rehabilitation programs the nurse works as a team member with other mental health professionals and nonprofessionals. Although the role and function of the nurse are always bounded by the nurse practice act of the state in which she is practicing, it varies from program to program, depending on the nature of the program and the available resources.

In some programs the nurse may be asked to function as "case manager" for a group of patients. This role cuts across professional boundaries and is based on two premises; that the chronically mentally ill have difficulty in establishing interpersonal relationships and that because of their many social, vocational, and health needs, services are likely to be needed from a variety of sources. At a minimum, the patient needs access or a link to family, friends, housing, and a source of income. Case managers are responsible for identifying, securing, and coordinating all the resources, from both folk and professional support systems, necessary for the patient's life in the community. When the patient is assigned a case manager, he does not have to independently negotiate relationships with the many individuals from whom services are needed. After an assessment process, the case manager is responsible for providing a 24-hour plan with links to activities and services for coordinating the activities of those involved, monitoring both the quality of service provided and the patient's response to the 24-hour plan, and functioning as an advocate, intervening on the patient's behalf when necessary.

The case manager role and the role of primary nurse are similar in that both have accountability and responsibility not only for the development of a 24-hour plan of care but also for its implementation and evaluation. They are also similar in that it is easier for the patient, especially for a chronically mentally ill patient, to organize his requests for assistance around one person, rather than negotiating individual requests with a variety of persons. However, unlike the role of primary nurse, the case manager role, as generally conceived, is also concerned with the development of a social network, an area of responsibility typically associated with the social worker. A nurse fulfilling this function can enlarge the scope of the 24-hour plan to include a plan for meeting nursing and health care needs as well.

■ Acute care settings

Conceptualization of care of the chronically mentally ill as a shared responsibility between the community and residential inpatient facilities means that the focus of care is different in different settings. Because the chronically mentally ill are likely to disengage from community treatment programs, have ongoing difficulties in complying with a medication regimen, and are acutely vulnerable to stress, there may be periods of acute exacerbation of symptoms and the need for inpatient hospitalization. The goal of care in an acute

treatment setting then becomes crisis resolution, with control of acute symptoms. The patient is helped to return to a precrisis level of functioning as quickly as possible so that he can return to the community, where he can continue to receive support and treatment in a less restrictive environment.

As with any acutely ill psychiatric patient, the nurse, after completing a nursing assessment, makes a nursing diagnosis and plans nursing interventions that help the patient cope with his behavioral responses to his illness. Given that chronically mentally ill patients are admitted to inpatient units for crisis intervention, the nurse working in such a setting must have a thorough understanding of the theory of crisis intervention and be skilled in its implementation. The specific factors to be assessed as the nurse attempts to understand the nature of the crisis and its effect on the patient are those identified in Chapter 10. That is, assessment must be made of the precipitating event, the patient's strengths and previous coping mechanisms, and the nature and strength of the patient's support systems. Intervention may be in terms of any of the four levels of intervention: environmental manipulation; general support; generic intervention, especially in terms of what is known about grief work; and particularly in the area of individual intervention, which depends on an understanding of the meaning of the precipitating event to an individual at a certain moment in time and an awareness of the resources available to that patient at that point. An individual approach, by definition, is idiosyncratic in nature and depends on the development of a competent nurse-patient relationship for its implementation.

Primary nursing, one of several modalities of providing nursing care, has several advantages in terms of meeting the needs of chronically mentally ill patients hospitalized during periods of acute exacerbation of symptoms. The most obvious advantage is that once assigned a primary nurse, the acutely ill patient, who is likely to have difficulties establishing interpersonal relationships, knows who is responsible for his care and can focus his energies on developing a trusting relationship with one person who will look out for him and intercede on his behalf when necessary. And, because the chronically mentally ill patient is likely to have recurrent inpatient admissions, the same primary nurse can be assigned to him for each admission. Consistent assignment of patients to primary nurses for each admission has advantages for both patients and nurses. It is assumed that it would be easier for an acutely ill patient to feel safe when cared for by a nurse he already knows. Prior knowledge of the patient provides the nurse with a historical data bank about the patient, including the patient's past responses to particular nursing interventions. This should expedite nursing care on subsequent admissions; it certainly should facilitate family and community involvement in the patient's care in that the primary nurse, agency staff, and family members probably were involved with each other on previous admissions and already have working relationships established.

But perhaps an even more important consequence of primary nursing and consistency of assignment is the primary nurse's sense of the patient's progress over time. If the patient has been making incremental gains, however small, in a community rehabilitation program, the goal of crisis therapy during successive admissions would be return to a steadily increasing functional level. Thus rather than acknowledging only the repeated admissions of the chronically mentally ill, the primary nurse working in an acute care setting can document the successes and progress the patient experienced while in the community. These observations can then be used to combat the discouragement and sense of hopelessness occasionally experienced by both herself and the patient and find the energy needed to continue the rehabilitation process.

■ Developing patients' strengths and potentials

Rehabilitation has been conceptualized as the "process of actualizing the remaining potentialities and abilities of a handicapped person."[23] Psychosocial rehabilitation programs, such as Fountain House, attribute their success to focusing on the strengths patients bring with them. The rehabilitation model of care is as concerned with maximizing wellness as with the control of disease or pathological conditions. Nursing also accepts responsibility for the promotion of wellness and the improvement of patients' health status by the development of their health potentials. This view of nursing is consistently reflected in the models of nursing being developed by nursing scholars.

The following discussion focuses on nursing interventions that facilitate the development of patients' strengths and potentials, because of the importance of these interventions in the care of chronically mentally ill patients. Such interventions, however, do not occur in isolation, but as part of the implementation of the nursing process, with the development of an individual plan of care only after completion of a nursing assessment. The principles of developing and implementing nursing care plans for psychiatric patients, as described in this text, also apply in the care of chronically mentally ill patients.

The development of chronically mentally ill patients' strengths and potentials is important for several reasons. Nursing interventions that develop patients' strengths and potentials can help the chronically mentally ill develop their independent living skills, adequacy in interpersonal relationships, and coping resources and thus help meet their special needs. Such nursing interventions also help patients alter their motivational style, increasing their willingness to become involved in growth-producing situations. Ultimately the expected outcome of such interventions would be changes in the patient's self-concept and an increase in self-esteem.

Dr. Vallory Lathrop, a leader in forensic psychiatric nursing, remarked that she would be pleased to receive a nickel from every patient who, when asked to name one of his strengths, responded that he did not have any. The negative self-concept and low self-esteem that characterize the chronically mentally ill as a group interfere with their ability to experience themselves as individuals with strengths and potentials.

Rogers[44] wrote that a therapeutic experience was one in which experiences contradictory to the individual's self-concept were brought into awareness and accepted as part of oneself. Through environmental and interpersonal experiences of adequacy, self-concept can be altered and self-esteem increased. One nursing intervention that assists patients in altering their negative self-perceptions and thereby increases their health potential is to identify with patients their strengths as perceived by the nurse in the here-and-now experiences of patients' participation in the psychiatric milieu. Nursing interventions in which patients become aware of their strengths fall into two major categories: those which occur as a response to the patient's spontaneous participation in the milieu and those which occur as part of a structured intervention in which the nurse, or the nurse and the patient together, plan an experience in which the patient can mobilize his strengths and develop his potentials. The following clinical examples illustrate the nurse's use of two spontaneously occurring situations to increase a patient's awareness of her strengths.

Although the strengths identified in this sequence, caring and helping, are consistent with the altruistic-nurturing motivational pattern that is most characteristic of this population, they are not the only strengths which occur spontaneously in the milieu. Patients have many opportunities for demonstrating behaviors reflective of leadership strengths, strengths in problem solving, or in increased autonomy among others. A different kind of strength is evident in Clinical example 34-2. Nurses with general knowledge of the patients on a ward or in a psychosocial rehabilitation program can share with the patient their impression of his or her strengths, as they see them naturally occur. Nurses who have an ongoing therapeutic relationship with a smaller

CLINICAL EXAMPLE 34-1

During a 1-hour period a nurse made the following observations. Marie, a frightened 22-year-old young woman who was psychotic as the result of PCP use was sitting in the craft room. The nurse joined Marie. Janet, another patient, came in and heaped clothes that were still warm from the dryer in Marie's lap. (Janet had voluntarily done Marie's laundry when she noticed Marie having trouble with the dial on the washing machine.)

JANET: **Here are your clean clothes.**

MARIE: **Silence, continues drawing.**

NURSE: **Do you want some help folding these clothes? It looks hard to draw with such a full lap.**

MARIE: **No, I'm fine, except my head gets dizzy.**

JANET: **That's from your medicine. Didn't you just start on your medicine?**

MARIE: **Yes.**

JANET: **It'll get better soon. It takes a few days to get used to your medicine. You're drawing a Christmas picture. Merry Christmas and Happy New Year. You're thinking about wanting to be home for Christmas aren't you?**

MARIE: **Shakes her head yes.**

JANET: **Your picture sure makes me think of how nice home is at Christmas, except we don't have a fireplace. But having a fireplace doesn't make Christmas. Being home with a family you love does.** (Janet continues showing the nurse other artwork that Marie has done, praising her ability.)

Another patient and the recreational therapist came into the room. The therapist changed the music from soul music to a classical symphony. Both Janet and Marie disapproved of the new music. Marie began to look more tense. Janet put her arm around her and said, "Come on. Let's go walk in the hall." They left together.

Later, when the nurse saw Janet in the dayroom, the nurse shared with Janet that she saw her as having been very helpful to Marie. Janet grinned broadly and said "Yeah, I'm a real friend to her. It feels good."

CLINICAL EXAMPLE 34-2

A nurse walking down the hall saw a patient who had made a serious suicide attempt 2 days earlier alone in the kitchen furiously cleaning out the refrigerator. The nurse joined the patient and began helping the patient clean the refrigerator. As they talked, the patient expressed concern that many of the feelings which led to the previous suicide attempt were returning. She had initiated the cleaning project to attempt to control her feelings. The nurse defined the cleaning as a strength in that it was more adaptive than another suicide attempt. As the nurse shared this observation with the patient the patient momentarily looked surprised and then said, "I hadn't thought of it that way. Maybe I am better than I was before."

group of patients can reflect to these patients very individualized observations of strengths in areas that are uniquely relevant to these patients. These interventions may be in response to behaviors that occur spontaneously. They may also be in response to a structured growth experience that was arranged as an intervention for a nursing diagnosis which was formulated from a careful and thorough nursing assessment. The structured nursing interventions in Clinical example 34-3 occurred in a community-based psychosocial rehabilitation program.

An initial research project by Bell[12] provided some support for the premise that identification and education of the chronically mentally ill about their strengths increase their self-esteem. Another finding was that it is important for nurses to understand the meaning of observed behaviors to their patients, rather than making interpretations from the nurses' own outside perspective. For example, one woman who had been out of the hospital for 2 months, after having lived there 20 years, was seen as continually helping others. When the nurse shared this observation with the patient, the patient responded, "Helping's good, but what really counts is that when I say I'll do something to help someone else, I can count on myself to do what I say." The nurse then redesigned her nursing care plan to include more opportunities for development of the patient's autonomy and independence. As the patient's early efforts at independence and autonomy were acknowledged and supported by staff, the patient set increasingly complex goals for herself. As she achieved these goals, she expressed how good it made her feel to be able to maintain herself in an independent living situation after so many years in a state institution.

The power of nursing interventions as described depends on the nurse maintaining professional identity and setting priorities that include participation in the milieu with the patient. Within the context of a competent caring nurse-patient relationship, psychiatric–mental health nurses can make significant contributions to the care of the chronically mentally ill as they support

CLINICAL EXAMPLE 34-3

Theresa, a woman in her 50s, had been in and out of psychiatric hospitals for 30 years and had been living in a supervised apartment in the community for 1 year. One of her nursing diagnoses was difficulty in dealing with interpersonal conflict because of her fear of her aggressive impulses. Theresa shared the apartment with two roommates. She was a talented musician and had her own baby grand piano. Despite her love for classical music, she only played the "oldies and goodies" her roommates preferred. She said that she didn't want to upset her roommates by practicing classical music. She was afraid that if she brought the issue out in the open she might get so upset she would hurt someone. She offered as evidence the numerous times she'd been placed in seclusion rooms for violent behavior. Clearly, keeping peace was her priority.

The nurse and Theresa discussed her strengths as a peacemaker, as well as ways in which she might calmly express her own needs to her roommates. The nurse offered to be with Theresa during the discussion. Declining the nurse's offer, Theresa said that even though she was somewhat anxious, she had a clearer understanding of the abilities she had to use in the situation, and she wanted to try to "pick up" for herself in a situation of interpersonal conflict. She carried out her plan and expressed surprise that her roommates accepted her need and quickly arranged 2 hours a day for her to practice. As she told of her success, Theresa smiled, saying she wondered what would have happened if she had tried expressing her needs many months earlier.

Cindy, in her early 20s, had recently moved into the supervised apartment with Theresa and one other roommate. One of Cindy's nursing diagnoses was ineffective individual coping related to low self-esteem and feelings of inadequacy. Cindy arrived at the day treatment program crying because she had had a seizure while at her nursing home job the evening before. She felt that in addition to having been embarrassed, she had failed to live up to the trust invested in her by the director of the nursing home. She had decided to quit her job.

The nurse explored with Cindy the meaning of these events in terms of her many strengths in caring for others. Her sensitivity to anticipated criticism and rejection from the director was related to the same sensitivity that allowed her to respond creatively to others' needs. Cindy, at this point, firmly stated that the job was important to her sense of being needed. The nurse encouraged her to call the nursing home, express both her embarrassment and sense of failure, yet, state that she wanted to continue working there. Cindy made the phone call with the nurse present for support. Her pleasure at finding out the job was still hers, that she was not viewed unfavorably by the director of nursing, and her sense of personal achievement at having taken a risk and won was so visible and contagious that the other patients staged an impromptu celebration.

them with one hand and with the other hand invite them to expand their horizons by involvement in growth-producing experiences. As Minkoff[37] stated, "It is only when rehabilitation is not attempted, that hope is truly lost."

Clinical case analysis

Clinical example 34-4 illustrates the "career" and development of increasing disability in a chronically mentally ill man. It focuses attention on several characteristics of chronically mentally ill patients: their low self-esteem, social isolation, involvement with the legal system as a consequence of the secondary symptoms of their illness, and poor coping resources. The example also provides a glimpse of the effect of his illness on his family. Particular attention is given to the nursing care he received when he was admitted to a state psychiatric hospital following a serious suicide attempt.

CLINICAL EXAMPLE 34-4

Abdul, the only son of a large and wealthy Middle Eastern family, came to the United States to pursue a graduate degree in engineering at a prominent university. He had been an outstanding student before coming to the United States but struggled all through his graduate education. He gravitated toward other international students and most of his social activities were with this group of people. He became involved with Ingrid, a graduate student from Germany. When Ingrid became pregnant, they married. Both Abdul and his wife described the discovery of Ingrid's pregnancy as a crisis, but by the time their daughter, Begum, was born, they had reconciled themselves to their situation and, in fact, were excited by the baby's arrival.

Despite the precipitous nature of their marriage, the early years together were pleasant with Abdul and Ingrid enjoying each other and their daughter. Both parents finished their graduate education, with Abdul finding work as an electrical engineer, and his wife finding employment as an assistant professor in the history department of a 4-year college.

By the time the baby, Begum, was 5 years old, Ingrid's parents were living in the United States; there was much visiting between the two families. Since Abdul had not yet introduced Ingrid and Begum to his family, they planned a trip to the Middle East the summer Begum was 5. Abdul's father had a sudden heart attack and died before Abdul and his family arrived. The visit home did not go well. Abdul's family expressed much disappointment in him. They were disappointed that he did not meet the family's standards for material wealth and were even more disappointed that he had not married a Moslem woman. Despite the family's disappointment in Abdul, they exerted much pressure on him to change his plans to return to the United States and remain in the Middle East to assume his proper role as the only son, now the head of the family. At the same time, Ingrid, who was experiencing both culture shock and a feeling of nonacceptance by Abdul's family, insisted on an immediate return to the United States. Abdul returned to the United States feeling disappointed in himself because he had not met his family's expectations and also because he had not been able to speak out in defense of his wife and American daughter.

Life began to deteriorate for Abdul and his family after their return to the United States. Abdul resigned from his engineering position because he believed he wasn't being promoted quickly enough. Although he soon found a position with another reputable company, his work record was increasingly spotty. Some days, Abdul just couldn't make himself get up and go to work. On other days, he'd set out for work, but by midmorning would call Ingrid and tell her he was going to a movie or a museum, followed by a visit to his favorite bar and grill. Abdul found alcohol comforting and began drinking more and more. As Ingrid pressured Abdul to be more responsible about working, Abdul increasingly withdrew and spent much of the time he was home, alone, watching television in his bedroom. Partly in response to her loneliness and sense of helplessness as she watched her husband change, Ingrid overate and began a rapid weight gain, which was accompanied by other physical problems.

After 7 years of university teaching, Ingrid lost her job because she did not meet the requirements for tenure. She began job hunting, but before finding another job, she was involved in a serious car accident and was hospitalized for several weeks. Tension between Abdul and Ingrid increased as a result of the accident. Abdul believed there had been a man in the car with his wife at the time of the accident and accused her of having an affair. This belief was never substantiated, yet Abdul held on to it tenaciously. While his wife was hospitalized, Abdul cared for 7-year-old Begum. However, the day Ingrid returned home from the hospital, Abdul took their car and left, not telling anyone where he was going. After 2 weeks of wandering across the United States, Abdul returned to find he had been fired.

Abdul made no pretense of looking for another job. Welfare funds became the family's sole income. He spent most days alone in his room "tinkering" with one invention or another, listening to Middle Eastern music, or sleeping. Increasingly he slept during the day and stayed up all night. Formerly a fastidious man, he paid little attention to his personal hygiene or nutrition and continued his alcohol consumption. Although he never again left home for any extended time, he periodically disappeared for 2- or 3-day intervals. He always took the family car and was arrested several times for driving without a license or for driving while intoxicated. Invariably Abdul called his wife to rescue him. Ingrid would somehow find money to pay his fine or post bail and would bring him home, where he would once again retreat to his bedroom.

Five years after his visit to the Middle East, Abdul became involved in an altercation with a policeman who stopped him for speeding. As a result

CLINICAL EXAMPLE 34-4—cont'd

ward his daughter. A loud argument followed. Abdul threatened his neighbor, telling him that if he ever saw him talking to his daughter again, he would come after him with a gun. As a result of this incident, Abdul and his family were ostracized and ignored by most of their neighbors. With no more help in outside home maintenance, Abdul and Ingrid's home, which was located in an upper middle class neighborhood, became increasingly run down. Abdul rarely went outside the house. Ingrid left home only to take care of essential errands and transport Begum. The years of impoverishment and dealing with chronic mental illness had taken their toll. Ingrid's world was that of her family, books, and television. No longer were there family outings or visits with friends. The concern had become that of getting through each day.

As she grew, Begum assumed more and more of the care of her parents. Yet, despite her many home responsibilities, Begum did well in school and talked of wanting to be a doctor when she grew up. Begum's physical education teacher took a special interest in her and helped her develop natural gymnastics abilities to the point where she applied for and won a scholarship to a first-rate gymnastics school. Begum quickly made friends with two girls who also attended her gymnastics school and developed strategies to spend time with her friends, away from her home.

The family's life followed much the same pattern until the Christmas Begum was 14. Ingrid and Begum planned to visit Ingrid's parents for several days. Although Abdul had been invited, he refused to accompany his family on their trip. Two days after Ingrid and Begum left, Abdul again made a serious suicide attempt. He cut both wrists and watched them bleed, as he waited to die. Several times, the blood clotted and he had to reopen the wounds for the blood to continue flowing. As he became weaker and started shaking, Abdul feared his suicide attempt would not be successful. He stated that he called the ambulance because he was too weak to hang himself. Abdul was taken to a general hospital for emergency treatment and, after his physiological condition stabilized, he was taken nonvoluntarily to the state psychiatric hospital that served his geographical area.

Immediately on arriving at the state hospital, Abdul was assigned to a nurse who would be his primary nurse for the period of time he was on the admission unit. After a first-level assessment, his nurse determined his immediate needs to be care of his bilateral wrist sutures, protection from further self-destructive behaviors, and maintenance of an adequate nutritional intake. Abdul was immediately given suicide precautions, meaning he was always within arm's reach of a nursing staff member, except at night when he slept in an open seclusion room across from the nursing station. The primary nurse was able to spend the first hour of his suicidal precaution time with him. She used this time to begin a relationship with Abdul, providing an initial orientation to her role as his primary nurse and to the ward, as well as finding out his immediate concerns. Abdul matter of factly expressed annoyance that measures such as suicide precautions were being used to keep him from trying to commit suicide. He stated he was disappointed in himself in that he had not succeeded in killing himself and was determined to succeed on his next attempt.

The nurse also discovered that Abdul had spoken with his wife, who was still out of state, only once since his suicide attempt. The nurse's offer to arrange a phone conversation between Abdul and his wife was met with a positive response and a slight smile from Abdul. Before the nurse left that evening, she had discovered that Abdul, who had barely touched his lunch, preferred small meals to three large ones. In addition to leaving the nursing order that Abdul's nutritional intake he recorded, she requested that he be offered a snack at midafternoon and bedtime. The nurse also alerted the night staff to the possibility that Abdul might have difficulty sleeping because of his history of sleeping during the day and staying awake at night. If he did have difficulty sleeping, his primary nurse requested that staff stay with him and offer him hot chocolate or warm milk.

In the next few days, the primary nurse, in consultation with Abdul and the treatment team, developed a plan of nursing care for Abdul (Table 34-3).

When the nurse first began spending time with Abdul in an effort to develop a trusting relationship he was unable to tolerate being in an office with her. He would either refuse to come into the office or, after 2 or 3 minutes, would become anxious and leave. The nurse, accepting him where he was, began sitting with him for periods of 10 to 15 minutes in the day hall. Sometimes they would work on a jigsaw puzzle together; sometimes they would carry on a conversation, essentially social in nature, and sometimes Abdul would use the time to sort out his reactions to living in a state hospital. Only rarely would

CLINICAL EXAMPLE 34-4—cont'd

of this altercation, Abdul was convicted of "assault" and served a brief jail sentence.

Ingrid was able to convince Abdul to seek psychiatric help after he was released from jail. He was admitted to an inpatient unit of a general hospital. He was given trifluoperazine (Stelazine), desipramine (Pertofrane), benztropine (Cogentin), and diazepam (Valium) and encouraged to participate in the ward milieu. He was not considered ready for discharge when his funds ran out 30 days later. At the encouragement of his psychiatrist, Abdul voluntarily admitted himself to the state mental hospital for continued treatment. Things did not go well for Abdul after his state hospital admission. Worried about Abdul's increasing nonresponsiveness to his environment, Ingrid supported and encouraged Abdul's leaving against medical advice after 3 weeks in the state hospital.

Abdul returned home still receiving medication. He was to attend a medication group at the local CMHC for regulation of his medication. However, he stopped taking his medication soon after he returned home because he did not like the side effects or the feeling that he was being controlled by the medications. He again withdrew to his room, lived a nocturnal existence, and occupied himself inventing electronic gadgets.

In the following year, Abdul made his first suicide attempt. He put a loaded gun into his mouth and pulled the trigger, but the gun didn't fire. He accused "men" who were always aware of his actions of coming into his house and making the gun nonfunctional by jamming it. Abdul was again hospitalized on a psychiatric unit in a general hospital in the community. He was once again given trifluoperazine (Stelazine), desipramine (Pertofrane), and benztropine (Cogentin) and was actively encouraged to participate in the ward milieu. After a month, his seclusive behavior had decreased enough that he was considered ready for discharge. The marital problems identified earlier had intensified sufficiently that couple group therapy was considered the aftercare treatment of choice, along with continuation of drug therapy. After discharge, Abdul unwillingly accompanied Ingrid to their appointments at the CMHC. He never actively participated in the sessions.

Ingrid occasionally sensed her husband's suffering and at those times felt compassion and caring for him. Generally, however, she felt anger toward Abdul and held him responsible for their predicament. She continued to deal with her frustrations by eating and now, because of her obesity, had difficulty getting around. She limited her trips outside the house to those absolutely essential. Because of health limitations and a general sense of despair about the family's situation, Ingrid became increasingly apathetic about the daily maintenance and upkeep of their home. Whenever possible, Begum, now 11, voluntarily accepted responsibility for family chores that her parents no longer performed. She cooked simple meals, did laundry, cleaned house, and cut the yard. The family received some support from the next-door neighbor who offered to help Begum with the heavy yardwork whenever he saw her struggling. Ingrid had long ago exhausted the support available from her friends and increasingly turned to Begum for companionship and emotional support.

In the next several years, Abdul and Ingrid were not involved in ongoing treatment. Ingrid would call a therapist at the CMHC at times of crisis, generally in response to her concern that Abdul was in physiological danger from not eating. In fact, during this 3-year time period, Abdul was admitted five times to general hospitals because of his extreme withdrawal that resulted in dehydration and other symptoms of malnourishment. Each time he was admitted because of these secondary symptoms, he also spent several weeks on psychiatric inpatient units where he received treatment for his withdrawal. Abdul's improvement after drug therapy with major tranquilizers or antidepressants was only moderate. Each time that Abdul was discharged with these medications, he immediately stopped taking them. Abdul, on discharge, would once again return to life in his bedroom and begin another sequence of isolation and progressive deterioration.

One of Abdul's discharge plans included a public health nursing referral. Home visits from the public health nurse helped monitor Abdul's condition but were ineffective in terms of helping him keep his appointments at the CMHC, comply with his medication regimen, and decrease his seclusive behavior. The public health nurse was helpful in arranging for health care for Ingrid and Begum, but was not able to help Ingrid alter her self-destructive behavior of using eating as a way of dealing with her own stress and frustration. By now Ingrid weighed over 250 pounds and was having serious health problems of her own.

The summer Begum turned 12, Abdul overheard a neighbor compliment her on her appearance. Abdul misinterpreted the neighbor's remark and accused the neighbor of making sexual advances to-

Continued.

TABLE 34-3

ABDUL'S ABBREVIATED NURSING CARE PLAN

Nursing diagnosis	Intervention	Expected outcome
Inadequate nutritional and fluid intake related to feelings of worthlessness and hopelessness	Monitor input; offer juices; offer snack at 3 and 9PM	Independent maintenance of adequate nutritional intake
Inadequate personal hygiene related to isolation and feelings of worthlessness and hopelessness	Help patient shave; remind him to bathe; have clean clothes available each day	Independent maintenance of personal hygiene
Sleep pattern disturbance related to withdrawal and isolation	Involve patient in ward activities so he stays awake during day; provide at least one exercise period a day; decrease stimuli and offer bath and warm milk at bedtime	Sleeps at night; stays awake during day
Self-destructive behavior related to feelings of worthlessness and hopelessness	Observe patient closely; be alert for suicidal thoughts; offer hope that future can be different	Investment in future
Social withdrawal related to distrust of others and feelings of inadequacy	Establish therapeutic nurse-patient relationship; invite patient to participate in structured activities, such as cards, chess, walks; help him transfer learnings from nurse-patient relationship to other relationships	Development of relationships with staff and patients
Misinterprets meaning of events in his environment related to social isolation and inadequate feedback	Listen for disorders in logical thinking; matter of factly offer alternate interpretations of events; listen to meaning behind distortions and idiosyncratic interpretation of events	Decrease in idiosyncratic interpretation of events; independence in seeking feedback regarding his interpretation of events
Negative self-concept and low self-esteem related to failure in meeting own and others' expectations	Identify personal strengths with patient; offer alternate view of self based on experiences of patient in milieu; develop nurse-patient relationship to help patient explore his feelings of worthlessness and make choices about future	Self statements reflecting realistic sense of abilities and limitations; willingness to make more productive choices in future

CLINICAL EXAMPLE 34-4—cont'd

he speak of his past life or personal concerns other than his adjustment to the hospital environment.

As Abdul began to trust the nurse, he accepted her invitation to meet at regular times in her office. Although he was only able to stay for 15 to 20 minutes before getting up and saying "I have to go now," he began to talk about his life and especially about his sense of humiliation at having failed in every area important to him. Despite the nurse's identifying growth he had made in the hospital, Abdul continued to believe there was no hope for the future, and suicide was the only alternative to a life as bleak as his.

Abdul had requested that he not be given medication. Because his history documented a poor response to psychotropic medication, the psychiatrist did not order medication. However, after Abdul had been hospitalized 6 weeks, he shared with his primary nurse his belief that during one of his hospitalizations, in a procedure that left no scars, an electrode had been implanted through his nostril into his brain. He believed that his behavior was controlled by laser beams from a radio tower 20 miles away. Because his behavior was under external control, he considered himself to be a robot and thus was not responsible for his behavior. Once the psychiatrist was aware of Abdul's delusional system, intramuscular fluphenazine decanoate (Prolixin) was ordered for him. Seven days after his first injection, Abdul showed significant differences in behavior. He began to initiate conversations with other patients, voluntarily attended ward activities, began to take care of his own hygiene, and expressed an interest in being able to go out for walks. His talk of suicide decreased, and he began to doubt he was controlled by laser beams.

As part of Abdul's treatment plan, the primary nurse and a psychiatric nurse prepared at the master's degree level met with the family weekly to help the family become more functional and again enjoy being together. Interventions were directed toward inproving family communication and helping the family reorganize itself so that the parents would assume more parental authority and Begum would become more like the 14-year-old she was, rather than continuing to maintain her role as the third adult in the family.

Two critical incidents are shared as an illustration of the growth of Abdul, Ingrid, and Begum. The first incident occurred 3 months after Abdul's admission. In the family meeting, both Ingrid and Begum were speaking about the disrepair of their home. They focused on their inability, physically and financially, to maintain their home and their embarrassment that their home had become a neighborhood eyesore. Abdul told Begum he did not want her to undertake the heavy yardwork alone. He asked if he might return home to help with the yardwork and fix the plumbing. Although suicide precautions were only dropped recently and Abdul was not ready for a weekend pass, the primary nurse wanted to support Abdul's initiative in assuming family responsibility. Arrangements were made for the primary nurse and the family therapist to take Abdul home for an afternoon. A potluck supper was planned with both nurses and all three family members contributing to the effort. Abdul returned from the trip home with new-found energy and a feeling of self-worth that came from having been needed and the sense of a job well done. The primary nurse capitalized on this experience in that as she helped Abdul examine the sense of well-being, however fragile, that resulted from making a contribution, she suggested he become involved in the hospital work program. With much support, Abdul accepted her offer and began working the hospital horticulture program.

The second incident occurred indirectly as a result of the home visit. After the potluck supper, Ingrid asked the primary nurse to look at some "sores" on her legs. The nurse was concerned not only about the large skin ulcers Ingrid showed her but also about the respiratory distress Ingrid was having. The nurse consulted a social worker who served as a liaison between the hospital and community, and, through the social worker, arrangements were made for Ingrid to be seen by a physician. After her appointment, Ingrid was hospitalized with pulmonary edema and skin ulcers. An old friend, with whom Ingrid has recently reestablished contact, was able to keep Begum for several days, but there was no one for Begum to stay with over the weekend. Abdul rose to the occasion and said he did not want his daughter home alone. He then marshalled his arguments and asked for a pass to go home and care for Begum. After much consideration, the psychiatrist and the primary nurse decided to let Abdul go home to be with Begum, provided the three following conditions were met: (1) the gun in Abdul's home was to be removed and brought to the hospital for safekeeping; (2) a written contract that specified activities and structure for the time Abdul was home was to be signed by Abdul, the psychiatrist, and the nurse; and (3) Abdul was to return to the hospital

Continued.

CLINICAL EXAMPLE 34-4
cont'd

Monday morning on the bus. Abdul agreed to these conditions. He returned to the hospital grinning because the weekend had gone better than he had expected. He was especially proud that he had cooked dinner Saturday night and given Begum the best piece of meat.

Abdul's continued improvement was not without setbacks. However, after he had been hospitalized on the admission unit 5 months, he was transferred to an unlocked continued-care ward where rehabilitation would continue until he was ready for discharge. Abdul and his primary nurse met with the social worker who would be coordinating his treatment plan on the new ward to facilitate the transition. While Abdul was in the continued-care area, he worked with vocational rehabilitation and was judged capable of a sheltered workshop placement when he returned to the community. With an eye toward discharge and a desire to increase compliance with an eventual aftercare program, Abdul began making weekly visits home to attend family therapy sessions at the CMHC. On these visits home, he shared with Ingrid his fear that his life was destined to be one of limited functioning and recurrent hospitalizations.

On one of his last weekends before discharge, he had a longer than usual pass because he had a Monday afternoon appointment with the vocational rehabilitation center in the community. Tuesday morning, Ingrid called Abdul's primary nurse on the admissions unit. Abdul was dead. He had hanged himself the night before.

The primary nurse had her own personal grief to confront. Despite her caring and the best efforts of many professionals, the final choice was Abdul's. After struggling for many years, he chose the pain of death over the pain of life. The primary nurse was left with the hope that for a time, however brief, Abdul's life was less painful, that he had a momentary glimmer that life could be different, and that he had experienced the respect and positive regard she had for him. Out of her own grief, respect for Abdul, and continuing concern for his family, Abdul's primary nurse went to his funeral—and cried.

■ SUGGESTED CROSS-REFERENCES ■

The phases of the nursing process are discussed in Chapter 5. Tertiary prevention and rehabilitative psychiatric nursing are discussed in Chapter 11. Problems with self-esteem are discussed in Chapter 14. Legal issues, including commitment proceedings and patient rights, are discussed in Chapter 7. Crisis intervention is discussed in Chapter 10.

DIRECTIONS FOR FUTURE RESEARCH

The following are some of the nursing research problems raised in Chapter 34 that merit further study by psychiatric nurses:

1. Validation of the stages of the natural history of chronic illness from the patient's perception (Table 34-1)
2. Validation of the stages of the natural history of chronic illness from the family's perception (Table 34-1)
3. Psychiatric patients' understanding of their rights to refuse treatment
4. Psychiatric patients' understanding of the risk/benefit ratio of their treatments as a result of having participated in the informed consent process
5. Development of psychoeducation programs to increase chronically mentally ill patients' understanding of and participation in self-care related to health promotion
6. Comparison of the quality of life experienced by chronically mentally ill patients residing in institutions and in communities
7. Common nursing problems of the younger chronically mentally ill patient during episodic hospitalizations
8. The effectiveness of specific nursing interventions in increasing patients' perceptions of their strengths
9. Evaluation of the integration of principles of psychiatric rehabilitation into the inpatient milieu
10. Evaluation of the effectiveness of the nurse in the role of case manager
11. Comparison of the patient's and nurse's perception of the patient's strengths
12. Comparison of primary and other modalities of nursing care in decreasing hospital stay of the chronically mentally ill patient
13. Nurses' attitudes toward caring for the chronically mentally ill
14. Strategies used by family members in coping with the chronically mentally ill member living at home

SUMMARY

1. Chronically mentally ill individuals no longer reside primarily in large public psychiatric hospitals. It is estimated that as a result of "deinstitutionalization," the process of moving long-term mental patients into the community to be supported by formal and informal resources, 50% of the chronically mentally ill are now living in local communities.

2. As health policy directed that long-term psychiatric patients have alternatives to life in a public mental hospital, court decisions reflected increasing attention to protection of the rights of this population. Of particular importance to the chronically mentally ill are issues surrounding civil commitment, the right to treatment and protection from harm in the least restrictive environment, the right to refuse treatment, confidentiality, and employment.

3. Chronically mentally ill individuals have both primary and secondary symptoms of their illness. Primary symptoms are those associated with the intrinsic nature of their illness. Secondary symptoms develop over time as a consequence of the illness and perpetuate the illness's existence. Chronic mental illness, with its associated secondary symptoms is not a state or end point, but a process of progressive deterioration.

4. Elaboration of the special characteristics of the chronically mentally ill portrays a population with difficulties in activities of daily living, and maintaining interpersonal relations, a lack of coping resources, and a need for long-term treatment. Other characteristics influencing the course of their illness are their consistently low self-esteem and their preoccupation with avoiding failure rather than achieving success. As a group, the chronically mentally ill can also be characterized by their unique strengths and potentials.

5. The "young" chronically ill patient, 18 to 35 years old, differs from chronically mentally ill patients over 35 years old. Because of deinstitutionalization and the development of community-based treatment facilities, younger patients have not had to adapt to long-term residence in public psychiatric hospitals. They alternate between inpatient and community-based facilities and maintain age-appropriate role expectations for themselves. Not meeting these expectations, they are continually confronted with their sense of failure. They are likely to enter the mental health system nonvoluntarily, are unlikely to follow through with aftercare plans, have a high suicide rate, and are more likely to abuse drugs and/or alcohol. They are likely to be better educated and have more independent living skills than the older patient. Present treatment resources are inadequate in meeting the needs of this group of patients.

6. Psychosocial rehabilitation programs that incorporate elements of the medical model, rehabilitation model, and social support model have demonstrated their effectiveness in meeting the needs of chronically mentally ill patients. Fountain House, a psychosocial rehabilitation program in New York City, has been used as a prototype for the development of other psychosocial rehabilitation programs. These programs offer their residents choices in living and work situations, but most important offer a sense of being needed and a place to belong. Basic to the rehabilitation process is focusing on the strengths of new members.

7. The role and function of the nurse in caring for chronically mentally ill patients is influenced by the setting in which the care is given.
   a. Nurses working in community-based psychosocial rehabilitation programs have the opportunity for long-term ongoing relationships with patients and the mutual setting of long-term goals. In these programs nurses may also be asked to function as "case manager," a role that cuts across professional boundaries.
   b. Nurses working in acute care settings often care for chronically mentally ill patients when they are in crisis. Nurses must be able to quickly establish relationships with acutely ill patients and be skilled in applying the principles of crisis intervention. Primary nursing, as a modality of nursing care, offers several advantages when caring for chronically mentally ill patients in acute care settings.

8. In all settings, nurses are responsible for improving their patients' health status by developing the patients' health potentials. Nursing interventions that developing the strengths and potentials of chronically mentally ill patients help them become more competent in meeting the demands of everyday life. Ultimately, the expected outcome of each interventions is a change in the patient's self-concept and an increase in his or her self-esteem. Nursing interventions in which patients are helped to become aware of their strengths fall into two categories.
   a. Those which occur as a response to the patient's spontaneous participation in the milieu
   b. Those which occur as part of a structured intervention in which experiences are planned to mobilize patients' strengths or develop their potentials

REFERENCES

1. Anderson, S., and Bauwens, E.: Chronic health problems: concepts and application, St. Louis, 1981, The C.V. Mosby Co.
2. Anthony, W., Cohen, M., and Cohen, B.: Psychiatric rehabilitation. In Talbott, J., editor: The chronic mental patient: five years later, New York, 1984, Grune & Stratton, Inc.
3. Applebaum, P.: Legal issues. In Talbott, J., editor: The chronic mental patient: five years later, New York, 1984, Grune & Stratton, Inc.
4. Applebaum, P.: Special section on APA's model commitment law: an introduction, Hosp. Community Psychiatry **36**(9):966, 1985.
5. Bachrach, L.L.: Deinstitutionalization: an analytical review and sociological perspective, U.S. Department of Health, Education, and Welfare Pub. No. (ADM) 76-351, Washington, D.C., 1976, U.S. Goverment Printing Office.
6. Bachrach, L.L.: A note on some recent studies of released mental hospital patients in the community, Am. J. Psychiatry **133**:73, 1976.

7. Bachrach, L.L.: Deinstitutionalization: what do the numbers mean, Hosp. Community Psychiatry **37**(2):118, 1986.

8. Baldwin, D.: *O'Connor v. Donaldson:* involuntary civil commitment and the right to treatment, Columbia Human Rights Law Rev. 7:573, 1975-1976.

9. Barter, J.: Psychoeducation. In Talbott, J., editor: The chronic mental patient: five years later, New York: 1984, Grune & Stratton, Inc.

10. Bassuk, E.L., and Gerson, S.: Deinstitutionalization and mental health services, Sci. Am. **238**:46, Feb. 1978.

11. Bell, M., and Ryan, E.: Integrating psychosocial rehabilitation into the hospital psychiatric service, Hosp. Community Psychiatry **35**(10):1017, 1984.

12. Bell, R.: The effect of interpersonal strengths identification and education on the self-esteem of psychiatric day treatment programs, doctoral dissertation, Washington, D.C., 1981, Catholic University of America.

13. Bender, M.: Young adult chronic patients: visibility and style of interaction in treatment, Hosp. Community Psychiatry **37**(3):265, 1986.

14. Brown, B.: Responsible care of former mental patients. In New dimensions in mental health: report from the director, Washington, D.C., 1977, National Institute of Mental Health.

15. Caton, D.: The new chronic patient and the system of community, Hosp. Community Psychiatry **32**:475, 1981.

16. Chodoff, P.: The case for involuntary hospitalization of the mentally ill, Am. J. Psychiatry **133**:496, 1976.

17. Coopersmith, S.: The antecedents of self-esteem, San Francisco (1967) 1981, Consulting Psychologists Press.

18. Crossen, M.: Contemporary models in psychiatric care and rehabilitation: Fountain House, Hoffman-LaRoche Laboratories.

19. Cutler, D., et al.: Disseminating the principles of a community support program, Hosp. Community Psychiatry **35**(1):51, 1984.

20. Falloon, H., et al.: Family management in the prevention of exacerbations of schizophrenia, N. Engl. J. Med. **306**(24):1437, 1982.

21. Fitts, W.: Tennessee self-concept manual, Nashville, Tenn., 1965, Counselor Recording and Tests.

22. Fitts, W.: The self-concept and psychopathology, Nashville, Tenn., 1972, Counselor Recording and Tests.

23. Fitts, W., et al.: The self-concept and self-actualization, Monograph No. III, Nashville, Tenn., 1971, Counselor Recording and Tests.

24. Friedman, P., and Yohalem, J.: The rights of the chronic mental patient. In Talbott, J., editor: The chronic mental patient: problems, solutions, and recommendations for a public policy, Washington, D.C., 1978, The American Psychiatric Association.

25. Goldman, H.H.: Mental illness and family burden: a public health perspective, Hosp. Community Psychiatry **33**(7):557, 1982.

26. Goldman, H.: Epidemiology. In Talbott, J., editor: The chronic mental patient: five years later, New York, 1984, Grune & Stratton, Inc.

27. Goldman, H., Gattozzi, A., and Taube, C.: Defining and counting the chronically mentally ill, Hosp. Community Psychiatry **32**:21, Jan. 1981.

28. Gruenberg, E.: The social breakdown syndrome: some origins, Am. J. Psychiatry **123**:1481, 1967.

29. Heinrichs, D.: Recent developments in the psychosocial treatment of chronic psychotic illnesses. In Talbott, J., editor: the chronic mental patient: five years later, New York, 1984, Grune & Stratton, Inc.

30. Intagliata, J., and Baker, F.: A comparative analysis of the young adult chronic patient in New York State's community support system, Hosp. Community Psychiatry **35**(1):45, 1984.

31. Krauss, J.: The chronic psychiatric patient in the community: a model of care, Nurs. Outlook **28**:308, 1980.

32. Krauss, J., and Slavinsky, A.: The chronically ill psychiatric patient and the community, Boston, 1982, Blackwell Scientific Pub.

33. Lamb, H., and Goertzel, V.: The long term patient in the era of community treatment, Arch. Gen. Psychiatry **34**:679, 1977.

34. Leavitt, M.: The discharge crisis: the experience of families of psychiatric patients, Nurs. Research **24**:33, 1975.

35. Lemert, E.: Secondary deviance and role conceptions. In Farrell, R., and Swigert, V., editors: Social deviance, New York, 1975, J.B. Lippincott Co.

36. McCarrick, A., Manderscheid, R., and Bertolucci, D.: Correlates of acting-out behaviors among young adult chronic patients, Hosp. Community Psychiatry **36**(8):848, 1985.

37. Minkoff, K.: A map of the chronic mental patient. In Talbott, J., editor: The chronic mental patient: problems, solutions, and recommendations for a public policy, Washington, D.C., 1978, The American Psychiatric Association.

38. Otto, H.: The human potentialities of nurses and patients, Nurs. Outlook **8**:32, 1965.

39. Otto, H.: Guide to developing your potential, New York, 1967, Charles Scribner's Sons.

40. Pepper, B., Kirshner, M., and Ryglewicz, H.: The young adult chronic patient: overview of a population, Hosp. Community Psychiatry **32**:463, 1981.

41. Pepper, B., and Ryglewicz, H.: The young adult chronic patient: a new focus. In Talbott, J., editor: The chronic mental patient: five years later, New York, 1984, Grune & Stratton, Inc.

42. Peterson, R.: What are the needs of chronic mental patients? In Talbott, J., editor: The chronic mental patient: problems, solutions, and recommendations for a public policy, Washington, D.C., 1978, The American Psychiatric Association.

43. Porter, E., and Maloney, S.: Strength deployment inventory: manual of administration and interpretation, Pacific Palisades, Calif., 1967, Personal Strengths Assessment Service, Inc.

44. Rogers, C.: Client centered therapy: its current practice, implications, and theory, Boston, 1965, Houghton Mifflin Co.

45. Rose, L.: Understanding mental illness: the experience of families of psychiatric patients, J. Adv. Nurs., 8:507, 1983.

46. Ross, G.: Attribution retraining of the psychiatrically disabled, doctoral dissertation, Philadelphia, 1978, University of Pennsylvania.

47. Schwartz, S., and Goldfinger, S.: The new chronic patient: clinical characteristics of an emerging subgroup, Hosp. Community Psychiatry 32:470, 1981.

48. Segal, S., Baumohl, J., and Johnson, E.: Falling through the cracks: mental disorder and social margin in a young vagrant population, Soc. Probl. 24:387, 1977.

49. Turner, J., and TenHoor, W.: The NIMH community support program: pilot approach to needed social reform, Schizophr. Bull. 4:319, 1978.

■ ANNOTATED SUGGESTED READINGS ■

Andreasen, N.: The broken brain, New York, 1984, Harper and Row.

In this book written for the lay person, the reader is treated as an intelligent person who is capable of understanding accurate information about the biological revolution in psychiatry and its meaning for patients and their families. It is written with sufficient depth that it also serves as a comprehensive reference for health care personnel.

Bassuk, E.L., and Gerson, S.: Chronic crisis patients: a discrete clinical group, Am. J. Psychiatry 137:1513, 1980.

This study of psychiatric patients who made repeated visits to an emergency room in a general hospital focuses on their nonproductive interaction with the caregivers from whom they seek help. The authors suggest interventions based on an understanding of their help-seeking–help-rejecting behavior.

*Craig, A., and Hyatt, B.: Chronicity in mental illness: a theory on the role of change, Perspect. Psychiatr. Care 16:139, May-June 1978.

General systems theory is used to explain the perpetuation of symptoms in the chronically mentally ill. Chronic mental illness is defined as a family systems problem rather than an individual problem, and interventions are related to the authors' theoretical position.

Crossen, M.: Contemporary models in psychiatric care and rehabilitation: Fountain House, Hoffman-LaRoche Laboratories.

The author provides an overview of the Fountain House program. Her report is based on interviews with Fountain House staff and members.

Donaldson, K.: Insanity inside out, New York, 1976, Crown Publishers, Inc.

This autobiography portrays Kenneth Donaldson's 15-year struggle to be released from a Florida state mental hospital. Donaldson describes his experiences as a patient and tells the story behind the landmark court decision (O'Connor v. Donaldson, 1975).

Falloon, H., et al.: Family management in the prevention of exacerbations of schizophrenia, N. Engl. J. Med. 306(24):1437, 1982.

This often cited research examines the effectiveness of family psychoeducation in reducing family stress and preventing rehospitalization of schizophrenic patients living at home. The family treatment approach was found more effective than individual supportive care in preventing relapse.

Friedman, P., and Yohalem, J.: The rights of the chronic mental patient. In Talbott, J., editor: The chronic mental patient: problems, solutions, and recommendations for a public policy, Washington, D.C., 1978, The American Psychiatric Association.

Five clusters of rights that greatly affect the quality of life for the chronically mentally ill are described. As court rulings are presented, the authors derive implications for this patient population.

Goldman, H., Gattozzi, A., and Taube, C.: Defining and counting the chronically mentally ill, Hosp. Community Psychiatry 32:21, Jan. 1981.

These authors present the results of a national study with the purpose of identifying the chronically mentally ill, both descriptively and numerically. The findings provided a foundation to the development of the National Plan for the Chronically Mentally Ill.

*Kane, C.: The outpatient comes home: the family's response to deinstitutionalization, J. Psychosoc. Nurs. Ment. Health Serv. 22(11):19, 1984.

An overview of the development of deinstitutionalization as federal policy is followed by a discussion of the effect of this policy on families. Highlighted is the development of the National Alliance for the Mentally Ill, a self-help group which is expected to have increasing political clout.

*Krauss, J.: The chronic psychiatric patient in the community: a model of care, Nurs. Outlook 28:308, 1980.

The author, based on her experience of caring for chronically mentally ill patients in the community, describes the needs of this patient population and discusses nursing interventions useful in meeting these needs.

Krauss, J., and Slavinsky, A.: The chronically ill psychiatric patient in the community, Boston, 1982, Blackwell Scientific Publications.

These authors have provided a comprehensive text on the chronically mentally ill which provides an in-depth analysis of the many issues surrounding this population. While this text is of value to all disciplines involved in the care of the chronically mentally ill, the material on nursing care is most sensitive and thorough.

*Lenehan, G., et al.: A nurse clinic for the homeless, Am. J. Nurs. 85:1237, 1985.

In 1972 a group of Boston nurses began a nursing clinic in a large shelter for homeless men. This article traces the development of that clinic from early beginnings with volunteer staff to its current status with two clinics and paid staff. This clinic is a model for health care for the homeless.

---

*Asterisk indicates nursing reference.

Minkoff, K.: A map of the chronic mental patient. In Talbott, J., editor: The chronic mental patient: problems, solutions, and recommendations for a public policy, Washington, D.C., 1978, The American Psychiatric Association.

The author provides a demographic overview of chronically mentally ill patients. The facts and figures presented supply information as to the scope and magnitude of the problems of this patient population.

Pepper, B., Kirshner, M., and Ryglewicz, H.: The young adult chronic patient: overview of a population, Hosp. Community Psychiatry 32:463, 1981.

Based on a study of nearly 300 patients, 18 to 35 years old, the authors provide a beginning description of the characteristics of this emerging subgroup of the chronically mentally ill.

Peterson, R.: What are the needs of chronic mental patients? In Talbott, J., editor: The chronic mental patient: problems, solutions, and recommendations for a public policy, Washington, D.C., 1978, The American Psychiatric Association.

Ronald Peterson, a veteran of 10 years in a state mental hospital, wrote this paper when he was a staff member of Fountain House, a psychosocial rehabilitation program. He provides an "insider's view" of the experience of leaving a state hospital and adjusting to community life. The importance of programs like Fountain House in meeting the needs of the chronically mentally ill is highlighted.

*Rose, L.: Understanding mental illness: the experience of families of psychiatric patients, J. Adv. Nurs. 8:507, 1983.

This article reports the results of a qualitative study describing families' experiences when a mentally ill relative is hospitalized for the first time. The process by which the family interpreted and assigned meaning to this experience is described. The process described parallels the stages of the natural history of chronic illness as described in this chapter. Nursing implications are derived.

Rubin, J.: The national plan for the chronically mentally ill: a review of financing proposals, Hosp. Community Psychiatry 32:704, 1981.

The author summarizes and analyzes fiscal recommendations in the National Plan for the Chronically Mentally Ill.

Schwartz, S., and Goldfinger, S.: The new chronic patient: clinical characteristics of an emerging subgroup, Hosp. Community Psychiatry 32:470, 1981.

The authors describe their impressions, based on 2 years' clinical work in a general hospital, of the characteristics of younger chronically mentally ill patients. They analyze the interaction of this patient group with present treatment resources and make recommendations for future development of treatment resources.

Sheehan, S.: Is there no place on earth for me? Boston, 1982, Houghton Mifflin Co.

This journalistic account of the life history of a chronically schizophrenic woman reveals the nature of the mental health care system, including changes initiated by the community mental health movement. The frustration of the patient and her family as they try to find help is clearly communicated to the reader. This book would be particularly worthwhile to the nurse who has had limited contact with chronically mentally ill patients.

Talbott, J.: The national plan for the chronically mentally ill: a programmatic analysis, Hosp. Community Psychiatry 32:699, 1981.

The author summarizes and analyzes the program recommendations in the National Plan for the Chronically Mentally Ill.

Torrey, E.F.: Surviving schizophrenia: a family manual, New York, 1983, Harper and Row.

This book was written for families with the hope that information about schizophrenia, its etiology and treatment, the process and characteristics of psychiatric hospitalization, aftercare, and legal and ethical dilemmas would counteract myths and facilitate family coping. This is a good resource of the beginning psychiatric nurse as well as the family.

Toward a national plan for the chronically mentally ill, U.S. Department of Health and Human Services Pub. No. (ADM)81-1077, Washington, D.C., 1980.

This federal report, originally requested by President Carter's Commission on Mental Health, describes the needs of the chronically mentally ill, analyzes problems in the implementation of deinstitutionalization, and makes recommendations to improve services to this group of patients. Attention is given to fiscal considerations in meeting the needs of the chronically mentally ill.

*Ulin, P.: Measuring adjustment in chronically ill clients in community mental health care, Nurs. Res. 30:229, July-Aug. 1981.

This study examines the usefulness of the Psychological Mental Health Index (PMHI) in assessing the psychological well-being of chronically ill psychotic patients being cared for in the community.

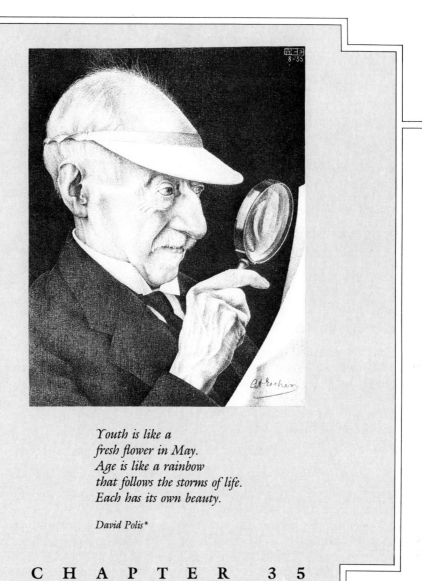

*Youth is like a
fresh flower in May.
Age is like a rainbow
that follows the storms of life.
Each has its own beauty.*

David Polis*

C H A P T E R   3 5

GERONTOLOGICAL PSYCHIATRIC NURSING

Beverly A. Baldwin

LEARNING OBJECTIVES

After studying this chapter, the student should be able to:

- describe psychiatric disorders associated with aging relative to the demographic characteristics of the population.

- identify the role and functions of the gerontological psychiatric nurse.

- critique the major biological, psychosocial, and personality theories of aging.

- assess the nursing care needs of the gerontological psychiatric patient.

- assess the nursing care needs of the family of the gerontological psychiatric patient.

- discuss the advantages and disadvantages of a variety of assessment tools that may be used by the nurse as one component of data collection.

- formulate nursing diagnosis consistent with observed patient behaviors and identified predisposing factors and precipitating stressors.

- analyze the interrelationship between physiological and psychological stressors as they affect the behavior of the aging patient.

- compare and contrast several intervention strategies that may be implemented with gerontological psychiatric patients.

- describe areas of intervention using patient and family education.

- identify directions for future nursing research.

- select appropriate readings for further study.

The fastest growing minority in the United States is the over-65 age-group, which now comprises almost 12% of the population. One in every nine Americans is 65 years of age or older; in the next half century, one in six or perhaps one in five Americans will be over 65 years old. By 2030, it is estimated that there will be 60 million persons over age 65—17% to 20% of the total United States population.[1]

Stereotypes and myths surrounding this age-group often portray a homogeneous profile of the elderly. To the contrary, the older adult represents the culmination of multiple interpersonal, developmental, and situational experiences. The complex and interactive nature of the needs and problems of old age is frequently underestimated and often understated. Mental health in later years depends on a number of factors, including one's physiological and psychological status, personality, social support system, economic resources, and prevailing life-style. It has been estimated that of the persons over 65, approximately 4 million have suffered moderate to severe psychiatric impairment secondary to either cerebral arteriosclerosis, senile dementia, functional psychosis, alcoholism, or other disease conditions. The elderly account for approximately 25% of the reported suicides, the highest rate occurring in white males in their 80s.[3] The extent of mental disorders in old age appears to be considerable; therefore nurses and other health care professionals will realize an increasing responsibility in the prevention and care of the older adult with mental and emotional health problems. Assisting the older adult to maximize his potential can be a challenging and rewarding experience for the nurse. This chapter will address selected aspects of the psychiatric–mental health needs of the geriatric patient and his or her family.

The problem of defining aging and the geriatric patient is complicated. Individual variations exist in how different people age, both psychologically and physiologically; therefore, it is recognized that the chronological demarcation of age 65 is an arbitrary one. To provide a base for understanding the aging phenomenon and the impact of individual variations, an overview of selected theories of aging is presented. A format for applying the theories of aging is the examination of components of the mental health evaluation of older adults. Although it is acknowledged that the assessment of mental health status is but one aspect of assessment of the total person, for purposes of this chapter, emphasis will be placed on the mental and emotional evaluation. By integrating current research findings with the role of the nurse in the care of the geriatric patient, the purpose, criteria, and uses of standardized instruments for evaluating mental status are compared with functional and other behaviorally focused measures.

Data obtained from the mental status evaluation, along with a profile of the patient's general status, offer the nurse an opportunity to develop a working nursing diagnosis and to plan intervention strategies. Memory loss, confusion, or disorientation may represent behavioral responses of the older adult to stress, whether originating from internal or external processes. Knowledge and skill are required of the nurse in determining the extent to which the stress is a negative or positive force in the observed behavioral responses of the patient. Comprehensive evaluation is the first step in making that determination.

The next step in the process of care is selection of intervention strategies to meet the needs of the patient. An overview of the current techniques being used in prevention and care of the mentally impaired (or potentially impaired) will focus on clinical research findings that indicate the effectiveness or ineffectiveness of selected interventions. The past two decades have witnessed a new interest in the treatment of the institutionalized geriatric patient by health professionals. Once the predictable victim of widespread neglect, the geriatric patient is now viewed in a more favorable light. The discussion of these intervention strategies will focus on the role of the nurse in implementing and assessing the impact on the patient, whether in an individual or group setting.

Evolution of the role of the gerontological psychiatric nurse

Prior to World War II, the sick elderly were found in general hospitals, their homes, and clinics, but the nurse attending them never thought of herself as a geriatric nurse. The passage of the Social Security Act of 1935 had profound effects on the status of the aged citizen in this country. Public assistance funds became available to the needy aged. It hastened the development of profit-making homes, since recipients receiving monthly stipends could not live in a public institution. Many retired and widowed nurses converted their homes into boarding houses which became, in practice, the first of our present-day nursing homes.[14] Care in the boarding houses for the aged deteriorated as the clients became ill and their needs grew in number and complexity. After World War II, each state established minimum standards for nursing home care, and licensing of homes was introduced. Many of the boarding house nurse-landladies became the administrators of the new federally subsidized nursing homes. With the increase in the number and needs of the patients, it became necessary to employ additional nursing personnel to provide the care.[15] The nurse administrator assumed the role of supervisor or manager of nonprofessional personnel, in addition to the duties of running the home.

■ Creation of a professional organization

The early practitioner in geriatric nursing experienced professional isolation from other nurses and felt a lack of prestige from physicians, nurses, and the general public. In fact, these nurses were completely outside the focus of concern in nursing's striving for professionalization. Continuing education for nurses was not available to geriatric nurses, and nursing literature on the care of the aged was nonexistent. As more nurses entered geriatric nursing, they sought to overcome their alienation by appealing to the American Nurses' Association.[7] In 1961, a committee within the association recommended the formation of a group whose main interest would be geriatric nursing. A year later, a conference called by this group became the forerunner of the Division on Geriatric Nursing Practice of the American Nurses' Association.

To meet criteria for constituting a separate nursing practice division, this group was charged with "providing evidence that a substantial number of nurses are practicing in a field with a well-defined and unique body of nursing knowledge and/or evidence that a significant health problem exists in which nursing is involved."[14] Certainly, there was sufficient evidence that the care of the aged was a major health problem involving nurses. In January 1967, 1 month after the first meeting of the Executive Committee of the Geriatric Nursing Division, over 2,000 nurses registered to become members of the division. The number of nurses identifying with care of the aged has continued to increase since the inception of the division. The division is charged with assessing the nursing needs of older people, planning and implementing nursing care to meet those needs, and evaluating the effectiveness of such care to achieve and maintain a level of health consistent with the limitation imposed by the aging process.[14] It was the first of the practice divisions to establish and publish standards of practice and to certify superior practitioners. The enthusiasm and momentum of this group merit attention from all areas of nursing. Although it is the newest of the practice divisions and probably the smallest, significant progress in upgrading nursing care in this area of practice has been made. The division voted, in 1974, to change the name to Gerontological Nursing Practice, to more accurately reflect the focus of this group. The term *geriatric* refers to the study of diseases of old age and *gerontology* refers to the study of the phenomenon of aging.[9] Since a primary function of the nurse is to assist the individual to reach and maintain optimum function throughout the process of aging, the term gerontological was considered to more appropriately reflect this function.

■ Future prospects

The prospects for the future of gerontological/geriatric nursing are encouraging for nurses seeking greater autonomy and control over their practice, in addition to increasing responsibility for decision making in the care of the aged. Several factors account for the potential for change within this field of nursing. Esther Lucille Brown,[6] in a study of nursing practice in hospitals, extended care facilities, and nursing and retirement homes, notes that except for a few specialists in geriatrics and chronic diseases, the medical profession is largely uninvolved in the problems of aging and care of the older patient who cannot be cured. The functional requirements of physicians in institutions devoted to chronic disease and rehabilitation are minimal. Most of the needs of the elderly in these settings, and in community and home care settings, are a result of chronic disability with multiple etiology. It is in these settings that the nursing domain may develop and expand.

■ **FUTURE ROLES.** Internally, the field of gerontological/geriatric nursing is changing rapidly. Stone[48] predicts this specialty promises virtually unlimited progress for the nurse in the future. Furthermore, she suggests five major roles for nurses specializing in care of the aged: (1) patient-care managers in nursing homes; (2) health assessors with a focus on the physical, mental, and functional assessment rather than medical assessment; (3) primary care providers in both institutional and community agencies; (4) independent practitioners in private or group practices with other nurses or other health professionals; and (5) researchers, involved in both nursing and interdisciplinary clinical studies.

■ **EDUCATIONAL PREPARATION.** As the role of the gerontological/geriatric nurse continues to expand and grow, the educational preparation for this specialist must expand. Presently, there are 32 graduate programs in nursing offering a concentration or specialty in this area. Preparation at the graduate level includes the clinical specialization, administration, education, and nurse practitioner roles. Also included is preparation of the beginning nurse researcher, the first step toward preparation at the doctoral level. Increasingly, faculty are including more content on gerontological/geriatric nursing in undergraduate curricula. Recognition of the need to prepare nurses to care for the aged continues to grow as the number of elderly persons grows. It is estimated that even in acute care settings, the number of patients over the age of 65 may range from 20% to 60%.[4]

■ Council of Nursing Home Nurses

In the spring of 1979, the Council of Nursing Home Nurses was established within the American Nurses' Association. Some of the areas of involvement for the new council include enhancing the visibility and influence of the nursing home nurse, influencing the quality and delivery of nursing care in the nursing home at the local, state, and national levels, and promoting effective utilization of gerontological nursing concepts to the consumer and health care community.[2]

Theories of aging

Approaches to defining aging and explaining the causes and consequences of the aging process constitute the basis for the numerous theories of aging. Theories are proposed based on two major conceptual approaches to aging: (1) the causes of the biological and psychological process of aging or (2) the psychosocial results of aging. It is clear that there is little consensus among gerontologists regarding the etiology and adaptation to aging, and it is unlikely that consensus will be sought. No one theory can take into account all the variables that influence aging and the individual's response to it, which include cultural and ethnic factors, genetic makeup and heritage, physiological conditions at conception and birth, growth and maturation, the environment, the family system, and relationships to significant others. Theories of aging are difficult to differentiate from changes over time that are considered to be secondary to the aging process. Distinctions between stress, disease processes, and specific age-related changes in relation to individual variation and uniqueness are tentative and will probably remain so for a long time to come. Selected theories will be discussed from the perspective of increasing understanding of the interaction of biopsychosocial manifestations of later life. The major theories are summarized in Table 35-1. Explanations for aging may further enhance knowledge of the physiological and mental changes experienced by the geriatric patient with whom the nurse will work.

■ Psychobiological theories

■ **DELIBERATE BIOLOGICAL PROGRAMMING.** Deliberate biological programming is one theory of aging that has received considerable attention over the last two decades. This theory holds that the memory and capacity for terminating the life of a cell is stored within the cell itself. Through laboratory studies, Hayflick and co-workers[26] demonstrated that normal human fibroblasts, when cultured, underwent a finite number of population doublings and then died. The number of doublings is not different in male and female cells. The theory of a human biological clock represents an entropic approach to the explanation of aging. The decline of biological, cognitive, and psychomotor function is viewed as inevitable and irreversible, even though mod-

TABLE 35-1

THEORIES OF AGING

Psychobiological theories		Psychosocial theories		Personality theories	
Biological program-ming	Cell stores memory and capacity for terminating life. Represents entropic explanation of aging.	Disengagement	Elderly people and society mutually withdraw from active exchange with each other. See older adults as homogeneous group.	Ego integrity	Eight stages of humans with specific phases and tasks present at each age. Ego integrity is the last stage and provides a point for reflection on one's life and accomplishments. Assumes normal progression from stage to stage.
Wear-and-tear	Changes occur due to abuse and/or care. Represents decremental model of aging, irreversible decline.	Activity	Aging is but one phase in the developmental process. Recognizes the heterogeneity of all age-groups	Stability of personality	Personality is established by early adulthood and remains fairly stable thereafter.
Stress-adaptation	Stress has both positive and negative consequences for the organism. Represents adaptive-coping model of aging.	Life review	Reminiscence is viewed as a normal life review process. Recognizes need for reintegration of life experiences as preparation for the final stage of life.		

ification of diet and prolonged hypothermia may slow up the terminal process. The notion of programmed aging, while answering some of the questions regarding longevity, does not address questions regarding the intrinsic and external influences on individual variations in aging.

■ **THE WEAR-AND-TEAR THEORY.** The wear-and-tear theory suggests that structural and functional changes occur which may be accelerated by abuse and decelerated by care.[39] From a physiological standpoint, aging is viewed ontogenetically, beginning with conception and leading to decline and death. The pathological consequences of aging are the result of an accumulation of stress, trauma, injuries, infections, nutritional inadequacies, metabolic and immunological disturbances, and prolonged abuse. Although less popular than some of the current theories, it illustrates the decremental model of aging, leading to irreversible decline. This concept of aging is often popularized by

widely accepted myths and stereotypes regarding the aged, as noted in phrases like, "He is doing well for his age" or "What can you expect at that age?" Newer research on the value of exercise and cognitive stimulation in later years refutes the basic premise of this theory in that the body and mind might benefit from use and stimulation.

■ **THE STRESS-ADAPTATION THEORY.** The stress-adaptation theory suggests the positive and negative aspects of stress on the physiological and psychological development of the individual. Eisdorfer[19] points out that stress is not always a negative experience, as is usually implied in many of the writings on the subject. Stress may stimulate a person to try new and more effective ways of adapting. Although it is presumed by some that stress actually accelerates the aging process, there is little evidence to substantiate that conclusion. Stress may deplete the reserve capacity of individuals, either physiologically or psychologically, thereby placing them in a vulnerable position for illness or disability to occur. Some of the assumptions regarding stress and adaptation are important for the understanding of the nature of emotional and mental problems in the aged. Although the link between stress and the development of mental illness is unclear, the effect and perception of stress by an individual plays a major role in his ability to cope and remain flexible in adverse situations.

■ Psychosocial theories

■ **DISENGAGEMENT THEORY.** This controversial theory evolved from studies conducted by the University of Chicago Committee on Human Development.[13] It postulated that older adults and society mutually withdrew from active exchange with each other as part of the normal process of aging. The withdrawal was assumed to be characterized by psychological well-being and adjustment on the part of the elder. This theory did not take into account heterogeneity of the elders and the personality variables important to coping with change. Stereotypes reinforced by this theory include the notion that older people enjoy the company of people their own age exclusively and that retirement facilities should promote homogeneous age cohorts and prohibit intergenerational living arrangements. Although many elders may desire this type of arrangement, others find themselves isolated and out of the mainstream of society.

■ **ACTIVITY THEORY.** Disputes over the reliability of the disengagement theory led to the development of the current and prevailing view that activity produces the most positive psychological climate for older adults. The activity theory[34] developed as a reaction to the negativistic perspective of disengagement. Many gerontologists champion the notion that aging is but one phase in the developmental process; others contend that old age is only an extension of the middle years and can be modified or abolished by increased activity levels. The activity theory maintains that the aged should remain active as long as possible. When work and comminuiy activities and affiliations must be curtailed or given up, substitutes should be found. The positive influence of activity on the older person's personality, mental health, and satisfaction with life are heralded, expressing the value of an active versus a passive role in relationships and in society.

■ **THE LIFE REVIEW.** The life review was postulated in 1961 by Robert Butler.[8] Reminiscence in the aged is viewed as part of a normal life review process brought about by the realization of approaching dissolution and death. Characteristic of the life review is the progressive return to consciousness of past experiences and the resurgence of unresolved conflicts that are examined and reintegrated. Successful reintegration can give meaning to one's life and prepare one for death by alleviating anxiety and fear. This process is believed to occur universally and represents a functional preparation for the final stage of life. Although seen in all age groups to a certain degree, the emphasis and focused concentration are evidenced more in the later stage of life. The aged appear to have a vivid memory for past events and can recall early life experiences with clarity and imagination. The person appears to be reviewing and sorting previous life events to better understand his present circumstances.

The life review process may result in either positive or negative consequences. Anxiety, guilt, fear, and depression may surface if the person finds himself unable to deal with, resolve, or accept unchanged old problems. On the other hand, the righting of earlier wrongs can aid in the establishment of a sense of serenity, pride in working through old conflicts, and acceptance of mortal life. Reflective activity becomes a positive approach to aging. In addition to offering an explanation for the consequences of aging, reminiscence and the life review have potential for psychotherapeutic intervention. Further discussion of this process will be found in the section on strategies for intervening in the mental health problems of the older adult.

■ Personality theories

■ **ERIKSON'S STAGE OF EGO INTEGRITY.** Erikson's eight stages of man[20] delineate specific developmental tasks present at each age, based on Freudian dynamics. The last stage of life that provides a point for reflection on one's life and accomplishments is one of ego integrity. Erikson maps out a predetermined structural order to development and maturation, progression by critical or crisis periods, and dependence on chronological timing and sequence. The rationale for the progression from one stage to the next is unclear; one must assume that there are biological or psychosocial forces that initiate and propel the movement. The concept of ego integrity leaves unanswered many questions regarding the consequences of fixation at one stage of development and the individual variation in the complex process of development and maturation.

■ **STABILITY OF PERSONALITY.** Costa and McCrae[18] as cited by Ehrman, contend that personality is established by early adulthood and remains fairly stable thereafter. Stability of personality has been observed in longitudinal studies of aging individuals at the National Institutes of Health Gerontology Research Center in Baltimore (the intramural research center for the National Institute on Aging). Usually no decline or change in personality, compared with other cognitive changes, is evident. If radical changes in personality do occur in older persons, it may be indicative of brain disease. Costa and McCrae found that periods of psychological crisis in adulthood do not occur at regular intervals, contradicting some theories, such as Erikson's, regarding the constancy and stability of stages of adult development. Persons with a long history of emotional instability are therefore more likely to encounter more crises. Costa and McCrae refute the conclusion that, according to their theory, individuals remain firmly locked into rigid behavior patterns. They note, to the contrary, that changes in roles, attitudes, and situational demands create the need for new behavioral responses and the majority of elderly persons in their studies appear to adapt effectively to those demands.

Assessment

The assessment process offers an opportunity for the nurse to collect data essential to the development of a nursing diagnosis. The interview and health history constitute a first step in the process. The use of selected standardized assessment tools augments the data obtained through interviewing the patient or family.

■ The interview

Establishing a supportive and trusting relationship is essential to a positive interview with the geriatric patient. Since the first encounter between the nurse and patient may be uncomfortable for the patient, the nurse must make every effort to put the patient at ease and offer reassurance and positive feedback. It may take repeated contacts and frequent explanations to allay fears and reduce anxiety. The geriatric patient may feel uneasy, vulnerable, and confused in new surroundings or in the presence of strangers. Patience and attentive listening promote a sense of security for the patient. The more comfortable the patient, the better able he will be to respond to the purpose and direction of the interview. Respect should be acknowledged by addressing the patient by his last name. The nurse opens the interview by introducing herself and describing in a short concise manner the purpose and length of the interview. The patient will respond best when he feels the nurse is interested and concerned about his welfare. The patient should not be rushed or pressed for answers. Direct questions may have to be rephrased or asked in a more indirect less intimidating manner.

■ **THERAPEUTIC COMMUNICATION SKILLS.** Specifying the time allotted and the topic to be discussed at the beginning of the interview orients the patient to the purpose and scope of the interaction. Reinforcing the amount of time remaining in the interview may facilitate redirection of wandering discussion and give the patient the security of knowing the nurse is in control of the situation. Older persons may be slow in responding to questions, since their reaction time to verbal stimuli is lengthened with age. It is important to give the patient sufficient time to formulate a response. Assuming the patient does not know the answer to a question, does not remember, or does not understand because he does not respond immediately can lead the interviewer to false conclusions regarding the patient's status and mental capabilities.

The manner in which the patient is questioned is important to the outcome. Older persons often have their own vocabulary, and may not be familiar with new words, slang, or contemporary colloquialisms. Avoid medical abbreviations, terminology, or jargon. Ask short concise questions, particularly if the patient indicates that he has difficulty with abstract thinking and conceptualization. Techniques such as clarification and summarization are important in validating information. Rephrase a question if the patient fails to answer appropriately or hesitates when answering.

Concentrated verbal interaction may be uncomfortable for the older person. The nurse can demonstrate interest and support by giving nonverbal cues and responses, such as direct eye contact, sitting close to the patient, and using touch appropriately. Touching the shoulder, arm, or hand of the patient in a firm purposeful manner conveys support and interest. Avoid stroking or patting the patient, since alterations in tactile perception and cultural orientation may result in misinterpretation.

The ability of the nurse to elicit useful relevant data in the assessment interview will depend, to a great degree, on her comfort and, ease in the intereview situation. The nurse's negative stereotypes and bias regarding the aged will surface in the interview setting. Older people are sensitive to others' disinterest and impatience.

Although older persons differ in their willingness to reveal life histories and personal experiences, most geriatric patients greatly desire relationships with others and are anxious to share information with interested persons. Elderly patients have much to tell and may offer more information than the nurse needs at a particular time. Reminiscence is common and should be reinforced and encouraged when possible. The patient is concerned with life review or integration of past events with current situations. The life review process may serve as an excellent source of data relevant to the patient's current health problems and support resources. Reminiscence and life review may present problems in keeping the patient focused on the topic at hand; however, it provides an opportunity to assess subtle changes in the patient, such as long-term memory, decision-making ability, judgment-making patterns, affect, and orientation to time, place, and person.

Many geriatric patients are aware of changes in their physical or psychological functioning; however, they may be hesitant to have some of their fears confirmed. Consequently, they may minimize symptoms or ignore them entirely, assuming they are age related and not relevant to current problems. Denial of changes in one's ability to function, remember, concentrate, or attend to personal needs is a common reaction among some older persons. Many geriatric patients consider alterations in functional ability, cognitive function, or emotional stage concomitant with aging and unimportant to maintenance of health and well-being. Often these misconceptions are reinforced by myths about aging and the false assumption by many health professionals that many of the presenting problems of the older person are irreversible or untreatable.

Contrary to popular myths, most older people do not dwell unrealistically on their health and usually have a physical problem when describing their health as poor. However, some older persons are preoccupied with their bodies and will dwell on the physical decline occurring with progressing age. It is essential that the nurse observe and listen carefully to clues that indicate the extent to which the patient's perception indicates individual personality factors developed over a lifetime of experience or represents a current distress.

The geriatric patient may misunderstand the purpose of the nurse's questions and fail to see the relevance to current health status of questions regarding habits, previous life experience, or social supports. Careful and repeated explanations are necessary if the patient is to cooperate with the nurse. The nurse should never assume the patient understands the purpose or protocol for the assessment interview. It is wiser to overstate than to increase the patient's anxiety and stress by omitting information. The nurse should take cues from the response of the patient by listening carefully and observing constantly.

■ **THE INTERVIEW SETTING.** The unfamiliar or new surroundings of the hospital setting or outpatient clinic may impede the progress of the initial interview by distracting the patient and increasing his fear of the unknown. The physical environment should be altered as much as possible to promote comfort. Many older persons are unable to sit for long periods of time because of arthritis or other joint disabilities. Chairs should be comfortable, and the patient should be encouraged to move about as desired. Changing positions and range-of-motion exercises stimulate circulation and prevent stiffness caused by limited mobility.

Most older persons experience some form of sensory deficit, particularly diminished high-frequency hearing or changes in vision as a result of cataracts or glaucoma. The environment should be modified as needed to decrease the impact of those deficits. The setting for the interview should be quiet and away from peripheral noises. The patient, already under a great deal of stress, may be easily distracted and annoyed by extraneous stimulation. The nurse should address the patient in a slow, low-pitched voice. Shouting raises the pitch of the noise and makes hearing more difficult. Because fatigue may contribute to diminished mental functioning in the elderly, the morning is the best time for the interview. Patients not only experience fatigue as the day progresses, but may experience a phenomenon known as **sundown syndrome**[10] in which cognitive ability diminishes in the late afternoon or early evening. Some patients become disoriented, confused, or apathetic.

The reliability of the data obtained from the assessment interview should be carefully evaluated. If the nurse questions some aspects of the patient's responses, family or others knowledgeable of the patient should be consulted. Consideration should be given to the physical condition of the patient at the time of the interview and other variables that may influence his status, such as medications, nutritional state, or level of anxiety.

■ **Functional assessment**

Functional assessment of the gerontological psychiatric patient is not limited to parameters of mental health. Rather, the ability to function emotionally and cognitively depends, to a great degree, on the older person's overall functional capability. Although not considered in this chapter, a comprehensive assessment is considered necessary for an accurate diagnosis. The present discussion emphasizes the aspect of the functional assessment that has the greatest potential for determining present mental and/or emotional status.

■ **MOBILITY.** The loss of mobility and independence are real fears among the elderly. The degree to which the gerontological psychiatric patient can move about unassisted should be determined early in the assessment process. Restriction of joints may limit ambulation. A plan for range-of-motion exercises or other activity may be needed to assure that the activity level of the patient remains functional. Patients in wheelchairs and/or walkers need assistance in moving from the bed or chair to standing or walking positions. Orthostatic hypotension is a possibility when patients move rapidly from a lying to a standing position. Secure footwear should be provided for the ambulating patient because gait may be unsteady and perception of spatial limits altered because of visual impairments.

In addition to changes in functional ability because of changes in physical and/or psychological status, many of the medications routinely taken by geriatric patients may alter perception and make ambulation and mobility difficult. Of particular significance are the sedatives/hypnotics, tranquilizers, and cardiovascular and hypertensive drugs.[21] Patients should be cautioned about side effects of the medications and encouraged to take plenty of time when ambulating and moving from one position to another. Many falls in the elderly occur because the patient did not have enough time to adjust to changes in the physical environment (e.g., lighting, texture, or grading of the floor or sidewalk).

■ **NUTRITION.** Many geriatric patients remain self-sufficient and do not require assistance with eating or in identifying nutritional needs. However, some of the psychosocial problems encountered in the gerontological psychiatric patient that precipitate the need for assistance in eating and monitoring of nutritional intake include

1. Patients who are depressed or lonely, with a consequent decrease in appetite
2. Patients experiencing changes in cognitive function, such as confusion or disorientation
3. Patients who are suicidal
4. Patients removed from their familiar ethnic/cultural patterns of eating
5. Patients fearful of hospital routines or procedures

The range of physical problems varies greatly from individual to individual, but some of the areas to be assessed include

1. The degree of mobility and strength to open cartons of milk, cut meat, handle utensils
2. The presence of neurological deficits or joint conditions that interfere with hand and/or arm coordination
3. The presence of visual problems
4. Edentulousness and other losses of chewing ability
5. Problems in swallowing or shortness of breath
6. The presence of ulcerations in the mouth or on the tongue
7. Periodontal disease
8. Dry mouth because of side effects of medications

Careful evaluation of the needs of the patient in eating should be made routinely, since nutritional needs of the elderly present one of the most significant problems in institutionalization and can precipitate other problems, such as skin breakdown, inadequate absorption of medications, and diminished wound healing.

■ **ACTIVITIES OF DAILY LIVING.** The assessment of self-care needs and activities of daily living (ADLs) is essential for establishing baseline data on the patient's potential for independence. Activity may be limited because of dysfunctional physical status or psychosocial impairment. ADLs include preparing meals, shopping, eating, bathing, toileting, dressing and other grooming procedures, mobility (e.g., walking, standing, bending, climbing stairs, moving objects from place to place, using a pen or pencil, or other fine motor skills), and housekeeping chores (e.g., making a bed and washing dishes or clothes). Although geriatric patients should be encouraged to move toward greater independence in self-care, it is unrealistic to expect that all patients can function totally independently. The very process of hospitalization and conformity to the routine and procedures of the hospital environment fosters dependence on the part of the patient. Encouraging patients to become involved in their own care is important, since the more interdependent the patient is, the more his self-esteem will be enhanced. Realistic goals should be established and reevaluated periodically.

■ **SOCIAL SUPPORT SYSTEMS.** Positive support systems constitute one of the more critical factors in maintaining a sense of well-being throughout life. Nowhere is this more important than with the gerontological psychiatric patient. Two fifths of all elderly persons are not spending their final years with a spouse.[27] Therefore, as the number of significant contacts diminishes, it is important that the remaining support systems are consistent and meaningful. The ethnic background of the patient may be an important factor in the determination of support systems and identification of significant others. Strong family and ethnic ties promote feelings of security. The elderly who live in isolation and are also without family ties generally encounter more serious problems in later life. These problems are not limited to financial instability, but may impact on the patient's desire to get well, be happy and content with his life, and maintain self-care activities whenever possible. Assessment of the support systems, to sustain the patient while in the hospital and on return home or to another institution, should be made on admission. Family/or friends can assist in reducing the shock and stress of hospitalization and offer reassurance and comfort to the distressed elder. Studies have shown that relocation of the elderly is often a traumatic event. High mortality has been recorded for patients moved from one facility to another or from their familiar home environment to a nursing home or other long-term care facility.[10] The stress of relocation should be identified and anticipated for all geriatric patients and intervention should be planned to reduce the impact. Allowing the patient to have his own belongings, liberal visiting hours for family or friends, and careful explanations regarding the purpose and procedures of the hospital are but a few of the ways in which the stress of hospitalization can be minimized. Establishing an effective support system within the hospital environment may prevent the negative behavioral responses often observed in isolated elders: apathy, depression, aggression, or hostility.

■ Mental status

Systematic and comprehensive assessment of cognitive function and psychiatric symptoms provides data for drawing diagnostic conclusions and planning intervention strategies. The appropriate use of standardized assessment instruments is an adjunct to the nursing history and interview.

■ **THE MENTAL STATUS QUESTIONNAIRE.** The Mental Status Questionnaire (MSQ)[30] has been extensively used in geriatric research and practice. The questionnaire contains ten questions of orientation regarding place, date, day of the week and month, age, and birthdate. The last two items cover current events and more distant events by questioning the patient's knowledge of the current and past presidents of the United States. Critics of this instrument suggest that the questions regarding the presidents are irrelevant and inappropriate for some elderly, particularly those in institutional settings and those isolated from the news of everyday happenings. The number of errors made by the patient in responding to the questions indicates the severity of the brain syndrome, which ranges from none or minimal to severe impairment. The MSQ was not designed to be used alone or as the only indicator of impairment. The instrument provides a gross measure of mental status and change in cognitive function. High reliability has been recorded with other measures of cognitive impairment.

■ **THE SHORT PORTABLE MENTAL STATUS QUESTIONNAIRE.** The Short Portable Mental Status Questionnaire (SPMSQ)[16] is also a ten-item questionnaire that tests orientation, remote and recent memory, practical skills (recalling a telephone number or street address), and mathematical ability (serial subtraction from 20 by 3s). Developed as part of the Older Americans Resources and Services (OARS) program at the Duke University Center for the Study of Aging and Human Development, the SPMSQ has high test-retest reliability. The instrument has been administered on both institutionalized and community-based elders. Scores range from 0 to 10 with four levels of disability (intact, mild, moderate, severe impairment) defined.

Score adjustments are made for race and for education.

■ **THE FACE-HAND TEST.** The Face-Hand Test[22] is a test of organicity which has been widely used in gerontological research and practice for the last 20 years. The instrument was developed to distinguish patients with brain damage from those who are psychotic without an organic cause. The test requires that the individual recognize tactile stimulation on the cheek and back of the hand. A rehearsal is allowed so that the individual can become familiar with the procedure. The last four of ten paired stimuli count for the score. The individual sits facing the examiner, with the hands resting on the knees and the feet flat on the floor. The individual is touched simultaneously on one cheek and the dorsum of one hand in a specified order. The test is administered twice, once with the individual's eyes closed, then repeated with the individual's eyes open. Some degree of concentration and attention to the procedure must be tolerated by the patient. Anxiety and distraction from peripheral activities may prevent the patient from following the instructions. The accompanying box describes the order of stimulation used in the Face-Hand Test.

■ **THE MINI-MENTAL STATE EXAMINATION.** The Mini-Mental State Examination[23] is a portable test of orientation (year, season, date, day, month, state, country, hospital, floor), registration (individually and collectively naming three objects), attention and calculation (counting backward by 7s from 100 or spelling "world" backward), recall (repeating three objects

---

Order of Stimulation Used in Face-Hand Test

1. Right cheek—left hand
2. Left cheek—right hand
3. Right cheek—right hand
4. Left cheek—left hand
5. Right cheek—left cheek
6. Right hand—left hand
7. Right cheek—left hand
8. Left cheek—right hand
9. Right cheek—right hand
10. Left cheek—left hand

Modified from Bender, M.B., Fink, M., and Green, M.: *Archives of Neurology and Psychiatry* **66**:355–362, 1951.

named earlier), and language (naming objects, repeating phrases, obeying three-step commands, writing a sentence, and copying a design). This test is presented in the accompanying box. Measurement of cognitive function is the primary focus of the examination, and it is thorough in that area. Requiring only 5 to 10 minutes to administer, it is not tiring to the patient. Difficulty in writing or reading may necessitate adjustments by the nurse administering the tool (e.g., use large bold print when writing out sentences or instructions). Extensive use of this test has been made in distinguishing between patients with diagnoses of dementia, psychosis, and affective disorders (e.g., depression).

■ **THE ZUNG SELF-RATING DEPRESSION SCALE.** The Zung Self-Rating Depression Scale[56] has the advantage of being a self-report test and the dis-

---

Mini-Mental State Examination

	Maximum score	Score
Orientation		
What is the (year) (season) (date) (day) (month)?	5	(_____)
Where are we (state) (county) (town) (hospital) (floor)?	5	(_____)
Registration		
Name 3 objects: 1 second to say each. Then ask the patient all 3 after you have said them. Give 1 point for each correct answer. Then repeat them until he learns all 3. Count trials and record. _____ Trials	3	(_____)
Attention and calculation		
Serial 7s. 1 point for each correct. Stop after 5 answers. Alternatively spell "world" backwards.	5	(_____)
Recall		
Ask for the 3 objects repeated above. Give 1 point for each correct.	3	(_____)
Language		
Name a pencil, and a watch. (2 points) Repeat the following "No ifs, ands, or buts." (1 point) Follow a 3-stage comment: "Take a paper in your right hand, fold it in half, and put it on the floor." (3 points) Read and obey the following: Close your eyes. (1 point) Write a sentence. (1 point) Copy design. (1 point)	9	(_____)
	TOTAL SCORE	_____

Assess level of consciousness along a continuum

Alert	Drowsy	Stupor	Coma

From Folstein, M.F., Folstein, S.E., and McHugh, P.R.: J. Psychiatr. Res. **12**:189–198, 1975. Copyright 1975, Pergamon Press, Ltd.

advantage of provoking wide interpretation and sensitivity on the part of the patient. The 20-item instrument consists of 10 negatively stated items (e.g., "I feel downhearted and blue") and 10 positively stated items (e.g., "My mind is as clear as it used to be"). The Likert-type scale ranges from "a little of the time" to "most of the time" and requires the individual to distinguish a choice on each item. Visual or language problems result in the test having to be administered orally. Although criticized by some researchers and clinicians as a potentially threatening test because of the sensitivity of the items, the scale takes minimal time to complete and provides an opportunity for the individual to participate in the assessment process by self-report.

■ **THE SANDOZ CLINICAL ASSESSMENT—GERIATRIC.** The Sandoz Clinical Assessment—Geriatric (SCAG)[45] specifies a rating of the patient on 18 dimensions and an overall impression score. Developed as part of psychopharmaceutical research, the SCAG necessitates interpretation and rating of the patient's presenting behavior and response to stimuli. Based on observations of the patient's behavior, the scale covers a broader area of assessment of mental status than the SPMSQ or the MSQ. Advanced clinical skill and experience are necessary for effective use of this instrument. As a supplement to other measurements of mental status, it provides data about mood, motivation, social ability, fatigue, and anxiety.

■ **THE NURSES' OBSERVATION SCALE FOR INPATIENT EVALUATION.** The Nurses' Observation Scale for Inpatient Evaluation (NOSIE)[28] was developed for use with a chronic institutionalized schizophrenic population and is based on nursing observation of patient behavior over a 3-day interval. Observable responses of the patient, such as "talks freely with visitors," "hoards things," and "has temper outbursts," are objectively scored using Likert-type choices ("never" to "always"). Factors of social competence, social interest, cooperation, and psychotic depression represent some of the dimensions on the scale. Although only recently used to any extent with a nonpsychiatric geriatric population, the instrument has potential for providing systematic objective ratings of patient behavior. Interrater reliability is high, based on selected studies, compared to the SCAG and other more subjective rating scales.

■ **Activities of daily living**

Measures of physical functioning in the elderly vary in scope and emphasis. The use of measures of ADL, along with measures of cognitive function and psychiatric symptoms, enables the nurse to develop a comprehensive data base on the patient. One or more of these instruments may constitute one component of the initial assessment interview in addition to being used throughout the intervention-evaluation phases of the nurse-patient relationship.

■ **THE KATZ INDEX OF ACTIVITIES OF DAILY LIVING.** The Katz index[31] consists of dichotomous rating of six ADL functions: bathing, dressing, toileting, transfer, continence, and feeding. One point is assigned for each item of dependency observed. The dichotomous dependent-independent categories for each function are defined in observable terms ("gets clothes from closets and drawers"). This widely known and used instrument has the advantage of measuring change in ADL functions over time and as a result of rehabilitation.

■ **PACE II.** PACE II[50] focuses on evaluation of physical health of nursing home patients. Checklists are used to identify the presence of defined conditions (diagnosed), abnormal laboratory or other findings, risk factors, and other impairments and disabilities. Under each medically defined condition, the duration, type, or location of the problem is specified. Thoroughness of observations is necessary in this patient–care-planning tool, in addition to review and inclusion of the medical history and examination. PACE II has the advantage of providing for interdisciplinary assessment and planning for care.

■ **Family-patient interaction**

The manner in which family members relate to and support (or fail to support) each other has a profound influence on individuals within the family structure and the group as a whole.[5] Nowhere is this influence more evident than when an older adult becomes the central focus of conflict or dysfunction for the family unit. Behavioral problems in the elderly may result from the family's lack of ability to deal with the losses and increasing dependence of an older member.

The importance of the inclusion of family members or significant others in the patient's life in the overall assessment process cannot be underestimated. In addition to verifying information supplied by the patient during the initial assessment process, the family's perceptions of their relationship with the patient add yet another dimension to the understanding of the response of the patient to his own aging and disability.

The format for assessment of patient-family dynamics varies, depending on the setting (e.g., community clinic, home, or institution) and the behavior and needs of the patient. Two instruments for consideration in collection of data relevant to this area of assessment are described here.

■ **THE FAMILY APGAR.** The family APGAR[47] is designed to assist clinicians in systematically assessing an impression of family function from the perception of individual family members. Categories for rating include adaptation, partnership, growth, affection, and resolve. Sample questions for the categories include the following: "I am satisfied with the help that I receive from my family when something is troubling me" (adaptation), "I find that my family accepts my wishes to take on new activities and make changes in my life-style" (growth), and "I am satisfied with the way my family and I share time together" (resolve). Each family member indicates his degree of satisfaction or dissatisfaction with each item on a Likert-type 0 to 2 scale ("almost always, hardly ever"), or the clinician can verbally administer each question and score the response. A score of 3 or less (out of 10) indicates high dysfunction for the individual; a score of 4 to 6 would indicate moderate dysfunction. Discrepancies or low scores obtained by individual family members are indicators of problem areas and require further exploration and assessment. This usable practical tool was not developed specifically for assessing families dealing with an older member. As an indication of the patient's and his family's perceptions of each other, this instrument has potential for understanding the dynamics of the family's structure and function.

■ **THE SOCIAL BEHAVIOR ASSESSMENT SCHEDULE.** The Social Behavior Assessment Schedule[40] utilizes the patient's significant relative or friend to elicit information regarding the patient's social functioning ability. The instrument consists of a semistructured interview schedule focusing on the patient's behavior and psychosocial status. Adverse or dysfunctional effects on family function are explored. Patient behavior, such as withdrawal, forgetfulness, and indecisiveness are included in the inventory. Rating of the behavior consists of evaluation of the response as moderate to severe, frequency of occurrence, and time of onset. Twelve areas of social performance, such as household tasks, household management, and decision making, make up the social functioning rating. The onset of diminished performance and dysfunction observed are rated in a fashion similar to the rating of patient behavior. Additional categories in the instrument query adverse effects of others on the patient's behavior, concurrent events (e.g., physical illness, medications), and support to the informant from neighbors, friends, and other family members. Nurses working with families in the home or community setting may find this instrument an important measure of baseline function of the patient as perceived by those involved in his care.

To date, nursing's use of standardized instruments in the data collection phase of the nursing process has been minimal. The selection of a tool depends on the setting, patient population, and purpose of the nursing assessment. The degree to which these tools are used alone or in conjunction with other forms of assessment (e.g., physical assessment and evaluation) varies with the presenting problems of the patient. Although skills required in the use of the instruments described here are easily learned, practice and verification with others providing care for the patient are necessary to develop confidence in the findings yielded by these measurement tools.

 # Nursing diagnosis

The nursing diagnosis is the culmination of the process of data collection and analysis regarding the patient's functional ability and resources. Behavioral interpretation of the patient's presenting needs and problems facilitates the nurse's role as intervenor in dysfunctional or disruptive processes. Both objective and subjective data are required to determine the extent of the patient's functional ability. Selective use of the data depends on the resources available to the patient and the nurse in collaboratively working toward resolution of the problem or problems.

The medical diagnosis is based on identification of the disease contributing to the patient's dysfunctional behavior. The medical diagnosis is complementary to the nursing diagnosis, since psychopathological conditions prevent the patient from functioning at his maximum potential. The relationship between the disease process and the behavioral response of the patient is not always clear because some of the same behaviors may be a result of different pathological processes.[42] For example, mood swings and alterations in mood may be present in patients who are depressed and patients who are experiencing disruptions in cognitive function because of organic changes, as seen in Alzheimer's disease and related diseases.

Although the older adult may experience a wide range of psychiatric problems, consideration is given to those problems of greatest significance to the nurse and patient in the development of a healing therapeutic relationship.

■ Alteration in thought processes

■ **MEMORY LOSS.** One of the most distressing and often frustrating aspects of aging is the potential for progressive memory loss. Although memory loss may be the result of organic brain disease or depression, the onset does not necessarily imply an inherent disease process. With age, loss of short-term memory, recall for recent events, is more likely to occur than loss of remote memory, recall for events that occurred in the distant past. The conceptual network of past thoughts, images, ideas, and experiences that make up memory and remembering develops and matures over one's lifetime. Primary memory comprises the conscious control system for memory and appears stable over the life span. It is believed that few differences exist between ages in relation to primary memory. The speed of access appears to slow with increasing age.[46] Long-term memory (secondary memory) is the storage system for what is commonly understood as memory. Failure in retrieval, original acquisition, or learning may account for some of the loss experienced in secondary memory.[46]

Many factors contribute to alterations in memory in older adults. Stress or confrontation with crisis, depression, and a sense of worthlessness, loss of interest in present events, cerebrovascular changes that affect cerebral function, loss of neural cells because of disease or trauma, and sensory deprivation or isolation from verbal interactions are all situations or events one experiences with advancing age.[37] Sensory loss, including changes in vision and hearing, makes the older person vulnerable to the environment and to those around him, often resulting in avoidance of the situation at hand and withdrawal into a less threatening world. Comfort may be sought in old memories and experiences, replacing the need and desire to remain in touch with the present.

Institutionalized elders appear to have more difficulty in memory than older adults living at home or in other community settings. The institutional geriatric patient is portrayed as dull, listless, and uncommunicative. The environment often promotes this response and reinforces the "compliant," "cooperative" patient. A stimulating environment and therapeutic regimen can counteract and, in many situations, reverse withdrawal behavior in the gerontological psychiatric patient and revive interest in recall and participation in the present.

■ **WITHDRAWAL.** Withdrawal "is an adaptive or coping mechanism . . . involving physically pulling away from or psychologically losing interest in an anxiety-producing situation, person or stressful environment."[37] Multiple losses or fear of loss may precipitate withdrawal. Prolonged grief and hesitation about returning to an active life after the loss of a spouse, sibling, or child predisposes the elder to dysfunctional and nonresponsive behavior. The introverted adult may find adjusting to change and flexibility in response to new situations more difficult with advancing age, therefore it is important to understand the personality of the patient and his previous adaptive styles.

Sudden withdrawal and refusal to invest in relationships with others should alert the nurse to the possibility of physiological factors as potential causes; low-grade infection, pain, and toxicity or side effects of medications are but a few of the many precipitating events that could initiate changes in behavior. Careful assessment and evaluation are necessary.

The geriatric patient experiencing organic intellectual impairment (e.g., Alzheimer's disease and related disorders) frequently withdraws from social contacts, daily routines, and ADLs. He may deny the possibility of a problem, or because of difficulties with memory, fear the consequences of these changes. Withdrawal can become a defense mechanism, reinforcing the denial of perceived disability and further loss of functional ability.

■ **CONFUSION.** Confusion is a phenomenon only recently studied systematically by nurses. The term is used by nurses "to describe a constellation of client behaviors, including inattention and memory deficits, inappropriate verbalizations, disruptive behavior, noncompliance, and failure to perform activities of daily living."[55] Frequently, confusion is a nonspecific label imposed by staff on apathetic, withdrawn, or uncooperative patients. Wolanin and Phillips[54] suggest several categories of patients as particularly vulnerable to being perceived and labeled as confused: the problem patient, the patient with communication problems (slurred speech, expressive dysphasia), the patient who challenges personal values of the staff, the physically unattractive patient, the depressed patient, and the "troublemaker" (e.g., does not improve despite nursing interventions and ministrations).[53]

Institutionalized elders are at particular risk for confusion. From 30% to 80% of these patients suffer from organic brain disease to some degree with concomitant disorientation regarding time, place, and person, gross remote and recent memory loss, and inability to execute simple calculations. In many nursing homes and other long-term care facilities, over 30% of the patients experience severe confusion.[24] The precipitating factors in confusion vary and depend on both the physiological and psychological status of the patient.

Early morning confusion, appearing as a type of **sunrise syndrome,** may be due to the hangover effects of sedatives-hypnotics or other nighttime medications that interact with drugs for sleep. Sleep disruptions and insomnia are particularly bothersome to the elderly. Adverse reactions to drugs prescribed for sleep are not uncommon and should be considered. Increasing disorientation or confusion at night, resulting from loss of visual accommodation, is known as **sundown syndrome.** Anticipation of the potential threats to the patient's safety during these times should alert the nurse to take special precautions to prevent falls and other mobility hazards.

The nurse should never assume that confusion and disorientation are natural consequences of changes in cognitive or physiological status. On the contrary, confusion is reversible in over half of the patients experiencing it. It is usually transient or of short duration and is one area in which the nurse has primary responsibility. The carefully planned, therapeutic nurse-patient relationship can be a significant factor in preventing and intervening in this distressing condition.

Although disorientation is often used interchangeably with confusion, care should be taken to differentiate between them. A disoriented patient is not necessarily confused, and a confused patient does not necessarily experience disorientation in all spheres. The mental status tests discussed earlier in the chapter differentiate disorientation in place, person, and time from components of confusion, such as alterations in memory, judgment, decision making, and problem solving.

■ **PARANOIA.** Paranoia and fear are reactions by some older persons to loss, isolation, and loneliness. Classic psychopathological paranoia, demonstrated by a well-organized and elaborate system of superiority, is rare in older persons. Delusions and disturbances in mood, behavior, and thinking may be a transient condition experienced by the geriatric patient in reaction to sensory deprivation or sensory loss, imposed or voluntary isolation from social contacts, or as an adverse reaction to psychotropic or other drugs.[33]

Paranoid symptoms appear as diffuse or specific. The geriatric patient may perceive threat from certain persons (e.g., family, friends, neighbors) or at stressful times (e.g., night). Relocation to a new home, new room in the hospital or nursing home, or strange environment devoid of familiar belongings precipitates fears, anxiety, and for some, paranoid ideation.

The personality of the aging paranoid patient is characterized by withdrawal, aloofness, fearfulness, over-sensitivity, and often secretiveness. As long as the patient does not call attention to himself or pose a threat to himself or others, he may go undetected for a long time. Once he is recognized as a potential threat to himself or others, institutionalization becomes a consideration. Older persons suffering from transient or chronic paranoia are at high risk for victimization by others, self-neglect, and abuse (e.g., refusal to eat, take prescribed medications, or attend to hygiene needs). Anticipation and assessment of the influence of paranoia on the patient's welfare constitutes an important aspect of the care of the patient.

■ Changes in affect

Disturbances in mood, mood swings, or oversensitive emotional reactions represent behaviors of older adults that are common to all age groups at one time or another. The reaction of an older person to physical limitations or disabilities, psychological loss (particularly a spouse or other significant other), or the possibility of institutionalization depends on previous coping styles, support systems, especially family, and present psychological and physiological strength.

Radical or abrupt alterations in mood indicate reaction to internal or external stress or inadequate coping mechanisms required to deal with progressive loss or dependency. When this behavior is evident in otherwise content, happy, and adjusted elderly people, physiological factors, including side effects of cardiovascular or psychotropic drugs, should be considered. Reassurance and support during evaluation are essential to reducing the anxiety and diminishing the threat perceived by the patient.

■ **DYSFUNCTIONAL GRIEVING.** Depression and sadness are viewed by some as a natural phenomenon of aging, and depression is essentially a disorder of later life. Comfort[12] suggests scores on the Zung Self-Rating Depression Scale may reflect mild depression in many older people because of the bias of the instrument. The questionnaire emphasizes social usefulness and activity, which may be limited in some older adults. Although not limited to social impositions, depression, grief, and loss are common in later life.

Prolonged grief and mourning over a real or imagined loss should be recognized as depression and responded to as such. Symptoms common to the depressed geriatric patient include, but are not limited to: weight loss; anorexia; undue fatigue; apathy; loss of interest in friends, family, and usual activities; and psychomotor retardation. None of the symptoms are precipitated by increasing age and should be considered problematical.[51]

The older person's attitude toward his own aging and toward death and dying may greatly influence the degree to which the depression can be successfully treated. The "loss of hope" expressed by some older persons, particularly in the face of increasing disabilities, may precipitate or stem from a depressive reaction.

Undiagnosed depression may have serious consequences for the elderly, since the problem is always manifested in physical behavior. Many of the medications routinely prescribed for the older person may potentiate or enhance a depression. Examples include tranquilizers (major and minor), barbiturates, cardiotonics (digoxin), and steroids. A medication history is part of the evaluation and assessment.

When considering mood changes, grief, and depression in the geriatric patient, it is important to recognize and understand the significance of the patient's and family's attitude toward death and dying. The old differ from the young in facing death in several ways: older persons tend to integrate attitudes of death with their formal religious training, tend to have more experience with death (e.g., peers, spouse), tend to be more accepting of death, and tend to approach problems primarily from an internal focus of activity. The state of the older person's health, in addition to the cues from observing peers or spouse who have died or are dying, signal that his life may be coming to an end. Awareness of the older person's "stage of dying" is important to understanding his needs and concerns.

■ **SUICIDE IN THE ELDERLY.** Intentional deaths among the elderly are not uncommon. Of all suicides committed in this country annually 25% are persons over the age of 65 years. White males over the age of 85 are at particular risk. Other high-risk persons include the isolated elderly, experiencing loss of family or friends through death; elderly with changes in body function and decreased independence because of pain, weakness, immobility, and shortness of breath; elderly with changes in body structure because of surgery or stroke; or those with the prospect of a terminal illness. Examples of intentional deaths include excessive risk taking, imprudence in the management of ordinary affairs, refusal to eat, overuse or misuse of alcohol or drugs, and noncompliance with life-sustaining medical regimens, such as refusal to take insulin or digoxin, when these activities take place with the expectation that death will occur.

Elizabeth Kübler-Ross[32] has described five stages of the dying process that represent the coping mechanisms of dying. Her model is described in detail in Chapter 15. The family and significant others in the patient's life play an important role in the dying process. Nurses can encourage and support increased involvement of these support groups in the care of the patient. Assessment should be indirect and based on the cues from the patient that there is readiness to talk. Attentive listening alerts the nurse to the patient's need to express feelings or ventilate fears. Covert or overt references to death or thoughts concerning dying are early cues the patient may be making preparations for his own death.

Over 60,000 "living wills" have been distributed by America's Euthanasia Educational Council.[10] This reflects an increasing interest by consumers in how one's death will occur. It represents a person's choice in participating in the final decision to refuse heroic measures after there is no reasonable expectation for recovery. On admission, the existence of a "living will" should be ascertained, from either the patient, family, or guardian. The nurse should be well acquainted with the hospital's policy regarding the acknowledgment of this document and the procedures for sharing with all staff and for ensuring the patient's wishes are recognized.

■ Somatic responses

■ **HYPOCHONDRIASIS.** There is much overlap and interaction between hypochondriasis and depression. Overconcern and preoccupation with one's physical and emotional health and expression through body complaints are common with depressive feelings and introspection but may be present in the absence of a depressed mood.

The rationale underlying hypochondriasis characterizes the needs being expressed by the patient. As a symbol of the geriatric patient's sense of defectiveness and deterioration, somaticism communicates the distress surrounding and displacement of a diminished sense of worth. Escape into the "sick" role is a legitimate and socially acceptable way to deal with stress and anxiety. Support, concern, and interest are conveyed to the patient and he experiences a sense of control.

One of the real problems encountered by the elder with a history of hypochondriasis is the tendency by health professionals to label the patient as a "crock" and dismiss complaints, even if based on organic pathological conditions. All complaints of the patient should be taken seriously and investigated thoroughly. One must never assume the problem is "just a response to some emotional distress" and can be dismissed. Whatever the reasons, the problem is real and the patient's discomfort is real.

■ **SLEEP PATTERN DISTURBANCE.** Insomnia may be a symptom or problem for the gerontological psychiatric patient. Many older adults experience chronic or semichronic sleep problems. Complaints of interrupted sleep, loss of sleep, or "poor sleep" with frequent awakenings and morning exhaustion are common. Daytime napping and drowsiness add to the problem.

Opinions regarding what is normal sleep with aging and the nature of normal sleep patterns in older adults vary and are often controversial. Some researchers suggest that older people need less sleep with increasing age. Chronic fatigue, physical illness, pain, and decreased mobility may result in a requirement for more sleep. Often, the geriatric patient expresses distress over the inability to sleep or stay asleep. Perceived lack of sleep becomes a cyclical reaction. Worry over the lack of sleep prevents the elder from falling asleep. Fatigue, the most common physical complaint of adults over the age of 75, contributes to much of the insomnia of this age group. Lack of exercise, limited mobility and side effects of drugs are the potential factors contributing to insomnia.

The emotional effects of insomnia vary with the individual, but reinforcement of fatigue and depression is common. Recognition of insomnia as a reaction to

TABLE 35-2

NURSING DIAGNOSIS

Alterations in thought processes		Changes in affect		Somatic responses	
Behaviors	Etiologies	Behaviors	Etiologies	Behaviors	Etiologies
Memory loss Recent and/or long-term	Stress, crisis, depression, low self-esteem, cerebrovascular alterations, disease, trauma, sensory deprivation	Disturbed mood Mood swings Overreactions Dysfunctional grieving	Internal or external stress, loss of independence, side effects of drugs, grief, mourning, depression, physiological imbalances	Preoccupation with one's physical and emotional health	Depression, distress, and diminishing sense of worth, sleep pattern disturbance, fatigue, physical illness, alteration in nutrition: less than body requirements, alteration in comfort: pain.
Withdrawal	Multiple losses or fear of loss, grief, resistance to change, infection, pain, toxicity, side effects of drugs, organic impairment				
Confusion	Medication "hangover" (sunrise syndrome), loss of visual accommodation (sundown syndrome), multiple physiological and emotional problems, relocation, loss of family, friends				
Paranoia	Loss, isolation and loneliness, sensory deprivation/loss, adverse drug reactions/toxicity				

emotional and physical disruptions and as a potential precipitator of other problems is the first step to an assessment of the nature of the problem.

■ **ALTERATION IN NUTRITION: LESS THAN BODY REQUIREMENTS.** Anorexia is common in depression but may be seen in confused or disoriented patients. Forgetting to eat or the inability to prepare one's meals may reinforce loss of appetite. Side effects of some drugs (e.g., dry mouth, change in taste) contribute to disinterest in food. The edentulous patient or the patient with gum disease avoids chewing when pos-

sible. The interaction of anorexia and emotional dysfunction should always be considered and included in the nutritional evaluation. Poor nutrition contributes to fatigue, listlessness, and immobility. Table 35-2 summarizes the categories of nursing diagnosis applicable to the psychogeriatric population.

♣ Planning and implementation

Nursing care strategies have been introduced throughout the chapter as part of the assessment and data collection process. Specific interventions will be considered as part of the total milieu for the patient. The elderly respond well to both individual and group psychotherapy. They need the opportunity to talk, have support in their efforts to deal with day-to-day problems, and plan for a meaningful future.

■ Approaches to intervention

■ **LIFE REVIEW THERAPY.** Life review therapy was first described by Butler.[8] It has a positive psychotherapeutic function, providing an opportunity for the individual to reflect on his life to resolve, reorganize, and reintegrate troubling or disturbing concerns. The life review works well in both group and individual settings. Chubon[11] describes an innovative approach to life review with a 65-year-old woman who had experienced multiple disabilities. Using a novel describing people with lives similar to that of the patient's, the therapist assisted the patient in identifying with the characters, thereby reducing the emotional impact of reliving old conflicts and experiences. In a group setting, members may positively reinforce each other and stimulate the mutual learning process. Developing individual autobiographies to share within the group is one way to introduce commonalities among the members and to put the individuals at ease with sharing personal histories. The group cohesiveness and sharing can build self-esteem and a feeling of belonging, in addition to the cathartic atmosphere of the review itself.

■ **REMINISCING GROUPS.** Reminiscing groups resemble life review groups in that the focus is on recounting earlier life experiences and events. In reminiscence, sharing perceptions, historical life events, and generational attributes provides a common theme for the interaction. Individual reminiscing should be encouraged as much as possible and supported as an effort to assist the patient in discharging emotional and cognitive energy. Rambling does not constitute a therapeutic reminiscing experience, since the preoccupation with the dissociated thoughts may actually increase anxiety. Reminiscing is both a way of holding on to the past and letting go.[17] Initiation of reminiscence may be stimulated by formal story telling or sharing of news events from an earlier time. Asking group participants to share experiences related to a specific event (e.g., D-Day, Lindbergh's flight) or a personal event (e.g., marriage, birth of first child, first day in school) provides a basis for the reminiscence process.

■ **REALITY ORIENTATION.** Reality orientation was developed as a specific therapeutic program for institutionalized geriatric patients by James C. Folsom and colleagues in 1958.[49] Both 24-hour and classroom (structured) reality orientation have potential for preventing confusion, keeping patients oriented to time, place, person, and situation. The structure of the environment reinforces contact with reality, the here and now, when it is kept simple and focused. Physical props can assist by the inclusion of clocks, directional signs, calendars, and orientation boards (season of the year, weather, etc.). The classroom reality orientation consists of an intensive small group experience, especially effective for the moderate to severely impaired elderly. It provides an opportunity to reinforce time, place, and person orientation with patients who have a short attention span and need extra verbal and visual stimulation. Reality orientation, along with a discussion of current events, stimulates the patient to maintain contact with reality and the outside world and his place in it. Current events discussions, used alone, may be more flexibly structured with sharing of newspaper headlines, special articles, or group viewing of television news programs. The scope and depth of the groups depend on the abilities of the patients and the other therapeutic modalities at hand.

■ **COGNITIVE TRAINING.** Much research is underway using cognitive training and stimulation.[55] Problem-solving situations, formal or didactic memory training, and memory exercises have proven effective in increasing attention span, efficiency of recall, and the ability to learn new skills (e.g., mathematical calculations, vocabulary). Intelligence does not decline with progressive age but may be dulled by depression, drugs, or lack of use. Cognitive training has promise for providing methods for keeping older adults active mentally, which in turn will enhance emotional well-being. The "use it or lose-it" adage holds as true for maintenance of intelligence as it does for physical functioning. Stimulating cognitive skills can challenge the nurse's creativity in relating to gerontological psychiatric patients. To be able to capitalize on the patient's interests and skills the nurse must be familiar with the patient's past occupation, hobbies, and leisure activities. The nursing interview should focus on gathering as much of that information as possible on admission and adding to the data base as the nurse builds a trusting relationship with the patient.

■ **RELAXATION THERAPY.** Relaxation therapy is another therapeutic modality receiving increasing interest and research. In addition to promoting a sense of physical well-being, relaxation has the potential for releasing tension and reducing stress, which are often viewed as barriers to relating with others. The steps in simple relaxation exercises are described in detail by Wolanin and Phillips and are presented in Chapter 12 of this text.[54] Relaxation, combined with mild isometric exercises, increases cardiovascular output, energy, and mobility and reduces stress. Relaxation and exercise strategies, used in group or individual contexts, do not require advanced skills of the nurse or the patient. They may begin with simple, basic tension-releasing muscle exercises, coupled with verbal instructions regarding breathing and concentration.

■ **SUPPORT AND COUNSELING GROUPS.** These groups offer therapeutic outlets for patients and families. Using a nondirective or unstructured format, the members can ventilate feelings, try out problem-solving approaches, and resolve conflicts in a rational systematical manner. Older adults respond well to a supportive group structure, increasing self-esteem, self-confidence, risk taking, and empathy for others. Caregiver groups are becoming very popular, since 80% of the older adults living at home are cared for by a spouse, sibling, or child.[52] Many community agencies, clinics, and senior citizen centers are responding to the need of this group with special activities, training classes, and supportive groups.

■ **USE OF HUMOR.** The ability to laugh at oneself and see the irony in everyday events provides an effective outlet for frustration, anger, stress, and anxiety. Promoting humor via jokes, joke-telling, story-telling, and cartoons can be therapeutic in both group settings and with individual patients. Expressions of humor and active laughter allow the older adult an opportunity to step out of his or her situation, thereby releasing some of the psychic energy required in coping with changes accompanying aging.

■ **Patient and family education**

As patients and families become more knowledgeable consumers of health services, the need for an increased emphasis on education will impact nursing care.

Older adults frequently question both physiological and cognitive (memory) changes which occur naturally in aging. Slowed response time, benign memory loss, alterations in gait, and interrupted sleep patterns represent a few of the normal changes of aging which can be interpreted as pathological. The nurse has an opportunity to teach patients about their own developmental changes during the assessment phase of the nurse-patient relationship. Expelling myths and stereotypes related to the aging process represents a primary goal for patient education.[25,35,44]

The depressed older adult is particularly receptive to the educative process, since it is in the depressive state that they are most vulnerable and open to suggestion. Exercises for promoting positive thoughts and images, visualization, and repetitive cognitive games can be used as a basis for teaching patients new patterns of behavior.

Family members often view nurses as the most appropriate group for understanding family relationships, conflicts, needs, and resources. Family education related to the normal aging process, family dynamics and family systems, and stress inherent in the caregiver role can be integrated easily into counseling sessions with family members, referral conferences, or as part of the family history on admission of the patient.

A more formal approach to family education can be developed utilizing the numerous books now available commercially which address the caregiving role with older adults.[35,43] These materials provide practical, step-by-step guides to handling common problems of the frail elderly, including agitation, wandering, withdrawal, resistance, anxiety, insomnia, incontinence, anorexia, and restlessness. These books, written specifically for the consumer, supply the text for nurse-family teaching sessions as well as excellent resource materials for the home.[25,29,35,41]

Evaluation and future trends

Specific nursing interventions designed to promote optimum cognitive function and emotional well-being have been considered as part of the role of the gerontological psychiatric nurse. Increasingly, research is being initiated to determine the most appropriate strategy for the needs of the patient and the most effective modality for implementing the strategy.

Gerontological psychiatric nursing offers an exciting and challenging future for nurses interested in working with patients responsive to knowledgeable and creative care. In one sense, most nurses today practice gerontological/geriatric nursing without recognizing it as such, since a growing proportion of patients in all health care settings are elderly. The significance of this growing population will become even more evident as we move toward the twenty-first century. The establishment of chronic disease and other long-term care facilities will supercede the growth of acute care hospitals.[36] The reliance on home care and the use of community resources to meet the health needs of all ages, but particularly the elderly, will grow in the next two decades. Advanced technology will permit shorter stays in acute care hospitals, quicker recovery periods, and less complicated disease courses.

Research in gerontological nursing has grown in the last 12 years. Without research, the direction and impact of practice remain unclear. Burnside[7] suggests several areas for research that stem from problems of concern to nurses working with the aged person: continence, sensory simulation and deprivation, drug abuse, the use of touch and other communicative strategies with the elderly, effectiveness of treatment modalities in senile dementia, and promotion of wellness, to mention a few. The influence of nursing research on nursing practice will depend on the ability of clinicians and researchers to work together in identifying clinical problems of importance and designing projects collaboratively to investigate those problems. Only through collaboration will a body of nursing knowledge develop and grow.

Interprofessional activities in gerontology and geriatrics offer yet another avenue for nurses to impact on the care of the elderly. The funding by private and federal sources of teaching nursing home demonstration projects with a combined academic, clinical, and research focus promises greater cooperation between nursing, medicine, dentistry, pharmacy, and social work. The extent to which the academic nursing home is successful depends, to a great degree, on the strength of the individual groups participating in the effort.

The concept of a nursing home without walls has grown in popularity over recent years.[38] The idea is to use the nursing home as a base for services for the elderly rather than a final resort, as it is now conceived. Maintenance of the patient in his home or other community setting as long as possible will become a reality by offering supportive and comprehensive services to the elder and his family. Patients will move into and out of the nursing home for intensive and episodical nursing care or as a respite for family members from their caregiver responsibilities.

The growing interest in and focus on gerontological/geriatric nursing in nursing education is promising and will assure the nurse of the future an opportunity to offer quality care to this age group.

■ SUGGESTED CROSS-REFERENCES ■

The phases of the nursing process are discussed in Chapter 5. The mental status examination is discussed in Chapter 6. Primary prevention and identification of the elderly as a high-risk group are discussed in Chapter 9. Disturbances of mood are discussed in Chapter 15. Nursing care of the patient with impaired cognition is discussed in Chapter 19.

■ SUMMARY ■

1. Sociodemographic factors of aging were presented with projections for the increase in this minority group over the next 20 years. Psychiatric and related disorders were defined, and the statistical significance was emphasized.

2. The evolution of the role of the gerontological psychiatric nurse was traced, beginning with changes in age distribution after World War II and the needs of an aging society. The gerontological nurse may function in a variety of roles, including patient-care manager in nursing homes or other long-term care settings, health assessor, primary care provider, independent practitioner, and researcher.

DIRECTIONS FOR FUTURE RESEARCH

The following are some of the nursing research problems raised in Chapter 35 that merit further study by psychiatric nurses:

1. The relationship between personality factors and coping with loss in increasing age
2. Differentiating depression from dementia
3. Factors contributing to sundown syndrome
4. The effectiveness of nursing actions with agitated elderly
5. Comparison of interventions with confused elderly
6. Preventive measures for disoriented elders
7. The relationship between family stress and elder self-esteem
8. The effectiveness of reminiscence with moderately confused elders
9. The relationship between functional ability and cognitive function
10. Supportive measures to reduce anxiety in the dementia patient
11. The effectiveness of physical exercise with depressed elders
12. The relationship between cognitive function and elder abuse
13. The effectiveness of humor in a regressed group of elders
14. The relationship between elder relocation and changes in recent memory
15. The effectiveness of cognitive therapy with paranoid elders
16. The relationship between staff attitudes toward the elderly and the elderly person's adjustment to an institutional setting
17. The relationship between mental status and cardiovascular response (B/P, P & R)
18. Factors that contribute to withdrawal of the elderly

---

3. Several theories of aging and the consequences of aging were presented. Biological theories attempt to explain the reasons the body ages over time. Deliberate biological programming theory suggests that humans have a biological time clock in which the memory and capacity for terminating the life of a cell is stored in the cell itself. The wear-and-tear theory posits the notion that structure and function change over time; these changes are accelerated by abuse and decelerated by care. The stress-adaptation theory presumes stress accelerates the aging process. Psychosocial and personality theories of aging focus on emotional response to the aging process. Disengagement theory postulates that mutual withdrawal by older adults and society is a normal and positive benefit of aging. Critics reacting to disengagement developed the activity theory, maintaining that active, involved elders are healthier and happier. The life review, postulated by Butler, involves reminiscence and recall of past life events with resulting release of anxiety, reduction of fear of the future, and successful reintegration of one's meaningful life experiences. Erikson's concept of ego integrity delineates the last developmental stage of life, in which one reflects on accomplishments and failures. Stability of personality (Costa and McRae) persists over the life span regardless of external or internal stressors.

4. Nursing assessment of the gerontological psychiatric patient is a multifaceted process, consisting of the interview, functional assessment, and evaluation of mental status.

5. Standardized measurement tools for assessing the older adult were presented, including the Mental Status Questionnaire, the Short Portable Mental Status Questionnaire, the Face-Hand Test, the Mini-Mental State Examination, the Zung Self-Rating Depression Scale, the Sandoz Clinical Assessment—Geriatric, the Nurses Observation Scale for Inpatient Evaluation, the Katz Index of Activities of Daily living, PACE II, the Family APGAR, and the Social Behavior Assessment Schedule. Discussion centered on the advantages and disadvantages of each of the tools as adjuncts to other assessment techniques.

6. Nursing diagnosis was differentiated from medical diagnosis. Behavioral approaches to nursing diagnosis with assessment and intervention strategies for each included consideration of memory loss, withdrawal, confusion, paranoia, mood swings, grief, loss, depression, perceptions of death and dying, hypochondriasis, insomnia, and anorexia. Emphasized throughout the discussion was the interrelationship between physiological and psychological factors impacting on optimum functioning.

7. The life review, as a therapeutic intervention, stressed the notion of context (group versus individual) and innovative approaches to the technique. The similarity of reminiscence groups and the purpose of reminiscence as a therapeutic strategy were discussed.

8. Examples of therapeutic interventions with the elderly include reality orientation, cognitive training, and relaxation therapy.

9. Families and caregivers of the home-bound and home-care elderly respond well to supportive and counseling groups and are receiving increasing attention from nurses and other health care professionals.

10. Humor is an important strategy for use with the elderly, since it both relieves anxiety and stress and provides an acceptable psychological outlet for frustration, anger, and hostility.

11. Patient and family education are important aspects of the gerontological psychiatric nursing role. Both formal and informal teaching should be provided to elders and their families in areas such as normal aging, differentiating normal from pathological states, family dynamics, and relationships.

12. New and innovative approaches to care of the elderly characterizes the future of gerontological nursing. The need for clinical research to build a body of nursing knowledge in gerontology is recognized by researchers and practitioners alike. Emphasis is being placed on interprofessional practice approaches to the care of the geriatric patient.

■ REFERENCES ■

1. Abdellah, F.G.: Nursing care of the aged in the United States of America, J. Gerontol. Nurs. 7:657, 1981.
2. American Nurses' Association: The American nurse, Kansas City, Mo., Apr. 20, 1979, The Association.
3. Atchley, R.: Aging and suicide: reflection of the quality of life? In Haynes, S.G., and Feinleib, M., editors: Epidemiology of aging, second conference, U.S. Department of Health and Human Services, Washington, D.C., July 1980.
4. Brehm, H.P.: Organizations and financing of health care for the aged: future implications. In Haynes, S.G., and Feinleib, M., editors: Epidemiology of aging, second conference, U.S. Department of Health and Human Services, Washington, D.C., July 1980.
5. Brody, E.M.: Parent care as a normative experience, Gerontologist **25**:19–29, 1985.
6. Brown, E.L.: The professional role in community nursing. II. Nursing reconsidered: a study of change. Philadelphia, 1971, J.B. Lippincott Co.
7. Burnside, I., editor: Nursing and the aged, New York, 1981, McGraw-Hill, Inc.
8. Butler, R.N.: Re-awakening interest, Nurs. Homes **10**:8, Jan. 1961.
9. Butler, R.N.: Why survive? being old in America, New York, 1975, Harper & Row, Publishers, Inc.
10. Butler, R.N., and Lewis, M.R.: Aging and mental health: psychosocial and biomedical approaches, ed. **3**, St. Louis, 1981, The C.V. Mosby Co.
11. Chubon, S.: A novel approach to the process of life review, J. Gerontol. Nurs. **6**:543, 1980.
12. Comfort, A.: Practice of geriatric psychiatry, New York, 1980, American Elsevier Publishing, Inc.
13. Cumming, E., and Henry, W.E.: Growing old: the process of disengagement, New York, 1961, Basic Books, Inc.
14. Davis, B.: A coming of age: a challenge for geriatric nursing, J. Am. Geriatr. Soc. **16**:1100, 1966.
15. Davis, B.: ANA and the geriatric nurse, Nurs. Clin. North Am. **3**:741, 1968.
16. Duke University Center for the Study of Aging and Human Development: Multidimensional functional assessment: the OARS methodology, Durham, N.C., 1978, Duke University.
17. Ebersole, P.P.: A theoretical approach to the use of reminiscence. In Burnside, I.M., editor: Working with the elderly: group processes and techniques, North Scituate, Mass., 1978, Duxbury Press.
18. Ehrman, J.: Elderly personalities remain stable over time, NIH Record **33**:3, Aug. 4, 1981.
19. Eisdorfer, C., and Feidel, R.O.: Cognitive and emotional

disturbance in the elderly: clinical issues, Chicago, 1977, Year Book Medical Publishers, Inc.

20. Erikson, E.H.: Identity and the life cycle: psychological issues, New York, 1959, International Universities Press, Inc.

21. Fielo, S., and Rizzolo, M.A.: The effects of age on pharmacokinetics, Geriatr. Nurs. **6**:6, 328–331, Nov.–Dec. 1985.

22. Fink, M., et al.: Face-hand test as a diagnostic sign of organic mental syndrome, Neurology **2**:46, Jan.–Feb. 1952.

23. Folstein, M.F., et al.: Mini-mental state: a practical method for grading the cognitive states of patients for the clinician, J. Psychol. Res. **12**:189, 1975.

24. Goldfarb, A.I.: Institutional care of the aged. In Busse, E.W., and Pfeiffer, E., editors: Behavior and adaptation in late life, Boston, 1977, Little, Brown & Co.

25. Hawranik, P.: Caring for aging parents: divided allegiances, J. Gerontol. Nurs. **11**:10, 19–22, Oct. 1985.

26. Hayflick, L., et al.: The serial cultivation of human diploid cells, Exp. Cell Res. **25**:585, 1961.

27. Hendricks, J., and Hendricks, C.D.: Aging in mass society, ed. 2, Cambridge, Mass., 1981, Winthrop Publishers, Inc.

28. Honigfeld, G., and Klett, C.J.: The nurses' observation scale for inpatient evaluation: a new scale for measuring improvement in chronic schizophrenia, J. Clin. Psychol. **21**:65, Jan. 1965.

29. Horne, J.: Caregiving: helping an aging loved one, Washington, D.C., 1985, American Association of Retired Persons.

30. Kahn, R.L.: Brief objective measure for the determination of mental status in aged, Am. J. Psychiatry **117**:326, 1960.

31. Katz, S., et al.: Studies of illness in the aged. The index of ADL; a standardized measure of biological and psychosocial function, J.A.M.A. **185**:914, 1963.

32. Kübler-Ross, E.: On death and dying, London, 1980, Tavistock Publications, Ltd.

33. Lamy, P.P.: Prescribing for the elderly, Littleton, Mass., 1980, PSG Publishing Co., Inc.

34. Lowenthal, M.F., et al.: Four stages of life: a comparative study of women and men facing transitions, San Francisco, 1975, Jossey-Bass, Inc., Publishers.

35. Mace, N.L., and Rabins, P.V.: The 36-hour day, New York, 1984, Warner Books.

36. Mace, N.: Do we need special care units for dementia patients? J. Gerontol. Nurs. **11**:10, 37–38, Oct. 1985.

37. Murry, R., et al.: The nursing process in later maturity, Englewood Cliffs, N.J., 1980, Prentice-Hall, Inc.

38. National Institute on Aging: National Advisory Council Meeting Minutes, Bethesda, Md., Oct. 1981, U.S. Department of Health and Human Services.

39. Ochsner, A.: Aging, J. Am. Geriatr. Soc. **24**:385, 1976.

40. Platt, S., et al.: Social behavior assessment schedule (SBAS): rationale, contents, scoring and reliability of a new interview schedule, Soc. Psychiatry **15**:43, 1980.

41. Powell, L.S., and Courtice, K.: Alzheimer's disease,

Menlo Park, Calif., 1983, Addison-Wesley Co.

42. Radar, J., et al.: How to decrease wandering, a form of agenda behavior, Geriatr. Nurs., July–Aug., 1985.

43. Reisberg, B.: A guide to Alzheimer's disease: for families, spouses and friends, New York, 1981, Free Press.

44. Schwab, Sr. M., et al.: Relieving the anxiety and fear in dementia, J. Gerontol. Nurs. **11**:5, 8–15, 1985.

45. Shader, R.I., et al.: A new scale for clinical assessment in geriatric populations: Sandoz Clinical Assessment—Geriatric (SCAG), J. Am. Geriatr. Soc. **12**:107, Mar. 1974.

46. Siegler, I.C.: The psychology of adult development and aging. In Busse, E.W., and Blazer, D.G., editors: Handbook of geriatric psychiatry, New York, 1980, VanNostrand Reinhold Co.

47. Smilkstein, G.: The family APGAR: a proposal for a family function test and its use by physicians, J. Fam. Pract. **6**:1231, 1978.

48. Stone, V.: The nurse and the aged, R.N. **39**:21, Feb. 1976.

49. Taulbee, L., and Folsom, J.: Reality orientation for geriatric patients, Hosp. Community Psychiatry **17**:133, May 1966.

50. U.S. Department of Health, Education and Welfare: Working-document on patient care management, Washington, D.C., 1978, U.S. Government Printing Office.

51. Waxman, H.M., et al.: A comparison of somatic complaints among depressed and non-depressed older persons, Gerontologist **25**:5, 501–507, 1985.

52. Who's taking care of our parents? Newsweek (Special Issue), 61–70, May 6, 1985.

53. Wolanin, M.O., and Phillips, L.R.F.: Who's confused here? Geriatr. Nurs. **1**:122, July–Aug. 1980.

54. Wolanin, M.O., and Phillips, L.R.F.: Confusion: prevention and care, St. Louis, 1981, the C.V. Mosby Co.

55. Yesavage, J.A., et al.: Senile dementia; combined pharmacologic and psychologic treatment, J. Am. Geriatr. Soc. **29**:164, Apr. 1981.

56. Zung, W.W.K.: A self-rating depression scale, Arch. Gen. Psychiatry **12**:63, Jan. 1965.

■ ANNOTATED SUGGESTED READINGS ■

Alzheimer's disease: Report of the Secretary's Task Force on Alzheimer's disease, Washington, D.C., 1984, U.S. Department of Health and Human Services.

Report of a presidential multi-agency Task Force on Alzheimer's Disease which covers areas of epidemiology, etiology, diagnosis, clinical course, treatment, family involvement, systems of care, projected needs for personnel and future research.

*Britnell, J., and Mitchell, K.: Inpatient group psychotherapy for the elderly, J. Psychiatr. Nurs. **19**:19, May 1981.

This is one of the few articles in the nursing literature on group psychotherapy for the elderly. It describes a theoretical framework and applies it to case examples.

*Burnside, I.M., editor: Working with the elderly: group processes and techniques, North Scituate, Mass., 1978, Duxbury Press.

This volume of papers provides an overview of group work with the elderly, including reminiscence, reality orientation, remotivation, music, and art therapy. A practical "how to" approach is utilized.

Busse, E.W., and Blazer, D.G., editors: Handbook of geriatric psychiatry, New York, 1980, Van Nostrand Reinhold Co.

A multiauthored volume that provides an eclectic perspective to the field of geriatric psychiatry. The authors integrate basic biological and psychosocial knowledge into the diagnosis and clinical treatment of psychiatric disorders of late life.

Comfort, A.: Practice of geriatric psychiatry, New York, 1980, American Elsevier Publishing, Inc.

A practical approach to geropsychiatry includes an overview and systematic discussion of every major category of geriatric mental disease. Both diagnostic and therapeutic data are included throughout the text.

Covell, M.: The home alternative to hospitals and nursing homes, New York, 1985, Holt, Rinehart and Winston.

The author presents some facts that relate to the impact of home health care on the health care system. A practical guide to care in the home, including care for a mentally ill relative and home care of the older adult. Provides examples of physical and emotional care for teaching families and other caregivers of the home care patient.

Department of Health, Education and Welfare, The Federal Council on the Aging: Mental health and the elderly: recommendations for action, Washington, D.C., 1979, U.S. Government Printing Office.

Two reports, The President's Commission on Mental Health: Task Panel on the Elderly and The Secretary's Committee on Mental Health and Illness of the Elderly, give an overview of the needs and resources for the elderly with mental health problems. Recommendations for action in the public and private sector are cited in areas of assessment, treatment, and health care service.

*Ernst, P., and Shaw, J.: Touching is not taboo, Geriatr. Nurs. **1**:193, Sept.–Oct. 1980.

The physician/nurse co-authors suggest that touch provides a therapeutic intervention in treating disturbed or regressed elderly patients. Findings from clinical research studies provide the premise for examining the therapeutic elements of touch.

*Hewes, C.J.: Role of the nursing coordinator on a geropsychiatric unit, J. Gerontol. Nurs. **7**:607, 1981.

The author is a nurse coordinator of a large neuropsychiatric institute in Southern California. Experimental role modeling for staff and patient advocacy are two of the many components of the role that are examined in this article.

Kane, R.A., and Kane, R.L.: Assessing the elderly: a practical guide to measurement, Lexington, Mass., 1981, Lexington Books.

The authors focus on specific areas of measurements addressing the particular needs of the aging individual. Criteria are included for instrument selection and for evaluating the reliability and validity of measurements presented.

Kra, S.: Aging myths: reversible causes of mind and memory loss, New York, 1986, McGraw-Hill Book Co.

Based on scientific findings, the author confronts some of the myths regarding age and memory loss. Using a case study approach, the reversible causes of dementia and memory loss are examined, concluding that senility is not an inevitable consequence of growing old.

Maclay, E.: Green winter, New York, 1977, McGraw-Hill Book Co.

A book of poems whose pages surprise with wit, with the unexpected turn of thought and the grit and tenderness of human spirit. A book of celebrations of old age.

*National League for Nursing: Overcoming the bias of ageism in long-term care, New York, 1985, NLN.

This volume contains a collection of papers presented at the Second Invitational Conference on Long-Term Care. Contains thoughts on recruiting and retaining nurses in long-term care, core content in gerontological and geropsychiatric nursing, and research in long-term care.

*Pavkov, J.R., and Walsh, J.: For nursing homes: a mental health charting instrument, J. Gerontol. Nurs. **7**:13, Jan. 1981.

This article describes a standardized charting tool developed in a geriatric outpatient service unit of a community mental health center. The purpose of the tool is to define the role of the mental health consultant in the nursing home and to assist medical and nursing staff in the development of treatment plans.

Seuss, Dr., and Geisel, A.S.: You're only old once! New York, 1986, Random House.

Theodor Seuss Geisel, better known as Dr. Seuss, celebrated his 82nd birthday on March 2, 1986, the publication date of this book. Filled with laughter typical of Dr. Seuss's books, we follow our hapless hero through his checkup with the experts at the Golden Years Clinic.

Shraberg, D.: An overview of neuropsychiatric disturbances in the elderly, J. Am. Geriatr. Soc. **28**:422, 1980.

A brief overview of the relationship between neurology and psychiatry in geriatric medicine. Included are some of the myths regarding aging, normal changes in the aging nervous system, and criteria for differential diagnosis of dementia and pseudodementia.

*Wahl, P.R.: Therapeutic relationships with the elderly, J. Gerontol. Nurs. **6**:260, 1980.

Components of a helping therapeutic relationship are posed. Special consideration of the needs of the elderly constitute the discussion of the phases of the relationship, goals, and outcome.

*Wolanin, M.O., and Phillips, L.R.F.: Confusion: prevention and care, St. Louis, 1980, The C.V. Mosby Co.

This 1982 American Journal of Nursing Book of the Year for gerontological nursing focuses on confusion in the elderly. Using a multidimensional approach to assessment and intervention, the authors emphasize the impact of the diagnosis or misdiagnosis of confusion on the treatment selection and outcome for the elderly client.

*Wolanin, M.O., and Phillips, L.R.F.: Who's confused here? Geriatr. Nurs. **1**:122, July–Aug. 1980.

The authors use case examples to illustrate how premature and biased labeling of patient behavior may lead to misinterpretation of the patient's problem and misdiagnosis. The consequence of misdiagnosis of confusion in the elderly is addressed, along with suggestions for more accurate assessment and nursing management.

Yesavage, J.A., Westphal, J., and Rush, L.: Senile dementia: combined pharmacologic and psychologic treatment, J. Am. Geriatr. Soc. **29**:164, Apr. 1981.

The authors introduced either supportive counseling or cognitive training as adjuncts to pharmacological treatment of geriatric patients with moderate dementia. Multidimensional outcome measures were used to assess changes in cognitive function (memory and learning), behavioral responses, and depression. Despite the improved effect on memory in the group receiving cognitive training, there was no difference between the two experimental groups on measures of overall behavioral change or on depression. The implications of these findings are discussed in relationship to previous studies on cognitive function and behavior and affective disorders of the elderly.

---

*Asterisk indicates nursing reference.

APPENDIXES

PSYCHOSOCIAL ASSESSMENT TOOL

Facility _____

Assessor _____

Date _____

Socialpsychologic Assessment Form

1. Assessor's immediate thoughts, feelings, impressions of client on first meeting

Demographic and vital data

2. Name:
3. Present address:
4. When did you move to that address?
5. From where did you move?
6. Why did you move?
7. When were you born?
8. Where were you born?
9. Marital status: (circle) S M D W Sep.
10. Sex: (circle) F M
11. Facial group: (circle)
    Caucasian   Mongoloid   Negro

Presenting data

12. Why are you here? (Voluntary or involuntary, referred, accompanied by whom, at whose urging, presenting difficulty whose perception?)
13. When did it all start?

Sociologic data

Now about your family . . .

14. Name the members and give their ages. Start with the oldest member. (Family is defined as whomever client perceives it to be.)

Name	Age	Relationship to client

15. Do you see them often? Where do they live?
16. Who talks to whom, about what, most of the time?

17. How open is your family to new ideas and new people?
18. Describe, in a few words, each family member.

Member	Description

19. How is your family reacting to your present difficulty?
20. In your family, who is more dependent and who is more independent in terms of money and emotionally (or psychologically)?

Now about your family's communication . . .

21. What problems or issues are discussed most in your family?
22. Are there members of the family who feel they are misunderstood? Explain.
23. Does your family seem to understand each other's hidden messages, i.e., can they read between the lines?
24. What patterns of nonverbal behavior have you noticed in the family, i.e., touch, facial grimaces, etc.?
25. Are there persons in your family who typically say one thing, but mean another?
26. Is there anyone in your family who tells you to do opposite things at the same time?
27. What topics are hardest to talk about in your family?

Now about your family's togetherness . . .

28. Is your family close?
29. Do you like it that way?

30. Is this present difficulty bringing the family closer together or causing problems?
31. How does your family view you, e.g., wild, bookworm type, or what? Do *you* think you act your age?
32. How do *you* view your family?
33. What is the *central concern* in your family, e.g., success, education, or what?
34. Does your present difficulty interfere with that central concern in any way?
35. Are your family experiences broad or narrow, e.g., have they traveled much?
36. What illness or hospitalization has there been in other members of your family?
37. When there are problems in the family do the members seem to get focused on you?

Now about you and your family's resources for crises . . .

38. Do you feel that you cannot cope with your present situation or difficulty? (If "no" skip to item 46.)
39. Have you been in a crucial or decisive situation like this before?
40. How did you handle it?
41. How do you feel about this situation?
42. How will you handle those feelings?
43. Are you hopeful about solving the present situation? Why or why not?
44. What will you do about it?
45. Are there family or friends who will help you? How will they help?
46. What roles do different members of your family play generally? For example, is there a boss, a peacemaker, etc.?

        Member   *Role*

47. Do they like those roles? Do they play them well?
48. Do your family members seem to work against one another?
49. Are your physical needs met by your family?
50. Are your emotional needs met by your family?
51. Are there family goals which all members work toward?
52. Do you feel free to pursue an individual goal with which the family is in disagreement?

Now about you and your family's response to illness . . .

53. Is this the first time you have had these symptoms? If "no" discuss previous times.

54. How long have you had this difficulty before seeking help?
55. Are you the only family member with some difficulty at the present time?
56. Have you had other major illnesses or hospitalizations?
57. What jobs do you do in your family?
58. What jobs do the other family members do in the family?
59. Who does your family jobs when you cannot do them?
60. What occupations do your family members work at presently outside the home?

        Member   *Occupation*

61. Does your family see itself as a healthy family or a sick family?

Now about your occupation . . .

62. Describe the work you do. (If unemployed skip to item 70.)
63. How long have you been on the job?
64. Do you like it? Can you advance? Do you feel secure in it?
65. Do you get along with the people you work for and with?
66. Is the job what you pictured yourself doing when you were younger?
67. What does your family think of the job?
68. What effect will this present difficulty have on your job?
69. Do you think the job is in any way related to your present symptoms (go to item 73)?
70. Why are you *not* working?
71. Are you satisfied not to be working?
72. What does your family say about not working?
73. What have your jobs been since you left school?
74. Why did you leave them?

Now about your education . . .

75. How far did you go in school or college?
76. Are you satisfied with your education?
77. Are you in any educational program now, and how are you doing?
78. Are you studying on your own or teaching yourself anything now? Describe it.
79. How does your education compare with members of your family? If it is different, does it cause problems?
80. What made you decide to seek professional assistance?

81. Do you have suggestions for how your present difficulty can be managed?

Now about your leisure time . . .

82. How much leisure time do you have?
83. What are your favorite recreational pastimes? Can you afford them?
84. Are you satisfied with the way you spend your leisure time?
85. Do you and your family engage in recreational activities together, or is there disagreement on what you will do?

Now about where you live . . .

86. In what section of the city (county) is your home?
87. Do you like your neighborhood? Describe it.
88. Do you like your home? Is it big enough? Does it require a lot of work? Describe it.
89. How long have you lived there?
90. Have you moved much in your life and why?
91. How far do you live from here, and is getting here a problem?
92. Are there certain illnesses or health problems that seem to occur a lot in your neighborhood?

Now about your family's income . . .

93. What was your total family income last year? (Use a card and have client identify category if there is hesitancy.)

_____ Under $5,000	_____ $15,000 to $20,000
_____ $5,000 to $9,999	_____ Over $20,000
_____ $10,000 to $14,999	

94. Who contributes most of this?
95. Is the income enough to live on? Are you satisfied with it?
96. Are other family members satisfied with it?
97. Who pays the bills and makes the decisions about big expenditures?
98. Where do you usually go for professional health care?
99. Will this difficulty affect your family income in any way?
100. Did concern about the cost keep you from getting assistance sooner?

Now about your ethnic background . . .

101. Where did your parents or ancestors come from and when?
102. Was a language other than English spoken at home? What?
103. Do you hold to the values and customs of your ethnic group?
104. Do you have specific practices for treating sickness that you learned from your ethnic group? What are they?

Now about your religious background . . .

105. Are you a member of a church? What denomination?
106. Would you say you are a religious person? Why or why not?
107. Do your parents belong to your church? If not why the difference?
108. (If married and/or children) Do you all go to the same church? If not, why not? Does it create problems?
109. Are you satisfied with your church and religious life? If not, why not?
110. How do you view illness generally? Do you feel you have any control over it?
111. Do you have any religious beliefs or practices about the treatment of illness?

Now your beliefs about illness . . .

112. What do you think caused your present difficulty? Did you have anything to do with it? Could someone else have caused it?
113. Did you try to treat yourself before coming here?
114. Did you seek treatment (relief) from others before coming here? If "yes" describe it.
115. What are some of the home remedies you routinely use for illness?
116. Have you ever engaged in faith healing?
117. What do you think is the major cause of illness generally?

Now about your attitudes toward life . . .

118. What do you think about life in general?
119. Are you glad to be alive now? If not when would you liked to have lived?
120. Has life become better or worse as you have grown older? Why?
121. Are you generally a pessimist or an optimist?
122. Do you believe you could have prevented some of your difficulty if you had behaved differently? Why?

Socialpsychologic Assessment Form—cont'd

Now about your standard of living . . .

123. Describe your life-style, or how you live.
124. Do you think any of your possessions or behavior are extravagant? Why or why not?
125. Can you rank order the amount of your income spent on:

Housing _____   Religion and
Recreation and   charity _____
   socializing _____   Health and
Shopping _____   illness _____
Education _____

Now about your habits . . .

126. What and how much do you eat in a typical day?
127. Do you consider yourself a big, an average, or a small eater?
128. Where and with whom do you generally eat your meals?
129. What foods do you like and dislike most?
130. Do you have medical or religious food or drink restrictions?
131. Do you have any food or beverage allergies?
132. Do you get enough to eat?
133. Do you have any difficulty eating?
134. What beverages and how much of them do you drink each day?
135. How much alcohol do you drink in a day and when do you drink it? (If client does not drink alcohol skip to item 143.)
136. What is your favorite alcoholic beverage?
137. Do you usually drink alone or with others?
138. Do you find yourself drinking more when you are under stress?
139. Do you get intoxicated? How often? Do you black out?
140. Have you injured yourself or others while drinking?
141. Has your drinking ever interfered with your job?
142. Do you or your family worry about your drinking?
143. Do your family members drink alcohol? How much? Any problem drinkers?
144. What patent medications do you take routinely? Why?
145. Do you have prescriptions from physicians? What are they for?
146. Do any of the medicines cause discomfort or do things they are not meant to do?

147. Have you been taking any medicine routinely for over a year? Why?
148. Do you smoke? How much? (If client does not smoke skip to item 151.)
149. When do you smoke?
150. Have you tried to stop smoking?
151. Do you feel as though you are dependent on coffee, tea, soft drinks, or alcohol?
152. Have you ever taken a narcotic drug for pain? How long?
153. Have you ever taken drugs to help you fall asleep or perk you up?
154. Have you taken drugs for depression?
155. Have you taken drugs for "kicks," or for the heck of it?
156. Have you taken medicine to control your appetite?
157. Have you been treated for taking too much of a drug, an overdose?
158. Have you ever gotten into trouble with the law from selling or using illegal drugs? What happened?
159. Do you believe that any of the medicines or drugs you have taken, or are taking now, are bad for your health?
160. Tell me about your bathing habits. How often do you bathe?
161. How often do you shampoo your hair?
162. Tell me about your sleeping habits. When do you go to bed? When do you get up?
163. Do you have difficulty falling asleep or waking up?
164. Do you sleep soundly or awaken a lot during the night? What awakens you?
165. Do you take naps during the day?
166. Do you feel you get enough sleep?
167. Have your sleeping patterns changed recently?
168. Do you wear glasses, contact lenses, or a hearing aid, and how do feel about it?
169. Does your job present a danger to your sight or hearing? How do you protect yourself?
170. Do you have any problems with taste, smell, or touch?

Now some questions about your sexual behavior . . .

171. How do you see yourself as a man (woman)?
172. Do you ever wish you were a (the opposite sex)? What would the advantages be?

Socialpsychologic Assessment Form—cont'd

173. Have you ever felt discriminated against because you are a man (woman)?
174. Have you ever had to do things you did not want to do because you are a man (woman)?
175. Who was most influential in teaching you how to be a man (woman)?
176. Where and when did you learn about sexual behavior?
177. Do you know any of your parents' beliefs about sexual behavior?
178. In what ways are your beliefs and attitudes about sex different from your parents?
179. Tell me about your earliest sexual experiences. When did they occur? How did you feel about them?
180. (If above experiences were heterosexual) Have you had any homosexual experiences? Tell me about them.
181. Do you have any worries or difficulties about sex?
182. Do you and your (primary) sexual partner agree on the frequency and nature of your sexual activities? (Ask about masturbation.)
183. How frequently do you engage in sexual activity? Who initiates it?
184. (If male) Do you have difficulty maintaining an erection or with premature ejaculation?
185. Do you have difficulty reaching a climax or orgasm?
186. (If married) Do you engage in sexual activities with persons other than your spouse? Does it cause problems?
187. (If single) Do you engage in sexual activities? With more than one person?
188. Are you satisfied with your sexual behavior?
189. Have the difficulties that brought you here interfered with your sexual life?

Psychologic data

Now some questions about you as an individual, specifically your thinking . . .

Consciousness

190. Tell me again about your situation. What is the difficulty? How did you get here and what can I do for you?
191. Do you know or have you been told that you have dreamlike periods when you do things that you do not remember afterwards?
192. Do you believe or feel that you are another person doing things sometimes?
193. Do you walk in your sleep or write things automatically as though another person was doing it?

Orientation

194. What is today's date?
195. Tell me about your activities since you got up this morning.
196. Where are you now . . . exactly?
197. Who are you, and who are some of the persons close to you?

Attention

198. Do you ever find yourself concentrating on something so much that you cannot get on with other things?
199. Do you find yourself so excited sometimes that you cannot concentrate or pay attention to anything for very long?
200. Do you ever find you are in the middle of a sentence and forgot what you wanted to say?

Perception

201. Do you experience things differently from the way others say they are? Is there something there, but it appears different from what it is?
202. Do you see or hear things that others say are not there?
203. Do you ever smell or taste things that others say are imaginary?
204. Do you ever feel you are being touched when no one is there?
205. Do you believe you have ESP powers?

Apperception

206. I will ask you a question now. Tell me what I am asking, then answer it. (Ask, "Have you learned anything from the interview session so far?")

Thought content

207. Tell me, what sorts of things do you think about a lot?

Socialpsychologic Assessment Form—cont'd

208. Do you think about or dwell too much on one idea sometimes?
209. Do you have trouble falling asleep because you go over and over some thought?
210. Do you ever think about something so much and so long that you lose track of where you are and what you are doing?

Thought form

211. Do you spend a lot of time daydreaming so that you do not get the things done you should get done?
212. Do you ever have crazy thoughts that others laugh at, such as something you believe that no one else believes?
213. Do you have thoughts that run through your mind all the time that you cannot get out? Do they interfere with your life?
214. Do you have fears of certain things that bother you?

Thought progress

215. Do your thoughts ever come out so fast or so slow that you have difficulty making people understand you?
216. Does your thinking ever wander so much that you have trouble getting to the point?

Memory

217. Have you ever lost, or been told you lost, your memory for a while?
218. Is there a specific event in your life for which you have no memory?
219. (If older ask) Do you remember things from way back better than you remember things from yesterday?
220. Is there an event in your life that you remember extremely well and in great detail that you will never forget?
221. Do you ever get mixed up between what is real and what is not real, like thinking a dream is real?
222. Describe the person who spoke with you when you first came in here today.
223. Do you often believe or get the feeling that something you are experiencing has happened before?

Self-concept

224. What kind of a person would you say you are? Describe yourself.
225. Are your views of yourself mostly positive, mostly negative, or are you mixed up about how you see yourself?
226. Do you like yourself?
227. Do you seem to influence others, or do they usually influence you?
228. Are you more of a leader or a follower?
229. What was your life like generally during high school (13 to 18 years of age)?
230. Would you say you have reached or are reaching your life dreams and goals?
231. Has life been good to you?

Body image

232. What do you think of your body? Do you like it?
233. What part of your body displeases you the most?
234. Have you lost any part of your body (even teeth) that bother you?
235. (If not deformed from arthritis) Would deforming arthritis threaten you?
236. Have you ever thought that some part of your body was in the wrong place or somehow different from what it should be?
237. If you could change your body how would you change it?

Now some questions about how you feel and your moods . . .

238. Have you ever felt strangely unreal and separated from the real world so that you could sort of watch yourself as you would watch someone else?
239. Have you ever been so depressed that you gave up and wanted to die?
240. Have you ever been unusually depressed following some sort of loss?
241. Have you ever lost something or someone dear to you, but could not grieve over it?
242. Do you tend to get mild blue spells?
243. Have you experienced a lot of guilt throughout your life?
244. Do you have "ups" and "downs" a lot?
245. Are you a "moody" person?
246. Do you often feel two ways about something and cannot decide which way to go?

Socialpsychologic Assessment Form—cont'd

247. Do you often feel apathetic, detached, and indifferent to things?
248. Have you ever felt different from everyone else in a situation, such as thinking something was funny when everyone else was sad?
249. Do you experience a lot of anxiety, nervousness, or restlessness? When is it worse and what do you do about it?
250. Do you have any physical complaints that could be related to your anxiety or nervousness?
251. Would you say you are a nervous person?
252. Are your feelings easily hurt?

Aspects of conation (appearance, facies, voluntary and automatic motor activity, and communication) are to be observed and recorded in the space provided at the end of the interview session.

Antecedent data

Now some questions about what you remember of your early years . . .

253. Do you know anything about your family situation when you were born? Were they able to take care of you? Who was there?
254. Are your parents still living and married to one another?
255. What do you know of your grandparents when you were born?
256. Do you believe you got any special attention or perhaps neglect?
257. Do you wish you had been born at a different time or into a different family?
258. Do you have any idea about what your parents thought or felt about you when you were born? Did they want you?
259. Do you remember your thoughts and feelings toward your parents? Are there positive memories of whomever raised you as far back as you can go?
260. (If brothers and sisters) How did you feel about your brothers and sisters when you were a child; how did they feel about you? Did you get along with them?
261. (If older siblings) Did you have to wear and play with a lot of hand-me-downs?
262. Do you remember any other stories about yourself before you started school?

263. Has trusting people ever been a problem for you?
264. Do you know anything of when you learned to walk or were toilet trained?
265. Have you tended to doubt yourself a lot, or feel ashamed or embarrassed about yourself?
266. Do you know with whom you identified as a child?
267. Who was your favorite older person as you were growing up?
268. What do you remember of grade school? Did you do well? Did you make friends?
269. What was it like at home during your grade school years?
270. Did people tease you?
271. What are your most vivid memories of childhood?
272. Do you remember junior high school (middle school)? What was it like?
273. What was important during those years (hobbies, scouts, church)?
274. Were you satisfied with your grades and accomplishments?
275. Did you miss a lot of school? Why?
276. Did you get in trouble because of your behavior?
277. Did you learn anything about health or sex? Has it influenced you?
278. (If female) Tell me about your first menstrual period. Were you prepared? (If male) Do you remember your first ejaculations and painful testicles?
279. (If female) Do you remember when your breasts started to develop? Were you embarrassed?
280. Do you remember getting interested in boys (girls)? What were your earliest experiences with them? How did you feel about it?
281. What were your senior high school years like (dating, work)?
282. If you could sum up your whole school experience in a few words, what would they be?
283. How did you feel about your parents during high school years?
284. What about the years right after school, were you mixed up and undecided?
285. Was sex a problem area for you during that time? (Ask about pregnancies.)

Socialpsychologic Assessment Form—cont'd

286. Did you leave home, when and why?
287. Describe your first living arrangements away from home.
288. Describe your major relationship during that time.
289. Did you find it difficult to give and share? (If client never married skip to item 299. If client has no children skip to item 303.)
290. When and how did you meet your husband (wife)?
291. What attracted you to him (her)? Is that attraction still there?
292. What made you decide to marry? Who suggested it? How did he (she) respond?
293. Have either of you been married before? Are there children from previous marriages?
294. What did each set of in-laws think about the marriage? Do you all get along with each other?
295. Were there obstacles or problems surrounding the marriage?
296. Were your early expectations of one another met?
297. Have your plans for the future been working out?
298. Do you have any problems with your marriage now? (If client has no children skip to item 303.)
299. Tell me about your children. (If female ask about father of children.)
300. What do you believe about raising children? Have you been able to carry it out?
301. Were the children easy or hard to raise?
302. Are you satisfied with the way the children are turning out?
303. Describe a typical day in your life.
304. How much time do you spend with family members and relatives?
305. What has your biggest accomplishment been in life?

306. What major events have occurred in your life in the last 5 years; for example, has there been a(n):
    Death _____
    Divorce _____
    Marital separation _____
    Someone in jail _____
    Injury or illness _____
    Marriage _____
    Job loss _____
    Marital reconciliation _____
    Retirement _____
    Other _____
307. What was most stressful in life? How did you cope with it?
308. How do you feel about your life? Are you satisfied as you look back?

Observed conation data

309. Describe the appearance *and* expression of the client's face, noting traces of past action:
310. Describe the client's dress, noting jewelry.
311. Describe the client's posture.
312. Describe the client's motor activity noting whether underactive, overactive, and/or stereotypic:
313. Comment on the client's verbal communication generally:
314. Describe any nonverbal behavior (physical appearance, dress, facial expression, gestures, posture, and gait) and state your impression of messages you believe were being communicated:
315. Discussion and clinical judgment:

*From Francis, G., and Munjas, B.: Manual of social-psychologic assessment, New York, 1976, Appleton-Century-Crofts.

MEDICATION AND DRUG ASSESSMENT TOOL

Facility _____

Assessor _____

Date _____

Medication and Drug Assessment

1. Psychiatric medications (for *each* medication *ever* taken by the patient obtain the following information):
   a. Name of drug
   b. Reason prescribed
   c. Date started
   d. Length of time taken
   e. Highest daily dose
   f. Prescribed by whom
   g. Summarize effects
   h. Side effects or adverse reactions
   i. Was it taken as prescribed? If not, explain.
   j. Other family members prescribed this drug
   k. If so, reason prescribed and effectiveness

2. Prescription (nonpsychiatric) medications (for *each* medication taken by the patient in the past 6 months and for major medical illnesses if more than 6 months ago obtain the following information):
   a. Name of drug
   b. Reason prescribed
   c. Date started
   d. Highest daily dose
   e. Prescribed by whom
   f. Summarize effects
   g. Side effects or adverse reactions
   h. Was it taken as prescribed? If not, explain.

3. Over-the-counter (nonprescribed) medications (for *each* medication taken by the patient in the past 6 months obtain the following information):
   a. Name of drug
   b. Reason taken
   c. Date started
   d. Frequency of use
   e. Summarize effects
   f. Side effects or adverse reactions

4. Alcohol and street drugs (see Appendix E for common street names of abused substances)
   a. Name of substance
   b. Date of first use
   c. Frequency of use
   d. Summarize effects
   e. Adverse reactions

PHYSICAL ASSESSMENT TOOL

Facility _____

Assessor _____

Date _____

Physical History

Biographical data

1. Name
2. Age
3. Race
4. Culture
5. Address
6. Marital status
7. Children and family in home
8. Occupation
9. Means of transportation to health care facility, if pertinent
10. Description of home; size and type of community

Reason for visit

One statement that describes the reason for the client's visit, or the chief complaint. State in the client's own words.

Present health status

1. General health status of the client in the past 1 year, 5 years, now
2. Client's current major health concerns
3. If illness is present, include (symptom analysis) history
   a. When was client last well
   b. Date of problem onset
   c. Character of complaint
   d. Nature of problem onset
   e. Course of problem
   f. Client's hunch of precipitating factors
   g. Location of problem
   h. Relation to other body symptoms, body positions, and activity
   i. Patterns of problem
   j. Efforts of client to treat
   k. Coping ability

4. Current medications
   a. Type (prescription, over-the-counter drugs, vitamins, etc.)
   b. Prescribed by whom
   c. Amount per day
   d. Problems

Current health statistics

1. Immunization status (note dates or year of last immunization)
   a. Tetanus, diphtheria
   b. Mumps
   c. Rubella
   d. Polio
   e. Tuberculosis tine test
   f. Influenza
2. Allergies (describe agent and reactions)
   a. Drugs
   b. Foods
   c. Contact substances
   d. Environmental factors
3. Last examinations (note physician/clinic, findings, advice, and/or instructions)
   a. Physical
   b. Dental
   c. Vision
   d. Hearing
   e. ECG
   f. Chest radiograph
   g. Pap smear (females)

Past health status

Although each of the following is asked separately, the examiner must summarize and record the data *chronologically*.

1. Childhood illnesses: rubeola, rubella, mumps, pertussis, scarlet fever, chickenpox, strep throat

Physical History—cont'd

2. Serious or chronic illnesses: scarlet fever, diabetes, kidney problems, hypertension, sickle cell anemia, seizure disorders, blood infections
3. Serious accidents or injuries: head injuries, fractures, burns, other trauma
4. Hospitalizations: elaborate, reason for, location, primary care providers, duration
5. Operations: what, where, when, why, by whom
6. Emotional health: past problems, help sought, support persons
7. Obstetrical history
   a. Complete pregnancies: number, pregnancy course, postpartum course, and condition, weight, and sex of child
   b. Incomplete pregnancies: duration, termination, circumstances (including abortions and stillbirths)
   c. Summary of complications

Family history

Family members include the client's blood relatives, spouse, and children. Specifically the interviewer should inquire about the client's maternal and paternal grandparents, parents, aunts, uncles, spouse, and children, as well as about the general health, stress factors, and illnesses of other family members. Questions should include a survey of the following:

Cancer	Retardation
Diabetes	Alcoholism
Heart disease	Endocrine diseases
Hypertension	Sickle cell anemia
Epilepsy (or seizure disorder)	Kidney disease
Emotional stresses	Unusual limitations
Mental illness	Other chronic problems

The most concise method to record these data is by a family tree.

Review of physiological systems

The purpose of this component of the data base is to collect information about the body regions or systems and their function.

1. General—reflect from client's previous description of current health status
   a. Fatigue patterns
   b. Exercise and exercise tolerance
   c. Weakness episodes
   d. Fever, sweats
   e. Frequent colds, infections, or illnesses
   f. Ability to carry out activities of daily living
2. Nutritional
   a. Client's average, maximum, and minimum weights during past month, 1 year, 5 years
   b. History of weight gains or losses (time element; specific efforts to change weight)
   c. Twenty-four-hour diet recall (helpful to mail client chart to fill in prior to visit)
   d. Current appetite
   e. Who buys, prepares food?
   f. Who does client normally eat with?
   g. Is client able to afford preferred food?
   h. Does client wear dentures? Is chewing a problem?
   i. Client's self-evaluation of nutritional status
3. Integumentary
   a. Skin
      (1) Skin disease or skin problems or lesions (wounds, sores, ulcers)
      (2) Skin growths, tumors, masses
      (3) Excessive dryness, sweating, odors
      (4) Pigmentation changes or discolorations
      (5) Pruritus (itching)
      (6) Texture changes
      (7) Temperature changes
   b. Hair
      (1) Changes in amount, texture, character
      (2) Alopecia (loss of hair)
      (3) Use of dyes
   c. Nails
      (1) Changes in appearance, texture
4. Head
   a. Headache (characteristics, including frequency, type, location, duration, care for)
   b. Past significant trauma
   c. Dizziness
   d. Syncope
5. Eyes
   a. Discharge (characteristics)
   b. History of infections, frequency, treatment
   c. Pruritus (itching)
   d. Lacrimation, excessive tearing
   e. Pain in eyeball

Physical History—cont'd

f. Spots (floaters)
g. Swelling around eyes
h. Cataracts, glaucoma
i. Unusual sensations or twitching
j. Vision changes (generalized or vision field)
k. Use of corrective or prosthetic devices
l. Diplopia (double vision)
m. Blurring
n. Photophobia
o. Difficulty reading
p. Interference with activities of daily living

6. Ears
   a. Pain (characteristics)
   b. Cerumen (wax)
   c. Infection
   d. Hearing changes (describe)
   e. Use of prosthetic devices
   f. Increased sensitivity to environmental noise
   g. Vertigo
   h. Ringing and cracking
   i. Care habits
   j. Interference with activities of daily living

7. Nose, nasopharynx, and paranasal sinuses
   a. Discharge (characteristics)
   b. Epistaxis
   c. Allergies
   d. Pain over sinuses
   e. Postnasal drip
   f. Sneezing
   g. General olfactory ability

8. Mouth and throat
   a. Sore throats (characteristics)
   b. Lesions of tongue or mouth (abscesses, sores, ulcers)
   c. Bleeding gums
   d. Hoarseness
   e. Voice changes
   f. Use of prosthetic devices (dentures, bridges)
   g. Altered taste
   h. Chewing difficulty
   i. Swallowing difficulty
   j. Pattern of dental hygiene

9. Neck
   a. Node enlargement
   b. Swellings, masses
   c. Tenderness
   d. Limitation of movement
   e. Stiffness

10. Breast
    a. Pain or tenderness
    b. Swelling
    c. Nipple discharge
    d. Changes in nipples
    e. Lumps, dimples
    f. Unusual characteristics
    g. Breast examination: pattern, frequency

11. Cardiovascular
    a. Cardiovascular
       (1) Palpitations
       (2) Heart murmur
       (3) Varicose veins
       (4) History of heart disease
       (5) Hypertension
       (6) Chest pain (character and frequency)
       (7) Shortness of breath
       (8) Orthopnea
       (9) Paroxysmal nocturnal dyspnea
    b. Peripheral vascular
       (1) Coldness, numbness
       (2) Discoloration
       (3) Peripheral edema
       (4) Intermittent claudication

12. Respiratory
    a. History of asthma
    b. Other breathing problems (when, precipitating factors)
    c. Sputum production
    d. Hemoptysis
    e. Chronic cough (characteristics)
    f. Shortness of breath (precipitating factors)
    g. Night sweats
    h. Wheezing or noise with breathing

13. Hematolymphatic
    a. Lymph node swelling
    b. Excessive bleeding or easy bruising
    c. Petechiae, ecchymoses
    d. Anemia
    e. Blood transfusions
    f. Excessive fatigue
    g. Radiation exposure

14. Gastrointestinal
    a. Food idiosyncrasies
    b. Change in taste
    c. Dysphagia (inability or difficulty in swallowing)

Physical History—cont'd

d. Indigestion or pain (associated with eating?)
e. Pyrosis (burning sensation in esophagus and stomach with sour eructation)
f. Ulcer history
g. Nausea/vomiting (time, degree, precipitating and/or associated factors)
h. Hematemesis
i. Jaundice
j. Ascites
k. Bowel habits (diarrhea/constipation)
l. Stool characteristics
m. Change in bowel habits
n. Hemorrhoids (pain, bleeding, amount)
o. Dyschezia (constipation due to habitual neglect to respond to stimulus to defecate)
p. Use of digestive or evacuation aids (what, how often)

15. Urinary
    a. Characteristics of urine
    b. History of renal stones
    c. Hesitancy
    d. Urinary frequency (in 24-hour period)
    e. Change in stream of urination
    f. Nocturia (excessive urination at night)
    g. History of urinary tract infection, dysuria (painful urination, urgency, flank pain)
    h. Suprapubic pain
    i. Dribbling or incontinence
    j. Stress incontinence
    k. Polyuria (excessive excretion or urine)
    l. Oliguria (decrease in urinary output)
    m. Pyuria

16. Genital
    a. General
       (1) Lesions
       (2) Discharges
       (3) Odors
       (4) Pain, burning, pruritus (itching)
       (5) Venereal disease history
       (6) Satisfaction with sexual activity
       (7) Birth control methods practiced
       (8) Sterility
    b. Males
       (1) Prostate problems
       (2) Penis and scrotum self-examination practices

c. Females
   (1) Menstrual history (age of onset, last menstrual period [LMP], duration, amount of flow, problems)
   (2) Amenorrhea (absence of menses)
   (3) Menorrhagia (excessive menstruation)
   (4) Dysmenorrhea (painful menses); treatment method
   (5) Metrorrhagia (uterine bleeding at times other than during menses)
   (6) Dyspareunia (pain with intercourse)

17. Musculoskeletal
    a. Muscles
       (1) Twitching
       (2) Cramping
       (3) Pain
       (4) Weakness
    b. Extremities
       (1) Deformity
       (2) Gait or coordination difficulties
       (3) Interference with activities of daily living
       (4) Walking (amount per day)
    c. Bones and joints
       (1) Joint swelling
       (2) Joint pain
       (3) Redness
       (4) Stiffness (time of day related)
       (5) Joint deformity
       (6) Noise with joint movement
       (7) Limitations of movement
       (8) Interference with activities of daily living
    d. Back
       (1) History of back injury (characteristics of problems, corrective measures)
       (2) Interference with activities of daily living

18. Central nervous system
    a. History of central nervous system disease
    b. Fainting episodes
    c. Seizure
       (1) Characteristics
       (2) Medications
    d. Cognitive changes
       (1) Inability to remember (recent vs. distant)
       (2) Disorientation

Physical History—cont'd

      (3) Phobias
      (4) Hallucinations
      (5) Interference with activities of daily living
    e. Motor-gait
      (1) Coordinated movement
      (2) Ataxia, balance problems
      (3) Paralysis (partial vs. complete)
      (4) Tic, tremor, spasm
      (5) Interference with activities of daily living
    f. Sensory
      (1) Paresthesia (patterns)
      (2) Tingling sensations
      (3) Other changes
19. Endocrine
    a. Diagnosis of disease states (thyroid, diabetes)
    b. Changes in skin pigmentation or texture
    c. Changes in or abnormal hair distribution
    d. Sudden or unexplained changes in height and weight
    e. Intolerance to heat or cold
    f. Exophthalmos
    g. Goiter
    h. Hormone therapy
    i. Polydipsia (↑ thirst)
    j. Polyphagia (↑ food intake)
    k. Polyuria (↑ urination)
    l. Anorexia (↓ appetite)
    m. Weakness
20. Allergic and immunological (Optional; use if client indicates allergic history. Note precipitating factors in each case.)
    a. Dermatitis (inflammation or irritation of skin)
    b. Eczema
    c. Pruritus (itching)
    d. Urticaria (hives)
    e. Sneezing
    f. Vasomotor rhinitis (inflammation and swelling of mucous membrane of nose; nasal discharge)
    g. Conjunctivitis (inflammation of conjunctiva)
    h. Interference with activities of daily living
    i. Environmental and seasonal correlation
    j. Treatment techniques
21. Does client have any other physiological problems or disease states not specifically discussed? If so, explore in detail (e.g., fatigue, insomnia, nervousness).

Health maintenance efforts

1. General statement of client's own physical fitness
2. Exercise (amount, type, frequency)
3. Dietary regulations; special efforts (describe in detail)
4. Mental health; special efforts such as group therapy, meditation, yoga (describe in detail)
5. Cultural or religious practices
6. Frequency of physical, dental, and vision health assessment

Environmental health

1. General statement of client's assessment of environmental safety and comfort
2. Hazards of employment (inhalants, noise, heavy lifting, psychological stress, machinery)
3. Hazards in the home (concern about fire, stairs to climb, inadequate heat, open gas heaters, inadequate toilet facilities, concern about pest control, inadequate space)
4. Hazards in neighborhood (noise, water, and air pollution, inadequate police protection, heavy traffic on surrounding streets, isolation from neighbors, overcrowding)
5. Community hazards (unavailability of stores, market, laundry facilities, drugstore; no access to bus line)

From Thompson, J., and Bowers, A.: Clinical manual of health assessment, St. Louis, 1980, The C.V. Mosby Co.

FAMILY ASSESSMENT TOOL

Facility _____

Assessor _____

Date _____

Guide to Family Analysis

Family genogram

1. Names, ages, ethnic and religious affiliation of all family members
2. Exact dates of birth, marriage, separation, divorce, death, and other significant life events
3. Notations with dates about occupation, grade in school, places of residence, illness, and changes in life course on the genogram itself
4. Information on three or more generations
5. Notation about frequency and type of contact (mail, telephone, visit, marriage, and funerals only)
6. Notation about closest and most distant relationships

Description of home environment

1. Characteristics of neighborhood, type of housing, ownership of housing, car
2. Adequacy of housing (safe, healthy, privacy, food preparation, temperature, space for children to play, yard)
3. Family satisfaction with housing, community
4. How does the family perceive the community's "attitude" toward it?
5. What are the private and public transportation facilities for the family? Are they a help or hindrance to their way of living?
6. What beauty exists in their environment? What efforts have they made to add beauty to the home?

Health and related factors

1. Physical level of growth and development, including developmental lags in the past
2. Past physical problems, including genetic and accidents
3. Current physical problems

4. Status of immunizations
5. Special physical abilities or hobbies, i.e., mechanical, gardening, sewing
6. What treatment does he rely upon before calling a physician?
7. How does he utilize medical resources (episodic or preventive)?
8. What is the family's usual source of health care, single or multiple?
9. What does the family's nutritional assessment reveal?
10. How susceptible to illness does the identified patient think he is? Does the family agree?
11. What is the identified patient's theory about his illness, i.e., to what does he attribute it? What is the family's theory?
12. How has the identified patient's illness changed the family's functioning? Who has been most involved in the care? Who has been most affected?
13. Mental abilities (social and/or academic performance, particular philosophical outlook, thought or language disorder)
14. Sense of self-esteem of family members
15. Sense of humor of family members
16. Personal appearance and hygiene of family members

Financial status

1. What is the family's annual income? Who earns it? Where?
2. What work and homemaking skills are available to each person?
3. How is money managed in this family?
4. If the family doesn't have an adult who is working, why isn't the adult able to work and

earn a living? (There is usually more than one reason.)

5. What consumer skills are available in the family? (Do they know how to comparison shop?) (Do they know how to determine what they need?) (Can they do home repair, sew, can food?)

6. Are there financial constraints on seeking health care?

Developmental state in family life cycle

1. Is the family in a normative crisis of transition?

2. Are there outstanding emotional tasks from previous stages unsuccessfully completed and impeding current family functioning?

3. What are the major emotional tasks confronting the family at this stage in the family life cycle?

4. How is the identified patient's illness influencing the emotional process of the family life cycle?

Family structure

1. Are the boundaries in the family clearly delineated or diffuse between the following:
   a. The marital subsystem
   b. The parental subsystem
   c. The sibling subsystem
   d. Individual subsystems
   e. The grandparent subsystem
   f. The sexes

2. Are there identifiable coalitions or alliances? What are the key family triangles?

3. Are authority and responsibility clearly defined and/or delegated? Does the responsibility to the delegated member exceed his physical or maturational capacities?

4. Are subsystem functions being performed and subsystem interpersonal skills being developed?

Intrafamily relationships

1. How do family members converse with each other? Is communication direct, clear, tangential, amorphous, covert? What kind of information is communicated? Is there a "central switchboard"?

2. How are decisions made (about vacations, discipline, large purchases, personal problems)?

3. How do they have fun together? Do they share time, space, money?

4. How do family members encourage separateness, recognize privacy, among members?

5. How is nurturance, recognition, support given to each other?

6. How is the marital relationship (emotionally and sexually satisfying or distant and conflictual)?

7. How does each parent relate to the children? What child-rearing skills do the parents have or lack?

8. How are children being taught to problem solve, to develop independence and self-reliance?

9. How do family members interact with the outside world (neighbors, schools, work, agencies, church)?

10. What is the nature of extended family relationships? (Is one side or both distant or cut off? Is contact formal and obligatory? Is contact open, regular, and emotionally meaningful even if infrequent?)

11. Who are the most significant members in the extended families? How are they significant?

Sociocultural family context

1. What is the ethnic or cultural background of the family? In what ways is this apparent in their way of living? In household furnishing?

2. Is there a religious belief? Affiliation? How does this influence each one or the family?

3. Have members in any way altered the cultural, ethnic, or religious practices or beliefs? What has been the result of these changes?

4. What are the dominant attitudes toward health, the community, achievement in school and career, toward life?

5. What dominant stereotyped sex-role expectations are expressed or demonstrated between husband and wife, between parents and children?

Strengths and weaknesses of the family

1. As seen by the family
2. As seen by the nurse

Problems identified

1. By the family
2. By the nurse
3. Solutions tried by the family to resolve the problems

From Helm, P.E.: Guide to family analysis, New Haven, Conn., 1982, Yale University School of Nursing.

DRUG ABUSE TERMS

This glossary* contains street language regarding the drugs of abuse. The same term may have different meanings in different areas.

a-boot Under the influence of drugs

Acapulco gold Mexican marijuana that contains about 1% or less of tetrahydrocannabinol (THC)

ace A marijuana cigarette

acid LSD (lysergic acid diethylamide)

acid head A user of LSD

ad Refers to an addict

all lit up Under the influence of a drug

amys Amyl nitrite ampules

angel dust Parsley leaves covered with phencyclidine, finely powdered hashish

Are you anywhere? Do you use marijuana?

around the turn Having gone through withdrawal period

artillery Equipment used for injecting and dissolving a powdered drug, or a solution of drugs

baby Marijuana

bad trip/bad acid An unpleasant reaction caused by a hallucinogenic drug, usually LSD; may be caused by taking a mixture of chemicals, resulting from an attempt at synthesis; emotions are dreadful and horrible; the images can be terrifying

bag (1) A package of drugs, usually marijuana or heroin; (2) a person's favorite "thing" or drug

bagman A person who supplies narcotics or other drugs; a pusher

ball Absorption of stimulants and cocaine through the genitalia

balloon A penny balloon that contains narcotics

bambita Desoxyn or amphetamine derivative

bammies A poor quality of marijuana

bang The injection of narcotics, usually heroin

banging Under the influence of drugs

barb(s) Barbiturates

barrels LSD tablets

batted out Apprehended by law

bean A capsule containing drugs

beat the gong Smoke opium

bedbugs Fellow addicts

behind the iron house Staying in jail

belongs On the habit

belted Under the influence of a drug

bending and bowing Under the influence of drugs

*From the Office of Training and Education for Addiction Services of the Maryland Department of Health and Mental Hygiene.

bennies Benzedrine tablets (amphetamines)

Bernice Cocaine

Bernie's flake Cocaine

bhang Marijuana

big bloke Cocaine

big C Cocaine

big D LSD

big John Police; law

big man A person who supplies drugs

big O Opium

bindle A package of narcotics (usually contains an ounce)

bingle A supplier of drugs

bingler A person selling narcotics

bingo The injection of drugs

biz Utensils used in dissolving and injecting narcotics and other drugs

black beauties Biphetamine capsules (amphetamines)

black magic LSD

black stuff Opium

blank Container of nonnarcotic powder that is sold as heroin

blast (1) Party, (2) a strong effect resulting from drug usage

blasted Under the influence of a drug

blow (1) To miss a vein when injecting, (2) to move from a place

blow Charlie or snow Sniff cocaine

blow horse Sniffing heroin

blow (pot) Smoke a cigarette that contains marijuana

blow your mind (1) To be high from a hallucinogenic drug, (2) to achieve a particular ecstatic mental level or high

blue acid LSD

blue angels, blue clouds, blue devils, blue heaven Amytal (amobarbital sodium) capsules

blue cheer LSD, methamphetamine, and strychnine tablets

blue heaven LSD

blue morphine Numorphan tablets (no longer made)

blue velvet (1) A mixture of Terpin Hydrate and Codeine Elixir and Pyribenzamine (tripelennamine) (antihistamine), (2) a mixture of Paregoric and antihistamine

bluebirds Amytal (amobarbital sodium) capsules

blues Amytal (amobarbital sodium)

bo bo bush Marijuana

bomb Heroin that is highly potent and relatively undiluted

bombida Methamphetamine

bombita An amphetamine injection, occasionally with heroin

boost Robbery

boxed Confined in jail

boy Heroin

brain pills Amphetamines

bread Money

brick Compressed block made of marijuana

broker A person who peddles dope to addicts

brown dots LSD

browns Multicolored capsules that are long-acting amphetamine sulfate

bull (1) A federal narcotics agent, (2) a police officer

bum trip A bad experience with psychedelics

bummer Another word for a "bad trip"

burn transaction Selling a substance as a certain drug when actually it is something else, e.g., goldenrod for marijuana

burned Getting cheated during a drug transaction

bush Marijuana

business Equipment used when injecting drugs

businessman's trip Dimethyltryptamine (DMT)

busted Arrested for possession of drugs

buttons Peyote buttons

buy A purchase of drugs

buzz Mild euphoric reaction to a drug

C Cocaine

C-joint A place where cocaine can be bought

cabbage head An individual who will use or experiment with any kind of drug

caca (1) Heroin; (2) an inferior quality of hashish, heroin, or LSD; (3) imitation or counterfeit heroin

cadet A new addict

California sunshine LSD

can A container that holds marijuana

candy Barbiturates

candy man A pusher

cannabis Marijuana

cap A gelatinous capsule that contains heroin or other drugs (usually one ounce or less)

Carrie Cocaine

cartwheels Amphetamine tablets

cashing a script Obtaining drugs by getting an illegal prescription filled

catch up A process of withdrawal

caught in a snow storm Being drugged by cocaine

CB Doriden (glutethimide) tablet

Cecil Cocaine

charge A quick drug effect

charged up Under the influence of drugs

chicken powder Some amphetamine powder

chief LSD

chip Use small injections occasionally

chipping Irregular use of small amounts of drugs

chocolate chips LSD

Cholley Cocaine

Christmas trees Tuinal (secobarbital sodium and amobarbital sodium) or Eskatrol (dextroamphetamine sulfate and prochlorperazine)

Cibas Doriden (glutethimide)

Cibees Doriden (glutethimide)

clean Not using drugs any longer

cleared up A withdrawal method

clipped Getting arrested

coasting Under the influence of drugs

coast-to-coast Long-acting amphetamines

coffee habit A beginner in the use of narcotics

coke Cocaine

cokie Cocaine addict

cold turkey Sudden withdrawal from narcotics

coming down Recovering from a drug experience or trip

connect To make a purchase of drugs

connection A drug supplier

contact lens LSD found on round gelatin flakes

cooker Bottle cap or spoon needed for heating and dissolving heroin in preparation for injection

cop To obtain drugs

cop a deuceway To buy a $2 pack of narcotics

cop man A supplier

cop out (1) Running away, (2) to leave, (3) to inform, (4) not participating, (5) to defect

cop-a-sneak To leave a place

co-pilots Amphetamine tablets

Corrine Cocaine

cotton shot When water is added to cotton to attempt to get remaining heroin out

crank Methamphetamine crystals

crashing Withdrawing from a drug experience

crashing pad Place where a user recovers from amphetamine use

crinic, cris, Cristina Methamphetamine

croaker A physician

croaker joint A hospital

crossroads Amphetamine tablets

crusher A police officer

crutch A device for holding a marijuana cigarette butt

crystal Methamphetamine (Methedrine); cocaine

crystal palace A room, location, or house where methamphetamine is injected

cube juice Morphine

cubehead A person who uses LSD frequently

cupcakes LSD

cut (1) To dilute a powder drug, usually a narcotic; (2) to dilute the potency of marijuana

cut out To leave a certain place

D Doriden (glutethimide) tablets

dabble To use small amounts of drugs infrequently

dead on arrival Phencyclidine base

dealer (1) A person who supplies drugs, (2) a pusher

deck A package of narcotics (usually an ounce)

dexies Dexedrine (dextroamphetamine sulfate) tablets or capsules (amphetamines)

diet pills Include amphetamine tablets or capsules

dime bag $10 purchase, usually marijuana

dirty Have drugs on you; can be arrested if searched

do a bit To spend time in jail

do righters Nonaddicts

DOA Phencyclidine base

doin' Using some kind of drug, such as "He is doin' cocaine"

dollies Dolophine (methadone) tablets

DOM STP (2,5-dimethoxy-4-methylamphetamine)

domes LSD tablets

domino To complete a purchase of drugs

doojee Heroin

dope Includes any narcotics, sometimes extended to other drugs

dope fiend A heroin addict

doper Someone who uses drugs regularly

double trouble Tuinal (secobarbital sodium and amobarbital sodium) capsule

down, downer, downie (1) Barbiturates, (2) tranquilizers

down it To swallow a pill or capsule

dream Cocaine

dried up Off drugs, especially heroin

dripper Eyedropper

drop To take a capsule or tablet orally

drop acid To take LSD

drop out To leave a place

dujie Heroin

dummy (1) A purchase in which there are no narcotics, (2) a poor quality of merchandise

dust Heroin, cocaine

dust of angels Phencyclidine base

dynamite (1) A high quality of heroin and cocaine taken together, (2) a strong drug

eighth Heroin (⅛ ounce) that is diluted with some inert powder

emsel Morphine

eye openers Amphetamines

factory The equipment used when injecting drugs

fall To be arrested

fall out When an addict nods or falls asleep on and off after injecting

far out (1) Out of touch with reality, (2) under the influence of drugs

Feds Federal agents

fine stuff Marijuana that is finely cut or manicured

fix An injection of a narcotic

fixed Under the influence of a drug

flake Cocaine

flash A euphoric feeling following an injection

flashback When a previous drug user hallucinates without taking the drug again

flats LSD tablets

flea powder Poor-quality heroin or heroin that is greatly diluted

flip Become psychotic

floating Under the influence of drugs

flying high Under the influence of marijuana

fold up A withdrawal procedure

folding stuff Money

foolish powder Heroin

footballs Amphetamine tablets or capsules that are oval shaped

freak A regular user of a particular drug, e.g., acid freak

freak out An experience that is unpleasant and frightful, resulting from the use of a drug

freeze When a sale is turned down

fresh and sweet A person coming out of jail

front of the bread The money is put up first for a drug purchase

fu Marijuana

Fuzz (1) A policeman, (2) a detective

Fuzzy tail Police

gage Marijuana

garbage A poor-quality drug

gazer A federal agent

GBs Seconal (secobarbital), Tuinal (secobarbital and amobarbital), or Doriden (glutethimide)

gear Refers to drugs in general

gee head A person who uses paregoric

geetis Money

geezer A needle shot of any type of narcotic

get beat To buy a package that does not contain any heroin

get a gift To obtain some narcotics

get high To smoke a cigarette containing marijuana

get off To inject or use drugs

get the wind To leave a place or area

gimmicks Equipment with which a person injects drugs

girl Cocaine

give wings Give the first heroin injection to a friend

glad rag A handkerchief or cloth saturated with substances to be inhaled

glass eyes A narcotic addict

glued Arrested

gluey An individual who sniffs glue vapors

G-man A federal agent

go in sewer Inject a drug into a vein

gold A Mexican marijuana that has 1% or less of tetrahydrocannabinol (THC)

gold dust Cocaine

good go Purchase a fair amount of narcotics for the money

good trip Psychedelic drugs that cause good emotional feelings and pleasant imagery

goods (1) Narcotics, (2) includes any drugs

goofball Barbiturate

gorilla pills Doriden (glutethimide)

gow head Addict

gram The cube form of hashish

grape parfait LSD

grass Marijuana

green domes LSD tablets

greenies The mixture of barbiturates and amphetamines found in a green heart-shaped tablet

griefo Marijuana

gun (1) Eyedropper, (2) syringe, (3) hypodermic needle

H Heroin

hack Physician

hairy Heroin

half spoon Half a teaspoonful of heroin

hand-to-hand Paying for drugs when they are delivered

hang-up (1) A personal problem or personality problem, (2) a withdrawal

happy dust Cocaine

hard narcotics Includes all addicting narcotics

hard stuff Includes any addicting narcotic, e.g., heroin, morphine

harness bull Police

Harry Heroin

hash Hashish

hassle The procedure of buying drugs, preparing them, and taking the injection

Hawaiian sunshine LSD

hay Marijuana

head A person who depends on drugs

hearts Amphetamine tablets that are heart shaped

heat The police

heaven dust Cocaine

heavenly blue Morning glory seeds

heavy man Someone who possesses narcotics

hemp Marijuana

high Under the influence of drugs

hit To make a purchase of drugs

hitting the pipe, hitting the steam Smoking opium

hitting the stuff Under the influence of drugs

hitting up The act of injecting drugs

hocus Morphine

hog Vegetable material that has phencyclidine in it

holding To have drugs in one's possession

hooked Dependent on drugs

hop Opium

hop head A narcotic addict, mainly an opium addict

hoppie A narcotic addict

horner One who sniffs narcotics

horse Heroin

hot (1) Sought by police, (2) stolen articles, merchandise

hotshot A fatal injection of heroin, that may have been intentional

hot sticks Marijuana cigarettes

hustle (1) Prostitution, (2) any activity used to obtain money for heroin

hustler Prostitute

hype Addict

ice-cream habit Nonregular drug use

iced In jail

I'm beat I need a marijuana cigarette

I'm holding I am carrying drugs

I'm way down I need a marijuana lift

in high Under the influence of drugs

in a jam Wanted by the police

Indian bay, Indian hay Marijuana

into Involved with a drug, e.g., "She is into acid"

jab (1) To inject a drug, (2) a hypodermic shot

jag (1) Under the influence of drugs, (2) under the influence of amphetamines

jay Marijuana cigarette

jelly beans Tuinal (secobarbital sodium and amobarbital sodium)

jive Marijuana

jive sticks, joints Marijuana cigarettes

jolly beans Pep pills

Jones A habit

joy popping (1) Subcutaneously injecting a drug, (2) irregular drug habit

joy powder Cocaine

jump skid To leave a place

junk (1) Heroin, (2) can denote any drug

junker, junkie Addict (heroin)

kee A kilogram of a drug, usually heroin

keif Hashish

kick To get rid of a habit

kick the habit To stop using narcotics or drugs in general

kick sticks Marijuana cigarettes

kicking A withdrawal process

kicking the gong To be around an area where narcotics are sold

kilo A kilogram of drugs equivalent to 2.2 pounds

kit Equipment used when injecting drugs

knocking on the door When an addict is trying to stay away from other addicts while attempting to quit a habit

LA turnabouts Various colored capsules that are long-acting amphetamine sulfate

lay out (1) Equipment for injecting drugs, (2) opium smoker's outfit

laying on the hip Smoking opium

laying the hypo Receiving or taking a shot of narcotics

LBJ-336-JB-336 Methyl piperidyl benzilate (hallucinogen)

leader User of cocaine

leaping Under the influence of drugs

lemonade Poor-quality heroin or any merchandise

lettuce Money

lid A measure of marijuana in a sale

lid poppers Amphetamines

lid proppers Amphetamines

lie down To smoke opium

light artillery A hypodermic addict

Lipton tea Poor-quality merchandise

lit up Under the influence of drugs

load A quantity of 25 bags of heroin

loco weed Marijuana

log Marijuana cigarette

long green Money

love drug (1) MDA (methylene dioxyamphetamine), (2) methaqualone (soapers)

love weed Marijuana

LSD Lysergic acid diethylamide

m Morphine

machinery Utensils used when injecting drugs

magic mushroom A mushroom containing psilocybin

magic pumpkin seed An STP (2,5-dimethoxy-4-methylamphetamine) tablet shaped like a pumpkin seed

mainlining Shooting or injecting a drug directly into a vein

maintaining Keeping a particular level of a drug effect

make a croaker To trick a physician into giving narcotics

make a meet To make a buy

make a reader To get a physician to fill out a prescription

make the turn A withdrawal process

man (1) Policeman, (2) detective

manicure Removal of seeds, dirt, and stems from dried marijuana

Mary Jane, Mary Warner Marijuana

merchandise Narcotics or any drug in general

mesc Mescaline (hallucinogenic drug from the peyote cactus)

meth (1) Methamphetamine, (2) methadone, (3) methedrine, (4) methaqualone

meth head A regular use of methamphetamine

meth run Constant intravenous injection of methamphetamine

Mexican horse Mexican (brown) heroin

Mexican reds Secobarbital capsules

mezz Marijuana

Mickey Chloral hydrate

Mickey Finn The mixture of chloral hydrate plus alcohol

micro dots LSD

mikes Micrograms (millionths of a gram)

mind benders, mind blowers Hallucinogens

Miss Emma Morphine

MJ Marijuana

monkey A drug habit in which there is a physical dependence

monster Methamphetamine

mootos Marijuana cigarettes

mor-a-grifa Marijuana

morph, morphie, morpho Morphine

mouth worker A narcotic addict who swallows his drugs

Mr. Whiskers Federal agents

mud Asthmador mixed with a carbonated cola beverage

muggles Marijuana cigarettes

mule A supplier of drugs

mutah Marijuana

nail Needle

nailed Arrested

narc, narco Federal, state, or local narcotic officer

needle The syringe for injecting drugs

needle freak A person who enjoys using a needle

nibies Nembutal (pentobarbital sodium)

nickel bag (1) A $5 purchase of marijuana, (2) a measure of heroin

nimby Nembutal (pentobarbital sodium)

noise Heroin

nose candy Cocaine

OD An overdose of drugs or narcotics, resulting in death or a coma

OJ Opium joint, a marijuana cigarette that has been dipped or smeared in opium

on ice In jail

on the beam Feeling good

on the blues Using Numorphan (oxymorphone hydrochloride)

on the bricks, on the ground Out of jail

on the nod The cycle of dozing and awakening when using heroin

on the street Out of jail

on a trip Under the influence of LSD

orange wedges LSD

oranges Heart-shaped amphetamine tablets containing Dexedrine (dextroamphetamine sulfate)

out of it Nonaddict

outfit Equipment used when injecting drugs

over the hump The completion of withdrawal

Owsley's acid LSD

pad A person's habitat or room

Pam freak Person who inhales aerosolized products

Panatella A large strong marijuana cigarette

panic man Addict who has lost his source of drugs

paper (1) A package of drugs (usually a quantity of 1 ounce), (2) prescription

PCP Phencyclidine

PCPA *p*-Chlorophenylalanine

peace (1) LSD tablets, (2) STP (2,5-dimethoxy-4-methylamphetamine)

peace pill Phencyclidine

peace tablet LSD tablets

peaches Benzedrine (amphetamine sulfate) tablets

peanuts Barbiturates

pearly gates Morning glory seeds

peddler Dealer in drugs

pee Heroin powder

pep pills Amphetamine capsules or tablets

Pepsi Cola habit A small habit

Peter Chloral hydrate

PG, PO Paregoric

pickup To buy drugs

piece (1) A measure of narcotics, (2) a holder of drugs

pig Policeman

piki A person who smokes opium

pillhead A person who often uses drugs, usually amphetamines and barbiturates

pillows Sealed polyethylene bags that contain drugs

pin yen Opium

pinks Seconal (secobarbital sodium) capsules

pipe (1) To look, (2) an opium utensil

plant A place to hide drugs

play around Irregular use of drugs

pod Marijuana

pop To inject drugs, usually below the skin

poppers Amyl nitrite ampules

pot Marijuana or hashish

pothead Marijuana user

product IV Combination capsules of PCP and LSD

purple barrels, purple haze, purple ozone LSD

purple rock A mixture of caffeine, barbiturates, heroin, and strychnine

push shorts To cheat a buyer of drugs; to sell short amounts of drugs

pusher A person who peddles drugs, narcotics, marijuana

R and R, ripple and reds Taking secobarbital capsules when drinking Ripple wine

rainbows Tuinal (secobarbital sodium and amobarbital sodium) capsules

red birds, red devils, red lilies, reds Secobarbital capsules

red rock Mixture of heroin and strychnine, barbiturates, and caffeine

reefer Marijuana cigarette

riding the wave Under the influence of narcotics

roach A marijuana cigarette butt

roach clip A device that holds a marijuana cigarette butt

robe Robitussin A-C cough syrup (guaifenesin and codeine phosphate)

robo, romo Codeine

rope Marijuana

roses Benzedrine (amphetamine sulfate) tablets

run Continuing the injection of methamphetamine

Sam Federal agent

satch cotton Cotton used to strain drugs before injection

sativa Marijuana

scag Heroin

scene Place where a person can buy drugs

schmack (1) Heroin, (2) cocaine

schoolboy Codeine

score To purchase drugs

scrap iron A bootleg drink made with a hypochlorite solution, alcohol, and mothballs

scratch Prescription

script Physician's prescription

script writer A person who forges prescriptions

seccy, seggy Seconal (secobarbital sodium) capsules

seeds Morning glory seeds

serenity, tranquility, and peace STP (2,5-dimethoxy-4-methylamphetamine)

sewer Vein

sex drug Methaqualone (soapers) or STP (2,5-dimethoxy-4-methylamphetamine)

sex juice An aphrodisiac

sharps Needles

shit (1) Heroin, (2) poor-quality heroin, hashish, or LSD, (3) drugs

shoot up To inject drugs

shooting gallery Location, room, or house where drugs are injected

shooting The injection of drugs

short go To take a small portion of narcotics

shot down Under the influence of drugs

shrink Psychiatrist

sizzling Sought by police

skee Opium

skid (1) Heroin, (2) to leave a place

skin popping The injecting of a narcotic underneath the skin

slammed In jail

sleepers, sleeping pills Barbiturates

sleigh ride Under the influence of drugs

smack (1) Heroin, (2) cocaine

smash Marijuana that has been cooked with acetone, the oil residue of which is added to hashish

smears LSD

smoke (1) Wood alcohol, (2) marijuana

snappers Amyl nitrite ampules

sniffer A narcotic addict who takes drugs through his nose

sniffing Inhaling solvents, cleaning fluid, etc.

snort The inhalation of cocaine or heroin through the nose

snorter A person who sniffs drugs through his nose

snow Cocaine crystals

snowbird Cocaine addict

soapers Methaqualone (sleeping pill)

sound Benactyzine

spaghetti sauce Robitussin A-C cough syrup (guaifenesin and codeine phosphate)

speed Amphetamines, usually methedrine

speed demon Methamphetamine user

speed freak Frequent methamphetamine user

speedball A mixture of heroin and cocaine that is taken intravenously

spike Hypodermic needle

splash Amphetamine powder

splim Marijuana

split To leave a place

splivins Amphetamine powder

spoon (1) A measure of heroin, (2) the spoon used for dissolving heroin over heat

spots Dextroamphetamine

square An individual who does not use drugs

squirrels LSD

star dust Cocaine

stash A safe place to keep drugs

station worker A user of narcotics who injects into his arms or legs

stick Marijuana cigarette

stinking Under the influence of drugs

stoned (1) Under the influence of drugs, (2) a relaxed, pleasant state of mind

stoolie Informer

stoppers Barbiturates

straight (1) Not using any drugs, (2) not having any drugs in one's possession

strawberry field LSD

street market Black market

strung out An amphetamine overdose

stuff Narcotics

stumblers (1) Barbiturates, (2) tranquilizers

sunshine LSD

superman pills Amphetamines

sweet Lucy Marijuana

swing man A supplier of drugs

syrup Codeine

TMA A combination of mescaline, LSD, and tetrahydrocannabinol

T-man A federal agent

take a powder, take the wind To leave a certain area

taking a main Injecting directly into the vein

tar Opium

taste A small amount of narcotics

tea Marijuana

tea pad The place where a group of people smoke marijuana

tea party A party where mostly everyone is smoking marijuana

teed up Intoxicated by a large quantity of drugs

Texas tea Marijuana

the bag The bag used to sniff airplane glue or cleaning fluid

the confidence drug Amphetamine

the one A material like hashish, supposedly natural tetrahydrocannabinol

thing A person's particular interest, often refers to a specific drug

three-day-habit The irregular use of drugs

TNT Heroin

toak (toke) A drag off a marijuana cigarette

to be off A process of withdrawal

toke pipe A short-stem pipe used for smoking marijuana

tooies Tuinal (secobarbital sodium and amobarbital sodium) capsules

tools Equipment used when injecting drugs

toy A small container of drugs

tracks Needle scars that result from frequent injecting of drugs

tranquility STP (2,5-dimethoxy-4-methylamphetamine)

travel agent LSD pusher

trey A purchase worth $3

trip A hallucinogenic drug experience

tripping out Under the influence of any hallucinogen

truck drivers Amphetamine tablets

tuies Tuinal (secobarbital sodium and amobarbital sodium)

turkey The absence of drugs or narcotics

turkey trots Scars and marks left from the use of a hypodermic needle

turn off To quit using drugs

turn on (1) To introduce a person to the use of drugs, (2) any stimulating experience caused by the use of drugs

turn up To feel the influence of a drug

turned on Under the influence of drugs

turps Terpin Hydrate and Codeine Elixir (a cough syrup)

twenty-five LSD

twist A marijuana cigarette

twisted Intense sedation caused by the use of drugs

uncle, Uncle Sam Federal narcotics agent

unkie Morphine

upper, ups Amphetamine tablets

viper's weed Marijuana

wake ups, washed ups Amphetamines

washed up A withdrawal process

wasted Under the influence of drugs

wedges (1) Dexedrine (dextroamphetamine sulfate) tablets, (2) LSD tablets

weed Marijuana

weekend habit The irregular use of drugs

wen shee Gum opium

whickers Federal agents

white junk Heroin

white lightening LSD

white merchandise, white stuff Morphine

whites Amphetamines

whiz bang A combination of morphine and cocaine, or heroin and cocaine, used by the old addicts

window glass A square gelatin flake that contains LSD

work the leather To leave an area

works Equipment used when injecting drugs

yellow birds Nembutal (pentobarbital sodium)

yellow dimples LSD

yellow jackets, yellow submarines, yellows Nembutal (pentobarbital sodium) capsules

yen hook The utensil used when smoking opium

yen shee The ashes from opium

yen sleep A period of restlessness and drowsiness during a withdrawal process

FREQUENTLY USED BEHAVIORAL RATING SCALES

The Beck Depression Inventory[1,4]

The Beck Depression Inventory consists of 13 multiple choice clinical items. This is a self-report scale, designed to measure the depth of depression as well as to rapidly screen depressed patients. The Beck is applicable to psychiatric and medical patients with depressive illness. It covers the time span at the rating session, i.e., "right now." The items measure sadness, pessimism, sense of failure, dissatisfaction, guilt, self-dislike, self-harm, social withdrawal, indecisiveness, self-image change, work difficulty, fatigability, anorexia.

Brief Psychiatric Rating Scale (BPRS)[4,8]

The 18 items of this rating scale provide rapid and efficient evaluation of treatment response in both clinical drug trials and routine clinical settings; its focus is primarily adult inpatient psychopathology, although it has been used in outpatient settings. It is designed to be scored after a 45-minute interview by a clinician on a Likert-type scale (0, not assessed, to 5, extremely severe). Span of 1 week between interviews is suggested. The scale items are: somatic concern, anxiety, emotional withdrawal, conceptual disorganization, guilt feelings, tension, mannerisms, grandiosity, depressive mood, hostility, suspiciousness, hallucinatory behavior, motor retardation, uncooperativeness, unusual thought content, blunted affect, excitement, disorientation.

Clinical Global Impressions (CGI)[4]

This rating scale consists of three global items which are for use in all research/psychiatric populations and designed to be administered by a clinician with at least some clinical experience. The first two items are rated on a 7-point scale, while the third item requires a rating of the interaction of drug therapeutic effectiveness and adverse reactions. The items of the CGI are 1) severity of illness (1, normal, not ill, to 7, among the most extremely ill patients); 2) global improvement: (1, very much improved, to 7, very much worse); and 3) efficacy index, rated on the basis of drug effect only (therapeutic improvement as compared with severity of side effects). Severity of illness is rated pre- and post-treatment and at the discretion of the clinician. It measures the time period of "now, or within the last week." Global improvement requires no pretreatment measurement; a post-treatment measurement is done, and more frequent measurements at the discretion of the clinician. It measures the time period "since admission to the study (program, or unit)." Efficacy index is rated like global improvement, but the time period is "now, or within the last week."

Hamilton Anxiety Scale (HAM-A)[4,6]

This 14-item scale was designed for use with patients already diagnosed as suffering from anxiety. The scale utilizes a 5-point Likert scale (0, not present, to 4, very severe), with the highest score rarely applicable in outpatient settings. The scale places great emphasis on the patient's subjective state, and the scale questions are answered by directly eliciting the patient's subjective feelings. In treatment, the patient's subjective state takes first place both as a criterion of illness, which brings the patient for treatment, and as a criterion of improvement. The scale items measure: anxious mood, tension, fears, insomnia, intellectual (cognitive) difficulty, depressed mood, general muscular somatic complaints, general sensory somatic complaints, cardiovascular symptoms, respiratory symptoms, gastrointestinal symptoms, genitourinary symptoms, autonomic symptoms, patient's behavior during interview. The HAM-A can be used as frequently as the clinician feels necessary.

Hamilton Psychiatric Rating Scale for Depression (HAM-D)[4,5]

The 21 items of this rating scale provide a simple way of quantitatively assessing the severity of an adult patient's condition, and for showing changes in that condition. It is not to be used as a diagnostic instrument. It is useful as both an inpatient and outpatient scale; it is designed to be scored after a 45-minute interview by a clinician. The scoring is multiple choice. A span of 3 to 7 days between interviews is suggested. It is desirable to supplement information the patient gives by questioning significant others and other staff. The scale items measure: depressed mood, guilt, suicide, insomnia, work and activities, retardation, agitation, anxiety, somatic symptoms, genital symptoms, hypochondriasis, weight loss, insight, diurnal variation, depersonalization and derealization, paranoid symptoms, and obsessive/compulsive symptoms.

Manic-State Rating Scale[2]

This rating scale is a quantitative measure of manic symptomatology. Each of 26 items is rated with a Likert-type scale on two parameters: frequency of observed behavior (0, none, to 5, all) and intensity of behavior (1, very minimal, to 5, very marked). The scale is designed to be used by clinical staff trained to work with manic patients and has good inter-rater reliability. Beigel and co-workers suggest that the scale can be used as frequently as every 8 hours on an inpatient service because it measures overt behavior, and manics frequently have mood swings. The items cover: looks depressed, talking, moving, threatening, poor judgment, inappropriate dress, happy and cheerful, seeks out others, distractable, grandiose, irritable, combative or destructive, delusional, verbalized depressed feelings, active, argumentative, talks about sex, angry, careless in dress and grooming, poor impulse control, suspicious, verbalizes feelings of well-being, makes unrealistic plans, demands contact with others, sexually preoccupied, jumps from one subject to another.

Nurses' Observation Scale for Inpatient Evaluation (NOSIE)[4,7]

This 30-item scale was designed for the assessment of adult and geriatric ward behavior by nursing personnel. It provides measures of the patient's strengths as well as pathology. It uses a five-point Likert-type scale (0, never, to 5, always). The items are written in simple language and ask for ratings based on the direct observation of behavior. The scale clusters into three positive factors: social competence, social interest, personal neatness, and four negative factors: irritability, manifest psychosis, retardation, depression. It is useful to include the observations of many ward personnel. A span of 3 to 7 days between ratings is suggested.

Self-report Symptom Check List— 90 (SCL—90)[3,4]

This 90-item scale was designed to be rated by the patient. It presents a list of problems and complaints that people sometimes have and it asks the patient to rate "how much that problem has bothered or distressed you during the past week, including today." This tool uses a 5-point Likert scale (0, not at all, to 4, extremely). Patients obviously have to be well enough to do the scale and should be encouraged not to take too long on any one item. The scale should take 15 minutes to complete. The items cluster into 9 subscales which measure: somatization, obsessive-compulsive, interpersonal sensitivity, depression, anxiety, anger-hostility, phobic anxiety, paranoid ideation, and psychoticism. The scale is designed for adults in psychiatric and nonpsychiatric outpatient settings, and should be utilized at least pre- and post-treatment. Many clinicians use it weekly.

■ REFERENCES ■

1. Beck, A.T., and Beamesderfer, A.: Assessment of depression: the depression inventory. In Pichot, P. (editor) Psychological measurements in psychopharmacology, Vol. 7, pp. 151–169, Karger, 1974, Basel, Switzerland.
2. Beigel, A., Murphy, M.D., Bunney Jr., W.E.: The Manic-state rating scale, Arch. Gen. Psychiatry **25**:256 Sept. 1971.
3. Derogatis, L.R., Lipman, R.S., Covi, L., et al.: Dimensions of outpatient neurotic pathology: comparison of a clinical vs. an empirical assessment. J. Consult. Clin. Psychol. **34**:102 1970.
4. Guy, W.: ECDEU assessment manual for psychopharmacology, revised. Rockville, Md., 1976, U.S. Department of Health, Education, and Welfare, National Institute of Mental Health, Psychopharmacology Research Branch, Division of Extramural Research Program.
5. Hamilton, M.: Development of a rating scale for primary depressive illness, Br. J. Soc. Clin. Psychol. **6**:278–296, 1967.
6. Hamilton, M.: Diagnosis and rating of anxiety. In Lader, M.D., editor: Studies of anxiety, Br. J. Psychiatry (Spec. and Pub.) **3**:76–79, 1969.
7. Honigfeld, G., and Klett, C.: The Nurses' Observation Scale for Inpatient Evaluation (NOSIE): a new scale for measuring improvement in chronic schizophrenia, J. Clin. Psychol. **21**:65–71, 1965.
8. Overall, J.E.: The Brief Psychiatric Rating Scale in psychopharmacology research, Psychometric Laboratory Reports, No. 29, Galveston, University of Texas, June 1972.

GLOSSARY

abreaction Ventilation of feelings that takes place as an individual verbally recounts emotionally charged areas.

absolute discharge A final and complete termination of the patient's relationship with the hospital.

abuse An act of misuse, exploitation, deceit; wrong or improper use or action so as to injure, damage, maltreat, or corrupt.

accountability Self-regulation and responsibility for the quality of one's nursing care.

acrophobia Fear of high places.

acting out Indirect expression of feelings through behavior, usually nonverbal, that attracts the attention of others.

action cues A category of nonverbal communication that consists of body movements and is sometimes referred to as *kinetics*.

activities of daily living When applied to the chronically mentally ill, refers to the skills necessary to live independently as an adult.

adolescence The period from the beginning of puberty to the attainment of maturity. The transitional stage during which the youth is becoming an adult man or woman. This period is described in terms of development in many different functions that may be reached at different times. Only conventional limits may be stated: 12 to 21 girls, 13 to 22 boys.

adventitious crisis Accidental, uncommon, and unexpected crisis that may result in multiple losses and gross environmental changes.

advocacy One method by which patients, mental health professionals, attorneys, and concerned citizens can work together to improve and protect the rights of all citizens to high-quality mental health care that is clinically and constitutionally appropriate.

affect Feeling; mood.

aggression Mental drive to action that encompasses both constructive and destructive activities.

agonist In pharmacology, a substance that acts with, enhances, or potentiates a specific activity.

agoraphobia Overwhelming symptoms of anxiety, often leading to a panic attack in a variety of everyday situations (i.e., standing in line, eating in public, being in crowds of people, on bridges, in tunnels, or driving) in which a person might have an attack and be unable to escape, get help, or be embarrassed.

akathisia Motor restlessness ranging from a feeling of inner disquiet, often localized in the muscles, to inability to sit still or lie quietly; a side effect of some antipsychotic drugs.

alcoholic hallucinosis A medical diagnosis referring to an alcohol withdrawal syndrome that is characterized by auditory hallucinations in the absence of any other psychotic symptoms.

alcohol withdrawal delirium A medical diagnosis for a serious alcohol withdrawal syndrome that is characterized by delirium and autonomic hyperactivity occurring within 1 week of reduction of alcohol intake.

alcoholism Any degree of dependency, physical or psychological, on alcohol to the extent that it interferes with normal life activities.

alexithymia The inability to consciously experience and communicate feelings.

alliance A relationship based on shared common interests.

altruism A sense of concern for the welfare of others that can be expressed at the level of the individual or the larger social system.

ambivalence An inability to make decisions based on double approach-avoidance conflict feelings.

amino acids Any organic acid containing one or more amino groups, they are integral parts of proteins and are precursors of brain neurotransmitters.

amnesia Loss of memory for a specific period of time or a loss of all past memories.

anaclitic depression A deprivational reaction in infants separated from their mothers in the second half of the first year of life. The reaction is characterized by apprehension, crying, withdrawal, psychomotor slowing, dejection, stupor, insomnia, anorexia, and gross retardation in growth and development.

anger A feeling that is an expression of the anxiety aroused by a real or perceived threat to one's rights, possessions, values, or significant others.

anorexia nervosa An eating disorder in which the person experiences hunger, but refuses to eat based on a distorted body image leading to a self-perception of obesity. Starvation ensues.

antagonist A substance or a drug that reduces or blocks the action of another substance or drug; by competing with another substance for the same receptor site, one of the substances is prevented from binding to the receptors and thus its effects are prevented.

anticipatory guidance Information and advice given to patients for future therapeutic purposes.

antisocial personality A personality disorder characterized by manipulativeness, disregard for social norms, and a lack of concern for others.

anxiety A diffuse apprehension that is vague in nature and is associated with feelings of uncertainty and helplessness. It is an emotion without a specific object, is subjectively experienced by the individual, and is communicated interpersonally. It occurs as a result of a threat to the person's being, self-esteem, or identity.

ascribed role An assigned role, such as age and sex, about which the individual has no choice.

assertiveness Behavior that is directed toward claiming one's rights without denying the rights of others.

assertiveness training An application of the behavioral model of psychiatric care. The patient is taught to stand up for his rights while not infringing on the rights of others.

assessment A phase of the nursing process in which information about the health status of a patient is systematically obtained, communicated, and recorded. Also known as the *nursing assessment.*

associationist model of learning A theory which defines learning as behavioral change that is a result of reinforced practice.

assumed role Role the individual selects or achieves by choice, such as occupational or marital roles.

attachment State of being emotionally attracted to a person and highly dependent upon that person for emotional satisfaction.

attention The element of cognitive functioning that refers to the maintenance of mental focus on a specific issue, activity, or object.

authority A relation between two or more persons such that the commands, suggestions, or ideas of one of them influence the other(s).

authority figure Person(s) who by virtue of status, role, or recognized superiority in knowledge, strength, etc., exerts influence in the authority relation.

autism A preoccupation with the self and with inner experiences.

autistic thought Ideation that has a private meaning to the individual.

autonomy The socially sanctioned condition that allows for the definition and control over one's work domain, achieved through a negotiated process.

autonomy drive The tendency for the individual to attempt to master the environment and to impose his purposes on it.

aversion therapy An application of the behavioral model of psychiatric care. A painful stimulus is given to create an aversion to another stimulus that leads to a behavior the individual wishes to change.

baseline behavior (or operant level) Specified rate (frequency and form) of a particular behavior during preintervention or preexperimental conditions.

baseline condition Environmental condition during which a particular behavior reflects a stable rate of responding, prior to the introduction of intervention or experimental conditions.

battered wife Any woman who is beaten by her mate, regardless of the legality of the marital relationship.

behavior Any observable, recordable, and measurable act, movement, or response of an individual.

behavior hierarchy A graded list of behavioral segments, beginning with the baseline behavior and gradually moving up to the terminal behavior.

behavior modification Changing and controlling behavior through the application of techniques derived from learning theory.

benzodiazepines A group of chemically related antianxiety drugs.

biofeedback A method of tension reduction in which electrodes are attached to the person's forehead, and he is then instructed to concentrate on relaxing, which will reduce the pitch of the biofeedback tone created by his tension. The lower the tone, the greater the muscle relaxation.

biological psychiatry A school of psychiatric thought that emphasizes physical, chemical, and neurologic causes and treatment approaches.

bipolar affective disorder A subgroup of the affective disorders that is characterized by at least one episode of manic behavior, with or without a history of episodes of depression.

bisexuality Sexual attraction to persons of both sexes and engagement in both homosexual and heterosexual activities.

blocking An interruption in the flow of speech due to the intrusion of distracting thoughts.

blood levels The concentration of a drug in the plasma, serum, or blood. In psychiatry, the term is most often applied to levels of lithium or some tricyclic antidepressants. Maximum clinical responses to these agents have been correlated with specific ranges of blood levels.

board and care home A site for housing discharged patients which may provide a shared room, three meals a day, the dispensing of medication, and minimal staff supervision.

body image Sum of the conscious and unconscious attitudes the individual has toward his body. It includes present and past perceptions, as well as feelings about size, function, appearance, and potential.

body language The transmission of a message by body position or movement.

borderline personality An individual with instability of mood, interpersonal relationships, and self-image, with a marked lack of a sense of identity.

buccolinguomasticatory triad A complex of lips, tongue, jaw, and head movements that are associated with tardive dyskinesia.

bulimia An eating disorder that is characterized by uncontrollable binge eating, alternating with vomiting or dieting.

burnout A syndrome of physical and emotional exhaustion, involving the development of negative self-concept, negative job attitudes, and loss of concern and feeling for clients. It may lead to physical illness, irritability, cynicism, fatigue, and withdrawal from one's nursing work.

butyrophenones A group of chemically related antipsychotic drugs.

camisole restraint A straitjacket; a shirtlike garment that restrains the arms.

case management The assignment of a mental health care provider to assist a patient in assessing the health care and social services systems and to assure that all required services are obtained.

case manager A clinician who accepts responsibility for identifying, securing, and coordinating all the resources necessary for a mentally ill client to live in the community.

catatonic A state of psychologically induced immobilization at times interrupted by episodes of extreme agitation.

catatonic excitement A state of extreme agitation that occurs when a person is unable to maintain catatonic immobility.

catatonic stupor An apparently unresponsive state that is related to a fear of loss of impulse control.

catharsis Release that occurs when the patient is encouraged to talk about things which bother him most. Fears, feelings, and experiences are brought out into the open and discussed.

cathexis Freud's term for the attachment of psychic energy (libido) to an object or mental construct.

certification The successful outcome of a formal review process of the clinical practice of a nurse who is required to show a high degree of proficiency in interpersonal skills, use of the nursing process, and psychiatric, psychological, and milieu therapies.

child An individual who is prepubescent (in infancy, of preschool age, of school age, or preadolescent).

child abuse Physical injury or sexual or emotional abuse that occurs when children are ignored, isolated, or continually shamed and demeaned.

chronic illness The process of progressive deterioration, with increasing symptoms, functional impairment, and disability over time.

chronic mental disability A label applied to an individual who has had either one continuous psychiatric hospitalization within the past 5 years or two or more psychiatric hospitalizations in a 12-month period.

circumstantial speech Inclusion of many nonessential details in a response.

clang association A speech pattern characterized by rhyming.

claustrophobia A fear of closed places.

client-centered mental health consultation A format through which the consultant focuses on helping the consultee find the most effective treatment for a client.

clinical nurse specialist A master's degree prepared nurse with a concentration in a specific area of clinical nursing.

coalition A power relationship composed either of two like partners joined together against an unlike opponent or an unlike partner joined together against an opponent who is like one of the partners. Partners can be differentiated by gender or generation.

cognition The ego function that relates to the process of logical thought.

cognitive model of learning A theory that defines learning as behavioral change based on the acquisition of information about the environment.

cohesiveness Force that attracts members to a group and causes them to remain in the group.

coitus Sexual intercourse with a partner of the opposite sex.

cold, wet sheet pack A form of somatic therapy in which the patient is swathed in cold, wet sheets, which then are warmed by body heat. The warmth and immobilization are soothing to very agitated people.

collective bargaining The use of collective action in negotiating patient care and economic issues with one's employer, including wages, hours, and conditions of work.

commitment Involuntary admission in which the request for hospitalization did not originate with the patient. When he is committed, he loses the right to leave the hospital when he wishes. It is usually justified on the grounds that the patient is dangerous to self or others and needs treatment.

community mental health A treatment philosophy based on the social model of psychiatric care that advocates a comprehensive range of mental health services that are to be made readily available to all community members.

compensation Process by which a person makes up for a deficiency in his image of himself by strongly emphasizing some other feature that he regards as an asset.

competent community A population that is aware of resources and alternatives, can make reasoned decisions about issues facing them, and can cope adaptively with problems. It parallels the concept of positive mental health.

compromise A task-oriented coping reaction that involves changing one's usual way of operating, substituting goals, or sacrificing aspects of one's personal needs. Compromise reactions are usually constructive and are frequently employed in approach-approach and avoidance-avoidance situations.

compulsion A recurring irresistible impulse to perform some act.

concrete operation A thought process based on a concrete rather than abstract point of reference.

concreteness Use of specific terminology rather than abstractions in the discussion of the patient's feelings, experiences, and behavior.

conditional discharge A specified leave of absence or liberty from a psychiatric hospital in which certain things are expected from the patient and during which the commitment order is still in effect.

confabulation The manufacture of a response that is inaccurate but sounds appropriate. This is done to avoid embarrassment about memory loss.

confidentiality The ethical principle in the nurse-patient relationship, founded on trust and respect, that prohibits disclosure of privileged information without the patient's informed consent.

conflict Clashing of two opposing interests. The person experiences two competing drives and must choose between them.

confrontation An expression by the nurse of perceived discrepancies in the patient's behavior. It is an attempt by the nurse to bring to the patient's awareness the incongruence in his feelings, attitudes, beliefs, and behaviors.

confusion Constellation of behaviors, including inattention, memory deficits, inappropriate verbalizations, disruptive behavior, noncompliance, and failure to perform activities of daily living.

congruent communication A communication pattern in which the sender is communicating the same message on both the verbal and nonverbal levels.

consensual validation Assuring understanding of the communication of another person by reaching agreement on the meaning of the message.

consequences Stimulus events following a behavior that strengthen or weaken the behavior. These are either reinforcers or punishers.

consultation A process of interaction between two professional persons—the consultant who is a specialist and the consultee.

context Setting in which an event takes place.

continuous reinforcement A schedule of reinforcement in which each emission of a response is followed by the reinforcer.

conversion disorder A somatoform disorder characterized by a loss or alteration of physical functioning without evidence of organic impairment.

coping mechanisms Any effort directed at stress management. They can be task-oriented and involve direct problem-solving efforts to cope with the threat itself or be intrapsychic or ego defense–oriented with the goal of regulating one's emotional distress.

coping resources Characteristics of the person, group, or environment that are helpful in assisting individuals in adapting to stress.

coping style The cognitive, affective, or behavioral response of a person to a problematic or traumatic life event.

coprolalic A person who obtains sexual pleasure from using filthy language.

countertransference An emotional response of the nurse that is generated by the qualities of the patient and is inappropriate to the content and context of the therapeutic relationship or inappropriate in the degree of intensity of emotion.

criminal prosecution The filing of a complaint in a criminal court for an alleged criminal or felonious act against a perpetrator; a guilty or not guilty verdict is delivered by either a judge or a jury, and the perpetrator, if convicted, is sentenced for the offense.

crisis An internal disturbance that results from a stressful event or perceived threat to self.

crisis intervention A short-term active mode of therapy that focuses on solving the patient's immediate problem and reestablishing psychological equilibrium.

cult A specific complex of beliefs, rites, and ceremonies maintained by a social group in association with some particular person or object. Cult is usually considered as having magical or religious significance.

cultural relativism The idea that health and normality emerge within a social context and that the content and form of mental health and mental illness will vary greatly from one culture to another. Differences are due to variations in stressors, symbolical interpretation, acceptance of expression and repression, and cohesion of social groups and their tolerance of deviation.

cunnilingus Oral stimulation of the female genitalia.

data base Sum total of information from which the patient's problems can be identified.

date/acquaintance rape The perpetration of a sexual assault or rape on a person by someone known to the victim; may include dates, casual acquaintances, therapists, employers, friends, etc.

daydream A reverie while awake; usually the unfulfilled wishes of the dreamer are imagined as fulfilled. Wishes are not disguised and fulfillment is imagined as direct, without repression. Not inherently pathological.

defense mechanisms Coping mechanisms of the ego that attempt to protect the person from feelings of inadequacy and worthlessness and prevent awareness of anxiety. They are primarily unconscious in nature and involve a degree of self-deception and reality distortion.

deinstitutionalization At the individual patient level, the transfer to a community setting of a patient who has been hospitalized for an extended period of time, generally many years; at the mental health care system level, a shift in the focus of mental health care from the large long-term institution to the community, accomplished by discharging long-term patients and by avoiding unnecessary admissions.

delayed treatment seeker A person who delays seeking mental health intervention for a problematic life event (e.g., sexual assault/rape) and seeks treatment months or years after the event, usually following a precipitating event.

deliberate biological programming Memory and the capacity for terminating the life of a cell is stored within the cell itself (one theory of psychobiological aging).

delinquency A relatively minor violation of legal or moral codes especially by children or adolescents. Juvenile delinquency is such behavior by a young person (usually under 16 or 18) as to bring him to the attention of a court.

delirium The medical diagnostic term that describes an organic mental disorder characterized by a cluster of cognitive impairments with an acute onset and the identification of a specific precipitating stressor.

delirium tremens A medical diagnostic term that has been replaced with the diagnosis of alcohol withdrawal delirium.

delusion A fixed false belief. It may be persecutory, grandiose, nihilistic, or somatic in nature.

delusion of grandeur The false belief that one has great money, power, and prestige. It is frequently manifested in the belief that the individual is a famous person.

delusion of poverty The false belief that one is impoverished.

dementia The medical diagnostic term that describes an organic mental disorder characterized by a cluster of cognitive impairments that are generally of gradual onset and irreversible. The predisposing and precipitating stressors may or may not be identifiable.

denial Avoidance of disagreeable realities by ignoring or refusing to recognize them.

depersonalization A feeling of unreality and alienation from oneself. It is associated with a panic level of anxiety that produces a blocking off of awareness and a collapse in reality testing. The individual has difficulty distinguishing self from others, and one's body has an unreal or strange quality about it. It is the subjective experience of the partial or total disruption of one's ego and the disintegration and disorganization of one's self-concept.

depot injection Intramuscular injection of medication in an oil suspension that results in sustained release over a period of several days.

depression An abnormal extension of overelaboration of sadness and grief. The term "depression" can be used to denote a variety of phenomena—a sign, symptom, syndrome, emotional state, reaction, disease, or clinical entity.

detoxification The removal of a toxic substance from the body, either naturally through physiological processes, such as hepatic or renal functions, or medically by the introduction of alternative substances and gradual withdrawal.

developmental tasks Hierarchy of age-appropriate behaviors to be mastered as an individual matures.

deviancy Failure to comply with a social norm.

differentiation Sufficient separation between intellect and emotions so that one is not dominated by the reactive anxiety of the family's emotional system.

direct nursing care functions Liaison nurse activities that are focused on a particular client and his family or on a group for whom the nurse is directly responsible and accountable.

direct self-destructive behavior (DSDB) Suicide behavior.

disability Impairment of instrumental role performance in at least three of the following areas: self-care, receptive and expressive language, learning, mobility, self-direction, capacity for independent living, and self-sufficiency.

discharge plan A formal written document that describes in detail the transition of the patient from one level of the mental health care system to another.

disengaged A transactional style in a family reflecting inappropriately rigid boundaries requiring a high level of individual stress to activate family response.

disengagement theory Individuals and society mutually withdraw as part of normal aging.

disorientation Inability to correctly identify the self in relation to time, place, or person.

displacement Shift of an emotion from the person or object toward which it was originally directed to another usually neutral or less dangerous person or object.

dissociation The separation of any group of mental or behavioral processes from the rest of the person's consciousness or identity.

dissociative reaction Process by which a person blocks off part of his life from conscious recognition because of the threat of overwhelming anxiety.

diurnal mood variation Changes in mood that are related to the time of day.

divorce therapy A type of counseling that attempts to help couples disengage from their former relationship and malicious behavior toward each other or their children.

double bind Simultaneous communication of conflicting messages in the context of a situation that does not allow escape. *(See incongruent communication.)*

dream analysis A psychoanalytical therapeutic technique that requires the patient to report his dreams to the analyst who then interprets the meaning of the dream symbolism to assist the patient in understanding his unconscious mental functioning.

drug abuse Use of any chemical substance for reasons other than medical treatment.

drug-induced parkinsonism A reversible syndrome resembling the disease parkinsonism, resulting from the dopamine-blocking action of antipsychotic drugs.

drug interaction The effects of two or more drugs being taken simultaneously, producing an alteration in the usual effects of either drug taken alone. The interacting drugs may have a potentiating or additive effect and serious side effects may result.

drug tolerance Repeated use of some substance or drug (e.g., narcotics) so that larger and larger doses are required to produce the same physiologic and/or psychologic effect obtained previously by a smaller dose.

drug trial The time it takes to administer a drug at adequate therapeutic doses for a long enough period of time to determine its efficacy for a particular patient. The trial culminates with: 1) acceptable clinical result; 2) intolerable adverse effects; 3) poor response after an appropriate blood level is reached or the drug is administered for a time period specific for the illness (3 weeks for antidepressants; 3 to 6 weeks for antipsychotics).

DSM-III Diagnostic and Statistical Manual of Mental Disorders—standard nomenclature of emotional illness used by all health-care practitioners; DSM-III-R is a revised version published in 1987; it updates and classifies mental illnesses, as well as presents guidelines and diagnostic criteria for various mental disorders.

dyspareunia Recurrent or persistent genital pain occurring before, during, or after intercourse (male or female).

dystonia Acute tonic muscle spasms, often of the tongue, jaw, eyes, and neck, but sometimes of the whole body. Sometimes occurs during the first few days of antipsychotic drug administration.

echolalia Repeating exactly whatever is heard.

echopraxia Imitation of the body position of another.

ego The I, self, or individual which is postulated as the "center" to which all of a person's psychological activities and qualities are referred. That aspect of the psyche which is conscious and most in touch with external reality. An aspect of the personality that is in contact with the external world by means of perception, thought, and reality.

ego boundaries An individual's perception of the boundaries between himself and the external environment.

ego defense mechanisms Coping mechanisms of the ego that attempt to protect the person from feelings of inadequacy and worthlessness and prevent awareness of anxiety. They are primarily unconscious in nature and involve a degree of self-deception and reality distortion.

ego deficit/strength The inability or ability of the ego to test reality and maintain that function under stress and anxiety.

ego interpretive techniques A milieu management technique that helps the child gain ego strength through insight into his maladaptive behavior.

ego state A transactional analysis term that refers to the role behaviors an individual assumes in a particular unit of communication. They may be adult, parent, or child.

ego supportive techniques A milieu management technique for dealing with a child in the early phase of treatment in which the child is helped to regain self-control and reenter the daily routine from a panic-aggressive state.

ejaculatory incompetence Inability of a man to ejaculate intravaginally. It is also known as retarded ejaculation.

electroconvulsive therapy (ECT) Artificial induction of a grand mal seizure by passing a controlled electrical current through electrodes applied to one or both temples. The patient is anesthetized and the seizure attenuated by administration of a muscle relaxant medication.

empathic understanding Ability to view the patient's world from his internal frame of reference. It involves the nurse's sensitivity to the patient's current feelings and the verbal ability to communicate this understanding in a language attuned to the patient.

enabler The role that is frequently assumed by the significant others of substance abusers, characterized by covert support of the substance-abusing behavior.

encopresis Repeated voluntary or involuntary passage of feces of normal or near-normal consistency into places not appropriate for that purpose, and not caused by any physical disorder.

encounter group therapy An application of the existential model of psychiatric care in a group setting. The focus is on here-and-now experience and the expression of real feelings verbally and nonverbally as members react to events in the group.

endorphins Naturally occurring peptides that have been found in the central nervous system and have a physiological effect similar to that of opiates.

endogenous Developing or originating within the organism, or arising from causes within the organism.

enkephalins Naturally occurring peptides that have been found in the central nervous system and have a physiological effect similar to that of opiates.

enmeshed A transactional style in a family reflecting diffuse subsystem boundaries resulting in stress in one family member emotionally reverberating quickly and intensely throughout the family system.

enuresis Repeated involuntary voiding of urine during the day or at night, after an age at which continence is expected, that is not due to any physical disorder.

environment The circumstances, objects, or conditions that surround and have an internal influence on the life and effective functioning of the family and its members.

environmental change Activities that have a social setting focus and require the modification of an individual's or group's immediate environment or the larger social system.

ethic A standard of valued behavior or beliefs adhered to by an individual or group. A goal to which one aspires.

ethical dilemma An issue for which moral claims conflict with one another. It can be defined as 1) a difficult problem that seems to have no satisfactory solution or 2) a choice between equally unsatisfactory alternatives.

ethnocentrism A threat to the therapeutic relationship by imposing one's own views and standards on other cultural groups and desiring to change the way of life of others to be consistent with one's own.

evaluation A phase of the nursing process in which the patient's progress or lack of progress toward goal achievement is determined by the patient and nurse. This determination directs reassessment, reordering of priorities, new goal setting, and revision of the plan of nursing care.

exhibitionism Intense sexual arousal or desire, and acts, fantasies, or other stimuli involving exposing one's genitals to an unsuspecting stranger.

existentialism A school of philosophical thought that focuses on the importance of experience in the present and the belief that man finds meaning in life through his experiences.

exogenous Developing or originating outside the organism.

extinction Witholding reinforcement that was previously provided.

expert witness A person qualified by experience and/or education to form a definition and objective opinion based on scientific opinion or medical theory.

extrapyramidal syndrome A variety of signs and symptoms, including muscular rigidity, tremors, drooling, shuffling gait (parkinsonism); restlessness (akathisia); peculiar involuntary postures (dystonia); motor inertia (akathisia); and many other neurologic disturbances. Results from dysfunction of the extrapyramidal system. May occur as a reversible side effect of certain psychotropic drugs, particularly antipsychotics.

face-hand test A psychomotor test used to assess the presence of organic mental disorders.

family A group of people living in a household, who are attached emotionally, interact regularly, and share concerns for the growth and development of individuals and the family.

family APGAR An evaluation tool that focuses on family function as viewed by each member.

family projection process Transmission of anxiety of one or both parents onto a target child establishing an overly protective or conflictual relationship with the child, resulting ultimately in impairment of the child.

family structure The way in which the family is organized according to roles, rules, power, and hierarchies, including generational boundaries.

family style Those pervasive patterns characteristic of the family's interaction—e.g., chaotic, rigid, enmeshed, conflictual.

family system Those individuals who contribute to the functional state of the family as a unit.

family therapy The focus of family therapy is to treat as the primary unit a social system, rather than an individual member who has been defined as a "patient."

family violence The physical, psychological, sexual, material, or social violation or exploitation of a person by a family member or their delegate; the mode by which a given family system expresses its dysfunction.

fellatio Oral stimulation of the male genitalia.

female orgasmic dysfunction Inability of a female to achieve orgasm that may be primary or situational in origin.

female sexual arousal disorder Either 1) persistent or recurrent partial or complete failure to attain or maintain the lubrication-swelling response until completion of sexual activity or 2) persistent or recurrent lack of a subjective sense of sexual excitement and pleasure in a female during sexual activity.

fetishism Intense sexual arousal or desire, and acts, fantasies, or other stimuli involving nonliving objects by themselves.

fixation A psychoanalytical term that refers to a failure to resolve the conflicts inherent in a particular stage of psychosocial development. Psychological energy (libido) is invested in these conflictual areas, thus inhibiting the person's ability to grow beyond that point.

fixed interval (FI) reinforcement Specific lapse of time required for reinforcement.

fixed ratio (FR) reinforcement Specific number of responses required for reinforcement.

flashback A phenomenon experienced by individuals who have taken hallucinogenic drugs in which they unexpectedly reexperience the effects of the drug.

flight of ideas A pattern of speech characterized by a rapid transition from one topic to another, frequently without completing the original thought. This behavior is characteristic of manic states.

Food and Drug Administration (FDA) One of a number of health administrations under the Assistant Secretary of Health of the U.S. Department of Health, Education and Welfare (in April 1980, Department of Health and Human Services) to set standards for, to license the sale of, and in general to safeguard the public from the use of dangerous drugs and food substances.

free association A psychoanalytical therapeutic technique that requires the patient to repeat all his thoughts without censorship, drifting naturally from one thought to the next.

freebasing A chemical process that is applied to cocaine to amplify the effect of the drug. The cocaine is then smoked.

frotteurism Intense sexual arousal or desire, and acts, fantasies, or other stimuli involving rubbing against a nonconsenting person.

frustration A feeling that results when something interferes with one's ability to attain a desired goal, satisfaction, or security.

functional disorder A mental or emotional impairment that is believed to be psychosocial in origin.

fusion A blurring of self-boundaries in a highly reactive emotional relationship with another.

game In the context of transactional analysis, repetitive sets of ulterior transactions that are psychologically gratifying.

genuineness A quality of the nurse characterized by openness, honesty, and sincerity. The nurse is self-congruent and authentic and relates to the patient without a defensive facade.

geriatric patient Chronologically, 65 years of age or older adult recipient of health care services.

gerontology The study of the phenomenon of aging.

gestalt therapy A therapeutic approach based on the existential model of psychiatric care. It was developed by Perls and focuses on the development of enhanced self-awareness.

grief An individual's subjective response to the loss of a person, object, or concept that is highly valued. Uncomplicated grief is a healthy, adaptive, reparative response.

group A collection of three or more individuals who have a relationship with one another, are interdependent, and who may share some common norms.

group maintenance Group functions directed toward satisfaction of members' psychosocial or emotional needs.

group-centered mental health consultation A format through which the consultant meets with a group to provide guidance regarding the consultees' work encounters.

group therapy A form of psychiatric treatment in which six to eight patients attend a specified number of meetings that are conducted by a therapist. Examples of some common inpatient groups are: remotivation groups; problem solving groups; supportive groups; and, reeducation groups.

habeas corpus A right retained by all psychiatric patients that provides for the release of an individual who claims he is being deprived of his liberty and detained illegally. The hearing for this determination takes place in a court of law, and the patient's sanity is at issue.

half-life The amount of time it takes the body to excrete approximately half of an ingested drug; after this time the effects of the drug usually begin to deteriorate.

hallucination A sensory experience that is not the result of an external stimulus; it may be visual, auditory, tactile, olfactory, or gustatory.

hallucinogens A class of abused drugs that cause a psychotic-like experience.

health education A nursing intervention that involves increasing a person's awareness of health issues, understanding of the dimensions of possible stressors and outcomes, knowledge of how to acquire needed resources; and actual coping responses.

helplessness A person's belief that no one will do anything to aid him.

homicide The illegal killing of one human being by another.

homosexual One who is motivated in adult life by a definite preferential erotic attraction to members of the same sex and who usually (but not necessarily) engage in overt sexual relations with them.

homosexual panic A state of extreme agitation resulting from fear related to awareness of previously repressed homosexual impulses.

hopelessness An individual's belief that neither he nor anyone else can do anything to aid him.

hostility A feeling of anger and resentment characterized by destructive behavior.

hyperactive Unusually or excessively active.

hypoactive sexual desire disorder Persistently or recurrently deficient or absent sexual fantasies and desire for sexual activity.

hypochondriasis A somatoform disorder characterized by the belief that one is ill without evidence of organic impairment.

hypomania A clinical syndrome that is similar to, but less severe than, that described by the term mania or manic episode.

id Element of the personality described by Freud that represents one's instinctual drives and primitive impulses and is largely unconscious in nature.

identification Process by which a person tries to make himself like someone else whom he admires by taking on the thoughts, mannerisms, or tastes of that individual.

identity Organizing principle of the personality system that accounts for the unity, continuity, uniqueness, and consistency of the personality. It is the awareness of the process of "being oneself" that is derived from self-observation and judgment and is

identity confusion Lack of clarity and consistency in one's perception of the self, resulting in a high degree of anxiety.

identity diffusion An individual's failure to integrate various childhood identifications into a harmonious adult psychosocial identity.

identity foreclosure Premature adoption of an identity that is desired by significant others without coming to terms with one's own desires, aspirations, or potential.

idiopathic pain disorder A somatoform disorder characterized by pain as its only symptom and no evidence of organic impairment.

illusion Misinterpretation of a sensory input.

immediacy State that occurs when the current interaction of the nurse and the patient is focused on.

implementation A phase of the nursing process in which nursing actions are carried out that assist the patient to maximize his health capabilities and provide for patient participation in health promotion, maintenance, and restoration.

impotence Failure to achieve an erection.

incest Act of having sexual relations with a close relative, such as one's mother, daughter, or son.

incompetency A legal status that must be proved in a special court hearing. As a result of the hearing the person can be deprived of many of his civil rights. Incompetency can be reversed only in another court hearing that declares the person competent.

incongruent communication A communication pattern in which the sender is communicating different messages on the verbal and nonverbal levels and the listener does not know to which level he should respond. (See *double bind*.)

indirect nursing care functions Liaison nurse activities used to problem solve with consultee who is responsible and accountable for implementing and evaluating any recommended changes to effect problem resolution.

indirect self-destructive behavior (ISDB) Any activity that is detrimental to the well-being of the person and potentially has the outcome of death, accompanied by lack of conscious awareness of the self-destructive nature of the behavior.

individual psychotherapy A formal one-to-one therapeutic relationship in which the patient is encouraged to develop insights into the sources of his thoughts, feelings, perceptions, and behavior. By developing these insights, the patient is better able to deal with stress and maintain effective interpersonal relationships.

informal admission A type of admission to a psychiatric hospital in which there is no formal or written application and the individual is free to leave at any time.

informed consent Disclosure of a certain amount of information to the patient about the proposed treatment and the attainment of the patient's consent, which must be competent, understanding, and voluntary.

inhibited female orgasm Persistent or recurrent delay in or absence of orgasm in a female following a normal sexual excitement phase during sexual activity that is judged by the clinician to be adequate in focus, intensity, and duration.

inhibited male orgasm Persistent or recurrent delay in or absence of ejaculation in a male following a normal sexual excitement phase during sexual activity that is judged by the clinician to be adequate in focus, intensity, and duration.

insanity defense Legal defense proposing that a person who has committed an act that in a usual situation would be criminal should be held not guilty by reason of "Insanity."

institutionalism syndrome Characterized by lack of initiative, apathy, withdrawal, and submissiveness to authority.

insulin shock therapy Induction of a coma by administration of insulin. The comatose state is allowed to last up to an hour and is then reversed by the administration of glucose or glucagon.

intellectualization Excessive reasoning or logic used to avoid experiencing disturbing feelings.

intermittent reinforcement Noncontinuous reinforcement in which not every response is reinforced. Some emissions of a particular behavior are reinforced; others are not.

interpersonal strength A behavioral characteristic of an individual that when used in an interpersonal relationship, enhances mutual enjoyment of the relationship, without interfering with the integrity of either person.

introjection An intense type of identification in which the person incorporates qualities or values of another person or group into his own ego structure.

involuntary admission See *commitment*.

involuntary patient A patient admitted to a psychiatric facility through the commitment process.

isolation Splitting off of the emotional component of a thought. It may be temporary or long term.

joining The process of the therapist gaining entry into a family system by recognizing family strengths, respecting existing hierarchies and values, and confirming individual members in their sense of self.

judgment The ability to make logical, rational decisions.

judicial discharge A discharge granted by the courts.

Katz Index of Daily Living An instrument that is used to measure the individual's ability to bathe, dress, toilet, transfer, and feed himself and remain continent.

la belle indifference Term used to describe the patient's lack of concern or anxiety regarding his physical illness. It is used to describe the bland attitude characteristic of hysteria or conversion reactions.

labile Subject to frequent or unpredictable changes.

latency Psychosexual stage of development first identified by Freud in which the child's ego has developed considerable impulse control and energy is focused on learning and more organized play.

learned helplessness A behavioral state and personality trait of a person who believes that he is ineffectual, his responses are futile, and he has lost control over the reinforcers in his environment.

learning A relatively stable, observable change in the frequency or form of behavior resulting from interaction with environmental antecedent and consequences.

least restrictive alternative Providing patients with the greatest freedom from restriction, especially that of long-term hospitalization.

legal responsibilities Include expectations of a mental health professional in: 1) documenting the signs and symptoms of a person in response to a life event, and 2) testimony in criminal and civil litigation proceedings.

lesbian A woman whose sexual preference is for another woman.

lethality An estimation of the probability that a person who is threatening suicide will succeed based on the method described, the specificity of the plan, and the availability of the means.

liaison nurse A master's degree prepared nurse clinician, who provides psychiatric nursing services in nonpsychiatric settings.

liaison nursing A professional process between two systems in which one of the systems (the user) has a current work-related problem and voluntarily requests help from an outside system (the provider) who is perceived to have a specialized competency in a defined area.

libido Freud's term for psychic energy.

life review Progressive return to consciousness of past experiences.

life space interview An interaction between a child and adult that takes place outside the context of individual therapy. The focus is on improving the child's sense of self-identity and ego functioning with the developmental process.

limbic system An area in the brain associated with the control of emotion, eating, drinking, and sexual activity.

limit setting Act of making a person aware of his rights and responsibilities, while communicating the expectation that he will respect the rules. Also, the application of appropriate sanctions if the person does not obey the rules.

living will Determining in advance one's participation in heroic measures during the dying process.

logotherapy An approach to psychotherapy based on the existential model and developed by Frankl. The focus is on the search for meaning in present experiences.

loose associations A communication pattern characterized by lack of clarity of connection between one thought and the next.

male sexual arousal disorder Either 1) persistent or recurrent partial or complete failure in a male to attain or maintain erection until completion of the sexual activity or 2) persistent or recurrent lack of a subjective sense of sexual excitement and pleasure in a male during sexual activity.

malingering Deliberate feigning of an illness.

malpractice Failure of a professional person to give the kind of proper and competent care that is given by members of his profession in the community, which causes harm to the patient.

mania A condition that is characterized by a mood that is elevated, expansive, or irritable.

manipulation Controlling the behavior of others to achieve one's own goals.

marital rape The perpetration of a sexual assault or rape on a partner by one's spouse.

masochism Intense sexual arousal or desire, and acts, fantasies, or other stimuli involving being humiliated, beaten, bound or otherwise made to suffer (real or simulated).

masturbation The induction of erection and the obtaining of sexual satisfaction in either sex, from manual or other artificial stimulation of the genitals. Usually is self-induced.

maturational crisis Transitional or developmental periods within a person's life when his psychological equilibrium is upset.

mechanical restraints Any of several means of restricting a patient's freedom of movement. Includes camisoles, wrist and ankle restraints, sheet restraints, and sheet packs.

medical diagnosis The independent judgment of a physician of the health problems or disease states of the patient.

meditation A technique of tension reduction in which the person closes his eyes, relaxes the major muscle groups, and repeats a cue word silently to himself each time he exhales.

memory The ability to recall past events.

menarche First menstruation of a woman, which indicates that she may be capable of conceiving.

mental health consultation nurse A master's degree prepared nurse whose scope of practice includes the health-illness continuum as it applies to psychosocial aspects of health care.

mental status examination A formal exploration of data relative to a patient's mental functioning in which information is collected about the patient's sensorium and intelligence, thought processes, mood and affect, and insight.

message A unit of communication.

metacommunication Messages about a communication pertaining to both the relationship and informational aspects.

milieu therapy A scientific manipulation of the environment aimed at producing changes in the personality of the patient.

Mini-Mental State Examination A brief psychological test designed to differentiate between dementia, psychosis, and affective disorders.

model A means of organizing a complex body of knowledge.

monoamine oxidase (MAO) inhibitors A group of chemically related antidepressant medications.

mood A prolonged emotional state that influences one's whole personality and life functioning.

mourning Includes all the psychological processes set in motion within the individual by a loss. The process of mourning is resolved only when the lost object is internalized, bonds of attachment are loosened, and new object relationships are established.

multidisciplinary health care team A group of health care workers who are members of different disciplines with each one providing specific services to the patient.

multigenerational transmission process The repetition of relationship patterns and anxiety associated with toxic issues passed through generations in a family.

multiple personality The existence within an individual of two or more distinct personalities or personality states, each having its own pattern of perceiving, feeling, and thinking.

mutual support groups A type of group in which members organize themselves to solve their own problems. They are led by the group members themselves who share a common experience, work together toward a common goal, and use their own strengths to gain control over their lives.

myth A false belief not supported by empirical facts.

narcissism An exaggerated sense of self-importance manifested as extreme self-absorption.

narcotics A class of drugs that have powerful analgesic and euphoria-inducing properties.

National Institute of Mental Health (NIMH) Responsible for programs dealing with mental health, NIMH is an institute within the Alcohol, Drug Abuse, and Mental Health Administration (ADAMHA). ADAMHA, an agency in the U.S. Department of Health and Human Services, provides leadership, policies, and goals for the federal effort to assure the treatment and rehabilitation of persons with alcohol, drug abuse, and mental health problems; this agency is also responsible for administering grants to advance and support research, training, and service programs.

National Organization of Victims Assistance A private, nonprofit organization of victim and witness assistance practitioners, criminal justice professionals, researchers, former victims, and others committed to the recognition of victims' rights; four purposes are: national advocacy, victims aid, service to local programs, and membership support.

necrophile A person who is sexually aroused by thoughts of death or sexual activity with a dead person.

need-fear dilemma An approach-avoidance conflict related to the need to experience closeness coupled with fear of the experience.

negative identity Assumption of an identity that is at odds with the accepted values and expectations of society.

negative punishment Removal of something following operant, decreasing probability of operant's recurrence.

negative reinforcement Refers to the procedure whereby the removal or termination of an aversive stimulus contingently follows the emission of a response and results in an increase in the rate of responding.

negative reinforcer A stimulus which, when presented immediately following the occurrence of a particular behavior, will decrease the rate of responding of that behavior. If antecedent to the emission of a particular behavior and terminated by that response, it will increase the rate of responding of that behavior.

neglect Condition that occurs when a parent is unable to or fails to provide minimal emotional and physical care to a child.

neologisms Words that are invented by the person and understood only by him.

networking A process of linking individuals or agencies with mutual interests to form a coalition and thereby more effectively bring about social change.

neurasthenia A type of disorder characterized by chronic mental and physical fatigue and a variety of vague aches and pains, including weakness, headaches, and back pain. This reaction is not caused by overwork but is an attempt to reduce or mask areas of conflict.

neuron Nerve cell; both an electrical and chemical unit; neurons are separated from each other by spaces called synapses. They are the basic function units of the nervous system.

neurotic behavior A behavioral dysfunction that is characterized by anxiety, but in which there is no distortion of reality.

neurotic disorders A category of health problems that are distinguished by the following characteristics: symptoms that are distressing and unacceptable to the individual, grossly intact reality testing, behavior that does not violate gross social norms, a disturbance that is relatively enduring or recurrent without treatment, and no demonstrable organic etiology.

neurotransmitter A chemical found in the nervous system (e.g., norepinephrine, serotonin, dopamine) that facilitates the transmission of impulses across synapses between neurons. Disorders in the brain physiology of neurotransmitters have been implicated in the pathogenesis of several psychiatric illnesses, particularly affective disorders and schizophrenia.

nihilistic delusion The false belief that the self, part of the self, or another object has ceased to exist.

noncompliance The failure of the individual to carry out the self-care activities prescribed in a health care plan.

nonverbal communication Transmission of a message without the use of words. It involves all of the five senses.

norm A culturally defined standard of behavior.

nuclear family emotional system Patterns of interaction between family members and the degree to which these patterns promote fusion.

nurse practice act A state law that defines the legal limits of nursing practice and that must be adhered to by all licensed nurses.

nurses' observation scale for inpatient evaluation (NOSIE) A systematical, objective behavioral rating scale applied by nurses to patients' behavior.

nursing The diagnosis and treatment of human responses to actual or potential health problems.

nursing audit A type of clinical evaluation of nursing care that may focus on a nursing activity (process audit) or on the behavior of a patient in response to the nursing care that has been provided (outcome audit).

nursing diagnosis The independent judgment of a nurse of the patient's behavioral response to stress. It is a statement of the patient's nursing problems, which may be overt, covert, existing, or potential, and includes both the behavioral disruption or threatened disruption and contributing stressors.

nursing problems Aspects of the patient's health that may need to be promoted or with which the patient needs held in his biopsychosocial adaptation to stress.

nursing process An interactive problem-solving process used by the nurse as a systematical and individualized way to fulfill the goal of nursing care. It includes the components of data collection, formulation of the nursing diagnosis, planning, implementation, and evaluation.

nursing therapeutic process The process by which the nurse strives to promote and maintain the adaptive coping responses of the patient that involves the establishment of a therapeutic nurse-patient relationship and the use of the nursing process.

obesity A condition in which the individual weighs at least 20 percent more than his ideal weight.

object cues A category of nonverbal communication that includes the speaker's intentional and nonintentional use of all objects, such as dress, furnishings, and possessions.

observers Individuals who are adults or children in the nuclear and extended family who neither perpetrate nor are victims of the family abuse or violence by an offender.

obsession A recurring thought that is unwanted but which cannot be voluntarily excluded from consciousness.

oculogyric crisis A side effect of antipsychotic medication that is characterized by the uncontrollable rolling upward of the eyes.

offenders Adults or children who perpetrate any type or form of abuse or violence on family members of other persons.

operant Behavior maintained or changed by its consequences.

operant behavior Behavior whose strength is controlled by the stimulus events that precede and follow it.

operant conditioning Modification of operant behavior by systematical manipulation of antecedents and consequences.

operant level Frequency or form of a performance under baseline conditions before any systematical conditioning procedures are introduced.

organic disorder A mental or emotional impairment that is believed to be physiological in origin.

orientation The ability to correctly relate the self to time, place, and person.

orthostatic hypotension A drop in blood pressure related to change in position. A common side effect of psychotropic medications.

PACE II An evaluation tool that focuses on the physical health of nursing home patients.

panic An attack of extreme anxiety that involves the disorganization of the personality. Distorted perceptions, loss of rational thought, and an inability to communicate and function are evident.

paranoia A behavioral manifestation representative of the unconscious operation of the mechanism of projection whereby the person attributes his ego-alien thoughts and impulses to others; a feeling of extreme suspicion.

paranoid delusion The false belief that one is being persecuted.

paraphilias Characterized by sexual arousal in response to objects or situations that are not normally arousing for affectionate sexual activities with human partners, i.e., pedophilia, exhibitionism, zoophilia, etc.

parent education Any educational experience geared toward the thoughtful conveyance of information enabling the parent to provide quality childrearing.

parkinsonian equivalents Side effects of antipsychotic medications that are behaviors characteristic of Parkinson's disease, including fine tremors, pill-rolling tremor of the fingers, drooling, and petit pas gait.

passive Behavior that subordinates the individual's own rights to the demands of others.

passive-aggressive Term describing indirect expression, verbal or nonverbal, of angry feelings.

paternalism The ethical principle that provides for the regulation of the activities of another in the same manner in which a benevolent parent regulates the activities of a child.

pedophilia Intense sexual arousal or desire, and acts, fantasies or other stimuli involving one or more children 13 years of age or younger.

peer A person deemed an equal for the purpose at hand. A companion or associate on roughly the same level of age or endowment, an age mate.

peer group The group with whom a child associates on terms of approximate equality. Usually very heterogenous.

peer review Review of clinical practice with peers, supervisors, and/or consultants.

perception Sensory reception of a stimulus; meaning one attributes to a situation.

perseveration Repetition of a single word or phrase over and over.

pharmacokinetics The study of the process and rates of drug distribution, metabolism, and disposition in the organism.

phenothiazines A group of chemically related antipsychotic medications.

phobic reaction A persistent fear of some object or situation that presents no actual danger to the person or in which the danger is magnified out of proportion to its actual seriousness.

physical dependence A characteristic of drug addiction that is present when withdrawal of the drug results in physiological disruptions.

physical restraint Limitation of the individual's freedom of movement by immobilizing all or part of the body or by restricting the person to a confined space.

planning A phase of the nursing process in which goals are derived from the nursing diagnosis, priorities are set, and nursing approaches or measures to achieve the goals are prescribed.

play therapy The utilization of child's play as a mode of self-expression and communication to work through conflicts with an adult therapist.

polypharmacy Use of combinations of psychoactive drugs in a patient at the same time; more than one drug may not be more effective than a single agent, can cause drug interactions, and may increase the incidence of adverse reactions.

positive punishment A punishment procedure in which the presentation of an aversive stimulus immediately following the occurrence of a particular behavior results in a decrease in the rate of responding of that behavior.

positive reinforcement Presentation of environmental event as a consequence of operant, increasing probability of operant's recurrence.

possession The belief that one has been taken over by some spirit or person.

postvention Therapeutic intervention with the significant others of an individual who has committed suicide.

pre-adolescence The arbitrarily distinguished period of 10 to 12 years of age, the 2 years before puberty.

predisposing factors Conditioning factors that influence both the type and amount of resources that the individual can elicit to cope with stress. They may be biological, psychological, and sociocultural in nature.

premature ejaculation Ejaculation occurring with minimal sexual stimulation, or before, upon, or shortly after penetration, and before the individual wishes it.

primary appraisal of stressor An evaluation of the significance of an event for one's well-being that takes place on the cognitive, affective, physiological, behavioral, and social levels.

primary gain A decrease in anxiety resulting from the individual's efforts to cope with stress.

primary nursing A modality of care delivery characterized by the assignment of one nurse to coordinate the total nursing care of a patient from admission to discharge.

primary prevention Biological, social, or psychological intervention that promotes health and well-being or reduces the incidence of illness in a community by altering the causative factors before they have an opportunity to do harm.

primary process thought Primitive thought process that is normally kept unconscious by use of the coping mechanism of repression; impulsive infantile ideation.

primary symptoms Symptoms that are intrinsically associated with the disease process.

privileged communication A legal term that applies only in court-related proceedings and means that the right to reveal information belongs to the person who spoke, and the listener cannot disclose the information unless the speaker gives permission. It exists between a patient and health professional only if a law specifically establishes it.

professionalization Evidence of a continuous attempt of a group in any community or society to gain more and more control over certain resources related to an occupational area.

program-centered consultation A format through which the consultant focuses on broader organizational and program areas in an attempt to help the consultee solve institution-wide issues.

projection Attributing one's own thoughts or impulses to another person. Through this process the individual can attribute his own intolerable wishes, emotional feelings, or motivations to another person.

pseudodementia A depressive condition of the elderly that is characterized by impaired cognitive functioning.

psychiatric nursing An interpersonal process that strives to promote and maintain behavior that contributes to integrated functioning. It employs the theories of human behavior as its science and purposeful use of self as its art. Psychiatric nursing is directed toward both preventive and corrective impacts on mental disorders and their sequelae and is concerned with the promotion of optimum mental health for society, the community, and those individuals who live within it.

psychoanalysis A therapeutic approach based on the belief that behavioral disorders are related to unresolved, anxiety-provoking childhood experiences that are repressed into the unconscious. The goal of psychoanalysis is to bring repressed experiences into conscious awareness and to learn healthier means of coping with the related anxiety.

psychobiological resilence A concept that proposes that there is a recurrent human need to weather periods of stress and change throughout life. The ability to successfully weather each period of disruption and reintegration leaves the person better able to deal with the next change.

psychodrama A modality of therapy that uses structured and directed dramatizations of a patient's emotional problems and experiences.

psychoeducation The use of the principles and methods of education to facilitate the rehabilitation and treatment of the mentally ill.

psychogenic amnesia Temporary inability to recall important personal information that is too extensive to be explained by ordinary forgetfulness.

psychogenic fugue Sudden, unexpected travel away from home or one's customary place of work, with an inability to recall one's past.

psychological autopsy A retrospective review of the individual's behavior for the time preceding his death by suicide.

psychological dependence A characteristic of drug addiction that is manifested in a craving for the abused substance and a fear that it will not be available in the future.

psychological factors affecting physical condition A category of psychophysiological disruptions in which organic impairment is evident. Examples include migraine headache, asthma, hypertension, colitis, and duodenal ulcer.

psychological testing A diagnostical tool used by the psychologist to aid in assessment of the patient. It includes administration of a battery of cognitive and projective tests.

psychomotor retardation A slowing of motor activity related to a state of severe depression.

psychoneuroimmunology The scientific field exploring the relationship between psychological states and the immune response.

psychopharmacology Drugs that treat the symptoms of mental illness, and whose actions in the brain provide us with models to better understand the mechanisms of mental disorders.

psychosocial rehabilitation The process of development of the many skills necessary for the chronically mentally ill patient to live independently.

psychosomatic reactions Disorders in which the emotional tension is not discharged outwardly but is instead unconsciously channeled through the visceral organs.

psychosurgery Surgical interruption of selected neural pathways that involve the transmission of emotional impulses in the brain.

psychotherapy group A group developed for the purpose of treating emotional distress and disorder through means of a group method and group process.

psychotic behavior Severely dysfunctional behavior characterized by a panic level of anxiety, personality disintegration, and regressive behavior. The person experiences a reduced level of awareness and has great difficulty functioning adequately.

psychotic disorders A category of health problems that are distinguished by the following characteristics: severe mood disorder, regressive behavior, personality disintegration, reduced level of awareness, great difficulty in functioning adequately, and gross impairment in reality testing.

psychotomimetic Imitating a psychosis; refers to the effects of hallucinogenic drugs.

puberty The period during which the generative organs become capable of functioning and the person develops secondary sex characteristics—in the female, its onset is marked by the beginning of menstruation; in males, one fairly reliable sign is the pigmenting of underarm hair.

punishment Procedures that decrease probability that operant will recur.

quality assessment measures Formal, systematic, organizational evaluation of overall patterns or programs of care, including clinical, consumer, and systems evaluation.

quality assurance activities Clinical evaluation of ongoing programs that include both evaluation and corrective action.

rape Legally defined as the forcible perpetration of the act of sexual intercourse on the body of a woman not one's wife. A more contemporary definition would include acts of oral and anal sodomy and allow for its occurrence within marriage as well.

rational-emotive therapy A therapeutic approach based on the existential model of psychiatric care and developed by Ellis. The emphasis is on risk taking and the assumption of responsibility for one's behavior.

rationalization Offering a socially acceptable or apparently logical explanation to justify or make acceptable otherwise unacceptable impulses, feelings, behaviors, and motives.

reaction formation Development of conscious attitudes and behavior patterns that are opposite to what one really feels or would like to do.

reality orientation Formal process of keeping an individual alert to events in the here-and-now.

reality testing The ego function of determining the objective reality of experience or a nursing action that validates objective reality for a patient who is unable to do so.

reality therapy A therapeutic approach based on the existential model of psychiatric care and developed by Glasser. The focus is on recognition and accomplishment of life goals with emphasis on development of the capacity for caring.

reasoning The ability to consider facts and arrive at a logical conclusion.

receptor A specialized area on a nerve membrane, a blood vessel, or a muscle that receives the chemical stimulation that activates or inhibits the nerve, blood vessel, or muscle.

reciprocal inhibition A behavior modification technique that attempts to substitute a more adaptive behavior for a symptom by learning an alternative means of reducing anxiety.

reframing To change the conceptual and/or emotional viewpoint in relation to which a situation is experienced and to place it in a different frame that fits the "facts" of the concrete situation equally well, and thereby changes its entire meaning; often imputing positive motivations behind undesirable behavior constitutes reframing.

regression A retreat in the face of stress to behavior characteristic of an earlier level of development.

reinforcer Consequence that increases probability that operant will recur.

reinforcement Process in which operant consequences increase probability operant will recur.

relatedness Process of establishing intimate relationships with others, including a meaningful balance among dependence, independence, and interdependence.

relaxation response A protective mechanism against stress that brings about decreased heart rate, lower metabolism, and decreased respiratory rate. It is the physiological opposite of the fight or flight, or anxiety, response.

relaxation therapy A behavior modification approach based on the principle of reciprocal inhibition. Consciously induced relaxation is experienced in conjunction with actual or fantasied anxiety-provoking experiences.

reminiscence Recounting early life experiences and events.

repression Involuntary exclusion of a painful or conflictual thought, impulse, or memory from awareness. It is the primary ego defense, and other mechanisms tend to reinforce it.

residual Remaining, or left behind; those symptoms that remain after treatment has reached its maximum effect.

resistance Attempt of the patient to remain unaware of anxiety-producing aspects within himself. Ambivalent attitudes toward self-exploration in which the patient both appreciates and avoids anxiety-producing experiences that are a normal part of the therapeutic process.

respect An attitude of the nurse that conveys caring for, liking, and valuing the patient. He is regarded as a person of worth and is accepted without qualification.

respite care The provision of temporary supervision in a community setting for a psychiatric patient who lives with his family to provide the family with relief from the demands of his care.

response Cost category of negative punishment in which reinforcer is lost or withdrawn following an operant.

reversible brain syndrome Also known as delirium, or acute brain syndrome, this disorder is related to a variety of biological stressors and is characterized by a disruption of cognition. Recovery is possible.

role ambiguity A type of role strain that occurs when shared specifications set for an expected role are incomplete or insufficient to tell the involved individual what is desired or how to do it.

role clarification Gaining the knowledge, information, and cues needed to perform a role.

role conflict Frustration experienced by the individual because of role demands that are incompatible or incongruent or confusing regarding appropriate role behavior.

role overload A type of role strain that occurs when a person is faced with a role set that is too complex or overwhelms available resources.

role playing Acting out of a particular situation. It functions to increase the person's insight into human relations and can deepen one's ability to see a situation from another point of view.

role strain Stress associated with expected roles or positions, experienced as frustration.

roles Set of socially expected behavior patterns associated with one individual's function in various social groups. Roles provide a means for social participation and a way to test out identities for consensual validation by significant others.

sadism Intense sexual arousal or desire, and acts, fantasies, or other stimuli involving the inflicting of real or simulated psychological or physical suffering.

Sandoz Clinical Assessment—Geriatric An examination of psychological functioning that is administered to the elderly to assist in the diagnostical process.

schizophrenia A manifestation of anxiety of psychotic proportions, primarily characterized by inability to trust other people and disordered thought process, resulting in disrupted interpersonal relationships.

school phobia A child's state of anxiety related to separating him from his parents by his attending school. It is a form of separation anxiety; the child is not afraid of school per se.

script A transactional analysis term that refers to a life plan which originates in childhood perceptions and experiences.

seclusion A form of physical restraint in which the individual is placed in a single room, which may be locked, to decrease stimuli and allow the agitated patient to gain control of his behavior.

secondary appraisal of coping resources An evaluation of one's coping resources or strategies that involves cognitive, affective, physiological, behavioral, and social responses.

secondary gain Advantages other than a decrease in anxiety that are associated with the sick role, e.g., dependency need gratification, relief from responsibilities.

secondary prevention A type of prevention that seeks to reduce the prevalence of illness by interventions that provide for early detection and treatment of problems.

secondary process thought Conscious thought processes that are under the control of the ego and are characterized by logic.

secondary symptoms Symptoms that are not intrinsically associated with the disease process but are a consequence of the illness process.

security operations A term related to the interpersonal model of psychiatric care that refers to mental mechanisms which are developed to deal with anxiety-provoking experiences.

self-actualization The process of fulfilling one's potential.

self-concept All the notions, beliefs, and convictions that constitute an individual's knowledge of himself and influence his relationships with others.

self-destructive behavior Any behavior, direct or indirect, that if uninterrupted, will ultimately lead to the death of the individual.

self-disclosure Revelation that occurs when a person reveals information about himself, his ideas, values, feelings, and attitudes.

self-esteem The individual's personal judgment of his own worth obtained by analyzing how well his behavior conforms to his self-ideal.

self-help group An organization of people who share a similar problem and meet to receive peer support and encouragement.

self-ideal The individual's perception of how he should behave based on certain personal standards. The standard may be either a carefully constructed image of the kind of person one would like to be or merely a number of aspirations, goals, or values that one would like to achieve.

self-system A term related to the interpersonal model of psychiatric care that refers to the self as perceived by the individual.

senility A nonspecific term that refers to impaired cognitive functioning in the elderly and is usually used in a derogatory sense.

sensitivity training group A group developed for the purpose of increasing self-awareness, increasing understanding of group process, or increasing awareness of the effects of one's behavior in groups.

separation-individuation A process whereby the child achieves a state of psychological separateness from the mother and develops a sense of identity.

set A predisposition to behave in a certain way.

sexual assault/rape The forcible perpetration of an act of sexual contact on the body (male or female) of another person without his or her consent; legal criteria vary among the states.

sexual aversion disorder Persistent or recurrent extreme aversion to and avoidance of all or almost all genital sexual contact with a partner.

sexuality Broadly defined as a desire for contact, warmth, tenderness, or love.

Short Portable Mental Status Questionnaire A short tool used to screen for cognitive impairment.

situational crisis Crisis that occurs when a specific external event upsets an individual's psychological equilibrium.

Social Behavior Assessment Scale A semistructured interview guide that elicits information from significant others regarding the patient's functioning.

social breakdown syndrome Progressive deterioration of social and interpersonal skills of long-term psychiatric patients.

social learning theory A theory that explains the development of aggressive behavior as part of the socialization process.

social margin The sum total of all the resources—material, personal, and interpersonal—available to assist an individual in coping with stress.

social networks See *social support systems.*

social support systems Those members of one's social environment who are perceived by the individual as "significant others" and who provide some degree of emotional support, task-oriented help, feedback and evaluation, social relatedness and integration, and access to new information.

society A nation, community or broad grouping of people who establish particular aims, beliefs, or standards of living and conduct.

somatic delusion The false belief that all or a part of the body is impaired in some way.

somatic therapies Treatment affecting one's physiological functioning.

somatization disorder A somatoform disorder characterized by multiple physical complaints with no evidence of organic impairment.

somatoform disorder A category of psychophysiological disruptions with no evidence of organic impairment.

somnambulism Dissociative manifestation of sleepwalking.

specialist in psychiatric and mental health nursing A psychiatric nurse who is characterized by graduate education, supervised clinical experience, and depth of knowledge, competence, and skill in practice.

splitting Viewing people and situations as either all good or all bad. Failure to integrate the positive and negative qualities of oneself.

steady state The body has reached a state of drug level equilibrium: a drug has been taken long enough that the amount of drug excreted equals the amount ingested. This occurs in approximately four to six half-lives.

stigma An irrational attribution of negative worth based on a person's behavior or experiences.

stimulus Any physical or environmental object, event, or condition, including one's own behavior and the behavior of others, that does or can influence.

strength An ability, skill, or interest an individual has previously used.

stress-adaptation theory Stress depletes the reserve capacity of individuals, thereby placing them in a vulnerable position for disease or illness.

stressors Stimuli that the individual perceives as challenging, threatening, or harmful. They require the use of excess energy and produce a state of tension and stress within the individual.

sublimation Acceptance of a socially approved substitute goal for a drive whose normal channel of expression is blocked.

substance abuse The use of any mind-altering agent to such an extent that it interferes with the individual's biological, psychological, or sociocultural integrity.

subsystems Smaller components of the larger system composed of individuals or dyads, formed by generation, gender, interest, or function.

suicide Self-inflicted death.

suicide attempt Any action deliberately undertaken by the individual that, if carried to completion, will result in his death.

suicide gesture A suicide attempt that is planned to be discovered in an attempt to influence the behavior of others.

suicide threat A warning, direct or indirect, verbal or nonverbal, that the individual plans to attempt suicide.

sundown syndrome Cognitive ability diminishes in the late afternoon or early evening.

sunrise syndrome Unstable cognitive ability upon rising in the morning.

superego Element of the personality described by Freud that represents one's conscience and culturally acquired restrictions.

supervision A process whereby a therapist is helped to become a more effective clinician. The nurse supervisor serves as a provider of theoretical knowledge and therapeutic techniques, validates the use of the nursing process, and supports the working through of transference and countertransference reactions.

suppression A process that is the conscious analogy of repression. It is the intentional exclusion of material from consciousness.

symptom-bearer The family member frequently seen as the psychiatric patient who is functioning poorly due to family dynamics that interfere with his functioning at a higher level.

synapse The gap between the membrane of one nerve cell and the membrane of another. The synapse is the point at which the transmission of nerve impulses occurs.

synergistic A reaction between two or more substances in which, after introduction into the body, the physiological effect of each is enhanced by the other.

systematical desensitization A technique of behavior therapy that involves the pairing of deep muscle relaxation with imagined scenes depicting situations that cause the patient to feel anxious. The assumption is that if the person is taught relaxation rather than anxiety while imagining such scenes, the real-life situation that the scene depicted will cause much less anxiety.

systems evaluation An evaluation of the organization of the health care delivery system that includes the components of systems analysis, economic analysis, and operations research. It is a supplement to clinical evaluation.

tangential speech Loss of goal direction in communication. Failure to address the original point.

tardive dyskinesia Literally, "late appearing abnormal movements"; a variable complex of choreiform or athetoid movements developing in patients exposed to antipsychotic drugs. Typical movements include tongue-writhing or protrusion, chewing, lip-puckering, choreiform finger movements, toe and ankle movements, leg jiggling, or movements of neck, trunk, and pelvis.

target symptoms Symptoms of an illness that are most likely to respond to a specific treatment, such as a particular psychopharmocologic drug.

tertiary prevention Measures designed to reduce the severity, disability, or residual impairment resulting from illness through rehabilitation.

testamentary capacity A person's competency to make a will, which requires that he knows he is making a will, the nature and extent of his property, and who his friends and relatives are.

thanatology The study of dying and death.

themes Underlying issues or problems experienced by the patient that emerge repeatedly during the course of the nurse-patient relationship.

therapeutic community A concept proposed by Maxwell Jones in which the patient's social environment would be used to provide a therapeutic experience for him by involving him as an active participant in his own care and the daily problems of his community.

therapeutic group A group developed for the purpose of preventing emotional turmoil or disturbances through prevention, education, and providing support.

therapeutic impasses Roadblocks in the progress of the nurse-patient relationship. They arise for a variety of reasons and may take different forms, but they all create stalls in the therapeutic relationship.

therapeutic nurse-patient relationship A mutual learning experience and a corrective emotional experience for the patient, in which the nurse uses herself and specified clinical techniques in working with the patient to bring about behavioral change.

therapeutic touch The nurse's laying of hands on or close to the body of an ill person for the purpose of helping or healing him.

third-party reimbursement Payment for health services by a government or private health insurance program.

time-out Category of negative punishment in which reinforcer is lost or withdrawn following an operant.

token economy A behavior modification approach that uses positive reinforcement in the form of a tangible object to promote positive behavioral change.

tolerance In pharmacology, progressive decrease of the effects of a drug during continued use of the same dose; this accounts for a decrease in some side effects, and also some therapeutic effects.

tort A civil wrong for which the injured party is entitled to compensation.

trance An altered state of consciousness with markedly diminished responsiveness to the environment.

transactional analysis A therapeutic modality based on the communications model of psychiatric care and developed by Berne. Therapy takes place through the identification and interpretation of communication units (transactions), leading to understanding of interpersonal games that underlie behavioral disturbances. The goal is to develop the ability to communicate directly without using games.

transference An unconscious response of the patient in which he experiences feelings and attitudes toward the nurse that were originally associated with significant figures in his early life.

transitional employment placement (TEP) A job which belongs to a psychosocial rehabilitation program rather than to an individual, and is assigned by program staff to a particular patient (member) for the time period that patient (member) needs it. When no longer needed by that patient (member), the TEP is assigned to someone else.

transsexual A person who is genetically an anatomical male or female, who expresses, with strong conviction, that he or she has the mind of the opposite sex, part time or full time, and seeks to change his or her sex legally and through hormonal and surgical sex reassignment.

transvestism Condition in which a male has a sexual obsession for or addiction to women's clothes.

triangle A predictable emotional process which takes place when there is difficulty in the relationship. Triangles represent dysfunctional efforts to reduce fusion or conflict in a relationship. The three corners of a triangle can be composed of three people, two people and an object or group or issue.

tricyclics A group of chemically related antidepressant medications.

undoing An act or communication that partially negates a previous one.

unidisciplinary health care team A group of health care workers who are all members of the same discipline.

urolognic A person who receives sexual stimulation from acts involving urine, such as watching people urinate or wishing to urinate on another.

vaginismus Involuntary contractions of the outer third of the vagina that prevent insertion of the penis.

value clarification A method whereby a person can assess, explore, and determine his personal values and what priority they hold in his personal decision making.

values The concepts that a person holds worthy in his own personal life. They are formed as a result of one's life experiences with family, friends, culture, education, work, and relaxation.

variable interval (VI) reinforcement Specific lapse of time required for reinforcement.

variable ratio (VR) reinforcement Various numbers of responses required for each reinforcement.

verbal communication Written or spoken transmission of a message.

victims Adults or children who are the target or scapegoat of family abuse or violence perpetrated by an offender and dysfunctional family system.

violence The exertion of extreme force or destructive action so as to injure or hurt; discordance, outrage, and sudden intense activity to the point of loss of control.

visualization The conscious programming of desired change with positive images.

vocal cues A category of nonverbal communication that includes all the noises and sounds that are extra-speech sounds. They are sometimes referred to as para-linguistic cues.

voluntary admission A type of admission to a psychiatric hospital in which the individual applies in writing and agrees to receive treatment and abide by the hospital rules. If the patient wishes to be discharged, he must give written notice to the hospital.

voluntary patient A patient who of one's own free will chooses to be admitted to a psychiatric facility.

voyerism Intense sexual arousal or desire, and acts, fantasies, or other stimuli involving observing unsuspecting people who are naked, in the act of disrobing, or engaging in sexual activity.

wear-and-tear theory Structural and functional changes of man may be accelerated by abuse and decelerated by care.

withdrawal An adaptive or coping mechanism that involves physically pulling away from or psychologically losing interest in others and the environment.

withdrawal syndrome Constellation of behaviors that occur when use of an abused substance is terminated. Behaviors are specific to the abused substance.

word salad A communication pattern characterized by a jumble of disconnected words.

working through Process by which repressed feelings are released and reintegrated into the personality.

young adult chronically mentally ill patient A chronically mentally ill person between 18 and 35 years of age.

zoophilia Intense sexual arousal or desire, and acts, fantasies, or other stimuli involving animals.

Zung Self-Rating Depression Scale An instrument administered to determine the presence of depression.

INDEX